BRAIN AND
VISUAL PERCEPTION

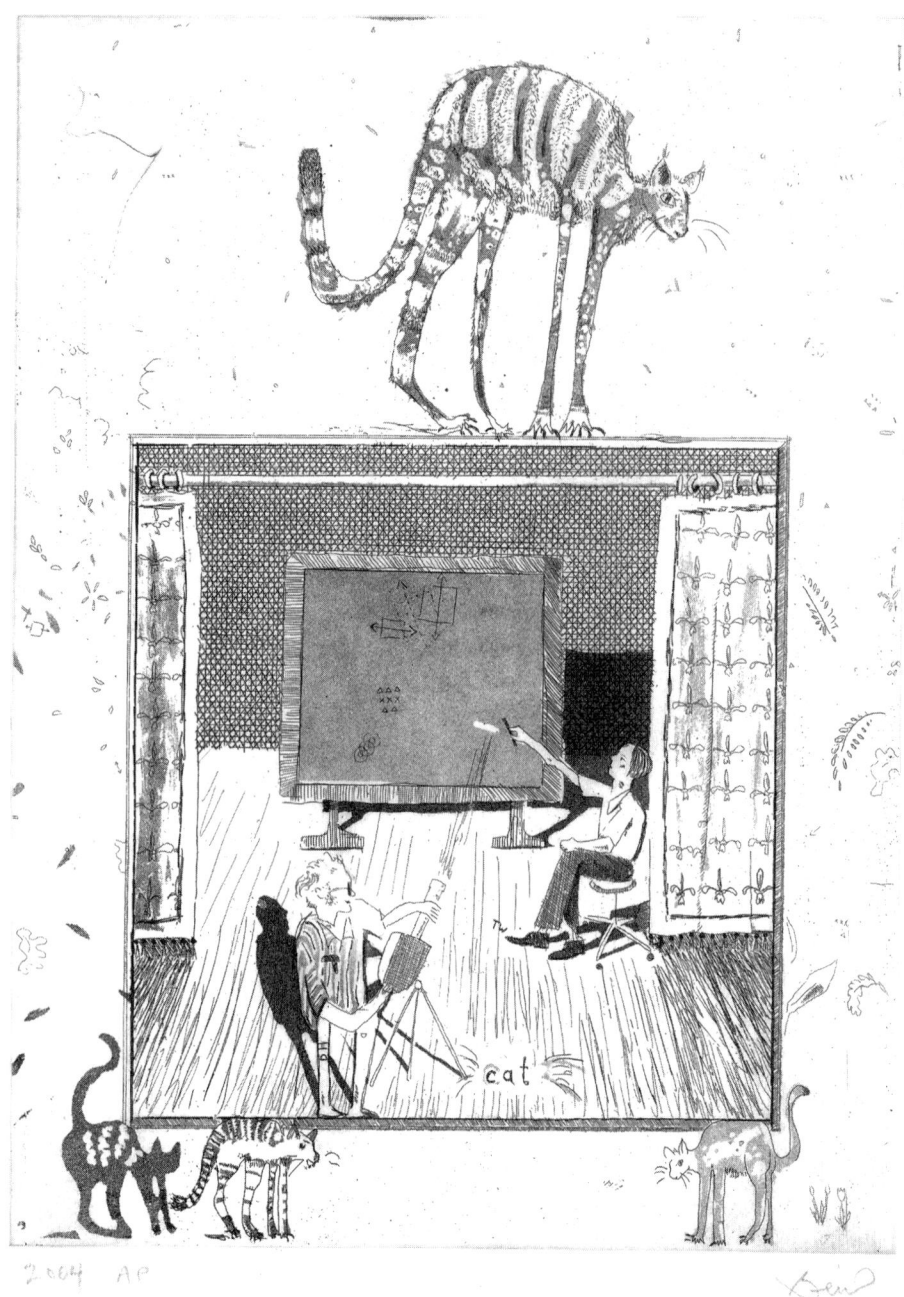

Bevil Conway, "Spots and Bars: David Hubel and Torsten Wiesel" (2004), Hardground etching and aquatint (edition:75).

I have depicted Hubel and Wiesel in the lab, in the early 1960s, at the peak of their exploration of the physiology of the early cat visual system. Hubel and Wiesel pulled back the metaphorical curtain on the black-box that was the visual system and established a firm foundation for our understanding of visual processing in all mammals including humans. Their discoveries have totally transformed the way in which we understand vision, a revolution that will have repercussions in all fields of knowledge, not least of which being the practice of art: just as understanding anatomy revolutionized the way renaissance artists made art, so too will an understanding of the neural mechanisms of visual processing profoundly affect art making. This frontispiece is a celebration of Hubel and Wiesel's achievement and serves as a reminder that science and art are constantly intertwined; in fact it is precisely at the interface of the two that the most exciting discoveries are made.

BRAIN AND VISUAL PERCEPTION

The Story of a 25-Year Collaboration

DAVID H. HUBEL
TORSTEN N. WIESEL

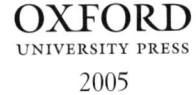

OXFORD

UNIVERSITY PRESS

2005

OXFORD

UNIVERSITY PRESS

Oxford   New York
Auckland   Bangkok   Buenos Aires   Cape Town   Chennai
Dar es Salaam   Delhi   Hong Kong   Istanbul   Karachi   Kolkata
Kuala Lumpur   Madrid   Melbourne   Mexico City   Mumbai   Nairobi
São Paulo   Shanghai   Taipei   Tokyo   Toronto

Copyright © 2005 by Oxford University Press, Inc.

Published by Oxford University Press, Inc.
198 Madison Avenue, New York, New York 10016
http://www.oup.com

Oxford is a registered trademark of Oxford University Press

Library of Congress Cataloging-in-Publication Data
Hubel, David H.
Brain and visual perception : the story of a 25-year collaboration / David H. Hubel,
Torsten N. Wiesel.
p. ; cm.
Includes index.
ISBN 0-19-517618-9
1. Visual pathways. 2. Visual perception. I. Wiesel, Torsten N. II. Title.
[DNLM: 1. Visual Perception—physiology—United States. 2. Biomedical
Research—history—United States. 3. History of Medicine, 20th Cent.—United States. WW
11 AA1 H877b 2005]
QP475.H815 2005
152.14—dc22   2004049553

2   4   6   8   9   7   5   3

Printed in the United States of America
on acid-free paper

To our wives and children,
who put up with so much.

CONTENTS

PART I

INTRODUCTION AND BIOGRAPHIES

This book is about a scientific collaboration that began in 1958 and lasted until 1983. It consists of reprints of papers we published over those years, with introductions and afterthoughts to each paper and an overall introduction and final summary. We had several motives for compiling it. Having put our writing energies into our main papers, avoiding as far as we could the temptation to write reviews or to contribute to symposia and book chapters, we hated to see our work get lost in bound journals on library shelves. But more than just that, we have always felt that scientific papers in the styles of today go out of their way to keep concealed the very things a reader may most want to know. What led the authors to ask the questions in the first place? In what order were the different parts of the research taken up? To what extent was luck involved? What were the surprises? Was it fun? How much competition was there? And above all, perhaps, who were the authors and what were their lives like? Papers written a century ago feel much more intimate than today's papers. One thinks of Wheatstone's introduction to the article in which he first described stereopsis, describing how Leonardo had almost, but not quite, made the discovery years before. Or Count Rumford's account of his discovery of colored shadows—how he "called two of my friends who happened to lodge in the house (Lord and Lady Palmerston) into the room, and without letting them into the secret simply asked them, with a feigned air of indifference, which of the two colours they saw in the centre of the circular piece of paper on the floor they thought the brightest". Today most papers seem dry, their juices sucked out, with little sense of the delight that can accompany discovery. Doubtless the authors have wanted to give the impression of scientific rigor, following a custom of scientific writing that treats science (with a capital S) as something with a separate existence that is independent of the humans who are responsible for it. We find the attitude unfortunate, but in our papers we have had to adhere to today's customs or face fierce editorial resistance. This book is in part an attempt to restore some of the juices.

Because this is the account of a collaboration between two people who contributed equally, we began it by referring to each of us in the third person. The result seemed stilted and awkward. Today our paths have diverged, leaving me (D.H.H.) with time for writing and research, while Torsten's time is occupied with running many scientific endeavors. Someone had to do the writing, so the bulk of the story, except for our separate biographies, will be told by me, in the first person. Nevertheless, what is said should be regarded as coming from the two of us in equal measure.

We apologize for not having led more adventurous lives. Neither of us climbed Mount Everest, took part in the French Resistance, or sailed around the world. Our purpose in the biographies is simply to give an impression of how we grew up and what kinds of people we are, things that are usually carefully kept out of scientific papers. Some will think that such things are unimportant, having nothing to do with science, where only facts are worth knowing. We simply don't agree. To take just two exalted examples, we wish we had a more vivid sense of what Bach and Galileo were like as humans, and find it even harder to imagine what many of the scientists of the past century were like.

Our experiences in science do constitute a kind of adventure, and above all we hope that this book will convey some slight impression of that adventure, and of the fun of doing science. For us, on the whole, aside from the late nights and the fatigue, it has been a wonderful journey, a bit like a ride on a roller coaster. We have especially enjoyed the variety of our lives in research: the experiments, involving surgery, electronics, and any number of toy-like gadgets; the fun and torture of writing, the teaching and advising of students, interactions with a huge range of technicians, administrators, and colleagues; the possibility of travel to all parts of the world (except Antarctica and Greenland); and the interacting with other scientists—some ordinary like ourselves and some giants. Above all else there has been the freedom, in choosing problems and projects, and even in deciding what to do from one hour to the next.

From our papers one might easily be led to think that the research was dogged, tedious, sedulous, demanding infinite patience. We are possibly guilty of encouraging that impression in order to keep down competition. People would surely crowd into a field if they had any idea how exciting the experiments can be. Finding a good cell and unlocking its secrets can be like fishing in richly populated streams without having to wait for the fish to bite, or playing with a wonderful new toy. Much of our time has been spent tinkering, playing with forms, colors, and rates of movement in an effort to learn what our cells need, in the way of stimuli, to make them react. When we succeed, and suddenly can make a cell fire like a machine gun, it can be thrilling, and on a good day the thrills may come every few hours. Unlike much of today's science, in which the actual work is done by technicians or graduate students, who pipette solutions from one column to another while the bosses write papers, raise money, or travel and talk about the graduate students' results, it is we who get to do the experiments—plus the other stuff! When it comes to sheer fun, our field is hard to beat. We try to keep that a secret.

It is hard to believe that we first began the project of collecting our reprints and comments one summer far back in the late 1960s, at the Salk Institute. We each had the loan of a beautiful studio-office, with floors covered by rugs with thick piles and views of the Pacific through teak-framed windows that would actually open, allowing us to hear the surf and distant tennis. The project did not take off, because it was so tempting either to lie on the rug and take a nap, or to escape to the tennis court or the beach. It was so tempting that we did only one experiment that summer. If you were brought up in Sweden or Canada and lived in Boston, La Jolla just wasn't the right place to get anything done. The ambiance was wrong. We missed the rain. So the writing of the book lapsed for a few years, to be taken up again, then lapse again, finally to be almost abandoned—but not quite. Here, at last, is the final result, and we hope you enjoy it.

Chapter 1 • David H. Hubel •

GROWING UP IN MONTREAL

My parents were American and grew up in Detroit. In the Depression my father, a chemical engineer, got a job as a chemist in Windsor, just across the border in Ontario, Canada. He soon tired of the daily commute and trips through customs, and finally moved permanently to Windsor, where I was born in 1926. At my birth my parents registered me as an American citizen, and so as a Canadian by birth and an American by derivation I grew up a dual citizen with all of the mixed loyalties that implies. In 1929 my father was transferred to Montreal, where I was brought up and educated and where I continued to live until the age of 28.

Our family lived in Outremont, a middle-class suburb of Montreal that was predominately French-speaking, and whose remaining English-speaking component was largely Jewish. English-speaking children attended the "Outremont Protestant Schools", "Protestant" meaning non-Catholic, which seems ironic given that on Jewish holidays out of a typical class of thirty pupils at my school I would find myself in a class of about five other Protestants. Our teachers were all English-speaking and non-Catholic because in Quebec, Catholics were not allowed to teach in "Protestant" schools. This had the strange and unfortunate result that French was taught either by English-speaking teachers or by Huguenots imported from France. No effort was made to teach us to speak or understand French as spoken with a French-Canadian accent, and after eight years of daily hour-long French lessons almost none of us could converse in French (Parisian or Canadian), nor could we understand the French spoken on a local radio station, or even read a French novel. At that time it was an economic necessity for the French to master English, and they did, but English-Canadians rarely bothered to learn French. We talked to our French neighbors in English, and were unable to buy a ticket on a streetcar without being laughed at by the French conductors. So the potential advantages of growing up in a bilingual society were largely lost.

We lived for the first seven years in the upper floor of a duplex, the lower floor of which was occupied by the French landlord's family. From the time I was three years old until I turned eight I played nonstop with the landlord's boy, Michael Fauteux, whom I first encountered on the day of our arrival, at a sandbox at the back of the house—so my first French word was *sable,* French for "sand" and pronounced in Canada "sawb". "Perhaps" was "p'tayt" (for peut-etre) and "I can't" was "poke-a-pab" (for "pas capable"). We gradually concocted a language of our own, part English and part French, jabbering away as our parents listened amazed, unable to understand a word.

At school (I attended Strathcona Academy until my high school graduation in 1943), the atmosphere was serious and encouraged hard work. Unfortunately, there was almost no emphasis on sports. Parents in the area were not wealthy, and they wanted their children to get ahead. To get into McGill College one needed a matriculation grade of 65, unless one was Jewish, and then the required grade was 75. The result was that Jewish children worked harder and generally got better grades. Everyone was ranked in class; for the first few years I averaged around fifteenth out of a class of 30. The top-ranking three or four pupils were always girls, but in Grade 6 all the classes became segregated by sex, and I began to rank first in my all-boys class, a rank I continued to hold till the end of high school. Of course I would rather have been in a mixed class and have ranked lower. (My wife, Ruth, was more fortunate. At her Montreal West school, pupils who got good grades were rewarded by being put in a mixed class.) Luckily for me my school was small, with about 150 pupils in each grade, divided into classes of about 28 each. Consequently the principal and the teachers knew most of the students in the school by name. Our library was not great and lab facilities were poor, but those things were probably far outweighed by our knowing our teachers and fellow students. Parents were not encouraged to butt into school affairs, something that must have saved the teachers much time and annoyance.

Most of our teachers were excellent. Schools in Canada were financed by the provinces rather than by the local communities, as they are in the United States, so that the quality of schools had nothing to do with the wealth of neighborhoods. In Montreal, the best English high school was in one of the poorest neighborhoods. My school was in a not-wealthy but not-poor part of Outremont, and ranked close to the top in the province. With high school matriculation examinations set by and graded by the province, one ended by knowing one's exact grade and standing. In the last year of high school I tied with a close friend for fourth place in Quebec province. I suppose I did well partly because I was bright, but mainly because I worked hard, probably harder than I ever have since.

In my final year of high school I was especially lucky in two of my teachers. A history teacher, Miss Julia Bradshaw, was famous in Quebec Province and vividly remembered and much loved by every graduate of my school. Tiny, short, thin, redheaded Irish with a temper to match, she assigned a weekly essay which she corrected with red ink, and was brutal in her comments, especially with the top students. I learned more about writing from her than from anyone before or since, perhaps partly because she was more concerned with original ideas than with sentence structure. My Latin teacher, Mr. Lindsay, was a mild-mannered man who had once taught in a university and had a profound knowledge of classics. With his encouragement and help I read an entire book of Caesar's *Gallic Wars*.

Unfortunately we were taught almost nothing about our neighbor to the south—literally nothing, if one happened to be home with a bad sore throat the one day U.S. history was covered. History was either British (and wonderful, with sovereigns like Henry VIII, Elizabeth I, and Edward II and the red-hot poker) or Canadian, which was boring. In the upper high school grades, world history in Miss Bradshaw's hands was superb, but tended to steer clear of matters involving the United States. English literature meant British literature, plus the little that there was of English Canadian literature, so we never heard of Walt Whitman or Mark Twain. And not a word about Tolstoy or Proust, to say nothing of French Canadian authors.

Neither of my parents was especially religious, though on my mother's side one great-grandparent was a Methodist minister. My father's father was born in Nördlingen, Bavaria, and came with his family to the United States at the age of four. This charming Protestant town, in the centre of an ancient meteorite crater, is separated from its strongly Catholic surroundings by a still-intact medieval wall. Both my parents were thus more anti-Catholic than simply Protestant. I was sent to Sunday school at a United Church (Methodist united with Presbyterian) in Outremont, but never got into the habit of regular church attendance. I finally began to attend the Unitarian Church in Montreal, attracted there because beliefs are completely up to the individual, and because my piano teacher was organist. In the years that followed, my wife and I continued to attend the Unitarian Church in Washington, D.C., where the minister, E. Powell Davies, was world-famous. Today we belong to the Wellesley Unitarian Church, though our attendance is irregular.

My mother's mild anti-Catholicism is well illustrated by an event that occurred years later. In 1992 I was invited along with all other living Nobel prize–winners to a celebration at the Vatican, at which the pope marked the 350th anniversary of the death of Galileo, and formally apologized (as it were) for the Church's treatment of him. After the pope's speech (which was for some reason in French) each prize-winner had the opportunity to be separately introduced and to exchange a few words with the Holy Father. Making the introductions was an Italian gentleman with a camera, and each of us was photographed shaking hands with the pope. On receiving copies of the picture, some months later, I proudly sent one to my mother, I suppose to show off the exalted company I was keeping. My mother without hesitation seized a pair of scissors, cut off the poor pope and threw that half picture in the wastebasket. All my relatives on my mother's side of the family, the Hunter side, have senses of humor that are rather special, and found this event hilarious in the extreme. Not all my friends have found the story quite so funny.

I became interested in science at a very early age. My grandfather on my father's side was part inventor and part businessman. He trained as a pharmacist, and became famous for devising the first process to mass-produce gelatine capsules. On retirement he sold his Detroit factory and patents to Park Davis Company. My mother's father and two of her brothers were architects, specializing in churches that still stand in Detroit and various towns in Ontario.

Part of my success in school I owe to my father, whom I plagued with incessant questions until I knew more chemistry than my teachers. For Christmas I was given my first chemistry set when I was five years old—a serious British-made set in the days before substances more interesting than salt and sugar were considered poisons. I vividly remember, that Christmas day, watching my father transform a glass of water into a bright purple-red solution with a single tiny crystal of potassium permanganate, and then make the color vanish by adding a pinch of sodium thiosulphate. In the years that followed I assembled a collection of chemicals and simple apparatus. In those days it was easy to obtain any chemicals one wanted. At age 14 I went downtown by streetcar and came back with two brown glass-stoppered one-pound bottles of concentrated sulphuric acid and nitric acid. My collection already included a four-ounce bottle of potassium cyanide.

I produced hydrogen by pouring hydrochloric acid over zinc carpet binding, and got the gas into a rubber balloon by looping its neck over the neck of a medicine bottle. I sent off many hydrogen balloons with attached notes, one of which brought an answer, after many months, in French, from a farmer's daughter 100 miles away in Sherbrooke, Quebec. I mixed potassium chlorate (which I bought by the pound) with sugar and a small amount of potassium ferrocyanide, put the mixture in a sturdy brass cannon replica inherited from my grandfather, and packed it with a rag. A match inserted into the Touch-hole produced a huge explosion that rattled the neighbors' kitchen pans, gave rise to a thin suspension of smoke over Outremont, and brought two burly French policemen to the house. I told them that I had put firecrackers in the cannon. They smiled and told me to stop doing that.

Of course I did not stop. On several occasions I climbed one of the Laurentian Mountains north of Montreal and fired off the cannon from the summit, listening to the echoes as they came back, one by one, from the other mountains in the area.

My father was an avid photographer and we set up a darkroom in the basement, where we developed film and made enlargements. I still keep up photography as a hobby, and have spent hours in the darkroom at the lab, photographing and reconstructing serial sections. Today black-and-white photography has largely given way to color, dark-room work at home has become impractical, and film is increasingly replaced by digital cameras.

Another hobby, electronics, was prompted by my hearing, on a crystal set, a radio amateur broadcasting from a station a few blocks away. I built several modest radios but had no one to advise me about electricity, and the few books I could find were of little use. My main text was the Radio Amateur's Handbook—a 1930s edition—which would have been opaque even to a college student, then or today. Nevertheless I did learn Ohm's Law and tried to understand L-C resonance. I built a more ambitious three-tube shortwave radio that never worked despite months of effort. It suffered from something called "motorboating", a series of loud clicks that drowned out any stations. Many years later I learned its cause—positive feedback though the power supply—which could have been eliminated by an expert in minutes. Discouraged, I lost interest in radio until in 1993, at age 67, my interest in radio revived and I passed five sets of ham radio exams, learned Morse code, and took on, or revived, a new hobby.

My interest in music went back to an early age. Like most of our neighbors' families we had a piano, which both my parents and my older sister played. I began to learn from my sister, who was three years older, and started formal lessons at the age of five. I acquired my first truly great music teacher, George Brewer, a pianist and the leading organist in Montreal, when I was midway through high school. Mr. Brewer was passionately fond of Bach and managed to impart that to me. I was only moderately talented and a hopelessly bad sight-reader: had it been otherwise I might have been tempted to go on with music as a career. I have wondered if my bad sight-reading, like my slow speed at ordinary reading, is related to my being left-handed.

A big advantage of growing up in Montreal was the easy availability of both skating—with rinks in almost every park—and skiing in the Laurentian Mountains 60 to 80 miles north of Montreal. One could take a train to some Laurentian town and ski back one or two stations, often mostly downhill, returning in the evening to the tune of riotous French-Canadian songs like "Alouette".

A large number of hobbies have been for me both a strength and a curse. Today I keep up interests in piano, flute, ham radio, weaving (rugs and blankets), amateur astronomy, photography, languages (French novels mainly, some German, Japanese), and tennis. I make up for the time those interests consume by reading as little as possible in my field of neurophysiology. Reading most papers today is like eating sawdust. I have been lucky in having co-workers who follow the literature compulsively and try to keep me informed.

In talking with young students I am impressed by the degree to which television and computers have replaced hobbies like chemistry (and explosives!), photography, and electronics. Our parents tended to leave us alone to develop our own interests; they did not chauffeur us from ballet or Hebrew lessons to Little League baseball. Few of my friends' families had cars, which were in any case useless in Montreal's snowy and frigid winter. With parents who didn't organize our lives it was much easier to reach the level of boredom necessary to think up things to do for ourselves.

As a twelve-year-old I found in a bookstore in Portland, Maine, a book called *The World of Science,* by an Englishman named F. Sherwood Taylor. It was written for adults, I suppose, but was lucid, readable, and a virtual encyclopedia of science. I read every one of its 1050 pages. In the 1930s, books that treated science on anything like an introductory level were almost nonexistent, and again and again I got caught up in puzzles to which I could not find answers. There was of course my father, but his field was chemistry and he knew very little physics. Any science books around the house were huge unreadable chemistry tomes by Mendeleeff and Mellor, so I spent days trying to figure out how electricity could go from positive to negative, when it consisted of electron flow and electrons were negative. All I needed was someone to tell me that it was a matter of an unfortunate convention, and that nothing actually went from positive to negative. That was long before the days when one had to consider holes as well as electrons; that would really have confused me!

Given that I ended up a biologist, it is ironic that I had almost no formal instruction in biology in grade school, high school, or college. In the final two years of high school our choice of concentration was between Latin, mathematics, and biology: Latin was recommended if one planned to go into medicine—oddly given that the only direct application of Latin to medicine was the few words that would crop up in prescriptions to help make them incomprehensible to the laity. Mathematics was for future engineers, and biology was chosen by the less ambitious students. The advanced math that was offered was easy enough for me to cover one evening in the bathtub. I had gotten to love Latin in the first two years of high school and chose that over biology, which I felt I could learn by myself or by reading *The World of Science*.

COLLEGE AND MEDICAL SCHOOL (1943–1951)

After high school I had hoped vaguely to go to MIT and even travelled to Boston for an interview, but that year (1939) World War II broke out, and plans to come to Boston had to be shelved. So I went to McGill College in Montreal, and lived at home. Socially, college was unexciting, partly because of living at home, without benefit of a car, with a daily round-trip commuting time of about two hours. I had developed a love for mathematics and physics, and enrolled in a combined honors course in those subjects. I spent much time doing problems, which I loved, with few facts to memorize and enough time to keep up some hobbies, to attend most of the concerts in Montreal, and to read many novels. Physics at McGill was almost defunct, much of the talent having been co-opted by the war. Mathematics was excellent, and although it did not turn out to be useful in any direct way in later work, it taught me the dangers of relying on reasoning that involves more than a very few steps.

Travel abroad during the war was impossible. Summers I spent mainly working on Quebec farms, where I learned to hitch a horse to a rake or a mowing machine, to milk cows, and to thin turnips. One summer I journeyed with some college friends to a job on the north shore of Lake Superior at a pulp-mill town called Red Rock. There I designed the town sewer system and worked as an electricians' helper. One summer I spent on a farm near the small town of Magog, which bordered a beautiful lake, Memphramagog. The farm was owned by a wealthy Montreal businessman who ran it as a hobby and owned a cottage on the lake. During the day I farmed, and in the evenings I danced with the teenagers who summered on the lake. I look back on that summer as an oasis in what was otherwise a social desert.

At the end of my final year in college (1947) I had to decide what to do next. I did not want to be a mathematician and doubtless lacked the virtuosity. Attending an international physics congress in Montreal in 1943 showed me how inadequate my physics training had been, but for want of an alternative I applied and was accepted to graduate school in physics at McGill. Almost on a whim I also applied to medical school, and to my horror was accepted there, too—so now I was faced with my first big career decision. I had no background or experience in medicine, but I suppose I had some vague ideas about applying physics to medical research, or else becoming a clinician, which sounded like fun. I also sensed that I was far from ready to make any final career decisions. The length of medical training would give me more time, and its breadth and greater range would ultimately give me more things to choose from.

By the time the registration date at the medical school rolled around I still had not made up my mind. I phoned the secretary, a Miss Mudge (who, as I later learned, virtually ran the school) and explained my predicament. She replied, "Take your time, there's no hurry; just let us know what you decide". I liked that generous attitude, and decided to give medicine a try. So in the fall of 1947 I found myself in the first-year medical class, in which half the students were newly returned World War II veterans, three to four years older than the rest of us, serious, and hard-working. Most of the students were of course men, in huge contrast with present-day medical classes.

Luckily medical school was not expensive. The fees at McGill were $400 a year, and by living at home and commuting I could end up debt-free. My father never breathed a word of protest at supporting me all those years, to say nothing of my parents' putting up with me around the house. But socially, compared to the lives led by most students today, life was pretty dry.

For me, medical school came as a shock. I had had almost no preparation in biology. To fulfil entrance requirements, the summer before medical school, I had taken the equivalent of a semester each of invertebrate zoology and botany, certainly an odd preparation for a future doctor. I looked on biology with the disdain that physicists often harbor. My worst disadvantage was being unused to memorizing facts—I assumed that if I could understand what I read or what a lecturer said I did not need to do anything further. The result was that in the first set of mid-term exams I received four Cs, a completely new experience. (C was in those pre-inflation days not a bad grade; it was just average.) Obviously I had to start working, and discovered to my surprise that if I worked at it even carbohydrate metabolism could be interesting. I later discovered that I could get enthusiastic over the more clinical subjects, even those almost devoid of intellectual content such as obstetrics. I enjoyed pediatrics because children were fun and case histories were mercifully short. I found neurology and neuroanatomy especially interesting because of their complexity and mystery. Neurophysiology was disappointing because so little was known.

At McGill, neurology and neuroanatomy were outstandingly well taught. The world-famous Montreal Neurological Institute was just a block away, with Herbert Jasper in clinical neurophysiology, Wilder Penfield in neurosurgery, and Francis MacNaughton in neurology and neuroanatomy. Penfield, who was easily the most celebrated doctor in Canada, surprised me by reading his lectures, but I was inspired the first time I heard him talk on epilepsy by the obvious passion he brought to the subject. Towards the end of my second year in medical school I screwed up my courage and called Penfield's secretary to ask for an interview. She said she would arrange it but that it would take some time. Months later the fatal moment arrived. I parked the family car on University Street and full of trepidation I approached the Great Man's office. I felt like a lowly monk going to an interview with the pope. Penfield, who turned out to be charming, listened attentively to my plans and interests. He quickly realized that I should be talking with Herbert Jasper and led me up the flight of stairs that separated their offices. So I met both Penfield and Jasper for the first time that day. Jasper, perhaps the leading neurophysiologist in Canada, was as friendly as Penfield had been. He asked me what I had read on the subject of neurophysiology. I answered that I had read *Cybernetics,* by Norbert Wiener. Looking a bit sceptical Jasper asked if I had understood it. I forget what I answered, but I hope that I was honest. Jasper introduced me to his electronics engineer and arranged for me to work summers at the Institute.

I must indeed have been nervous that day. When I arrived back at the parked family car I found that I had left it locked with the motor running and the keys in the ignition. Luckily there was still gas left when I finally arrived back one and a half hours later after the round-trip home by streetcar to pick up a spare set of keys. (Years later when I met the real pope, I was not nervous at all. One does get over stage fright.)

INTERN AND RESIDENT (1951–1955)

After graduating from medical school, at age 25, I did a rotating internship at Montreal General Hospital. For the first time I was not living at home. The year was intense and enormous fun. It was divided into four three-month rotations, which consisted of medicine, outpatient surgery (called "accident room" or "emergency room" in the United States), gynecology, and psychiatry at the mental hospital in Verdun. Rather to my surprise I found internal medicine dull, perhaps because it was skewed in the direction of geriatrics. Psychiatry and surgery tied for the most interesting. I loved sewing up lacerations and setting bones. Gynecology consisted of attending outpatient clinics, which I enjoyed, and assisting at hysterectomies, which after the first few operations was tedious. I did dozens of dilation-andcurettages. I found the psychiatric patients, who were mostly psychotic, fascinating even though they were a complete mystery and treatment was most unsatisfactory. The field seemed to lack theoretical underpinning, relying either on the ideas of Freud, which I found unconvincing, or on bland though well-meaning recipes for living that lacked the strength and wisdom of Ann Landers.

During my year of medical internship I started going out with Ruth (my future wife), whom I met at the McGill choral society. (In the United States of America it would be called a "glee club"). One of Ruth's closest friends was Ellen Simons, who was engaged to and later married Mario Duschenes, one of the leading flautists in Canada and also a consummate recorder player. Ruth and I soon joined a group of about 20 recorder enthusiasts, led by Mario. I began to work hard at the recorder, partly because no piano was available at the hospital. I practiced at the eye clinic, which was always deserted in the evenings. I got good enough to be invited by Mario to join his recorder quartet, probably the only such quartet in Canada. I joined the musician's union, and in addition to doing several concerts in Montreal we performed twice for the Canadian Broadcasting Company.

By 1952 I was eager to start doing research—being 26 years old and never having done a minute of research of any kind. But on Herbert Jasper's advice I decided to do some clinical neurology as a background for future research in neurophysiology. So I put in a year of neurology residency at the Montreal Neurological Institute (MNI), and followed that by a year of clinical neurophysiology (mostly electroencephalography [EEG]) with Herbert Jasper.

Students often ask me whether all that clinical training was really necessary. Would not a Ph.D. have been a more useful training for a research career in neurophysiology? My answer is that I really can't say. One cannot go back and do a control. But just out of college with a degree in mathematics and physics I was certainly in no position to choose a research career. I needed the perspective that the medical training gave, but whether I needed seven years of perspective is anyone's guess. The research Torsten and I did later, especially the work on visual deprivation, was clearly influenced by our clinical backgrounds.

I was married in June, 1953, on an incredibly hot day the summer after the first neurology residency year. I had been engaged to Ruth far too long, but marriage had had to be postponed for lack of an income. We were married at the Montreal West United Church. Mario Duschenes played one of our favorite pieces of music, the slow movement of the Bach solo flute partita. The reception that followed the wedding was marked by an incident that came close to a disaster. My sister, Joan, suddenly came up behind Ruth and began to slap her on the back vehemently. This unusual and seemingly not very friendly behavior was prompted by Joan's noticing that Ruth's wedding dress was on fire. It turned out that the fire had nothing to do with the heat of the day—Ruth had walked a bit too close to the candles that decorated the festive table. The back-slapping extinguished the fire and saved Ruth from a badly timed immolation. The guests must have thought that in supplying entertainment we were going a bit too far.

Our marriage had had to be postponed for financial reasons. As an intern and during the following year as a neurology resident I earned nothing, although the hospitals were generous enough to pay for our uniforms and our board and meals. The year after that, for reading so many electroencephalograms (EEGs), I was paid $1500 (per annum!), and during the final residency year at Hopkins I earned $35 a month. So for the first two years after we were married we lived on Ruth's slender earnings as research assistant at one or another hospital. I am most grateful to her for keeping us going—and I am certainly resentful towards the medical profession of that era for exploiting trainees the way it did. In the years that followed, Ruth was great to put up so cheerfully with my late nights, and trips abroad that were foreclosed to her because of having to take care of our children, and an often truculent and inconsiderate husband. Children would have to be postponed until I entered the army, when a captain's salary finally made that possible.

Today in medicine residents are paid infinitely more, given that then we were paid nothing. But at least our medical-school fees were far lower, compared with the astronomical fees of today. In the United States of America, graduates from medical schools typically have accumulated debts of a few hundred thousand dollars. For those who wish to do research, there may be additional years of training and little expectation of quick rewards at the end to help pay off the debts. At one point in my post-doctoral training I could easily have used the research I had done to obtain a Ph.D. but the effort of writing a thesis seemed daunting and a bore. The doctorate would have been for the work I did at Walter Reed, in Washington, and would have been granted by one of the few universities in the area. When I mentioned the possibility to Steve Kuffler, he remarked, "From some universities you are better *not* to have a Ph.D.!"

I began the EEG year (1953–1954) at the MNI as apprentice to Cosimo Ajmone-Marsan, who taught me for three months but then left to take a position as head of EEG at the labs that were just starting up at the National Institutes of Health (NIH), in Bethesda. So with that brief preparation I took over as Herbert Jasper's main assistant, being landed with all the institute's EEGs except for those of the Penfield service, which were read by Jasper himself. Reading EEGs was and probably still is largely empirical, with little understanding of what produces the electrical waves or why they change in conditions such as brain tumours or epilepsy. Turning the pages day after day gave me writer's cramp. At the end of that year I resolved never again to read an EEG, though next to Jasper I was possibly the world expert on the subject. I have stuck to that resolution.

During the EEG-fellowship year I took part in a course in which the Fellows were assigned topics on which they had to give talks. By some lucky chance I was given vision as my topic, a subject about which I knew almost nothing. In preparing, I happened to come across the 1952 Cold Spring Harbor symposium, which included papers by Keffer Hartline and Stephen Kuffler. That was my first exposure to the idea of a set of nerve cells receiving information from the environment and transforming it in a way that could be useful to an organism. I was hugely impressed. I could hardly have predicted that I would get to know both Hartline and Kuffler, and that I would one day become a close friend and associate of Kuffler's.

One day shortly after Ajmone-Marsan's departure, a young neurologist, Charles Luttrell, visited the Montreal Neurological Institute from Johns Hopkins Hospital to learn EEG, and it fell to me to teach him. Charles must have been impressed with the instruction, because a few days after his return to Baltimore he telephoned me, around 6:30 A.M., to ask if I would be interested in the neurology residency at Hopkins. I consulted Jasper, and remember his saying that Hopkins was not famous as a center for neurology, but was a major center for neurophysiology, with such people as Mountcastle and Kuffler. I had no other exciting prospects, and decided to accept. Up to then I had had all my training in Montreal, and wanted to see something new.

Baltimore was insufferably hot when Ruth and I arrived from Montreal in July, 1954, and it was hard to find much beauty in it. To get out of the heat we went to a movie the first night. It was cooler there, but the movie, *Gone with the Wind,* was the longest and most tedious I have ever been unlucky enough to sit through. (And as Canadians, we were not used to the reek of popcorn at movies.) We moved into an apartment on the ten hundred block of North Broadway, which was very nearly a slum area but had the advantage that most of our neighbors were Hopkins house staff. Our landlady, who was nice enough, tried to alleviate the smell of garbage in the front hall by liberally spraying it with cheap perfume. The combination of smells was unpleasant but interesting. We found the cockroaches unpleasant, especially the large variety that click as they scuttle along. We soon moved to a better apartment a bit closer to the hospital and in a safer area, with a tiny back yard, small enough that the grass could be cut with a pair of kitchen scissors. Ruth got a job as assistant in the lab of Curt Richter, a famous, ingenious, eccentric psychologist, with a feel for biology. Ruth's project was to study the history of the use of the rat as a laboratory animal. Richter had on the wall of his laboratory a map of Baltimore that showed, by shading, the incidence of rat bites, and it was clear that we were living in the very epicenter of such events. (Both species, rats and cockroaches, fall into what Kafka might have categorized as *Ungezieffer* in his novel *Metamorphosis.*) Ruth's job gave us a tiny income. My own contribution as a resident was $17 a month, which was augmented by the kind head of neurology, Jack Magladery, who managed to dig up an additional $18. Rents were of course much lower than they are today, around $70 a month.

At Hopkins the atmosphere was exhilarating, lively, and informal. At lunch everyone in fields related to neurology gravitated to the same table in the doctors' dining room, and I soon met and got to know both Stephen Kuffler and Vernon Mountcastle, whose friendliness and informality made it easy to forget that they were established high priests in neurophysiology.

Neurology at Hopkins was a branch of internal medicine, not a separate department, so the emphasis was quite different from what I had experienced Montreal, where it was closely related to, and dominated by, neurosurgery. I saw two great clinicians in action, the pediatric neurologist Frank Ford, and the neuro-ophthalmologist Frank Walsh. Their style of neurology was far from the obsessively interminable histories and physical examinations that neurologists of the Queen Square tradition were famous for. Ford seemed hardly to take a history or examine his patients, and yet in thinking about it later one realized he had asked every important question and missed nothing, and his diagnoses were almost always right. Walsh was dynamic and colorful, and introduced me to a field whose existence I had hardly even been aware of. That was important, considering that I ended up a neurophysiologist specializing in the visual system.

At Hopkins I found my previous clinical preparation no match for the high-powered training that was usual at the best clinical centers in the United States of America—except for my experience with epilepsy at the Montreal Neurological Institute. So I made my share of mistakes. These were to some extent eclipsed by two clinical coups that are fun to look back on. The chief of neurology, Jack Magladery, cultivated an eccentric bedside manner. He always began his neurological examination of a patient by listening to the eyes with a stethoscope, never hearing anything but always impressing onlookers. One night I was prowling around the medical wards looking for interesting cases when one of the medical interns brought me to see a patient who was a major puzzle, with a hemiparesis and an assortment of other symptoms that I can't remember, and in any case made no sense to anyone. I began examining him, and because a few house staff were looking on I started by listening to the eyes. To my amazement, from one of the eyes came a noise like a pulsating fire hose, a bruit the likes of which I had never heard before, and which made it immediately clear that this man's problem was a cerebral arteriovenous shunt. So suddenly there were crowds of interns and residents around the bed, and I had been catapulted to instant fame. That cancelled out any number of previous blunders. My second coup occurred when I was called to see a young man with obvious meningitis, with stiff neck, headache, and pain on straight-leg raising. The diagnosis was clear, and my job was to do the lumbar puncture so that the spinal fluid could be cultured to determine the organism. On a whim I decided to look at the spinal fluid myself instead of simply sending it to the bacteriology lab. I can still see the swarms of double bacteria swimming in that fluid like infinity signs. So I could return to the wards ten minutes later and announce that the patient had pneumococcal meningitis, cancelling out still more former blunders and adding to my local fame.

WALTER REED AND BEGINNING RESEARCH (1955–1958)

As a dual citizen I was subject to the American draft, which up to then I had escaped by never having resided in the United States. But I knew that on accepting the Hopkins residency I would have to register for the doctor's draft. There was no war on then—it was between World War II and Korea—but because of a shortage in the armed services, doctors continued to be called up for two years of service. I registered and was indeed called up, but was deferred until the end of the residency year at Hopkins. My choice was between the army and the Public Health Service, and I applied first to the U.S. Public Health Service, hoping to be assigned to a neurophysiology laboratory at the NIH in Bethesda—that would have fulfilled the service obligation—but they were not interested. I introduced myself to a group of neurophysiologists at Walter Reed Army Institute of Research, and probably because of my training in EEG they agreed to put in a request for me should I join the army. The Walter Reed people subsequently forgot to make the request, and had I not reminded them just in time, I would have ended up spending the two years of service in Japan examining recruits.

So I arrived at Walter Reed Army Institute of Research, in Washington, D.C., in August of 1955, as an army captain. We moved into a pleasant apartment (rat-free and roach-free) in Silver Spring, which we could afford because suddenly I was paid the huge annual salary of $10,000. At last we were solvent. Ruth got a job as research assistant at the Armed Forces Institute of Pathology, but worked there only up to the time of the birth of our first boy, Carl. He was born at Walter Reed Army Hospital in 1955, for which the bill, after a week's stay, was $18.00. I have to compliment the obstetrics service at Walter Reed: among other things, at Ruth's request, no anesthetic was used for the delivery, only mild sedation. The delivery was easy and uneventful. The experience for our second child, Eric, back in Baltimore in 1959, was equally smooth. Our youngest, Paul, was born at Boston Lying In, as it was then called. There the ultra-conservative obstetricians insisted on heavy anesthesia. Only at my urging was spinal anesthesia avoided. My training in neurology was not entirely wasted!

Our three years in suburban Washington were relatively uneventful I remember D.C. as populated mainly by civil servants, without much of a life or soul of its own. For amusement in the evening we would walk around the Silver Spring neighborhood looking into our neighbors' large apartment picture-living-room windows, which were then fashionable. We had the rare opportunity to go regularly to concerts at the Library of Congress, where the Budapest String Quartet was in residence, and people in the armed forces and their dependents could easily get tickets. Three years of regular attendance was the musical experience of a lifetime.

To be part of the Walter Reed neurophysiology group was a fantastic piece of luck. I had complete independence, the benefit of advice from my supervisor, the spinal cord neurophysiologist Mike Fuortes; from Robert Galambos, a well-known auditory neurophysiologist; and the neuroanatomist Walle Nauta, who was already one of the leaders of modern experimental neuroanatomy and famous for developing a stain for degenerating fibers that revolutionized that field. The entire group consisted of only about a dozen people and was part of the neuropsychiatry section of Walter Reed, led by the eminent psychiatrist and neuranatomist David Rioch. No one tried to influence what I did, though everyone was helpful and generous with advice. I could change direction of my research without consulting anyone. The first day it was made clear to me that they hoped I would be the local EEG expert. Feeling slightly guilty over having come to Walter Reed under false pretenses, I made my opinions about EEG clear. David Rioch seemed to sympathize, and the matter was dropped.

I was lucky to have Mike (Michelangelo) Fuortes as my immediate advisor. He was a young and vigorous Italian neurophysiologist with a wonderful biological sixth sense and a great sense of humor. The day I turned up, Mike wanted to know what, if anything, I had done in neurophysiology: Had I ever done any dissection? Had I ever anesthetized a cat? Had I ever made electrodes or run amplifiers? To all these questions the answers were "no". Mike, his face expressionless, turned and looked out the window for a while. He then announced a plan for the day. He had intended to do a cat spinal cord recording that morning, but decided that we should instead begin by setting up a frog sciatic-nerve recording so that I could learn about compound action potentials. We postponed the cat to the afternoon. That was my crash course in electrophysiology. In the next months we collaborated and completed a cat spinal cord project. Mike quickly composed and dictated a paper into some kind of dictaphone, the authors of which were to be Fuortes and Hubel. That was my first publication. What impressed me most was Mike's emphasizing to me that the order of authors had nothing to do with priority but reflected the policy of *The Journal of Physiology,* in which the order of authors was strictly alphabetical. I had not heard of that rule, and in any case had not dreamed that I should be first author, but it was typical of his generosity to point out the rule.

The time came to select a project of my own. Mike listed a few ideas for me to consider, one of which was to take fine insulated wires, cut them off with scissors, poke them into cat cortex, sew up the cat, and hope to record single cells when the animal recovered. I thought it worth trying, and so I began a project that was to last three years.

The first experiments were utter failures, and I soon realized that I would have to develop an electrode fine enough to record from single cells and stiff enough to push into the brain, and some way of advancing it in fine, controlled steps. So I began to work on developing a new electrode and a means of holding and positioning it.

It took months before I succeeded in sharpening tungsten wire electrolytically—I was lucky to have the help of Irvin Levin, the head of instrumentation, who had gotten his Ph.D. in electrochemistry. The use of potassium nitrite and removing metal with alternating current would never have occurred to me. The idea of electopolishing stainless steel wires had originated with Harry Grundfest in 1950, but tungsten was better than steel because it was far stiffer. The result was a point that looked sharp and smooth even under an electron microscope. Finding a suitable insulating material to coat the wires took even longer, but as the weeks went by no one ever expressed the least impatience. The electrodes finally worked, better than any metallic electrodes then available, and suddenly the other electrophysiologists in the group had all switched to using them, and the word began to spread to other laboratories. Preparing a paper on the electrode (in *Science**) took some time because I wanted to see if it could be used for intra-cellular work and for direct-current (DC) recordings. It turned out that the impedance to DC was astronomical, and the noise at low frequencies was consequently too high for it to be very useful. Like most others in the field, I must have thought that more prestige attached to intracellular work than to extracellular. I abandoned any thoughts of intracellular recording, and set about to record extracellularly from a wide sampling of different parts of the central nervous system. I put the electrode into the auditory cortex, cochlear nuclei (I had a free run of the auditory lab of Bob Galambos), the spinal cord, olfactory bulb, and lateral geniculate nucleus. One day, after a few months of this tour of the cat's central nervous system, Galambos gently asked if I wasn't losing sight of my original plan to develop a technique for recording from awake behaving cats. I took him seriously and buckled down to work.

Herbert Jasper, meanwhile, had gotten wind of the tungsten electrode and came down from Montreal to Washington to learn to make them. His group was also trying to develop a system for recording single cells from awake animals and had gotten as far as to plant a hollow screw in the cat skull, to which an advancer could be attached. That was clearly a good strat-egy, but there remained the problem of closing the cortex to the atmosphere, to dampen the millimeter-size up-and-down cortical movements that would otherwise occur with each vascular and respiratory pulsation, the impor-tance of which Phil Davies had established in Mountcastle's lab some years before. I decided that to get anywhere with the project I would have to design and develop the hardware myself. That meant learning to do machin-ing, so I got the head of the shop at a technical school in Washington, D.C., to agree to take me on as an apprentice. In a few sessions I learned to work a metal-turning lathe, to drill metal, and to turn, face, and cut threads. At Walter Reed I ordered and acquired a lathe and began to start work on my first advancer, a piston-cylinder combination made of brass, which could be attached to a 3/8-inch diameter nylon screw whose oversize threads sat solidly in the cat's skull. The first version worked well, but I slowly improved it so that after some months I had equipment that I could continue to use for the next few decades, at Walter Reed and later, with Torsten, at Hopkins and Harvard. (I love machining and continue to design and build equipment, almost as an additional hobby or as a form of occupational therapy. Had it not been for Torsten's ability to keep his eye on the ball I might have squan-dered all my time playing with and designing equipment, rather than stick-ing to biology.)

Within a few months of Galambos' remark I did my first recording of single cells from a cat that was looking around, purring, and unrestrained except for a chest harness. The very first attempt was successful, and I was so excited that I ran up and dragged David Rioch down to my lab to see the recording. It was not the first-ever such recording: Jasper's group had

Science (1957, 125:549–550)

already succeeded doing awake-alert recordings (to be sure, with the help of my electrode!), but I had the satisfaction of being the first to see cells in an alert cat respond to any kind of environmental stimulation.

I had chosen the visual cortex to record from, perhaps influenced by the Hartline and Kuffler Cold Spring Harbor papers that I had read some years before, and partly because there was less temporal muscle covering the part of the cat skull between the visual cortex and the outside world. (Big decisions can sometimes depend on trivial considerations!) I began by comparing spontaneous activity and responses of cells in visual cortex in sleeping and alert cats. There were clear differences, but nothing that shed light on the nature of sleep. There was also the slight difficulty that when asleep a cat closes its eyes, making visual stimulation problematic. My interests gradually shifted to vision itself, especially to understanding what the visual cortex (area 17) was doing with the information that it gets from prior stages. I soon confirmed the results obtained a few years before by Richard Jung and Günter Baumgartner, in Freiburg, that cortical responses to diffuse visual stimuli were of four types, "on," "off", "on-off", and an additional cell type that they called "Type A", which did not respond at all (Jung and Baumgartner, 1955, Pflügers Archiv. 261, 434–456).

Meanwhile, I had developed a way of making electrolytic lesions to mark recording sites so that they could be found microscopically. I was determined to do this partly as a result of a conversation I had with the neuroanatomist Jerzy Rose, on the steps of the Walter Reed Army Institute of Research. Jerzy was coming over regularly from Hopkins Medical School to collaborate with Bob Galambos on an auditory neurophysiology project. I asked him if he thought it necessary for neurophysiologists to monitor their recording sites histologically. He seemed a bit surprised at the question and replied emphatically that it was, indeed, absolutely essential. Grundfest had identified the tip positions of his steel electrodes by passing current and staining with the Prussian Blue reaction. I resolved to stick with tungsten because of its stiffness, and I was also afraid that depositing iron would turn the electrodes into windsocks. It seemed clear that I had to work out a way of making micro-lesions with my new electrodes.

I began by passing currents through egg white to get an idea of the appropriate current magnitude and time to produce a reasonable-sized spot of coagulation. The first trials in brain tissue were most encouraging; the lesions, about 100 microns in diameter, seemed perfect for assigning cells to layers and were easy to find. I made my first lesion, in a real experiment, after recording from a typical Jung "on" cell (type B, in their terminology), and was astounded on sectioning the brain to find it comfortably nestled in subcortical white matter. That was important because it showed that microelectrodes like mine could easily record from fibres (something the micropipettes of those days could not do) and in raising the suspicion that the "on", "off" and "on-off" cells of Jung's group were not really cortical cells at all, but fibers coming up to the cortex from the lateral geniculate body. This at once raised the further suspicion that many of the cells I was seeing, those that did not respond to turning on and off the room lights—the "unresponsive" cells that Richard Jung's group had observed and called "type A"—were in fact the cortical cells.

I slowly became convinced that cortical cells required for their activation fancier stimuli than simply turning on or off the room lights. I started casting about for ways to make them react. My first successes came one day when out of desperation I waved my hand back and forth in front of a cat. My electrode was lodged between two cortical cells that gave unequal-amplitude spikes that I could easily tell apart, neither of which reacted to turning on and off the room lights. But to my amazement they responded vigorously to the hand-waving, and my amazement increased when I saw that one of the cells was responding to left-to-right movement and the other to right-to-left. Clearly the cortex must be doing something interesting! I observed similar cells several times, but with the cat free to look around it was hard to stimulate any one part of the visual field for more than a few seconds. It was only a few years later that Torsten and I managed to learn more about how these cells were working.

I met Torsten Wiesel for the first time when he and his co-worker Ken Brown drove over to Walter Reed from Baltimore, from Steve Kuffler's lab at the Wilmer Institute, where they were post-docs, to learn to make tungsten electrodes. Little did I think then how well I would get to know Torsten. (For retinal work the electrode turned out to be useless because of the incredible toughness of the inner limiting membrane of the retina.) Torsten and I met subsequently at a small visual symposium in Washington, where we both presented our results, in Torsten's case recordings from the different retinal layers, and in my case recordings from cat cortex. This, my first public presentation of any kind, was when I was still having severe stage fright. I thought my presentation went well, but in the intermission that followed, the well-known NIH neurophysiologist Wade Marshall gave me a severe dressing down for implying that conventional central-nervous neurophysiology, with its anesthetics and respirators, might soon be passé. That taught me to be less brash and to have more respect for others' feelings. The entire symposium was later published in the *American Journal of Ophthalmology* (1958, 46:110–122). These were both brief encounters with Torsten, but it was at once clear that we had many of the same interests and biases. We were about the same age and at about the same stages in our careers.

Armed with a few results, such as the influence of sleep on cortical cells, and the responses to to-and-fro hand-waving, I visited Dr. Magladery (my previous chief, head of neurology at Hopkins), to show him what I had been doing. He immediately said, "You should be showing this stuff to Steve Kuffler, not me; let's go over and see him". The reaction from Steve could not have been more enthusiastic and encouraging—I can still hear him saying "Isn't that interesting!"—without any of the picky questions or objections that people often have when shown something new. As I was to learn, this was typical Kuffler, full of enthusiasm for the things he understood and liked, and simply vague and quiet when he found something boring.

My two years in the army at Walter Reed had gone so well that I decided to stay on for another year as a civilian. That gave me the chance to finish up the research and start writing it up for publication. Near the end of the third year I was attending one of the small informal conferences that were held regularly and jointly between people from Bethesda, Walter Reed, and Johns Hopkins, when Vernon Mountcastle came up to me and asked if I would be interested in returning to Baltimore to join the physiology department at Johns Hopkins, and to continue my work on vision. I was flattered, and accepted eagerly. In the field of cortical neurophysiology Vernon was the world leader. His discovery in 1957 of columns in cat somatosensory cortex was the most important landmark in cortical neurophysiology since topographic localization.

BACK TO BALTIMORE AND THE BEGINNINGS OF COLLABORATION WITH TORSTEN (1958)

When the time drew close for Ruth, Carl (our two-year-old), and me to move back from Washington (Silver Spring) to Baltimore, word came from Vernon that there would be a delay of at least six months before I would be able to set up a lab there, because the physiology department was remodeling their entire space. One day while I was wondering what I should do with the six months, Steve Kuffler telephoned to ask if I would be interested in working in the interim in his labs at the Johns Hopkins Wilmer Institute of Ophthalmology. Kenneth Brown, who had been collaborating with Torsten, was moving to San Francisco, and Torsten would welcome someone to work with. That seemed a perfect solution because it offered me the chance to learn visual physiology, in particular retinal physiology, from experts.

In 1958, a month before the projected time of the move, I drove over from Washington, D.C., to Johns Hopkins Hospital in Baltimore to meet with Stephen Kuffler and Torsten Wiesel for lunch. Torsten and I were to start working together in July, and we wanted to make plans. What we should set out to do seemed obvious. Torsten had the equipment and techniques for controlled stimulation of the retina. He had already succeeded in recording intracellularly from all the retinal layers and was an authority on retinal physiology, a subject in which I had no first hand experience. On the other hand I had the techniques that I had developed for recording from cortical cells in awake cats, which could easily be adapted for use in anesthetized animals.

That day we decided to try to map receptive fields of cells in the visual cortex, using some of the methods Stephen Kuffler had used so successfully in the retina. The optic nerve fibers do not project directly from the retina to the cerebral cortex but end in two nests of cells deep in the brain, called the "lateral geniculate bodies", and it is the geniculate cells that feed into the primary visual cortex. It was not clear what, if anything, the lateral geniculate might be doing with the retinal input before relaying it on to the cortex, but we decided to finesse that question and proceed right to the cortex. That of course was unsystematic, even unscientific, but it seemed to us more exciting. If we found interesting differences between the behavior of retinal ganglion cells and cells in the cortex, we could always go back and look at the lateral geniculate to see if any changes had occurred there.

We decided to revert to anesthetized animals because we had no hope of training cats to fix their gaze on a spot on a screen, in order to stimulate the retina in a controlled way. (Cats can be stubborn and unccooperative, and are notoriously hard to train to do anything that is against their nature. They are not good at visual tasks.) We had no guarantee that cortical cells in an anesthetized animal would respond to any kind of visual stimulation, given that anesthetics tend to suppress synaptic transmission, but that was a chance we had to take. I hated to give up the techniques I had taken such pains to develop for working with awake behaving chronically prepared cats, but the advantages of joining forces with someone already expert in receptive field studies were obvious, and I would soon be going back to the chronic studies—or so I thought.

We moved back to Baltimore in the early summer of 1958. We rented a rowhouse in an area of Baltimore called Rodgers Forge, which was attractive physically but turned out to be stultifying. Baltimore consists largely of rowhouses, red brick and of two types, older and newer, a million of each, like two species of fungus. The older ones included the houses around Hopkins Hospital, and we had occupied one of those, with its tiny back yard, during my first neurology-residency year at Hopkins. Our neighbors had mainly been Johns Hopkins Hospital house staff, and we had felt at home. Rodgers Forge, on the contrary, was an example of Baltimore at its most ethnically monotonous. It happened to be Roman Catholic, where a Presbyterian or Unitarian was a rank outsider and a Jew or black prospective buyer would not even be shown houses. As Unitarians we felt isolated. The houses were like peas in a pod. One night, coming back after a late experiment, I got to the front door before sensing vaguely that something was amiss. It turned out that the house number was right but the street was wrong. I discovered my mistake before trying the key, which for all I know might have worked. I had come close to invading a Catholic neighbor's privacy.

I soon settled in at the Wilmer Institute at Hopkins. Torsten and I shared a lab, about 15 feet by 15 feet, which included my office space. The time Torsten and I had to collaborate was to be short (or so it seemed then), and we felt pushed to get going. We did our first recording of cortical cells in July, 1958, within a few weeks of joining forces, and in a few more weeks we began to get the first glimmerings of what lay ahead. On returning home from our first experiment I remember telling Ruth that I thought that the new collaboration was going to work out well. It was clear that with similar outlooks in science and many common outside interests, we were going to enjoy working together. This became even clearer with the passage of time.

I had much to gain from Torsten's profound insight into science and people. As important as anything was his drive, his reluctance ever to put off experiments, in marked contrast to my tendency to seize any excuses to postpone them, especially when there was a chance of developing some new technique—to build some new gadget, even if we had no real need for it. Torsten had an ability to see what was important to our progress.

Chapter 2 • Torsten N. Wiesel •

I was born in 1924 in Uppsala, Sweden, the youngest of five children. My father, a psychiatrist, was appointed head of Långbro Hospital when I was four, and we lived on the enclosed grounds of the mental hospital that had been built around the turn of the century in a large stucco house with ivy covering its walls. The patients tended our garden of fruit trees, elms, white birches, and raspberry bushes. It was within this idyllic world that I spent my earliest years.

As a boy, I was struck by the unpredictability of human behavior, perhaps because I grew up in such an unusual environment. About a year after we had moved to Långbro, I recall watching a group of patients in striped hospital pants and jackets raking gravel on the path to our front door. There was one patient in particular, who was working intently, with great precision and concentration under the warden's supervision. Suddenly, I noticed that he was holding his rake upside down. Even though I could not put this episode into words at the time, his behavior struck me as a wonderful gesture of protest.

A few years later when I was nine, my father became the director of Beckomberga, a new mental hospital on the outskirts of Stockholm. It was the largest institution of its kind in Scandinavia, with twelve hundred patients and a staff of two hundred. Once again, we lived on the hospital grounds, and it was there that I would spend the rest of my boyhood and early adulthood.

Beckomberga was enclosed by a high fence with locked gates. The patients were housed in a dozen pink concrete, three-story buildings, while the doctors and their families lived in a separate area within the compound. At times we could hear agonized screams reverberating through the barred windows of the "storm building," as we children called it, where the most severely ill patients were kept. Although it was a strange world, I soon felt at home. There were many activities that appealed to me: a network of underground tunnels to play in, a big orchard that could be raided at night, a soccer field for me and my friends. It was a self-contained world with clear divisions and boundaries. I had my own key to the gates and felt more secure within the hospital grounds than I did in the world outside its borders.

Certain patients were allowed to move freely around the grounds, and it was not unusual to see them displaying odd behavior. Since such things were never discussed in my family, I accepted these incongruities without question; if I wondered about them, I sought to explain them to myself. One patient, who worked as a carpenter on the hospital grounds, fascinated me because he had the ability to speak backwards. I ran into him on an afternoon when he was doing some repairs in the attic of one of the buildings. As we were speaking, he took out an axe and hammer from his tool chest, and I realized suddenly that I was in a precarious situation. This man, towering over me with an axe, could cause me serious harm. How could I know what he was thinking? I thought of running away, but instead, I observed in myself a clash of emotions—respect and fear, all at once—and nonetheless I decided to stay.

Holidays, too, were colored by the circumstances in which I lived. On Christmas Eve, our father would take the five of us children into the wards to wish everyone *God Jul*. A Christmas tree glistened in each common room, and the patients were dressed up in their best clothes, but only a few had visitors. That evening, we would celebrate a traditional Swedish Christmas at our home, with my father dressing up as Santa Claus and handing out presents, followed by our dancing hand-in-hand around our tree. Even so, these festivities did not obscure the loneliness I had witnessed earlier in the day. Images of the sick and abandoned lingered in my mind.

After our move to Beckomberga, my parents enrolled me in Whitlock-ska Samskolan, a coeducational private day school in Stockholm. My favorite subject was history, taught by a dynamic woman instructor, but I was a poor student in most other courses. My parents divorced when I was fourteen, and, perhaps because of my distress, I had trouble concentrating on my homework. I excelled only in athletics, especially track and field, and this helped to provide me with a focus while so much else in my life seemed to be falling apart. One of my responsibilities as head of the athletic society that year was to give a short speech at the school's Christmas festivities. I wanted to look my best for the occasion, so I dressed up in a dark suit and bow tie. After my talk, a girl in my class approached me and said, "I see you've left your galoshes on". I've often thought of that humiliating moment: you go up on stage, your head puffed up with the illusion that you are somebody, but in reality, you're nothing but a chucklehead.

Given my interest in sports, I followed the 1936 Olympic Games closely. That was the year when Jesse Owens embarrassed Hitler and the Nazi party by winning four gold medals. It was my first real exposure to the depth of racial discrimination and to the nature of the Nazi regime. Around the same time, I began to follow the developments of the civil war in Spain, and felt the first stirrings in myself of opposition to fascism and communism. Among my soccer teammates, there were some whose parents were Social Democrats and belonged to Swedish labor unions. I learned from my teammates that the unions, which could enable the less powerful to protect themselves, were forbidden in totalitarian states. It had become clear by the summer of 1939 that Germany posed a serious threat to Europe; rumors were already spreading about the existence of concentration camps. Nevertheless, there was still significant pro-German sentiment in Sweden. And so I came of age in a country that was making compromises to survive.

During this period, it began to concern me that I still had no idea what I wanted to do with my life. Then one afternoon, soon after my seventeenth birthday, I realized that I wanted to be a doctor. In retrospect, it was an obvious choice, and certainly, my family experience and upbringing had influenced my decision. My father was a psychiatrist, my sister had nearly died of intestinal tuberculosis, one of my brothers had been diagnosed with a heart defect, and my eldest brother had begun to show early signs of schizophrenia. With new conviction, I applied myself to my schoolwork and managed to graduate with marks high enough so that I was accepted into medical school. At the same time, I began to read literature, history, and philosophy intensively and was especially influenced by the writings of Schopenhauer and Kant. What interested me in particular was the structure of the mind and its workings.

I was also introduced in this period to art by Curt Clemens, a painter who was well known in Sweden. Clemens, who was then in his mid thirties, was a dipsomaniac, and when he drank he sought treatment at Beckomberga. I was struck by how different he was from other people I knew. He called me periodically, and we would get together to speak about literature and music. Clemens asked me questions that no one else would think of asking, and he possessed a freedom of thought and expression that I found liberating. He was the first adult to take me seriously, the first to make me realize that I had an identity. I became concerned when he stopped calling and was deeply shaken to discover that he had fallen down a staircase while drunk and broken his neck.

In the fall of 1946, I began my studies at the Karolinska Institute in Stockholm. Starting medical school was like entering a strong current that guided me steadily through a series of interlocking channels. I was never good at taking lecture notes or memorizing by rote, so, out of necessity, I developed a more intuitive method by reading all the texts and papers that I could find on a particular subject. In a way, this process was not unlike the popular Swedish sport orienteering, a game in which the participants are given a map and compass, and then race through the forest, navigating a triangular course. No trail exists, and, to succeed, you must be both a strong runner and a skilled navigator. I have always enjoyed this sport—the feeling of running alone though the pine forest, finding my way—much like the approach I have taken to solve scientific questions.

In Sweden, at that time, it took seven years to graduate from medical school. The first two years were spent studying basic science; the remaining five were devoted to gaining practical experience in the various clinical disciplines. Our lives were strictly scheduled: as soon as we reached one target, another would be set. We were plugged into a system designed to produce doctors. For relief from the regimented training at medical school, I escaped every Saturday afternoon to chamber music performances at the Lilla Konsert Hallen in Stockholm, where I could hear classical music one week and contemporary music the next. My only other extravagance was to purchase first editions of contemporary Swedish poetry.

In my second year at the Karolinska, I began to focus on the nervous system and was fortunate to study with two exceptional professors in that field: Ulf von Euler, a professor of physiology and a future Nobel laureate, and Carl Gustav Bernhard, a professor of neurophysiology. Professor Bernhard was a brilliant and compassionate man who would have a crucial impact on my future in science. In those days, the typical Swedish professor pontificated from his pulpit like a bishop in a cathedral, but Bernhard sat informally on a bench facing the class and spoke without notes, explaining complex and intriguing facts about the brain. His spirited lectures gave me the courage to make my first presentation to the class: a ten-minute talk on the neural control of respiration. At the end of the term, I volunteered to work as a teaching assistant in the physiology department. My responsibilities kept me in contact with Bernhard's laboratory, and gradually I became part of his extended scientific family.

Around that time, I was finally able to leave my father's home at Beckomberga and move into a place of my own in Stockholm. After living for so many years on hospital grounds, it felt strange at first to be on the outside. I rented a tiny cold-water flat that my friend Lars Rolf, an artist, had painted a monastic white. The most notable feature of the dilapidated building was a row of outhouses in the inner courtyard. That summer, I hitchhiked to Paris with a girlfriend and, while there, picked up a few etchings for next to nothing by Bonnard, Toulouse Lautrec, and Segonzac.

To cover my living expenses, I began to work as a night nurse at Beckomberga, where my father was still director. Four nights a week, from 8 P.M. to 7 A.M., I admitted new patients and made the rounds through each ward, administering medications. Certain patients, who had violent episodes, were kept in padded cells with bars on the windows. It was in that hospital that I saw lobotomized patients for the first time. As a form of treatment, lobotomy was rather new at the time, and Beckomberga had brought in a surgeon who specialized in the procedure. I can still see those three lobotomized patients lying pale and lifeless under the sheets of their high-sided beds. I felt as if I had entered a camp in which a horrific act had been committed. There were individual protests against the procedure from doctors in several countries but most of the medical community approved of the treatment; patients who had been aggressive or hard to manage became docile. With hindsight, it is shocking that Egas Moniz, the Portuguese doctor who developed the psychosurgical procedure of lobotomy, received the Nobel Prize in 1949 for what he claimed was "a simple operation, always safe, which may prove to be an effective surgical treatment in certain cases of mental disorder". Moniz had been confined to a wheelchair in 1939 after he was shot eight times at close range in his office by one of his disturbed patients.

In the 1950s, a medical student in Sweden was permitted in his final year of training to practice as a doctor, which made it possible for me to accept a summer position as a surgeon in the main hospital of Sundsvall in the northern part of the country. There, I performed appendectomies and other minor operations. The work gave me a sense of purpose, and I felt that I could actually help patients, even cure them. On one occasion, a young man covered in blood was brought into the emergency ward. Both of his arms had been severed by a machine in the factory where he worked. The head of surgery looked at me and said, "Don't do too much. Let him go." It is strange, the thoughts one has at such moments. I knew right away that I wanted to do everything in my power to save the man; I felt it was my duty to help him. Even if he had to live without arms, his life could still be meaningful. Years later, I heard that he had gotten married, had children, and was able to paint by manipulating a brush with his lips and feet.

In the fall, I returned to Beckomberga and continued to work for six months as a doctor in a psychiatric ward for adult patients. Soon, it became clear to me that the prevalent methods of treatment, such as electroshock therapy and hypoglycemic coma, were inadequate to ameliorate the suffering of patients. I decided to try child psychiatry for a year in the pediatrics ward at the Karolinska Hospital, hoping that a child's brain might be more responsive to treatment. Although psychiatry in Sweden has always been biologically based, the head of child psychiatry at the Karolinska during that period took a psychoanalytic approach, and under her tutelage I learned about those methods. The drawings and paintings of the children under my care caught my interest, and I began to collect and analyze them for diagnostic purposes. Still, by the end of that year I had come to the conclusion that the psychoanalytic school was as much in the dark as the biological school in understanding how to treat mental illness. Before psychiatry could become a true medical science, I believed it was crucial to learn more about the basic functions of the brain.

Soon after graduating from medical school, I asked Professor Bernhard whether there might be an opening in his laboratory. I was poorly prepared for the type of research he did, but perhaps Bernhard, who knew me both as a student and teaching assistant, had seen some latent promise, since he agreed to appoint me as an instructor in the Department of Neurophysiology at the Karolinska Institute.

My first assignment in the lab was to test a large set of local anesthetics, some of which when injected intravenously had been found to prevent epileptic seizures in animal experiments. Professor Bernhard, in collaboration with the neurosurgeon Einar Bohm, wanted to explore the possibility of using a local anesthetic to halt status epilepticus, a condition of continuous epileptic activity that could occur during brain surgery. After six months of research, I found that lidocaine was the most effective anesthetic in preventing seizures induced in cats. The findings were published and eventually led to the use of lidocaine as a treatment for status epilepticus during brain surgery. Still, I felt that this research had little to do with my primary interest, which was to explore the possibility of doing neurophysiological research at a more advanced level. It was a stroke of luck that in June 1955, soon after I had completed the project, Professor Bernhard called me into his office and asked me, "What about going to America?"

I was then thirty-one years old, with a medical degree and no serious obligations to keep me in Sweden. As I stood in front of Bernhard's desk, he told me that a scientist named Stephen Kuffler was looking for a postdoctoral fellow to continue the study of the visual system that he had pioneered at the Johns Hopkins Medical School. Kuffler, according to Bernhard, was already an internationally renowned neurophysiologist, celebrated for having localized the neuromuscular junction. As a newcomer to the field, I was ignorant of his work, but intrigued when Professor Bernhard explained that Kuffler's work on the cat's visual system centered on studies of single neurons. That night, I went home and read Kuffler's classic paper on the center-surround receptive fields of retinal ganglion cells, which he had presented a few years earlier in June 1952 at the Cold Spring Harbor Symposium. I had never read a paper that documented such outstanding research, and I decided there was no reason to hesitate joining Kuffler's laboratory in Baltimore.

So, in July 1955, I boarded the *Van Dam,* a Dutch oceanliner bound for New York, and in early August arrived in Baltimore to begin my postdoctoral fellowship at the Wilmer Institute at Johns Hopkins Medical School. I found myself in a new land, a somewhat strange country, trying to learn its customs, its music, its ways of life. Even though I felt insecure about my ability as a researcher, I was eager to meet the demands of the new lab. I expected to return to Sweden at the end of my three-year fellowship, but, as it turned out, I would spend the next half-century in the United States.

Steve Kuffler was a master experimentalist who always worked with his own hands in the laboratory. He was forever in search of the ideal preparation with which to pursue the guiding question of his research: how nerve cells communicate across synapses. He had attracted a number of outstanding postdoctoral students to his lab at the Wilmer Institute: Edwin Furshpan, David Potter, Josef Dudel, and Taro Furokawa, among others. Together, they constituted a dynamic and interactive set of research groups. Steve created an informal tone and open style in the lab that all of us enjoyed. He hated pomposity, and never hesitated to use the needle of humor to deflate pretentious behavior. He remains my role model almost fifty years later.

Since the Wilmer Institute was an ophthalmologic clinic as well as an eye research institute, Steve wanted at least one of his research groups to work on vision, and that was his main reason for inviting me and another postdoctoral student, Kenneth Brown, to join his lab. My first task was to learn how to make different types of microelectrodes, which was a relatively new technique for recording impulse activity from single nerve cells. Ken Brown, who joined the lab a few weeks after me, was interested in pursuing the cellular origins of the electroretinogram. Although this topic was not paramount among my own interests, we collaborated on this problem for the three years that Ken worked there. In my spare time, I developed a few single-cell projects, focusing on the receptive field properties of retinal ganglion cells, which were published in *The Journal of Physiology* and in *Nature*. Steve must have appreciated the single-cell work I had done, because when my three-year fellowship came to an end, he asked me to continue in his lab.

About a year earlier, in the spring of 1957, I had attended a conference in Atlantic City of the Federation of Experimental Biologists and had been impressed by the sharp intellect of one of the speakers—a young scientist from Walter Reed Hospital named David Hubel. I had first met David in 1956 when Ken Brown and I visited him at his lab to learn how to make his newly developed tungsten microelectrode. It was clear to me then that David had a highly original approach to cortical neurophysiology. He had developed an elegant method for making single-cell recordings in the awake cat, noting that some cells fired when he waved his hand in front of the cat's eyes in one direction, while other cells fired when he waved his hand in the opposite direction. As David recounted his discoveries, I realized that cells in the visual cortex were much more sophisticated than the ganglion cells that Steve Kuffler had reported in the retina of the cat. In a sense, David's early studies in the visual cortex served to stake out the ground for our future collaborative work.

In the late spring of 1958, Steve invited David and me to lunch in the cafeteria at Johns Hopkins so we could discuss the possibility of a collaboration between the two of us. David and I realized that if we were to work together, we should start by adapting his approach to mapping receptive fields, recording from single cortical cells in anesthetized cats rather than in awake cats. And so began our collaboration, which would last for close to twenty years, first at Johns Hopkins, and then at Harvard.

David and I approached the visual cortex as explorers of a new world. Neither of us had any preconceived ideas about what we would find on our journey; instead, we let our discoveries dictate what questions to ask next. At times we felt more like naturalists of a bygone era. We made every effort to carry out experiments twice a week, beginning early in the morning and working late into the night. We communicated in a private shorthand, and most of our scientific ideas were developed through those fragmentary dialogues. I admired David's ability to communicate difficult concepts with clarity, a skill that was crucial to gaining recognition for our findings. To have such an imaginative partner in our scientific explorations was most fortunate, and our time together stands out as one of the most exciting and engrossing experiences of my life.

In 1973, I succeeded my mentor Steve Kuffler as chair of the Department of Neurobiology at Harvard Medical School and became increasingly occupied with administrative responsibilities. At the same time, David began traveling frequently to give talks about our work. Yet, there may have been a more profound reason that our partnership came to an end. The additional demands on our time sprang up during a period when we were investigating the properties of cells of higher visual areas beyond the primary

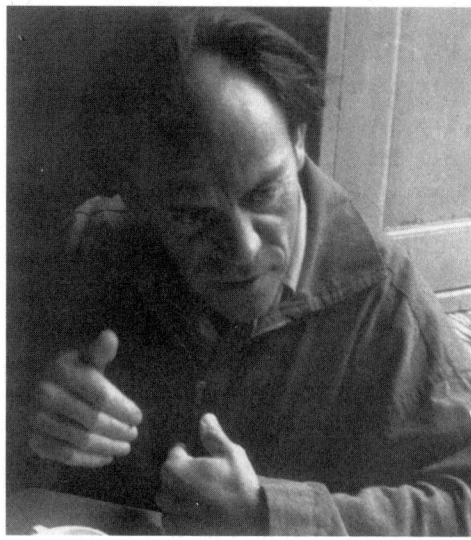

Torsten Wiesel, 1975.

visual cortex, an exploration that each of us eventually regarded as a failure. Perhaps we had been spoiled by the steady pace of new discoveries. The two naturalists, who for so long had journeyed together with a seemingly inexhaustible sense of wonder, were unaccustomed to the frustration that is the daily bread of so much scientific research. David and I had never spent much time together outside the lab; what developed between us, our special bond and private dialogues, took place while we carried out our experiments. When those explorations stalled, when the wonder faded, so did our collaboration. Perhaps it was necessary for each of us to turn to new partners and questions.

When my partnership with David ended, I continued my research on the visual cortex with Charles Gilbert, a former graduate student from Harvard Medical School, who had returned to my lab as a postdoctoral candidate. Charles and I decided to explore the new method of intracellular recordings with microelectrodes filled with horseradish peroxidase, which, when injected into the neuron, led to an intense, dark brown staining of the cell body, its dendrites and axonal branches. This approach led to our discovery of extensive and precise horizontal connections between cortical cells. My collaboration with Charles continued at The Rockefeller University, where we moved in 1983. My experimental work came to an end eight years later, in 1991, when the Rockefeller board of trustees appointed me president of the university, a responsibility that I found to be an interesting challenge.

Since leaving that position in 1998, I have been able to focus on issues that have long concerned me. While remaining at The Rockefeller University as director of the Shelby White and Leon Levy Center for Mind, Brain, and Behavior, I have assumed a number of advisory positions at organizations that support the training of students and investigators in the United

States and abroad. Since its initiation, I have participated in the Pew Charitable Trust program, which supports the training of Latin American postdoctoral students in the best laboratories in the United States. I have also been involved as chair of the Committee of Human Rights of the National Academies of Science in assisting colleagues who have been imprisoned or harassed for asserting their right to free speech or for their peaceful opposition to the policies of their governments. In the spring of 2000, I was appointed secretary general of the Human Frontier Science Program (HFSP), an organization which supports international and interdisciplinary collaboration between investigators in the life sciences and sponsors the training of post-doctoral students from different parts of the world in leading laboratories. All these endeavors have a common and quite simple theme: to provide young scientists with the opportunity that Steve Kuffler so generously gave to David and me, the freedom to explore, the freedom to fail, the freedom to follow where the experiments lead you.

Even now, I am struck by the complexity of the brain and how little we know about it. Can the brain really understand itself? Many of us in neuroscience assume there are no limits to what we can learn about the brain, but still we hesitate to make the claim that the richness of all human behavior and culture can be explained in biological and physical terms. In our quest, we can anticipate the benefits of new knowledge, but can we foresee the dangers that this knowledge might bring about in the future?

For now, most of us are not as concerned as we might be. I was taken aback not long ago on being asked, "When will you be able to control the human mind?" My immediate response was, "Never, I hope."

PART II
BACKGROUND TO OUR RESEARCH

Chapter 3 • Cortical Neurophysiology
in the 1950s •

Neurophysiology has changed radically since the late 1950s. The number of neurophysiologists was then a small fraction of what it is now, perhaps about one one-hundredth. The Society for Neuroscience, now with some 30,000 members, did not yet exist. (The National Eye Institute was founded only in the late 1960s). In the United States the important meetings were those of the Federation of Experimental Biologists. Known as the Federation Meetings, they covered all experimental biology and were held every spring in Atlantic City, of all charming places. The hundred or so neurophysiologists who gathered there each year formed only a small minority. The big international event in physiology was the meeting, every third year, of the International Union of Physiological Sciences. It would take place at some major city such as Brussels or Munich. The community of neurophysiologists who attended these meetings was small and intimate, and a beginner could expect to get to know and talk with most of the important figures in the field. Those working in basic nerve-synapse physiology formed a select group that included Hodgkin, Huxley, Eccles, Katz, and Kuffler, names associated with the beginnings of an ionic, molecular-level approach to neurons and synapses that was to become the foundation of the field of neurobiology. In the area that we now call "systems"—roughly speaking, the central nervous system—the main players of the previous generation had been the Spaniard Ramón y Cajal in neuroanatomy, and Charles Sherrington and E. D. Adrian, both from England, in physiology. In the early 1960s one of the most active fields in central-nervous physiology was spinal cord, in which some of the main players were John Eccles, Karl Frank, and my first advisor, M. G. F. Fuortes.

In the cerebral cortex, early work was mainly concerned with localization of function, essentially a type of neuroanatomy that used clinical neurology and electrical stimulation and electrical recording. Decades of clinical neurology, going back to the eighteen-hundreds, had indicated that the cortex was divided up into areas ranging in size from postage stamps to credit cards, each area devoted to a separate function, such as sensory or motor. In animals such as cats, these areas accounted for a fair percentage of the total cortical area, but in humans the sensory and motor areas comprised only a small part of the cortex, the rest of which remained terra incognita. Even when a given area could be designated as visual, somatic sensory (touch and so on), or motor, the details of the mapping were still vague. In the 1940s and 1950s the details began to be worked out, in humans in the operating room, using electrical stimulation and recording, in what was called clinical neurophysiology, and in the laboratory, using cats and monkeys. Some of the main names in clinical neurophysiology were Jasper and Penfield, and in animal studies Clinton Woolsey and Vernon Mountcastle.

Much of the early cortical mapping was done by the method of evoked potentials, a technique in which relatively crude (1 mm or larger) recording electrodes were placed on the surface of the cortex and brief sensory stimuli, such as touch, flashes of light, and auditory clicks, led to transient changes in surface potential. These "evoked potentials" are one form of what are known as "slow waves", as distinguished from single-cell action potentials. By the late 1950s the topographic maps of the primary and secondary visual, auditory, and somatosensory receiving areas had been delineated electrically, in humans, cats, and monkeys. In the mid-1950s, with major improvements in electrical equipment and electrodes, it became possible to record impulses from single cells, and the new methods began to be exploited in work such as that of Vernon Mountcastle in the somatosensory cortex.

Slow waves can occur spontaneously. In the electroencephalogram (EEG), the records are made by electrodes placed on the scalp; in the electrocorticogram (ECG) the electrodes are placed directly on the cortical surface.

In the 1950s and 1960s attempts to understand the nature of slow waves consumed much time and effort, in many laboratories. In retrospect these efforts would seem to have represented a cul-de-sac in the neurophysiology of that generation. One can understand why neurophysiologists were so preoccupied with slow waves given their usefulness in mapping sensory areas, and given the striking changes that occurred in the EEG when a human subject engaged in mental activity, became drowsy, or slept. But the techniques available to tackle the problem of the nature of the waves were far from adequate then and still seem inadequate now, despite the advent of the microelectrode and the possibility of correlating slow waves with events in single cells. The preoccupations of neurophysiologists gradually changed from studying slow waves to studying single cells, and the emphasis changed from trying to understand the waves and ever-enticing subjects such as sleep and consciousness, to learning how the cortex was handling sensory information.

In vision the most important topographic mapping had been done back in 1941 by Wade Marshall (the same Wade Marshall who had bawled me out after I gave my first paper) and Samuel Talbot, at Johns Hopkins. In a tour de force that was far ahead of its time, they stimulated the retina by having their anesthetized animal (rabbit, cat, or monkey) face a screen on which they projected small spots of light. They placed a millimeter-sized electrode on the cortical surface and flashed the spot on various parts of the screen, searching for the region that gave the maximum slow wave response. This produced the first mapping of the cortical projection of the visual fields.

To understand the importance of Talbot and Marshall in the visual cortex, Mountcastle's work in somatic sensory cortex, or Jasper and Penfield's mapping of human brain, one has to recall the uncertainties that prevailed in the 1940s and 1950s, even concerning the existence of topographic representation. Some psychologists had destroyed various parts of the rat brain and failed to detect specific behavioral defects—in retrospect not because none existed but because of the limitations of the behavioral methods—and they concluded that the brain must work in some rather mushy way, like a cauliflower rather than a computer. In vision, attempts at mapping the cortex sometimes failed because of the mistake of stimulating the retina in conditions of dark adaptation, using a very dim background light and flashing spots of light bright enough to scatter over the entire retina. Talbot and Marshall avoided this problem by having their animals face a projection screen on which they shone spots of light against a moderately bright background light. We, too, were lucky enough to avoid that pitfall, not out of any great insight but simply because working with dark-adapted animals made no sense to us, and groping about in very dim light is no fun.

In the mid-1950s, the first single-cell studies of the visual cortex came from a group led by Richard Jung and his collaborator Günter Baumgartner, in Freiburg. It is easy to forget what an accomplishment it was, at that time, to record a single cortical cell long enough to get any idea of its behavior in response to sensory stimulation. The main problem was instability, the up-and-down movements of the cortex relative to the recording electrode, caused by vascular pulsations and respiration. This was before the development of the closed chamber technique, which by walling off the cortex from the atmosphere served to dampen the pulsations almost completely. The Freiburg group stimulated by illuminating the retina diffusely, possibly to avoid the technical problems of obtaining a focused image on the retina. As already mentioned in the context of my hand-waving stimuli, it was natural to assume that illuminating the entire retina would be the most effective visual stimulus, rather than the least effective, as it turned out.

In the 1950s most of the single-cell recordings from sensory cortex were concerned with topography. Mountcastle's studies of somatosensory cortex, however, went far beyond questions of simple mapping and led to the discovery of columnar organization. He showed that cells are gathered into small groups a millimeter or so in cross-sectional area and extending through the entire 2-millimeter cortical thickness. Columns differed, one from the next, in the sensory submodality (to use Mountcastle's term) to which the cells responded, some being sensitive to light touch or bending of skin hairs, others to changes in joint position. This was a profound discovery, indicating the cortex was not uniform but diced up, perhaps like a checkerboard, into small regions that differed in the information feeding in from lower levels, and that these regions were basic units of cortical organization. Surprisingly, the cells seemed to respond in much the same way as cells at lower levels, in dorsal column nuclei or thalamus, and it was not clear what the cortex was doing to transform the information it received from these lower levels. This seemed quite different from the retina, where Stephen Kuffler had shown that ganglion cells' receptive fields, with their centers and surrounds, must surely represent a major transformation of the information coming from the rods and cones. One thought of a sensory cortex, visual or somatosensory, as "analyzing" the information it received from below, without specifying what the analysis might possibly consist of.

Chapter 4 • The Group at Hopkins •

The importance in science of what might be called *mentors* or *role models* can hardly be exaggerated. One can even trace genealogies of scientists, often back many generations, and speak of cousins, brothers, and the like. One can of course have several mentors in a lifetime: I can trace my own intellectual ancestry to three, all differing in the closeness of the relationships and the admiration, sometimes mixed with resentments and varieties of complexes. My first such father figure was Herbert Jasper, whose own mentor in-loco-parentis was certainly Wilder Penfield, whose very gestures and way of standing were said to derive from the famous neurosurgeon Harvey Cushing. Jasper could be extremely kind, but was subject to moods that ranged from irritable depression to buoyant effervescence. When I needed something, I waited for a buoyant day and almost felt guilty at his cheerful compliance. Mike Fuortes, my first mentor in research, was not at all moody; he had a slightly sardonic sense of humor and a profound sense of what was important in biology. (We became close friends, and went swimming every noon in the summer, at the Walter Reed officers' club.) And more than anyone else, Steve Kuffler played a role that was crucial for both Torsten and me, in terms both of its day-to-day importance and the fact that it was sustained over some thirty years.

For Steve, my third mentor, and the most important mentor to both Torsten and me, the scientific ancestry went back at least two generations. He was born in Austria-Hungary in what must have been a well-to-do family. He went to medical school in Vienna, finishing at about the time of the outbreak of World War II. He realized that Europe was no place for him and boarded a ship for Australia. He began as a post-doctoral fellow in pathology in Sydney, Australia, and met Jack Eccles on a tennis court. Eccles is supposed to have said, "You play tennis too well to stay in pathology. You must come and work with me in neurophysiology". Bernard Katz was one of Eccles' other trainees, and the three of them began to collaborate. Eccles, who won a Nobel Prize in 1963, had trained in England under Sir Charles Sherrington, who shared with E. D. Adrian the distinction of being one of the world's leading figures in neurophysiology. The two shared the Nobel

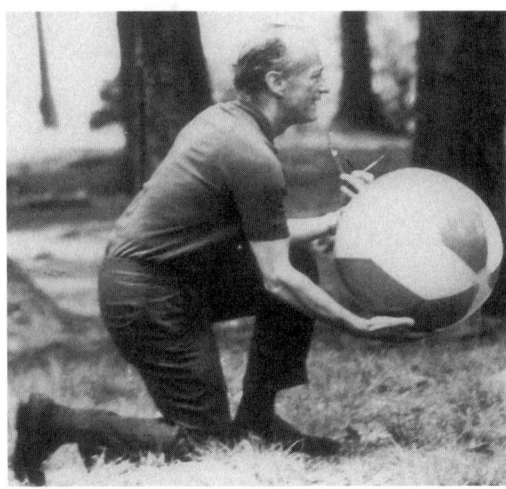

Steve Kuffler, at annual department picnic, early 1970s.

prize for Medicine/Physiology in 1932. So I suppose in some sense Torsten and I could be thought of as Sherrington's great grandchildren.

We have a picture that shows Eccles, Katz, and Kuffler striding along some street in Australia, probably from the mid-Forties. Another picture, taken probably in the United States of America about twenty years later, again shows them striding briskly along the street . . . as youthful and vigorous as ever (pp. 44, 45).

Eccles, at the time of Steve's arrival, was one of the main proponents of the widely held notion that synaptic transmission in the central nervous system was electrical. (Neuromuscular transmission was an exception, since it was known to be chemical.) I once asked Steve to make me a selection of his main reprints. As he leafed through his collection, he came upon one and said, "This is the paper that at last convinced Jack [Eccles] that synaptic transmission is chemical". That impressed me, because no one was less prone to boasting than Steve.

In the late 1940s, Steve left Australia and went to work for a brief time with Ralph Gerard in Chicago. In 1949 he took a position at the Wilmer Institute of Ophthalmology at the Johns Hopkins Hospital in Baltimore, and it was there that he began his studies of single retinal ganglion cells.

Steve (as he was known by everyone—no one who knew him at all would have dreamed of calling him "Dr. Kuffler", which would probably have hurt his feelings) once told us that when he left Austria-Hungary he had to decide whether he wanted to be called Stephen or William, and he chose Stephen because he did not want to be called "Bill". From then on Torsten and I called him Bill at every opportunity, and I still have a note from him, from Woods Hole, that reads "Gee it's nice here", signed "Bill". Steve's broad range of interests was reflected in the group that began to form around him in the late 1950s—first Torsten, who had already been there for several years when I arrived in 1958, and then Edwin Furshpan and David

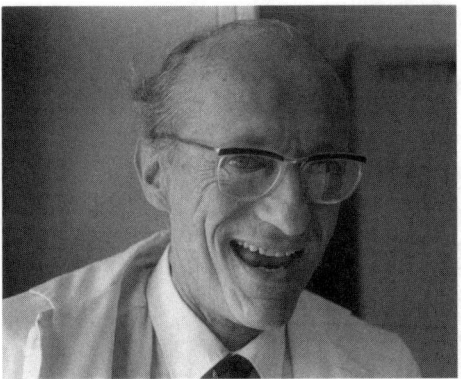

Steve Kuffler, 1975.

Potter, who arrived from Bernard Katz's lab in London, just having made a major contribution to synaptic physiology by discovering the first electrical synapse, in the squid. Furshpan was soon joined by the Japanese neurophysiologist Taro Furukawa, in a project on the goldfish Mauthner cell. Thus over a very few years Steve's group had grown from two or three people working together to four or five independent subgroups, each consisting of two or more collaborators.

Steve had a special and unusual style of working that largely determined the character of the group he slowly built around him. He worked alone with one colleague, or rarely with two. He loved doing experiments, especially the dissections. In the years that followed he had to put up with increasing amounts of administration work but never complained: he would come in to work early in the morning, clean up whatever letters he had to write, and be dissecting by 9:30.

On coming to the Wilmer around 1950, Steve first collaborated with Carlton Hunt, on cat muscle spindles and the small motoneurone system that regulated the spindles' sensitivity. That was a major contribution to mammalian spinal cord physiology. It was followed by the epoch-making visual study in cats: the discovery of the center-surround organization of the receptive fields of retinal ganglion cells, a subject that will come up again and again in this book, because more than any topic in vision it formed the basis of all our research. Then came work with Carlos Eyzaguirre on crayfish and lobster stretch receptors. Around 1957 he took Horace Barlow and Dick FitzHugh as postdoctoral fellows, and the work on vision resumed. They mapped receptive fields of retinal ganglion cells under conditions of dark adaptation and made a statistical analysis of the firing patterns. Steve's heart was probably not in those topics. When FitzHugh and Barlow left, he returned to studies of synaptic mechanisms, especially synaptic inhibition. With the German physiologist Josef Dudel, he took up the subject of presynaptic inhibition, and then went on to the role of gamma amino butyric acid (GABA) in synaptic inhibition, with David Potter and Ed Kravitz; and neuroglia, in the medicinal leech, with John Nicholls. It was his style to switch

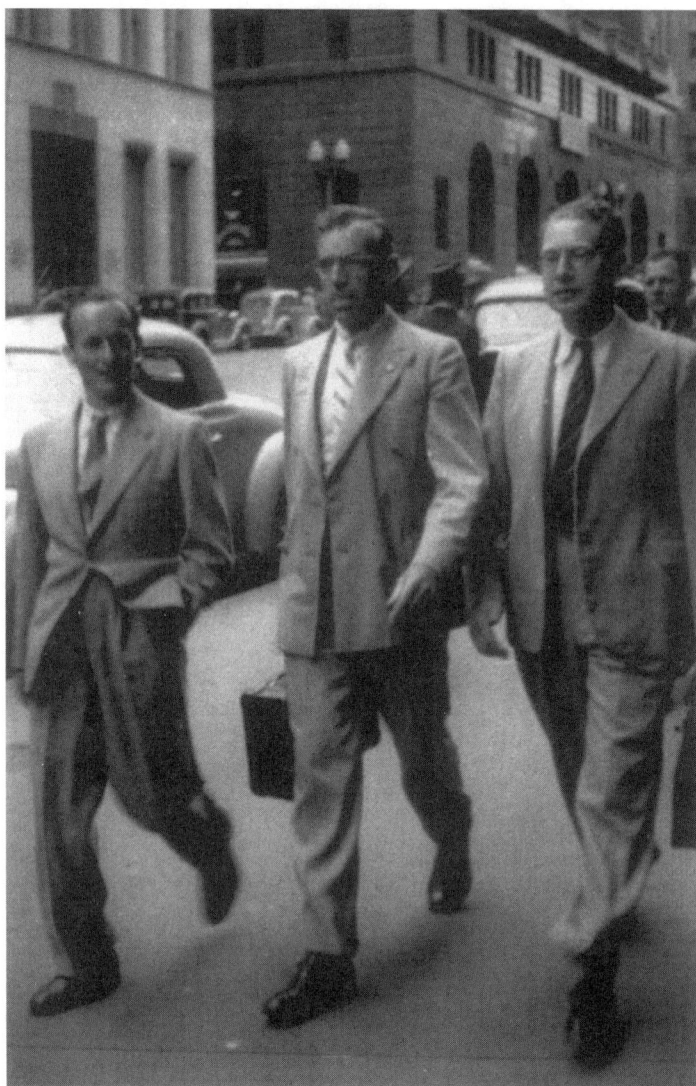

Steve Kuffler, Jack Eccles, Bernard Katz (from left to right), late 1940s.

over to an entirely new realm of neurophysiology every three or four years, often just after making a major contribution and opening up some other field. He would use whatever species seemed best suited to a problem, from crayfish and cats to leeches. Most scientists would have settled down to mining one problem for decades—as indeed we did—and most neurophysiologists would have assumed the role of leader of a team of disciples, ceasing to work actively in the lab.

Steve presumably felt he owed it to the Wilmer Ophthalmology Institute to keep up a laboratory in visual research, and after Horace Barlow and Dick FitzHugh left, the tradition was continued by Kenneth Brown and Torsten, working in collaboration. They undertook the difficult project of recording intracellularly from the retina, layer by layer. When in 1958 Torsten and I began to work together, Steve was studying presynaptic inhi-

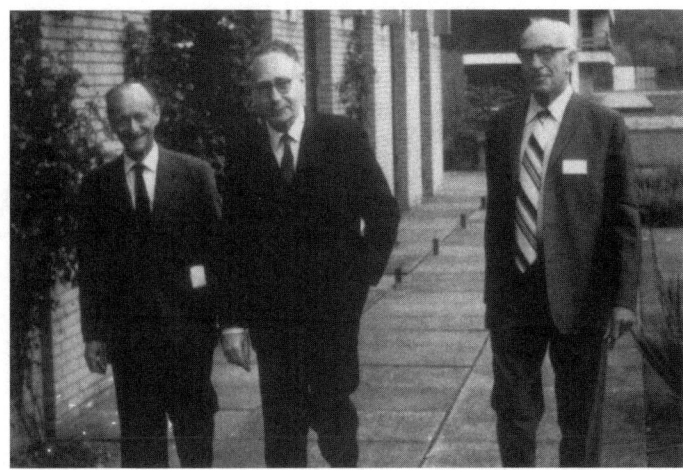

Steve Kuffler, Bernard Katz, Jack Eccles (from left to right), 1970s.

bition in the crayfish neuromuscular junction, collaborating with Joseph Dudel. One of the first things Steve asked me to do was to read critically three papers he and Dudel had just written. I was immensely flattered, and knowing nothing about that subject, I dug in and spent a full weekend covering the papers with red ink. Steve must have been impressed because he and Joseph rewrote the papers completely. They must have felt, as I did, that so important a work should be written so as to be understandable to non-experts. (Maybe Steve was getting back at us when some months later he tore into our first abstract—about which more later.)

Heavy-handed advising was definitely not Steve's style. Though everyone talked a lot about the work they were doing, Steve would not have thought of offering anything but questions and gentle suggestions. If he was impressed with something one of us was doing, he would let it be known through his buoyant enthusiasm, and would keep on re-expressing the enthusiasm day after day. The lab was a loose federation of small subgroups rather than a big group led by a chief who administered but did no experiments, as is the style in most laboratories today. Being technically in an ophthalmology department, he did no formal teaching, and seeking grants took very little of anyone's time in those happy days.

Space in the Wilmer basement was compressed, to put it mildly. All of us together occupied the amount of space generally allotted to one assistant professor today. This 15×15 foot vision lab (Torsten and myself) was in an inner room across the hall from Steve's office, and included my desk. Torsten's office was a tiny partitioned space across another hall. The other groups, including Steve's, each had about as much space as we did. The compression had its advantages: each group was completely independent, but there was much communication between the labs. Every time someone wrote a paper it was handed around for criticism, and since criticism was fierce (especially from Steve and Ed Furshpan), a manuscript ended up being written and rewritten many times. Our first paper, in 1959, went through 11 drafts, each of which, in those computerless days, had to be typed by one or

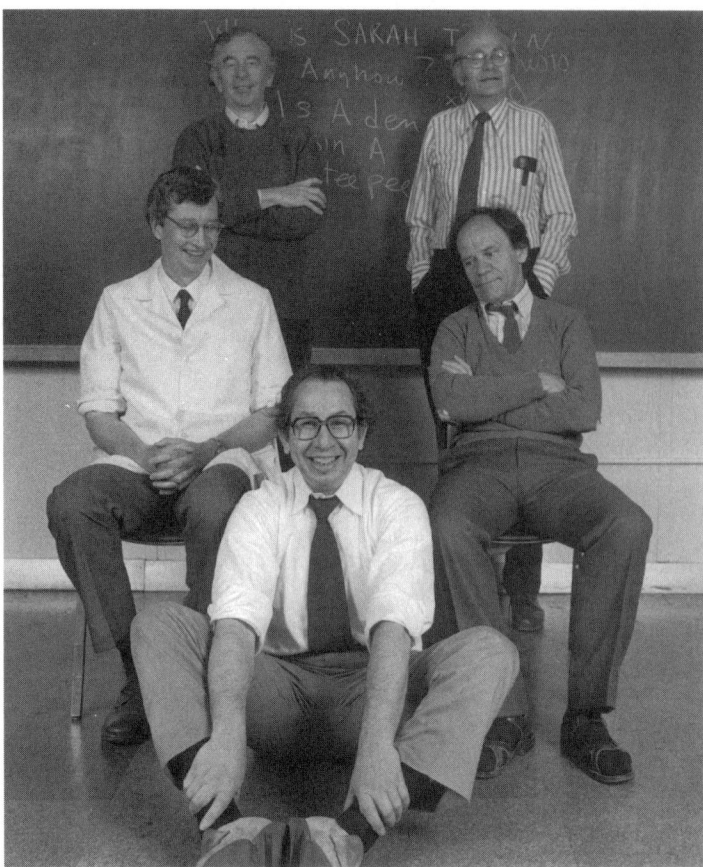

Neurobiology group, 1975. Back row: Ed Furshpan, David Hubel. Middle row: David Potter, Torsten Wiesel. Front: Ed Kravitz.

the other of us on an old Underwood non-electric typewriter. We cherished that typewriter (on which we wrote our experimental protocols), because being mechanical it gave no electrical interference to our recordings, and because we quickly discovered that we could not read each other's writing. We still have filing cabinets filled to bursting with 30 years' worth of protocols, one folder for each experiment.

The group was broad. The two of us (and of course Steve) represented central nervous physiology; Furshpan and Potter (and of course Steve) represented synaptic physiology; and Ed Kravitz, representing neurochemistry, arrived soon after our move to Harvard. This was a far cry from the inevitable specialization of today's big departments. We no longer try, or are asked, to read critically papers outside our immediate fields, and we all suffer for that.

The atmosphere in the lab was lighthearted and fun. In January, 1959, Baltimore experienced a sudden cold snap (a rare thing for Baltimore), and Torsten discovered that north of Baltimore a huge reservoir system with interconnecting rivers had frozen over to glass ice. The two of us took the day off and went skating. The next day we rather sheepishly told Steve, but far from being displeased over our taking the time off, he was obviously disappointed that we hadn't invited him to come along. So for the rest of that week everyone in the lab, together with all the families (including Steve, his wife and three children) went skating. Everyone obviously felt that first things should come first.

It is easy to look back 40 years with rose-tinted spectacles and forget the anxieties or hardships we must have had. Certainly it is the good things that stand out in our minds. We were not badly paid: each of our fellowship salaries that year amounted to about $10,000, which was a lot for postdocs in those days. There can be no question that in science many things were easier then. There was far less competition: journal editors provided little of the niggling criticism that they do today; a paper was usually either accepted or (rarely) rejected. The pressure to publish was less, and more than once Torsten and I wrote a paper and put it in a drawer for several months to let the ideas mature. The NIH had just come into being; suddenly funding had become more generous. It was hard to write a grant that was so bad it would not be funded. Steve used to say that Mrs. Hughes (his middle-aged, endearing secretary) would probably be the last person to read our grant requests. The time for applying for a job seemed far in the distance, and jobs seemed unlikely to be a problem in a field that was clearly taking off.

The prevailing spirit of lightheartedness was a matter, not just of the time, but also of the place. Johns Hopkins was informal and friendly, contrasting strongly, as we later found, with the rather pompous prevailing atmosphere at Harvard. This may have been partly because the medical school and hospital were so close to each other, geographically and spiritually, and medical schools and hospitals tend to be lively places. At Harvard the associated hospitals are scattered all over Boston, and the closest, the Peter Bent Brigham (now Brigham and Women's) is the one that always seemed to me to be the stuffiest. Our time at Hopkins seems in retrospect to have been a truly golden era.

Chapter 5 • The Move from Hopkins to Harvard •

At Harvard Medical School the Department of Pharmacology was led by Otto Krayer, a longtime friend of Stephen Kuffler. In 1958 one of the quadrangle buildings (then Building B) had just been remodeled, and pharmacology had suddenly come by more space than they knew what to do with. Dr. Krayer, sensing a weakness in neurophysiology at Harvard, decided to promote the idea of bringing in Steve as a full professor, and somehow persuaded the ultraconservative Harvard faculty to take such an unprecedented step. At that time there were no full professors at Harvard Medical School who were not also chairmen. (Then, as now, "chairpersons" were almost always men.) Steve justifiably felt neglected at Hopkins and decided to leave and to bring his entire group with him. (He once described to me how he had been promoted at Hopkins to a full professorship but, until he protested, any adjustment of his salary was forgotten. He doubtless felt out of place in the Department of Ophthalmology, since for years he had been working on almost every topic except for vision.) Everyone in the group knew of the impending move except me, probably because Steve assumed that I would be moving over to the Hopkins Physiology Department, as planned. Torsten often remarked that our time was limited, and that we should get going at writing up the results we had and press on with the work. That had puzzled me, because I would be only a few blocks away and we would surely be able to keep on collaborating at least part of the time.

One afternoon as Steve was driving me home he asked casually how strongly I was committed to going over to physiology at Hopkins. Would I be interested in moving to Boston, to Harvard, with Torsten, Ed Furshpan, David Potter, and all the rest? I was flabbergasted, having no idea such a move was in the works. This suddenly explained what the rush to publish was all about. In the end my decision was easy: our collaboration was proving so successful that any thought of breaking it up seemed ridiculous. (Ruth and I, thinking that we would be staying in Baltimore for years, had made an offer on a house just a few weeks before. Luckily at the last moment the offer fell through—otherwise it would have been a lot harder to leave.)

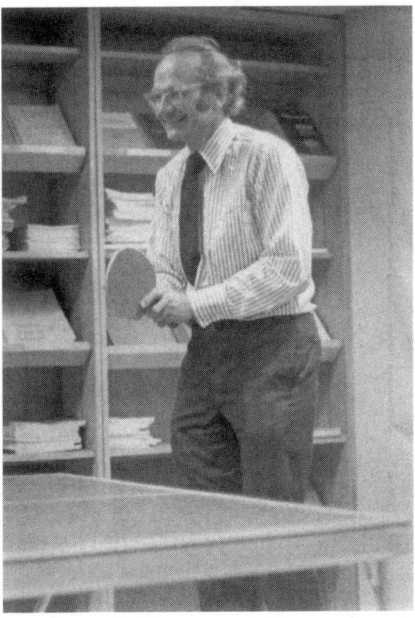

David Hubel, Neurobiology Christmas party, 1973.

So in the spring of 1959 nine families moved from Baltimore to Boston, to the Department of Pharmacology, of which we became in effect a subdepartment. At Hopkins, Torsten and I had just been promoted to assistant professorships, but the dean at Harvard Medical School said that we hardly qualified for such exalted positions at Harvard. Perhaps by the time the papers we had submitted were published Harvard might give the matter further thought. So we were demoted to the status of "Associates". The rest of the world, according to the administration, must surely know that an associate at Harvard was the equivalent of an assistant professorship anywhere else. Steve, and perhaps also we, found that amusing. In the newly remodeled Building B, the two of us started with a 20×20–foot room that was to contain our entire empire, including the lab and our two offices. We immediately ordered a large metal-turning lathe, which sat in the hall until Otto Krayer, our chairman, relented on space and let us have a second 20×20 room, where we put the lathe and set up benches for histology.

From the beginning, teaching was a major new item for the group. With Sandford Palay's group in neuroanatomy, we taught medical students for six weeks each spring. That was a full-time task, for us as well as for the first-year medical school class. It was the best teaching experience any of us ever had; we all went to one another's lectures, and the feedback we got from the students made it clear that our course was by far the most popular in the school. We taught it for about five years, when the medical school in its wisdom revamped the curriculum, as faculties do periodically, and our course disappeared.

Some things inevitably changed in our lives, at first slowly. Our work was becoming known, though for the first ten years we had the visual cortex almost to ourselves. We started to get invitations to speak and to travel. I suppose I was more at home in writing in English than Torsten, and I took an active part in teaching, which Torsten shunned in the interest of getting research done. I was asked to be on the medical school admissions committee, which was viewed as an important assignment and a step along the way to tenure. (We were indeed made assistant professors after the first year at Harvard!) We got busier, although until the mid-Seventies we were largely free of administrative chores.

One day early in January of 1964, I was sitting at my desk when the phone rang. "This is Jonas Salk" came the voice from the other end. "Yes . . . ?", I answered, " . . . I'm sorry, who did you say was speaking?" It was indeed Jonas Salk, calling to invite me to a meeting at the Salk Institute in La Jolla, the object of which was to inform a remarkable cast of molecular-biological celebrities, each more famous than the next, about the state of the field of neurobiology. The molecular people included Francis Crick, Sydney Brenner, Jacques Monod, Seymour Benzer . . . and so on. The neurobiologists were to include Roger Sperry, Rita Levi-Montalcini, Walle Nauta . . . and so on (including several neurobiological losers, if one may use that term). I was in the midst of teaching, travel, and experiments, and my first impulse was to decline. But the temptation was too great. One motivation for accepting had to do with a macromolecular theory of learning that was circulating in neurobiology circles at that time. Some neurobiologists were wedded to a theory that memories were encoded on macromolecules, and that the serum of an animal trained to a learning task, when injected into a naïve animal, could induce learning in that animal. We all thought the idea was nonsense, but many neurobiologists took it very seriously. I wanted to find out if the real molecular biologists gave the idea the time of day. But, more important, it seemed a great chance to meet some of the world's leading scientists. I decided to go, for one day only.

I was slated to talk for an hour, on Sunday, February 23. I talked for the hour, on cell categories in striate cortex, simple, complex, and so on. I was interrupted many times with questions, especially from a young man in the front row with a French accent, whom I took to be a very bright teenager, but who turned out to be Jacques Monod. When I finished, Francis Crick jumped up and said, "But you were supposed to tell us something about visual deprivation and learning". I pointed out that my hour was up, but that seemed to make no difference—so I went on for another hour. At which Crick again rose up and said, "But I heard that you and Wiesel had done work on color. Are you not going to tell us about that?" Time and schedules seemed to present no problems to these molecular biologists, so I went on for still another hour. I felt like Fidel Castro. Their enthusiasm seemed boundless, and I began to think that our work was not so boring after all.

In subsequent months it became clear that the Salk wanted to recruit me. Their offer was hugely tempting. But I made it clear that Torsten and I did not want to break up our collaboration; they would have to take both of us or neither. Torsten, after a visit, was enthusiastic, as were the Fellows at the Salk Institute, but Torsten did not want to come without Steve. Steve visited the Salk and became enthusiastic, but insisted that Ed Furshpan, David Potter, and Ed Kravitz be included. There were long discussions and negotiations, but finally, when the smoke cleared, it turned out that the Salk couldn't afford to bite off so much, and whole idea evaporated. For several summers various ones of us went out to La Jolla on mini-Sabbaticals, and it was during one of those, already mentioned, that the idea of the present book was born, and the project started.

On a two-month summer visit we made to the Salk a few years later, I was asked to give a lecture to the assembled Salk Fellows. Afterwards, Jonas Salk approached me and apologized that his wife, Françoise Gilot (of Picasso fame), had wanted to attend but could not. Would I mind repeating the lecture, the next day, for her? Of course I agreed—after all, I had had a dress rehearsal so it should be easy. In fact it was a sheer pleasure, because her questions were, for an outsider, brilliant and imaginative, and I began to appreciate how potentially interesting visual neurophysiology could be to an artist. That is the only time I have given a formal lecture to an audience of one—up to now.

In 1968 Torsten and I went together to Japan, to the International Physiological Congress in Tokyo. We stood the luxury of the Okura Hotel (it was wasted on us, and could have been in Chicago) for a day, and took the Gizna subway line to Asakusa and found a tiny ryokan recommended in *Japan on $5 a Day*. We made that our headquarters and travelled to Kyushu, where we visited many famous rural pottery studios. I was impressed with Japanese culture and hospitality and with the beauty of the country, and started to learn the language, continuing with lessons at Harvard for about five years. I seriously underestimated the problem of learning the 1,850 Chinese characters necessary just to read a Japanese newspaper. On my next trip to Japan I was able, with intensive coaching by Masanori Otsuka and his postdoctoral fellows, to give two lectures in Japanese. The audience seemed to have no trouble in understanding my Japanese, to judge from the questions that followed, and the laughter that greeted the jokes that I put in as controls.

I was asked to give three "Special Lectures" at University College, University of London, which took place on Monday, Wednesday, and Friday of the last week in January, 1965. I was amazed at the enthusiastic reception these received. (In England, approval of a lecture is expressed by the audience's banging on the seats or stamping, and my first talk, that Monday, was followed by an almost frightening noise.) On those three days I talked about cortical physiology in normal animals, columnar organization, and deprivation. On one of the intervening days I was invited to talk at Cambridge, and rather foolishly decided to talk on an entirely different topic, color—as if I didn't already have enough to do that week. I rode up on the train from London with Andrew Huxley, whom I knew only slightly and revered as one of the most famous figures in neurophysiology. The train was met by Mrs.

Huxley, who drove us over to William Rushton's house, where I was to stay overnight. When we arrived there the house was empty but unlocked, so we went in and made ourselves comfortable. Suddenly Mrs. Huxley exclaimed "Look, here is a note, now we'll see why William isn't here". The note said "One small brown"—obviously left for the baker! Finally William showed up, having been at a chamber-music gathering, playing the bassoon.

The Cambridge audience included my host, William Rushton, famous for his work in visual psychophysics, and, most frightening of all, Lord Adrian, easily the most revered neurophysiologist of that era. Rushton invited me to High Table Dinner at Trinity College and sat me down next to the Master, Adrian himself. It was a bizarre experience because I quickly realized that to talk about our common interests was simply not done in that august society—so we discussed such subjects as Queen Mary (not of Scots, but Bloody Mary, Elizabeth's half-sister) never once even mentioning neurophysiology, then or at any subsequent time.

I was beginning to take flute lessons. My recorder playing had lapsed since leaving Montreal, and the flute seemed to be a greater challenge. But I underestimated the difficulties of learning a new instrument as an adult. Japanese and the flute were enjoyable projects but I have to count them both as failures, in some sense. After about three years of flute and Japanese lessons I finally went back to German and French, and to my original instrument, the piano. What finally convinced me that I should give up the flute was trying the piano one day after a decade's interval and finding I was immediately far better at it than I would ever be with the flute.

Chapter 6 • The New Department •

By 1964, Steve's group had grown and multiplied exuberantly, so that as a sub-department of pharmacology we were like the tail wagging the dog. Harvard finally took the unheard-of step of creating a new department, which after some discussion we called "neurobiology". We think the term was new, and reflected a realization that our field was being held back by artificial academic boundaries. Neurophysiology, for example, had by then come to have much more in common with neuroanatomy and neurochemistry than it had with renal or cardiac physiology. So despite some resistance from the more conservative senior faculty (but with the strong support of an imaginative dean, Robert Ebert), the first-ever Department of Neurobiology was launched, in 1966, with Steve as our chairman. Suddenly we had graduate students, administration, more committees. But administration never seemed to bother Steve, who continued to be productive in research year after year despite major health problems that included glaucoma, diabetes, and advancing coronary disease.

Though our new department expanded greatly, Torsten and I kept our own subgroup small. At any one time, between about 1960 and 1980, we had two to four postdoctoral fellows and one or two graduate students. We did not go out of our way to encourage graduate students, partly because we felt we were ourselves somewhat narrowly trained, both having come from clinical backgrounds, with little to offer a beginning scientist by way of basic neurophysiology. Partly it was because we felt that only the most determined young people should be encouraged: those who hung around and would not go away. In the end our policy (if that is the right word) paid off handsomely, and we can credit ourselves with having had people like Jim Hudspeth and Carla Shatz as graduate students. We sometimes got beginners launched by sitting in with them on their first experiments, but we saved time by having the older graduate students and postdocs do much of whatever training was done. We shied away from giving emphatic advice on what projects a beginning student should undertake, feeling that it was a mistake to deprive anyone of the most important thing one can learn in research—to choose one's own projects. To a large extent students were free to do whatever they

53

wanted, and they worked independently. Doubtless they sometimes felt neglected, but we felt they should learn from their own mistakes, and we had our own work to do.

If Torsten and I had any problems in that otherwise wonderful period, in the 1960s and 1970s, they concerned the question of our continuing collaboration. Steve was puzzled over how to justify two senior (tenure) appointments to the rest of the faculty, especially two people working together in the same field. We wanted to continue collaborating because we enjoyed it and because the collaboration obviously was working—well enough, we thought, to justify two full professorships. To us a partnership between equals seemed ideal. Steve doubtless thought so, too: the problem was to persuade the heads of other departments at Harvard Medical School. When it came time to decide on tenure positions, Steve's solution was for me to be promoted in the department and for Torsten to be appointed to a professorship technically in the department of psychiatry, but without having to move. We would continue our partnership as before, within Steve's group. Practically this worked out well enough, though a professorship in psychiatry seemed a slightly contrived solution.

Around the time the new department was being formed, the dean of the medical school called me in and asked if I would be interested in being chairman of the Department of Physiology. I was astonished, to put it mildly, and enormously flattered to be offered the chair that had once been occupied by such figures as Henry Bowditch and Walter Cannon. But I was most reluctant to risk putting a damper on our research, which at that time was moving ahead in a wonderful way. I got lots of advice from colleagues and senior faculty, much of it to the effect that with a good secretary and a willingness to delegate responsibilities I could easily take on a chairmanship and keep pulling my weight in our collaboration. I could, that is, have my cake and continue eating it. I was also told that the least I could do was make a contribution to the school. Chairs at Harvard Medical School are like feudal fiefdoms; they are more or less lifetime jobs, with much power. Here, I was told, was a chance to build something important. I accepted, in large part because it seemed like an opportunity for Torsten and me to build up a group of our own, in parallel with Steve's department, and to obtain professorships and promotions for close colleagues such as Zach Hall and John Nicholls. Yet certain awkward aspects of the arrangement soon became evident. Torsten's and my backgrounds were in neurology and psychiatry, not in physiology. Whenever we had to choose between attending a seminar in the neurobiology department and one on renal physiology (for example) in the physiology department, the decision was easy. That tended to hurt the feelings of my colleagues in the physiology department. And contrary to the predictions of some of my friends, there was far from enough time to do justice to both the chairmanship and our research. Our experiments lasted all day and well into the night; they had to be planned, and the results evaluated and discussed. Also, I had not realized how much of a chairman's time had to be spent helping run the school. There were many lofty committees, with decisions on chairmanships of other departments, curriculum, and so on. One had to be hospitable to visitors. I found that while shaving in the morning my preoccupations were with the department and the school, rather than what to do next in our research. One day during an experiment, when I complained about some of this, Torsten suddenly said, "You are selling yourself too cheaply. There is no reason to keep on doing these things if you don't want to." Suddenly I felt the lifting of a great weight. At last I recognized that I had made a mistake, and I resigned the job before doing the Department of Physiology *and* our research irreparable harm. It was a good lesson: I was never again tempted to become chairman of anything, despite several opportunities. Luckily we had not yet physically moved over to physiology, which was housed in another building across the Medical School quadrangle, and the space we were slated to occupy had not yet been remodeled. My colleagues in neurobiology welcomed Torsten and me back to that department, heartily and cheerfully, for which I have always been grateful.

PART III
NORMAL PHYSIOLOGY AND ANATOMY

In reprinting our papers and discussing them, it has seemed to us most natural to take up separately the ones involving normal physiology and anatomy in adult animals, and those dealing with deprivation and development. To combine the two sets in strict chronological order would have been awkward, with inevitable breaks in continuity and for the reader the necessity of flipping back and forth from one set to the other. To include every last paper would have made the book far too long, and our choices have had to be somewhat arbitrary. We have found it especially hard to decide on some of the summary papers such as the Ferrier Lecture (published in 1977), but in the end we could not resist including it despite the obvious overlap with the original papers. The Ferrier Lecture was a major exception to our tendency to shy away from writing reviews, even reviews of our own work. That was mainly to save time, and to encourage people to read the original papers. The other question was whether to include the two Nobel lectures—another exception that we could hardly avoid. The problem was one of length and price versus completeness, but in the end it was hard to resist telling the story of the Nature versus Science contretemps (see p. 658).

Chapter 7 • Our First Paper, on Cat Cortex, 1959 •

FOREWORD

In getting started, that first week in the spring of 1958 at Johns Hopkins, we simply used whatever equipment we could assemble from Steve's old retinal setup, together with various gadgets I had made at Walter Reed and brought to Hopkins with me. We stimulated the retina with the same glorified two-beam ophthalmoscope that Steve had used for his retinal work. A picture of this apparatus is included in Steve's famous 1962 Cold Spring Harbor paper on retinal ganglion cells. Attached to the ophthalmoscope was a head holder that had the animal rotated so that it looked more or less straight up. For our purposes this arrangement was awkward to say the least. It was designed to deliver to the retina precisely calibrated stimuli for precise lengths of time, and allowed one to view the retina and the recording electrode directly. At that stage and for years after we had little use for such niceties. We were recording from the cortex, not the retina, and we needed to be able to stimulate both eyes, not just one. In generating our visual stimuli we needed flexibility, because we had no idea what cortical cells might require to make them respond. Latencies (the number of milliseconds between the light stimulus and the response of the cell) and carefully calibrated stimulus intensities were not uppermost in our minds.

For recording, we used a microelectrode advancer that I had designed and built with my lathe at Walter Reed. It consisted of a plexiglass cylinder the size and shape of a fountain-pen cap through whose top we introduced the mineral oil, which lowered the piston that held the microelectrode. To accomplish the electrode positioning with the atmosphere excluded (see p. 19), we drilled a 2 to 3 mm hole in the skull over the visual cortex, cut the dura (the thick membrane covering the brain), positioned a hollow steel guide tube in the hole, waxed in the space between skull and guide tube, lowered the tungsten electrode, and hoped for the best. I had designed and built this advancer system as part of my setup for recording from cats that were awake and moving around. For recording from anesthetized cats or mon-

59

keys it gave a stability that would have allowed us to continue recording from a cell even in the presence of an earthquake.

In our very first experiments we used circular spots of light, or black spots, because these had served Stephen Kuffler so well in delineating receptive fields of retinal ganglion cells. To produce a spot of light on the retina we inserted, into a slot in the light path of the ophthalmoscope, a small brass plate the size and shape of a microscope slide. In the brass plate a tiny hole had been drilled to determine the spot diameter. Dark spots on a light background were obtained with glass microscope slides on which small circles of metal of various sizes had been glued. The ophthalmoscope also supplied a background whose intensity could be varied.

Pessimists by nature, we were amazed when our system for advancing the electrode and recording worked well even from the beginning. We found it easy to record from single cells and observe their spontaneous all-or-none signals (as deflections on the oscilloscope and clicks on the audio monitor) for many hours. But for the very first day or so we had no success in getting any clear responses. It turned out that the early failures had nothing to do with the anesthetic but were a matter of finding the right stimulus. It was hard to know where to stimulate in the retina because of difficulties in keeping track of retinal position relative to the cat's retinal landmarks, the area centralis (equivalent to the primate fovea), and the optic disc. The break came one long day in which we held onto one cell for hour after hour. To find a region of retina from which our spots gave any hint of responses took many hours, but we finally found a place that gave vague hints of responses. We worked away, in shifts. Suddenly, just as we inserted one of our glass slides into the ophthalmoscope, the cell seemed to come to life and began to fire impulses like a machine gun. It took a while to discover that the firing had nothing to do with the small opaque spot—the cell was responding to the fine moving shadow cast by the edge of the glass slide as we inserted it into the slot. It took still more time and groping around to discover that the cell gave responses only when this faint line was swept slowly forward in a certain range of orientations. Even changing the stimulus orientation by a few degrees made the responses much weaker, and an orientation at right angles to the optimum produced no responses at all. The cell completely ignored our black and white spots. When finally we could think of nothing more to do with this cell, we discovered we had worked with it for nine hours. The 1959 paper of course gives no hint of our struggle. As usual in scientific reports we presented the bare results, with little of the sense of excitement or fun.

That cell was our first clear example of what we came to call *orientation selectivity,* which turns out to be the most striking attribute of cells in the primary visual cortex. But that day, in the spring of 1958, we had no reason to believe that the cell was not a strange and unusual exception—the great prevalence of orientation-selective cells only became clear in the months that followed. In retrospect, that first cell was almost certainly an example of the type that we finally came to term *complex.*

People hearing the story of how we stumbled on orientation selectivity might conclude that the discovery was a matter of luck. While never denying the importance of luck, we would rather say that it was more a matter of bullheaded persistence, a refusal to give up when we seemed to be getting nowhere. If something is there and you try hard enough and long enough you may find it; without that persistence, you certainly won't. It would be more accurate to say that we would have been *un*lucky that day had we quit a few hours before we did. It is hard to imagine that we would not, sooner or later, have found orientation selectivity, provided we kept on doing experiments. But just as important as stubbornness, in getting results, was almost certainly the simplicity, the looseness, of our methods of simulation. The incredible crudeness of our first slide projectors and the projection screens that soon replaced the ophthalmoscope, and our refusal to waste time bothering with measuring intensities, rates of movement and so on, or to spend time drawing graphs or histograms, all worked in our favor.

Despite our speed at getting started, everything did not always go smoothly in those early experiments. We examined histologically all the brains we recorded from, to verify that we had recorded from striate cortex and to determine if possible what layer each of our cells had been lodged in. So the last event in any experiment was to give the cat a lethal overdose of barbiturate and perfuse it with formalin, a preserving fluid consisting of dilute formaldehyde, which we injected through the heart. One night the rubber tubing coming from the huge overhead bottle of evil-smelling perfusion fluid broke loose and we were treated with our first formalin early-morning shower. We felt cleansed and chastened, went home smelling strongly of a funeral home. From then on we were more careful to see that the tubing was securely attached.

The time came when we had enough results to write a short paper. We had collected about a hundred cells, some of which we felt we understood and some of which we were sure we did not. By "understand" we mean that we could predict responses to slits, bars, or edges from the receptive fields mapped by turning on and off small stationary circular spots, in the way Kuffler had mapped his center-surround fields in the retina. We called these cells (or receptive fields) *simple*. Those that we did not understand in terms of excitatory and inhibitory subregions we kept aside, hoping to be able to make sense of them as time went on.

Jack Eccles, by then Sir John Eccles, under whom Steve Kuffler had trained in Australia, was a frequent visitor to Steve's lab and one of his closest friends. When Eccles visited, Steve usually brought him by to talk with us. On one of these visits we showed Sir John pictures of our first results. His reaction was to ask about the latency of the responses. Of course we had no idea. To which he commented: "You know, sooner or later you will have to start doing neurophysiology". We did not know whether to be annoyed or amused, and we suddenly realized how far apart our neurophysiological world was from his. In our experiments, as we repeatedly dragged the slit or edge across our cell's receptive field, the responses could vary in the time it took them to start to fire by periods of up to 1/4 second. In Eccles' world, with its electrical stimulation of entire nerve bundles, one more millisecond in the time it took for a cell to respond could point to an extra synapse in the circuit he was studying. We were clearly operating on very different wavelengths!

We were lucky to get into this field when we did, with the tools that we had, the relative absence of competition, and the conviction that we must be sitting on a gold mine. That conviction came from the recognition that anything as anatomically regular and beautiful as the striate cortex must surely be carrying out an interesting and impressive set of functions.

One day Vernon Mountcastle came over to visit Steve and wandered into our lab. The night before his visit we had decided to give up on the old ophthalmoscope and try a projection screen instead. We could shine our stimuli onto a screen, using a simple slide projector which we held by hand. We determined the positions on the screen that corresponded to the retinal area centralis and optic disc by viewing these with an ordinary ophthalmoscope to which we had attached a lamp that projected a spot back onto the screen. The day of Vernon's visit we had had to devise an overhead screen because our head holder had the cat looking straight up. We brought in bedsheets from home, and spread them across the many pipes that crisscrossed the ceiling of our lab. When Vernon walked in, our room must have seemed like a circus, complete with a tent and exotic animals. We were mapping the receptive fields of three simultaneously recorded cells, reaching up to make marks on pieces of paper pinned to the sheets. The receptive fields of the three cells, recorded by a single electrode tip and hence presumably next-door neighbors, lay side-by-side but not completely overlapping, all with the same orientation. The grouping of cells with common physiological properties into columns was of course Vernon's great discovery in the mid-1950s, and given the similar orientation selectivity of our three neighboring cells, the thought that they might be lodged in a column analogous to Vernon's somatosensory columns was surely in the backs of all three of our minds.

Vernon naturally asked how many such cells we had seen. He had just published a paper on the somatosensory cortex in which he had observed some 600 cells. To us that was an astronomical number, literally. We answered that in our series the three cells were numbers 3006, 3007, and 3008. In order to catapult ourselves into a league that came close to Vernon's, we had begun our series of cells with No. 3000, but we did not tell Vernon.

With the Talbot-Kuffler head-holder-and-ophthalmoscope combination we had the problem that it was only possible to stimulate one eye at a time. Consequently we had no idea whether our cells were binocular or monocular. (It was clear from the anatomy of the visual pathway that the striate cortex was the first place were the inputs from the two eyes *could* combine, but no one knew whether single cells would typically be influenced from the two eyes.) To be able to work with the two eyes, we obviously had to make radical changes in our system of stimulating the eyes. (It was impossible to imagine using *two* Talbot-Kuffler ophthalmoscopes—one was bad

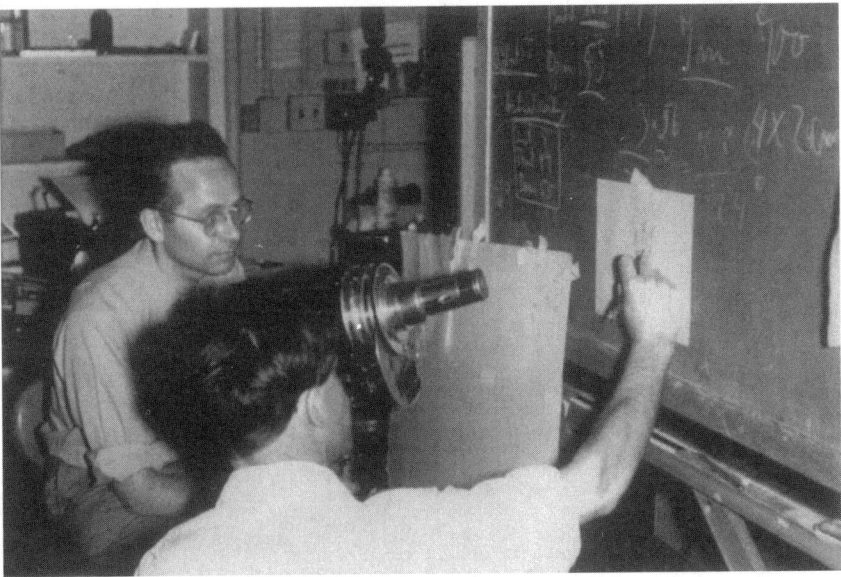

Wiesel and Hubel, 1959, mapping a receptive field with a crude projector and screen.

enough!) In the 1940s Talbot had designed a Horsley-Clarke stereotaxic apparatus that was not only beautifully made, entirely of stainless steel, but also sturdy and still very precise. (Some American neurobiologists tend to prefer the term *stereotax,* which makes me cringe. Horsley and Clarke were British neurosurgeons. I'm not sure if Americans prefer *stereotax* because of chauvinism, hatred of eponyms, or just a lack of feeling for the English language.) The instrument was unique in leaving the animal's visual fields completely unobstructed, an obviously important consideration for us. Engraved on it were the words "Physiological Optics" and "Wilmer Institute Johns Hopkins Hospital". This instrument was first used by Talbot and Marshall in their topographic evoked-potential mapping of the visual cortex, and is shown in one of their illustrations (*Am J Ophthal,* 1941, 24: 1255–1272, fig. 2). Steve had had no use for it in his retinal work and had lent it to Vernon, who used it for years in the department of physiology, mapping somatosensory representations, first in the thalamus and later in the cortex. Vernon had mentioned to us that he had just obtained and was now using a fancier stereotaxic instrument, and we concluded that the Talbot apparatus must be gathering dust. One day, to look official, we donned white lab coats (the only time we ever wore such garments) and screwing up our courage went over to the Hopkins medical school (one block away) to reclaim the Wilmer Horsley-Clarke. Vernon seemed less than pleased but had little choice. So we acquired a magnificent stereotaxic head holder, which we continued to use for the remaining 20 years of our collaboration. If one includes the visual mapping done by Talbot and Marshall and the subsequent somatosensory mapping by Mountcastle, that piece of stereotaxic equipment undoubtedly

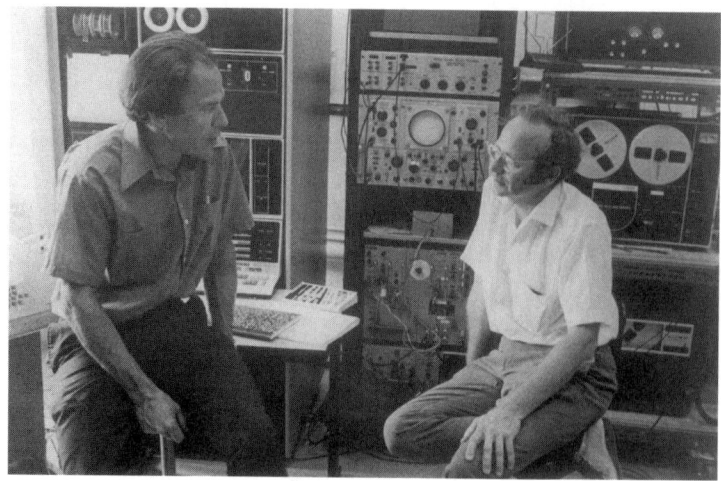

Hubel and Wiesel, 1970.

holds a record for longevity and distinction, and well deserves to end up in some museum.

Our new (as it were) head holder, with the cat facing forward, allowed us to arrange a sensible screen in the form of a freestanding school blackboard covered with white cardboard, and for once we could stimulate the two eyes. We quickly found that many (though not all) cat cortical cells could be influenced from both eyes, that many cells responded better to one eye than to the other, and that when stimulated together the two eyes showed mutual facilitation. That is described in the 1959 paper, minus of course the more interesting stories of how we retrieved the head holder, using the lab coats, and Vernon's possible dismay—to say nothing of formaldehyde shower-baths.

Clearly the cortex was doing something with the information it got from the eyes, and we could start to be concrete about what the "something" was, instead of the vague idea that it was "analyzing" things. We still had to show that lateral geniculate cells lacked the sophistication of cortical cells, so shortly we set about to record directly from the geniculate. The interest of the geniculate study was not just that the cells turned out to closely resemble retinal ganglion cells, but that they, too, showed a clear difference from the cells coming in from the retina. The difference, though clear, was far subtler than the difference between geniculate cells and cortical cells.

We first presented these results at a Federation Meeting, held as usual in Atlantic City, and the abstract we wrote for the occasion was our first literary effort. We labored over it and finally gave the result to Steve to look over. When I came into the lab the next day, Torsten, looking glummer than usual, complained that "Steve didn't think too much of our abstract". The original abstract, with Steve's comments, is reproduced here. It represents one of our first exposures to the kind of criticism that prevailed in Steve's community, in which a colleague dug in deeply, letting no lapses pass, whether in logic or in style. Steve liked to be able to read without being inter-

Single units were recorded extracellularly from (the) striate cortex of ~~the~~

lightly anesthetized cat. With the eye immobilized restricted light stimuli of

various shapes were shone on the light adapted retina, Most receptive fields

~~could be subdivided into excitatory and inhibitory regions, as found for~~

~~retinal ganglion cells (Kuffler, 1953).~~ These regions mutually interacted,

so that a large spot covering the entire field was usually ineffective. ~~However~~

Excitatory and inhibitory areas were arranged in several types of specialized

and complex patterns, and specific stimuli were required for effective driving.

oncentric recepetive fields described for retinal ganglion cells were not seen

in the cortex. For example, ~~frequently~~ an excitatory ~~xxx~~ inhibitory region was

long and narrow with areas of opposite type to either side only, ~~Such~~ fields

were oriented in a vertical, horizontal or oblique manner. The two ~~regions~~

regions were often but not always equally destibuted, ~~on the two sides of the~~

~~central area.~~ With this type of field a stationary slit of light, when flashed

onto the retina with appropriate position and orientation gave (the strongest)

responses. Responses to transverse movements of slits were also dependent on

the slit orientation . Many units could be binocularly activated, and when

mapped out in the two eyes separately, the receptive fields were found to have

a similar organization.

Our first abstract, with Steve Koffler's comments, 1958

rupted by difficulties of syntax or logic, and would mark any difficult passages, complaining when something "tripped me up". When one compares his criticisms with the kind of readings that can prevail in English courses at universities, in which the only comment may be a B- (or today, usually A-) at the top of the page, one can understand why graduate students and even postdoctoral fellows so often lack the ability to write coherently or logically. It is hard to imagine a book-length Ph.D. thesis being criticized in the detail that our abstract was subjected to by Steve, and a book-length thesis too often represents a beginning scientist's first efforts at serious writing. Steve took an interest in writing for its own sake, and he and the two of us spent much time reading and discussing books on English writing by Strunk and White, Gowers, and of course Fowler.

In our first attempt to write a full-length paper we proceeded sentence by sentence, discussing the wording as we went along. That clearly did not work—it was like two people trying to improvise music singing alto and bass. In later papers we ended by having one author write the first draft, which the other would then edit and criticize. The burden was shared more or less equally, though occasionally we differed in our enthusiasm or interest, in which case the one with the greater interest wrote the first draft. Papers were written and rewritten, and we gave each new draft to one of our group to criticize as harshly as possible. Criticism took every possible form, from interpretation of results, to sentence structure and semantics. This paper represented, for both of us, one of our first efforts to put scientific results into words. It was the first report that suggested any major reorganization of incoming information by the cerebral cortex, and we could see that it was important. We wanted to do the results justice, if we possibly could.

After 11 drafts, typing each draft ourselves our old Underwood typewriter (this was years before the trials and agonies of contending with Microsoft Word) we sent the final version to the *Journal of Physiology*. The response was gratifying. It began, "Congratulations upon a very fine paper . . ." and made no suggestions for revisions. We assumed, without proof, that the reviewer was William Rushton—the same famous psychophysicist who had sat me down at Trinity High Table next to Lord Adrian—partly because of his use of the word "upon". Meanwhile, we kept on doing experiments, recording more cells and trying to make sense of the more complex cells.

Still in the back of my mind was the feeling that my stay at the Wilmer was to be temporary, and that we had to make the most of the limited time we had left to collaborate.

Receptive Fields of Single Neurones in the Cat's Striate Cortex

D. H. HUBEL* AND T. N. WIESEL* • *Wilmer Institute, The Johns Hopkins Hospital and University,*

Baltimore, Maryland

In the central nervous system the visual pathway from retina to striate cortex provides an opportunity to observe and compare single unit responses at several distinct levels. Patterns of light stimuli most effective in influencing units at one level may no longer be the most effective at the next. From differences in responses at successive stages in the pathway one may hope to gain some understanding of the part each stage plays in visual perception.

By shining small spots of light on the light-adapted cat retina Kuffler (1953) showed that ganglion cells have concentric receptive fields, with an 'on' centre and an 'off' periphery, or vice versa. The 'on' and 'off' areas within a receptive field were found to be mutually antagonistic, and a spot restricted to the centre of the field was more effective than one covering the whole receptive field (Barlow, FitzHugh & Kuffler, 1957). In the freely moving light-adapted cat it was found that the great majority of cortical cells studied gave little or no response to light stimuli covering most of the animal's visual field, whereas small spots shone in a restricted retinal region often evoked brisk responses (Hubel, 1959). A moving spot of light often produced stronger responses than a stationary one, and sometimes a moving spot gave more activation for one direction than for the opposite.

The present investigation, made in acute preparations, includes a study of receptive fields of cells in the cat's striate cortex. Receptive fields of the cells considered in this paper were divided into separate excitatory and inhibitory ('on' and 'off') areas. In this respect they resembled retinal ganglion-cell receptive fields. However, the shape and arrangement of excitatory and inhibitory areas differed strikingly from the concentric pattern found in retinal ganglion cells. An attempt was made to correlate responses to moving stimuli with receptive field arrangements. Some cells could be activated from either eye, and in these binocular interaction was studied.

METHODS

In this series of experiments twenty-four cats were used. Animals were anaesthetized with intraperitoneal thiopental sodium (40 mg/kg) and light anaesthesia was maintained throughout the experiment by additional intraperitoneal injections. The eyes were immobilized by continuous intravenous injection of succinylcholine; the employment of this muscle relaxant made it necessary to use artificial respiration. Pupils of both eyes were dilated and accommodation was relaxed by means of 1% atropine. Contact lenses used with a suitably buffered solution prevented the corneal surfaces from drying and becoming cloudy. The lids were held apart by simple wire clips.

A multibeam ophthalmoscope designed by Talbot & Kuffler (1952) was used for stimulation and viewing the retina of the left eye. Background illumination was usually about 0.17 log. metre candles (m.c.), and the strongest available stimulus was 1.65 log. m.c. Many sizes and shapes of spots of light could be produced, and these were well focused on the retina. Stimulus durations were of the order of 1 sec.

For binocular studies a different method of light stimulation was used. The animal faced a large screen covering most of the visual field. On this screen light spots of various sizes and shapes were projected. The light source was a tungsten filament projector mounted on an adjustable tripod. Stimuli could be moved across the screen in various directions and with different speeds. Spots subtending an angle as small as 12 min of arc at the cat's eyes could be obtained, but generally 0.5–1° spots were used for mapping receptive fields. (Dimensions of stimuli are given in terms of equivalent external angles; in the cat 1 mm on the retina subtends about 4°.) Spots were focused on the two retinas with lenses mounted in front of the cat's eyes. Lenses for

J. Physiol. (1959) 148, 574–591

Received 22 *April* 1959.

* Present address, Harvard Medical School, 25 Shattuck St., Boston 15, Massachusetts.

focusing were selected by using a retinoscope. Spot intensities ranged from –0.76 to 0.69 log. cd/m^2. A background illuminance of –1.9 log. cd/m^2 was given by a tungsten bulb which illuminated the whole screen diffusely. Intensities were measured by a Macbeth Illuminometer. Values of retinal illumination corresponding to these intensities (Talbot & Kuffler, 1952, Fig. 4) were within the photopic range but were lower than those employed with the ophthalmoscope. Whenever the two methods of stimulation were checked against each other while recording from the same unit they were found to give similar results. This principle of projecting light spots on a screen was described by Talbot & Marshall (1941). Areas responsive to light were marked on sheets of paper fixed on the screen, in such a way as to indicate whether the responses were excitatory or inhibitory. The sheets of paper then provided permanent records of these responses, and showed the shape, size and orientation of the regions.

Single unit activity was recorded extracellularly by techniques described previously (Hubel, 1959). A hydraulic micro-electrode positioner was attached to the animal's skull by a rigidly implanted plastic peg. The cortical surface was closed off from the atmosphere to minimize respiratory and vascular movements of the cortex (Davies, 1956). This method gave the stability needed for thorough exploration of each receptive field, which often took many hours. Electrodes were electrolytically sharpened tungsten wires insulated with a vinyl lacquer (Hubel, 1957). Cathode follower input and a condenser-coupled pre-amplifier were used in a conventional recording system.

Recordings were made from parts of the lateral gyrus extending from its posterior limit to about Horsley-Clarke frontal plane 10. At the end of each penetration an electrolytic lesion was made (Hubel, 1959) and at the end of the experiment the animal was perfused, first with normal saline and then with 10% formalin. The borders of the trephine hole were marked with Indian ink dots and the brain was removed from the skull and photographed. Paraffin serial sections were made in the region of penetration and stained with cresyl violet. These sections showed that all units described were located in the grey matter of the striate cortex. Correlation between location of units in the striate cortex and physiological findings will not be dealt with in this paper. There is evidence that cortical cells and afferent fibres differ in their firing patterns and in their responses to diffuse light (Hubel, 1960). The assumption that the spikes recorded were from cell bodies is based on these differences, as well as on electrophysiologic criteria for distinguishing cell-body and fibre spikes (Frank & Fuortes, 1955; Hubel, 1960).

RESULTS

Several hundred units were recorded in the cat's striate cortex. The findings to be described are based on thorough studies of forty-five of these, each of which was observed for a period of from 2 to 9 hr. Times of this order were usually required for adequate analysis of these units.

In agreement with previous findings in the freely moving light-adapted cat (Hubel, 1959) single cortical units showed impulse activity in the absence of changes in retinal illumination. Maintained activity was generally less than in freely moving animals, and ranged from about 0.1–10 impulses/sec. The low rate was possibly due to light barbiturate anaesthesia, since on a number of occasions deepening the anaesthesia resulted in a decrease of maintained activity. This need not mean that all cortical cells are active in the absence of light stimuli, since many quiescent units may have gone unnoticed.

In most units it was possible to find a restricted area in the retina from which firing could be influenced by light. This area was called the receptive field of the cortical unit, applying the concept introduced by Hartline (1938) for retinal ganglion cells. The procedure for mapping out a receptive field is illustrated in Fig. 1. Shining a 1° spot (250 μ on the retina) in some areas of the contralateral eye produced a decrease in the maintained activity, with a burst of impulses when the light was turned off (Fig. 1a, b, d). Other areas when illuminated produced an increase in firing (Fig. 1c, e). The complete map, illustrated to the right of the figure, consisted of a long, narrow, vertically oriented region from which 'off' responses were obtained (triangles), flanked on either side by areas which gave 'on' responses (crosses). The entire field covered an area subtending about 4°. The elongated 'off' region had a width of 1° and was 4° long.

Most receptive fields could be subdivided into excitatory and inhibitory regions. An area was termed excitatory if illumination produced an increase in frequency of firing. It was termed inhibitory if light stimulation suppressed maintained activity and was followed by an 'off' discharge, or if either suppression of firing or an 'off' discharge occurred alone. In many units the rate of

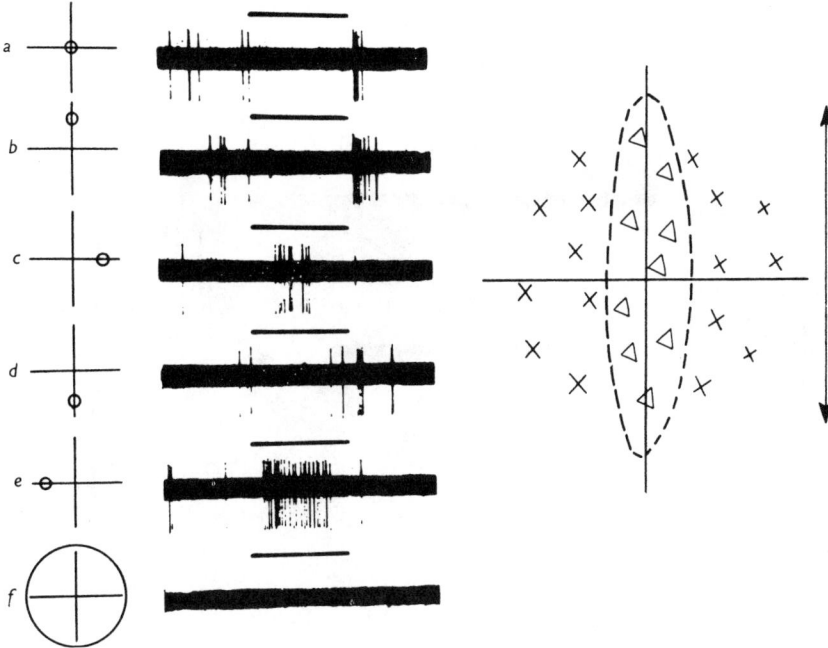

Fig. 1. *Responses of a cell in the cat's striate cortex to a 1° spot of light. Receptive field located in the eye contralateral to the hemisphere from which the unit was recorded, close to and below the area centralis, just nasal to the horizontal meridian. No response evoked from the ipsilateral eye. The complete map of the receptive field is shown to the right.* ×, *areas giving excitation;* △, *areas giving inhibitory effects. Scale, 4°. Axes of this diagram are reproduced on left of each record.* a, *1° (0.25 mm) spot shone in the centre of the field;* b–e, *1° spot shone on four points equidistant from centre;* f, *5° spot covering the entire field. Background illumination 0.17 log. m.c. Stimulus intensity 1.65 log. m.c. Duration of each stimulus 1 sec. Positive deflexions upward.*

maintained activity was too slow or irregular to demonstrate inhibition during illumination, and only an 'off' discharge was seen. It was, however, always possible to demonstrate inhibitory effects if the firing rate was first increased by stimulation of excitatory regions.

As used here, 'excitatory' and 'inhibitory' are arbitrary terms, since both inhibition and excitation could generally be demonstrated from both regions, either during the light stimulus or following it. We have chosen to denote receptive field regions according to effects seen during the stimulus. Furthermore, the word 'inhibition' is used descriptively, and need not imply a direct inhibitory effect of synaptic endings on the cell observed, since the suppression of firing observed could also be due to a decrease in maintained synaptic excitation.

When excitatory and inhibitory regions (used in the sense defined) were stimulated simultane-

ously they interacted in a mutually antagonistic manner, giving a weaker response than when either region was illuminated alone. In most fields a stationary spot large enough to include the whole receptive field was entirely without effect (Fig. 1f). Whenever a large spot failed to evoke responses, diffuse light stimulation of the entire retina at these intensities and stimulus durations was also ineffective.

In the unit of Fig. 1 the strongest inhibitory responses were obtained with a vertical slit-shaped spot of light covering the central area. The greatest 'on' responses accompanied a stimulus confined to the two flanking regions. Summation always occurred within an area of the same type, and the strongest response was obtained with a stimulus having the approximate shape of this area.

In the unit of Figs. 2 and 3 there was weak excitation in response to a circular 1° spot in the

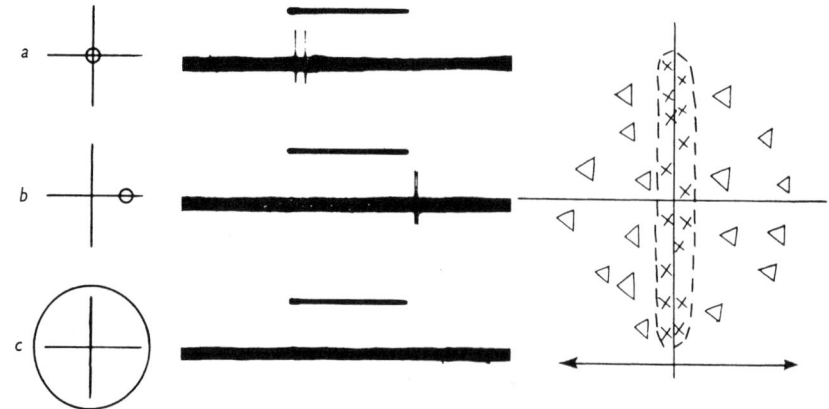

Fig. 2. *Responses of a unit to stimulation with circular spots of light. Receptive field located in area centralis of contralateral eye. (This unit could also be activated by the ipsilateral eye.) a, 1° spot in the centre region; b, same spot displaced 3° to the right; c, 8° spot covering entire receptive field. Stimulus and background intensities and conventions as in Fig. 1. Scale, 6°.*

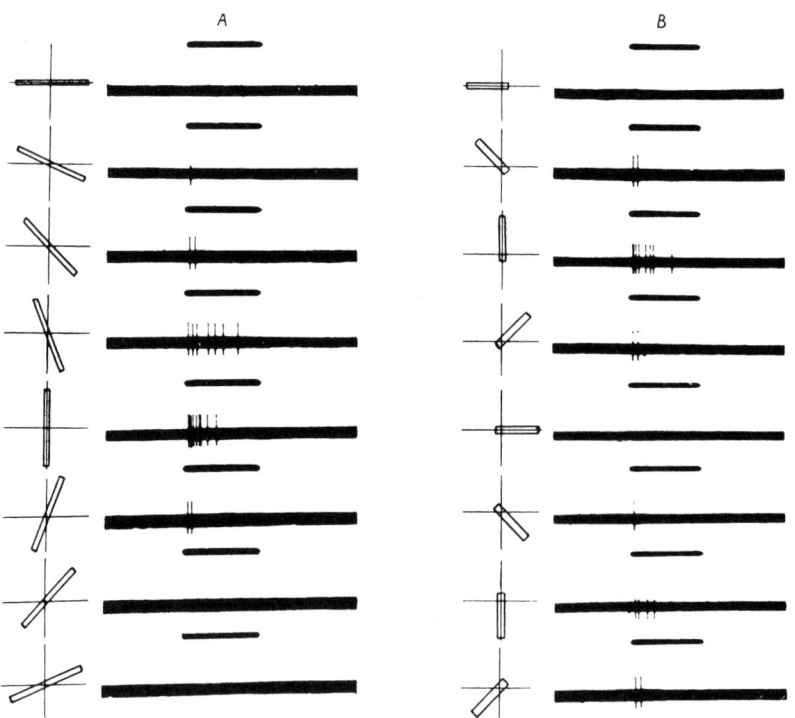

Fig. 3. *Same unit as in Fig. 2. A, responses to shining a rectangular light spot, 1° × 8°; centre of slit superimposed on centre of receptive field; successive stimuli rotated clockwise, as shown to left of figure. B, responses to a 1° × 5° slit oriented in various directions, with one end always covering the centre of the receptive field: note that this central region evoked responses when stimulated alone (Fig. 2a). Stimulus and background intensities as in Fig. 1; stimulus duration 1 sec.*

Fig. 4. Responses evoked only from contralateral eye. Receptive field just outside nasal border of area centralis. a, 1° spot covering the inhibitory region; b, right half of a circle 12° in diameter; c, light spot covering regions illuminated in a and b. Background and stimulus intensities and conventions as in Fig. 1. Scale, 12°.

central region. A weak 'off' response followed stimulation in one of the flanking areas (Fig. 2a,b). There was no response to an 8° spot covering the entire receptive field (Fig. 2c). The same unit was strongly activated by a narrow slit-shaped stimulus, measuring 1° by 8°, oriented vertically over the excitatory region (Fig. 3A). In contrast, a horizontal slit of light was completely ineffective, despite the fact that the central area was capable of evoking a response when stimulated alone (Fig. 2a). As the optimum (vertical) orientation of the slit was approached responses appeared and rapidly increased to a maximum.

These findings can be readily understood in terms of interacting excitatory and inhibitory areas. The strength of the response to a vertically oriented slit is explained by summation over the excitatory region and by the exclusion of inhibitory regions. When parts of the inhibitory flanking areas were included by rotating the slit, responses were reduced or abolished. Thus a horizontal slit was ineffective because it stimulated a small portion of the central excitatory area, and larger portions of the antagonistic regions.

Some units were not responsive enough to permit mapping of receptive fields with small light spots. In these the effective stimulus pattern could be found by changing the size, shape and orientation of the stimulus until a clear response was evoked. Often when a region with excitatory or inhibitory responses was established the neighbouring opposing areas in the receptive field could only be demonstrated indirectly. Such an indirect method is illustrated in Fig. 3B, where two flanking areas are indicated by using a short slit in various positions like the hand of a clock, always including the very centre of the field. The findings

thus agree qualitatively with those obtained with a small spot (Fig. 2a).

Receptive fields having a central area and opposing flanks represented a common pattern, but several variations were seen. Some fields had long narrow central regions with extensive flanking areas (Figs. 1–3): others had a large central area and concentrated slit-shaped flanks (Figs. 6, 9, 10). In many fields the two flanking regions were asymmetrical, differing in size and shape; in these a given spot gave unequal responses in symmetrically corresponding regions. In some units only two regions could be found, one excitatory and the other inhibitory, lying side by side. In these cases of extreme asymmetry it is possible that there was a second weak flanking area which could not be demonstrated under the present experimental conditions.

An interesting example of a field with only two opposing regions is shown in Fig. 4. The concentrated inhibitory region was confined to an area of about 1° (Fig. 4a). The excitatory area situated to the right of the inhibitory was much larger: a spot of at least 4° was required to evoke a response, and a very strong discharge was seen when the entire 12° excitatory area was illuminated (Fig. 4b). Despite the difference in size between excitatory and inhibitory areas, the effects of stimulating the two together cancelled each other and no response was evoked (Fig. 4c). The semicircular stimulus in Fig. 4b was of special interest because the exact position of the vertical borderline between light and darkness was very critical for a strong response. A slight shift of the boundary to the left, allowing light to infringe on the inhibitory area, completely cancelled the response to illumination. Such a boundary between light and darkness, when properly positioned and oriented, was often an effective type of stimulus.

Cortical receptive fields with central and flanking regions may have either excitatory (Fig. 2) or inhibitory (Figs. 1, 6, 7) centres. So far we have no indication that one is more common than the other.

The axis of a field was defined as a line through its centre, parallel to an optimally oriented elongated stimulus. For each of the field types described examples were found with axes oriented vertically, horizontally or obliquely. Orientations were determined with respect to the animal's skull. Exact field orientations with respect to the horizontal meridians of the retinas were not known, since relaxation of eye muscles may have caused slight rotation of the eyeballs. Within these limitations the two fields illustrated in Figs. 1–3 were vertically arranged: a horizontal field is shown in Fig. 6, 9 and 10, and oblique fields in Figs. 7 and 8.

All units have had their receptive fields entirely within the half-field of vision contralateral to the hemisphere in which they were located. Some receptive fields were located in or near the area centralis, while others were in peripheral retinal regions. All receptive fields were located in the highly reflecting part of the cat's retina containing the tapetum. So far, retinal ganglion cell studies have also been confined to the tapetal region (Kuffler, 1953).

It was sometimes difficult to establish the total size of receptive fields, since the outer borders were often poorly defined. Furthermore, field size may depend on intensity and size of the stimulus spot and on background illumination, as has been shown for the retina by Hartline (1938) and Kuffler (1953). Within these limitations, and under the stimulus conditions specified, fields ranged in total size from about 4° to 10°. Although in the present investigation no systematic studies have been made of changes in receptive fields under different conditions of stimulation, fields obtained in the same unit with the ophthalmoscope and with projection techniques were always found to be similar in size and structure, despite a difference of several logarithmic units in intensity of illumination. This would suggest that within this photopic range there was little change in size or organization of receptive fields. No units have been studied in states of dark adaptation.

Responses to Movement

Moving a light stimulus in the visual field was generally an effective way of activating units. As was previously found in the freely moving animal (Hubel, 1959), these stimuli were sometimes the only means by which the firing of a unit could be influenced. By moving spots of light across the retina in various directions and at different speeds patterns of response to movement could be outlined in a qualitative way.

Slit-shaped spots of light were very effective and useful for studies of movement. Here also the orientation of the slit was critical for evoking responses. For example, in the unit of Fig. 3 moving a vertical slit back and forth across the field evoked a definite response at each crossing (Fig. 5a), whereas moving a horizontal slit up and down was without effect (Fig. 5b). The vertical slit crossed excitatory and inhibitory areas one at a time and each area could exert its effect unopposed, but a horizontal slit at all times covered the antagonistic regions simultaneously, and was therefore ineffective. The response to a vertical slit moved horizontally was about the same for the two directions of movement.

In some units a double response could be observed at each crossing of the receptive field. The receptive field in Fig. 6 had an extensive inhibitory centre flanked by elongated, horizontally oriented, concentrated flanking regions. A horizontal slit moved slowly up or down over the receptive field evoked a discharge as each excitatory region was crossed. A further description of this unit is given in the binocular section of this paper (p. 584).

Many units showed directional selectivity of a different type in their responses to movement. In these a slit oriented optimally produced responses that were consistently different for the two directions of transverse movement. In the example of Fig. 7, the receptive field consisted of a strong inhibitory area flanked by two excitatory areas, of which the right was weaker than the left. Each region was elongated and obliquely oriented. As usual, a large spot was ineffective (Fig. 7c). A narrow slit, with its long axis parallel to that of the field, produced a strong response when moved transversely in a direction down and to the left, but only a feeble response when moved up and to the right (Fig. 7d). A tentative interpretation of these

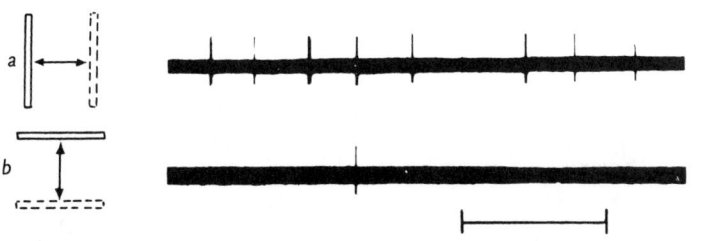

Fig. 5. *Same unit as in Figs. 2 and 3. Receptive field shown in Fig. 2. Responses to a slit (1° × 8°) moved transversely back and forth across the receptive field. a, slit moved horizontally. b, slit moved vertically. Background and stimulus intensities as in Fig. 1; time, 1 sec.*

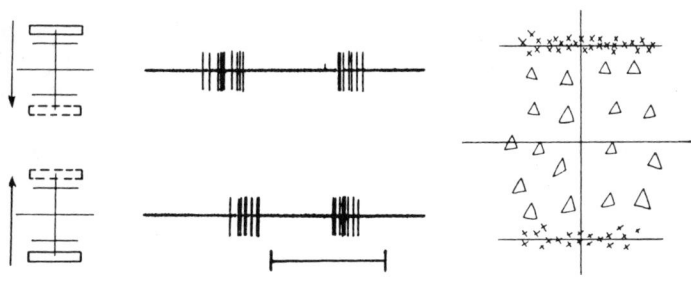

Fig. 6. *Slow up-and-down movements of horizontal slit (1° × 8°) across receptive field of left eye. Burst of impulses at each crossing of an excitatory region. For details see Fig. 9. ×, excitatory; △, inhibitory. Background illumination –1.9 cd/m²; stimulus intensity 0.69 cd/m²; time, 1 sec.*

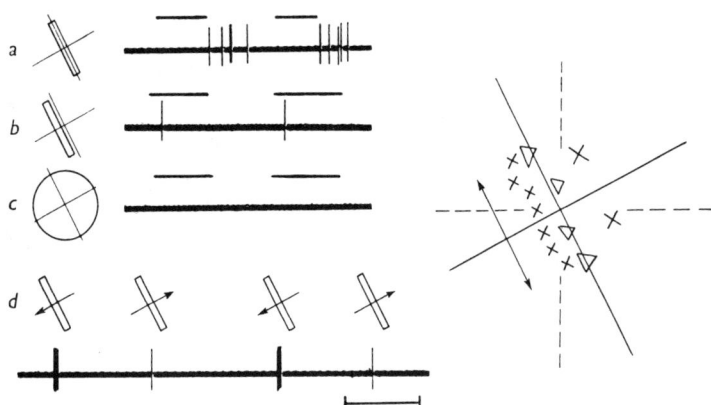

Fig. 7. *Unit activated from ipsilateral eye only. Receptive field just temporal to area centralis. Field elongated and obliquely oriented. Left excitatory flanking region stronger than right. a, 1° × 10° slit covering central region; b, 1° × 10° slit covering left flanking region; c, 12° spot covering entire receptive field; d, transverse movement of slit (1° × 10°) oriented parallel to axis of field—note difference in response for the two directions of movement. Background and stimulus intensities and conventions as in Fig. 6. Scale, 10°; time, 1 sec.*

findings on the basis of asymmetry within the receptive field will be given in the Discussion.

A number of units responded well to some directions of movement, but not at all to the reverse directions. An example of this is the unit of Fig. 8. Again a slit was moved back and forth transversely in a number of different directions. Only movements up and to the right evoked responses. As with many units, this one could not be activated by stationary stimuli; nevertheless, by using moving stimuli it was possible to get some idea of the receptive field organization—for example, in this unit, the oblique orientation.

Binocular Interaction

Thirty-six units in this study could be driven only from one eye, fifteen from the eye ipsilateral to the hemisphere in which the unit was situated, and

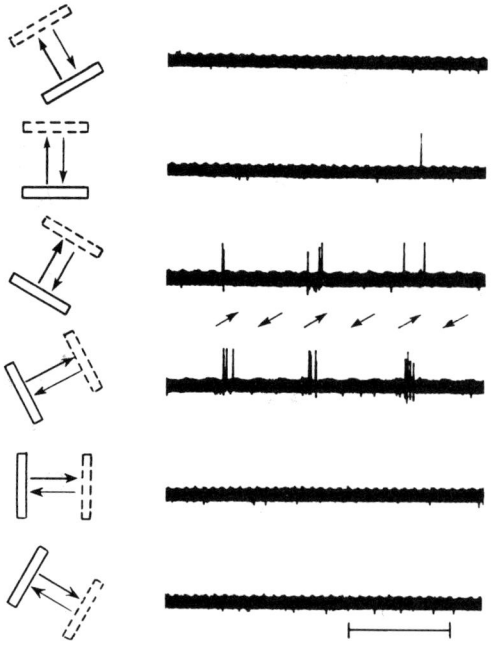

Fig. 8. Records from unit activated by ipsilateral eye only; unresponsive to stationary spots, influenced by movement in an area temporal to area centralis. A slit (0.5° × 8°) moved back and forth transversely with different orientations, as shown to the left. For slit orientations evoking responses only one direction was effective—up and to the right. Stimulus and background intensities as in Fig. 6; time, 1 sec.

twenty-one from the contralateral. Nine, however, could be driven from the two eyes independently. Some of these cells could be activated just as well from either eye, but often the two eyes were not equally effective, and different degrees of dominance of one eye over the other were seen. In these binocular units the receptive fields were always in roughly homologous parts of the two retinas. For example, a unit with a receptive field in the nasal part of the area centralis of one eye had a corresponding field in the temporal part of the area centralis of the other eye.

Receptive fields were mapped out on a screen in front of the cat. With the eye muscles relaxed with succinylcholine the eyes diverged slightly, so that receptive fields as charted were usually side by side, instead of being superimposed. Whenever the receptive fields of a single unit could be mapped out in the two eyes separately, they were similar in shape, in orientation of their axes, and in arrangement of excitatory and inhibitory regions within the field.

The receptive fields shown in Fig. 9 were obtained from a binocularly activated unit in which each field was composed of an inhibitory centre flanked by narrow horizontal excitatory areas. Responses of the same unit to a horizontal slit moved across the field have already been shown in Fig. 6, for the left eye.

Summation occurred between corresponding regions in the receptive fields of the two eyes (Fig. 9). Thus simultaneous stimulation of two corresponding excitatory areas produced a response which was clearly stronger than when either area was stimulated alone (Fig. 9A). As the excitatory flanks within one receptive field summed, the most powerful response was obtained with a stimulus covering the four excitatory areas in the two eyes (Fig. 9B). Similarly, summation of 'off' responses occurred when inhibitory areas in the two eyes were stimulated together (Fig. 9C).

Antagonism could also be shown between receptive fields of the two eyes (Fig. 10A). Stimulated alone the central area of the left eye gave an 'off' response, and one flanking area of the right eye gave an 'on' response. When stimulated simultaneously the two regions gave no response. The principles of summation and antagonism could thus be demonstrated between receptive fields of the two eyes, and were not limited to single eyes.

Finally, in this unit it was possible with a moving stimulus to show that opposite-type areas need not always inhibit each other (Fig. 10A), but may under certain circumstances be mutually reinforcing (Fig. 10B). The right eye was covered, and a spot was projected on the screen, over the centre (inhibitory) area of the left eye. Moving the spot as illustrated, away from the centre region of the left eye, produced an 'off' response (Fig. 10B, 1). When the left eye was covered and the right eye uncovered, making the same movement again evoked a response as the flanking excitatory region of the right eye was illuminated (Fig. 10B, 2). The procedure was now repeated with both eyes uncovered, and a greatly increased response was produced (Fig. 10B, 3). Here the movement was made in such a way that the 'off' response from the left eye apparently added to the 'on' response from the right, producing a response much greater than with either region alone. It is very likely that

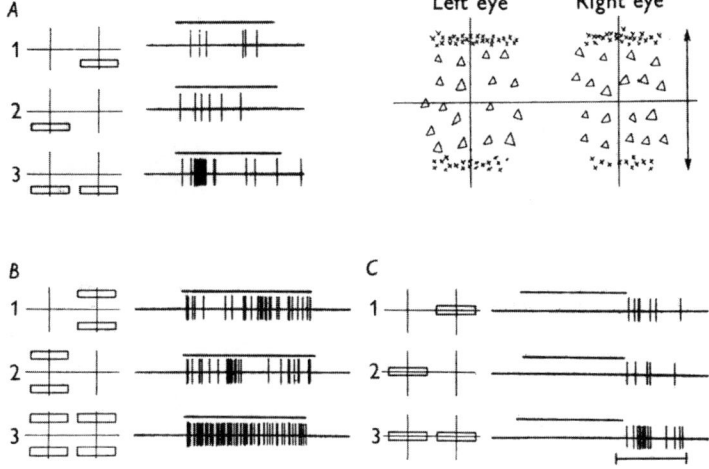

Fig. 9. *This unit was activated from either eye independently. The illustration shows summation between corresponding parts of the two receptive fields. Receptive field in the contralateral eye was located just above and nasal to area centralis; in the ipsilateral eye, above and temporal. Receptive fields of the two eyes were similar in form and orientation, as shown in upper right of the figure; scale 8°. The pairs of axes in the receptive field diagram are reproduced to the left of each record. Background and stimulus intensities and conventions as in Fig. 6. (Same unit as in Fig. 6.) A. 1, horizontal slit covering lower flanking region of right eye; 2, same for left eye; 3, pair of slits covering the lower flanking regions of the two eyes. B. 1, pair of horizontal slits covering both flanking regions of the right eye; 2, same for left eye; 3, simultaneous stimulation of all four flanking regions. C. 1, horizontal slit in central region of right eye; 2, same for left eye; 3, simultaneous stimulation of central regions of both eyes. Time, 1 sec.*

DISCUSSION

In this study most cells in the striate cortex had receptive fields with separate excitatory and inhibitory regions. This general type of organization was first described by Kuffler (1953) for retinal ganglion cells, and has also been found in a preliminary study of neurones in the lateral geniculate body (Hubel & Wiesel, unpublished). Thus at three different levels in the visual system a cell can be inhibited by one type of stimulus and excited by another type, while a stimulus combining the two is always less effective. Most retinal ganglion and geniculate cells give clear responses to a large spot of light covering the entire receptive field. At the cortical level the antagonism between excitatory and inhibitory areas appears to be more pronounced, since the majority of units showed little

within a single receptive field opposite-type regions may act in this synergistic way in response to a moving stimulus.

or no response to stimulation with large spots. Similar findings in the cortex of unanaesthetized, freely moving cats (Hubel, 1959) suggest that this is probably not a result of anaesthesia.

Other workers (Jung, 1953, 1958; Jung & Baumgartner, 1955), using only diffuse light stimulation, were able to drive about half the units in the cat striate cortex, while the remainder could not be activated at all. In recent studies (Hubel, 1960) about half the units recorded in striate cortex were shown to be afferent fibres from the lateral geniculate nucleus, and these responded to diffuse illumination. The remainder were thought to be cell bodies or their axons; for the most part they responded poorly if at all to diffuse light. The apparent discrepancy between our findings and those of Jung and his co-workers may perhaps be explained by the exclusion of afferent fibres from the present studies. On the other hand it may be that cells responsive to diffuse light flashes are more common in the cortex than our results would imply, but were not detected by our methods of

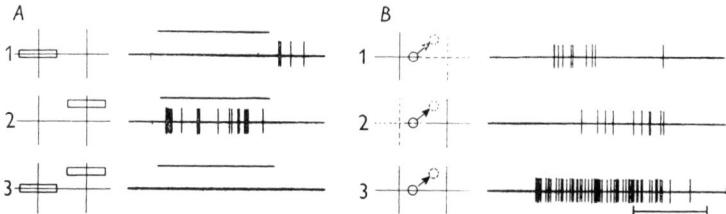

Fig. 10. Same unit as in Fig. 9. A. Antagonism between inhibitory region in the left eye and an excitatory region in the right eye; stationary spots. 1, horizontal slit in centre of left eye; 2, horizontal slit covering upper flanking region of right eye; 3, simultaneous stimulation of the regions of 1 and 2. B. Synergism between inhibitory region in left eye and an excitatory region in the right eye; moving spot of light. 1, right eye covered, spot moved from inhibitory region in left eye, producing an 'off' response; 2, left eye covered, spot moved into excitatory region in right eye, producing an 'on' response; 3, both eyes uncovered, spot moved from inhibitory region in left eye into excitatory region of right eye, producing a greatly enhanced response. Time, 1 sec.

recording and stimulating. However, cortical cells may not be primarily concerned with levels of diffuse illumination. This would be in accord with the finding that in cats some capacity for brightness discrimination persists after bilateral ablation of the striate cortex (Smith, 1937).

The main difference between retinal ganglion cells and cortical cells was to be found in the detailed arrangement of excitatory and inhibitory parts of their receptive fields. If afferent fibres are excluded, no units so far recorded in the cortex have had fields with the concentric configuration so typical of retinal ganglion cells. Moreover, the types of fields found in the cortex have not been seen at lower levels.

Spots of more or less circular (or annular) form are the most effective stimuli for activating retinal ganglion cells, and the diameter of the optimum spot is dependent on the size of the central area of the receptive field (Barlow *et al.* 1957). At the cortical level a circular spot was often ineffective; for best driving of each unit it was necessary to find a spot with a particular form and orientation. The cortical units described here have had in common a side-by-side distribution of excitatory and inhibitory areas, usually with marked elongation of one or both types of regions. The form and size of the most effective light stimulus was given by the shape of a particular region. The forms of stimulus used in these studies were usually simple, consisting of slit-shaped spots of light and boundaries between light and darkness. Position and orientation were critical, since imperfectly placed forms

failed to cover one type of region completely, thus not taking advantage of summation within that region, and at the same time could invade neighbouring, opposing areas (Fig. 3).

The phenomena of summation and antagonism within receptive fields seem to provide a basis for the specificity of stimuli, in shape, size and orientation. Units activated by slits and boundaries may converge upon units of higher order which require still more complex stimuli for their activation. Most units presented in this paper have had receptive fields with clearly separable excitatory and inhibitory areas. However, a number of units recorded in the striate cortex could not be understood solely in these terms. These units with more complex properties are now under study.

Other types of receptive fields may yet be found in the cortex, since the sampling (45 units) was small, and may well be biased by the microelectrode techniques. We may, for example, have failed to record from smaller cells, or from units which, lacking a maintained activity, would tend not to be detected. We have therefore emphasized the common features and the variety of receptive fields, but have not attempted to classify them into separate groups.

There is anatomical evidence for convergence of several optic tract fibres on to single geniculate neurons (O'Leary, 1940) and for a more extensive convergence of radiation fibres on to single cortical cells (O'Leary, 1941). Consistent with these anatomical findings, our results show that some single cortical cells can be influenced from relatively large retinal regions. These large areas, the receptive fields, are subdivided into excitatory and inhibitory regions; some dimensions of these may be very small compared with the size of the entire fields. This is illustrated by the fields shown in Figs. 1, 2 and 7, in which the central regions were long but very narrow; and by that of Fig. 9, in which both flanks were narrow. It is also shown by the field of Fig. 4, which had a total size of about 12° but whose inhibitory region was only about 1° in diameter. Thus a unit may be influenced from a relatively wide retinal region and still convey precise information about a stimulus within that region.

Movement of a stimulus across the retina was found to be a very potent way of activating a cell, often more so than a stationary spot. Transverse movement of a slit usually produced responses only when the slit was oriented in a certain direction. This was sometimes explained by the arrangement within the receptive fields as mapped out with stationary stimuli (Fig. 5).

In many units (Fig. 7) the responses to movement in opposite directions were strikingly different. Occasionally when the optimum direction of movement was established, there was no response to movement in the opposite direction (Fig. 8). Similar effects have been observed with horizontally moving spots in the unanaesthetized animal (Hubel, 1959). It was not always possible to find a simple explanation for this, but at times the asymmetry of strength of flanking areas was consistent with the directional specificity of responses to movement. Thus in the unit of Fig. 7 best movement responses were found by moving a slit from the inhibitory to the stronger of the two excitatory regions. Here it is possible to interpret movement responses in terms of synergism between excitatory and inhibitory areas. This is further demonstrated in Fig. 10*B,* where areas antagonistic when tested with stationary spots (Fig. 10*A*) could be shown to be synergistic with moving stimuli, and a strong response was evoked when a spot moved from an 'off' to an 'on' area.

Inhibition of unitary responses by stimulation of regions adjacent to the excitatory area has been described for the eccentric cell in the *Limulus* eye (Hartline, 1949) and for ganglion cells both in the frog retina (Barlow, 1953) and in the cat retina (Kuffler, 1953). Analogous phenomena have been noted for tones in the auditory system (dorsal cochlear nucleus, Galambos, 1944) and for touch and pressure in the somatosensory system (Mountcastle, 1957). In each system it has been proposed that these mechanisms are concerned with enhancing contrast and increasing sensory discrimination. Our findings in the striate cortex would suggest two further possible functions. First, the particular arrangements within receptive fields of excitatory and inhibitory regions seem to determine the form, size and orientation of the most effective stimuli, and secondly, these arrangements may play a part in perception of movement.

It is clear from stimulation of separate eyes with spots of light that some cortical units are activated from one eye only, either the ipsilateral or the contralateral, while others can be driven by the two eyes. In view of the small number of cells studied, no conclusion can be drawn as to the relative proportions of these units (ipsilaterally, contralaterally and bilaterally driven), but it appears that all three types are well represented.

Studies of binocularly activated units showed that the receptive fields mapped out separately in the two eyes were alike. The excitatory and inhibitory areas were located in homologous parts of the retinas, were similarly shaped and oriented, and responded optimally to the same direction of movement. When corresponding parts of the two receptive fields were stimulated summation occurred (Fig. 9). Assuming that the receptive fields as projected into the animal's visual field are exactly superimposed when an animal fixes on an object, any binocularly activated unit which can be affected by the object through one eye alone should be much more strongly influenced when both eyes are used. The two retinal images of objects behind or in front of the point fixed will not fall on corresponding parts of the fields, and their effects should therefore not necessarily sum. They may instead antagonize each other or not interact at all.

It is possible that when an object in the visual field exerts, through the two eyes, a strong influence on binocularly activated units, those influences may lead in some way to an increased awareness of the object. If that is so, then objects which are the same distance from the animal as the object fixed should stand out in relief. On the other hand such units may be related to mechanisms of binocular fixation, perhaps projecting to mid-brain nuclei concerned with the regulation of convergence.

SUMMARY

1. Recordings were made from single cells in the striate cortex of lightly anaesthetized cats. The retinas were stimulated separately or simultaneously with light spots of various sizes and shapes.

2. In the light-adapted state cortical cells were active in the absence of additional light stimulation. Increasing the depth of anaesthesia tended to suppress this maintained activity.

3. Restricted retinal areas which on illumination influenced the firing of single cortical units were called receptive fields. These fields were usually subdivided into mutually antagonistic excitatory and inhibitory regions.

4. A light stimulus (approximately 1 sec duration) covering the whole receptive field, or diffuse illumination of the whole retina, was relatively ineffective in driving most units, owing to mutual antagonism between excitatory and inhibitory regions.

5. Excitatory and inhibitory regions, as mapped by stationary stimuli, were arranged within a receptive field in a side-by-side fashion with a central area of one type flanked by antagonistic areas. The centres of receptive fields could be either excitatory or inhibitory. The flanks were often asymmetrical, in that a given stationary stimulus gave unequal responses in corresponding portions of the flanking areas. In a few fields only two regions could be demonstrated, located side by side. Receptive fields could be oriented in a vertical, horizontal or oblique manner.

6. Effective driving of a unit required a stimulus specific in form, size, position and orientation, based on the arrangement of excitatory and inhibitory regions within receptive fields.

7. A spot of light gave greater responses for some directions of movement than for others. Responses were often stronger for one direction of movement than for the opposite; in some units these asymmetries could be interpreted in terms of receptive field arrangements.

8. Of the forty-five units studied, thirty-six were driven from only one eye, fifteen from the ipsilateral eye and twenty-one from the contralateral; the remaining nine could be driven from the two eyes independently. In some binocular units the two eyes were equally effective; in others various degrees of dominance of one eye over the other were seen.

9. Binocularly activated units were driven from roughly homologous regions in the two retinas. For each unit the fields mapped for the two eyes were similar in size, form and orientation, and when stimulated with moving spots, showed similar directional preferences.

10. In a binocular unit excitatory and inhibitory regions of the two receptive fields interacted, and summation and mutual antagonism could be shown just as within a single receptive field.

We wish to thank Dr S. W. Kuffler for his helpful advice and criticism, and Mr R. B. Bosler and Mr P. E. Lockwood for their technical assistance. This work was supported in part by U.S. Public Health Service grants B-22 and B-1931, and in part by U.S. Air Force contract AF 49 (638)-499 (Air Force Office of Scientific Research, Air Research and Development Command).

References

Barlow, H. B. (1953). Summation and inhibition in the frog's retina. *J. Physiol.* **119**, 69–88.

Barlow, H. B., FitzHugh, R. & Kuffler, S. W. (1957). Change of organization in the receptive fields of the cat's retina during dark adaptation. *J. Physiol.* **137**, 338–354.

Davies, P. W. (1956). Chamber for microelectrode studies in the cerebral cortex. *Science,* **124**, 179–180.

Frank, K. & Fuortes, M. G. F. (1955). Potentials recorded from the spinal cord with microelectrodes. *J. Physiol.* **130**, 625–654.

Galambos, R. (1944). Inhibition of activity in single auditory nerve fibers by acoustic stimulation. *J. Neurophysiol.* **7**, 287–304.

Hartline, H. K. (1938). The response of single optic nerve fibers of the vertebrate eye to illumination of the retina. *Amer. J. Physiol.* **121**, 400–415.

Hartline, H. K. (1949). Inhibition of activity of visual receptors by illuminating nearby retinal areas in the *Limulus* eye. *Fed. Proc.* **8**, 69.

Hubel, D. H. (1957). Tungsten microelectrode for recording from single units. *Science,* **125**, 549–550.

Hubel, D. H. (1959). Single unit activity in striate cortex of unrestrained cats. *J. Physiol.* **147**, 226–238.

Hubel, D. H. (1960). Single unit activity in lateral geniculate body and optic tract of unrestrained cats. *J. Physiol.* (In the Press.)

Jung, R. (1953). Neuronal discharge. *Electroenceph. clin. Neurophysiol.* Suppl. **4**, 57–71.

Jung, R. (1958). Excitation, inhibition and coordination of cortical neurones. *Exp. Cell Res.* Suppl. **5**, 262–271.

Jung, R. & Baumgartner, G. (1955). Hemmungsmechanismen und bremsende Stabilisierung an einzelnen Neuronen des optischen Cortex. *Pflüg. Arch. ges. Physiol.* **261**, 434–456.

Kuffler, S. W. (1953). Discharge patterns and functional organization of mammalian retina. *J. Neurophysiol.* **16**, 37–68.

Mountcastle, V. B. (1957). Modality and topographic properties of single neurons of cat's somatic sensory cortex. *J. Neurophysiol.* **20**, 408–434.

O'Leary, J. L. (1940). A structural analysis of the lateral geniculate nucleus of the cat. *J. comp. Neurol.* **73**, 405–430.

O'Leary, J. L. (1941). Structure of the area striata of the cat. *J. comp. Neurol.* **75**, 131–164.

Smith, K. U. (1937). Visual discrimination in the cat: V. The postoperative effects of removal of the striate cortex upon intensity discrimination. *J. genet. Psychol.* **51**, 329–369.

Talbot, S. A. & Marshall, W. H. (1941). Physiological studies on neural mechanisms of visual localization and discrimination. *Amer. J. Ophthal.* **24**, 1255–1263.

Talbot, S. A. & Kuffler, S. W. (1952). A multibeam ophthalmoscope for the study of retinal physiology. *J. opt. Soc. Amer.* **42**, 931–936.

AFTERWORD

The idea that visual cells might be specialized to mediate complex forms was not new, having first been emphasized by Horace Barlow in 1953, in a study of the frog optic nerve, and followed by Lettvin and Maturana's description of optic fibers recorded in the frog tectum. Our first meeting with Jerry Lettvin took place shortly after we came to Harvard, when he came over from MIT to the Medical School to visit, bringing some simple equipment and a frog, which he proceeded to use to demonstrate his convex-edge detectors and other wonders. We were impressed. It was clear from such early work that cells in the frog retina responded to stimuli that were more sophisticated than anything found in cat or primate retinas, and possibly more complex than what we had so far seen in the cortex. We obviously had much in common with Lettvin and Maturana, especially our exploratory approach and freedom from complex apparatus, hypotheses, and so on. Jerry and Humberto Maturana carried their unusual approach to extremes, perhaps because they lacked an advisor like Steve, who insisted that we make at least a few measurements for the sake of scientific respectability. They published relatively seldom, sometimes in out-of-the-way places, and were often regarded with disbelief; quite unjustifiably, as the world came to realize.

The most flattering reaction to our paper was something we heard much later: that a few days after its publication in *Journal of Physiology,* E. D. Adrian walked into Alan Hodgkin's office holding the issue of the *Journal,* saying "Have you seen this paper?" To have the paper noticed by two of our all-time heroes was an undreamed-of compliment. The reaction was not necessarily shared by everyone, as can be appreciated by the story, mentioned above, of Eccles' first visit.

Our paper probably did not completely conceal our qualitative, descriptive approach to measurements. We could have expressed many more of our results as graphs of responses, or thresholds, plotted against all possible parameters—orientation, rate of movement, intensity, and so on. Today's referees would scream at our looseness. It is easy to forget that in the 1950s and 1960s it was much more common to present results in figures that told stories, such as Figures 3 and 8 of the 1959 paper. Graphs, especially ones with error bars, were uncommon in the days before computers made things all too easy. Steve's attitudes to quantification were refreshing. He never asked about latencies, but insisted that we measure the light intensities we were using. His argument was pragmatic—that if we did not make at least a few physical measurements we wouldn't be taken seriously.

All this was years before the appearance of computers as standard lab equipment. Within five years or so we finally did buy a monster called a "PDP12", but it was several more years before we used it to do anything except heat our lab at Harvard. (In those days Harvard did not have many thermostats.) At that stage of our work we wanted a qualitative description of how receptive fields changed as one went further and further into the nervous system. Measurements, we felt, could wait.

Our methods were undoubtedly homespun—our enemies might call them sloppy. The Talbot-Kuffler ophthalmoscope, together with some electronics that Steve's electronics assistant, Bob Bosler, had built for the retinal work, gave accurate stimulus timing, which we felt we did not need. The upward-facing head holder and circus-tent bedsheets were amusing but awkward, and it was impossible to stimulate both eyes. We needed something more practical even if crude. So we graduated to our blackboard—screen, and found a simple projector that resembled an old-fashioned child's (or Marcel Proust's) magic lantern—a bulb, a simple lens, and a reflector (see figure, p. 63). To vary orientation and speed of movement we had to tilt and move the entire projector by hand, and we produced our line stimuli by cutting out slits in pieces of cardboard that we stuck to a frame with masking tape. We turned the stimulus on and off by interposing our hand in front of the lens. We later learned that two competing groups had attempted to activate cortical cells by using more elaborate methods: the Freiburg group led by Jung had built a device that somehow projected horizontal lines onto the retina, whereas a group in Montreal had built a projecting device that was limited to vertical lines. Both methods were presumably used to locate receptive fields efficiently, but neither was capable of varying orientation, so that it was impossible to stumble on orientation selectivity. Our methods, though crude, were flexible, and paid off.

We see little to amend in this paper, perhaps because we were cautious in our conclusions. The main conclusions were clear. Stimuli that produced responses in retina were very different from those that were most effective in cortex. For "simple" cortical cells, the geometrical arrangement of on and off regions was usually all one needed to know to predict the responses to any stimulus, stationary or moving. Generally a moving stimulus would produce the asymmetrical responses to movement predicted from the asymmetries in inhibitory flanks. Reversing contrast by substituting a slit for a dark bar would then reverse any preference for left-right or up-down movement. There were occasional exceptions, which we excused by saying, "After all, this is biology".

In subsequent papers on striate cortex, in 1962 and 1968, we quietly dropped the cell type described here in Fig. 4; in talking about it we referred to it as the "palette cell", and never again saw anything like it. Either it exists but is a rare species, or, more likely, we were mistaken in our description.

At the time we wrote the 1959 paper, we had already collected and studied many cells that we felt we did not understand. For the time being we excluded these, reserving them for the next cortical paper, which appeared in 1962. We called them *complex,* and attempted to explain their behavior in terms of neuronal circuits. Probably we would have held off and published the entire story in one paper had we not felt pressured by the fear that our collaboration must soon end.

One of the most striking characteristics of the simple cells described in this paper (and also the complex cells that came later) was their failure to respond to changes in diffuse light levels. Both cell types required spatial gradations in illumination, or contours. The cells would blissfully ignore our turning the room lights on or off, and a flashlight directed into the animal's face produced little or no response, even though (and indeed *because*) such a stimulus could be expected to affect every rod or cone in the animal's retina. Steve's retinal ganglion cells responded, though weakly, to spots large enough to include the receptive-field surround: the ability of the surround to counteract the stimulation of the center is evidently far better developed in cortical cells. All these cells were evidently interested, not in changes in overall light levels, but in comparing the light level in one region with that in another.

What struck us forcibly in this early work was the precision of the interplay between excitation and inhibition, the outcome of which was to produce the progressive specialization and specificity of cells at higher and higher levels in the central nervous system. To get impressive responses from cells, one had to have the excitation without the counteracting inhibition, and that called for refinement in stimuli. Such refinement was of course already apparent in Steve's retinal ganglion cells, but it took time for us to realize that at both levels, the point of the inhibition was to produce the specialization.

At the time, the prevailing thought was that retinal ganglion cells and cortical cells "enhance contrast". While in some sense that is so, we look upon the changes that occur as one goes centrally, along the visual path, as representing an increase in cell specialization, a tendency for cells to ignore boring things such as diffuse light levels in favor of objects that contrast with their surroundings. The contrast is already there, and needs no enhancement. It took us some time to realize fully that these results could explain the very existence of black and white—that they were matters of contrast, not absolute energies, and that the whole point of the physiology was to free the viewer from a dependence on the energy in the light source. Only much later, when we became influenced by Edwin Land, and when we recorded from double opponent cells, did we realize that the freedom extended also to the exact spectral content of the light source.

The paper came out in 1959, by which time we had already moved from the Wilmer Institute at Johns Hopkins to the Department of Pharmacology at Harvard. In many ways we hated to leave Hopkins. The space there was certainly tight, but perhaps partly for that reason the relationships among the members of Steve's group were rich and lively. We had felt welcome at the Wilmer, though we had little contact with most of the ophthalmologists there. Years later our shabby old quarters, with its brick walls, pipes running around the ceiling, and the noise of the nearby eye clinic, were remodeled, and the ophthalmologists sent Torsten and me each a brick from the wall of our lab with an inscribed brass plaque saying, "To David [Torsten] from his friends at the Wilmer, where it all began."

Chapter 8 • Recordings from Fibers in the Monkey Optic Nerve •

We began our research using cats partly because in those days they cost almost nothing, being easily available as strays that were collected and taken to pounds. Because of this easy availability, cats were by far the most commonly used animals in central nervous neurophysiology, and there existed a rich background knowledge of cat anatomy and physiology. That was especially important for us because of the work of Steve on the cat retinal ganglion cell. For Steve, the cat had been a lucky choice of animal because the complex color-coded cells one finds in the macaque monkey were very nearly absent. That surely simplified things for him. It was only much later that Nigel Daw and Alan Pearlman, postdocs in our lab, managed to find a few rare color-coded cells in the geniculates of cats (*J Physiol* 1970, 211:125–137).

Perhaps because of our clinical backgrounds we were especially interested in humans, and monkeys obviously had much more in common with humans than cats did. This was especially true of the visual system. Cats have excellent audition, but vision is not their strong suit—their acuity is lower, their color vision and probably also their stereopsis are less important. We forget why, at first, we chose the spider monkey—perhaps because they were more easily available to us than macaques, and they are certainly far more endearing and easier to work with. Monkeys were of course much more expensive than cats, but were still orders of magnitude cheaper then than they are today.

Our first experience with a spider monkey was unforgettable. To anesthetize the animal we as usual prepared to give it an intraperitoneal injection (into the abdomen) of pentothal. Torsten held the animal's arms with one hand and the syringe with the other, while I held its legs. Suddenly the syringe flew out of Torsten's grasp, firmly wrapped around by a coil of the monkey's tail. We knew that the tail was prehensile, with ridges on its undersurface like our fingerprints, but we had no idea how skilfully it could be used. We decided that from then on it would take three people to anesthetize our spider monkeys.

Receptive Fields of Optic Nerve Fibres in the Spider Monkey

D. H. HUBEL AND T. N. WIESEL • *Neurophysiology Laboratory, Department of Pharmacology, Harvard Medical School, Boston, Mass.*

Our present knowledge of how mammalian retinal ganglion-cell receptive fields are organized is based mainly on findings in the cat by Kuffler (1953). These results have since been confirmed and extended (Barlow, FitzHugh & Kuffler, 1957; Hubel, 1960; Wiesel, 1960), but up to now similar studies have not been made in primates. The retina of the monkey is of interest, since in most species, including *Ateles* (spider monkey) and *Macaca mulatta*, it is deeply pigmented and has a well defined fovea. It appears to be much closer to the human retina than to that of the cat, which has a highly reflectile tapetum and lacks a fovea. The purpose of this report is to describe the receptive fields of single optic nerve fibres in the spider monkey. In view of the monkey's ability to discriminate colours, some observations were also made on ganglion cell responses to monochromatic stimuli.

METHODS

The four young spider monkeys (8–10 lb., 3.6–4.5 kg) in this study were prepared in a manner similar to that described for the cat (Hubel & Wiesel, 1959). An animal was anaesthetized with thiopental sodium and light anaesthesia was maintained throughout the experiment. The head was placed in a Horsley—Clarke stereotaxic instrument designed to permit stimulation of almost any part of the visual field (Talbot & Marshall, 1941). The eyes were immobilized with the muscle relaxant succinylcholine: this made it necessary to use artificial respiration. The eyelids were held open and contact lenses protected the corneas. The pupils were dilated and accommodation was relaxed with atropine. A slit retinoscope was used to determine the correct supplementary lenses for focusing the eyes on a screen at a given distance.

The animal faced a large tangent screen. This was generally placed 1.5 m from the monkey, but for the smallest stimuli it was moved to a distance of 10 m. A distant tungsten lamp supplied a diffuse background

light which produced on the screen a variable luminance of up to 2.0 $\log_{10}$ cd/m^2. Circular or annular spots provided by a tungsten projection lamp could be shone on different parts of the screen. The maximum spot luminance was 3.0 $\log_{10}$ cd/m^2. Stimulus spots were adjusted in intensity with an iris diaphragm so as not to exceed the background by more than 2 $\log_{10}$ units. At 10 m distance spots were obtainable subtending angles down to about 20 sec of arc, equivalent to about 2 μ on the retina. Fifteen interference filters (Farrand Optical Co., New York, N.Y.) ranging from 400 to 700 mμ with a band width at half maximum transmission of 25–50 mμ, were used to obtain coloured stimuli. The coloured lights were not calibrated for equal energy, but this was not necessary for the observations to be described.

By a projection method points corresponding to the optic disk and the fovea were mapped out on the screen. An ophthalmoscope was designed which permitted direct vision of the fundus by means of a small spot of light. This spot was directed through the centre of the pupil at the fovea or optic disk and the instrument was locked in position. The ophthalmoscope shone a second beam in a direction exactly opposite to the retinal beam, making a small spot on the screen. The position of this spot then corresponded to the illuminated retinal point. Points on the screen could thus be specified with reference to the fovea and the optic disk, and points on the retina were stimulated by illuminating the corresponding points on the screen. The correspondence could be verified by illuminating a point on the screen (e.g. that corresponding to the optic disk) and observing the retina directly with an ordinary ophthalmoscope through a half-silvered mirror placed at 45° in front of the eye.

Regions in the visual field which gave 'on' or 'off' (excitatory or inhibitory) responses to illumination were marked on sheets of paper fixed to the screen. These provided permanent records of the size and shape of the receptive fields and of their position with respect to the fovea and the optic disk.

Single fibres were recorded from the optic nerve with tungsten micro-electrodes (Hubel, 1957). Cathode-follower input and a condenser-coupled pre-amplifier were used in a conventional recording system. In pre-

J. Physiol. (1960), **154**, *pp.* 572–580.

Received 12 *July* 1960.

liminary experiments, not included in this series, the nerve was approached under direct vision from below by a transpharyngeal route and from above by removing one frontal lobe. Both procedures proved tedious, and neither gave good stability. The method finally adopted was a modification of a technique used for single-unit recording within the brain of the unrestrained animal (Hubel, 1960). The nerve was approached from above through the intact brain. A closed system was used to lessen vascular and respiratory pulsations. A hydraulic micro-electrode positioner was oriented by Horsley—Clarke stereotaxic methods. The co-ordinates of the optic nerve were determined from the position of the bony optic foramen, using the average from several spider monkey skulls. During the actual experiment a small hole was made in the skull and an 18-gauge steel tube attached to the positioner was lowered through the brain until its tip was several millimetres above the optic nerve. The space between the tube and the skull was sealed with dental-impression cement. The electrode, held within this outer tube by an insulated 26-gauge hollow needle, was then hydraulically advanced until it entered the optic nerve.

RESULTS

One hundred and twelve optic nerve fibres were studied. In the light-adapted state all fibres showed maintained activity; that is, they discharged impulses in the absence of any stimulus besides the steady uniform background light. No systematic observations were made in the dark-adapted state. Firing patterns resembled, at least superficially, those described for the cat's ganglion cell by Kuffler, FitzHugh & Barlow (1957).

If a small spot of light was projected on the screen one could always find a restricted area over which firing of a fibre could be influenced. This was termed the receptive field of the fibre. Receptive fields had the same general characteristics as those of the cat, described by Kuffler (1953). As in the cat, two main types could be distinguished, both concentrically arranged, one with an 'on' centre and an 'off' periphery, the other with an 'off' centre and an 'on' periphery. Records from an 'off' centre unit are shown in Fig. 1, and illustrate suppression of firing with an 'off' discharge in response to a centred spot, and an 'on' discharge in response to an annulus. Responses from the periphery of receptive fields were often difficult or impossible to elicit in the monkey when stimulus and background intensities were of the same order as those used in work on the cat's retina. However, if both the stimulus and the background luminances were increased by about 2 log units, peripheral responses could usually be obtained. The influence of peripheral parts of receptive fields could be demonstrated even with weaker stimuli, since it was always possible to decrease a centre response by simultaneous stimulation of regions outside the field centre. In Fig. 2 spots of successively larger size were used to stimulate an 'on' centre fibre. The smallest spot did not fill the centre (Fig. 2A), and it gave a response considerably weaker than that evoked by a second spot (B) which just filled the centre. A still larger spot invaded the periphery (C), and the response was now less marked than with the second.

The receptive fields studied were situated in various parts of the retina, ranging between 4° and 56° from the fovea. In any given penetration through the optic nerve from above there was a tendency for receptive fields of the first fibres recorded to be located in the lower quadrants of the visual field. As the electrode was lowered the receptive fields tended to be located higher and higher in the visual field. Otherwise, however, there was little order in the position of fields, and

Fig. 1. Responses of an 'off' centre unit to restricted light stimulation. In each example the upper line indicates when the stimulus light is on. A, ½° spot of light shone in the centre of the receptive field; B, annulus 5° in outside diameter, 2° inside diameter, with its centre over that of the receptive field. Receptive field located on the retina 28° above and 12° nasal to the fovea. Duration of stimuli, 1.5 sec.

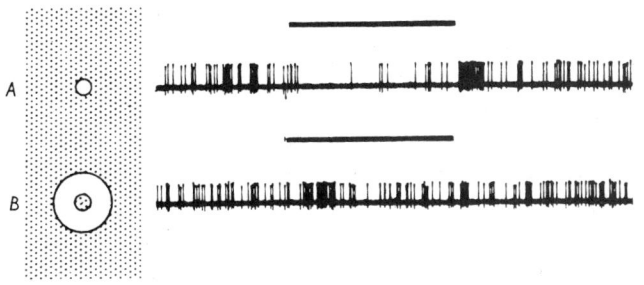

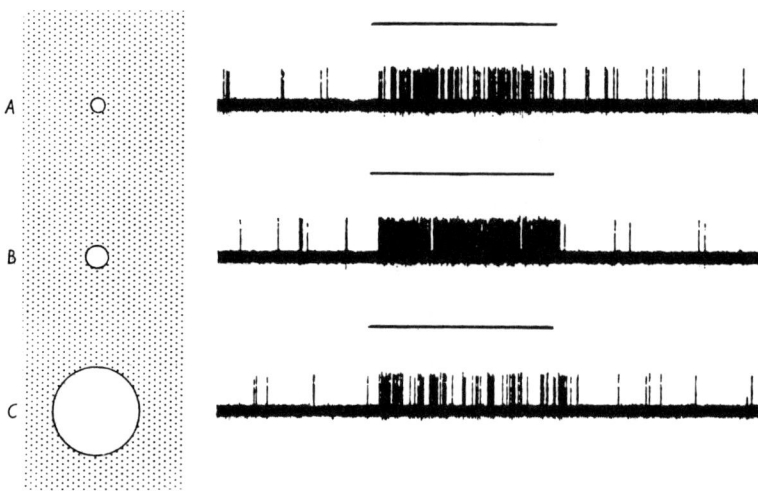

Fig. 2. 'On' centre unit with receptive field 11° above, 4° nasal to fovea. Responses to centred spots ⅛°, ½° and 4° in diameter. Duration of stimuli, 1.5 sec.

fields of successively recorded fibres were often separated by a considerable distance, in an unpredictable fashion. This is illustrated in Fig. 3 for a particular penetration in which 20 fibres were mapped. From this and other penetrations one had the impression that there was no very detailed topographical representation in this part of the optic nerve, but only a coarse segregation of fibres from the different quadrants.

The size of receptive field centres ranged from 4 min to 2° of arc. The centres were mapped out by using spots of light which for each field were chosen so as to be small relative to the size of the centre. Relatively high background illumination ($1.0 \log_{10}$ cd/m² or more) was used to minimize effects of scattered light. No attempt was made to determine accurately the total extent of each receptive field, but there was little doubt that for most fields the total diameter was many times that of the centre. There was a clear tendency for receptive field centres near the fovea to be smaller than those in the periphery, although there was considerable variation in centre size at any given distance from the fovea. In Fig. 4 the diameters of 65 field centres are plotted against distance from the fovea. Both 'on' and 'off' centre units were well represented in the series. The number of units is too small to justify any conclusions about the preponderance of one type of field over the other. In particular, the apparent predominance of 'on' centre units over

'off' centre in the region near the fovea is of interest, but again, conclusions can hardly be drawn from such a small sample.

In the present work there was no attempt to make a thorough study of responses to coloured stimuli. However, some preliminary results showed that there are ganglion cells which respond in specific ways to colour. An example is given in Fig. 5. In this unit a 2° spot of white light gave a weak response consisting of suppression of firing followed by a feeble 'off' discharge (Fig. 5A). A decrease in intensity of the white light produced even weaker 'off' responses. With the light source intensity set as in Fig. 5A, a blue interference filter was placed in front of the projector. Each time the blue spot of light was shone on the screen it produced a strong 'on' response (Fig. 5B). If a red filter was substituted for the blue the firing was strongly suppressed during the stimulus and this was followed by an 'off' discharge (Fig. 5C). It is clear that either filter greatly reduced the radiant flux of the light beam, yet the effects of the stimulus were much enhanced. Moreover, the responses to stimulation with the two different colours were of opposite type. This was true regardless of stimulus intensity or spot size. Two other units studied with monochromatic light gave 'on' responses to wave-lengths shorter than 498 mμ and inhibition with 'off' responses for longer wavelengths. With 498 mμ a very feeble 'off' response was produced.

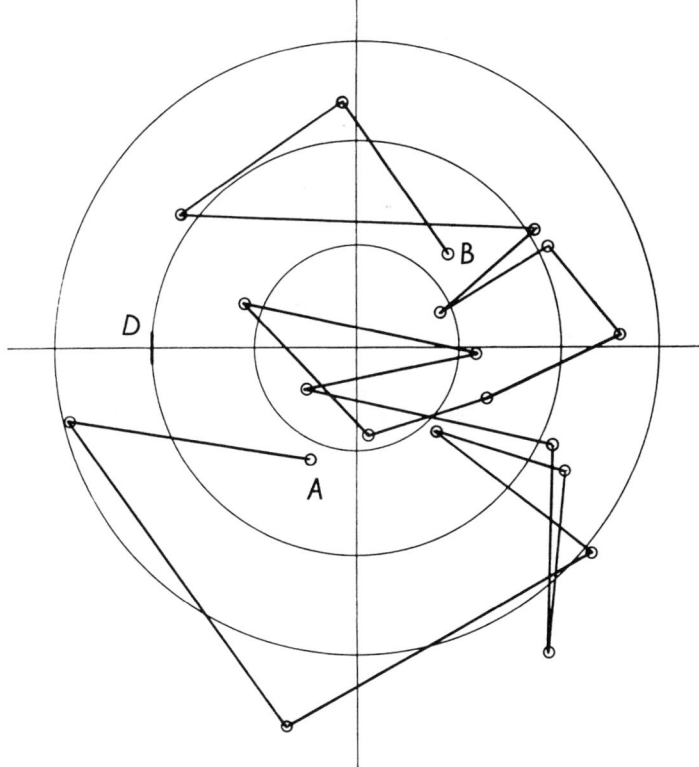

Fig. 3. Location on the visual field of receptive fields of 20 optic nerve fibres recorded in sequence as the electrode was advanced vertically from above through the left optic nerve. The vertical and horizontal lines represent the vertical and horizontal meridia; these cross at the fovea. The optic disk D *is situated in the temporal field 20° from the fovea. The first unit,* A, *had its receptive field in the lower temporal quadrant of the visual field; the last,* B, *in the upper nasal quadrant.*

It is likely that the units with specific colour responses described above form a small minority of the population of optic nerve fibres, since a number of additional units studied with monochromatic stimuli gave centre responses of constant type, either 'on' or 'off', for all wave-lengths. In these white light gave brisk responses. In this type of ganglion cell, however, there were indications of some variability in the position of spectral sensitivity peaks from one unit to the next, suggesting that they too, conveyed information on colour.

DISCUSSION

From the results presented in this paper it is clear that in the monkey, as in the cat, the receptive fields of retinal ganglion cells are of two main types, one with an 'off' centre and an 'on' periphery, the other with an 'on' centre and an 'off' periphery. The antagonism between centre and periphery of a receptive field is generally not so complete that diffuse light is ineffective.

Fields in the vicinity of the monkey fovea tend to have smaller centres than those in the periphery (Fig. 4). A similar finding has been reported for the cat (Wiesel, 1960). Differences between central and peripheral visual acuity in man may well be related to variations in receptive-field centre size similar to those found in the monkey and cat. In the present study the smallest centre was found for a receptive field 4° from the fovea; this had a diameter of less than 4 minutes of arc. No recordings were made from fibres with receptive fields in the fovea, but it is likely that even smaller field centres are present in this region, since there is less convergence in the pathway from receptors to ganglion cells in the foveal region than in other parts of the retina (Polyak, 1957). Our failure to find foveal fields is probably related to the small diameter of the macular fibres. Moreover, the macular bundle occupies a small part of the optic nerve, and could easily be missed in random penetrations.

The cat has a highly reflectile tapetum behind the retina; in contrast, the retina of the spider mon-

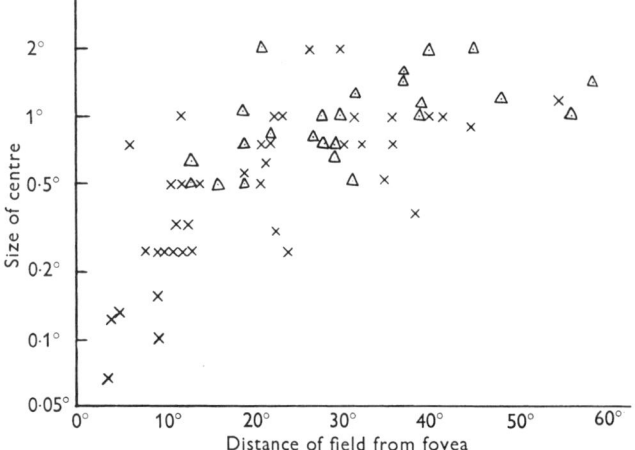

Fig. 4. Diameters of receptive field centres in degrees (logarithmic scale), plotted against distance in degrees of each field from the fovea. ×, *'on' centre units;* △, *'off' centre units.*

key is deeply pigmented. With identical stimulus conditions it was generally more difficult to produce a response from the receptive-field periphery in the spider monkey than in the cat. However, it was found that by increasing the stimulus and background luminance by two logarithmic units peripheral responses could consistently be obtained. It is probable that the tapetum of the cat increases the effectiveness of the background illumination, and this may be necessary for the production of a good response from the periphery of the receptive field.

It is known, for example, that the influence of the periphery on the centre response becomes more pronounced with increasing background illumination (Barlow *et al.* 1957).

Several authors have described responses of opposite type to stimulation with light of different colours. Svaetichin (1956) demonstrated membrane hyperpolarization with short wave-lengths and depolarization with long wave-lengths in recordings from cells in the inner nuclear layer of the fish retina (MacNichol & Svaetichin, 1958). Similar

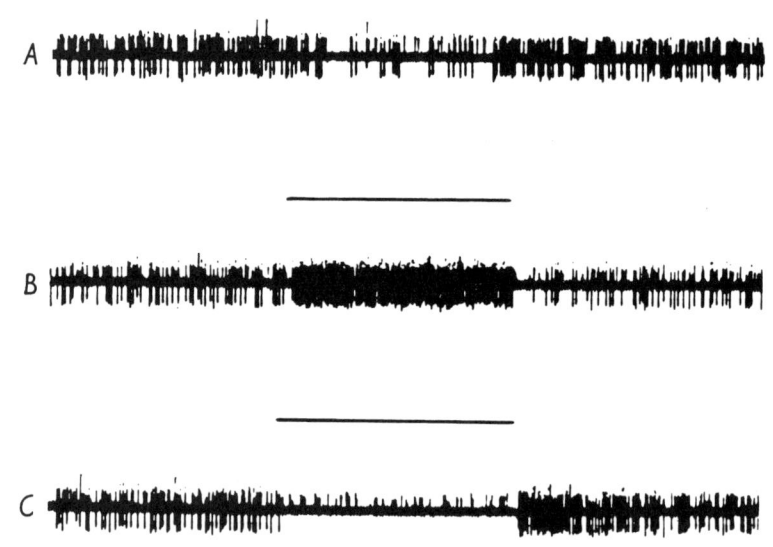

Fig. 5. Response of optic nerve fibre to 2° spot of light shone in centre of receptive field. Location of field, 7° below, 29° temporal to fovea. A, white light; B, same as A, but with blue interference filter (peak transmission 480 mμ) inserted between projector and screen; C, same as A, but with red interference filter (peak transmission 630 mμ) inserted between projector and screen. Duration of first stimulus, 1 sec.

results have been reported by other workers (Moto-kawa, Oikawa & Tasaki, 1957; Tomita, Tosaka, Watanabe & Sato, 1958). In the lateral geniculate body of the rhesus monkey de Valois, Smith, Kitai & Karoly (1958) described units responding with an 'on' discharge to blue light and an 'off' discharge to red light. Wagner, MacNichol & Wolbarsht (1960), recording spike discharges from ganglion cells in the goldfish retina, have since found similar discharge patterns to coloured stimuli.

In the present study of the spider monkey's extra-foveal retina three ganglion cells showed colour responses analogous to those described above. The presence of maintained discharges made it possible to demonstrate inhibitory effects during long wave-length stimuli, in addition to the excitatory responses to short wave-lengths. White light was less effective than monochromatic light, provided the wave-length was either longer or shorter than about 500 mμ. The decreased responsiveness to white light which has been noted also by de Valois (1960) is presumably due to the antagonistic effects of monochromatic light of short and long wave-lengths. This is strikingly similar to the way in which form specificity is obtained in the visual system; shining a restricted light on appropriate parts of a receptive field produces excitatory or inhibitory responses, and the effects tend to cancel when opposing regions are stimulated simultaneously, for instance with diffuse light. In both cases an unspecific stimulus produces less effect on the firing of a single cell than one restricted in form or wave-length, even though it contains more energy.

SUMMARY

1. Receptive fields of retinal ganglion cells were studied in the light-adapted spider monkey. All fields mapped with white light had a concentric arrangement similar to that of cat retinal ganglion cells, with a sharply demarcated 'on' centre surrounded by an antagonistic 'off' periphery, or the reverse.

2. The smallest receptive field centres were found near the fovea, and the size of centres tended to increase with increasing distance from the fovea. The smallest centre had a diameter of 4 minutes of arc (corresponding to about 20 μ on the retina) and was located 4° from the fovea; the largest centre had a diameter of 2°.

3. Three ganglion cells out of about 100 responded in a specific way to coloured stimuli. In these cells light of short wave-length produced an 'on' response and light of long wave-length evoked inhibition followed by an 'off' response. Transition between the two types of response occurred at about 500 mμ; light of this wave-length evoked only feeble 'off' responses. Very weak responses were obtained to white light, presumably owing to the antagonism between light of short and long wave-lengths.

This work was supported by research grants B-2251 and B-2260 United States Public Health Service, and by the United States Air Force Office of Scientific Research of the Air Research and Development Command under contract no. AF 49(638)-713.

References

Barlow, H. B., FitzHugh, R. & Kuffler, S. W. (1957). Dark adaptation, absolute threshold and Purkinje shift in single units of the cat's retina. *J. Physiol.* **137**, 327–337.

De Valois, R. L. (1960). Color vision mechanisms in the monkey. *J. gen. Physiol.* **43**, pt. 2, 115–128.

De Valois, R. L., Smith, C. J., Kitai, S. T. & Karoly, A. J. (1958). Response of single cells in monkey lateral geniculate nucleus to monochromatic light. *Science,* **127**, 238–239.

Hubel, D. H. (1957). Tungsten microelectrode for recording from single units. *Science,* **125**, 549–550.

Hubel, D. H. (1960). Single unit activity in lateral geniculate body and optic tract of unrestrained cats. *J. Physiol.* **150**, 91–104.

Hubel, D. H. & Wiesel, T. N. (1959). Receptive fields of single neurones in the cat's striate cortex. *J. Physiol.* **148**, 574–591.

Kuffler, S. W. (1953). Discharge patterns and functional organization of mammalian retina. *J. Neurophysiol.* **16**, 37–68.

Kuffler, S. W., FitzHugh, R. & Barlow, H. B. (1957). Maintained activity in the cat's retina in light and darkness. *J. gen. Physiol.* **40**, 683–702.

MacNichol, E. J. & Svaetichin, G. (1958). Electric responses from the isolated retinas of fishes. *Amer. J. Ophthal.* **46**, No. 3, Part II, 26–40.

Motokawa, K., Oikawa, T. & Tasaki, K. (1957). Receptor potential of vertebrate retina. *J. Neurophysiol.* **20**, 186–199.

Polyak, S. (1957). *The Vertebrate Visual System,* ed. Klüver, H. The University of Chicago Press.

Svaetichin, G. (1956). Spectral response curves from single cones. *Acta physiol. scand.* **39**, Suppl. **134**, 17.

Talbot, S. A. & Marshall, W. H. (1941). Physiological studies on neural mechanisms of visual localization and discrimination. *Amer. J. Ophthal.* **24**, 1255–1263.

Tomita, T., Tosaka, T., Watanabe, K. & Sato, Y. (1958). The fish EIRG in response to different types of illumination. *Jap. J. Physiol.* **8**, 41–50.

Wagner, H. G., MacNichol, E. F. & Wolbarsht, M. L. (1960). The response properties of single ganglion cells in the goldfish retina. *J. gen. Physiol.* **43**, pt. 2, 45–62.

Wiesel, T. N. (1960). Receptive fields of ganglion cells in the cat retina. *J. Physiol.* **153**, 583–594.

AFTERWORD

The first nine fibers we recorded in this entire project were all on-center, and we began to wonder if we were onto a new discovery, that primate optic nerves were all on-centers, unlike those in cats. It was a great disappointment (or perhaps relief) when the tenth one turned out to be off-center.

The surprising finding, that the optic nerve and tract fibers (between the eye and the geniculate) are scrambled for most of their extent, was contrary to accepted ideas about optic nerve organization, and was confirmed anatomically in 1979 by Horton, Greenwood, and Hubel (*Nature,* 282:720–722).

When we began this study, color was evidently not uppermost in our thoughts, and we had no elaborate equipment for generating colored stimuli. Ed Furshpan walked in one day just as we began using a yellow cardboard Kodak 35 mm film box, getting vigorous responses from a cell that was oblivious to changes in white light. Ed's comment was "That's *interesting!*" Up to that time we had never heard him express such enthusiasm, and we decided it must indeed be *very* interesting.

Chapter 9 • Recording from Cells in the Cat Lateral Geniculate •

This little paper is one of our favorites. It represented a rare opportunity to study directly the difference between the information entering a structure and the information leaving it, and thus to learn directly something about the function of that structure. Many of our colleagues spent years studying the superior cervical ganglion (to take one example) without ever asking what that structure might be contributing to the animal. There is of course nothing wrong with that: they were studying synapses and development and did not care at all about function. On the other hand, function was what we were studying and details of synaptic mechanisms could wait.

We began recording from the geniculate because we felt we had to know what was coming into the cortex. Having found that cortical cells were very different from optic nerve fibers, we had to be sure the transformations were indeed occurring in the cortex, rather than in the geniculate. It took only a few experiments to satisfy ourselves that the receptive fields of geniculate cells and retinal ganglion cells are indeed qualitatively very similar in having an antagonistic center-surround organization. We might have decided that our main objective had been met (as in the case of the 1991 first Gulf War) and that the lateral geniculate was, as many people thought then, just a passive relay that handed on information from the retina without changing it. But from the first we did see clear differences. Geniculate cells had slower spontaneous rates of firing; they responded much less well to diffuse light (i.e., to stimulation with large spots); and they often fired in short, high-frequency bursts that we called *clusters,* which we never saw in retinal ganglion cells. We knew from previous work in unrestrained cats that the clusters occurred only when the cat was drowsy or asleep, especially when the stimulus was such as to suppress the cell's firing (for example, an annulus in the case of an on-center cell). From this we concluded that the lateral geniculate body must be something more than a simple relay station, though in the beginning we failed to understand what use such changes might be to the animal. We could have left it at that, but luckily we pushed on.

If one looks only at the impulses recorded extracellularly from geniculate cells, the main feature is the slow firing rates, compared to the rapid buzzing that occurs in spontaneously firing optic-nerve fibers—plus the tendency, just mentioned, for geniculate cells to fire in clusters. On close scrutiny we could see, in our records, tiny all-or-none deflections that were dwarfed by the big geniculate-cell spikes. These little spikes occurred in rapid succession, but never in clusters. They responded just as actively to diffuse light as retinal ganglion cells did. Their behavior in fact resembled in every way that of retinal ganglion cells. As our electrode advanced, these tiny spikes usually increased in size and in duration, so that they came more and more to resemble typical, intracellularly recorded, excitatory post-synaptic potentials (EPSPs). We soon noticed that nearly every geniculate spike was preceded by one of these smaller spikes, which we termed *prepotentials*. There was one exception: when the geniculate cell fired a high-frequency burst (a cluster), only the very first spike was preceded by a prepotential. It was hard for us to swallow the idea that in our experiments each of these small all-or-none potentials could be an EPSP related to a single optic fiber. Each geniculate cell was known to receive input from a huge number of presynaptic optic-fiber endings, seemingly contradicting the idea that an impulse in a single optic nerve fiber could lead to an impulse in a geniculate cell. We were hesitant to accept that an EPSP from a single afferent fiber could be recorded extracellularly. Today it is clear that one optic nerve fiber breaks up into a huge number of branches, and that a single geniculate cell can receive most of its direct inputs from all or a large subset of these branches—and hence show huge EPSPs. In this way one optic nerve fiber can virtually monopolize one geniculate cell. Though in almost all of our work we tried to use natural stimulation, this was one case where graded electrical stimulation of the optic chiasm helped convince us that the prepotentials did indeed represent activity of single optic nerve fibers.

We often saw several EPSPs (to use the modern term) of different sizes, all associated with the spikes of one geniculate cell, and we tentatively concluded that one geniculate cell could sometimes receive major excitatory inputs from the branches of two or more such afferents. We did not emphasize this in the paper because Ed Furshpan could hardly make out the smaller of the tiny deflections in our records and forbade us to publish them, saying, in the margin, "bullshit!" We now know that Ed was too cautious, and haven't quite forgiven him.

We called the prepotentials *optic tract synaptic potentials*. Since then, they have become known by the more efficient but less self-explanatory term *s-potential*.

Integrative Action in the Cat's Lateral Geniculate Body

D. H. HUBEL AND T. N. WIESEL • *Neurophysiology Laboratory, Department of Pharmacology, Harvard Medical School, Boston 15, Massachusetts*

It has often been asked whether the lateral geniculate body contributes to the integration of incoming visual impulses or is a mere 'way-station' in the pathway from retina to cortex. While perhaps less complex than the retina or cortex, the geniculate is histologically far from the simple structure that the term 'way-station' would imply (O'Leary, 1940; Glees, 1941). The presence of extensive dendritic arborizations, the profuse ramifications of incoming optic-tract fibres, and the existence of short-axon cells, all suggest that there may be something more than a 1:1 transmission of impulses from optic nerve to optic radiations.

The retinal region over which a cell in the visual system can be influenced (excited or inhibited) by light is called the receptive field of that cell. Largely through the work of Kuffler (1953), retinal ganglion cells in the cat are known to have a well defined, concentric, receptive field arrangement. Up to now receptive fields of cells in the dorsal lateral geniculate have received very little attention, although recent work (Hubel, 1960) has suggested that they too, are concentrically arranged. In the present work receptive fields in the optic tract and lateral geniculate body are compared. This provides a sensitive means of detecting and studying any modification of the visual input to the lateral geniculate.

Details of stimulating and recording procedures have been described elsewhere (Hubel, 1960; Hubel & Wiesel, 1960). Receptive fields were mapped on sheets of paper attached to a screen which the cat faced from a distance of 1.5 m. Spots of light of maximum intensity 3.0 $\log_{10}$ cd/m^2 were shone on the screen and a light-adapted state was maintained by a uniform background luminance of up to 2.0 $\log_{10}$ cd/m^2. Spot intensities were varied with neutral density filters and an iris diaphragm.

Tungsten micro-electrodes were used (Hubel, 1957). Amplifiers were condenser-coupled. Horsley-Clarke co-ordinates for the lateral geniculate body were taken from a stereotaxic Atlas (Jasper & Ajmone-Marsan, 1954). Penetrations were made in a dorsoventral direction, and at one or more points in each penetration a 50–100 μ diameter electrolytic lesion was made (Hubel, 1960). A typical lesion is shown in Pl. 1. All brains were examined histologically in serial sections, and the location of any unit was determined either from the position of a lesion made during the recording, or by calculating the distance back from lesion along an electrode track, by means of readings of the hydraulic micrometer drive corresponding to the unit and the lesion. Because of the necessity for allowing for shrinkage in calculating distances along tracks, recording sites determined directly from lesions were considered more reliable. For this reason multiple lesions were often made in single penetrations; for example, each time a new layer was entered, as judged by ocular dominance. The presence of several lesions in a track was also useful for estimating brain shrinkage.

METHODS

About 300 units were recorded in 20 micro-electrode penetrations through the geniculate. Fifteen cats were used. The animals were anaesthetized with thiopental sodium and throughout the experiment light anaesthesia was maintained and monitored by observing the electrocorticogram. The eyes were immobilized with continuously injected succinylcholine; this made it necessary to use artificial respiration (Brown & Wiesel, 1959).

RESULTS

Lateral Geniculate Receptive Fields

ARRANGEMENT OF GENICULATE FIELDS. Receptive fields were mapped for 190 lateral geniculate units. 150 recordings were made within the nucleus; the remaining 40 were from geniculate axons encountered as the electrode was lowered through the

J. Physiol. (1961), **155,** *pp.* 385–398.
Received 3 October 1960.

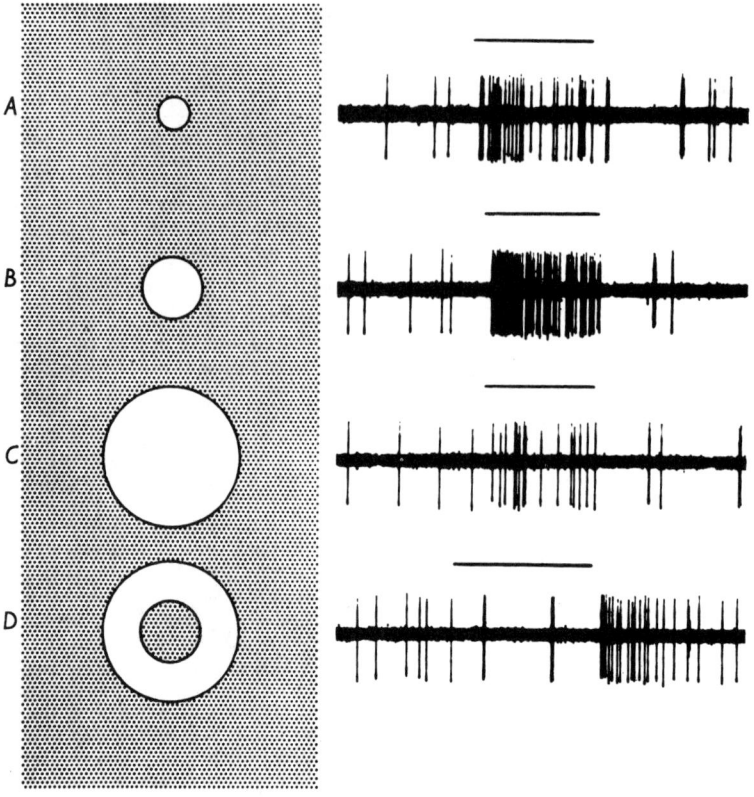

Fig. 1. Responses from an 'on'-centre cell recorded in layer A of the left lateral geniculate. Receptive field 25° to the left of and slightly above the area centralis of the right eye. A, B, and C, centred light spots 1°, 2° and 14° in diameter. D, annular stimulus with inner diameter 2° and outer diameter 14°. Upper line in each record indicates when the light is on. Positive deflexions upward. Duration of stimulus in A, 1 sec.

optic radiations just above the geniculate. For comparison, 75 optic-tract fibres (retinal ganglion cell axons) were studied, within the geniculate body as well as in the optic tract proper.

Criteria for distinguishing between recordings of optic-nerve fibres and geniculate cells have been dealt with in detail elsewhere (Hubel, 1960). Geniculate-cell records were recognized by the cell-type spikes and the characteristic 'clustered' pattern of firing. Optic-tract fibres showed axon-type spikes, which were never clustered. In two experiments these criteria were controlled by electrically stimulating the optic nerve near the chiasma; optic-nerve fibres could then be distinguished from geniculate units by their shorter latency and by their ability to follow stimulation at a more rapid rate (approximately 700/sec.).

In their general arrangement geniculate receptive fields resembled those of retinal ganglion cells, having an excitatory ('on') centre and inhibitory ('off') periphery, or the reverse. 'On' and 'off' centre units seemed to be about equally common. Records from a typical 'on'—centre cell are shown in Text-fig. 1. In this unit there was summation of the centre-type 'on'-response within a central area about 2° in diameter (Text-fig. 1 *A, B*); inclusion of the region surrounding this centre led to a reduction in the response (Text-fig. 1*C*). When the peripheral part of the receptive field was stimulated by itself the firing of the cell was suppressed, and an 'off'-response followed the stimulus (Text-fig. 1 *D*).

VARIATIONS IN GENICULATE RECEPTIVE FIELDS; BINOCULAR CONSIDERATIONS. In most penetrations the electrode advanced through the dorsal, middle, and ventral layers of the geniculate (layers A, A_1, and B) in sequence. A lesion made at the end of a penetration is shown in Pl. 1. All cells in the dorsal and ventral layers were driven exclusively by the contralateral eye, those in the middle layer by the ipsilateral eye. An electrode advancing through a layer in a direction approximately normal to it encountered cells whose receptive fields had almost identical positions on the retina. Successively recorded units were seldom separated by more than one degree of arc, and they generally overlapped or were superimposed. On passing into the next layer one encountered cells with receptive fields in the exactly homologous position in the other eye (see Hubel & Wiesel, 1960, for projection technique for determining homologous retinal points).

'On'-centre and 'off'-centre units were found in all three layers. Cells recorded from the two dorsal layers (A and A_1) had similar patterns of firing, and showed no systematic differences in size or organization of their receptive fields. In layer B, however, receptive field centres were, on the average, several times larger than those in layers A and A_1. Responses from this layer were more sluggish, with longer latencies and lower frequencies of firing. Anatomical differences between layer B and the two dorsal layers are discussed by O'Leary (1940) and Hayhow (1958).

Receptive field centres situated in or near the area centralis tended to be smaller than those in the retinal periphery. Furthermore, the suppression of a centre response on including the receptive field periphery (peripheral suppression) was more marked for cells near the area centralis. The tendency for area centralis units to have smaller field centres and to exhibit more suppression by the receptive field periphery has already been noted for retinal ganglion cells (Wiesel, 1960).

In some cells the antagonism exerted by the receptive field periphery on the centre was so great that a spot completely covering both portions, even if very bright, evoked no response at all. Using diffuse light exclusively, one might have been led to conclude that some geniculate units were unresponsive to light. On the contrary, all the geniculate cells in this series responded to a small spot appropriately placed. So far we have no evidence that there are nerve cells unresponsive to visual stimulation, either in the optic nerve, the lateral geniculate body, or in the striate cortex.

Attempts were made for each unit to determine whether firing was influenced from only one eye or from both eyes. After finding which eye projected to a cell, and outlining its receptive field, we explored the other eye carefully with small spots, concentrating especially on the region homologous to that containing the already mapped receptive field. However, no responses could be evoked; neither was there any effect on responses from the other eye. Between layers some cells were driven ipsilaterally and others contralaterally, and on several occasions two units were recorded simultaneously, one driven exclusively from one eye, and one exclusively from the other. Thus binocular interaction was not observed in any of the cells studied.

Hayhow (1958), using silver-impregnation methods on degenerating fibres, has shown that only the interlaminar regions of the lateral geniculate body receive fibre terminations from the two eyes. These are therefore the regions where one might expect to find binocularly influenced cells. In the cat single units driven by the two eyes have been reported by Erulkar & Fillenz (1958, 1960) and by Bishop, Burke & Davis (1959), but the exact position of these cells within the geniculate was not determined histologically. Our results suggest that even in the interlaminar regions not all cells are binocularly influenced. We conclude that binocular interaction in the lateral geniculate body as a whole must be relatively unimportant.

COMPARISON OF RETINAL GANGLION CELL AND GENICULATE CELL RECEPTIVE FIELDS SIMULTANEOUSLY RECORDED GENICULATE CELLS AND OPTIC-TRACT FIBRES. Optic-tract fibres and geniculate cells were often recorded simultaneously with the same electrode. Twenty-five pairs of units of this type were studied; in all these the two receptive fields either overlapped or were closely adjacent, with less than 1° separation. Responses from an 'on'-centre optic-tract fibre and an 'off'-centre geniculate cell are shown in Text-fig. 2. The two receptive fields were almost superimposed and had centres of about 1° diameter. A spot covering both centres gave strong responses from both units (Text-fig. 2*A*). An increase in spot size to 2° made little change in the response from the optic-tract fibre, but the 'off' response from the geniculate cell was much reduced (Text-fig. 2*B*). A further increase, to 8°, caused a definite reduction in the tract-fibre response; the 'off' discharge from the cell was now almost completely abolished (Text-fig. 2*C*). Enlarging the spot beyond

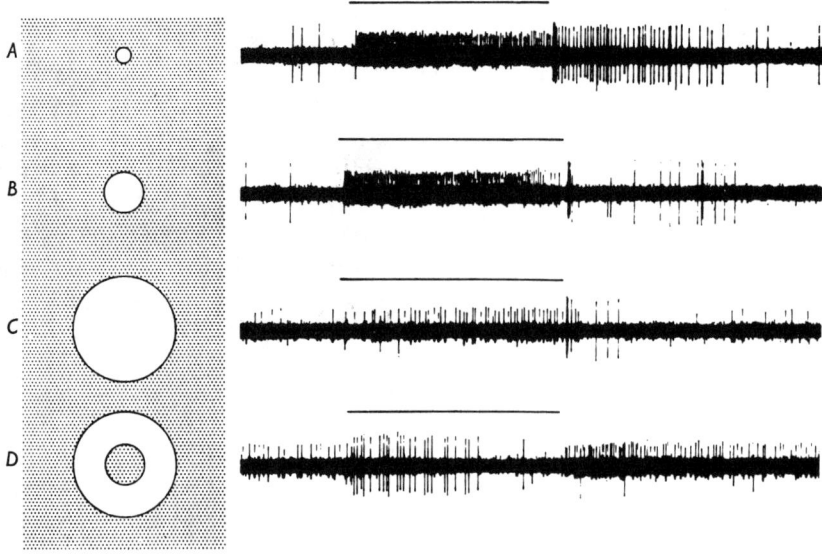

Fig. 2. Responses from an 'on'-centre optic-tract fibre (small positive spikes) and an 'off'-centre lateral genicu-late cell (large positive-negative spikes). Cell situated in layer A$_1$ of the right lateral geniculate body; receptive field 24° above and to the right of the area centralis of the right eye. A, B, and C, centred light spots 1°, 2° and 8° in diameter. D, annular stimulus with inner diameter 2° and outer diameter 8°. Duration of first stimulus, 1 sec.

8° had no further effect on either response. An annulus, as might be expected, evoked peripheral responses from both units, 'on' for the cell, 'off' for the fibre (Text-fig. 2D).

These two units illustrate a finding common to all simultaneous recordings of geniculate cells and optic-tract fibres, that the degree of suppression of centre responses on whole-field illumination appeared to be greater for geniculate cells than for optic-tract fibres. This observation was verified by comparing thresholds for different areas of stimulation. The difference in threshold between a geniculate cell and an optic-nerve fibre was very much less for small spots than for large ones (see also Text-fig. 5). Indeed, with the stimulus intensities available some geniculate cells could not be activated at all with large spots.

Optic-Tract Synaptic Potentials. In a number of recordings the great majority of geniculate spikes were immediately preceded by potentials which, by criteria given above (p. 386), were related to impulses in an optic-tract fibre. This suggested that the optic-tract fibre was an excitatory input to the geniculate cell. In Text-fig. 3A, several optic-tract potentials are superimposed in a single frame

by triggering the oscilloscope sweep by the potentials themselves. The slow time course of the potentials is discussed below. Geniculate spikes accompanied three of these potentials, and appear on the rising phase, on the peak, and on the falling phase. Thus the time elapsing between the optic-tract potential and the cell spike was, for a given pair of units, variable from one pair of impulses to the next. The generation of a spike on the falling phase was seen many times, often after an even greater time interval than the longest in this example (see Freygang, 1958). In an occasional geniculate spike no optic-tract potential could be discerned; presumably either the time interval of separation was too short to allow the two events to be distinguished, or the geniculate cell could at times fire in the absence of a preceding impulse in the tract fibre. In a few units there were several distinct sizes of optic-tract potentials, suggesting for these units the convergence of a number of excitatory tract fibres on a single cell.

An interesting though not easily interpreted aspect of these records concerns the sequence of events that occurred as the electrode was advanced. The cell spike showed the usual change from an initially negative to an initially positive shape,

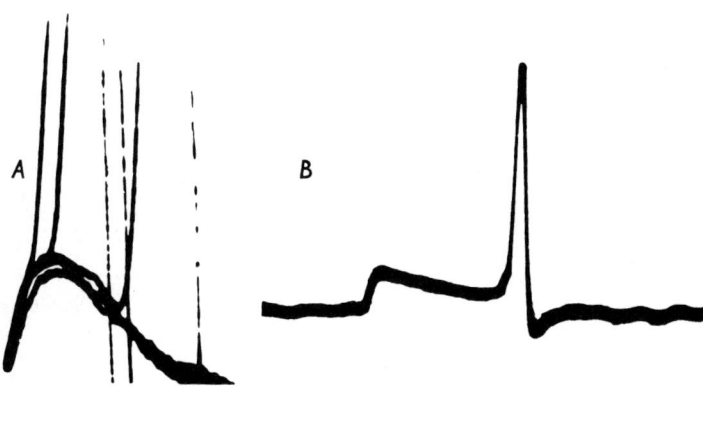

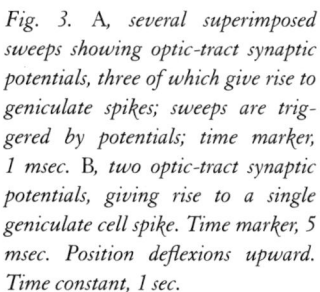

Fig. 3. A, several superimposed sweeps showing optic-tract synaptic potentials, three of which give rise to geniculate spikes; sweeps are triggered by potentials; time marker, 1 msec. B, two optic-tract synaptic potentials, giving rise to a single geniculate cell spike. Time marker, 5 msec. Position deflexions upward. Time constant, 1 sec.

finally becoming predominantly positive and often large (up to 20–30 mV) (see Hubel, 1960). The optic tract fibre impulse was first seen as a very small, brief, positive spike. This increased in amplitude as the electrode moved forward, at the same time becoming much longer in duration, so that in its final form it had an abrupt rising phase of less than 1 msec and a prolonged falling phase lasting up to 8 or 10 msec. The forms of the cell spike and the optic tract fibre potential are shown in Text-fig. 3B. Here a second afferent impulse arising in the falling phase of the first was successful in triggering the geniculate-cell spike, presumably owing to summation. Many similar examples of summation were observed.

Since no resting potentials could be measured with the metal electrode used, it was assumed that the electrode tips were extracellular. Freygang (1958) and Bishop, Burke & Davis (1958), on stimulating the severed optic nerve electrically, have recorded similar slow potentials extracellularly from lateral geniculate cells. Freygang has interpreted these potentials as resulting from extracellular current flow related to the post-synaptic potentials. It should be emphasized, however, that the main conclusions of this section depend only on the assumption that each of the small potentials was related to an impulse in an optic-nerve fibre, whether recorded pre- or post-synaptically. For the purposes of this paper we shall refer to these potentials as 'optic-tract synaptic potentials'.

Fifteen recordings were made of geniculate cells in which the spikes were immediately preceded by optic-tract synaptic potentials of the type described above. The receptive fields of a geniculate

cell and its associated optic-tract fibre were concentric, of about the same size and of the same type, both 'on' centre or both 'off' centre. Text-figure 4 shows the responses of an 'on' centre pair. A small (1°) low-intensity spot covering the centre of both receptive fields evoked a burst of optic-tract synaptic potentials, and many of these were followed by a geniculate-cell spike. A larger spot evoked no geniculate impulses, but only synaptic potentials at a lower frequency. If the intensity of the larger spot was now increased (Text-fig. 4B) the rate of the synaptic potentials could be made at least as great as in Text-fig. 4A, but even then no geniculate-cell spikes were evoked. Thus the failure of geniculate-cell discharges was certainly not due to decreased input from the particular excitatory fibre recorded here. The recorded optic-tract synaptic potential very likely represented an important excitatory input; its failure to generate geniculate-cell spikes when a large spot was used may have been due to a decrease in other excitatory inputs not seen here, or to a direct inhibition at the geniculate level.

Response characteristics of a geniculate cell and its associated optic-tract synaptic potential were further compared by plotting, for each unit, the threshold intensity of a centred stimulating spot against spot diameter (see Barlow, FitzHugh & Kuffler, 1957). Such a pair of curves is shown in Text-fig. 5. Thresholds decreased with increasing spot size, up to a diameter of about 1°, indicating summation of centre-type responses for both units over this area. With stimuli at or near threshold and confined to this central region, almost every optic-tract synaptic potential was followed by a geniculate spike, and thresholds for the two units

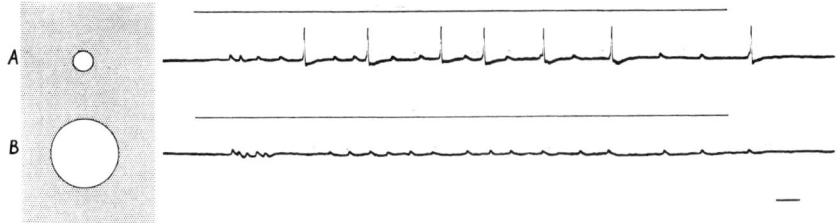

*Fig. 4. Responses of a geniculate cell and associated optic-tract synaptic potentials to centred spots of light. A, 1°
spot. B, 10° spot with brightness increased so as to make frequency of optic-tract synaptic potentials about equal
to that in A. Time constant, 5 msec. Time marker, 10 msec.*

were consequently identical. Spots larger than the
receptive-field centres invaded the antagonistic
peripheral portions, and the thresholds rose. The
rise was much more pronounced for the geniculate
cell than for the fibre, indicating once more, as in
Text-fig. 4, that peripheral antagonism is more
pronounced at the geniculate level than in the
retina. These findings of an increased peripheral
suppression at the geniculate level make it difficult
to avoid the conclusion that there are multiple
inputs to a geniculate cell.

Clustered Firing Patterns

Under certain conditions lateral geniculate cells
fire in high-frequency clusters of 2–8 or more
spikes. In a previous study (Hubel, 1960) clustered
firing was observed in the unrestrained animal
during natural sleep but not in the waking state.
During sleep the clusters were accentuated by
stimuli that tended to suppress firing and were
abolished by stimuli that activated the unit. It
seemed clear that clustered firing was not related to
injury of the cell, since it could be eliminated by

arousing the animal, and since it was seen at every
stage as the electrode was advanced during a
recording. Moreover, it was observed both in
geniculate cells and in optic-radiation fibres.

In the present work clustered firing was
observed with thiopental anaesthesia in the great
majority of geniculate cells and was most pronounced in moderate or deep anaesthesia, as
judged by the electrocorticogram. This type of firing was found in all three layers of the geniculate.
When clusters were rare or absent they could generally be brought on by a small additional intravenous injection of thiopental (3–5 mg/kg). Their
appearance was probably not due to a direct action
of anaesthetic on the geniculate-cell membrane,
since clusters also occur in natural sleep.

It is unlikely that the individual spikes of a
cluster could each be triggered by impulses in a single optic-tract fibre, since clustered firing does not
normally occur in retinal ganglion cells. Records of
geniculate-cell spikes preceded by optic-tract
synaptic potentials tended to support this. In Text-
fig. 6 three clusters and a single spike are shown

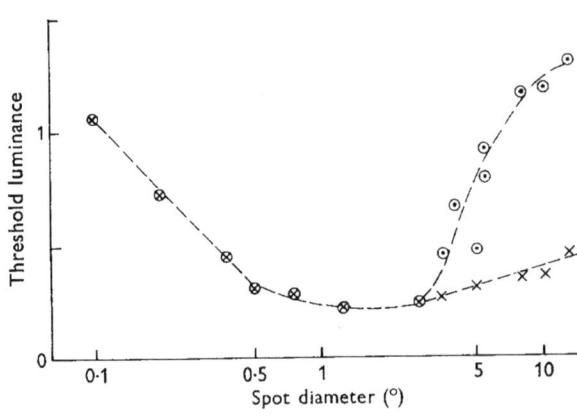

*Fig. 5. Thresholds of an 'off'-centre
geniculate cell ☉ and an associated
optic-tract synaptic potential (x),
measured for various spot diameters.
Ordinate, threshold luminance; relative log. scale, 0 corresponding to
screen luminance of –2.7 log. cd/m².
Abscissa, spot diameter in degrees.
Background luminance –2.5 log.
cd/m²; stimulus duration 1 sec.*

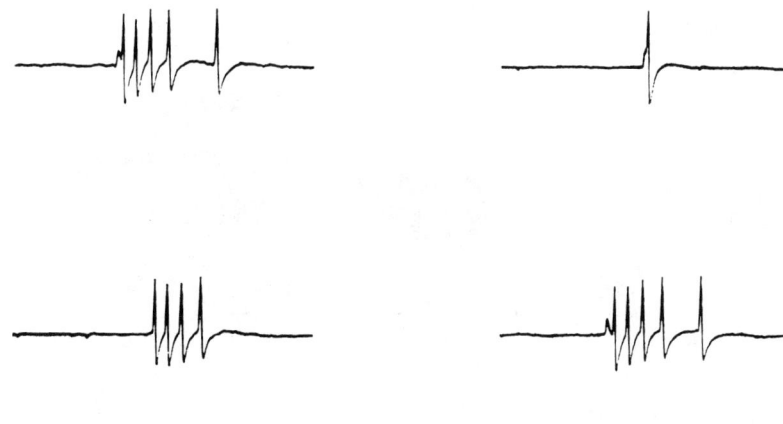

Fig. 6. Records of four randomly occurring discharges of a geniculate cell. Optic-tract synaptic potentials are seen preceding three of the discharges. Note clustered firing in three of the examples. Time constant, 5 msec. Time marker, 10 msec.

from a geniculate cell. An optic-tract synaptic potential preceded three of the four discharges, but none was seen before spikes other than the first in a cluster. Similar observations made in other units led to the impression that an entire cluster could be initiated by a single optic-tract synaptic potential. The presence of occasional clusters with no preceding optic-tract synaptic potentials suggested, as in the case of single spikes, that other inputs might contribute to this type of firing. However, as with single spikes, it is possible that a synaptic potential might be undetected owing to a short time interval between it and the first geniculate spike.

DISCUSSION

In combination with previous work in the retina and striate cortex, the present study makes it possible to compare receptive fields at three successive levels in the cat's visual system. Certain similarities are at once evident. At each stage receptive fields can be divided into excitatory and inhibitory ('on' and 'off') regions. Summation of responses occurs over regions of the same type, and antagonism between areas of opposite type. Diffuse light always leads to a response weaker than that obtainable from a suitably chosen restricted stimulus. These similarities hold for simple cortical receptive fields (Hubel & Wiesel, 1959), but not necessarily for more complex ones (Hubel & Wiesel, unpublished).

In the spatial arrangement of its receptive fields the lateral geniculate body clearly has more in common with retinal ganglion cells than with the striate cortex. In both retina and geniculate body the receptive fields are concentric, with an 'on' centre surrounded by an 'off' periphery, or the reverse. In the cortex, on the other hand, there is a much greater variety of receptive fields, and no types so far studied have the concentric, circularly symmetrical pattern found at lower levels. This marked increase in receptive field complexity is undoubtedly related to the greater variety of cell types and interconnexions in the cortex. Furthermore, binocular interaction would seem to be minimal at the lateral geniculate level, whereas the majority of striate cortical cells we have studied were influenced by both eyes (Hubel & Wiesel, unpublished).

The differences between retinal and geniculate receptive fields are more subtle. They may be seen when centre-periphery interaction is compared in simultaneous recordings of a geniculate cell and an optic tract fibre with closely adjacent receptive fields. One then finds that geniculate cells are less responsive to diffuse light than retinal ganglion cells. This can be interpreted as an increased antagonistic action of the receptive field periphery on the centre. Previous studies indicate that in the striate cortex the process is carried still further, and that with diffuse-light stimuli cortical cells are even less responsive than cells of the geniculate body. For example, in the striate cortical projection area for

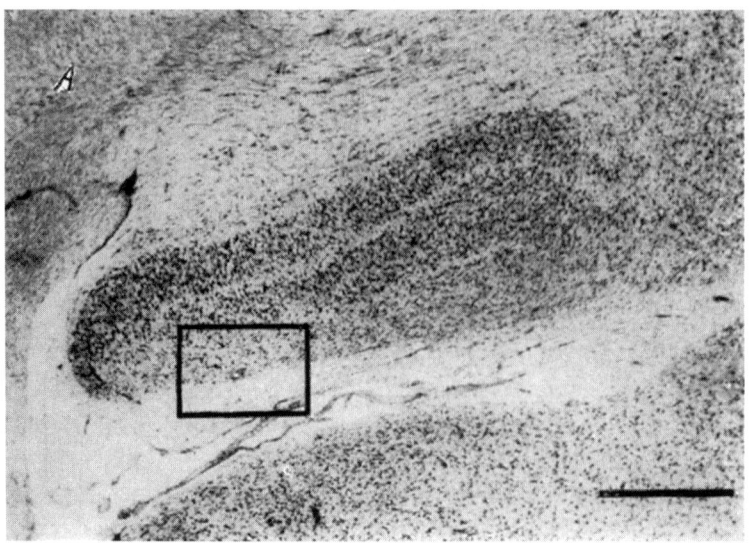

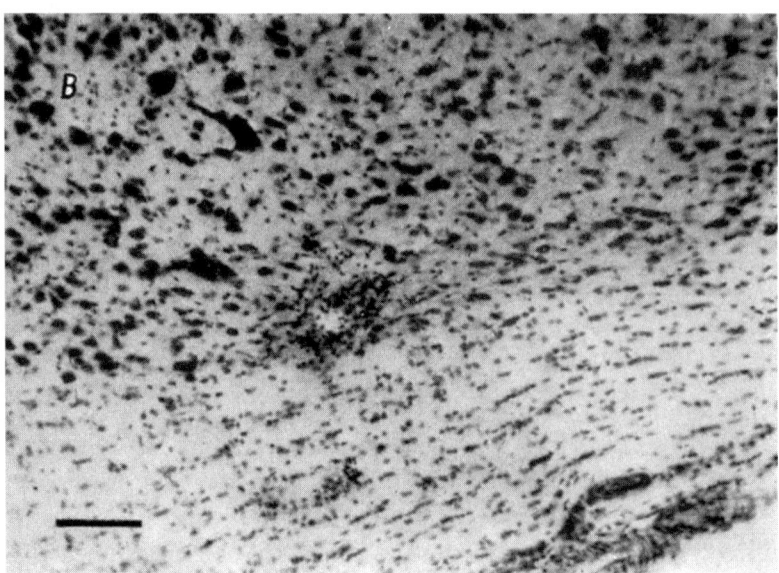

Plate 1   Coronal section (celloidin, cresyl violet stain) through left lateral geniculate body, showing a lesion at the ventral border of layer B, made at the end of a vertical micro-electrode penetration. Receptive fields encountered during this penetration were situated in the right visual field close to the horizontal meridian, 23° to the right of the centre of gaze. A, low power, scale 1 mm; B, outlined portion of A, high power, scale 0.1 mm.

central vision most cells seem to lack clear responses to diffuse illumination regardless of stimulus intensity. Thus at progressively higher levels in the visual system cells become less and less concerned with registering changes in total illumination.

The lateral geniculate body's ability to modify incoming signals was studied more directly in records showing both geniculate-cell spikes and optic-tract synaptic potentials. Here the two units were not as randomly picked, since one was an excitatory input to the other, and, under the right conditions was apparently able to trigger it. However, the geniculate cell's output was not simply a slavish copy of the optic-tract impulses: it was also influenced by other inputs which for some reason were not recorded. The changes introduced by the lateral geniculate were systematic, leading to a relative ineffectiveness of the optic-tract fibres when the receptive field periphery was included in the stimulus. A simple interpretation of this is to assume that the inclusion of the receptive field periphery evoked responses from optic-tract fibres with direct inhibitory endings on the geniculate cell. These would be 'on'-centre units if the geniculate cell was 'on'-centre in type, and 'off'-centre if the geniculate cell was 'off'-centre. One could equally well imagine that inclusion of the field periphery affected ganglion cells making excitatory synaptic contact with the geniculate cell. These would be 'off'-centre units if the geniculate cell was 'on'-centre, and conversely. Both mechanisms are plausible, since within the retinal area occupied by a geniculate cell's receptive field there are hundreds of ganglion cells with overlapping receptive fields of both types, 'on'-centre and 'off'-centre. Any of these ganglion cells could end on the geniculate cell, exciting or inhibiting it directly, or possibly indirectly by short-axon cells. Intracellular recording with micropipette electrodes may help to decide between the several alternatives.

The mechanisms demonstrated, leading to an increased selectivity in the responsiveness of a geniculate cell, almost certainly do not represent the only type of integration occurring in this structure. For example, some records showed several distinct sizes of optic-tract synaptic potentials, indicating probable convergence of several excitatory fibres on a single geniculate cell. This is consistent with Freygang's (1958) finding of a non-continuous gradation of synaptic potentials evoked in response to electrical stimulation of the optic nerve, from which he concluded that there were several fibres supplying the cells he studied. As a second example, the firing of geniculate cells can be influenced simply by changing the unanaesthetized animal's state of arousal (Hubel, 1960), which suggests that there are probably other fibres ending on geniculate cells besides those of the optic tract.

SUMMARY

1. Cells were recorded with tungsten electrodes in the dorsal lateral geniculate body of the cat. Receptive fields of these units were mapped out, in the light-adapted state, with small spots of light. In their general arrangement geniculate receptive fields resembled those of retinal ganglion cells, having an excitatory ('on') centre and inhibitory ('off') periphery, or the reverse. The two portions of a receptive field were mutually antagonistic; the decrease in centre responses caused by inclusion of peripheral portions of receptive fields was termed peripheral suppression.

2. Cells recorded in layers A and B of the lateral geniculate body were driven from the contralateral eye; cells in layer A_1 from the ipsilateral eye. In penetrations normal to the layers receptive fields of cells in a single layer were close together or superimposed, and from one layer to the next occupied exactly homologous positions in the two retinas. Binocular interaction was not observed in any of the cells studied.

3. All three layers of the lateral geniculate contained both 'on'-centre and 'off'-centre units. Cells in layers A and A_1 were similar both in their firing patterns and in average receptive field size. Cells in layer B were more sluggish in their responses to light stimuli, and tended to have larger receptive field centres.

4. Cells with receptive fields within or near the area centralis tended to have smaller field centres and stronger suppression by the receptive field periphery than cells with their fields situated in more peripheral regions of the retina.

5. In some recordings almost all geniculate cell spikes were immediately preceded by potentials related to impulses in a single optic-tract fibre, suggesting that the optic-tract fibre was an excitatory input to the geniculate cell. The long duration of these potentials, the presence of summation, and their apparent ability to trigger the geniculate cell, suggested that they were of synaptic origin. They were termed 'optic-tract synaptic potentials'.

6. In simultaneous records of geniculate cells and optic-tract fibres, and in particular in records showing optic-tract synaptic potentials, an increase in peripheral suppression at the geniculate level could be demonstrated (*a*) by comparing responses of the two units to small and large spots, and (*b*) by measuring threshold intensities of the two units at different spot diameters. These comparisons made it clear that the geniculate cell and the optic-tract fibre were not related in a strictly one-to-one manner, and that integration leading to increased per-

ipheral suppression occurred at the geniculate level.

7. Clustered firing in the form of brief bursts of spikes at high frequency, previously described in natural sleep, was observed under thiopental anaesthesia. From simultaneous records it appeared that a single impulse in an optic-tract fibre could give rise to a cluster of impulses in a geniculate cell.

We wish to thank Miss Sally Fox for participating in some of the experiments, and Mrs Jane Chen and Miss Jaye Robinson for their technical assistance. The work was supported in part by Research Grants B-2251 and B-2260 from United States Public Health Service, and in part by the United States Air Force through the Air Force Office of Scientific Research of the Air Research and Development Command under contract No. AF 49 (638)-713. The work was done during the tenure of a U.S. Public Health Service Senior Research Fellowship No. SF 304-R by D.H.H.

References

Barlow, H. B., Fitzhugh, R. & Kuffler, S. W. (1957). Change of organization in the receptive fields of the cat's retina during dark adaptation. *J. Physiol.* **137**, 338–354.

Bishop, P. O., Burke, W. & Davis, R. (1958). Synapse discharge by single fibre in mammalian visual system. *Nature, Lond.,* **182**, 728–730.

Bishop, P. O., Burke, W. & Davis, R. (1959). Activation of single lateral geniculate cells by stimulation of either optic nerve. *Science,* **130**, 506–507.

Brown, K. T. & Wiesel, T. N. (1959). Intraretinal recording with micropipette electrodes in the intact cat eye. *J. Physiol.* **149**, 537–562.

Erulkar, S. D. & Fillenz, M. (1958). Patterns of discharge of single units of the lateral geniculate body of the cat in response to binocular stimulation. *J. Physiol.* **140**, 6 P.

Erulkar, S. D. & Fillenz, M. (1960). Single unit activity in the lateral geniculate body of the cat. *J. Physiol.* **154**, 206–218.

Freygang, W. H. Jr. (1958). An analysis of extracellular potentials from single neurons in the lateral geniculate nucleus of the cat. *J. gen. Physiol.* **41**, 543–564.

Glees, P. (1941). The termination of optic fibres in the lateral geniculate body of the cat. *J. Anat., Lond.,* **75**, 434–440.

Hayhow, W. R. (1958). The cytoarchitecture of the lateral geniculate body in the cat in relation to the distribution of crossed and uncrossed optic fibers. *J. comp. Neurol.* **110**, 1–64.

Hubel, D. H. (1957). Tungsten microelectrode for recording from single units. *Science,* **125**, 549–550.

Hubel, D. H. (1960). Single unit activity in lateral geniculate body and optic tract of unrestrained cats. *J. Physiol.* **150**, 91–104.

Hubel, D. H. & Wiesel, T. N. (1959). Receptive fields of single neurones in the cat's striate cortex. *J. Physiol.* **148**, 574–591.

Hubel, D. H. & Wiesel, T. N. (1960). Receptive fields of optic nerve fibres in the spider monkey. *J. Physiol.* **154**, 572–580.

Jasper, H. H. & Ajmone-Marsan, C. (1954). *A Stereotaxic Atlas of the Diencephalon of the Cat.* Ottawa: The National Research Council of Canada.

Kuffler, S. W. (1953). Discharge patterns and functional organization of mammalian retina. *J. Neurophysiol.* **16**, 37–68.

O'Leary, J. L. (1940). A structural analysis of the lateral geniculate nucleus of the cat. *J. comp. Neurol.* **73**, 405–430.

Wiesel, T. N. (1960). Receptive fields of ganglion cells in the cat's retina. *J. Physiol.* **153**, 583–594.

AFTERWORD

This study gave us a rare opportunity to come to grips with the integrative functions of a structure by comparing directly the firing of a cell with the firing of its excitatory inputs. Because the surround of a stimulus had a much stronger suppressive effect on the center response for a geniculate cell, compared to the effect on an afferent optic tract fiber, it was clear that one major function of the geniculate was to beef up the effects of the receptive-field surround. The work was followed in 1971 by a study by Cleland, Dubin, and Levick (*Nature New Biology,* 231:191–192), who performed the tour de force of recording simultaneously from a single ganglion cell in the retina, and one of the geniculate cells it supplied. We would have thought that such an experiment would be well-nigh impossible and are still filled with admiration that anyone would have attempted it. The result confirmed our work and in addition supplied direct proof that geniculate cells can receive more than one direct excitatory afferent (and vindicating our interpretation of the tiny deflections).

We made one observation, or set of observations, that we never wrote up, and to our knowledge has not since been taken up. We noticed that during the course of a typical response, to a light turned on, say for one second and then off, the ratio of the firing frequency of the prepotentials (today's *s-potentials*) to the frequency of the geniculate spikes is continually changing. In an on-center cell, the proportion of s-potentials that trigger a geniculate spike (we coincidentally called this success rate "s") is highest just after the stimulus turns on, and lowest just after "off". It changes more or less in parallel with the firing rate, but not simply because of the changes in firing rate. So "s" is a function not only of the amount of the surround included in the stimulus, but also of time. We prepared figures and planned to write up the results, but other priorities must have been higher. The figures still languish in our file cabinet.

Chapter 10 • Our Major Paper on Cat Striate Cortex, 1962 •

FOREWORD

This was our first magnum opus, and of all our papers it is probably the one we would pick if we had to choose one paper to be remembered for. It took a long time to write, but we did not feel pressured to write quickly. We had the advantage of a vow we had taken early in our collaboration, that we must never (well, hardly ever) accept an invitation to a symposium in which a manuscript was required. Even when we were assured by those inviting us that a book was expected to come out of the meeting, but that we would be excused from contributing to it, we would decline rather than risk being seen later as poor sports and ending up feeling guilty. To write a paper at all was difficult for us, and we could see no point in writing up the same material more than once. Especially to be avoided, we thought, was the publishing of results in preliminary form at a symposium before they had been submitted in final form to a regular journal. That made the final, definitive paper an anticlimax. The policy of course reduced our total number of publications, and usually we felt happy if we produced a single paper each year. On the whole we suspect our careers did not suffer because of the slim list of publications. Perhaps that is a credit to our deans—given the tendency for deans to count papers rather than read them—and to Steve for his unwavering support.

We also tended to resist the temptation to publish every new finding in preliminary short papers in *Science* or *Nature*. Especially in the first years with fewer competitors there was little danger of being scooped. And we again avoided the anticlimax effect. Sometimes we yielded, but in retrospect we feel we gained little from the brief papers we did write. Several times the result was a lessening the pressure to write a full account of the research. The most important example was our failure to ever publish properly the prestriate stereoscopic depth material, which was only presented as a brief report to *Science* (see reprint no. 16). Consequently, we usually tried to discourage our postdocs from writing brief, preliminary, flashy papers—unless the results were earth-shaking, à la Watson and Crick.

The 1962 paper was a continuation of the 1959 paper, which purposely stopped short of the complex cells because in 1959 we did not yet feel we understood them. By writing a shorter paper confined to what we later called "simple cells", we took off some of the pressure at a time when we did not even know that we could continue to collaborate. It also allowed us to emphasize, in that first paper, the most important single point—that a major function of the striate cortex was to elaborate orientation selectivity.

In the 1962 paper we deliberately chose to make a single long paper out of what could easily have been three. We felt it was esthetically more pleasing not to subdivide it, and were saved the trouble of writing three introductions and three discussions. To have three separate papers in one year would have done more for us in terms of promotions, but we took a perverse pleasure in bucking the trend. Today it is unlikely that one would get away with such a strategy (if that is the right word), from the viewpoint either of promotions or of competition for grant money.

What made the 1962 paper such a pleasure to write was the articulation of the different parts: first the description of the different levels of complexity of the fields, then the columnar organization and topographic representation, including the scattering, and finally the climax in which one could conclude that the columns were serving the purpose of grouping together the very cells that one expected to be interconnected in the circuits we were proposing.

At that time we were hesitant about ocular dominance columns—in fact, it was only when we recorded from cats with artificial strabismus, a few years later, that we became convinced of their existence in cats. Also, as we later learned, they are far more conspicuous in macaque monkeys because of the prevalence of cells that strongly prefer one eye or the other, and the abruptness of the shifts as one crosses column boundaries, especially in layer 4. In 1962 we had just begun to record from macaque monkeys, and our first monkey-cortex paper appeared only in 1968.

Receptive Fields, Binocular Interaction and Functional Architecture in the Cat's Visual Cortex

D. H. HUBEL AND T. N. WIESEL • *Neurophysiology Laboratory, Department of Pharmacology Harvard Medical School, Boston, Massachusetts*

What chiefly distinguishes cerebral cortex from other parts of the central nervous system is the great diversity of its cell types and inter-connexions. It would be astonishing if such a structure did not profoundly modify the response patterns of fibres coming into it. In the cat's visual cortex, the

J. Physiol. (1962), **160,** *pp.* 106–154 *With 2 plates and 20 text-figures Printed in Great Britain*
Received 31 *July* 1961.

receptive field arrangements of single cells suggest that there is indeed a degree of complexity far exceeding anything yet seen at lower levels in the visual system.

In a previous paper we described receptive fields of single cortical cells, observing responses to spots of light shone on one or both retinas (Hubel & Wiesel, 1959). In the present work this method is used to examine receptive fields of a more complex type (Part I) and to make additional observations on binocular interaction (Part II).

This approach is necessary in order to understand the behaviour of individual cells, but it fails to deal with the problem of the relationship of one cell to its neighbours. In the past, the technique of recording evoked slow waves has been used with great success in studies of functional anatomy. It was employed by Talbot & Marshall (1941) and by Thompson, Woolsey & Talbot (1950) for mapping out the visual cortex in the rabbit, cat, and monkey. Daniel & Whitteridge (1959) have recently extended this work in the primate. Most of our present knowledge of retinotopic projections, binocular overlap, and the second visual area is based on these investigations. Yet the method of evoked potentials is valuable mainly for detecting behaviour common to large populations of neighbouring cells; it cannot differentiate functionally between areas of cortex smaller than about 1 mm². To overcome this difficulty a method has in recent years been developed for studying cells separately or in small groups during long micro-electrode penetrations through nervous tissue. Responses are correlated with cell location by reconstructing the electrode tracks from histological material. These techniques have been applied to the somatic sensory cortex of the cat and monkey in a remarkable series of studies by Mountcastle (1957) and Powell & Mountcastle (1959). Their results show that the approach is a powerful one, capable of revealing systems of organization not hinted at by the known morphology. In Part III of the present paper we use this method in studying the functional architecture of the visual cortex. It helped us attempt to explain on anatomical grounds how cortical receptive fields are built up.

METHODS

Recordings were made from forty acutely prepared cats, anaesthetized with thiopental sodium, and maintained in light sleep with additional doses by observing the electrocorticogram. Animals were paralysed with succinylcholine to stabilize the eyes. Pupils were dilated with atropine. Details of stimulating and recording methods are given in previous papers (Hubel, 1959; Hubel & Wiesel, 1959, 1960). The animal faced a wide tangent screen at a distance of 1.5 m, and various patterns of white light were shone on the screen by a tungsten-filament projector. All recordings were made in the light-adapted state. Background illumination varied from –1.0 to +1.0 $\log_{10}$ cd/m². Stimuli were from 0.2 to 2.0 log. units brighter than the background. For each cell receptive fields were mapped out separately for the two eyes on sheets of paper, and these were kept as permanent records.

Points on the screen corresponding to the area centralis and the optic disk of the two eyes were determined by a projection method (Hubel & Wiesel, 1960). The position of each receptive field was measured with respect to these points. Because of the muscle relaxant the eyes usually diverged slightly, so that points corresponding to the two centres of gaze were not necessarily superimposed. In stimulating the two eyes simultaneously it was therefore often necessary to use two spots placed in corresponding parts of the two visual fields. Moreover, at times the two eyes were slightly rotated in an inward direction in the plane of their equators. This rotation was estimated by (1) photographing the cat before and during the experiment, and comparing the angles of inclination of the slit-shaped pupils, or (2) by noting the inclination to the horizontal of a line joining the area centralis with the optic disk, which in the normal position of the eye was estimated, by the first method, to average about 25°. The combined inward rotations of the two eyes seldom exceeded 10°. Since the receptive fields in this study were usually centrally rather than peripherally placed on the retina, the rotations did not lead to any appreciable linear displacement. Angular displacements of receptive fields occasionally required correction, as they led to an apparent difference in the orientation of the two receptive-field axes of a binocularly driven unit. The direction and magnitude of this difference were always consistent with the estimated inward rotation of the two eyes. Moreover, in a given experiment the difference was constant, even though the axis orientation varied from cell to cell.

The diagram of Text-fig. 1 shows the points of entry into the cortex of all 45 microelectrode penetrations. Most electrode tracks went no deeper than 3 or 4 mm, so that explorations were mainly limited to the apical segments of the lateral and post-lateral gyri (LG and PLG) and a few millimetres down along the adjoining medial and lateral folds. The extent of the territory covered is indicated roughly by Text-figs. 13–15. Although the lateral boundary of the striate cortex is not always sharply

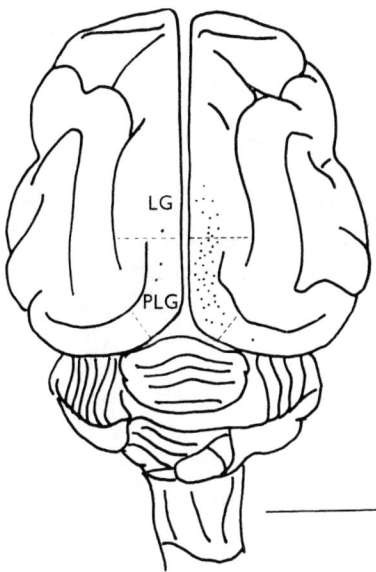

Fig. 1. Diagram of dorsal aspect of cat's brain, to show entry points of 45 micro-electrode penetrations. The penetrations between the interrupted lines are those in which cells had their receptive fields in or near area centralis. LG, lateral gyrus; PLG, post-lateral gyrus. Scale, 1 cm.

defined in Nissl-stained or myelin-stained material, most penetrations were well within the region generally accepted as 'striate'(O'Leary, 1941). Most penetrations were made from the cortical region receiving projections from in or near the area centralis; this cortical region is shown in Text-fig. 1 as the area between the interrupted lines.

Tungsten micro-electrodes were advanced by a hydraulic micro-electrode positioner (Hubel, 1957, 1959). In searching for single cortical units the retina was continually stimulated with stationary and moving forms while the electrode was advanced. The unresolved background activity (see p. 129) served as a guide for determining the optimum stimulus. This procedure increased the number of cells observed in a penetration, since the sampling was not limited to spontaneously active units.

In each penetration electrolytic lesions were made at one or more points. When only one lesion was made, it was generally at the end of an electrode track. Brains were fixed in 10% formalin, embedded in celloidin, sectioned at 20 μ, and stained with cresyl violet. Lesions were 50–100 μ in diameter, which was small enough to indicate the position of the electrode tip to the nearest cortical layer. The positions of other units encountered in a cortical penetration were determined by calculating the distance back from the lesion along the track, using

depth readings corresponding to the unit and the lesion. A correction was made for brain shrinkage, which was estimated by comparing the distance between two lesions, measured under the microscope, with the distance calculated from depths at which the two lesions were made. From brain to brain this shrinkage was not constant, so that it was not possible to apply an average correction for shrinkage to all brains. For tracks marked by only one lesion it was assumed that the first unit activity was recorded at the boundary of the first and second layers; any error resulting from this was probably small, since in a number of penetrations a lesion was made at the point where the first units were encountered, and these were in the lower first or the upper second layers, or else at the very boundary. The absence of cell-body records and unresolved background activity as the electrode passed through subcortical white matter (see Text-fig. 13 and Pl. 1) was also helpful in confirming the accuracy of the track reconstructions.

Part I
Organization of Receptive Fields in Cat's Visual Cortex: Properties of 'Simple' and 'Complex' Fields

The receptive field of a cell in the visual system may be defined as the region of retina (or visual field) over which one can influence the firing of that cell. In the cat's retina one can distinguish two types of ganglion cells, those with 'on'-centre receptive fields and those with 'off'-centre fields (Kuffler, 1953). The lateral geniculate body also has cells of these two types; so far no others have been found (Hubel & Wiesel, 1961). In contrast, the visual cortex contains a large number of functionally different cell types; yet with the exception of afferent fibres from the lateral geniculate body we have found no units with concentric 'on'-centre or 'off'-centre fields.

When stimulated with stationary or moving patterns of light, cells in the visual cortex gave responses that could be interpreted in terms of the arrangements of excitatory and inhibitory regions in their receptive fields (Hubel & Wiesel, 1959). Not all cells behaved so simply, however; some responded in a complex manner which bore little obvious relationship to the receptive fields mapped with small spots. It has become increasingly apparent to us that cortical cells differ in the complexity of their receptive fields. The great majority of fields seem to fall naturally into two groups, which we have termed 'simple' and 'complex'. Although the fields to be described represent the commonest subtypes of these groups, new varieties are continually appearing, and it is unlikely that the ones we have listed give anything like a complete picture of the striate cortex. We have therefore avoided a rigid system of classification, and have designated receptive fields by letters or numbers only for convenience in referring to the figures. We shall concentrate especially on features common to simple fields and on those common to complex fields, emphasizing differences between the two groups, and also between cortical fields and lateral geniculate fields.

RESULTS

Simple Receptive Fields

The receptive fields of 233 of the 303 cortical cells in the present series were classified as 'simple'. Like retinal ganglion and geniculate cells, cortical cells with simple fields possessed distinct excitatory and inhibitory subdivisions. Illumination of part or all of an excitatory region increased the maintained firing of the cell, whereas a light shone in the inhibitory region suppressed the firing and evoked a discharge at 'off'. A large spot confined to either area produced a greater change in rate of firing than a small spot, indicating summation within either region. On the other hand, the two types of region within a receptive field were mutually antagonistic. This was most forcefully shown by the absence or near absence of a response to simultaneous illumination of both regions, for example, with diffuse light. From the arrangement of excitatory and inhibitory regions it was usually possible to predict in a qualitative way the responses to any shape of stimulus, stationary or moving. Spots having the approximate shape of one or other region were the most effective stationary stimuli; smaller spots failed to take full advantage of summation within a region, while larger ones were likely to invade opposing regions, so reducing the response. To summarize: these fields were termed 'simple' because like retinal and geniculate fields (1) they were subdivided into distinct excitatory and inhibitory regions; (2) there was summation within the separate excitatory and inhibitory parts; (3) there was antagonism between excitatory and inhibitory regions; and (4) it was possible to predict responses to stationary or moving spots of various

shapes from a map of the excitatory and inhibitory areas.

While simple cortical receptive fields were similar to those of retinal ganglion cells and geniculate cells in possessing excitatory and inhibitory subdivisions, they differed profoundly in the spatial arrangements of these regions. The receptive fields of all retinal ganglion and geniculate cells had one or other of the concentric forms shown in Text-fig. 2A, B. (Excitatory areas are indicated by crosses, inhibitory areas by triangles.) In contrast, simple cortical fields all had a side-to-side arrangement of excitatory and inhibitory areas with separation of the areas by parallel straight-line boundaries rather than circular ones. There were several varieties of fields, differing in the number of subdivisions and the relative area occupied by each subdivision. The commonest arrangements are illustrated in Text-fig. 2C–G: Table 1 gives the number of cells observed in each category. The departure of these fields from circular symmetry introduces a new variable, namely, the orientation of the boundaries separating the field subdivisions. This orientation is a characteristic of each cortical cell, and may be vertical, horizontal, or oblique. There was no indication that any one orientation was more common than the others. We shall use the term *receptive-field axis* to indicate a line through the centre of a field, parallel to the boundaries separating excitatory and inhibitory regions. The *axis orientation* will then refer to the orientation of these boundaries, either on the retina or in the visual field. Axes are shown in Text-fig. 2 by continuous lines.

Two common types of fields, shown in Text-fig. 2C, D, each consisted of a narrow elongated area, excitatory or inhibitory, flanked on either side by two regions of the opposite type. In these fields the two flanking regions were symmetrical, i.e. they were about equal in area and the responses obtained from them were of about the same magnitude. In addition there were fields with long narrow centres (excitatory or inhibitory) and asymmetrical flanks. An example of an asymmetrical field with an inhibitory centre is shown in Text-fig. 2E. The most effective stationary stimulus for all of these cells was a long narrow rectangle ('slit') of light just large enough to cover the central region without invading either flank. For maximum centre response the orientation of the slit was critical;

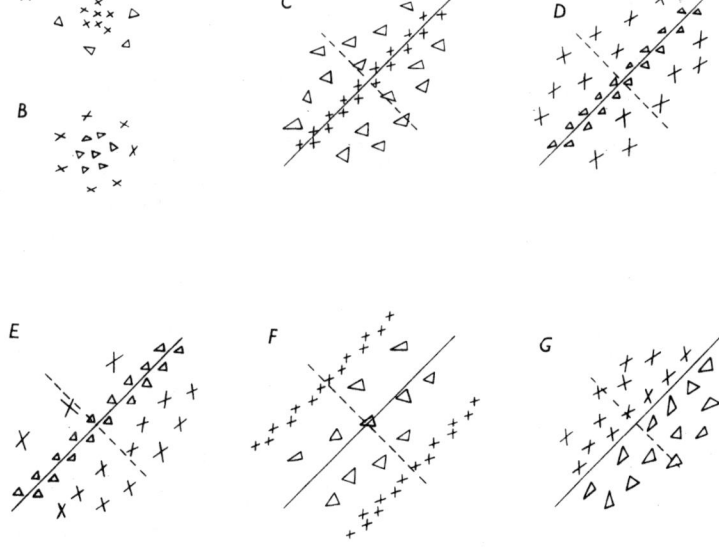

Fig. 2. *Common arrangements of lateral geniculate and cortical receptive fields. A. 'On'-centre geniculate receptive field. B. 'Off'-centre geniculate receptive field. C–G. Various arrangements of simple cortical receptive fields. ×, areas giving excitatory responses ('on' responses); △, areas giving inhibitory responses ('off' responses). Receptive-field axes are shown by continuous lines through field centres; in the figure these are all oblique, but each arrangement occurs in all orientations.*

changing the orientation by more than 5–10° was usually enough to reduce a response greatly or even abolish it. Illuminating both flanks usually evoked a strong response. If a slit having the same size as the receptive-field centre was shone in either flanking area it evoked only a weak response, since it covered only part of one flank. Diffuse light was ineffective, or at most evoked only a very weak response, indicating that the excitatory and inhibitory parts of the receptive field were very nearly balanced.

In these fields the equivalent but opposite-type regions occupied retinal areas that were far from equal; the centre portion was small and concentrated whereas the flanks were widely dispersed. A similar inequality was found in fields of type *F*, Text-fig. 2, but here the excitatory flanks were elongated and concentrated, while the centre was relatively large and diffuse. The optimum response was evoked by simultaneously illuminating the two flanks with two parallel slits (see Hubel & Wiesel, 1959, Fig. 9).

Some cells had fields in which only two regions were discernible, arranged side by side as in Text-fig. 2G. For these cells the most efficient stationary stimulus consisted of two areas of differing brightness placed so that the line separating them fell exactly over the boundary between the excitatory and inhibitory parts of the field. This type of stimulus was termed an 'edge'. An 'on' or

Table 1. *Simple Cortical Fields*

	Text-fig.	No. of cells
(*a*) Narrow concentrated centres		
(i) Symmetrical flanks		
Excitatory centres	2C	23
Inhibitory centres	2D	17
(ii) Asymmetrical flanks		
Excitatory centres	—	28
Inhibitory centres	2E	10
(*b*) Large centres; concentrated flanks	2F	21
(*c*) One excitatory region and one inhibitory	2G	17
(*d*) Uncategorized	—	117
Total number of simple fields		233

an 'off' response was evoked depending on whether the bright part of the stimulus fell over the excitatory or the inhibitory region. A slight change in position or orientation of the line separating the light from the dark area was usually enough to reduce greatly the effectiveness of the stimulus.

Moving stimuli were very effective, probably because of the synergistic effects of leaving an inhibitory area and simultaneously entering an excitatory area (Hubel & Wiesel, 1959). The optimum stimulus could usually be predicted from the distribution of excitatory and inhibitory regions of the receptive field. With moving stimuli, just as with stationary, the orientation was critical. In contrast, a slit or edge moved across the circularly symmetric field of a geniculate cell gave (as one would expect) roughly the same response regardless of the stimulus orientation. The responses evoked when an optimally oriented slit crossed back and forth over a cortical receptive field were often roughly equal for the two directions of crossing. This was true of fields like those shown in Text-fig. 2*C, D* and *F*. For many cells, however, the responses to two diametrically opposite movements were different, and some only responded to one of the two movements. The inequalities could usually be accounted for by an asymmetry in flanking regions, of the type shown in Text-fig. 2*E* (see also Hubel & Wiesel, 1959, Fig. 7). In fields that had only two discernible regions arranged side by side (Text-fig. 2*G*), the difference in the responses to a moving slit or edge was especially pronounced.

Optimum rates of movement varied from one cell to another. On several occasions two cells were recorded together, one of which responded only to a slow-moving stimulus (1°/sec or lower) the other to a rapid one (10°/sec or more). For cells with fields of type *F*, Text-fig. 2, the time elapsing between the two discharges to a moving stimulus was a measure of the rate of movement (see Hubel & Wiesel, 1959, Fig. 5).

If responses to movement were predictable from arrangements of excitatory and inhibitory regions, the reverse was to some extent also true. The axis orientation of a field, for example, was given by the most effective orientation of a moving slit or edge. If an optimally oriented slit produced a brief discharge on crossing from one region to another, one could predict that the first region was inhibitory and the second excitatory. Brief re-

sponses to crossing a very confined region were characteristic of cells with simple cortical fields, whereas the complex cells to be described below gave sustained responses to movement over much wider areas.

Movement was used extensively as a stimulus in experiments in which the main object was to determine axis orientation and ocular dominance for a large number of cells in a single penetration, and when it was not practical, because of time limitations, to map out every field completely. Because movement was generally a very powerful stimulus, it was also used in studying cells that gave little or no response to stationary patterns. In all, 117 of the 233 simple cells were studied mainly by moving stimuli. In Table 1 these have been kept separate from the other groups since the distribution of their excitatory and inhibitory regions is not known with the same degree of certainty. It is also possible that with further study, some of these fields would have revealed complex properties.

Complex Receptive Fields

Intermixed with cells having simple fields, and present in most penetrations of the striate cortex, were cells with far more intricate and elaborate properties. The receptive fields of these cells were termed 'complex'. Unlike cells with simple fields, these responded to variously-shaped stationary or moving forms in a way that could not be predicted from maps made with small circular spots. Often such maps could not be made, since small round spots were either ineffective or evoked only mixed ('on-off') responses throughout the receptive field. When separate 'on' and 'off' regions could be discerned, the principles of summation and mutual antagonism, so helpful in interpreting simple fields, did not generally hold. Nevertheless, there were some important features common to the two types of cells. In the following examples, four types of complex fields will be illustrated. The numbers observed of each type are given in Table 2.

The cell of Text-fig. 3 failed to respond to round spots of light, whether small or large. By trial and error with many shapes of stimulus it was discovered that the cell's firing could be influenced by a horizontally oriented slit ⅛° wide and 3° long. Provided the slit was horizontal its exact positioning within the 3°-diameter receptive field was not critical. When it was shone anywhere above the

Table 2. *Complex Cortical Receptive Fields*

	Text-fig.	No. of cells
(*a*) Activated by slit—non-uniform field	3	11
(*b*) Activated by slit—uniform field	4	39
(*c*) Activated by edge	5–6	14
(*d*) Activated by dark bar	7–8	6
Total number of complex fields		70

centre of the receptive field (the horizontal line of Text-fig. 3) an 'off' response was obtained; 'on' responses were evoked throughout the lower half. In an intermediate position (Text-fig. 3C) the cell responded at both 'on' and 'off'. From experience with simpler receptive fields one might have expected wider slits to give increasingly better responses owing to summation within the upper or lower part of the field, and that illumination of either half by itself might be the most effective stimulus of all. The result was just the opposite: responses fell off rapidly as the stimulus was widened beyond about ⅛°, and large rectangles covering the entire lower or upper halves of the

receptive field were quite ineffective (Text-fig. 3F, G). On the other hand, summation could easily be demonstrated in a horizontal direction, since a slit ⅛° wide but extending only across part of the field was less effective than a longer one covering the entire width. One might also have expected the orientation of the slit to be unimportant as long as the stimulus was wholly confined to the region above the horizontal line or the region below. On the contrary, the orientation was critical, since a tilt of even a few degrees from the horizontal markedly reduced the response, even though the slit did not cross the boundary separating the upper and lower halves of the field.

In preferring a slit specific in width and orientation this cell resembled certain cells with simple fields. When stimulated in the upper part of its field it behaved in many respects like cells with 'off'-centre fields of type *D*, Text-fig. 2; in the lower part it responded like 'on'-centre fields of Text-fig. 2C. But for this cell the strict requirements for shape and orientation of the stimulus were in marked contrast to the relatively large leeway of the stimulus in its ordinate position on the retina. Cells with simple fields, on the other hand, showed very little latitude in the positioning of an optimally oriented stimulus.

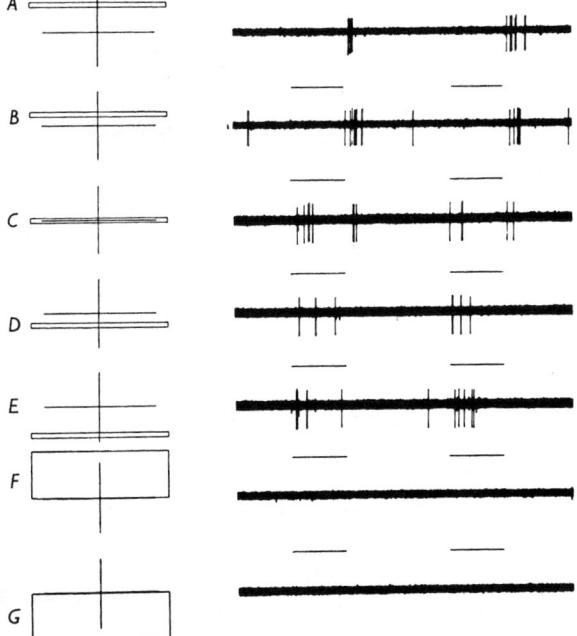

Fig. 3. *Responses of a cell with a complex receptive field to stimulation of the left (contralateral) eye. Receptive field located in area centralis. The diagrams to the left of each record indicate the position of a horizontal rectangular light stimulus with respect to the receptive field, marked by a cross. In each record the upper line indicates when the stimulus is on. A–E, stimulus ⅛ × 3°, F–G, stimulus 1½ × 3° (4° is equivalent to 1 mm on the cat retina). For background illumination and stimulus intensity see Methods. Cell was activated in the same way from right eye, but less vigorously (ocular-dominance group 2, see Part II). An electrolytic lesion made while recording from this cell was found near the border of layers 5 and 6, in the apical segment of the post-lateral gyrus. Positive deflexions upward; duration of each stimulus 1 sec.*

The upper part of this receptive field may be considered inhibitory and the lower part excitatory, even though in either area summation only occurred in a horizontal direction. Such subdivisions were occasionally found in complex fields, but more often the fields were uniform in this respect. This was true for the other complex fields to be described in this section.

Responses of a second complex unit are shown in Text-fig. 4. In many ways the receptive field of this cell was similar to the one just described. A slit was the most potent stimulus, and the most effective width was again ⅛°. Once more the orientation was an important stimulus variable, since the slit was effective anywhere in the field as long as it was placed in a 10 o'clock–4 o'clock orientation (Text-fig. 4A–D). A change in orientation of more than 5–10° in either direction produced a marked reduction in the response (Text-fig. 4E–G). As usual, diffuse light had no influence on the firing. This cell responded especially well if the slit, oriented as in A–D, was moved steadily across the receptive field. Sustained discharges were evoked over the entire length of the field. The opti-

mum rate of movement was about 1°/sec. If movement was interrupted the discharge stopped, and when it was resumed the firing recommenced. Continuous firing could be maintained indefinitely by small side-to-side movements of a stimulus within the receptive field (Text-fig. 4H). The pattern of firing was one characteristic of many complex cells, especially those responding well to moving stimuli. It consisted of a series of short high-frequency repetitive discharges each containing 5–10 spikes. The bursts occurred at irregular intervals, at frequencies up to about 20/sec. For this cell, movement of an optimally oriented slit was about equally effective in either of the two opposite directions. This was not true of all complex units, as will be seen in some of the examples given below.

Like the cell of Text-fig. 3 this cell may be thought of as having a counterpart in simple fields of the type shown in Text-fig. 2C–E. It shares with these simpler fields the attribute of responding well to properly oriented slit stimuli. Once more the distinction lies in the permissible variation in position of the optimally oriented stimulus. The variation is small (relative to the size of the receptive field) in

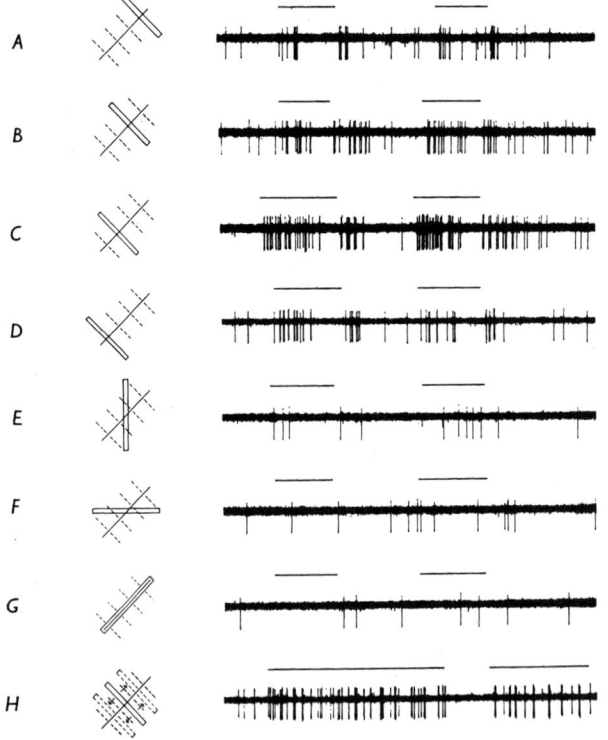

Fig. 4. Responses of a cell with a complex field to stimulation of the left (contralateral) eye with a slit ⅛ × 2½°. Receptive field was in the area centralis and was about 2 × 3° in size. A–D, ⅛° wide slit oriented parallel to receptive field axis. E–G, slit oriented at 45 and 90° to receptive-field axis. H, slit oriented as in A–D, is on throughout the record and is moved rapidly from side to side where indicated by upper beam. Responses from left eye slightly more marked than those from right (Group 3, see Part II). Time 1 sec.

the simple fields, large in the complex. Though resembling the cell of Text-fig. 3 in requiring a slit for a stimulus, this cell differed in that its responses to a properly oriented slit were mixed ('on-off') in type. This was not unusual for cells with complex fields. In contrast, cortical cells with simple fields, like retinal ganglion cells and lateral geniculate cells, responded to optimum restricted stimuli either with excitatory ('on') responses or inhibitory ('off') responses. When a stimulus covered opposing regions, the effects normally tended to cancel, though sometimes mixed discharges were obtained, the 'on' and 'off' components both being weak. For these simpler fields 'on-off' responses were thus an indication that the stimulus was not optimum. Yet some cells with complex fields responded with mixed discharges even to the most effective stationary stimuli we could find. Among the stimuli tried were curved objects, dark stripes, and still more complicated patterns, as well as monochromatic spots and slits.

A third type of complex field is illustrated in Text-figs. 5 and 6. There were no responses to small circular spots or to slits, but an edge was very effective if oriented vertically. Excitatory or inhibitory responses were produced depending on whether the brighter area was to the left or the right (Text-fig. 5*A, E*). So far, these are just the responses one would expect from a cell with a vertically oriented simple field of the type shown in Text-fig. 2*G*. In such a field the stimulus placement for optimum response is generally very critical. On the contrary, the complex unit responded to vertical edges over an unusually large region about 16° in length (Text-fig. 6). 'On' responses were obtained with light to the left (*A–D*), and 'off' responses with light to the right (*E–H*), regardless of the position of the line separating light from darkness. When the entire receptive field was illuminated diffusely (*I*) no response was evoked. As with all complex fields, we are unable to account for these responses by any simple spatial arrangement of excitatory and inhibitory regions.

Like the complex units already described, this cell was apparently more concerned with the orientation of a stimulus than with its exact position in the receptive field. It differed in responding well to edges but poorly or not at all to slits, whether narrow or wide. It is interesting in this connexion that exchanging an edge for its mirror equivalent re-

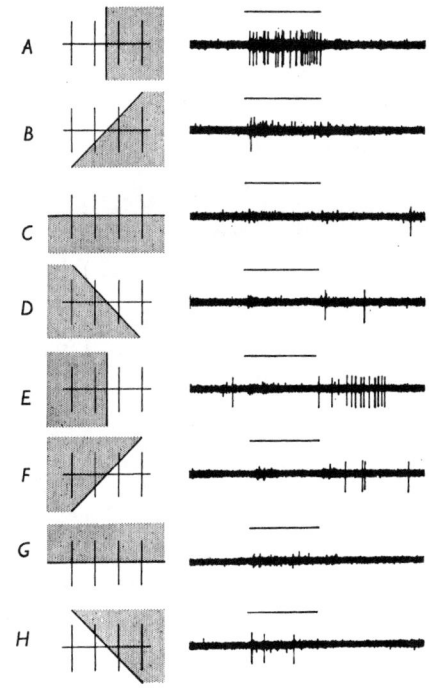

Fig. 5. Responses of a cell with a large (8 × 16°) complex receptive field to an edge projected on the ipsilateral retina so as to cross the receptive field in various directions. (The screen is illuminated by a diffuse background light, at 0.0 log_{10} cd/m². At the time of stimulus, shown by upper line of each record, half the screen, to one side of the variable boundary, is illuminated at 1.0 log_{10} cd/m², while the other half is kept constant.) A, vertical edge with light area to left, darker area to right. B–H, various other orientations of edge. Position of receptive field 20° below and to the left of the area centralis. Responses from ipsilateral eye stronger than those from contralateral eye (group 5, see Part II). Time 1 sec.

versed the response, i.e. replaced an excitatory response by an inhibitory and vice versa. The ineffectiveness of a slit might therefore be explained by supposing that the opposite effects of its two edges tended to cancel each other.

As shown in Text-fig. 6, the responses of the cell to a given vertical edge were consistent in type, being either 'on' or 'off' for all positions of the edge within the receptive field. In being uniform in its response-type it resembled the cell of Text-fig. 4. A few other cells of the same general category showed a similar preference for edges, but lacked this uniformity. Their receptive fields resembled

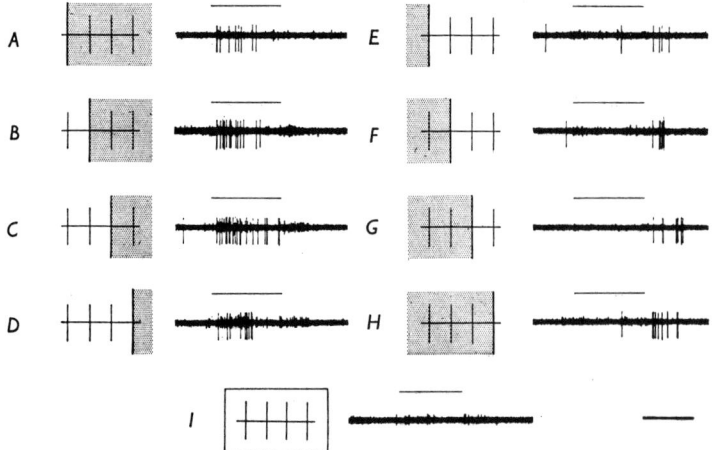

Fig. 6. Same cell as in Text-fig. 5. A–H, responses to a vertical edge in various parts of the receptive field: A–D, brighter light to the left; E–H, brighter light to the right; I, large rectangle, 10 × 20°, covering entire receptive field. Time, 1 sec.

the field of Text-fig. 3, in that a given edge evoked responses of one type over half the field, and the opposite type over the other half. These fields were divided into two halves by a line parallel to the receptive-field axis: an edge oriented parallel to the axis gave 'on' responses throughout one of the halves and 'off' responses through the other. In either half, replacing the edge by its mirror image reversed the response-type. Even cells, which were uniform in their response-types, like those in Text-fig. 4–6, varied to some extent in the magnitude of their responses, depending on the position of the stimulus. Moreover, as with most cortical cells, there was some variation in responses to identical stimuli.

A final example is given to illustrate the wide range of variation in the organization of complex receptive fields. The cell of Text-figs. 7 and 8 was not strongly influenced by any form projected upon the screen; it gave only weak, unsustained 'on' responses to a dark horizontal rectangle against a light background, and to other forms it was unresponsive. A strong discharge was evoked, however, if a black rectangular object (for example, a piece of black tape) was placed against the brightly illuminated screen. The receptive field of the cell was about 5 × 5°, and the most effective stimulus width was about ⅓°. Vigorous firing was obtained regardless of the position of the rectangle, as long as it was horizontal and within the recep-

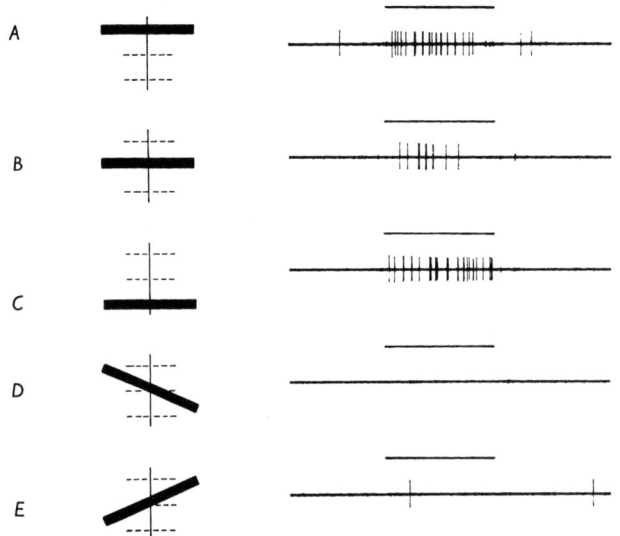

Fig. 7. Cell activated only by left (contralateral) eye over a field approximately 5 × 5°, situated 10° above and to the left of the area centralis. The cell responded best to a black horizontal rectangle, ⅓ × 6°, placed anywhere in the receptive field (A–C). Tilting the stimulus rendered it ineffective (D–E). The black bar was introduced against a light background during periods of 1 sec, indicated by the upper line in each record. Luminance of white background, 1.0 $\log_{10}$ cd/m²; luminance of black part, 0.0 $\log_{10}$ cd/m². A lesion, made while recording from the cell, was found in layer 2 of apical segment of post-lateral gyrus.

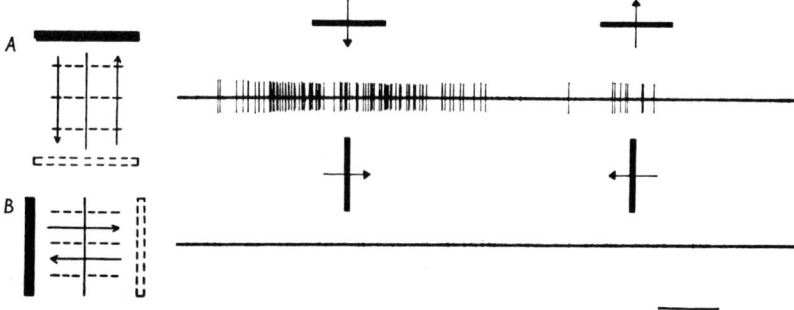

Fig. 8. Same cell as in Text-fig. 7. Movement of black rectangle ⅓ × 6° back and forth across the receptive field: A, horizontally oriented (parallel to receptive-field axis); B, vertically oriented. Time required to move across the field, 5 sec. Time, 1 sec.

tive field. If it was tipped more than 10° in either direction no discharge was evoked (Text-fig. 7D, E). We have recorded several complex fields which resembled this one in that they responded best to black rectangles against a bright background. Presumably it is important to have good contrast between the narrow black rectangle and the background; this is technically difficult with a projector because of scattered light.

Slow downward movement of the dark rectangle evoked a strong discharge throughout the entire 5° of the receptive field (Text-fig. 8A). If the movement was halted the cell continued to fire, but less vigorously. Upward movement gave only weak, inconsistent responses, and left-right movement (Text-fig. 8B) gave no responses. Discharges of highest frequency were evoked by relatively slow rates of downward movement (about 5–10 sec to cross the entire field); rapid movement in either direction gave only very weak responses.

Despite its unusual features this cell exhibited several properties typical of complex units, particularly the lack of summation (except in a horizontal sense), and the wide area over which the dark bar was effective. One may think of the field as having a counterpart in simple fields of type D, Text-fig. 2. In such fields a dark bar would evoke discharges, but only if it fell within the inhibitory region. Moreover, downward movement of the bar would also evoke brisker discharges than upward, provided the upper flanking region were stronger than the lower one.

In describing simple fields it has already been noted that moving stimuli were often more effec-

tive than stationary ones. This was also true of cells with complex fields. Depending on the cell, slits, edges, or dark bars were most effective. As with simple fields, orientation of a stimulus was always critical, responses varied with rate of movement, and directional asymmetries of the type seen in Text-fig. 8 were common. Only once have we seen activation of a cell for one direction of movement and suppression of maintained firing for the opposite direction. In their responses to movement, cells with complex fields differed from their simple counterparts chiefly in responding with sustained firing over substantial regions, usually the entire receptive field, instead of over a very narrow boundary separating excitatory and inhibitory regions.

Receptive-Field Dimensions

Over-all field dimensions were measured for 119 cells. A cell was included only if its field was mapped completely, and if it was situated in the area of central vision (see p. 135). Fields varied greatly in size from one cell to the next, even for cells recorded in a single penetration (see Text-fig. 15). In Text-fig. 9 the distribution of cells according to field area is given separately for simple and complex fields. The histogram illustrates the variation in size, and shows that on the average complex fields were larger than simple ones.

Widths of the narrow subdivisions of simple fields (the centres of types C, D and E or the flanks of type F, Text-fig. 2) also varied greatly: the smallest were 10–15 minutes of arc, which is roughly the diameter of the smallest field centres we have

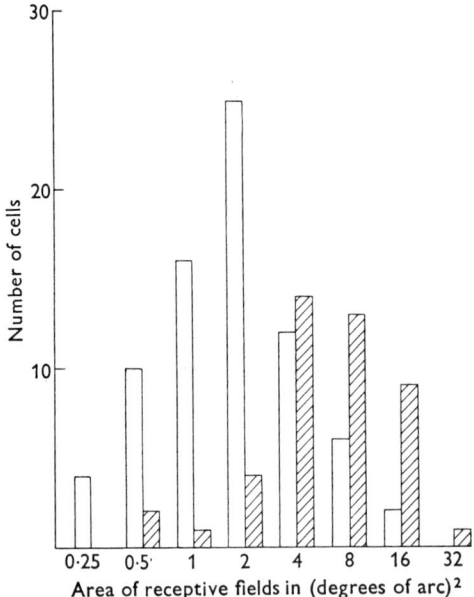

Fig. 9. Distribution of 119 cells in the visual cortex with respect to the approximate area of their receptive fields. White columns indicate cells with simple receptive fields; shaded columns, cells with complex fields. Abscissa: area of receptive fields. Ordinate: number of cells.

found for geniculate cells. For some cells with complex fields the widths of the most effective slits or dark bars were also of this order, indicating that despite the greater overall field size these cells were able to convey detailed information. We wish to emphasize that in both geniculate and cortex the field dimensions tend to increase with distance from the area centralis, and that they differ even for a given location in the retina. It is consequently not possible to compare field sizes in the geniculate and cortex unless these variations are taken into account. This may explain the discrepancy between our results and the findings of Baumgartner (see Jung, 1960), that 'field centres' in the cortex are one half the size of those in the lateral geniculate body.

Responsiveness of Cortical Cells

Simple and complex fields together account for all of the cells we have recorded in the visual cortex. We have not observed cells with concentric fields. Except for clearly injured cells (showing extreme spike deformation or prolonged high-frequency bursts of impulses) all units have responded to visual stimulation, though it has occasionally taken several hours to find the retinal region containing the receptive field and to work out the optimum stimuli. Some cells responded only to stimuli which were optimum in their retinal position and in their form, orientation and rate of movement. A few even required stimulation of both eyes before a response could be elicited (see Part II). But there is no indication from our studies that the striate cortex contains nerve cells that are unresponsive to visual stimuli.

Most of the cells of this series were observed for 1 or 2 hr, and some were studied for up to 9 hr. Over these periods of time there were no qualitative changes in the characteristics of receptive fields: their complexity, arrangements of excitatory and inhibitory areas, axis orientation and position all remained the same, as did the ocular dominance. With deepening anaesthesia a cell became less responsive, so that stimuli that had formerly been weak tended to become even weaker or ineffective, while those that had evoked brisk responses now evoked only weak ones. The last thing to disappear with very deep anaesthesia was usually the response to a moving form. As long as any responses remained the cell retained the same specific requirements as to stimulus form, orientation and rate of movement, suggesting that however the drug exerted its effects, it did not to any important extent functionally disrupt the specific visual connexions. A comparison of visual responses in the anaesthetized animal with those in the unanaesthetized, unrestrained preparation (Hubel, 1959) shows that the main differences lie in the frequency and firing patterns of the maintained activity and in the vigour of responses, rather than in the basic receptive-field organization. It should be emphasized, however, that even in light anaesthesia or in the attentive state diffuse light remains relatively ineffective; thus the balance between excitatory and inhibitory influences is apparently maintained in the waking state.

Part II
Binocular Interaction and Ocular Dominance

Recording from single cells at various levels in the visual system offers a direct means of determining the site of convergence of impulses from the two eyes. In the lateral geniculate body, the first point at which convergence is at all likely, binocularly influenced cells have been observed, but it would seem that these constitute at most a small minority of the total population of geniculate cells (Erulkar & Fillenz, 1958, 1960; Bishop, Burke & Davis, 1959; Grüsser & Sauer, 1960; Hubel & Wiesel, 1961). Silver-degeneration studies show that in each layer of the geniculate the terminals of fibres from a single eye are grouped together, with only minor overlap in the interlaminar regions (Silva, 1956; Hayhow, 1958). The anatomical and physiological findings are thus in good agreement.

It has long been recognized that the greater part of the cat's primary visual cortex receives projections from the two eyes. The anatomical evidence rests largely on the observation that cells in all three lateral geniculate layers degenerate following a localized lesion in the striate area (Minkowski, 1913). Physiological confirmation was obtained by Talbot & Marshall (1941) who stimulated the visual fields of the separate eyes with small spots of light, and mapped the evoked cortical slow waves. Still unsettled, however, was the question of whether individual cortical cells receive projections from both eyes, or whether the cortex contains a mixture of cells, some activated by one eye, some by the other. We have recently shown that many cells in the visual cortex can be influenced by both eyes (Hubel & Wiesel, 1959). The present section contains further observations on binocular interaction. We have been particularly interested in learning whether the eyes work in synergy or in opposition, how the relative influence of the two eyes varies from cell to cell, and whether, on the average, one eye exerts more influence than the other on the cells of a given hemisphere.

RESULTS

In agreement with previous findings (Hubel & Wiesel, 1959) the receptive fields of all binocularly influenced cortical cells occupied corresponding positions on the two retinas, and were strikingly similar in their organization. For simple fields the spatial arrangements of excitatory and inhibitory regions were the same; for complex fields the stimuli that excited or inhibited the cell through one eye had similar effects through the other. Axis orientations of the two receptive fields were the same.

Indeed, the only differences ever seen between the two fields were related to eye dominance: identical stimuli to the two eyes did not necessarily evoke equally strong responses from a given cell. For some cells the responses were equal or almost so; for others one eye tended to dominate. Whenever the two retinas were stimulated in identical fashion in corresponding regions, their effects summed, i.e. they worked in synergy. On the other hand, if antagonistic regions in the two eyes were stimulated so that one eye had an excitatory effect and the other an inhibitory one, then the responses tended to cancel (Hubel & Wiesel, 1959, Fig. 10*A*).

Some units did not respond to stimulation of either eye alone but could be activated only by simultaneous stimulation of the two eyes. Text-figure 10 shows an example of this, and also illustrates ordinary binocular synergy. Two simultaneously recorded cells both responded best to transverse movement of a rectangle oriented in a 1 o'clock–7 o'clock direction (Text-fig. 10*A*, *B*). For one of the cells movement down and to the right was more effective than movement up and to the left. Responses from the individual eyes were roughly equal. On simultaneous stimulation of the two eyes both units responded much more vigorously. Now a third cell was also activated. The threshold of this third unit was apparently so high that, at least under these experimental conditions, stimulation of either eye alone failed to evoke any response.

A second example of synergy is seen in Text-fig. 11. The most effective stimulus was a vertically oriented rectangle moved across the receptive field from left to right. Here the use of both eyes not only enhanced the response already observed with a single eye, but brought into the open a tendency that was formerly unsuspected. Each eye mediated a weak response (Text-fig. 11*A*, *B*) which was greatly strengthened when both eyes were used in parallel (*C*). Now, in addition, the cell gave a weak response to leftward movement, indicating that this had an excitatory effect rather than an inhibitory one. Binocular synergy was often a useful means of bringing out additional information about a receptive field.

In our previous study of forty-five cortical cells (Hubel & Wiesel, 1959) there was clear evidence of convergence of influences from the two eyes in only one fifth of the cells. In the present series 84% of the cells fell into this category. The

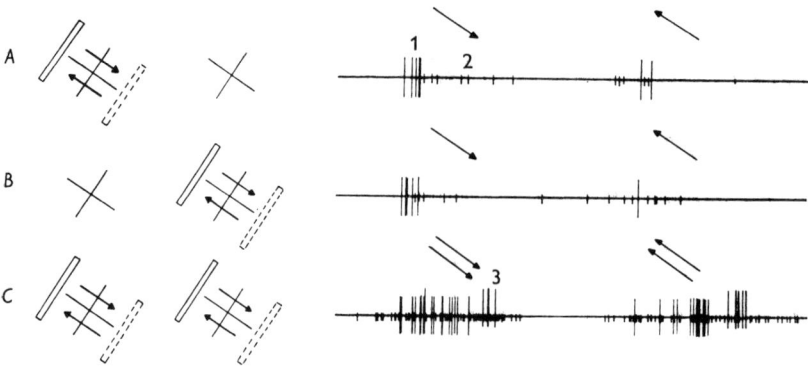

Fig. 10. Examples of binocular synergy in a simultaneous recording of three cells (spikes of the three cells are labelled 1–3). Each of the cells had receptive fields in the two eyes; in each eye the three fields overlapped and were situated 2° below and to the left of the area centralis. The crosses to the left of each record indicate the positions of the receptive fields in the two eyes. The stimulus was ⅛ × 2° slit oriented obliquely and moved slowly across the receptive fields as shown; A, in the left eye; B, in the right eye; C, in the two eyes simultaneously. Since the responses in the two eyes were about equally strong, these two cells were classed in ocular-dominance group 4 (see Text-fig. 12). Time, 1 sec.

difference is undoubtedly related to the improved precision in technique of binocular stimulation. A field was first mapped in the dominant eye and the most effective type of stimulus determined. That stimulus was then applied in the corresponding region in the other eye. Finally, even if no response was obtained from the non-dominant eye, the two eyes were stimulated together in parallel to see if their effects were synergistic. With these methods, an influence was frequently observed from the

non-dominant eye that might otherwise have been overlooked.

A comparison of the influence of the two eyes was made for 223 of the 303 cells in the present series. The remaining cells were either not sufficiently studied, or they belonged to the small group of cells which were only activated if both eyes were simultaneously stimulated. The fields of all cells were in or near the area centralis. The 223 cells were subdivided into seven groups, as follows:

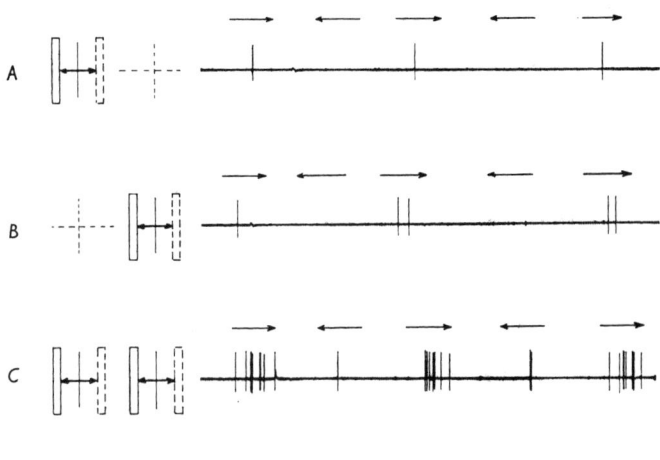

Fig. 11. Movement of a ¼ × 2° slit back and forth horizontally across the receptive field of a binocularly influenced cell. A, left eye; B, right eye; C, both eyes. The cell clearly preferred left-to-right movement, but when both eyes were stimulated together it responded also to the reverse direction. Field diameter, 2°, situated 5° from the area centralis. Time, 1 sec.

Group	Ocular Dominance
1	Exclusively contralateral
2*	Contralateral eye much more effective than ipsilateral eye
3	Contralateral eye slightly more effective than ipsilateral
4	No obvious difference in the effects exerted by the two eyes
5	Ipsilateral eye slightly more effective
6*	Ipsilateral eye much more effective
7	Exclusively ipsilateral

* These groups include cells in which the non-dominant eye, ineffective by itself, could influence the response to stimulation of the dominant eye.

A histogram showing the distribution of cells among these seven groups is given in Text-fig. 12. Assignment of a unit to a particular group was to some extent arbitrary, but it is unlikely that many cells were misplaced by more than one group. Perhaps the most interesting feature of the histogram is its lack of symmetry: many more cells were dominated by the contralateral than by the ipsilateral eye (106 vs. 62). We conclude that in the part of the cat's striate cortex representing central vision the great majority of cells are influenced by both eyes, and that despite wide variation in relative ocular dominance from one cell to the next, the contralateral eye is, on the average, more influential. As the shaded portion of Text-fig. 12 shows, there is no indication that the distribution among the various dominance groups of cells having complex receptive fields differs from the distribution of the population as a whole.

A cortical bias in favour of the contralateral eye may perhaps be related to the preponderance of crossed over uncrossed fibres in the cat's optic tract (Polyak, 1957, p. 788). The numerical inequality between crossed and uncrossed tract fibres is generally thought to be related to an inequality in size of the nasal and temporal half-fields, since both inequalities are most marked in lower mammals with laterally placed eyes, and become progressively less important in higher mammals, primates and man. Thompson *et al.* (1950) showed that in the rabbit, for example, there is a substantial cortical region receiving projections from that part of the peripheral contralateral visual field which is not represented in the ipsilateral retina (the 'Temporal Crescent'). Our results, concerned with more central portions of the visual fields, suggest that in

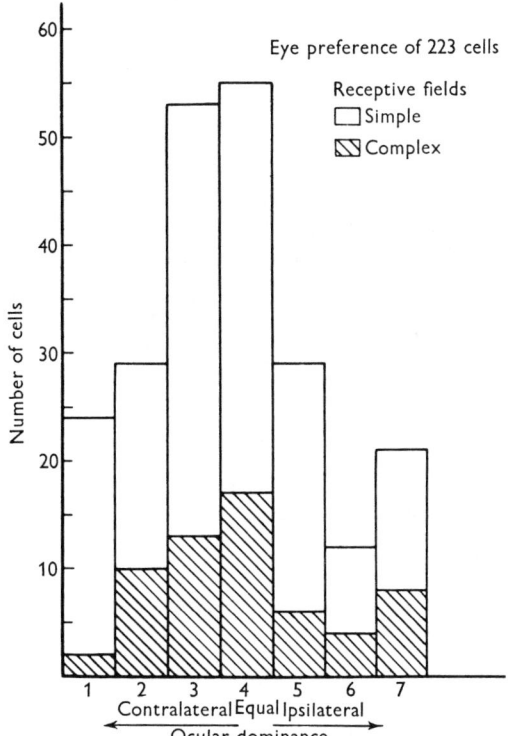

Fig. 12. *Distribution of 223 cells recorded from the visual cortex, according to ocular dominance. Histogram includes cells with simple fields and cells with complex fields. The shaded region shows the distribution of cells with complex receptive fields. Cells of group 1 were driven only by the contralateral eye; for cells of group 2 there was marked dominance of the contralateral eye, for group 3, slight dominance. For cells in group 4 there was no obvious difference between the two eyes. In group 5 the ipsilateral eye dominated slightly, in group 6, markedly; and in group 7 the cells were driven only by the ipsilateral eye.*

the cat the difference in the number of crossed and uncrossed fibres in an optic tract is probably not accounted for entirely by fibres having their receptive fields in the temporal-field crescents.

Part III
Functional Cytoarchitecture of the Cat's Visual Cortex

In the first two parts of this paper cells were studied individually, no attention being paid to their grouping within the cortex. We have shown that the number of functional cell types is very large, since cells may differ in several independent physiological characteristics, for example, in the retinal position of their receptive fields, their receptive-field organization, their axis orientation, and their ocular-dominance group. In this section we shall try to determine whether cells are scattered at random through the cortex with regard to these characteristics, or whether there is any tendency for one or more of the characteristics to be shared by neighbouring cells. The functional architecture of the cortex not only seems interesting for its own sake, but also helps to account for the various complex response patterns described in Part I.

RESULTS

Functional architecture of the cortex was studied by three methods. These had different merits and limitations, and were to some extent complementary.

(1) Cells Recorded in Sequence. The most useful and convenient procedure was to gather as much information as possible about each of a long succession of cells encountered in a micro-electrode penetration through the cortex, and to reconstruct the electrode track from serial histological sections. One could then determine how a physiological characteristic (such as receptive-field position, organization, axis orientation or ocular dominance) varied with cortical location. The success of this method in delineating regions of constant physiological characteristics depends on the possibility of examining a number of units as the electrode passes through each region. Regions may escape detection if they are so small that the electrode is able to resolve only one or two cells in each. The fewer the cells resolved, the larger the regions must be in order to be detected at all.

(2) Unresolved Background Activity. To some extent the spaces between isolated units were bridged by studying unresolved background activity audible over the monitor as a crackling noise, and assumed to originate largely from action potentials of a number of cells. It was concluded that cells, rather than fibres, gave rise to this activity, since it ceased abruptly when the electrode left the grey matter and entered subcortical white matter. Furthermore, diffuse light evoked no change in activity, compared to the marked increase caused by an optimally oriented slit. This suggested that terminal arborizations of afferent fibres

contributed little to the background, since most geniculate cells respond actively to diffuse light (Hubel, 1960). In most penetrations unresolved background activity was present continuously as the electrode passed through layers 2–6 of the cortical grey matter.

Background activity had many uses. It indicated when the cells within range of the electrode tip had a common receptive-field axis orientation. Similarly, one could use it to tell whether the cells in the neighbourhood were driven exclusively by one eye (group 1 or group 7). When the background activity was influenced by both eyes, one could not distinguish between a mixture of cells belonging to the two monocular groups (1 and 7) and a population in which each cell was driven from both eyes. But even here one could at least assess the relative influence of the two eyes upon the group of cells in the immediate neighbourhood of the electrode.

(3) Multiple Recordings. In the series of 303 cells, 78 were recorded in groups of two and 12 in groups of three. Records were not regarded as multiple unless the spikes of the different cells showed distinct differences in amplitude, and unless each unit fulfilled the criteria required of a single-unit record, namely that the amplitude and wave shape be relatively constant for a given electrode position.

In such multiple recordings one could be confident that the cells were close neighbours and that uniform stimulus conditions prevailed, since the cells could be stimulated and observed together. One thus avoided some of the difficulties in evaluating a succession of recordings made over a long period of time span, where absolute constancy of eye position, anaesthetic level, and preparation condition were sometimes hard to guarantee.

Regional variations of several physiological characteristics were examined by the three methods just outlined. Of particular interest for the present study were the receptive-field axis orientation, position of receptive fields on the retina, receptive-field organization, and relative ocular dominance. These will be described separately in the following paragraphs.

Orientation of Receptive-Field Axis

The orientation of a receptive-field axis was determined in several ways. When the field was simple the borders between excitatory and inhibitory regions were sufficient to establish the axis directly. For both simple and complex fields the axis could always be determined from the orientation of the most effective stimulus. For most fields, when the slit or edge was placed at right angles to the optimum position there was no response. The receptive-field axis orientation was checked by varying the stimulus orientation from this null position in order to find the two orientations at which a response was only just elicited, and by bisecting the angle between them. By one or other of these procedures the receptive-field orientation could usually be determined to within 5 or 10°.

One of the first indications that the orientation of a receptive-field axis was an important variable came from multiple recordings. Invariably the axes of receptive fields mapped together had the same orientations. An example of a 3-unit recording has already been given in Text-fig. 10. Cells with common axis orientation were therefore not scattered at random through the cortex, but tended to be grouped together. The size and shape of the regions containing these cell groups were investigated by comparing the fields of cells mapped in sequence. It was at once apparent that successively recorded cells also tended to have identical axis orientations and that each penetration consisted of several sequences of cells, each sequence having a common axis orientation. Any undifferentiated units in the background responded best to the stimulus orientation that was most effective in activating the cell under study. After traversing a distance that varied greatly from one penetration to the next, the electrode would enter an area where there was no longer any single optimum orientation for driving background activity. A very slight advance of the electrode would bring it into a region where a new orientation was the most effective, and the succeeding cells would all have receptive fields with that orientation. The change in angle from one region to another was unpredictable; sometimes it was barely detectable, at other times large (45–90°).

Text-figure 13 shows a camera lucida tracing of a frontal section through the post-lateral gyrus. The electrode track entered normal to the surface, passed through the apical segment in a direction parallel to the fibre bundles, then through the white matter beneath, and finally obliquely through half the thickness of the mesial segment. A lesion was made at the termination of the penetration. A composite photomicrograph (Pl. 1) shows the lesion and the first part of the electrode track. The units recorded in the course of the penetration are indicated in Text-fig. 13 by the longer lines crossing the track; the unresolved background activity by the shorter lines. The orientations of the most effective stimuli are given by the directions of the lines, a line perpendicular to the track signifying a vertical orientation. For the first part of the penetration, through the apical segment, the field orientation was vertical for all cells as well as for the background activity. Fibres were recorded from the white matter and from the grey matter just beyond it. Three of these fibres were axons of cortical cells having fields of various oblique orientations; four were afferent fibres from the lateral geniculate body. In the mesial segment three short sequences were encountered, each with a different common field orientation. These sequences together occupied a distance smaller than the full thickness of the apical segment.

In another experiment, illustrated in Text-fig. 14 and in Pl. 2, two penetrations were made, both in the apical segment of the post-lateral gyrus. The medial penetration (at left in the figure) was at the outset almost normal to the cortex, but deviated more and more from the direction of the deep fibre bundles. In this penetration there were three different axis orientations, of which the first and third persisted through long sequences. In the lateral track there were nine orientations. From the beginning this track was more oblique, and it became increasingly so as it progressed.

As illustrated by the examples of Text-figs. 13 and 14, there was a marked tendency for shifts in orientation to increase in frequency as the angle between electrode and direction of fibre bundles (or apical dendrites) became greater. The extreme curvature of the lateral and post-lateral gyri in their apical segments made normal penetrations very difficult to obtain; nevertheless, four penetrations were normal or almost so. In none of these were there any shifts of axis orientation. On the other hand there were several shifts of field orientation in all oblique penetrations. As illustrated by Text-fig. 14, most penetrations that began nearly normal to the surface became more and more oblique with increasing depth. Here the distance traversed by the electrode without shifts in receptive-field orientation tended to become less and less as the penetration advanced.

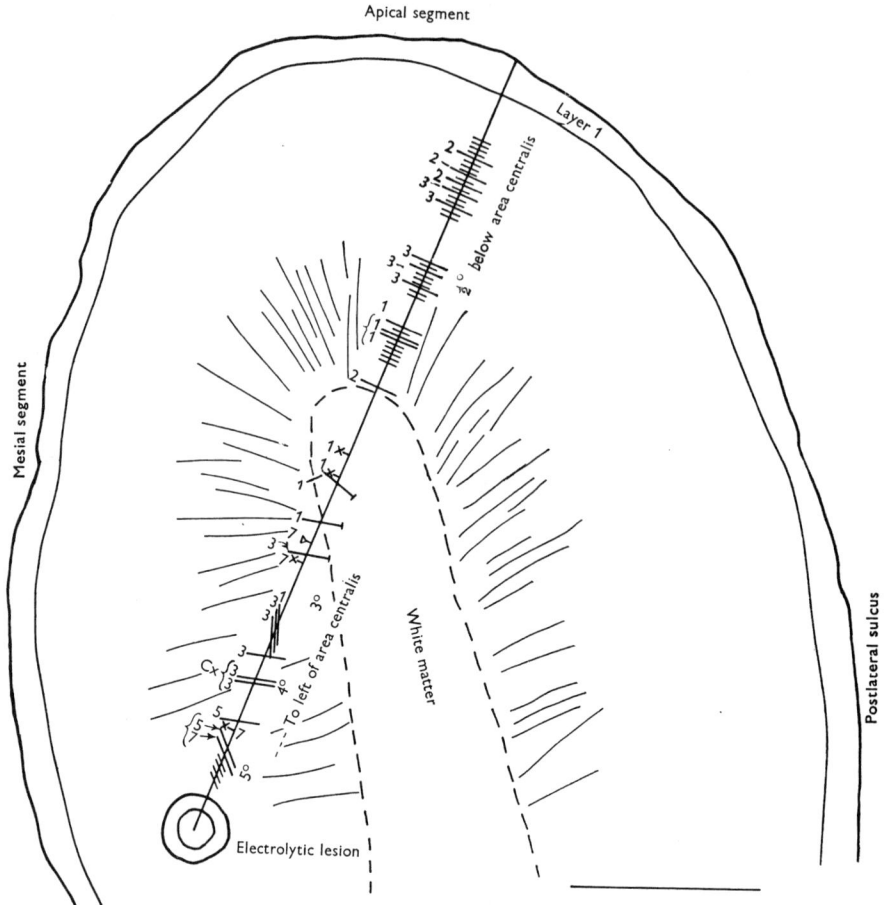

Fig. 13. Reconstruction of micro-electrode penetration through the lateral gyrus (see also Pl. 1). Electrode entered apical segment normal to the surface, and remained parallel to the deep fibre bundles (indicated by radial lines) until reaching white matter; in grey matter of mesial segment the electrode's course was oblique. Longer lines represent cortical cells. Axons of cortical cells are indicated by a crossbar at right-hand end of line. Field-axis orientation is shown by the direction of each line; lines perpendicular to track represent vertical orientation. Brace-brackets show simultaneously recorded units. Complex receptive fields are indicated by 'Cx'. Afferent fibres from the lateral geniculate body indicated by ✗, for 'on' centre; △, for 'off' centre. Approximate positions of receptive fields on the retina are shown to the right of the penetration. Shorter lines show regions in which unresolved background activity was observed. Numbers to the left of the penetration refer to ocular-dominance group (see Part II). Scale 1 mm.

It can be concluded that the striate cortex is divided into discrete regions within which the cells have a common receptive-field axis orientation. Some of the regions extend from the surface of the cortex to the white matter; it is difficult to be certain whether they all do. Some idea of their shapes may be obtained by measuring distances between shifts in receptive-field orientation. From these measurements it seems likely that the general shape is columnar, distorted no doubt by any cur-

vature of the gyrus, which would tend to make the end at the surface broader than that at the white matter; deep in a sulcus the effect would be the reverse. The cross-sectional size and shape of the columns at the surface can be estimated only roughly. Most of our information concerns their width in the coronal plane, since it is in this plane that oblique penetrations were made. At the surface this width is probably of the order of 0.5 mm. We have very little information about the cross-

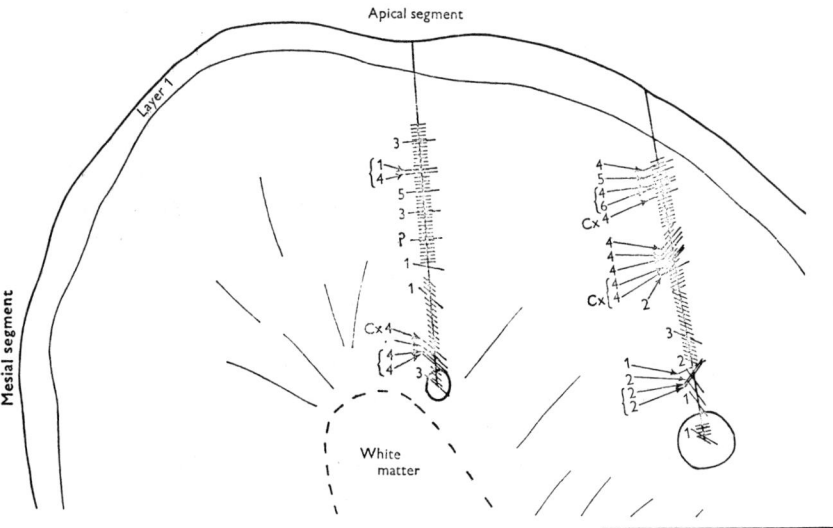

Fig. 14. Reconstructions of two penetrations in apical segment of post-lateral gyrus, near its anterior end (just behind anterior interrupted line in Text-fig. 1, see also Pl. 2). Medial penetration is slightly oblique, lateral one is markedly so. All receptive fields were located within 1° of area centralis. Conventions as in Text-fig. 13. Scale 1 mm.

sectional dimension in a direction parallel to the long axis of the gyrus. Preliminary mapping of the cortical surface suggests that the cross-sectional shape of the columns may be very irregular.

Position of Receptive Fields on the Retina

GROSS TOPOGRAPHY. That there is a systematic representation of the retina on the striate cortex of the cat was established anatomically by Minkowski (1913) and with physiological methods by Talbot & Marshall (1941). Although in the present study no attempt has been made to map topographically all parts of the striate cortex, the few penetrations made in cortical areas representing peripheral parts of the retina confirm these findings. Cells recorded in front of the anterior interrupted lines of Text-fig. 1 had receptive fields in the superior retinas; those in the one penetration behind the posterior line had fields that were well below the horizontal meridian of the retina. (No recordings were made from cortical regions receiving projections from the deeply pigmented non-tapetal part of the inferior retinas.) In several penetrations extending far down the mesial (interhemispheric) segment of the lateral gyrus, receptive fields moved

further and further out into the ipsilateral half of each retina as the electrode advanced (Text-fig. 13). In these penetrations the movement of fields into the retinal periphery occurred more and more rapidly as the electrode advanced. In three penetrations extending far down the lateral segment of the post-lateral gyrus (medial bank of the post-lateral sulcus) there was likewise a clear progressive shift of receptive-field positions as the electrode advanced. Here also the movement was along the horizontal meridian, again into the *ipsilateral* halves of both retinas. This therefore confirms the findings of Talbot & Marshall (1941) and Talbot (1942), that in each hemisphere there is a second laterally placed representation of the contralateral half-field of vision. The subject of Visual Area II will not be dealt with further in this paper.

Cells within the large cortical region lying between the interrupted lines of Text-fig. 1, and extending over on to the mesial segment and into the lateral sulcus for a distance of 2–3 mm, had their receptive fields in the area of central vision. By this we mean the area centralis, which is about 5° in diameter, and a region surrounding it by about 2–3°. The receptive fields of the great majority of cells were confined to the ipsilateral halves of the two retinas. Often a receptive field covering several degrees on the retina stopped short in the area centralis right at the vertical meridian. Only rarely did a receptive field appear to spill over into the contralateral half-retina; when it did, it was only by 2–3°, a distance comparable to the possible error in determining the area centralis in some cats.

Because of the large cortical representation of the area centralis, one would expect only a very slow change in receptive-field position as the electrode advanced obliquely (Text-fig. 13). Indeed, in penetrations through the apex of the post-lateral gyrus and extending 1–2 mm down either bank there was usually no detectable progressive displacement of receptive fields. In penetrations made 1–3 mm apart, either along a parasagittal line or in the same coronal plane (Text-fig. 14) receptive fields again had almost identical retinal positions.

RETINAL REPRESENTATION OF NEIGHBOURING CELLS. A question of some interest was to determine whether this detailed topographic representation of the retina held right down to the cellular level. From the results just described one might imagine that receptive fields of neighbouring cortical cells should have very nearly the same retinal position. In a sequence of cells recorded in a normal penetration through the cortex the receptive fields should be superimposed, and for oblique penetrations any detectable changes in field positions should be systematic. In the following paragraphs we shall consider the relative retinal positions of the receptive fields of neighbouring cells, especially cells within a column.

In all multiple recordings the receptive fields of cells observed simultaneously were situated in the same general region of the retina. As a rule the fields overlapped, but it was unusual for them to be precisely superimposed. For example, fields were often staggered along a line perpendicular to their axes. Similarly, the successive receptive fields observed during a long cortical penetration varied somewhat in position, often in an apparently random manner. Text-figure 15 illustrates a sequence of twelve cells recorded in the early part of a penetration through the cortex. One lesion was made while observing the first cell in the sequence and another at the end of the penetration; they are indicated in the drawing of cortex to the right of the figure. In the centre of the figure the position of each receptive field is shown relative to the area

centralis (marked with a cross); each field was several degrees below and to the left of the area centralis. It will be seen that all fields in the sequence except the last had the same axis orientation; the first eleven cells therefore occupied the same column. All but the first three and the last (cell 12) were simple in arrangement. Cells 5 and 6 were recorded together, as were 8 and 9.

In the left-hand part of the figure the approximate boundaries of all these receptive fields are shown superimposed, in order to indicate the degree of overlap. From cell to cell there is no obvious systematic change in receptive-field position. The variation in position is about equal to the area occupied by the largest fields of the sequence. This variation is undoubtedly real, and not an artifact produced by eye movements occurring between recordings of successive cells. The stability of the eyes was checked while studying each cell, and any tendency to eye movements would have easily been detected by an apparent movement of the receptive field under observation. Furthermore, the field positions of simultaneously recorded cells 5 and 6, and also of cells 8 and 9, are clearly different; here the question of eye movements is not pertinent.

Text-figure 15 illustrates a consistent and somewhat surprising finding, that within a column defined by common field-axis orientation there was no apparent progression in field positions along the retina as the electrode advanced. This was so even though the electrode often crossed through the column obliquely, entering one side and leaving the other. If there was any detailed topographical representation within columns it was obscured by the superimposed, apparently random staggering of field positions. We conclude that at this microscopic level the retinotopic representation no longer strictly holds.

Receptive-Field Organization

MULTIPLE RECORDINGS. The receptive fields of cells observed together in multiple recordings were always of similar complexity, i.e. they were either all simple or all complex in their organization. In about one third of the multiple recordings the cells had the same detailed field organization; if simple, they had similar distributions of excitatory and inhibitory areas; if complex, they required identical stimuli for their activation. As a rule these fields

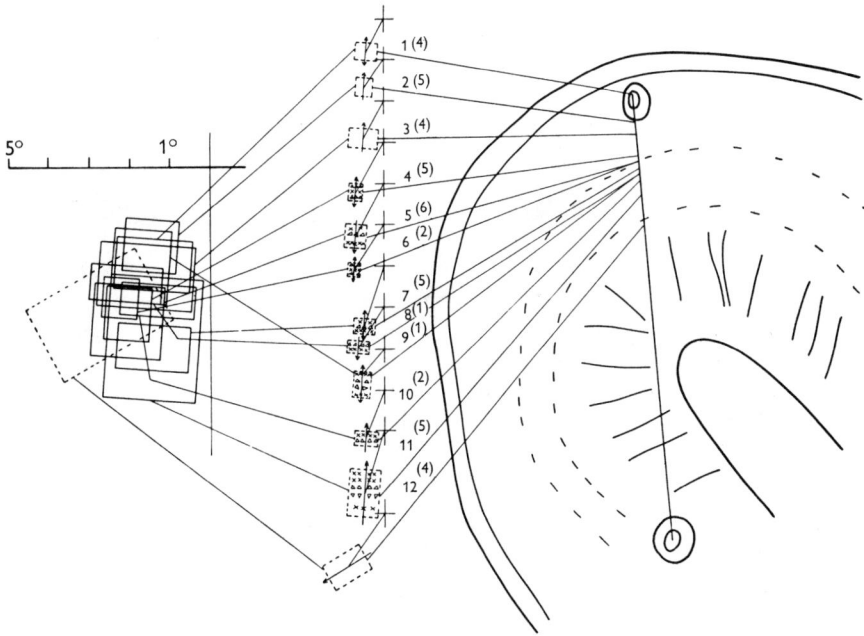

Fig. 15. *Reconstruction of part of an electrode track through apical and mesial segments of post-lateral gyrus near its anterior end. Two lesions were made, the first after recording from the first unit, the second at the end of the penetration. Only the first twelve cells are represented. Interrupted lines show boundaries of layer 4.*

In the centre part of the figure the position of each receptive field, outlined with interrupted lines, is given with respect to the area centralis, shown by a cross. Cells are numbered in sequence, 1–12. Numbers in parentheses refer to ocular-dominance group (see Part II). Units 5 and 6, 8 and 9 were observed simultaneously. The first three fields and the last were complex in organization; the remainder were simple. ✕, areas giving excitation; △, areas giving inhibitory effects. Note that all receptive fields except the last have the same axis orientation (9.30–3.30 o'clock). The arrows show the preferred direction of movement of a slit oriented parallel to the receptive-field axis.

In the left part of the figure all of the receptive fields are superimposed, to indicate the overlap and variation in size. The vertical and horizontal lines represent meridia, crossing at the area centralis. Scale on horizontal meridian, 1° for each subdivision.

did not have exactly the same retinal position, but were staggered as described above. In two thirds of the multiple recordings the cells differed to varying degrees in their receptive field arrangements. Two types of multiple recordings in which field arrangements differed seem interesting enough to merit a separate description.

In several multiple recordings the receptive fields overlapped in such a way that one or more excitatory or inhibitory portions were superimposed. Two examples are supplied by cell-pairs 5 and 6, and 8 and 9 of Text-fig. 15. Their fields are redrawn in Text-fig. 16. The fields of cells 5 and 6 are drawn separately (Text-fig. 16 *A*) but they actually overlapped so that the reference lines are to be

imagined as superimposed. Thus the 'on' centre of cell 6 fell directly over the upper 'on' flank of 5 and the two cells tended to fire together to suitably placed stimuli. A similar situation existed for cells 8 and 9 (Text-fig. 16 *B*). The field of 9 was placed so that its 'off' region and the lower, weaker 'on' region were superimposed on the two regions of 8. Again the two cells tended to fire together. Such examples suggest that neighbouring cells may have some of their inputs in common.

Cells responded reciprocally to a light stimulus in eight of the forty-three multiple recordings. An example of two cells responding reciprocally to stationary spots is shown in Text-fig. 17. In each eye the two receptive fields were almost superimposed.

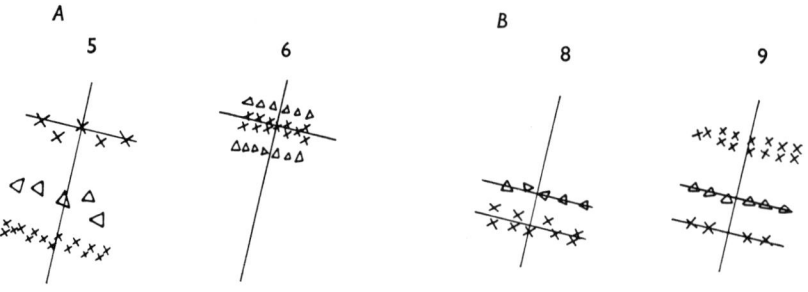

Fig. 16. Detailed arrangements of the receptive fields of two pairs of simultaneously recorded cells (nos. 5 and 6, and 8 and 9, of Text-fig. 15). The crosses of diagrams 5 and 6 are superimposed as are the double crosses of 8 and 9. Note that the upper excitatory region of 5 is superimposed upon the excitatory region of 6; and that both regions of 8 are superimposed on the inhibitory and lower excitatory regions of 9. Scale, 1°.

The fields consisted of elongated obliquely oriented central regions, inhibitory for one cell, excitatory for the other, flanked on either side by regions of the opposite type. Instead of firing together in response to an optimally oriented stationary slit, like the cells in Text-fig. 16, these cells gave opposite-type responses, one inhibitory and the other excitatory. Some cell pairs responded reciprocally to to-and-fro movements of a slit or edge. Examples have been given elsewhere (Hubel, 1958, Fig. 9; 1959, Text-fig. 6). The fields of these cell pairs usually differed only in the balance of the asymmetrical flanking regions.

RELATIONSHIP BETWEEN RECEPTIVE FIELD ORGANIZATION AND CORTICAL LAYERING. In a typical penetration through the cortex many different field types were found, some simple and others complex. Even within a single column both simple and complex fields were seen. (In Text-fig. 13 and 14 complex fields are indicated by the symbol 'Cx'; in Text-fig. 15, fields 1–3 were complex and 4–11 simple, all within a single column.) An attempt was made to learn whether there was any relationship between the different field types and the layers of the cortex. This was difficult for several reasons. In Nissl-stained sections the boundaries between layers of the cat's striate cortex are not nearly as clear as they are in the primate brain; frequently even the fourth layer, so characteristic of the striate cortex, is poorly demarcated. Consequently, a layer

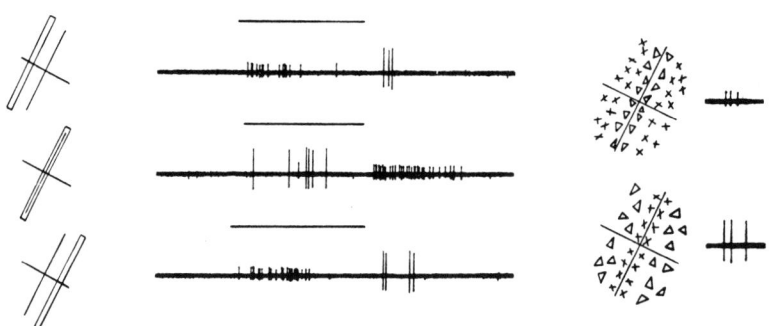

Fig. 17. Records of two simultaneously observed cells which responded reciprocally to stationary stimuli. The two receptive fields are shown to the right, and are superimposed, though they are drawn separately. The cell corresponding to each field is indicated by the spikes to the right of the diagram. To the left of each record is shown the position of a slit, ¼ × 2½°, with respect to these fields.

Both cells binocularly driven (dominance group 3); fields mapped in the left (contralateral) eye; position of fields 2° below and to the left of the area centralis. Time, 1 sec.

could not always be identified with certainty even for a cell whose position was directly marked by a lesion. For most cells the positions were arrived at indirectly, from depth readings and lesions made elsewhere in the penetrations: these determinations were subject to more errors than the direct ones. Moreover, few of the penetrations were made in a direction parallel to the layering, so that the distance an electrode travelled in passing through a layer was short, and the error in electrode position correspondingly more important.

The distribution of 179 cells among the different layers is given in the histograms of Text-fig. 18. All cells were recorded in penetrations in which at least one lesion was made; the shaded portions refer to cells which were individually marked with lesions. As shown in the separate histograms, simple-field cells as well as those with complex fields were widely distributed throughout the cortex. Cells with simple fields were most numerous in layers 3, 4 and 6. Especially interesting is the apparent rarity of complex fields in layer 4, where simple fields were so abundant. This is also illustrated in Text-fig. 15, which shows a sequence of eight cells recorded from layer 4, all of which had simple fields. These findings suggest that cells may to some extent be segregated according to field complexity, and the rarity with which simple and complex fields were mapped together is consistent with this possibility.

Ocular Dominance

In thirty-four multiple recordings the eye-dominance group (see Part II) was determined for both or all three cells. In eleven of these recordings there was a clear difference in ocular dominance between cells. Similarly, in a single penetration two cells recorded in sequence frequently differed in eye dominance. Cells from several different eye-dominance categories appeared not only in single penetrations, but also in sequences in which all cells had a common axis orientation. Thus within a single column defined by a common axis orientation there were cells of different eye dominance. A sequence of cells within one column is formed by cells 1–11 of Text-fig. 15. Here eye dominance ranged from wholly contralateral (group 1) to strongly ipsilateral (group 6). The two simultaneously recorded cells 5 and 6 were dominated by opposite eyes.

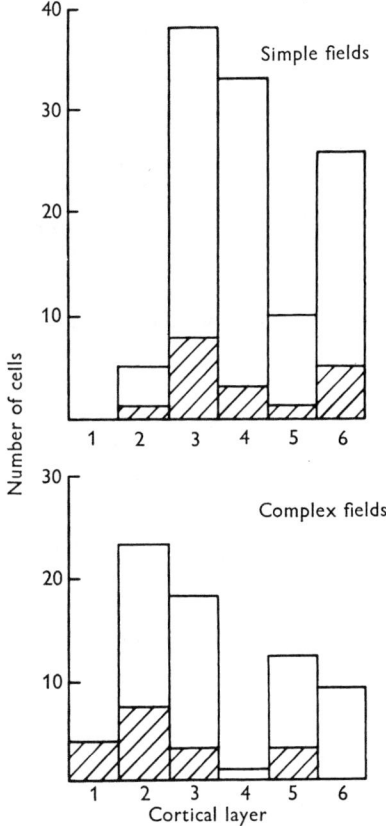

Fig. 18. Distribution of 179 cells, 113 with simple fields, 66 with complex, among the different cortical layers. All cells were recorded in penetrations in which at least one electrolytic lesion was made and identified; the shaded areas refer to cells marked individually by lesions. Note especially the marked difference in the occurrence, in layer 4, between simple and complex fields.

While these results suggested that cells of different ocular dominance were present within single columns, there were nevertheless indications of some grouping. First, in twenty-three of the thirty-four multiple recordings, simultaneously observed cells fell into the same ocular-dominance group. Secondly, in many penetrations short sequences of cells having the same relative eye dominance were probably more common than would be expected from a random scattering. Several short sequences are shown in Text-fig. 13 and 14. When such sequences consisted of cells with extreme unilateral dominance (dominance groups 1, 2, 6, and 7) the undifferentiated background activity was usually also driven predominantly by one eye, suggesting that other neighbouring units had similar eye preference. If cells of common eye dominance are in fact regionally grouped, the groups would seem to be relatively small. The cells could be arranged in nests, or conceivably in very narrow columns or thin layers.

In summary, cells within a column defined by a common field-axis orientation do not necessarily all have the same ocular dominance; yet neither do cells seem to be scattered at random through the cortex with respect to this characteristic.

DISCUSSION

A Scheme for the Elaboration of Simple and Complex Receptive Fields

Comparison of responses of cells in the lateral geniculate body with responses from striate cortex brings out profound differences in the receptive-field organization of cells in the two structures. For cortical cells, specifically oriented lines and borders tend to replace circular spots as the optimum stimuli, movement becomes an important parameter of stimulation, diffuse light becomes virtually ineffective, and with adequate stimuli most cells can be driven from the two eyes. Since lateral geniculate cells supply the main, and possibly the only, visual input to the striate cortex, these differences must be the result of integrative mechanisms within the striate cortex itself.

At present we have no direct evidence on how the cortex transforms the incoming visual information. Ideally, one should determine the properties of a cortical cell, and then examine one by one the receptive fields of all the afferents projecting upon that cell. In the lateral geniculate, where one can, in effect, record simultaneously from a cell and one of its afferents, a beginning has already been made in this direction (Hubel & Wiesel, 1961). In a structure as complex as the cortex the techniques available would seem hopelessly inadequate for such an approach. Here we must rely on less direct evidence to suggest possible mechanisms for explaining the transformations that we find.

The relative lack of complexity of simple cortical receptive fields suggests that these represent the first or at least a very early stage in the modification of geniculate signals. At any rate we have found no cells with receptive fields intermediate in type between geniculate and simple cortical fields. To account for the spatial arrangements of excitatory and inhibitory regions of simple cortical fields we may imagine that upon each simple-type cell there converge fibres of geniculate origin having 'on' or 'off' centres situated in the appropriate retinal regions. For example, a cortical cell with a receptive field of the type shown in Text-fig. 2C might receive projections from a group of lateral geniculate cells having 'on' field centres distributed throughout the long narrow central region designated in the figure by crosses. Such a projection system is shown in the diagram of Text-fig. 19. A slit of light falling on this elongated central region would activate all the geniculate cells, since for each cell the centre effect would strongly outweigh the inhibition from the segments of field periphery falling within the elongated region. This is the same as saying that a geniculate cell will respond to a slit with a width equal to the diameter of its field centre, a fact that we have repeatedly verified. The inhibitory flanks of the cortical field would be formed by the remaining outlying parts of the geniculate-field peripheries. These flanks might be reinforced and enlarged by appropriately placed 'off'-centre geniculate cells. Such an increase in the potency of the flanks would appear necessary to explain the relative indifference of cortical cells to diffuse light.

The arrangement suggested by Text-fig. 19 would be consistent with our impression that widths of cortical receptive-field centres (or flanks, in a field such as that of Text-fig. 2F) are of the same order of magnitude as the diameters of geniculate receptive-field centres, at least for fields in or near the area centralis. Hence the fineness of discrimination implied by the small size of geniculate receptive-field centres is not necessarily lost at the cortical level, despite the relatively large total size of many cortical fields; rather, it is incorporated into the detailed substructure of the cortical fields.

In a similar way, the simple fields of Text-fig. 2 D–G may be constructed by supposing that the afferent 'on'- or 'off'-centre geniculate cells have their field centres appropriately placed. For example, field-type G could be formed by having geniculate afferents with 'off' centres situated in the region below and to the right of the boundary, and 'on' centres above and to the left. An asymmetry of flanking regions, as in field E, would be produced if the two flanks were unequally reinforced by 'on'-centre afferents.

The model of Text-fig. 19 is based on excitatory synapses. Here the suppression of firing on illuminating an inhibitory part of the receptive field is presumed to be the result of withdrawal of tonic excitation, i.e. the inhibition takes place at a lower level. That such mechanisms occur in the visual system is clear from studies of the lateral geniculate body, where an 'off'-centre cell is suppressed on illuminating its field centre because of suppression of firing in its main excitatory afferent (Hubel & Wiesel, 1961). In the proposed scheme one should, however, consider the possibility of direct inhibitory connexions. In Text-fig. 19 we may replace any of the excitatory endings by inhibitory ones, provided we replace the corresponding geniculate cells by ones of opposite type ('on'-centre instead of 'off'-centre, and conversely). Up to the present the two mechanisms have not been distinguished, but there is no reason to think that both do not occur.

The properties of complex fields are not easily accounted for by supposing that these cells receive afferents directly from the lateral geniculate body. Rather, the correspondence between simple and complex fields noted in Part I suggests that cells with complex fields are of higher order, having cells with simple fields as their afferents. These simple fields would all have identical axis orientation, but would differ from one another in their exact retinal positions. An example of such a scheme is given in Text-fig. 20. The hypothetical cell illustrated has a complex field like that of Text-figs. 5 and 6. One may imagine that it receives

afferents from a set of simple cortical cells with fields of type *G,* Text-fig. 2, all with vertical axis orientation, and staggered along a horizontal line. An edge of light would activate one or more of these simple cells wherever it fell within the complex field, and this would tend to excite the higher-order cell.

Similar schemes may be proposed to explain the behaviour of other complex units. One need only use the corresponding simple fields as building blocks, staggering them over an appropriately wide region. A cell with the properties shown in Text-fig. 3 would require two types of horizontally oriented simple fields, having 'off' centres above the horizontal line, and 'on' centres below it. A slit of the same width as these centre regions would strongly activate only those cells whose long narrow centres it covered. It is true that at the same time a number of other cells would have small parts of their peripheral fields stimulated, but we may perhaps assume that these opposing effects would be relatively weak. For orientations other than horizontal a slit would have little or no effect on the simple cells, and would therefore not activate the complex one. Small spots should give only feeble 'on' responses regardless of where they were shone in the field. Enlarging the spots would not produce summation of the responses unless the enlargement were in a horizontal direction; anything else would result in invasion of opposing parts of the antecedent fields, and cancellation of the responses from the corresponding cells. The model would therefore seem to account for many of the observed properties of complex fields.

Fig. 19. Possible scheme for explaining the organization of simple receptive fields. A large number of lateral geniculate cells, of which four are illustrated in the upper right in the figure, have receptive fields with 'on' centres arranged along a straight line on the retina. All of these project upon a single cortical cell, and the synapses are supposed to be excitatory. The receptive field of the cortical cell will then have an elongated 'on' centre indicated by the interrupted lines in the receptive-field diagram to the left of the figure.

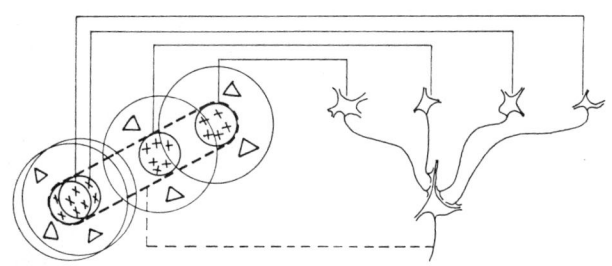

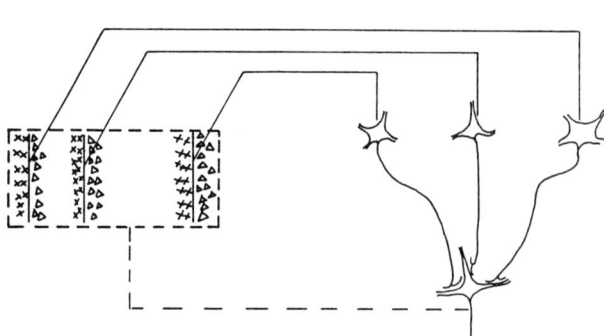

Fig. 20. Possible scheme for explaining the organization of complex receptive fields. A number of cells with simple fields, of which three are shown schematically, are imagined to project to a single cortical cell of higher order. Each projecting neurone has a receptive field arranged as shown to the left: an excitatory region to the left and an inhibitory region to the right of a vertical straight-line boundary. The boundaries of the fields are staggered within an area outlined by the interrupted lines. Any vertical-edge stimulus falling across this rectangle, regardless of its position, will excite some simple-field cells leading to excitation of the higher-order cell.

Proposals such as those of Text-figs. 19 and 20 are obviously tentative and should not be interpreted literally. It does, at least, seem probable that simple receptive fields represent an early stage in cortical integration, and the complex ones a later stage. Regardless of the details of the process, it is also likely that a complex field is built up from simpler ones with common axis orientations.

At first sight it would seem necessary to imagine a highly intricate tangle of interconnexions in order to link cells with common axis orientations while keeping those with different orientations functionally separated. But if we turn to the results of Part III on functional cytoarchitecture we see at once that gathered together in discrete columns are the very cells we require to be interconnected in our scheme. The cells of each aggregate have common axis orientations and the staggering in the positions of the simple fields is roughly what is required to account for the size of most of the complex fields (cf. Text-fig. 9). That these cells are interconnected is moreover very likely on histological grounds: indeed, the particular richness of radial connexions in the cortex fits well with the columnar shape of the regions.

The otherwise puzzling aggregation of cells with common axis orientation now takes on new meaning. We may tentatively look upon each column as a functional unit of cortex, within which simple fields are elaborated and then in turn synthesized into complex fields. The large variety of simple and complex fields to be found in a single column (Text-fig. 15) suggests that the connexions between cells in a column are highly specific.

We may now begin to appreciate the significance of the great increase in the number of cells in the striate cortex, compared with the lateral geniculate body. In the cortex there is an enormous digestion of information, with each small region of visual field represented over and over again in column after column, first for one receptive-field orientation and then for another. Each column contains thousands of cells, some cells having simple fields and others complex. In the part of the cortex receiving projections from the area centralis the receptive fields are smaller, and presumably more columns are required for unit area of retina; hence in central retinal regions the cortical projection is disproportionately large.

Complex Receptive Fields

The method of stimulating the retina with small circular spots of light and recording from single visual cells has been a useful one in studies of the cat's visual system. In the pathway from retina to cortex the excitatory and inhibitory areas mapped out by this means have been sufficient to account for responses to both stationary and moving patterns. Only when one reaches cortical cells with complex fields does the method fail, for these fields cannot generally be separated into excitatory and inhibitory regions. Instead of the direct small-spot method, one must resort to a trial-and-error system, and attempt to describe each cell in terms of the stimuli that most effectively influence firing. Here there is a risk of over- or under-estimating the complexity of the most effective stimuli, with corresponding lack of precision in the functional description of the cell. For this reason it is encouraging to find that the properties of complex fields can be interpreted by the simple supposition that they receive projections from simple-field cells, a supposition made more likely by the anatomical findings of Part III.

Compared with cells in the retina or lateral geniculate body, cortical cells show a marked increase in the number of stimulus parameters that must be specified in order to influence their firing. This apparently reflects a continuing process which has its beginning in the retina. To obtain an optimum response from a retinal ganglion cell it is generally sufficient to specify the position, size and intensity of a circular spot. Enlarging the spot beyond the size of the field centre raises the threshold, but even when diffuse light is used it is possible to evoke a brisk response by using an intense enough stimulus. For geniculate cells the penalty for exceeding optimum spot size is more severe than in the retina, as has been shown by comparing responses of a geniculate cell and an afferent fibre to the same cell (Hubel & Wiesel, 1961). In the retina and lateral geniculate body there is no evidence that any shapes are more effective than circular ones, or that, with moving stimuli, one direction of movement is better than another.

In contrast, in the cortex effective driving of simple-field cells can only be obtained with restricted stimuli whose position, shape and orientation are specific for the cell. Some cells fire best to a moving stimulus, and in these the direction and even the rate of movement are often critical. Diffuse light is at best a poor stimulus, and for cells in the area of central representation it is usually ineffective at any intensity.

An interesting feature of cortical cells with complex fields may be seen in their departure from the process of progressively increasing specificity. At this stage, for the first time, what we suppose to be higher-order neurones are in a sense less selective in their responses than the cells which feed into

them. Cells with simple fields tend to respond only when the stimulus is both oriented and positioned properly. In contrast, the neurones to which they supposedly project are concerned predominantly with stimulus orientation, and are far less critical in their requirements as regards stimulus placement. Their responsiveness to the abstraction which we call orientation is thus generalized over a considerable retinal area.

The significance of this step for perception can only be speculated upon, but it may be of some interest to examine several possibilities. First, neurophysiologists must ultimately try to explain how a form can be recognized regardless of its exact position in the visual field. As a step in form recognition the organism may devise a mechanism by which the inclinations of borders are more important than their exact visual-field location. It is clear that a given form in the visual field will, by virtue of its borders, excite a combination of cells with complex fields. If we displace the form it will activate many of the same cells, as long as the change in position is not enough to remove it completely from their receptive fields. Now we may imagine that these particular cells project to a single cell of still higher order: such a cell will then be very likely to respond to the form (provided the synapses are excitatory) and there will be considerable latitude in the position of the retinal image. Such a mechanism will also permit other transformations of the image, such as a change in size associated with displacement of the form toward or away from the eye. Assuming that there exist cells that are responsive to specific forms, it would clearly be economical to avoid having thousands for each form, one for every possible retinal position, and separate sets for each type of distortion of the image.

Next, the ability of some cells with complex fields to respond in a sustained manner to a stimulus as it moves over a wide expanse of retina suggests that these cells may play an important part in the perception of movement. They adapt rapidly to a stationary form, and continuous movement of the stimulus within the receptive field is the only way of obtaining a sustained discharge (Text-fig. 4 *H*). Presumably the afferent simple-field cells also adapt rapidly to a stationary stimulus; because of their staggered fields the moving stimulus excites them in turn, and the higher-order cell is thus at all times bombarded. This seems an elegant means of overcoming a difficulty inherent in the problem of movement perception, that movement must excite receptors not continuously but in sequence.

Finally, the above remarks apply equally well to displacements of retinal images caused by small eye movements. The normal eye is not stationary, but is subject to several types of fine movements. There is psychophysical evidence that in man these may play an important part in vision, transforming a steady stimulus produced by a stationary object into an intermittent one, so overcoming adaptation in visual cells (Ditchburn & Ginsborg, 1952; Riggs, Ratliff, Cornsweet & Cornsweet, 1953). At an early stage in the visual pathway the effect of such movements would be to excite many cells repeatedly and in turn, rather than just a few continuously. A given line or border would move back and forth over a small retinal region; in the cortex this would sequentially activate many cells with simple fields. Since large rotatory movements are not involved, these fields would have the same axis orientations but would differ only in their exact retinal positions. They would converge on higher-order cells with complex fields, and these would tend to be activated continuously rather than intermittently.

Functional Cytoarchitecture

There is an interesting parallel between the functional subdivisions of the cortex described in the present paper, and those found in somatosensory cortex by Mountcastle (1957) in the cat, and by Powell & Mountcastle (1959) in the monkey. Here, as in the visual area, one can subdivide the cortex on the basis of responses to natural stimuli into regions which are roughly columnar in shape, and extend from surface to white matter. This is especially noteworthy since the visual and somatic areas are the only cortical regions so far studied at the single-cell level from the standpoint of functional architecture. In both areas the columnar organization is superimposed upon the well known systems of topographic representation—of the body surface in the one case, and the visual fields in the other. In the somatosensory cortex the columns are determined by the sensory submodality to which the cells of a column respond: in one type of column the cells are affected either by light touch or by bending of hairs, whereas in the other the cells respond to stimulation of deep fascia or manipulation of joints.

Several differences between the two systems will at once be apparent. In the visual cortex the columns are determined by the criterion of receptive-field axis orientation. Presumably there are as many types of column as there are recognizable differences in orientation. At present one can be sure that there are at least ten or twelve, but the number may be very large, since it is possible that no two columns represent precisely the same axis orientation. (A subdivision of cells or of columns into twelve groups according to angle of orientation shows that there is no clear prevalence of one group over any of the others.) In the somatosensory cortex, on the other hand, there are only two recognized types of column.

A second major difference between the two systems lies in the very nature of the criteria used for the subdivisions. The somatosensory cortex is divided by submodality, a characteristic depending on the incoming sensory fibres, and not on any transformations made by the cortex on the afferent impulses. Indeed we have as yet little information on what integrative processes do take place in the somatosensory cortex. In the visual cortex there is no modality difference between the input to one column and that to the next, but it is in the connexions between afferents and cortical cells, or in the interconnexions between cortical cells, that the differences must exist.

Ultimately, however, the two regions of the cortex may not prove so dissimilar. Further information on the functional role of the somatic cortex may conceivably bring to light a second system of columns, superimposed on the present one. Similarly, in the visual system future work may disclose other subdivisions cutting across those described in this paper, and based on other criteria. For the present it would seem unwise to look upon the columns in the visual cortex as entirely autonomous functional units. While the variation in field size from cell to cell within a column is generally of the sort suggested in Text-figs. 9 and 15, the presence of an occasional cell with a very large complex field (up to about 20°) makes one wonder whether columns with similar receptive-field orientations may not possess some interconnexions.

Binocular Interaction

The presence in the striate cortex of cells influenced from both eyes has already been observed by several authors (Hubel & Wiesel, 1959; Cornehls & Grüsser, 1959; Burns, Heron & Grafstein, 1960), and is confirmed in Part II of this paper. Our results suggest that the convergence of influences from the two eyes is extensive, since binocular effects could be demonstrated in 84% of our cells, and since the two eyes were equally, or almost equally, effective in 70% (groups 3–5). This represents a much greater degree of interaction than was suggested by our original work, or by Grüsser and Grüsser-Cornehls (see Jung, 1960), who found that only 30% of their cells were binocularly influenced.

For each of our cells comparison of receptive fields mapped in the two eyes showed that, except for a difference in strength of responses related to eye dominance, the fields were in every way similar. They were similarly organized, had the same axis orientation, and occupied corresponding regions in the two retinas. The responses to stimuli applied to corresponding parts of the two receptive fields showed summation. This should be important in binocular vision, for it means that when the two images produced by an object fall on corresponding parts of the two retinas, their separate effects on a cortical cell should sum. Failure of the images to fall on corresponding regions, which might happen if an object were closer than the point of fixation or further away, would tend to reduce the summation; it could even lead to mutual antagonism if excitatory parts of one field were stimulated at the same time as inhibitory parts of the other. It should be emphasized that for all simple fields and for many complex ones the two eyes may work either synergistically or in opposition, depending on how the receptive fields are stimulated; when identical stimuli are shone on corresponding parts of the two retinas their effects should always sum.

Although in the cortex the proportion of binocularly influenced cells is high, the mixing of influences from the two eyes is far from complete. Not only are many single cells unequally influenced by the two eyes, but the relative eye dominance differs greatly from one cell to another. This could simply reflect an intermediate stage in the process of mixing of influences from the two eyes; in that case we might expect an increasing uniformity in the eye preference of higher-order cells. But cells with complex fields do not appear to differ, in their distribution among the different eye-dominance groups, from the general population of cortical cells (Text-fig. 12). At present we have no clear notion of the physiological significance of this incomplete mixing of influences from the two eyes. One possible hint lies in the fact that by binocular parallax alone (even with a stimulus too brief to allow changes in the convergence of the eyes) one can tell which of two objects is the closer (Dove, 1841; von Recklinghausen, 1861). This would clearly be impossible if the two retinas were connected to the brain in identical fashion, for then the eyes (or the two pictures of a stereo-pair) could be interchanged without substituting near points for far ones and vice versa.

Comparison of Receptive Fields in the Frog and the Cat

Units in many respects similar to striate cortical cells with complex fields have recently been isolated from the intact optic nerve and the optic tectum of the frog (Lettvin, Maturana, McCulloch & Pitts, 1959; Maturana, Lettvin, McCulloch & Pitts, 1960). There is indirect evidence to suggest that the units are the non-myelinated axons or axon terminals of retinal ganglion cells, rather than tectal cells or efferent optic nerve fibres. In common with complex cortical cells, these units respond to objects and shadows in the visual field in ways that could not have been predicted from responses to small spots of light. They thus have 'complex' properties, in the sense that we have used this term. Yet in their detailed behaviour they differ greatly from any cells yet studied in the cat, at any level from retina to cortex. We have not, for example, seen 'erasable' responses or found 'convex edge detectors'. On the other hand, it seems that some cells in the frog have asymmetrical responses to movement and some have what we have termed a 'receptive-field axis'.

Assuming that the units described in the frog are fibres from retinal ganglion cells, one may ask whether similar fibres exist in the cat, but have been missed because of their small size. We lack exact information on the fibre spectrum of the cat's optic nerve; the composite action potential suggests that non-myelinated fibres are present, though in smaller numbers than in the frog (Bishop, 1933; Bishop & O'Leary, 1940). If their fields are different from the well known concentric type, they must have little part to play in the geniculo-cortical pathway, since geniculate cells all appear to have concentric-type fields (Hubel & Wiesel, 1961). The principal cells of the lateral geniculate body (those that send their axons to the striate cortex) are of fairly uniform size, and it seems unlikely that a large group would have gone undetected. The smallest fibres in the cat's optic nerve probably project to the tectum or the pretectal region; in view of the work in the frog, it will be interesting to examine their receptive fields.

At first glance it may seem astonishing that the complexity of third-order neurones in the frog's visual system should be equalled only by that of sixth-order neurones in the geniculo-cortical pathway of the cat. Yet this is less surprising if one notes the great anatomical differences in the two animals, especially the lack, in the frog, of any cortex or dorsal lateral geniculate body. There is undoubtedly a parallel difference in the use each animal makes of its visual system: the frog's visual apparatus is presumably specialized to recognize a limited number of stereotyped patterns or situations, compared with the high acuity and versatility found in the cat. Probably it is not so unreasonable to find that in the cat the specialization of cells for complex operations is postponed to a higher level, and that when it does occur, it is carried out by a vast number of cells, and in great detail. Perhaps even more surprising, in view of what seem to be profound physiological differences, is the superficial anatomical similarity of retinas in the cat and the frog. It is possible that with Golgi methods a comparison of the connexions between cells in the two animals may help us in understanding the physiology of both structures.

Receptive Fields of Cells in the Primate Cortex

We have been anxious to learn whether receptive fields of cells in the monkey's visual cortex have properties similar to those we have described in the cat. A few preliminary experiments on the spider monkey have shown striking similarities. For example, both simple and complex fields have been observed in the striate area. Future work will very likely show differences, since the striate cortex of the monkey is in several ways different morphologically from that of the cat. But the similarities already seen suggest that the mechanisms we have described may be relevant to many mammals, and in particular to man.

SUMMARY

1. The visual cortex was studied in anaesthetized cats by recording extracellularly from single cells. Light-adapted eyes were stimulated with spots of white light of various shapes, stationary or moving.

2. Receptive fields of cells in the visual cortex varied widely in their organization. They tended to fall into two categories, termed 'simple' and 'complex'.

3. There were several types of simple receptive fields, differing in the spatial distribution of excitatory and inhibitory ('on' and 'off') regions. Summation occurred within either type of region; when the two opposing regions were illuminated together their effects tended to cancel. There was generally little or no response to stimulation of the entire receptive field with diffuse light. The most effective stimulus configurations, dictated by the spatial arrangements of excitatory and inhibitory regions, were long narrow rectangles of light (slits), straight-line borders between areas of different brightness (edges), and dark rectangular bars against a light background. For maximum response the shape, position and orientation of these stimuli were critical. The orientation of the receptive-field axis (i.e. that of the optimum stimulus) varied from cell to cell; it could be vertical, horizontal or oblique. No particular orientation seemed to predominate.

4. Receptive fields were termed complex when the response to light could not be predicted from the arrangements of excitatory and inhibitory regions. Such regions could generally not be demonstrated; when they could the laws of summation and mutual antagonism did not apply. The stimuli that were most effective in activating cells with simple fields—slits, edges, and dark bars—were also the most effective for cells with complex fields. The orientation of a stimulus for optimum response was critical, just as with simple fields. Complex fields, however, differed from simple fields in that a stimulus was effective wherever it was placed in the field, provided that the orientation was appropriate.

5. Receptive fields in or near the area centralis varied in diameter from ½–1° up to about 5–6°. On the average, complex fields were larger than simple ones. In more peripheral parts of the

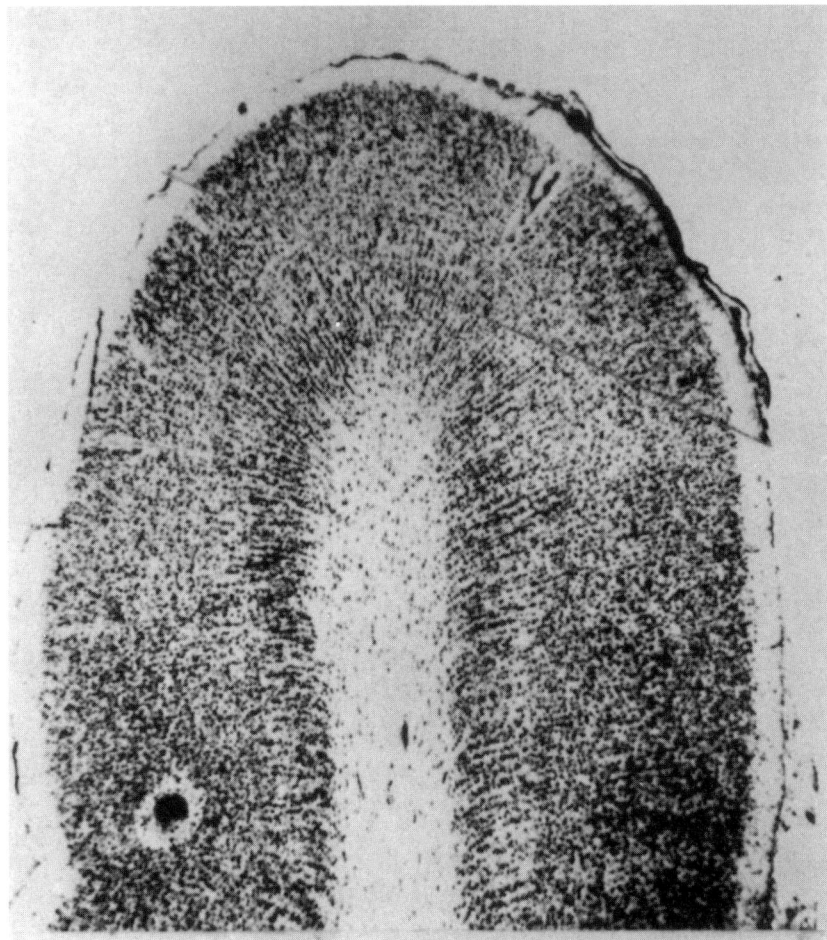

Plate 1. Coronal section through post-lateral gyrus. Composite photomicrograph of two of the sections used to reconstruct the micro-electrode track of Text-fig. 13. The first part of the electrode track may be seen in the upper right; the electrolytic lesion at the end of the track appears in the lower left. Scale 1 mm.

retina the fields tended to be larger. Widths of the long narrow excitatory or inhibitory portions of simple receptive fields were often roughly equal to the diameter of the smallest geniculate receptive-field centres in the area centralis. For cells with complex fields responding to slits or dark bars the optimum stimulus width was also usually of this order of magnitude.

6. Four fifths of all cells were influenced independently by the two eyes. In a binocularly influenced cell the two receptive fields had the same organization and axis orientation, and were situated in corresponding parts of the two retinas. Summation was seen when correspon-

ding parts of the two retinas were stimulated in identical fashion. The relative influence of the two eyes differed from cell to cell: for some cells the two eyes were about equal; in others one eye, the ipsilateral or contralateral, dominated.

7. Functional architecture was studied by (*a*) comparing the responses of cells recorded in sequence during micro-electrode penetrations through the cortex, (*b*) observing the unresolved background activity, and (*c*) comparing cells recorded simultaneously with a single electrode (multiple recordings). The retinas were found to project upon the cortex in an orderly fashion, as described by previous authors. Most record-

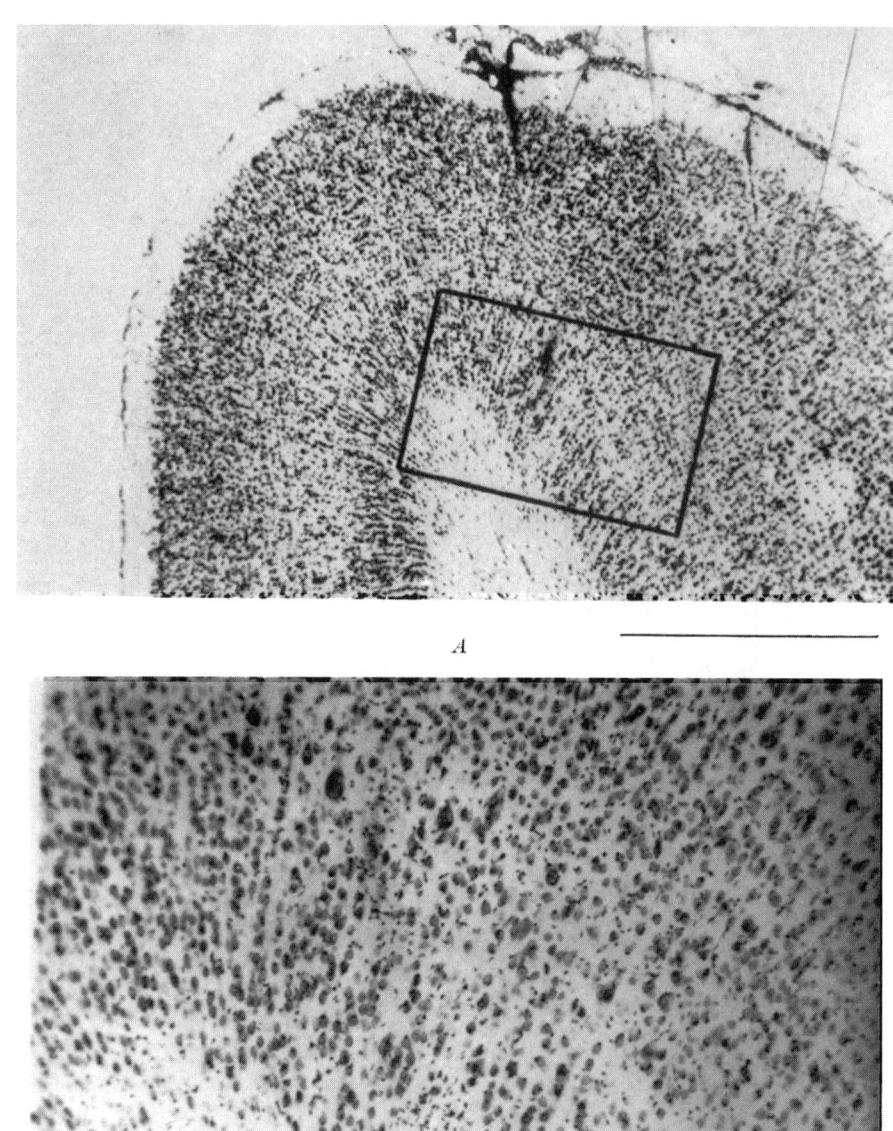

A

B

Plate 2. A, coronal section through the anterior extremity of post-lateral gyrus. Composite photomicrograph made from four of the sections used to reconstruct the two electrode tracks shown in Text-fig. 14. The first part of the two electrode tracks may be seen crossing layer 1. The lesion at the end of the lateral track (to the right in the figure) is easily seen; that of the medial track is smaller, and is shown at higher power in B. Scales: A, 1 mm, B, 0.25 mm.

ings were made from the cortical region receiving projections from the area of central vision. The cortex was found to be divisible into discrete columns; within each column the cells all had the same receptive-field axis orientation. The columns appeared to extend from surface to white matter; cross-sectional diameters at the surface were of the order of 0.5 mm. Within a given column one found various types of simple and complex fields; these were situated in the same general retinal region, and usually overlapped, although they differed slightly in their exact retinal position. The relative influence of the two eyes was not necessarily the same for all cells in a column.

8. It is suggested that columns containing cells with common receptive-field axis orientations are functional units, in which cells with simple fields represent an early stage in organization, possibly receiving their afferents directly from lateral geniculate cells, and cells with complex fields are of higher order, receiving projections from a number of cells with simple fields within the same column. Some possible implications of these findings for form perception are discussed.

We wish to thank Miss Jaye Robinson and Mrs Jane Chen for their technical assistance. We are also indebted to Miss Sally Fox and to Dr S. W. Kuffler for their helpful criticism of this manuscript. The work was supported in part by Research Grants B-2251 and B-2260 from United States Public Health Service, and in part by the United States Air Force through the Air Force Office of Scientific Research of the Air Research and Development Command under contract No. AF 49 (638)-713. The work was done during the tenure of a U.S. Public Health Service Senior Research Fellowship No. SF 304-R by D.H.H.

References

Bishop, G. H. (1933). Fiber groups in the optic nerve. *Amer. J. Physiol.* **106**, 460–474.

Bishop, G. H. & O'Leary, J. S. (1940). Electrical activity of the lateral geniculate of cats following optic nerve stimuli. *J. Neurophysiol.* **3**, 308–322.

Bishop, P. O., Burke, W. & Davis, R. (1959). Activation of single lateral geniculate cells by stimulation of either optic nerve. *Science,* **130**, 506–507.

Burns, B. D., Heron, W. & Grafstein, B. (1960). Response of cerebral cortex to diffuse monocular and binocular stimulation. *Amer. J. Physiol.* **198**, 200–204.

Cornehls, U. & Grüsser, O.-J. (1959). Ein elektronisch gesteuertes Doppellichtreizgerät. *Pflüg. Arch. ges. Physiol.* **270**, 78–79.

Daniel, P. M. & Whitteridge, D. (1959). The representation of the visual field on the calcarine cortex in baboons and monkeys. *J. Physiol.* **148**, 33P.

Ditchburn, R. W. & Ginsborg, B. L. (1952). Vision with stabilized retinal image. *Nature, Lond.,* **170**, 36–37.

Dove, H. W. (1841). Die Combination der Eindrücke beider Ohren und beider Augen zu einem Eindruck. *Mber. preuss. Akad.* **1841**, 251–252.

Erulkar, S. D. & Fillenz, M. (1958). Patterns of discharge of single units of the lateral geniculate body of the cat in response to binocular stimulation. *J. Physiol.* **140**, 6–7P.

Erulkar, S. D. & Fillenz, M. (1960). Single-unit activity in the lateral geniculate body of the cat. *J. Physiol.* **154**, 206–218.

Grüsser, O.-J. & Sauer, G. (1960). Monoculare und binoculare Lichtreizung einzelner Neurone im Geniculatum laterale der Katze. *Pflüg. Arch. ges. Physiol.* **271**, 595–612.

Hayhow, W. R. (1958). The cytoarchitecture of the lateral geniculate body in the cat in relation to the distribution of crossed and uncrossed optic fibers. *J. comp. Neurol.* **110**, 1–64.

Hubel, D. H. (1957). Tungsten microelectrode for recording from single units. *Science,* **125**, 549–550.

Hubel, D. H. (1958). Cortical unit responses to visual stimuli in nonanesthetized cats. *Amer. J. Ophthal.* **46**, 110–121.

Hubel, D. H. (1959). Single unit activity in striate cortex of unrestrained cats. *J. Physiol.* **147**, 226–238.

Hubel, D. H. (1960). Single unit activity in lateral geniculate body and optic tract of unrestrained cats. *J. Physiol.* **150**, 91–104.

Hubel, D. H. & Wiesel, T. N. (1959). Receptive fields of single neurones in the cat's striate cortex. *J. Physiol.* **148**, 574–591.

Hubel, D. H. & Wiesel, T. N. (1960). Receptive fields of optic nerve fibres in the spider monkey. *J. Physiol.* **154**, 572–580.

Hubel, D. H. & Wiesel, T. N. (1961). Integrative action in the cat's lateral geniculate body. *J. Physiol.* **155**, 385–398.

Jung, R. (1960). Microphysiologie corticaler Neurone: Ein Beitrag zur Koordination der Hirnrinde und des visuellen Systems. *Structure and Function of the Cerebral Cortex,* ed. Tower, D. B. and Schadé, J. P. Amsterdam: Elsevier Publishing Company.

Kuffler, S. W. (1953). Discharge patterns and functional organization of mammalian retina. *J. Neurophysiol.* **16**, 37–68.

Lettvin, J. Y., Maturana, H. R., McCulloch, W. S. & Pitts, W. H. (1959). What the frog's eye tells the frog's brain. *Proc. Inst. Radio Engrs, N.Y.,* **47**, 1940–1951.

Maturana, H. R., Lettvin, J. Y., McCulloch, W. S. & Pitts, W. H. (1960). Anatomy and physiology of vision in the frog (*Rana pipiens*). *J. gen. Physiol.* **43**, part 2, 129–176.

Minkowski, M. (1913). Experimentelle Untersuchungen über die Beziehungen der Gross-hirnrinde und der Netzhaut zu den primären optischen Zentren, besonders zum Corpus geniculatum externum. *Arb. hirnanat. Inst. Zürich,* **7**, 259–362.

Mountcastle, V. B. (1957). Modality and topographic properties of single neurons of cat's somatic sensory cortex. *J. Neurophysiol.* **20**, 408–434.

O'Leary, J. L. (1941). Structure of the area striata of the cat. *J. comp. Neurol.* **75**, 131–164.

Polyak, S. (1957). *The Vertebrate Visual System,* ed. Klüver, H. The University of Chicago Press.

Powell, T. P. S. & Mountcastle, V. B. (1959). Some aspects of the functional organization of the cortex of the postcentral gyrus of the monkey: a correlation of findings obtained in a single unit analysis with cytoarchitecture. *Johns Hopk. Hosp. Bull.* **105**, 133–162.

Riggs, L. A., Ratliff, F., Cornsweet, J. C. & Cornsweet, T. N. (1953). The disappearance of steadily fixated visual test objects. *J. opt. Soc. Amer.* **43**, 495–501.

Silva, P. S. (1956). Some anatomical and physiological aspects of the lateral geniculate body. *J. comp. Neurol.* **106**, 463–486.

Talbot, S. A. (1942). A lateral localization in the cat's visual cortex. *Fed. Proc.* **1**, 84.

Talbot, S. A. & Marshall, W. H. (1941). Physiological studies on neural mechanisms of visual localization and discrimination. *Amer. J. Ophthal.* **24**, 1255–1263.

Thompson, J. M., Woolsey, C. N. & Talbot, S. A. (1950). Visual areas I and II of cerebral cortex of rabbit. *J. Neurophysiol.* **13**, 277–288.

von Recklinghausen, F. (1861). Zum körperlichen Sehen. *Ann. Phys. Lpz.* **114**, 170–173.

AFTERWORD

In the decade that followed this paper, we had few comments from other neurophysiologists, perhaps partly because so few people were doing single-cell studies in the cortex. But slowly this changed: papers appeared that elaborated, extended, and to an extent complicated what we had thought was a fairly clean picture. Our main interlocutors in the beginning were Peter Bishop and his colleagues, and the main problem was his redefining our terms *simple* and *complex* on the basis of recordings made almost exclusively with moving stimuli. To qualify as a simple cell, by our definition, one had to show a clear segregation of the receptive field into regions that responded to stationary stimuli with excitation or inhibition (for example, with on or off responses). One could not object to the use of moving stimuli, only to the terminological confusion. It was hard for us to be sure that Bishop's simple cells did not include cells we would have classed as complex. We did not write rebuttals, but over the years we simply continued to use the terms *simple* and *complex* in the way we originally defined them. Much of the same confusion arose again in subsequent work in macaque monkeys, though here the quarrel (much too strong a word!) was with a different Peter (in this case, Schiller). In our opinion there was again the problem of using moving stimuli in defining simple and complex cells. If those terms were to be used, it seemed to us important to show beyond doubt that they were being used to refer to same cell categories—or else invent new terms. (Some authors did invent new terms, such as *s* for *simple,* but we thought that only perpetuated the confusion.)

In a book of his collected papers on audition, von Békésy stresses the importance and usefulness of enemies in keeping one honest, and he emphasizes the distinction between good enemies and bad ones. Both Peters were good enemies, of the highest quality, but in a field as complex as ours it would be strange if there had been no differences. With time, this problem of definition seems to have receded, and our original definitions of simple and complex cells seem to have prevailed. What is gratifying is the possibility of having scientific differences with one's contemporaries, and yet maintaining close friendships and lively dialogues with them.

Charles Gilbert, one of our first graduate students, and later a close colleague of Torsten's at Harvard and then at the Rockefeller Institute, devoted his graduate thesis to a close layer-by-layer examination of receptive fields of cells in the cat striate cortex. Compared to his thorough study, our results in this 1962 paper can only be regarded as "preliminary".

We can perhaps be forgiven for missing the hypercomplex cells (later called *end-stopped*) in these our first ventures into the striate cortex. We missed them partly because they are less common in cat striate cortex, and probably partly because we failed to try short slits when cells failed to respond to longer ones. Cells that are injured often show it by failing to respond to otherwise effective stimuli, so that an unresponsive cell can be hard to assess. The story of our discovery of hypercomplex cells, first in cat cortical area 19, then in cat visual 2, and finally by Charles Gilbert in striate cortex, will be told in the context of our long 1965 paper (Chapter 11).

Our proposals as to how simple cells are built up from center-surround cells, and complex from simple (immortalized in Figs. 19 and 20) have been the subject of much debate in the ensuing decades, and numbers of alternative circuits have been proposed. Our schemes were merely the simplest we could think of, and neither of us would have been heartbroken had they needed radical amendment or been proven completely wrong. Our main point was that the cells' behavior must surely be the product of *some* circuit involving excitation or inhibition, or both. The commonest proposed alternative circuits have involved inhibition, perhaps because of a wistful hope (still largely unfulfilled) of finding a use for the inhibitory synapses said by neuroanatomists to be so prevalent in cortex.

One the first of these invokers of inhibition was Otto Creutzfeldt, in Munich and later Göttingen. He proposed that for a simple cortical cell with an excitatory center strip, the center should be determined by an excitatory input from a single incoming geniculate on-center cell, and the orientation selectivity be supplied by inhibitory inputs from other on-center geniculate cells, with fields cutting in at either side. We felt that this ingenious idea was made less likely by our observation that, for any given eccentricity, the widths of the center strips of simple fields were about the same as the diameters of the centres of geniculate fields, and that the lengths of the strips were many times greater. Another set of proposals, championed mainly by Colin Blakemore, was based in part on the psychophysical phenomenon known as the *tilt effect:* that a set of parallel vertical lines is seen as tilted after prolonged viewing of parallel lines that are not quite vertical. Here the idea was that a cell's orientation selectivity should be sharpened if it received inhibitory connections from other cells whose optimal orientations were slightly different. Against that, we felt, was our failure to see any marked differences in degree of orientation selectivity between simple and complex cells. The possibility that preparing tuning curves of hundreds of simple and complex cells might bring out such differences did not bother us, because we could hardly get excited about an effect so feeble as to require statistics for its demonstration.

An inhibitory mechanism to explain orientation selectivity was felt by some to be supported by the lessening or elimination of the selectivity by antagonists of inhibition such as bicuculline (Sillito, A. M. 1975, *J Physiol* 250, 305–329). We had for years observed that orientation selectivity can be impaired by any form of injury, and suspected that the effects Sillito had described were the result of nonspecific injury by the bicuculline.

Meanwhile subsequent work has served to justify our original scheme, especially the work of Clay Reid (Reid and J. M. Alonso [1995] *Nature,* 378:281–284) and David Ferster (Ferster, Chung & Wheat, 1996, *Nature,* 380, 249–252). We are sure that the last word has not been said on this topic, but we continue to be interested, if relaxed. In a *Nature* "News and Views" commentary on Ferster's paper (*Nature,* 1996; 380:197–198), I remarked that the evidence supporting our original scheme for the geniculate-to-simple cell projection scheme had been 35 years in coming, and hoped that it wouldn't take until A.D. 2031 for the simple- to complex circuit to be vindicated or disproved.

Chapter 11 • Recordings from Cat Prestriate Areas, 18 and 19 •

FOREWORD

This is one of our all-time longest papers, so long, indeed, that neither of us had carefully reread it until writing the present book made that necessary. Our readers must have shared our enthusiasm, because we still have hundreds of reprints left over. It is probably more a monograph than a paper in the usual sense, and shares with monographs its tiny readership. Its range is wide, encompassing topography, columnar architecture, physiological mapping, conventional Nissl, myelin, and silver-degeneration (Nauta-method) histology, and receptive-field analysis. It contains the first description of end-stopped (hypercomplex) cells. It represents our first use of single-cell recordings combined with electrolytic lesions and Nauta silver-degeneration anatomy, a combination we were to exploit further a few years later in examining geniculo-cortical connexions in monkeys.

Had we split the paper into three or four shorter papers it might have had more impact—or more readers.

Obviously our main purpose in this research was to continue the quest the two of us and Steve had outlined that morning at the Hopkins canteen, to learn what happens to visual information as one goes farther and farther along the visual path. The next place to look was visual 2, which had already been mapped retinotopically in the cat by Talbot, way back in 1942 (*Fed Proc* 1:84)—not in 1941 by Talbot and Marshall, as our references suggest. Our paper was thus a followup of Talbot's work, all of 23 years later. Between those dates the only study of visual area 2 was that of Thompson, Woolsey, and Talbot, in 1950, with a more thorough description of the topography in the rabbit.

Receptive Fields and Functional Architecture in Two Nonstriate Visual Areas (18 and 19) of the Cat[1]

DAVID H. HUBEL AND TORSTEN N. WIESEL • *Neurophysiology Laboratory, Department of Pharmacology,*

Harvard Medical School, Boston, Massachusetts

To understand vision in physiological terms represents a formidable problem for the biologist. It amounts to learning how the nervous system handles incoming messages so that form, color, movement, and depth can be perceived and interpreted. One approach, perhaps the most direct, is to stimulate the retina with patterns of light while recording from single cells or fibers at various points along the visual pathway. For each cell the optimum stimulus can be determined, and one can note the characteristics common to cells at each level in the visual pathway, and compare a given level with the next.

From studies carried out in the cat it is clear that visual messages undergo considerable modification, within the retina and the lateral geniculate body, and especially within the striate cortex (16, 12, 10, 13). Retinalganglion and geniculate cells respond optimally to an appropriately placed spot of light of just the right size; a smaller or larger spot is less effective. Cells at these levels therefore register not simply the illumination of a region on the retina, but also the difference in illumination between a region and its surround. In the striate cortex cells are far more complex and diverse in their response properties. The great majority respond best to straight-line stimuli: for a given cell the optimum stimulus may be a white or dark line, or an edge separating light from dark. A line stimulus is effective only when shone in an orientation that is characteristic for the cell; there is typically no response when the stimulus is shone at 90° to the optimum orientation, and the range of orientations over which a response is evoked may be 30° or even less. Some cells prefer one inclination, others another, and we have no evidence that any one orientation, such as vertical or horizontal, is more common than another. For some cells, termed "simple," the exact position of the stimulus is critical: even a slight displacement of the line to a new position, without changing its orientation, produces a dramatic decrease in the response. These properties of simple cells are dictated by the arrangement of excitatory and inhibitory regions of the receptive field, as mapped with small-spot stimulation (10). The simplest assumption is that each of the simple cortical cells receives its input directly from a specific group of cells in the lateral geniculate body (13, text-Fig. 19). Other cells, termed "complex," respond to an appropriately oriented stimulus regardless of where in the receptive field it is positioned. These cells behave as though they received projections from a large number of simple cortical cells, all having the same receptive-field arrangement and orientation, but differing in the exact retinal positions of these fields (13, text-Fig. 20).

All of this suggests a highly specific and intricate set of cortical connections, first between the incoming geniculate axons and the simple cortical cells, and then between certain simple cells and certain complex ones. Strong indirect support for the specific connections between simple and complex cells comes from a study of cortical functional architecture. From single long microelectrode penetrations and from multiple short penetrations it can be shown that neighboring cells in the striate cortex usually have the same receptive-field orientation, and roughly the same receptive-field position. In fact, cells having the same receptive-field orientation are aggregated into regions of columnar shape extending from surface to white matter,

From *J. Neurophysiol.* (1965) 28, 229–289

Received for publication August 24, 1964.

[1]This work was supported in part by Research Grants NB-02260-05 and NB-02253-06 from the National Institutes of Health, and in part by Research Grant AF-AFOSR-62-76 from the U.S. Air Force.

with walls perpendicular to the cortical layers (13, 14). Such an arrangement means that the very cells that are supposed to be interconnected on physiological grounds—simple and complex cells with the same receptive-field orientation, and a certain small variation in receptive-field position—are in fact grouped together, and are therefore highly likely to be interconnected also on anatomical grounds. This columnar system presumably makes for great economy in length and number of interconnections.

A given small region of retina is thus represented in the striate cortex many times, first in a column representing one orientation, then in a column representing another. For the entire visual field such an analysis must require a very large number of columns, and an even greater number of cells. One can now begin to understand the dramatic increase in the number of cells as one goes from geniculate to striate cortex.

To pursue this work further it is obviously necessary to learn where the next steps in integration occur. The efferent connections of the cat striate cortex have not been worked out in any great detail, but a number of results in the cat and other species suggest that there are multiple projections, both cortical and subcortical. We have begun by looking at the cortex itself, first examining the cortical regions just lateral to the striate. These areas have long been suspected, on various grounds, of being involved in vision. The strongest physiological evidence for this was presented in 1941 by Talbot and Marshall (27). Stimulating the retinas with small spots of light, and recording evoked potentials, they mapped out in each hemisphere of the cat cortex two orderly topographic projections of the contralateral half-field of vision. The more medial of the two areas, which they termed "visual area I," seems from their maps to correspond roughly to the anatomically defined striate cortex; the lateral area, termed "visual II," has not yet been correlated with cytoarchitecture.

In the present study we explored the cortex from medial to lateral in successive penetrations, crossing from visual I into Talbot and Marshall's visual II, and then continuing into what has proved to be a third distinct topographically organized visual area lying lateral to the second. We have called this region "visual area III."

In analyzing visual II and III we have followed our usual procedure of describing cells in terms of their responses to visual stimulation, attempting at the same time to build up a picture of cortical architecture by comparing the behavior of neighboring cells, and of cells recorded in sequence, in long penetrations. Our hope has been to learn how the next stages of integration make use of the input from cells of the striate cortex, and to find out whether the columnar plan of architecture that is present in the primary visual area holds also for higher areas. Finally, we have made a correlation of the three physiologically defined visual areas with the histological variations of the cortex as seen on Nissl- and myelin-stained sections, and have used the Nauta technique to establish that visual areas II and III actually receive direct projections from visual I.

METHODS

Seventeen cats were used. Procedures for preparing the animal, including anesthesia, immobilization of eyes, correction of refractive errors, and mapping of area centralis and optic discs on the projection screen, have all been described elsewhere (10, 11, 13). The retinas were stimulated by shining spots or patterns of light from a tungsten filament projector onto a wide movable tangent screen at 1.5 m. distance. Recordings were made in the light-adapted state. Background illumination was about 1.0 cd/m^2, and stimuli were 0.5–1.5 log units brighter than the background. All recordings were made with tungsten microelectrodes (8). In nine experiments (11 penetrations) a small hole was drilled in the skull over the right hemisphere, the dura incised, and a 19-gauge hollow stainless steel needle cemented into the hole with its lumen close to the cortex, to form a closed chamber; the electrode was hydraulically introduced through the needle. In each of the remaining eight experiments a number of penetrations were made through a modified Davies chamber (4) which was cemented onto the skull (14); the brain was photographed through a dissecting microscope and an enlarged print was used to indicate the points of entry of the electrode relative to cortical blood vessels. Forty-two penetrations were made in these mapping experiments. At the end of each experiment the brain was perfused with saline followed by formol-saline, the calvarium removed, and the brain photographed again. All brains were imbedded in celloidin, sectioned serially at 26 μ., and stained with cresyl violet (Nissl) or Loyez stain (myelin). In each penetration one or several lesions were made by passing direct current through the electrode (about 5 μA. for 5 sec.). The lesions were used to reconstruct electrode tracks (9, 13). Destructive lesions for silver-degeneration studies by the Nauta method (22) were made in four cats with coarse electrodes (30–35 μ. from end of insulation to tip); currents of the order of 10 μA. were passed for 10 sec. In two cats lesions were made by stabbing the cortex with a 25-gauge hypodermic needle.

RESULTS

Part I. Visual Areas I, II, and III: Physiological Mapping and Correlation with Histology

Topographical Representation[2]

All of the 53 penetrations of the present experiments were made from the lateral, postlateral, and middle and posterior suprasylvian gyri, at levels close to the junction or region of overlap of the lateral and postlateral sulci (Horsley-Clarke coordinates P 4.0-A 4.0). Topographic mapping was thus confined to regions of cortex in and lateral to the striate representation of the area centralis and parts of the visual field a few degrees below it. We have shown previously that in the course of a long penetration down the mesial (interhemispheric) segment of the lateral or postlateral gyrus parallel to the surface, the receptive fields of successively recorded cells tend gradually to move out into the contralateral half-field of vision (13: Text-fig. 13 and p. 134). The visual I representation of the midline (the vertical meridian) is located deep in the lateral bank of the postlateral gyrus at posterior levels, while more anteriorly it appears on the surface of the lateral gyrus close to where the postlateral sulcus ends, and then crosses the gyrus obliquely from lateral to medial. This line forms the lateral border of visual area I (compare the boundary between 17 and 18 in Fig. 37).

The cortical region lateral to visual I was first explored by making deep microelectrode penetrations along both walls of the postlateral sulcus. In the experiment illustrated in Fig. 1 the electrode tip passed obliquely along the entire medial wall of the sulcus, crossed the underlying white matter, and ended in the upper bank of the splenial sulcus. The positions of the receptive fields in the contralateral visual field are shown to the left of the figure. Each diagram shows one or several receptive fields in relation to the center of gaze (the area centralis projection), which is re-represented in each diagram

by the crossing of the short horizontal lines and the long common vertical line. Fields of successive cells are shown on the same diagram if their orientations are the same, i.e., if they are located in the same column (see below). At the outset the cells had their receptive fields very close to the vertical meridian. As the electrode advanced from one cell to the next there were slight, more or less random fluctuations in field positions. Superimposed on these fluctuations one could detect a gradual trend outward, into the contralateral half-field of vision, so that deep in the postlateral sulcus the fields had moved out about 8–10°. In the white matter a few geniculate axons were recognized by their clustered firing pattern (9, 12), and by the concentric center-surround arrangement of their receptive fields; some of the fields were located near the center of gaze, others in the far periphery. Finally, four cells recorded from suprasplenial striate cortex (i.e., from visual I) had their receptive fields 35–50° out in the contralateral visual field, close to the horizontal meridian.

In another experiment the postlateral sulcus was explored in its lateral bank at a slightly more posterior level (Fig. 2). The first cells had their receptive fields 15–20° out in the contralateral field of vision close to the horizontal meridian. As the electrode advanced down the bank there was a rapid inward drift in field position, so that halfway down the fields were about 5–10° from the center of gaze. The electrode then crossed the sulcus to the opposite bank; here the fields of six cells were only about 5° out, and there was little or no detectable over-all drift as the full thickness of cortex was traversed, undoubtedly because this part of the penetration was almost perpendicular to the cortical layering. Several geniculate axons were recorded from white matter: their fields (not illustrated) were near the area centralis. Finally, a single cell recorded from the interhemispheric gray matter had its receptive field 17° out from the midline.

These two experiments suggest that as one proceeds laterally along the cortex, starting at the lateral margin of the primary visual area, the receptive fields of cells move out from the vertical meridian into the contralateral half-field of vision. This, together with other experiments to be illus-

---

[2]Names of gyri and sulci used in this study are generally those of Winkler and Potter (31); they are illustrated in Fig. 37.

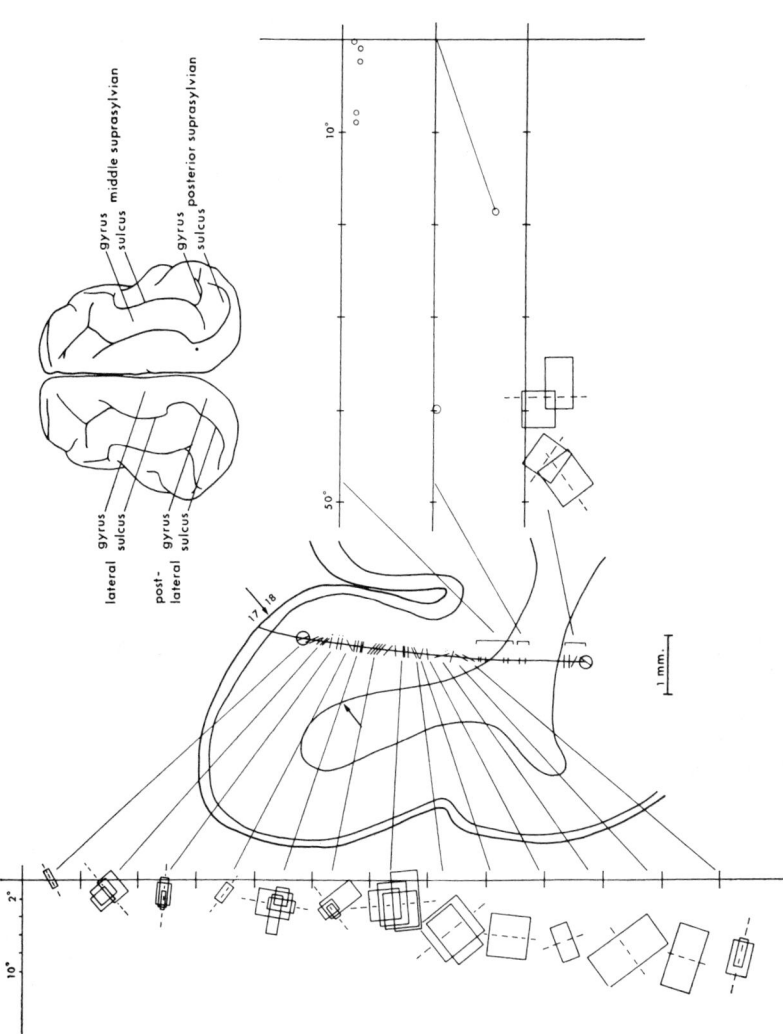

Fig. 1. Reconstruction of an electrode track which passed down along the medial wall of the right postlateral sulcus. Tracing of a coronal section through the postlateral gyrus is shown near the center of the figure. To the upper right is a tracing of a photograph of the dorsal view of the brain (anterior is to the top of the figure): point of entry of electrode is indicated by a dot. Electrode entered cortex close to the 17–18 boundary (i.e., the visual I–visual II boundary); and a lesion was made at the point where the first cells were recorded (indicated by a circle). A second lesion was made at the end of the penetration, in the upper bank of the splenial sulcus. Lines intersecting the electrode track indicate single units; the longer lines, cells; the shorter, axons. Orientations of receptive fields of cells are indicated by the directions of these lines: a line perpendicular to track represents a vertical orientation; a line-plus-dot perpendicular to track represents a horizontal orientation. To the left, the position of each receptive field in the visual field is given with respect to the area centralis (center of gaze), which is indicated separately for every change of receptive-field orientation, by the intersection of the long common vertical line (the vertical meridian) and the short horizontal crossbars. Receptive-field orientations are shown by interrupted lines.

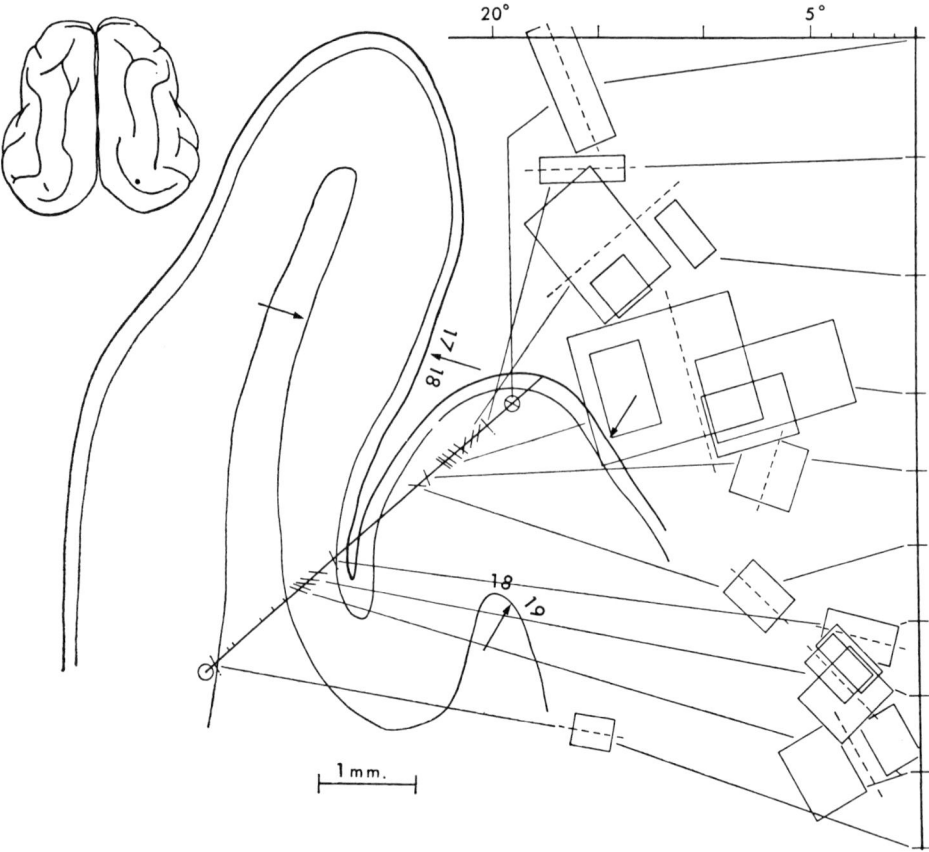

Fig. 2. Reconstruction of an electrode track that passed down the lateral bank of the postlateral sulcus, then through gray matter deep in the postlateral sulcus, and finally ended in area 17 (visual I) after crossing white matter. Of five axons recorded from white matter, four were from geniculate cells, and one was from a complex cortical cell. For conventions see legend of Fig. 1. Note how receptive fields move in toward the vertical meridian as the electrode moves medially across the cortex of visual II.

trated below (Figs. 3, 29, 32), confirms the finding of Talbot and Marshall (27) that there is a topographically organized second visual area lateral to the primary one. Other characteristics of cells in visual II, such as field size and response properties, will be discussed below.

We were naturally interested in establishing the lateral boundaries of visual II, and in learning what lay beyond that area. The first of eight mapping experiments is illustrated in Fig. 3A. A series of four microelectrode penetrations was made at the level of the posterior end of the lateral gyrus,

Fig. 1. (continued)
The field of the first cell, oriented at 2:00, was thus about 5° below the area centralis, near the vertical meridian. (For technical reasons one cannot be sure that this field actually crossed into the ipsilateral field.) The next three cells had overlapping fields oriented at 1:30, slightly to the left of the first field, and overlapping it. Note the gradual drift of receptive fields away from the midline, so that the final ones recorded from area 18 lie almost 10° in the contralateral (left) visual field. All of the fields in 18 were complex. Geniculate axons in white matter, and cells in the suprasplenial gyrus, have fields whose positions are indicated in the same way, to the right of the figure. For convenience, fields of cortical cells are shown as rectangles; their precise borders were not always determined, but the diagrams by their width and length show accurately the optimum stimulus length, and the distance over which the stimulus was effective.

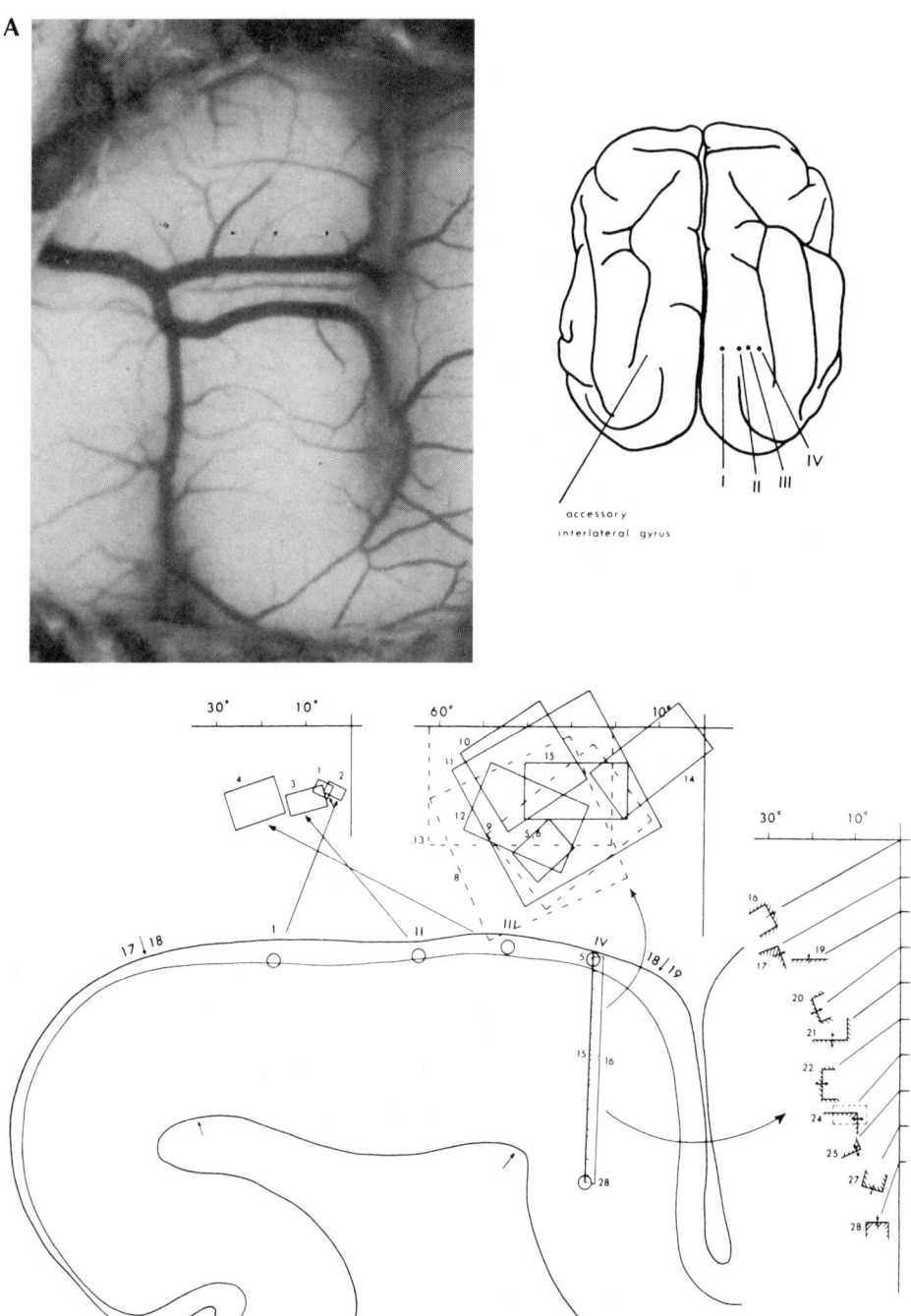

Fig. 3. A: *four microelectrode penetrations through the right lateral gyrus near its posterior end. Points of entry are shown in brain tracing (upper right) and in a photograph of the exposed brain surface made at the beginning of the experiment (upper left; width of photograph, 8 mm.). Penetrations I, II, and III are superficial; in each of these a lesion was made at the positions of the first units recorded, and the electrode was then removed. Note that there was a progressive movement out into the contralateral visual field as the electrode moved laterally across 18. Penetration IV passed down along the lateral bank of the lateral gyrus. Fields 1–15 of track IV illustrate the large size and wide scattering seen far out in 18. At cell 16 of track IV, the 18–19 (visual II-visual III)*

(continued)

147

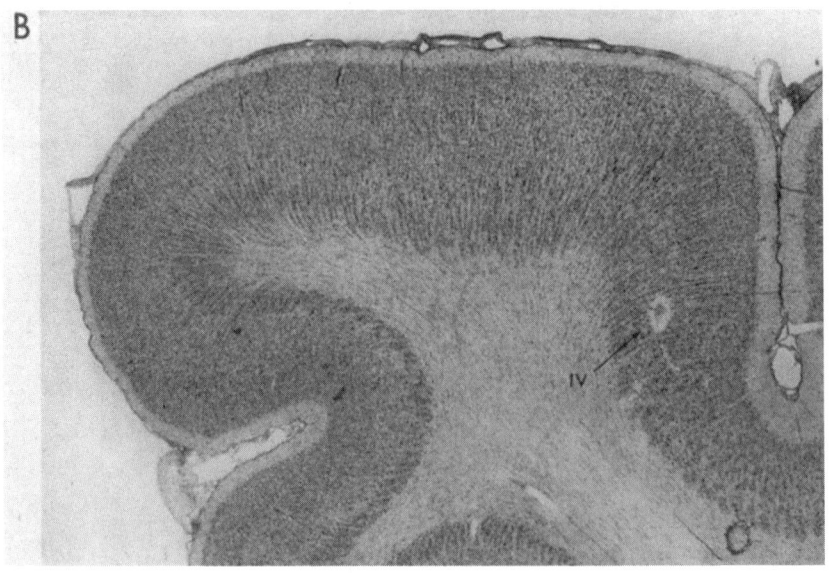

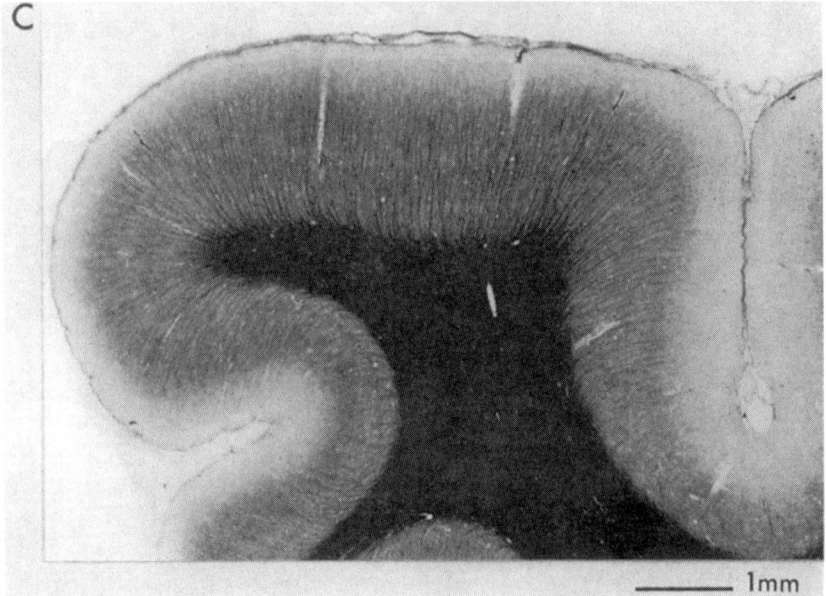

1mm

Fig. 3. (continued)
boundary, the fields began to move back toward the midline, and a high proportion were hypercomplex. Dia-
grams of fields 16–28 show the positions of the fields, and the optimum stimulus shape, orientation, and direc-
tions of movement. Cells 16, 20, and 22 responded to a light tongue on a dark background (a double-stopped
edge); 27 and 28, to a dark tongue; 17, 24, and 25 to a dark corner on a light background; 21 to a light corner;
and 19 (a complex cell) to an edge. The area over which a cell was driven was mapped carefully only for cell 24,
and is shown by the interrupted rectangle. B and C: same experiment as Fig. 3A. Coronal sections through lat-
eral gyrus; Nissl stain (cresyl violet) and myelin stain (Loyez). Same scale as coronal tracing in Fig. 3A. Arrow
in Nissl section indicates second lesion of penetration IV. Note the lack of any dramatic transition in Nissl archi-
tecture between 17 and 18, and the very coarse myelination of radial fibers in 18.

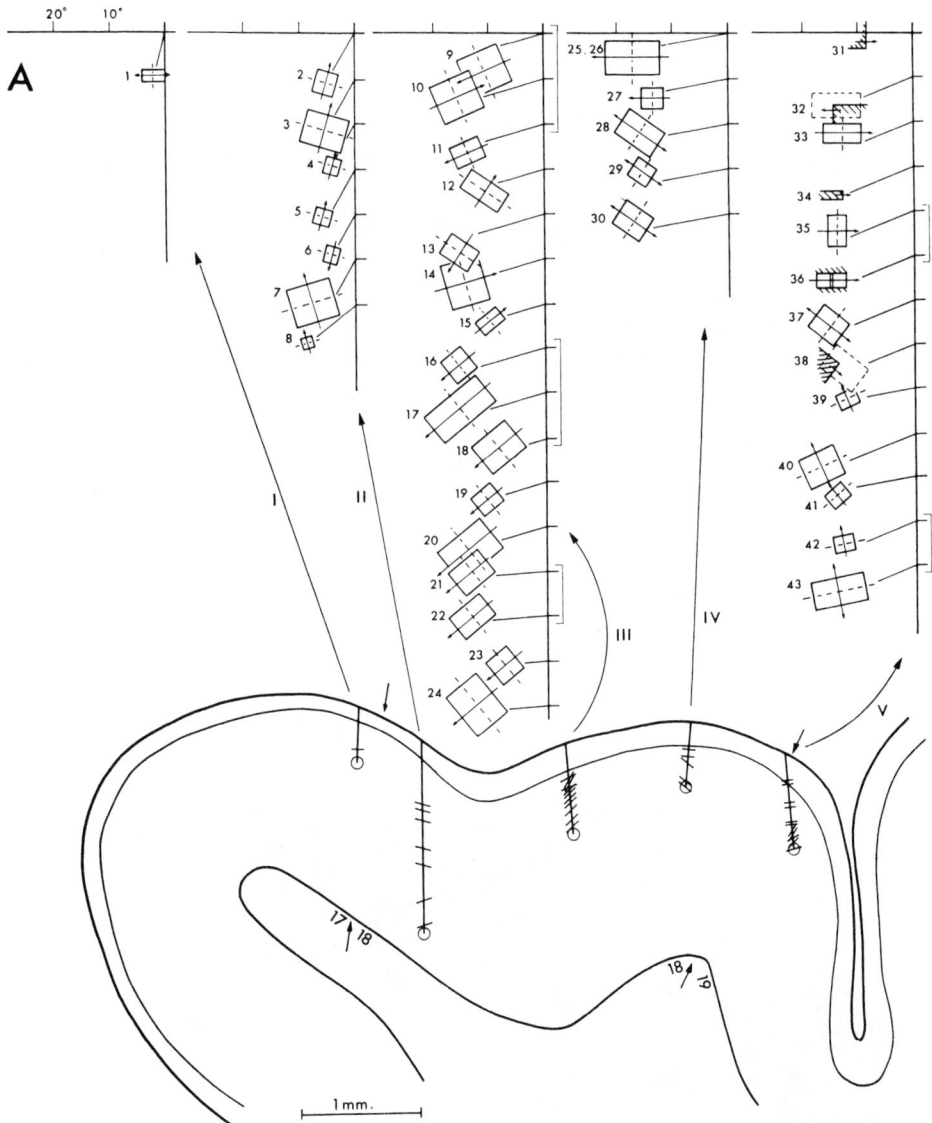

Fig. 4. A: *reconstructions of five microelectrode penetrations in the lateral gyrus, from a single experiment. Conventions as in Figs. 1 through 3. Lines perpendicular to track represent a vertical receptive-field orientation for all penetrations except IV, where they indicate horizontal orientation. Note 1) how fields move progressively out as one moves laterally in area 18, but apparently no further, in this experiment, than 15–20° (penetration IV); 2) the relatively long sequences of cells with the same receptive-field orientations, in penetration III, which was almost perpendicular to the cortical surface; 3) the mixture of complex cells (rectangles) and hypercomplex cells (drawn with crosshatching) in area 19. Cells 31, 32, and 38 responded to dark corners; 34 to a dark tongue (double-stopped edge); 36 to a double-stopped slit. Areas over which cells 32 and 38 responded are indicated by interrupted rectangles: the activating portion of field 36 is shown by the continuous rectangle. Arrow through receptive field indicates most effective direction of movement. B and C: Nissl-stained and myelin-stained coronal sections of lateral gyrus in experiment of Fig. 4A. The Nissl section shows part of the electrode track and the lesion of penetration V. Note in the myelin section the coarse pattern formed by the radial fibers in area 18. D: left, photograph of cortical surface, showing entry points of the five penetrations. Right, tracing from photograph of brain surface; anterior is up. (continued)*

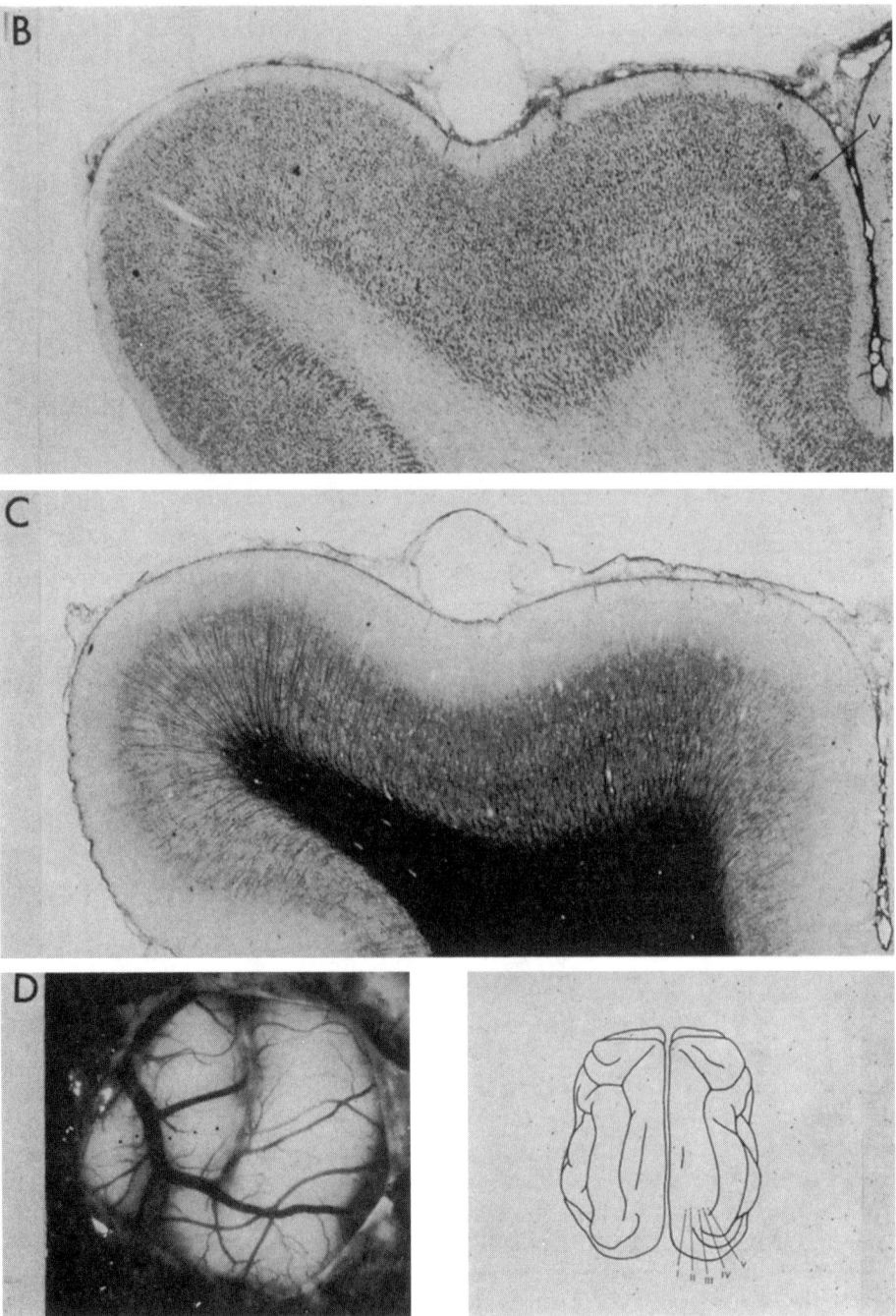

Fig. 4. (continued)

beginning about 2.5 mm. from the midline and working laterally. In the first penetration, two cells had receptive fields situated in the contralateral half-field of vision about 5° out from the midline. The second and third penetrations showed a clear progressive outward movement, establishing that these two penetrations (and probably also the first) were in visual II. In the fourth penetration most of the first 15 cells had tremendous receptive fields, some extending out as far as 60°. From cell 16 on, however, as the electrode advanced down the lateral bank of the gyrus, the receptive fields came to occupy positions closer and closer to the midline, indicating a reversal of the outward trend. At the same time there was an abrupt change in receptive field size and response characteristics (to be discussed below). This experiment, which was subsequently confirmed in similar mapping experiments in 7 other animals (see for example, Fig. 31), indicates that there is a third topographically organized visual area lateral to the second. We term this area "visual III."

Some notion of the regions of cortex explored so far can be obtained from Fig. 37. The area centralis representation in visual III appears to be quite large, including much of the knee-like junction of the middle and posterior suprasylvian gyri. There is little doubt that visual III is arranged in a manner similar to visual I, in that as one proceeds forward along the cortex the receptive fields occupy progressively lower positions in the visual field. We have made no attempt to define physiologically the lateral borders of visual III, though in several short penetrations along the medial bank of the suprasylvian gyrus at the levels of Figs. 3 and 4 we failed to record responses to visual stimuli. At these levels, visual III would thus seem to occupy the entire lateral bank of the lateral gyrus (see area marked 19 in Fig. 37). A little further back visual III occupies the lateral half of the accessory interlateral gyrus (Fig. 37B), and extends over to the medial bank of the suprasylvian gyrus (see Fig. 29). Still further back (Fig. 37C; also Figs. 30 and 31) visual III begins in the medial wall of the posterior suprasylvian gyrus and extends laterally for an unknown distance.

In a few experiments involving a succession of penetrations from medial to lateral we failed to move far out into the periphery of the contralateral visual field while crossing visual II and III in succession. Figure 4 provides an illustration of this. Here as we proceeded laterally across the posterior part of the lateral gyrus the fields moved out in the usual manner, except that none of them extended further than about 15°; it seems unlikely that the entire remaining periphery could have been represented in the small unexplored area between penetrations IV and V. A similar experiment is illustrated in Fig. 29. It is thus our impression that the extreme lateral parts of the visual field may sometimes have no representation at these antero-posterior levels. It is as if the large regions of visual I, II,

and III devoted to area centralis had crowded the lateral representations into more anterior and posterior parts of the cortex.

Correlation of the Three Visual Areas with Microscopic Anatomy

An obvious question concerns the correlation of these three physiologically defined areas with cytoarchitectural subdivisions. The borders of areas 17, 18, and 19 were, accordingly, determined in Nissl- and myelin-stained sections of all the experimental brains, using slides that showed the electrode tracks and lesions. The criteria used were those given in a recent comprehensive study of the visual areas of the cat by Otsuka and Hassler (23). For determining both the medial and lateral borders of area 18 we have found especially useful the presence of large third-layer pyramidal cells in 18, and, in myelin-stained sections, the coarse, irregular, and often oblique pattern of fibers in the deeper cortical layers. In Figs. 1 through 4 and 29 through 32 the designations 17, 18, and 19 are based entirely on histological criteria.

A comparison of the physiologically defined visual areas I, II, and III with the anatomically determined 17, 18, and 19 has shown a remarkably exact correspondence. An example is shown in Fig. 3, where the border between visual II and III is precisely defined physiologically as occurring between cells 15 and 16. The correlation between this and the border between 18 and 19 seen on the myelin-stained section (Fig. 3B) is quite striking. In no case has there been any disagreement between physiological and anatomical findings. Moreover, our composite picture of the borders between visual I, II, and III from all experiments coincides well with the gross borders shown by Otsuka and Hassler (23: Fig. 8b), which are based on their own microscopic analysis.

Part II. Responses of Single Cells in Visual Areas II and III

General Comments

For every spontaneously firing cell in visual II and III, it was sooner or later possible to find a visual stimulus that evoked a response, unless the cell was badly injured or the cortex was in a pathologic state. By continuously stimulating the retina as the electrode advanced one could even activate and hence study a number of otherwise quiescent cells. There may, of course, be cells that neither fire spontaneously nor respond to visual stimuli. As in visual I (13), deepening the level of anesthesia suppressed spontaneous activity and made responses more sluggish, without, however, lowering the response specificity.

Outside of visual I no simple cells were found, and no axons with geniculate properties were encountered in gray matter. In visual II and III one can distinguish several distinct categories of cells. The first group contains cells that resemble complex cells of the striate cortex. A second large group consists of cells with more elaborate properties. All cells that exceed the complex type in the intricacy of their behavior we have called "hypercomplex," and within this group we distinguish lower order and higher order cells. The types of cells found in visual II and III are summarized in Table 1.

Complex Cells

Complex cells were common both in visual II and visual III. In visual II they were in the overwhelming majority, forming 96% of the cells studied. This figure may, however, be misleading, since it includes cells recorded in early experiments done at a time when hypercomplex cells had not been recognized: 90% would probably be a closer estimate. In visual III, of 109 cells recorded, 46 (42%) were complex and 63 (58%) were hypercomplex.

Complex cells in visual II and III closely resembled those in visual I in their responses to retinal stimulation. Diffuse light or small circular spots evoked little or no response. A given cell was affected most by a line regardless of its precise position in the receptive field, provided the orientation was optimal; at 90° to the best orientation no responses were evoked. The preferred orientation differed from one cell to another, and there was no indication that any one orientation was more common than the others. If the adequate stimulus was a slit or a dark bar, its width was usually important: making it narrower or wider than some optimum usually rendered it ineffective. In the present context it is particularly worth emphasizing the effects of varying the stimulus *length*. A maximum response was obtained when the full length of a receptive field was covered; making the stimulus even longer had no additional effect, a result that is implicit in the term "receptive field," since we use this term in the sense of the entire region of the retina functionally connected with the cell. There was, in other words, simple summation of stimulus effects over the entire receptive field along the direction of the field orientation. This was not true of the higher order cells to be described below.

Movement of an optimally oriented line stimulus in a direction perpendicular to the orientation was usually the most powerful way of activating a cell. The two directions of movement were not

Table 1. *290 cells recorded in areas 18 and 19*

Cell Type	Activated by	Visual II	Visual III
Complex	Edge	38	6
	Dark bar	12	12
	Slit	72	23
	Mixed	17	0
	Uncategorized	34	5
Total		173	46
Hypercomplex*	Edge		
	single-stopped (corner)	6	18
	double-stopped (tongue)	0	33
	Slit (double-stopped)	2	5
	Dark bar (double-stopped)	0	3
	Uncategorized	0	4
Total		8	63
Totals		181	109

*Eleven of the cells in visual III were classed as higher order hypercomplex.

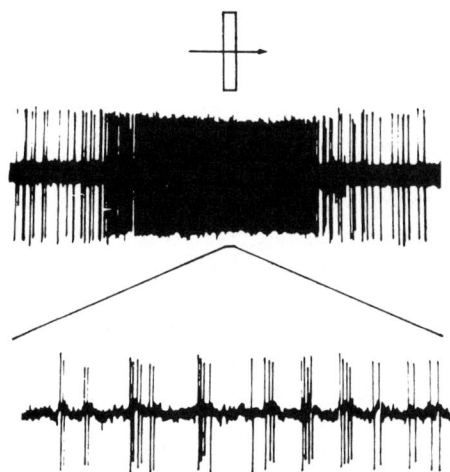

Fig. 5. Response of a complex cell, recorded from visual II, to a vertical 1° × 4° slit moved slowly to the right at a speed of about 2°/sec. Stimulation of right (ipsilateral) eye; ocular-dominance group 5. Receptive field extended from the center of gaze out into the contralateral visual field for about 10°. A portion of the same response is shown with a faster sweep in the lower record, to illustrate the pattern of firing. Time, upper sweep, 10 sec., lower sweep, 200 msec. Background intensity, 0 $\log_{10}$ cd/m²; slit, 1.3 $\log_{10}$ cd/m².

Figure 5 illustrates a type of cell commonly seen in both visual I and II. These cells fired rapidly, and in a characteristic pattern of very brief high-frequency bursts, as a line stimulus slowly crossed the receptive field. The cell of Fig. 5 was typical in that it responded when a slit was moved in one direction, but was neither excited nor inhibited by the reverse movement. (Edges or dark bars evoked only feeble responses). It was rare for a cell to be activated by movement in one direction and inhibited by movement in the reverse direction; one of the few convincing examples is shown in Fig. 6. Here the cell responded to a slit, bar, or either type of edge, with excitation to movement up and suppression of firing to movement down. Inhibition of this sort would, of course, tend to be overlooked in cells with a slow maintained rate of firing, and may be more common than our results suggest.

In visual II complex receptive fields tended to be larger than those in visual I. As in visual I, field size was loosely correlated with distance from the area centralis, a relationship that is illustrated in Fig. 7, where the area of each field is plotted against the distance of its geometric center from the area centralis. In some experiments in which visual II was explored from medial to lateral, receptive fields of successively recorded cells expanded in such a way, as they moved into the periphery, that their inner borders continued to extend medially almost to the vertical meridian. A field whose center was 30–40° out thus came to occupy a large part of the contralateral visual field. As in visual I, all fields were confined entirely or almost entirely to the contralateral half-field of vision; many in fact

necessarily equally effective, and sometimes one direction of movement produced no response at all. The rate of movement was usually an important variable, since the cell's firing frequency tended to fall off sharply if the rate was less or greater than some optimum. The most effective rates of movement varied from cell to cell, from about 0.1°/sec. up to about 20°/sec.

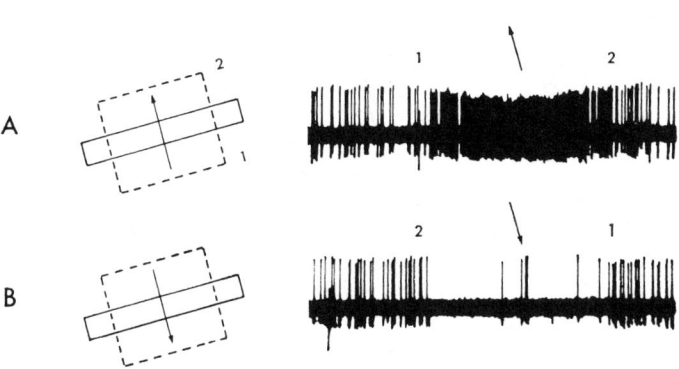

A

B

Fig. 6. Responses of another complex cell recorded in visual II, in the same penetration as the cell of Fig. 5. Stimulation of left (contralateral) eye, ocular-dominance group 3. Size of receptive field 3° × 4°. Upper record, optimally oriented slit, 6° × 1°, moved up across receptive field. Lower record, same slit, moved downward; note inhibition of resting discharge, beginning at 2, when slit enters field, and ending at 1, when it leaves. Rate of movement 0.5°/sec. Duration of sweeps, 10 sec. Stimulus intensities as in Fig. 5.

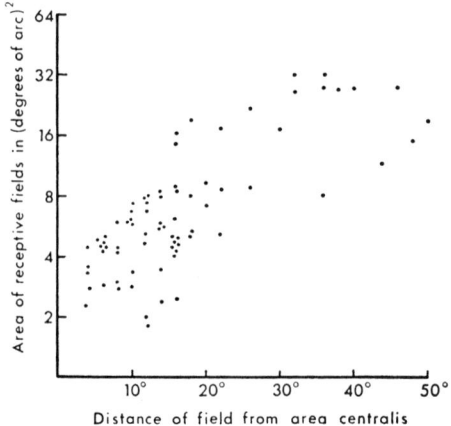

Fig. 7. Receptive-field areas in (degrees of arc)^2 of 72 cells in visual II, plotted against distance of the geometric center of each field from the area centralis.

stopped abruptly at the vertical meridian, and those that extended across it did so for such a small distance as to make it doubtful whether this represented a genuine encroachment on the ipsilateral field, or whether it was an artifact related to an error in estimation of the vertical meridian (see DIS-CUSSION).

Complex cells in visual III were similar in all respects to those found in the striate cortex. While no analysis was made of receptive-field size, as was done for visual II cells, we have the impression that the complex fields of visual III were similar in size to those of visual I.

Hypercomplex Cells

Cells even more specialized than complex cells were present in both visual II and III. In visual II they formed about 5–10% of the population. In visual III they were much more numerous, comprising about half of the cells in some penetrations and almost all of them in others. A useful indication that an electrode had passed from visual II to visual III was the abrupt increase in the numbers of higher order cells. This is shown particularly well in Fig. 3, penetration IV.

We term these more complicated cells of areas 18 and 19 "hypercomplex." Cells in this group showed certain common features, but varied widely in other respects, both in the types of stimuli they responded to and in their apparent order of complexity. These common features and differ-

ences can best be described by several examples, and we shall begin by describing the responses of four lower order hypercomplex cells, and shall follow this with two examples of cells of higher order.

LOWER ORDER HYPERCOMPLEX CELLS. Records of a hypercomplex cell in visual II are shown in Figs. 8 through 11 (see Fig. 32, unit 7). This cell responded best to a 2:00–8:00 edge with dark below, moved upward at about 2°/sec. over a circumscribed region as shown in Fig. 8C. The area over which responses were evoked, about 2° × 2°, is indicated roughly by the left half of the interrupted rectangle. As more and more of this area was stimulated the response steadily improved (Fig. 8, A through C). The orientation of the edge was critical, since changing it by more than 10°–15° produced a marked decrease in the response, and a 30° change made the stimulus ineffective. Downward move-

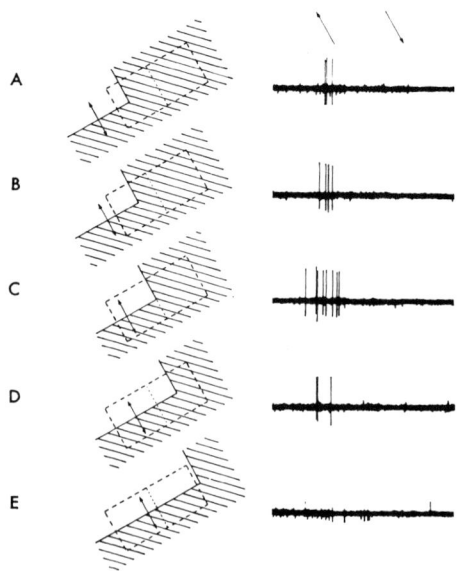

Fig. 8. Records from a hypercomplex cell in visual II (see Fig. 32, unit 7). Stimulation of right (ipsilateral) eye, ocular-dominance group 6. Receptive field, 2° × 4°, indicated by interrupted rectangle. Stimulus consisted of an edge oriented at 2:00, with dark below, terminated on the right by a second edge intersecting the first at 90°. Brighter regions, 1.3 log_{10} cd/m^2; dark areas, 0.0 log_{10} cd/m^2. A through C: up-and-down movement across varying amounts of the activating portion of the field; D–E: movement across all of the activating portion and varying amounts of the antagonistic portion. Rate of movement 4°/sec. Each sweep 2 sec.

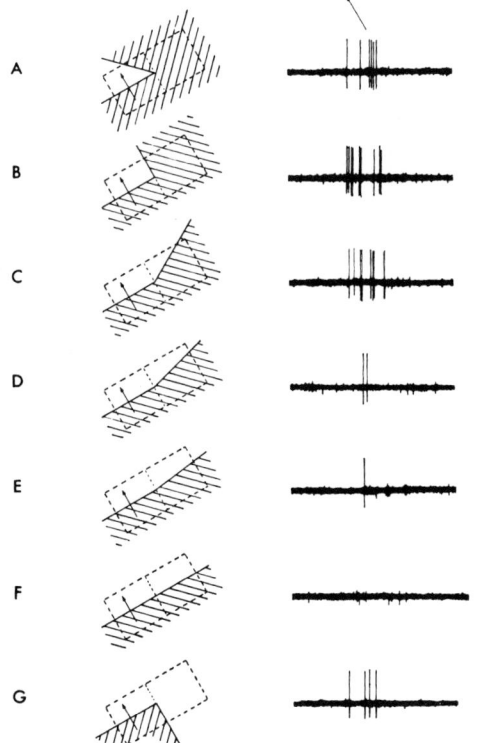

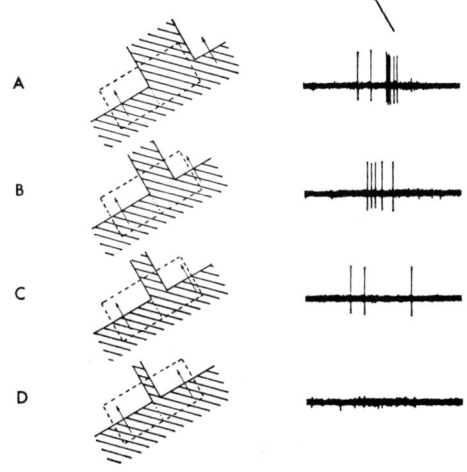

Fig. 10. Same cell as in Figs. 8 and 9. Each time an optimally oriented stopped edge is moved up across the activating (left) part of the receptive field at optimal speed (2°/sec.), a second edge is simultaneously moved up to the right of the first, at varying distances. The antagonistic effect, first noted about 2° from the boundary between the two parts of the field, increases the closer the edge is to this boundary. Sweep duration, 2 sec.

Fig. 9. Same cell as in Fig. 8. Stimulation with two intersecting edges moved up across the receptive field as shown. Inhibition is maximum when the right (antagonistic) half of the receptive field is stimulated with an edge having the same orientation as the optimum edge for the left (activating) half (F). Duration of each sweep, 2 sec.

ment was entirely ineffective, as were small circular spots, diffuse light, or up-and-down movement of an edge with dark above. The cell was driven by both eyes, the ipsilateral one giving the better responses (group 5).

From these responses alone one would conclude that this was an ordinary complex cell, responding to an edge at 2:00 with dark below, moved up. The situation was more complicated than that, however. The remainder of Fig. 8 shows that as more and more of the right half of the interrupted rectangle was included in the stimulus, simply by extending the edge further to the right, the response became progressively weaker, until it failed completely when the entire rectangular area was stimulated.

It would seem from Fig. 8 that this cell required as a stimulus an edge crossing the left half of the rectangular field, but also required that a similar edge should *not* simultaneously cross the right half. There are, however, several possible alternatives. Perhaps it was important to have the 11:00–5:00 edge come somewhere near the boundary between the two halves. Or perhaps it was necessary to have some kind of interruption in the continuity of the 2:00 edge at the boundary. The records of Figs. 9 through 11 allow one to eliminate some of these possibilities. In all of the records of Fig. 9, the left half of the interrupted rectangle was stimulated in the most powerful way; the orientation of the stimulus to the right was meanwhile varied through all possible angles. From the selection of records shown it is clear that the closer the orientation was to that of the left edge, the weaker was the response. Stimulating the right ("antagonistic") region thus effectively suppressed the response, provided the orientation of the edge crossing that region was not more than about 15° or so from the inclination that was optimal for the left half. This represents an orientation specificity comparable to that of the left ("activating") region.

By stimulating the left and right subdivisions of the field separately, and varying the length of the right-hand stimulus, as shown in Fig. 10, it was found that the antagonistic region had roughly the same length as the activating. Records 10C and 10D suggest, moreover, that merely having a discontinuity near the dotted line dividing the rectangles, even in the form of an 11:00–5:00 edge, was not enough to make the 2:00 edge effective. This is further supported by the experiment of Fig. 11, in which a notch of varying width interrupted the edge. Here, moreover, one could map roughly the extent of the antagonistic area in the 11:00–5:00 direction, and show that it was roughly equal to the extent of the activating region.

From these experiments the essential property of the cell seems to have been its responsiveness to a specifically oriented edge, provided the edge was limited in its length at one end (in this case the right). As to the extent of the edge to the left, the longer it was the better was the response, until it passed the left boundary of the interrupted rectangle; beyond that point the length made no difference. For convenience we shall refer to cells of this type as responding to a "stopped edge." A term such as "corner cell" has the disadvantage that the cell responded not to all corners, but to a particular class of corners (those of Fig. 9, B and G) over a narrow range of orientations and positions.

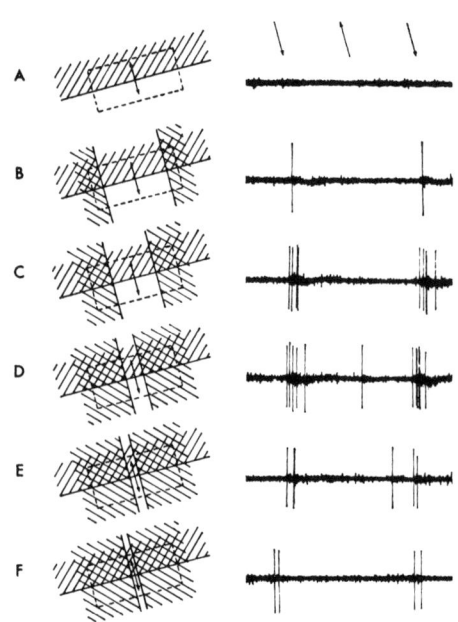

Fig. 12. Recordings from a cell in area 19 of the right hemisphere; stimulation of left eye. Receptive field about 8° below the center of gaze, about 13° long and 6° wide. Rapid (30°/sec.) up-and-down movement of a long edge with dark above evoked no response (A). Responses to downward movement began to appear when the stimulus was limited in its length (B, C), and became maximal when a 2½°-wide region in the center was stimulated (D), at which point an occasional response occurred even to upward movement. Further narrowing made the response weaker (E and F). Duration of each sweep, 1 sec.

A hypercomplex cell of a second type, this one recorded from visual III, is described in Figs. 12 through 15. It was driven from the contralateral eye only (group 1). It responded to an edge moved very rapidly down and to the right, but only if the region stimulated was restricted on both sides. In Fig. 12A, for example, moving a very long edge down gave no response. The edge became effective when it was shortened by blocking out both ends of the region being stimulated, and the responses increased until all but the center 2½° was eliminated (Fig. 12, B and D). At this point there was not only a brisk response to movement down, but also a weak response to movement up. Further narrowing of the area stimulated reduced the response.

The 2½° stimulus of Fig. 12D was most potent when it was oriented in a 2:00 direction. As shown in Fig. 13, a 30° change in either direction all but eliminated the response.

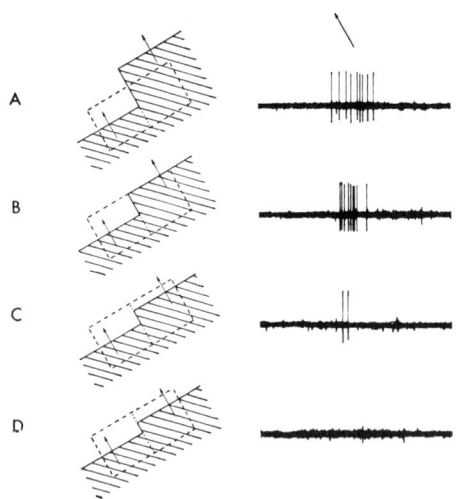

Fig. 11. Same cell as in Figs. 8 through 10. The two halves of the field are stimulated simultaneously by two edges separated by a step of varying height; antagonistic effects are first seen when the step equals the width of the field, and increase as the step is narrowed, to about 1/2°, after which no change is seen. Each sweep, 2 sec.

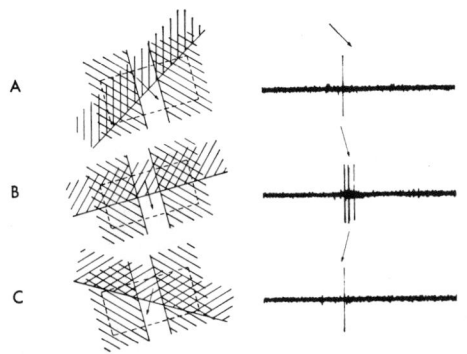

Fig. 13. Same cell as in Fig. 12. Effects of varying the orientation of the edge. Duration of each sweep, 1 sec.

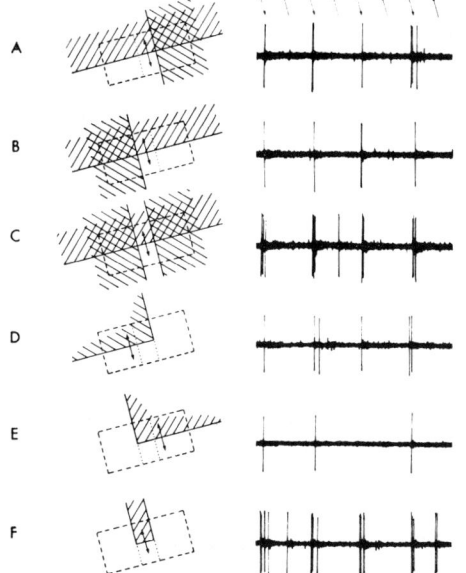

Fig. 14. Same cell as in Figs. 12 and 13. In A and B portions of the field to the right and left of the 21/2°-wide center are blocked separately, to show that the more important antagonistic region is to the right. The equivalent experiment is repeated in D and E, using dark corners. In F, which corresponds to C, a dark tongue is used instead of an edge blocked to either side: a dark tongue moved in from above (F) is equivalent to a light tongue moved out from below (C). Duration of each sweep, 2 sec.

To assess the relative effectiveness of the end zones of the interrupted rectangle in interfering with the response, each end was blocked off in turn (Fig. 14, *A* and *B*). Both end regions were clearly capable of antagonizing the responses, the right one somewhat more so than the left, and eliminating both produced the best response, with even an

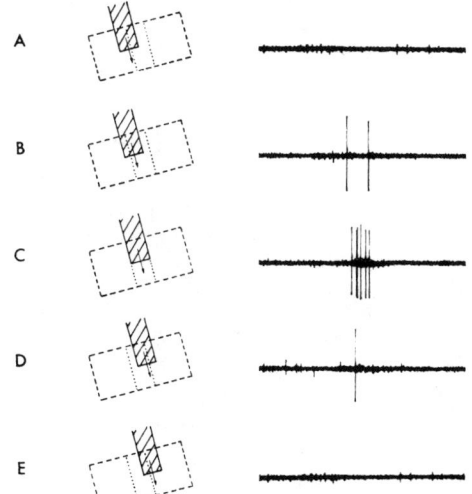

Fig. 15. Same cell as in Figs. 12 through 14. A dark tongue 2½°-wide crosses receptive field from above downward, in different positions. Maximum excitation occurs when the central (activating) strip of field is stimulated. Varying the position by 1/2° either way greatly reduces the response. Duration of each sweep, 1 sec.

occasional impulse in response to upward movement. One can say that this field was "stopped" at both ends. The region stimulated could be constricted either by blocking off the end regions (as in Figs. 12 and 13; or 14, *A* through *C*) or by reducing the length of the edge (Fig. 14, *D* through *F*); when the length was reduced the optimum stimulus became a 21/2° tongue moved rapidly into the activating part of the field in a 11:00–5:00 orientation (Fig. 14*F*). The exact positioning of the stimulus was then highly critical, since introducing it even slightly to the left or right of the central region presumably meant reducing the activating area covered and at the same time including some of the antagonistic. This is shown in Fig. 15.

For this cell and the previous one the receptive field, defined as the entire area functionally connected with the cell, is outlined by the interrupted rectangles. The fields so defined are subdivided into activating and antagonistic regions in a manner analogous to the excitatory and inhibitory parts of simple fields we have described in previous papers (10, 13). The terms "excitatory" and "inhibitory," if used for hypercomplex fields, must be understood in a more abstract way, since the effects of the regions do not add or subtract in any simple spatial sense, but only along a line parallel to the

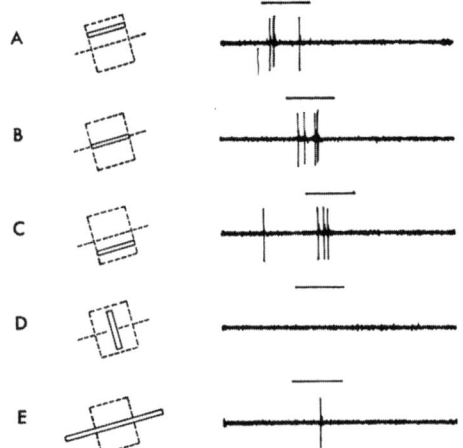

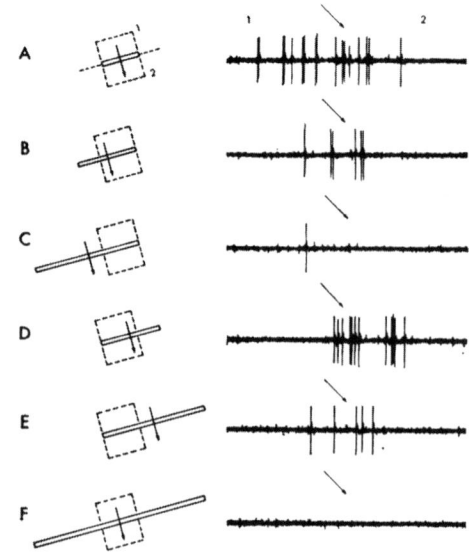

Fig. 16. Responses of a cell recorded in area 19, right hemi-sphere (see cell 22, penetration V, Fig. 29). Receptive field was 10° below and to the left of the center of gaze. Excitatory portion roughly 2°×2°, represented by interrupted rectangle. A through C, stimulation with an optimally oriented slit, 1/8° × 2°, in various parts of receptive field in right (ipsilat-eral) eye. D: same slit, shone at 90° to optimum orientation. E: optimally oriented slit 5 1/2° long, extending beyond exci-tatory region on both sides. For each record upper line shows when stimulus light was on. Duration of each sweep, 1 sec. Intensity of slit, 1.0 $\log_{10}$ cd/m²; background, 0.0 $\log_{10}$ cd/m².

Fig. 17. Same cell as in Fig. 16. Responses to 1/8°-wide slits of various lengths moved downward across receptive field at about 3°/sec. A: stimulation of activating part only; B through F: stimulation of activating part, as well as varying portions of the antagonistic flanks. Right flank is weaker than left. Sweep duration, 1 sec.

receptive-field axis (see DISCUSSION). For the cells described below (Figs. 16 through 20), interrupted rectangles are used to outline the excitatory (or activating) subdivision of receptive fields and the antagonistic regions are not shown.

The two cells just described responded best to edge stimuli. Two examples of cells responding to slits and dark bars are shown in Figs. 16 and 17 and Figs. 18 through 20. These cells were recorded in sequence from a single penetration of visual III in the right hemisphere (see Fig. 29, units 21 and 22). Unit 22, illustrated in Figs. 16 and 17, responded best to a slit 1/8° wide and 2° long, oriented about 15° to the horizontal. It was driven by both eyes, but preferred the ipsilateral (group 5). Brisk responses were evoked with stationary stimuli: shining the slit anywhere within a 2° × 2° region evoked an "on" response (Fig. 16, *A* through *C*), provided the orientation was within about 20–30° of the optimum. At 90° to the optimum there was no response (Fig. 16*D*). A slit 1/8° wide, as used in *A* through *C*, was clearly optimal, and this dimen-

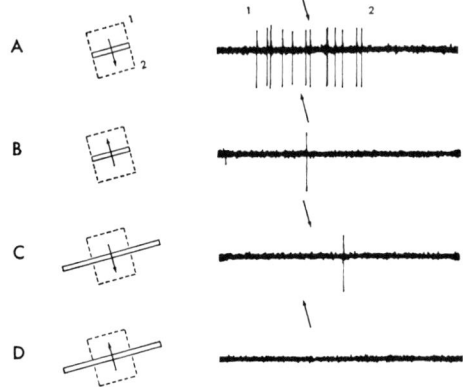

Fig. 18. Cell recorded near that of Fig. 16 and 17 (see Fig. 29, cell 21, penetration V). Receptive field 8° below and to the left of the center of gaze; activating portion, roughly 4° long and 3–4° wide, denoted by the interrupted rectangle. Responses to up-and-down movement of a slit 1/8° × 3° (A and B), and 1/8° × 8° (C and D). Intensity of slit, 1.3 $\log_{10}$ cd/m²; background, 0.0 $\log_{10}$ cd/m². Rate of movement about 3°/sec.; sweep duration 2 sec.

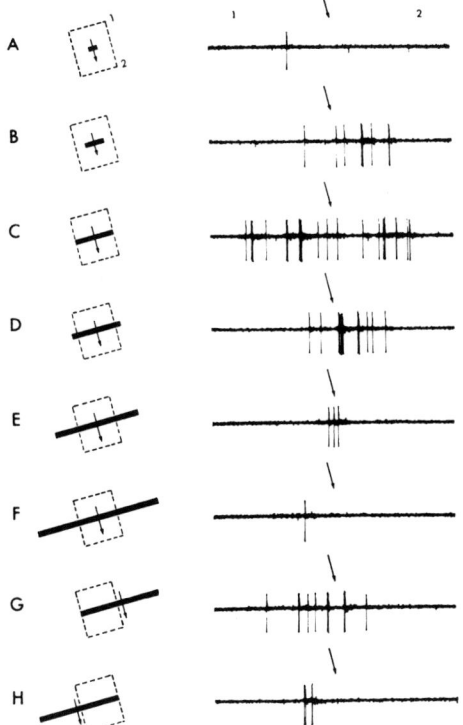

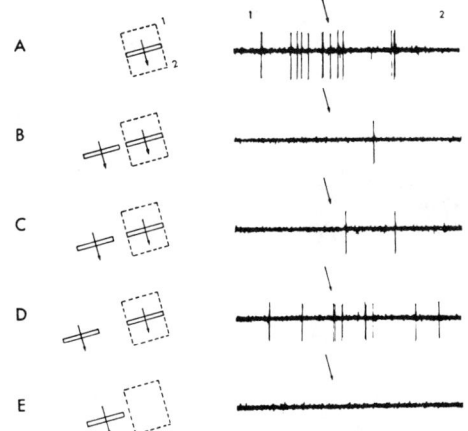

Fig. 20. Same cell as in Figs. 18 and 19. A: *responses to slit 1/8° × 3° moved down across the activating region.* B *through* D: *responses to two slits, 1/8° × 3°, one moved down across the activating region, the second moved simultaneously in the left flank, at varying distances from the first;* E: *second slit moved in flank, unaccompanied by the first. Sweep duration, 2 sec.*

Fig. 19. Same cell as in Fig. 18. Responses to black bars, 1/8° wide and of various lengths, moved down over various parts of the receptive field, as indicated to the left. Rate of movement about 2°/sec. Intensity of bar, 0.0 log₁₀ cd/m²; surround, 1.3 log₁₀ cd/m². Sweep duration, 2.5 sec.

sion was critical, since 1/16° and 1/4° evoked distinctly weaker responses, and 1/2° was ineffective. Taken by themselves, these results would be typical for an ordinary complex cell. This cell, however, responded weakly or not at all to a 1/8° slit extending several degrees beyond the excitatory region in both directions (Fig. 16E).

Responses to moving stimuli are shown in Fig. 17. Upward movement, not illustrated in Fig. 17, was about as effective as downward. The optimum rate was of the order of 3°/sec. By stimulating with slits extending beyond the excitatory region in one or both directions and for various distances, it was possible to compare the inhibitory capabilities of the two outlying regions and form some idea of their extent. From the responses shown in Fig. 17 we concluded that inhibitory areas were present at both ends, extending 2–3° beyond the ends, with

the left stronger than the right (Fig. 17, cf. *B* with *D*, or *C* with *E*).

Another cell, recorded just prior to the one described above, had many similar properties but several interesting differences (Figs. 18 through 20). Like the last cell, it was driven from both eyes, but preferred the contralateral (group 3). It responded to a slit, and again the optimum width was 1/8° and the orientation was about 15° to the horizontal. A moving stimulus was far more effective than a stationary one, and downward movement was more effective than upward over a range of about 4°. The optimum length was about 3° (Fig. 18, *A* and *B*). Extending the slit in both directions made it virtually ineffective (Fig. 18, *C* and *D*), showing that this cell, like the last, was no ordinary complex one. Unlike the cell just described, it responded to a black bar at least as well as to a slit; the optimum dimensions were the same, as was the directional preference for downward movement. Figure 19 demonstrates summation within the confines of the activating part of the field and antagonism from the outlying parts, and it emphasizes how critical the optimum length can be. From Fig. 19, *G* and *H,* it seems that for this cell the left-hand antagonistic region was more powerful than the right-hand one.

The experiment of Fig. 20 was designed to measure how far the left antagonistic area extended, by stimulating the activating area with a downward-moving slit, at the same time moving down a second slit at varying distances to the left of the first. It would seem that most of the antagonistic region was within about 2–3° of the activating region. In Fig. 20E we show that stimulation of the flanking region by itself was without effect. Perhaps this was because there was too little spontaneous activity for any inhibition to be apparent. A failure to respond to stimulation of an antagonistic region alone has been observed in all hypercomplex cells so far studied.

The four cells just described had in common a close resemblance to complex cells, except that their receptive fields were stopped at one or both ends. Hypercomplex fields, like complex ones, occurred in all orientations, with no indication that one orientation was more common than any other. From these and other examples we find that the main types of ordinary complex cells—distinguished by whether they respond to slits, edges or dark bars, or any combination of these—all have their counterparts among the hypercomplex cells. A hypercomplex cell driven by edges may have its field stopped at one end (Figs. 8 through 11) or at both ends (Figs. 12 through 15). So far, hypercomplex cells activated by slits or bars (Figs. 16 through 20) have all had fields stopped at both ends. The frequency with which these various cell types were observed is shown in Table 1.

HIGHER ORDER HYPERCOMPLEX CELLS. Twelve hypercomplex cells recorded in visual III had properties that could not be described in these relatively simple terms. We have called such cells "higher order hypercomplex."

One of the main characteristics of higher order cells was an ability to respond to two sets of stimuli with orientations 90° apart. Figures 21 and 22 show records of unit 2 in the experiment of Fig. 30. This cell responded to stimulation of either eye (group 5), to a 2:00 edge with dark above. With a stimulus stopped to the left (Fig. 21B) the cell responded to movement down or up throughout an oval area indicated roughly by the left interrupted rectangle. With the edge stopped to the right (Fig. 21D) the cell responded over a separate region suggested by the right interrupted rectan-

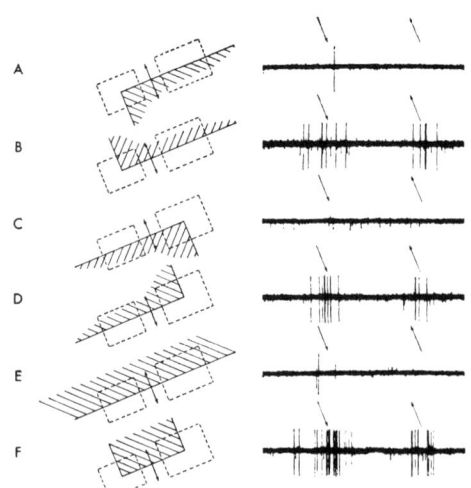

Fig. 21. Responses of a cell recorded in area 19, right hemisphere (see cell no. 2, Fig. 31). Receptive field 6° from center of gaze. Regions from which responses were evoked are indicated roughly by the two interrupted rectangles, of which the right was 3° × 4° in size. A right-angled corner with dark up and to the right (B) evoked responses when moved down or up over the left-hand region; no response was evoked in the right-hand region. A corner with darkness up and to the left evoked responses to up-and-down movement only over the right-hand region (D). Little or no response was obtained with corners with dark below (A and C), or with unstopped edges (E). A tongue (F), combining stimuli B and D, gave the most powerful responses. Rate of movement, about 0.5°/sec. Duration of each sweep, 20 sec. Intensities, shaded areas 0.0 log₁₀ cd/m²; background, 1.0 log₁₀ cd/m².

gle. Corners made from an edge with dark below were almost ineffective (Fig. 21, A and C), as was an unstopped edge with dark above (Fig. 21E). A dark tongue 5° wide, combining the two corners of Fig. 21, B and D, evoked a very brisk response when it was moved in from above (Fig. 21F). The responses shown in B, D, and F were highly sensitive to the orientation of the stimulus, and fell off quickly if the orientation was changed by more than 10–15°. Up to this point, then, the cell behaved in many respects like a lower order hypercomplex cell responsive to a double-stopped edge, such as that of Figs. 12 through 15. Considered in that way, the field would have a central activating region, presumably including most of the two rectangular areas and the region between them, flanked on both ends by antagonistic areas. It seems doubtful, however, whether such a simple arrangement could explain the properties of this cell. The relatively large regions over which corners evoked responses indicate that the points at which the edges were stopped were not very critical. This was not generally true for a lower order hypercomplex cell (cf. Fig. 15): usually the more of the activating region the stimulus covered the more active was the response, with a sharp dropoff in response as soon as the inhibitory region was invaded. In this cell the responses to each corner were, on the contrary, surprisingly vigorous and uniform over its own entire rectangle, suggesting a complexity of organization greater than that of any hypercomplex cells described up to now. A better example of this kind of behavior is provided by the cell to be described next (Figs. 23 through 26).

That the cell just described was complex in still another way is shown in Fig. 22. The cell responded vigorously when the corner used in Fig. 21*D* was moved down and to the left or up and right (Fig. 22*A*). Sidewise movement, like downward movement, evoked responses only when the stimulus corner was oriented as shown in Fig. 22, *A* and *B*; a change of 15–20° was enough to abolish the response. The range over which a response was evoked was very nearly the same as before, and is indicated by the same interrupted rectangle. The corner of Fig. 21*B* similarly evoked a brisk response when moved sidewise over the left-hand

rectangular area, as shown in Fig. 22*B*. Combining the two stimuli by using a wide bar produced a very powerful response (Fig. 22*D*), whereas there was no response when the bar extended below the excitatory regions (Fig. 22*C*).

This cell would seem to combine the attributes of two sets of lower order hypercomplex cells, one set having a 2:00 receptive-field orientation, the other a 5:00 orientation. Such complicated cells, combining characteristics of two groups of lower order hypercomplex cells with orientations 90° apart, seem to be much less common than ordinary lower order hypercomplex cells, in that we have seen only 11 of a total of 63 hypercomplex cells in visual III, and have found none in visual II. A high proportion (8 cells) were recorded in two of the penetrations (see Figs. 30 and 31), both of which were in the region of area centralis representation. The behavior of these cells can be better understood by considering responses of other neighboring cells recorded simultaneously or in the same penetration, a topic that is taken up in a later section (p. 261).

A second example of a higher order cell is shown in Figs. 23 through 26. Recorded in the

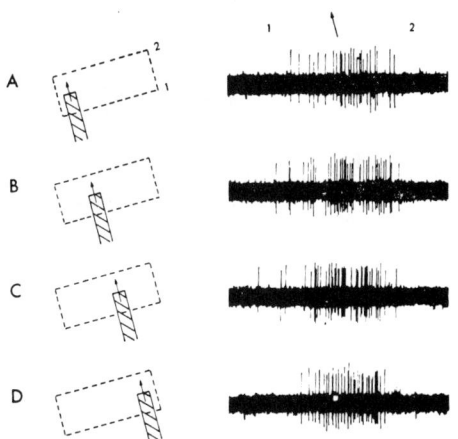

Fig. 23. *Responses of a cell recorded in area 19, right hemisphere (see cell no. 6 of Fig. 31). Region from which responses were evoked, 4° × 1½°, are indicated approximately by the interrupted rectangle. Responses to a dark tongue 1/2° wide introduced from below in four different positions, at a rate of about 0.5°/sec. Intensities as in Fig. 21. Duration of each sweep, 5 sec.*

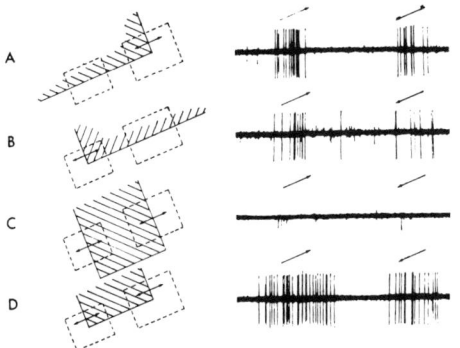

Fig. 22. *Same cell as Fig. 21. Responses to movement down and to the left, and up and to the right, of corners with dark above (A and B); failure to respond to an unstopped dark bar (C); strong response to a dark bar stopped below (D), combining stimuli (A) and (B). Sweep duration, 20 sec.*

same penetration as the last cell (see Fig. 30, unit 6), its receptive field was in roughly the same region, and measured 4° × 1½°. A powerful response was evoked by an edge with dark below, inclined at 15° to the horizontal, stopped at both ends, and introduced into the field from below at a rate of about 1°/sec. The response was markedly reduced by changing the orientation by 20–30°. Although the field itself was 4° long, the optimum length of the stimulus edge was only 1/2°. Indeed, the most interesting feature of this cell was its ability to respond regardless of where along the 4°-long lower border of the field the stimulus was introduced (Fig. 23)—this despite the fact that an edge only slightly longer than 1/2° was distinctly less effective, and a 2° edge evoked no response (Fig. 24). Active responses were evoked not only to a 1/2°-long double-stopped edge, but also to a double-stopped slit or dark bar, whose optimal length

was again 1/2°: the thickness of the stimulus was not critical provided it exceeded 1/4°.

This cell, then, had many features similar to the cell of Figs. 12 through 15, in responding to an appropriately oriented edge stopped at both ends: it differed in that it responded over a wide area of receptive field, whereas with the other cell there was a well-defined region from which responses were evoked, flanked by regions from which responses could be suppressed. Indeed, it is as if properties like those of the previous cell had been generalized over a considerable expanse of retina. This generalization was probably also a feature of the last cells (Figs. 21 and 22), though in that case it was perhaps not so clear. These two cells were also similar in their ability to respond to either of two stimuli 90° apart. A powerful response was obtained with a 1/4°-wide slit or dark bar, oriented at 2:30 and introduced into the receptive field from the right at a rate of about 1°/sec. (Fig. 25); left-to-right movement gave a much weaker response. The stimulus worked regardless of the exact level at which it crossed the field (Fig. 25, A through C). Yet a slit or dark bar 1° wide evoked no response (Fig. 25D). The orientation was again critical to within 15–20°; but, surprisingly, changing the orientation of the 11:30 leading edge by using instead a sharply pointed slit or bar did not lessen the potency of the stimulus, so that the important thing

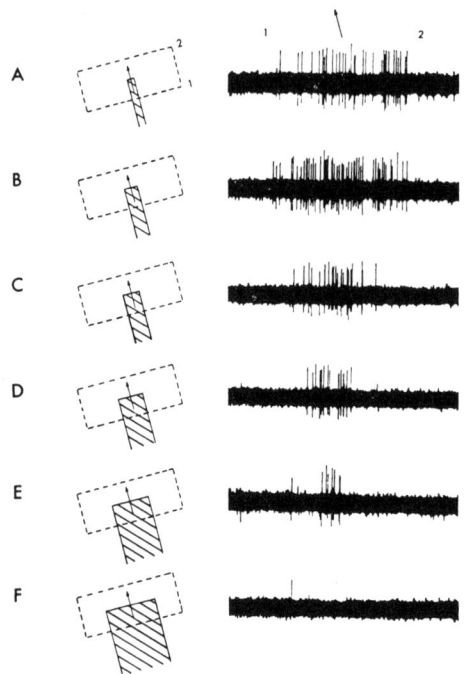

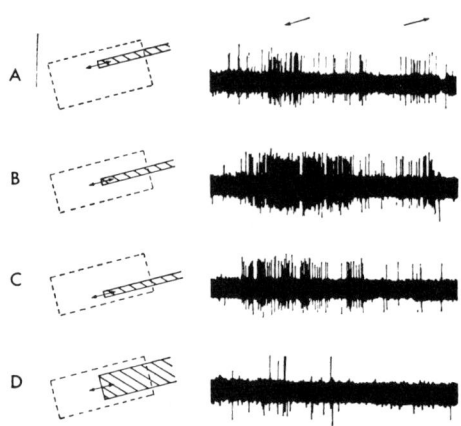

Fig. 24. Effects of varying the width of tongue, in cell of Fig. 23. Movement from below up over center of field at rate of 0.5°/sec. Widths, A through F, are ¼°, ½°, ¾°, 1°, 1½°, and 2°; optimum width (B), ½°. Duration of each sweep, 5 sec.

Fig. 25. Same cell as in Figs. 23 and 24. A through C: responses to a dark 1/4° tongue moved across the field from right to left in various positions as shown, at a rate of 1°/sec. D: response to a 1° tongue moved across field. Duration of each sweep, 10 sec.

was probably the direction of movement of the stimulus, and not the orientation of the leading edge.

Finally, this cell showed a phenomenon that we have occasionally seen in complex cells as well as hypercomplex ones. As a stimulus was repeated time after time at intervals of 2–3 sec. it tended to become progressively less effective, until finally the cell failed to respond. For example, in Fig. 26 a 1/2° tongue was brought in from below and moved up slowly through the field, and this was repeated once every 3 sec. After four stimuli the response began to fail, and after nine stimuli the cell had virtually stopped responding. Now no stimulus was delivered for about 10 sec. A new stimulus (10) introduced after this resting period was once more quite effective. If the dark bar was introduced each time in a different part of the field, there was no progressive decline in the response. If it was reintroduced repeatedly in the same place, as in Fig. 26, until the response faded, a brisk response occurred when it was suddenly introduced in a new place.

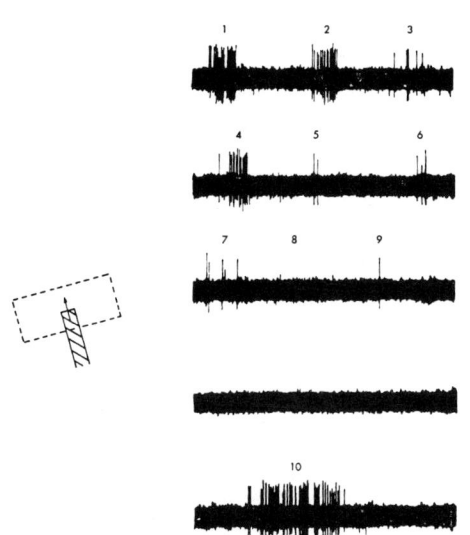

Fig. 26. Same cell as in Figs. 23 through 25. Continuous record. Dark tongue 1/4° wide is moved up and down over center of field at 1°/sec., and the stimulus is repeated every 2–3 sec. By the eighth or ninth repetition the cell is failing to respond. No stimulus is given for 10 sec. The tenth stimulus is then highly effective. Each sweep, 10 sec.

This kind of progressive decline in responsiveness has often been seen in complex cells in visual I and II. For example, many cells are strongly influenced by a critically oriented stationary line stimulus regardless of its position within the receptive field (13: Text-fig. 7). Such cells often fail to respond after several applications of the stimulus in the same place; changing the part of the field stimulated revives the response. In cells of this type, moving the stimulus generally produces a vigorous discharge, perhaps because new regions of the receptive field are being stimulated successively.

Binocular Interaction

For most cells in visual II and III the receptive-field characteristics were worked out separately for each eye, and then both eyes were stimulated together. The results were very similar to those we have previously reported for cells in visual I (13). Most cells, though not all, were influenced independently from the two eyes. A cell that could be driven from both eyes always had receptive fields in corresponding positions in the two retinas, at least to within the limits of accuracy of the method: the two receptive fields thus occupied the same position in the contralateral visual field. The two receptive fields were of the same size and arrangement, so that whatever stimulus was the most effective in one eye—in form, orientation, and direction and rate of movement—was also the most effective in the other eye. Both stimuli together gave more vigorous responses than either applied alone. For a given cell the two eyes were not necessarily similar in their ability to evoke responses. Some cells responded equally well to the two eyes, others favored the ipsilateral eye, still others the contralateral. A few cells responded only to one eye. Thus all shades of relative ocular dominance were found, from cells driven exclusively by the contralateral eye to those driven exclusively by the ipsilateral one. As in previous studies (13), we have divided cells into seven groups according to relative ocular dominance; these groups are defined in Fig. 28.

In Fig. 27 the relative influence of the two eyes was determined for two cells recorded simultaneously in visual area III. One cell was driven almost equally well from the two eyes, and was classed as group 4 (Fig. 27, *A* and *B*). The second

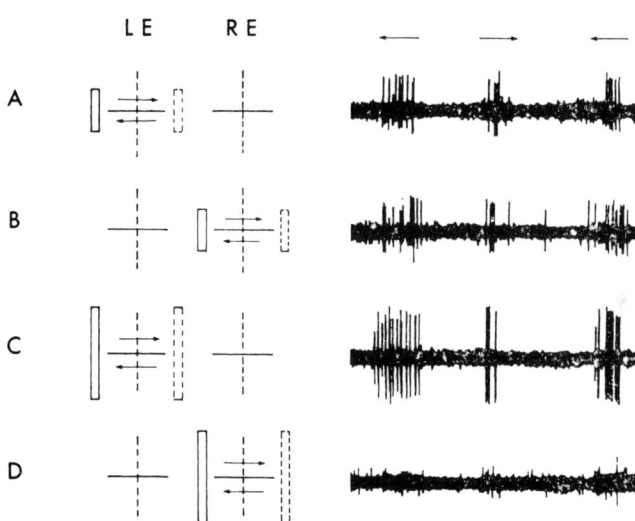

Fig. 27. Two cells simultaneously recorded from area 19; these were cells 35 (complex, large spikes) and 36 (hypercomplex, small spikes), in Fig. 4, penetration V. A and B: responses of the hypercomplex cell (no. 36) to a vertical slit, 1/2° × 2°, moved rapidly back and forth across the receptive field of the left eye (A), and the right eye (B); no response from the complex cell. C and D: movement of a slit 1/2° × 12° produces no response from the hypercomplex cell, but a brisk response from the complex cell (no. 35), in the left eye only. Intensity of stimulus, 1.0 log_{10} cd/m²; background, 0.0 log_{10} cd/m². Rate of movement about 20°/sec. Sweep duration, 1 sec.

cell, on the other hand, responded only from the left or contralateral eye and was placed in group 1. This record is an example of a simultaneous recording from a complex and a hypercomplex cell and will be referred to again.

One hundred and forty-nine of the cells in visual area II, and 89 of those in visual III, were categorized as to ocular dominance. The distribution of these cells among the seven different groups is given in Fig. 28, B and C. It will be seen that for both

visual areas, cells driven by the two eyes (groups 2 through 6) form the great majority, and that cells favoring the contralateral eye (groups 1 through 3) exceed those favoring the ipsilateral (groups 5 through 7). Comparison with Fig. 28A shows a marked similarity between these histograms and the one obtained previously for visual I. In the histograms for visual II and III the shaded area represents hypercomplex units. While one can say little about the ocular-dominance distribution of hyper-

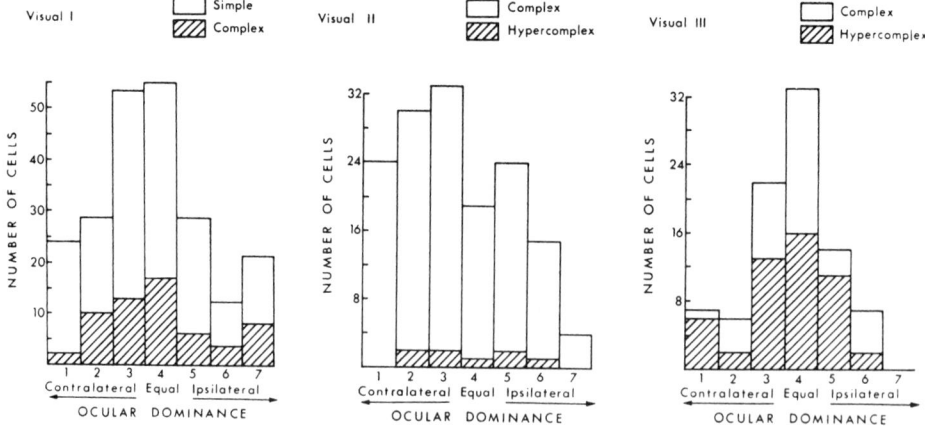

Fig. 28. Distribution according to ocular dominance of (A), 223 cells in visual I (13: text-Fig. 12), (B), 149 cells in visual II, and (C), 89 cells in visual III. Cells of group 1 are driven only by the contralateral eye; for cells of group 2 there is marked dominance of the contralateral eye; for group 3, slight dominance. For cells in group 4 there is no obvious difference between the two eyes. In group 5 the ipsilateral eye dominates slightly, in group 6, markedly; and in group 7 the cells are driven only by the ipsilateral eye.

complex cells in visual II, in visual III the distribution of these cells seems to run parallel to that of the general population. It seems surprising that the functional separation of the two eyes should persist with so little change from one level to the next in the hierarchy, beginning with simple and then complex cells in visual area I, and proceeding to complex and then hypercomplex cells in visual III.

Part III. Functional Architecture of Visual Areas II and III

In this section we examine similarities between neighboring cortical cells, with the object of learning whether there are discrete regions of cortex throughout which the cells share certain receptive-field characteristics. As in previous studies (13, 14) we have proceeded by studying *1)* sequences of cells in single penetrations, *2)* unresolved background activity, and *3)* multiple-unit recordings. The advantages and limitations of these three approaches have already been discussed (13).

Receptive-Field Orientation

Columns with Single Orientation. We were anxious to examine the receptive-field orientations of neighboring cells in visual areas II and III, since in visual I the relative constancy of receptive-field orientation from cell to cell forms the basis for the entire columnar system. Remarkably similar results were found in both areas of nonstriate visual cortex. At any stage in a penetration through gray matter the background activity of unresolved single units was driven best by a line stimulus in a specific orientation, and was silent if the stimulus was oriented at 90° to that orientation. When a single cell was isolated its receptive-field orientation and the optimum orientation for the unresolved background activity almost always coincided. In all multiunit recordings (16 two-unit and 3 three-unit recordings) the cells studied together had identical receptive-field orientations. As the electrode advanced the optimum stimulus orientation for unresolved background activity and for isolated cells would remain constant for varying distances, and would then change abruptly. At the transition point there was either no clear preferred orientation or there were two preferred orientations, that of the cells in the region the electrode was leaving,

and that of cells in the new region. Like area 17, areas 18 and 19 are thus subdivided into discrete regions in which cells have similar receptive-field orientations.

By observing distances between shifts in orientation as the electrode advanced in various directions through gray matter it was possible to assess the size and shape of these regions. In visual area II, examples of two oblique penetrations are seen in Figs. 1 and 2. The short sequences of cells between shifts in orientation—here the longest sequences contained only four to five cells—were typical of such oblique penetrations. On the other hand, in penetrations that were almost normal to the surface the sequences of cells with a similar orientation tended to be much longer. In the experiment of Fig. 4, penetration III was almost perpendicular to the cortex of area 18: here after three short sequences there was a relatively long one, containing all cells from no. 15 to no. 24. Other examples of penetrations more or less normal to the surface can be seen in Fig. 4, penetration II, where a sequence of five cells occupies a large part of the cortical thickness, and Fig. 29, penetration IV, with a sequence of four cells. From these and other experiments we conclude that visual area II, like visual I, is subdivided into discrete regions within which cells have a common receptive-field orientation. The variation of sequence lengths with obliquity of electrode path makes it very likely that here also the regions are columnar in shape and extend from surface to white matter, with walls perpendicular to the radial fiber bundles.

Similar results were found in visual III. Figure 4 shows an oblique penetration (V) containing four shifts of orientation and no very long sequences. Figure 29, on the other hand, shows a particularly long sequence of 15 cells occupying an entire penetration (V) that was very nearly perpendicular to the cortical layers. Thus here too there seems to be a distribution of cells in columns according to receptive-field orientation. (One important exception to this principle for columns in visual III will be discussed in the next section.)

In the striate cortex one finds within a single column both simple cells and complex cells in large numbers (13). In areas 18 and 19 there were both complex cells and hypercomplex cells in a single column. Examples of both types of cells in a single sequence can be found in Fig. 29, penetration IV (visual II), and penetration V (visual III). A clear

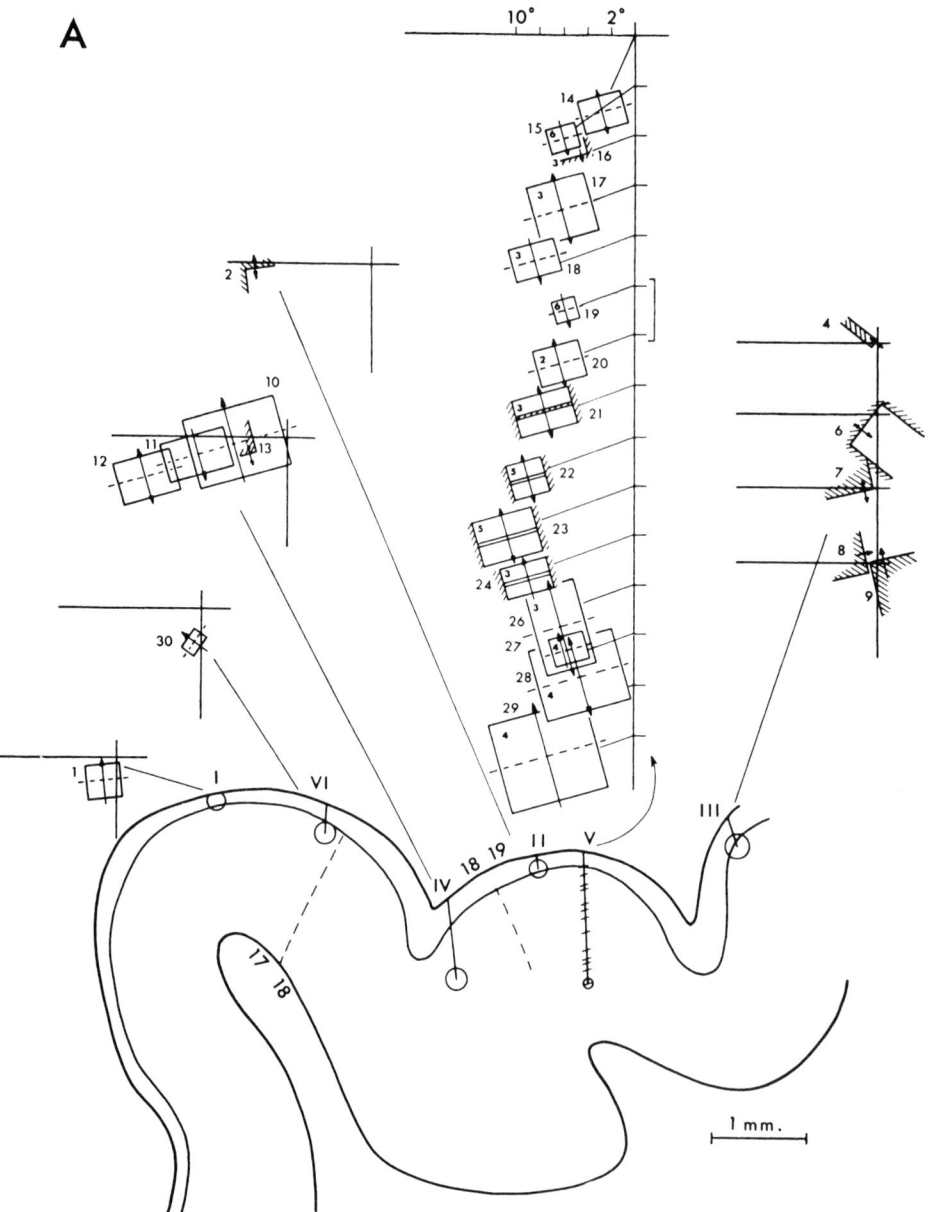

Fig. 29. A: *six microelectrode penetrations through the right postlateral, accessory interlateral, and suprasylvian gyri, at a level indicated in the brain tracing (B, upper right). Points of entry were originally marked on the photograph of the exposed brain surface taken at the beginning of the experiment (B, upper left). Two of the lesions (IV and V) can be made out in the photomicrograph of a Nissl-stained section through this area (B, below); other lesions and electrode tracks appeared on adjacent sections. Conventions as in Figs. 1 through 4. Position and size of complex receptive fields are indicated by rectangles. In penetration V, ocular-dominance groups are indicated in the upper left of each receptive field. Hypercomplex cells 7, 8, 9, and 13 responded to dark corners; 2 and 16 to light corners; 4 to a dark tongue; 6 to a light tongue; 21 responded to a double-stopped dark bar or slit; and 22–24 to double-stopped slits. For cells 21–24 the rectangles indicate the activating portion of the receptive fields. In this experiment note especially 1) the apparent absence of any far peripheral visual-field representation; 2) single columns traversed by penetrations IV and V; 3) cells 8 and 9 simultaneously recorded, fields oriented 90° apart.*

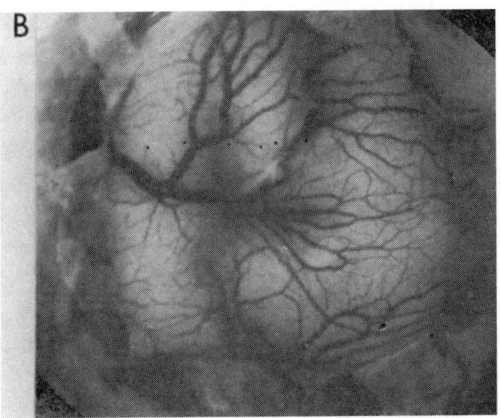
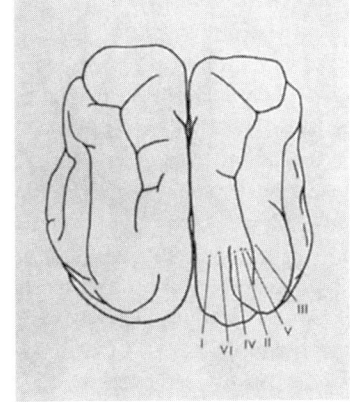

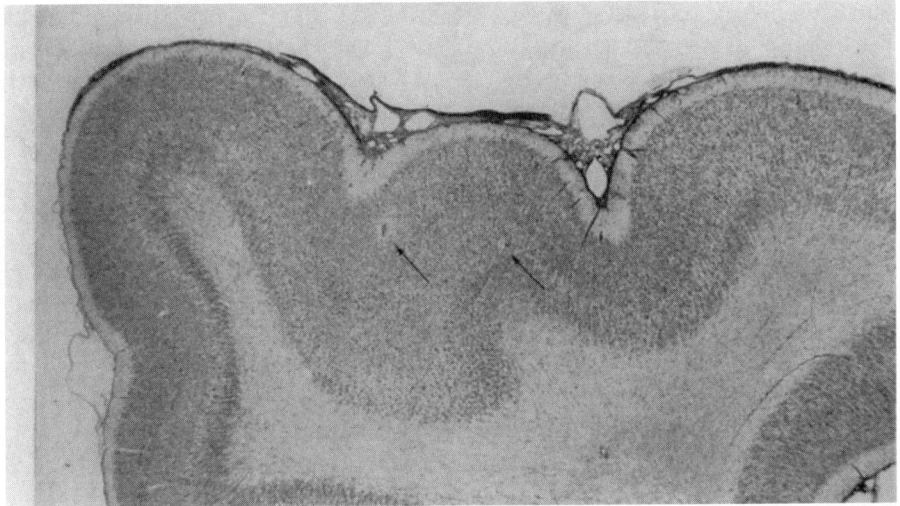

Fig. 29. (continued)

demonstration can also be seen in Fig. 27, in which a complex cell and a hypercomplex one were recorded simultaneously. A short slit, covering the entire activating portion of the hypercomplex cell's field, evoked a strong response from that cell (small spikes, *A* and *B*), but failed to activate the complex cell, presumably because it crossed only a small part of the complex cell's field. A long slit (*C* and *D*), on the contrary, crossed most or all of the complex cell's field and evoked a strong response from the complex cell; in so doing it crossed both the activating and antagonistic portions of the hypercomplex cell's field, and consequently evoked no response.

In visual I there was an indication that simple and complex cells were to some extent segregated by layers, since complex cells seemed to be virtually absent from layer 4 (13: Text-fig. 18). So far we have insufficient material to make a similar analysis of visual II and III, though from examples like that of Fig. 29 it seems that there is no strict segregation of complex and hypercomplex cells by layers.

Figure 29 illustrates one further point, that within a single column one can find representatives of all ocular-dominance groups; in this case the two cells belonged to groups 1 and 4. In penetration V of Fig. 29 the ocular-dominance groups of all of the cells (except 14, for which the grouping was not determined) are noted inside each receptive-field diagram; all groups from 2 to 6 were represented in the one column.

COLUMNS WITH DUAL ORIENTATION. In PART II we have described hypercomplex cells of higher order that responded to stimuli in either of two orientations 90° apart. The relationship of these cells to neighboring ones, especially to complex and lower order hypercomplex cells, obviously presents a special case, since columns so far described have contained cells with a single common receptive-field orientation. The three penetrations in which cells with dual orientation were found were particularly interesting in that some of the lower order neighboring cells responded to one of the two orientations, while others responded to the other. A good example of this type of cell sequence can be seen in Fig. 30. Four of the first nine cells were hypercomplex, and each responded to two stimulus orientations, 2:30 and 11:30. Of the remaining five cells, no. 5 and no. 6 were hypercomplex and responded to dark bars with an 11:30 orientation, but not to stimuli oriented at 2:30. On the other hand, no. 7 (complex) and no. 8 (hypercomplex), responded to stimuli oriented in a 2:30 direction, but not to an 11:30 stimulus. Cells no. 6 and no. 7 were recorded simultaneously and had fields oriented 90° apart, an event that is exceedingly rare in visual I, occurring only at the boundary between two columns.

Another example is to be seen in the short sequence formed by cells 4 through 6 of Fig. 31. Here cell no. 4 responded to a 2:30 edge moved downward: the cell was hypercomplex, with the field stopped at both ends. Cell no. 5 responded to an edge oriented at 11:30 (i.e., 90° to the previous stimulus), and the field was stopped above and below. Cell no. 6, whose records are illustrated in Figs. 23 through 26, responded to *both* stimulus orientations (though it will be recalled that here there was some doubt as to just what it was about the horizontal tongue that activated this cell). In the same figure a similar sequence is formed by cells no. 1 to no. 3: cell no. 1 had a complex field oriented at 2:00, no. 2 was hypercomplex and responded to 2:00 and 11:00 orientations (described in Figs. 21 and 22), and no. 3, recorded simultaneously with no. 2, responded only to a 2:00 edge stopped on the left.

The few dual-orientation hypercomplex cells that we have studied (11 in all) have all occurred in sequences of this type. Such sequences may thus represent a different type of column, containing complex and hypercomplex cells with either of two

receptive-field orientations 90° apart, and also higher order complex cells responding to both stimulus orientations. If these columns are a distinct kind within visual III, it would be interesting to know whether they are scattered among the ordinary visual III columns, or are grouped together, as Figs. 30 and 31 would seem to suggest.

RELATIONSHIP BETWEEN NEIGHBORING COLUMNS. In most penetrations through visual areas II and III there was no obvious relation between receptive-field orientations of cells in neighboring columns. Just as in visual I, however (14), there were a few startling exceptions. In the experiment of Fig. 32 the electrode passed obliquely down the lateral bank of the postlateral gyrus, with the usual very gradual outward drift of receptive fields, typical for visual II, beginning in this case at about 10° and ending some 20° out from the area centralis. The shifts in orientation were meanwhile highly regular. Each shift was small and clockwise, except for the brief reversal in direction between cells 15 and 16, and the large shift in orientation between 13 and 14. We conclude that at least some groups of columns in visual II are organized in a regular way.

In this example one is struck by the minute widths of the columns, at least in the coronal plane: it is unusual to find a shift of orientation at almost every new unit (cf. Figs. 1 and 2, for example). It therefore seemed worth asking whether there might not be some relation between the shifts in orientation and the radial fiber bundles. Close examination of Nissl sections in the region between the middle and lower lesions suggested that there were in the order of 30 radial fiber bundles and associated cell fascicles. Within this area, between cells 15 and 25 (a distance of ca. 0.6 mm.), about 10 clockwise shifts in orientation were detected. Since there may have been more shifts in orientation than were actually observed, it is at least possible that each of the radially oriented anatomical subdivisions represented a column. The columns may thus be no more than about 20 μ. across, though it is not known whether this would represent the diameter of a more or less circular cylinder, or, as seems more likely, the width of a slab-shaped structure of long, narrow cross section (14). No surface mapping has been done in visual II or III, but to judge from oblique microelectrode penetrations, the columns in these two areas, like those in visual

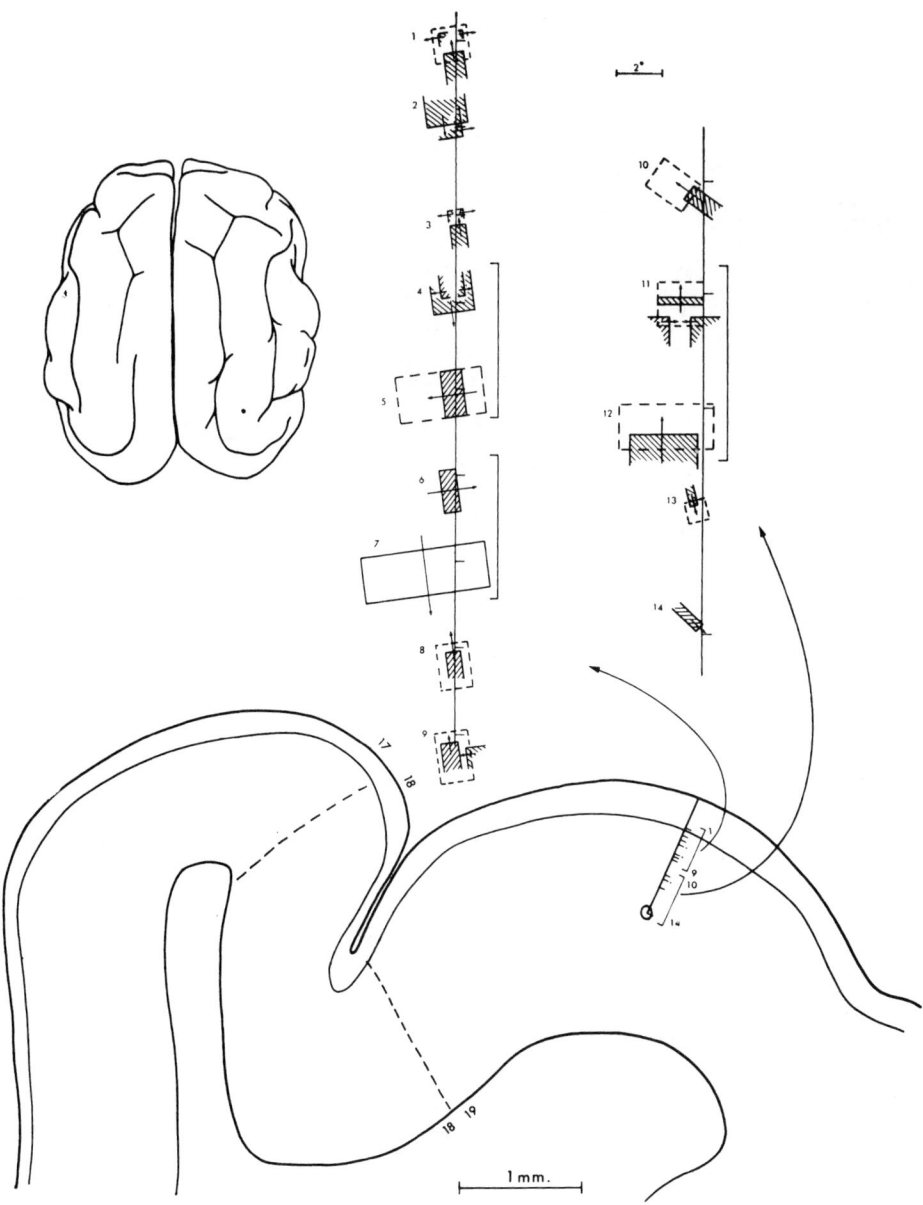

Fig. 30. Single penetration part way through visual III. All cells were hypercomplex, with double-stopped fields, except for no. 7, which was complex. First nine cells were apparently in the same column, within which orientations 2:30 and 5:30 were both represented. For hypercomplex cells, interrupted rectangles indicate roughly the regions from which responses were evoked, where these were mapped. Cells 1–4, 8–10, and 12–14 responded best to dark tongues; 5, 6, and 11 to double-stopped dark bars. Cells 4 and 5, 6 and 7, and 11 and 12 were simultaneously recorded pairs. All receptive fields were located in or near the area centralis. Whether any of these fields extended beyond the vertical meridian into the ipsilateral half visual field is uncertain.

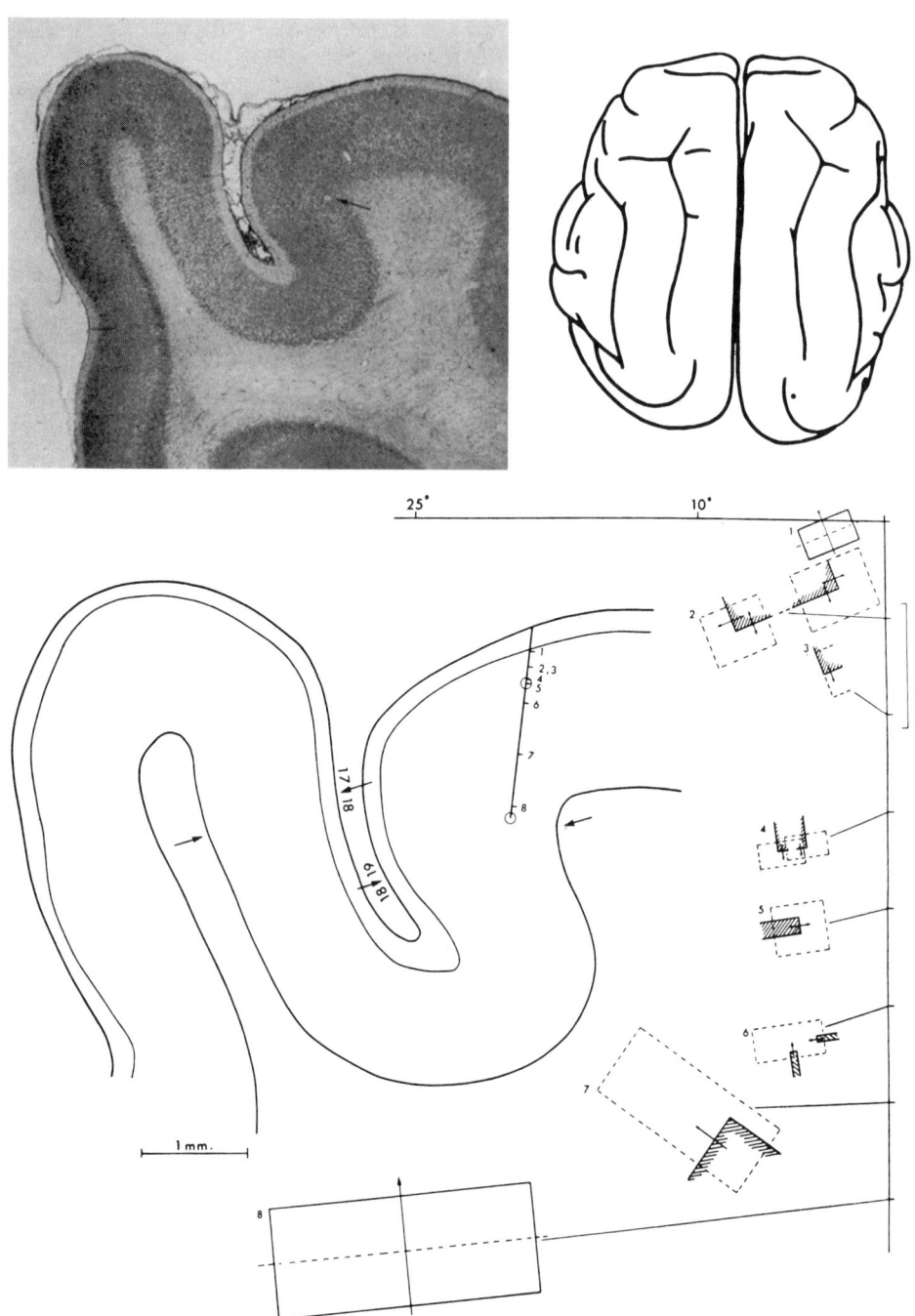

Fig. 31. Single oblique penetration through visual III. The deeper of the two lesions is shown in the Nissl section in upper left. Cells 1 and 8 were complex, 2–7 hypercomplex. Units 2 and 3 were recorded simultaneously. Conventions as in previous figures.

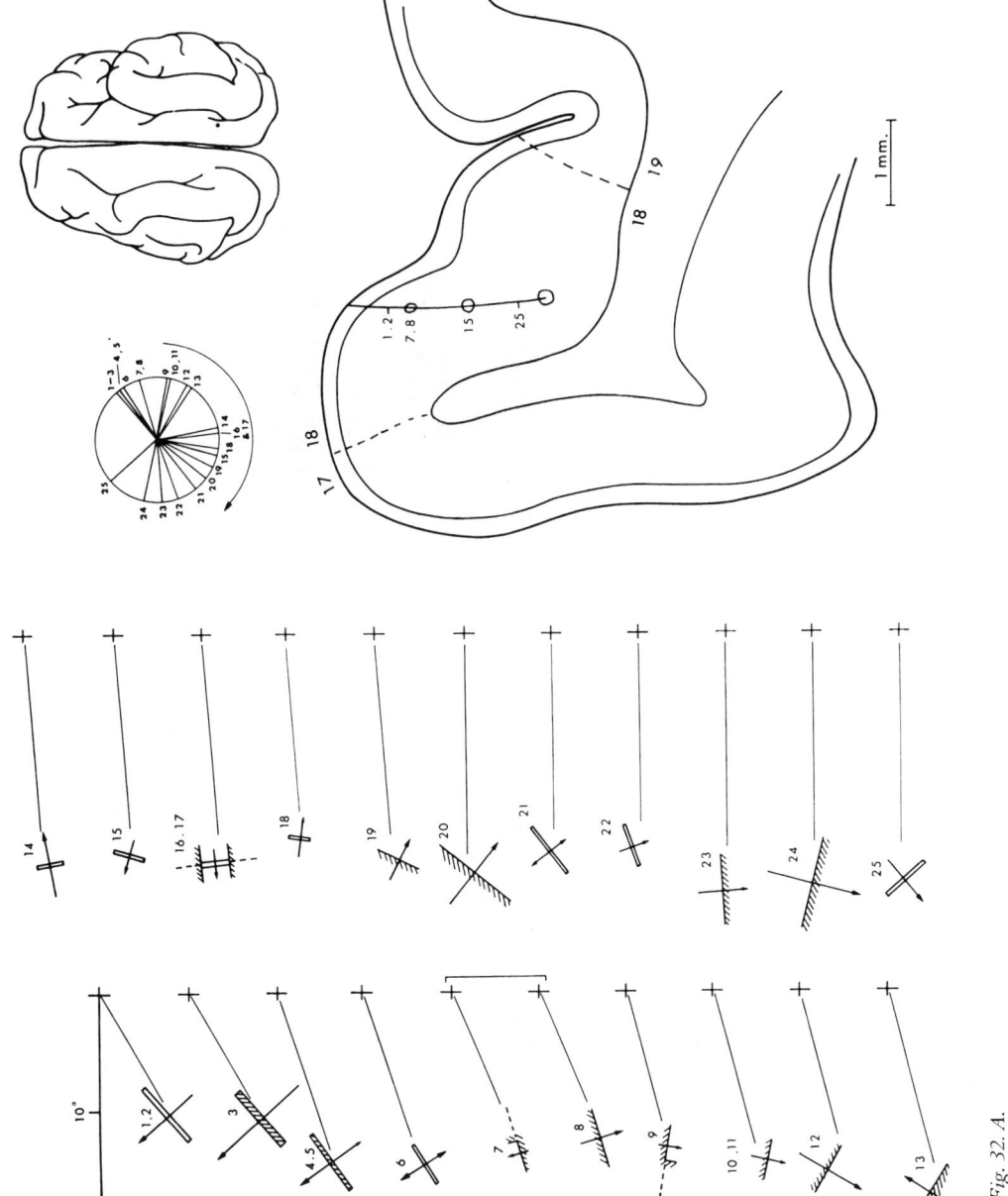

Fig. 32. A.

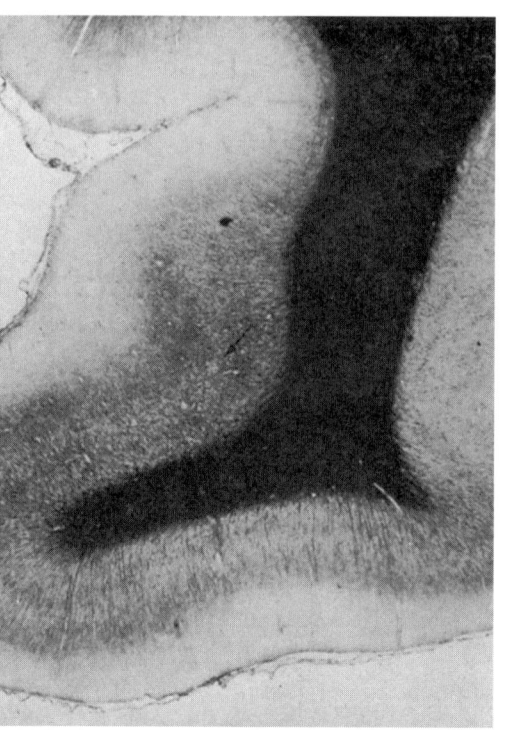

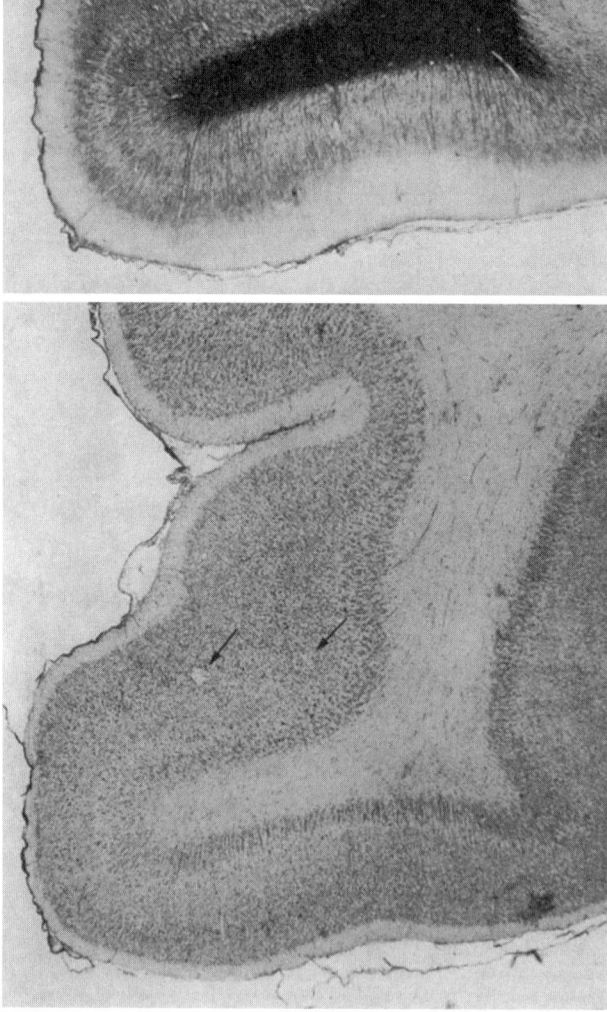

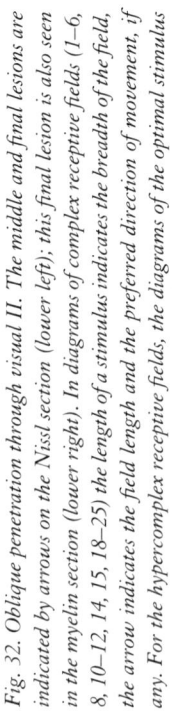

Fig. 32. Oblique penetration through visual II. The middle and final lesions are indicated by arrows on the Nissl section (lower left); this final lesion is also seen in the myelin section (lower right). In diagrams of complex receptive fields (1–6, 8, 10–12, 14, 15, 18–25) the length of a stimulus indicates the breadth of the field, the arrow indicates the field length and the preferred direction of movement, if any. For the hypercomplex receptive fields, the diagrams of the optimal stimulus suggest the breadth of the excitatory part of the field; the interrupted line, the breadth of the inhibitory area; the arrow, the field length and the preferred direction of movement. Note 1) the gradual tendency of fields to move out toward the periphery; 2) the steady systematic clockwise rotation of receptive-field orientation, illustrated in the circular diagram to the left of the tracing of the brain surface.

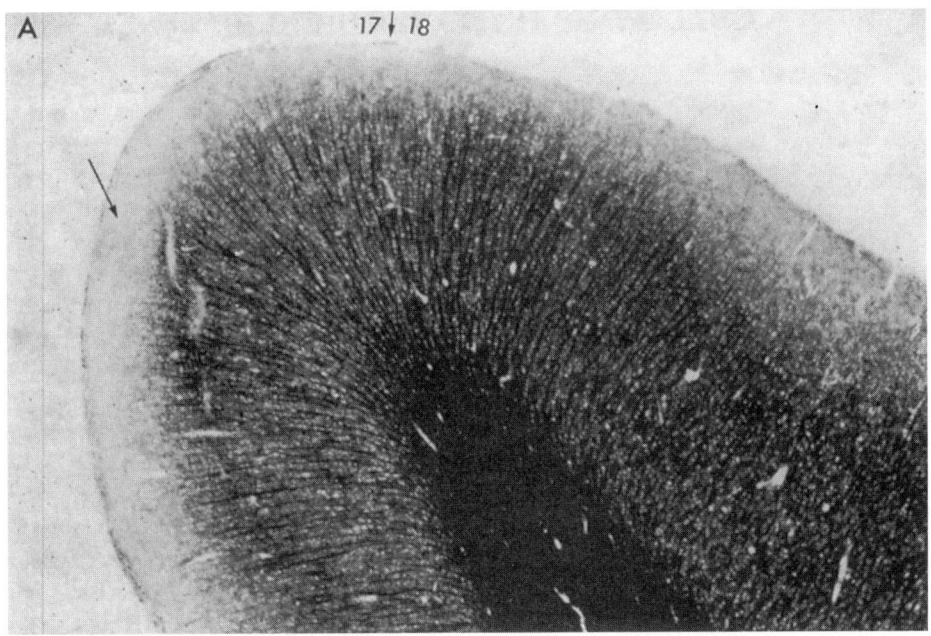

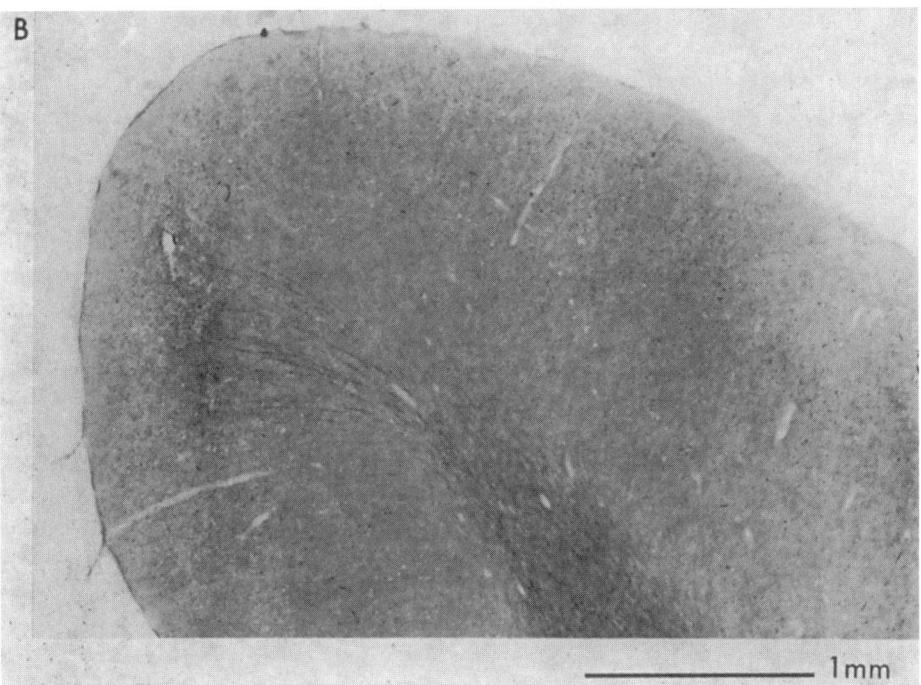

Fig. 33. A: *myelin-stained section showing lesion in area 17, made for the purpose of studying degenerating fibers. Stab wound made by needle can be seen extending down medial aspect of lateral gyrus (arrow). Note also the transition between 17 and 18, indicated by coarser pattern of myelinated fibers. (Loyez stain.) B: Nauta stain of a section close to A, showing degenerating fibers leaving in the radial fiber bundles. Brain perfused 10 days after lesion was made.*

CONTRALATERAL IPSILATERAL

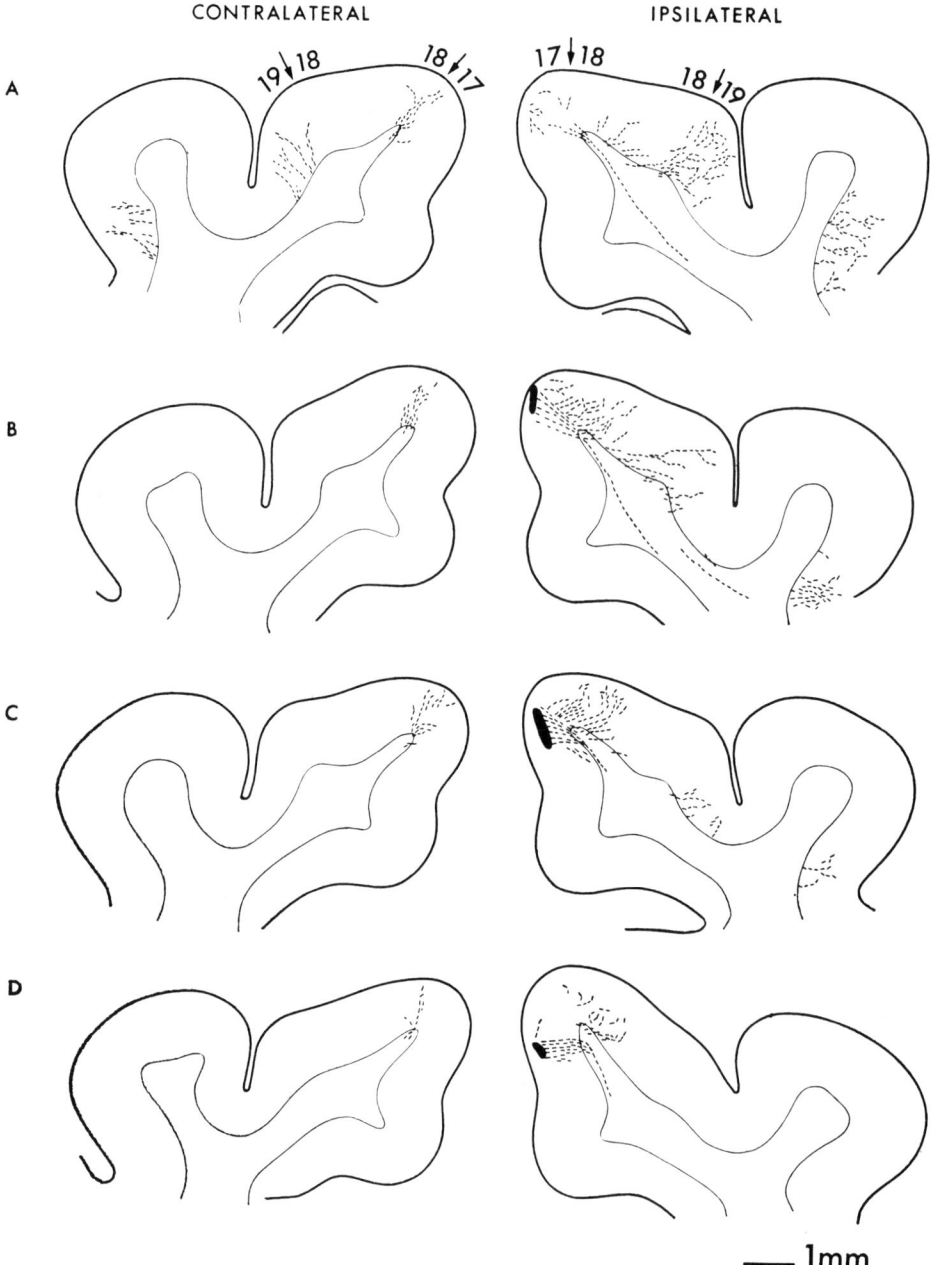

Fig. 34. Same brain as in Fig. 33. Camera-lucida tracings of degenerating fibers (broken lines) in lateral and suprasylvian gyri. Lesion is shown in B, C, and D as the black area in the right hemisphere. The four sections are taken approximately 750 μ. apart.

I, can have cross-sectional diameters of up to about 0.5 mm.

Receptive-Field Position

As described in PART I, during an oblique penetration or in a penetration parallel to the cortical lay-

ers, the receptive fields of successively recorded cells tended to drift across the retina in an orderly fashion, in accordance with the topographical mapping of visual fields onto the cortex. In visual II and III, as in visual I (13), this topographic orderliness did not hold down to the cellular level. In proceeding from cell to cell in a single penetration the positions of successively mapped receptive fields were instead staggered in an apparently random way (Figs. 1 through 4, 29 through 31). Even in crossing a single column or several columns there was never any clear change in average receptive-field position. Only in very long penetrations (Figs. 1 through 3, etc.), traversing many columns, was a net change in receptive-field position seen against the otherwise random staggering. In a penetration perpendicular to the surface, as the electrode advanced from surface to white matter, there was no net change in receptive-field position. When two or three cells were recorded simultaneously they had receptive fields in the same general part of the retina, differing slightly in their positions, but usually overlapping. The area over which fields of cells in a single column were dispersed in this apparently random way was of the same order as the area occupied by the largest receptive fields in the column. For a column in the part of the cortex representing the area centralis, the upper limit of receptive-field size was small (perhaps about 3°), and so was the variation in position; whereas in regions representing peripheral retina, field size and variation in position both tended to be larger. The correlation between field size and dispersion was especially impressive in visual area II, where peripheral receptive fields tended to be very large and widely scattered (see Fig. 3, upper part of penetration IV).

In summary, a column is defined as a region within which cells have a common receptive-field orientation (with the one exception described above). These cells differ in their ocular dominance, in the details of the organization of their fields, and, to a small extent, in the retinal positions of their fields. A given region of retina must be represented by a number of columns, corresponding to the different possible orientations. In experiments like that of Fig. 32 one can distinguish at least 10–15 orientations, so that this would be a possible lower limit for the number of columns required to represent any given small retinal area.

Part IV. Projections from Striate Cortex to Other Cortical Areas

The findings of the preceding sections are difficult to interpret without information on the intercon- nections of areas 17, 18, and 19. It would be especially desirable to know, for example, whether area 17 sends direct connections to 18 and 19. To learn more about the projections of 17 to other cortical areas we accordingly made small lesions in area 17 in six cats, and subsequently traced degenerating fibers by the method of Nauta and Gygax (22). In three cats the lesions were made in the interhemispheric segment of the lateral gyrus; in the other three they were made further back, in the medial aspect of the exposed part of the postlateral gyrus. To determine the boundaries of 17, 18, and 19, sections were stained at 1/2-mm. intervals with myelin and Nissl stains.

The results of an anterior lesion are illustrated in Figs. 33 and 34. In this experiment the cortex was simply stabbed with a 25-gauge hypodermic needle. The track began 1–2 mm. medial to the boundary between 17 and 18 (as determined from adjacent Nissl- and myelin-stained sections; Fig. 33A), and extended for about 3 mm. in a direction almost tangential to the layers of the cortex. Silver stains showed degenerating axons in large numbers fanning out from the site of the lesion, many following the direction of the radial fiber bundles and proceeding toward white matter (Fig. 33B), many others streaking through the cortex toward area 18, seemingly by as direct a route as possible (Fig. 34, *B* and *C*). In serial sections some of the axons could be followed down through the white matter as far as the corpus callosum, and then across and up the other side; others were lost deep in white matter, and were presumed to be bound for subcortical structures. On the side of the lesion large numbers of degenerating axons were found in three areas: *1*) A region confined to 18, extending laterally from a point close to the boundary between 17 and 18, along the lateral gyrus for about 1–2 mm.; axons could often be traced directly in single sections from the lesion to this area. *2*) A region in the lateral wall of the lateral gyrus, well within area 19. *3*) A region confined to the lateral wall of the suprasylvian gyrus, chiefly in its lower half. In each of these three areas the degeneration was maximal a few millimeters anterior to the site of the lesion, and extended for only several millimeters in an anterior-posterior direction. The fibers entered the cortex obliquely or even almost tangentially, showing no tendency to assume the orderly radial pattern that might be expected from examining Nissl- or myelin-stained sections of these regions. This contrasted strongly with the pronounced radial pattern of the fibers leaving area 17, shown in Fig. 33B. In the contralateral hemisphere degenerating fibers were found in the most medial millimeter or so of area 18. The border between 17 and 18 was not sharp enough, even in the myelin-stained sections, to exclude the possibility of some projections to contralateral 17. If any fibers did reach 17, they were confined to a small area near the 17–18 border; no fibers were seen on the medial (interhemispheric) segment. Thus there is no evidence for a set of connections linking homologous regions of 17 on the two sides (see DISCUSSION). Some contralateral projections were also found in 19 and in the lateral wall of the suprasylvain gyrus.

In the experiment of Figs. 35 and 36 an electrolytic lesion was made with a microelectrode deep in the cortex of the interhemispheric segment of the postlateral gyrus, in layers 5 and 6, well within area 17, probably in a portion receiving projections from the contralateral visual field 4–8° out along the horizontal meridian (13: Text-fig. 13). No recordings were made, and the electrode was withdrawn immediately after the current was passed. The resulting lesion was roughly 125 μ. in diameter (Fig. 35A). Compared with acutely made electrolytic lesions (9), those in which several days elapsed before the death of the animal showed a dense infiltration with phagocytes and glial cells. At the level of the lesion there was again a massive outpouring of fibers directed radially toward white matter, and a much sparser group of fibers coursing through 17 in all directions for about 1–2 mm. tangentially and obliquely, extending superficially at least to the second layer. A few fibers heading down obliquely along the medial wall of the hemisphere appeared bound for white matter; otherwise there were no degenerating fibers in distant parts of area 17.

Again three discrete regions of cortex were found in the ipsilateral hemisphere, in area 18, area 19, and along the medial wall of the suprasylvian sulcus (Fig. 36). It is interesting to notice how the projection to 19 moves, in sections taken at progressively more posterior levels, from the lateral bank of the lateral gyrus (Fig. 36A) to the crest of the interlateral accessory gyrus (B), and finally to the medial part of the posterior suprasylvian gyrus (C). These are precisely the areas occupied by visual III in physiological experiments (Fig. 37). Thus studies of Nissl-stained and myelin-stained mate-

rial and experiments with silver degeneration all correlate well with the physiological findings.

In posterior sections, fibers projecting to the lateral bank of the suprasylvian gyrus came to occupy a higher position in the sulcus, and the gap between this area and the degeneration in 19 narrowed so that the two almost coalesced. In both these regions the degeneration was again at a level slightly anterior to the lesion, and extended over an area of cortex only a few millimeters in diameter. In this brain, stains of the contralateral hemisphere were unsatisfactory.

Almost identical results were obtained from the other four experiments. In summary, then, a given small region of area 17 gives cortical projections to at least three small discrete regions in the ipsilateral and contralateral hemispheres; one in area 18, one in 19, and a third in a region of cortex occupying the lateral bank of the suprasylvian gyrus.

These results appear to be similar to those given in a preliminary account by Polley and Dirkes (25), except that they found degeneration in area 17 of the contralateral hemisphere. The findings are difficult to compare, however, without more detailed information on where their lesions were placed.

The projection to the lateral wall of the suprasylvian gyrus seems to involve precisely the area from which Clare and Bishop (1) recorded responses to stimulation of the optic nerve and the striate cortex (see also 5, 29). As to areas 18 and 19, we conclude that these are "higher" visual areas, in which messages from 17 are further elaborated. Whether 18 and 19 are interconnected, or whether they receive projections from other parts of the visual pathway (tectum, thalamus, etc.), are matters for future anatomical studies.

DISCUSSION

Cortical Visual Areas

To casual inspection one of the striking features of the cerebral cortex is its relative anatomical uniformity. It is true that there are occasional abrupt and obvious transitions, such as occur between somatic sensory and motor cortex, or in primates between areas 17 and 18. On the other hand, there are large areas in which variations in structure as seen with Nissl or myelin stains are more subtle, requiring

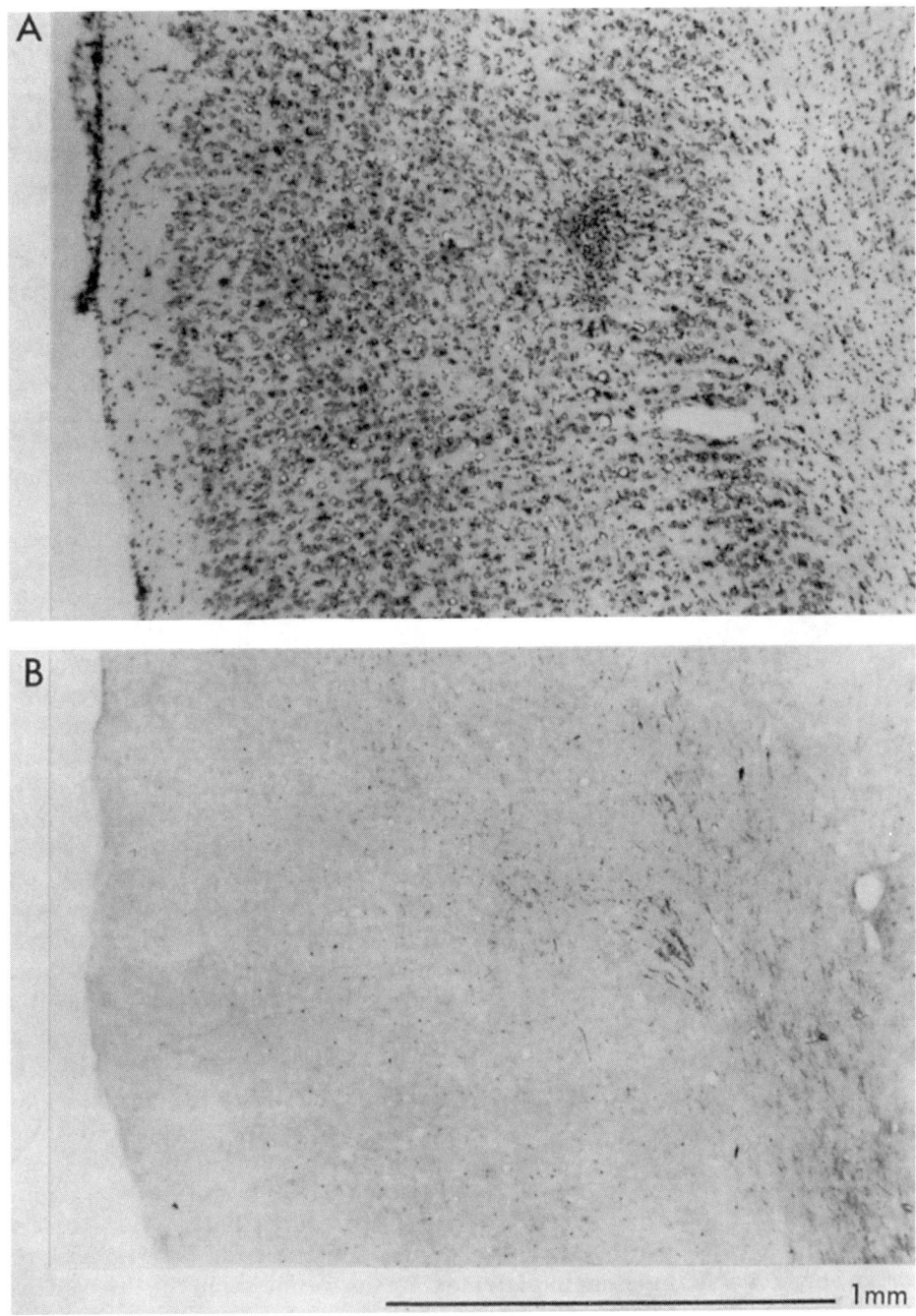

Fig. 35. A: *Nissl-stained section showing electrolytic lesion in area 17, made for the purpose of tracing degenerating fibers. Eight days elapsed between making lesion and perfusing the animal. (Cresyl violet.)* B: *Nauta stain of section close to* A, *showing degenerating fibers leaving lesion along radial fiber bundles.*

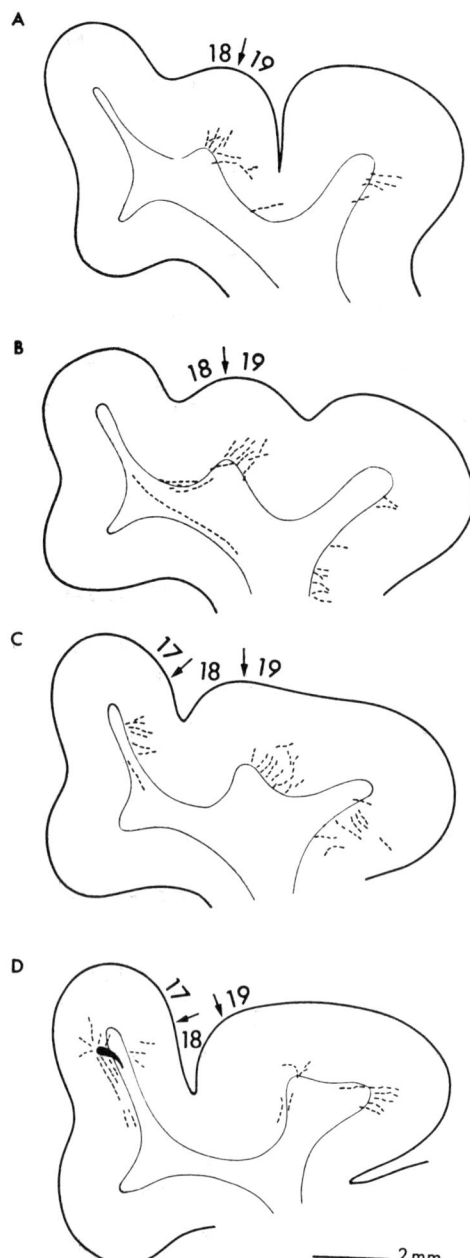

Fig. 36. Same brain as in Fig. 35. Camera-lucida tracings of degenerating fibers at four levels approximately 1.25 mm. apart. Levels A, B,—C and D correspond roughly to levels A, B, and C in Fig. 37.

considerable experience to distinguish genuine architectural variations from those produced by changes in cortical curvature, or small differences in the angle at which a gyrus or sulcus is sectioned. For this reason, the extent to which the cortex can

be justifiably subdivided has been a matter of some dispute.

From the present study it is clear that some architectural subdivisions, subtle though they may be, are quite valid, reflecting differences both in connections and in function. We began by showing that in each hemisphere of the cat brain there are at least three precisely organized topographical projections of the contralateral half-field of vision. It turns out that these three physiologically defined areas, visual I, II, and III, are identical to the areas defined anatomically as 17, 18, and 19. Furthermore, from silver-degeneration studies it seems that two of the cortical areas to which 17 projects coincide with visual areas II and III. The boundaries between 17, 18, and 19 can thus be assessed by four independent methods, the Nissl-stain, the myelin-stain, silver-degeneration techniques (Nauta method), and physiological mapping. In the areas examined, the boundaries determined by all four methods are identical. These are summarized in Fig. 37, for three different antero-posterior levels.

In this paper we have used the terminology, "visual I, II, and III" and "areas 17, 18, and 19" more or less interchangeably, favoring the former when the context was a physiological one, and the latter when the context was anatomical. The designations 17 through 19 refer specifically to the regions anatomically defined by Otsuka and Hassler for the cat (23). The terms "occipital" and "pre-occipital" have been avoided, since they seem inappropriate to the cat brain. "Peristriate" and "parastriate" are terms too easily confused to be useful. We use "area 17" and "striate cortex" interchangeably, since, even though this part of the cortex is not particularly striated compared with the primate area 17, there seems to be no doubt about the homology between the areas in cat and primate. The relationship between areas 18 and 19 in the cat, and the regions so designated in primates, is less clear; at present it would seem to depend mainly on the proximity of the regions to area 17, and on the large pyramidal cells in layer 3 of area 18. Future studies of anatomy and physiology should help to clarify the extent to which the areas in the two species are homologous. From preliminary experiments in spider monkeys (unpublished) it seems that area 18 is precisely arranged topographically, with the vertical-meridian representation bordering that of area 17, just as it does in the

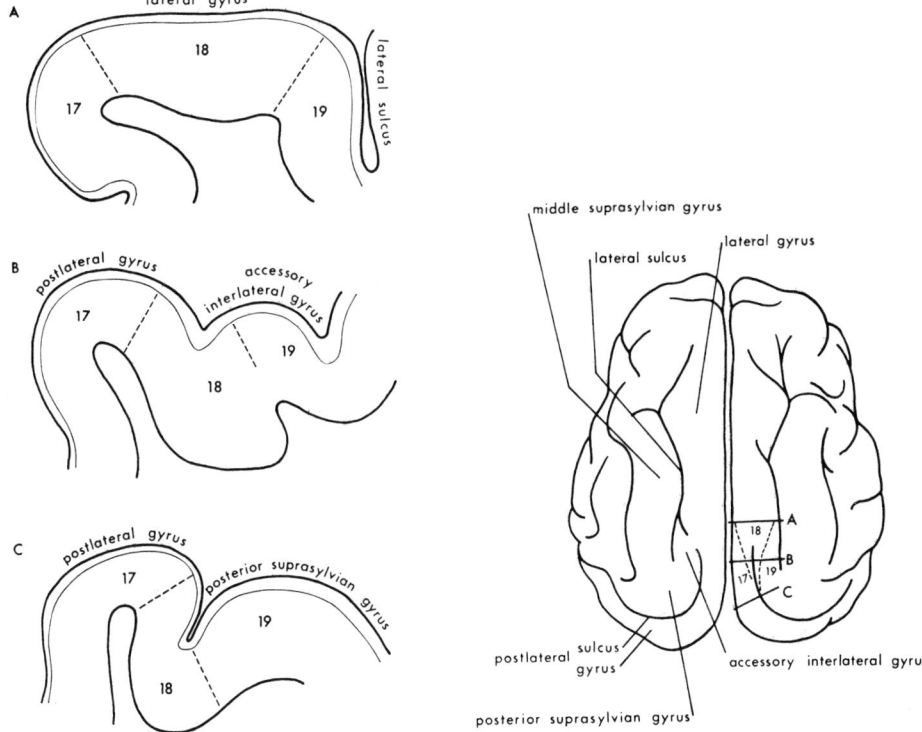

Fig. 37. *Composite diagram showing coronal sections at three antero-posterior levels through visual areas I, II, and III (or 17, 18, and 19). Boundaries are based on several criteria, including histology as studied in Nissl- and myelin-stained sections, distribution of projections from area 17 to nonstriate visual cortex by the silver-degeneration technique, and physiological recordings.*

cat. Similar results have been reported for the squirrel monkey and the rhesus monkey by Cowey (2).

In the rabbit, visual areas I and II have been precisely mapped by the method of evoked potentials by Thompson, Woolsey, and Talbot (28). So far the two visual areas have not been correlated with cytoarchitectonics. As in the cat, visual II was situated anterolateral to visual I, with the vertical meridian projecting to the boundary between the two. Visual II was more extensive in the rabbit than in the cat, and there was a smaller region of binocular projection, reflecting the more lateral position of the rabbit's eyes.

We have limited our comparison between physiological mapping and cytoarchitecture to the part of the cat cortex indicated in Fig. 37. No studies were made of the posterior portions of 17, 18, and 19, where the superior visual fields presumably have their representation. Neither have we any

information on the cortical area that adjoins 17 deep in the splenial sulcus, a region that Otsuka and Hassler designate as 19. For the present we tentatively assume that the entire visual II lies lateral to visual I; whether, as the cytoarchitectural studies suggest, some of visual III lies next to visual I in the splenial sulcus—i.e., whether some parts of the visual fields have their visual III representation there and not lateral to visual II—remains to be determined.

As many authors have stressed (20, 23), the lateral boundary of area 17 in the cat is often difficult to define sharply, especially in Nissl sections. Myelin stains are usually helpful, for in these the transition is seen as an abrupt coarsening of the radial efferent fibers (23; see also Figs. 3, 4, 32), and as an increase in the proportion of obliquely running fibers. The difficulty in pinpointing this 17–18 border, added to possible variations from cat to cat, probably accounts for the differences in position assigned to it by various neuroanatomists (cf., e.g., Figs. 2 and 3 in ref. 20). It is nevertheless agreed by most authorities, and can indeed be considered as established by Otsuka and Hassler (23), that the part of area 17 that extends over the dorsal surface of the brain occupies only a part of the width of the lateral gyrus, probably 1/3–1/4 depending on the antero-posterior level.

That such a small part of the lateral gyrus is striate cortex is worth emphasizing, because the region of maximal cortical evoked potential in response to a visual stimulus is probably *outside* area 17, as first pointed out by Doty (5). This area of maximum response appears to lie in 18, in the area of projection of the inferior visual fields, and cannot therefore be used as a guide to the position of the striate cortex. Studies involving stimulation or ablation of the visual areas, or recording from them, are therefore of limited value if the regions worked upon are not precisely determined by gross and microscopic anatomy.

The position of the lateral border of 19 is not clear, either from anatomical studies (23) or from the physiological mapping done so far. Our mapping of visual II agrees fairly well with the rough sketch of Talbot and Marshall (27), except for a few crosses which they show extending over to the exposed part of the posterior suprasylvian gyrus. The region designated as visual II in the diagrams of Woolsey (32), based, presumably, on the map of Talbot and Marshall, seems to include most or all of what we would term visual III (area 19).

An additional comment may be made here concerning possible functions of visual II. For technical reasons related to difficulties in defining the area centralis to an accuracy of less than 1° or so, we cannot be sure whether or not the fields of cells in either 17 or 18 extend into the ipsilateral field of vision. Assuming for argument's sake that receptive fields of area 17 are entirely confined to the contralateral half-field, the fact that 18 receives projections from 17 of the opposite hemisphere suggests that some cells in 18 should have at least part of their receptive fields in the ipsilateral visual field. This would mean that 18 might have an important function in correlating the two half-fields of vision along the vertical meridian. In crossing the 17–18 border from medial to lateral there should thus be a slight additional movement of receptive fields past the midline and into the

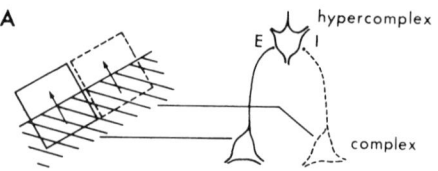

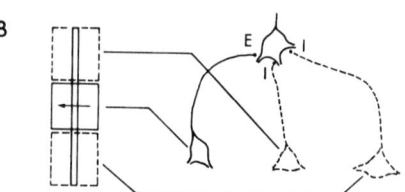

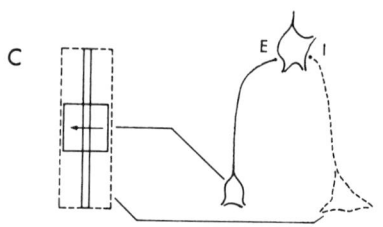

Fig. 38. Wiring diagrams that might account for the properties of hypercomplex cells. A: hypercomplex cell responding to single stopped edge (as in Figs. 8 through 11) receives projections from two complex cells, one excitatory to the hypercomplex cell (E), the other inhibitory (I). The excitatory complex cell has its receptive field in the region indicated by the left (continuous) rectangle; the inhibitory cell has its field in the area indicated by the right (interrupted) rectangle. The hypercomplex field thus includes both areas, one being the activating region, the other the antagonistic. Stimulating the left region alone results in excitation of the cell, whereas stimulating both regions together is without effect. B: scheme proposed to explain the properties of a hypercomplex cell responding to a double-stopped slit (such as that described in Figs. 16 and 17, except for the difference in orientation, or the hypercomplex cell with small spikes in Fig. 27). The cell receives excitatory input from a complex cell whose vertically oriented field is indicated to the left by a continuous rectangle; two additional complex cells inhibitory to the hypercomplex cell have vertically oriented fields flanking the first one above and below, shown by interrupted rectangles. In an alternative scheme (C), the inhibitory input is supplied by a single cell with a large field indicated by the entire interrupted rectangle. In either case (B or C), a slit covering the entire field of the hypercomplex cell would be ineffective. Scheme C requires that a slit covering but restricted to the center region be too short to affect the inhibitory cell.

ipsilateral field, prior to a movement in the reverse direction. We have no evidence yet that this occurs. An absence of projections linking corresponding parts of area 17 in the two hemispheres would make good sense, especially for parts of 17 not adjoining 18, since it is difficult to imagine why cells having receptive fields in a particular part of the visual field should have connections with other cells in the contralateral hemisphere, with fields in a mirror position in the other half-field of vision. Previous studies of this subject, anatomical (26) and physiological (3, 6), have been somewhat contradictory, and it is hard to evaluate them because of changing notions about the exact definition and location of 17, 18, and 19 in the cat.

Schemes for Elaboration of Hypercomplex Fields

With areas 18 and 19 well established as anatomical and physiological entities, and with the evidence that area 17 sends strong projections to both of them, it is natural to ask what further processing of the visual messages takes place in 18 and 19. In both areas a proportion of cells seem to have properties identical to those of higher order cells of area 17—i.e., they have complex properties. Complex cells are in the great majority in visual II, and seem to form about half the population in visual III. In visual II the very large size of some receptive fields suggests that one cell may receive input from a number of fibers from the striate cortex. These incoming fibers would presumably all have the same receptive-field orientation and a similar preference as to form of stimulus (slit vs. bar, etc.); they would only need to differ from one another in their precise receptive-field positions. In visual III, on the other hand, complex cells did not differ in any obvious way from cells of visual I, so that one need not propose any extensive convergence of afferents onto complex cells.

Since the next step in complexity is represented by the hypercomplex cell, it seems reasonable to try to interpret hypercomplex properties by assuming that these cells receive their afferents from complex cells. To see how this might work, it may be useful to contrast complex properties with hypercomplex. With complex cells the responses are more vigorous the longer the stimulus line, until the stimulus reaches the boundaries of the receptive field. Beyond this it makes no difference

how long the stimulus is. There is, in other words, summation across the entire receptive field in the direction of the receptive-field orientation. With hypercomplex cells of lower order (Figs. 8 through 27) a similar summation occurs in one portion of the field, which can be loosely termed excitatory. If the stimulus extends beyond this part into inhibitory regions the response no longer increases, but, on the contrary, is suppressed, and a line crossing the entire receptive field is indeed usually ineffective. Here one can speak of excitatory and inhibitory subdivisions of a hypercomplex field, or perhaps better, an activating region and an antagonistic one, provided it is clearly understood that it is not simple illumination of these regions that determines whether the cell is excited or its response prevented. Each region by itself is typically complex, i.e., a cell responds when an appropriately oriented line (slit, bar, or edge) is shone or moved anywhere within the activating area, and the response is prevented with similar and simultaneous stimulation of the antagonistic region. Summation occurs in each region, in the sense that within one region the longer the line the greater its effect; mutual antagonism occurs in the sense that adequate stimulation of the activating region is offset by adequate stimulation of the opposing one. Summation and mutual antagonism thus occur only along the direction of the receptive-field orientation, and not in any simple spatial sense, as is so for simple cortical cells and cells at lower levels. In hypercomplex cells it is of course the similarity of the orientation of the two opposing subdivisions of the field that makes a long straight line ineffective, and a stopped line, properly placed and oriented, the most effective stimulus.

It is perhaps worth emphasizing this distinction between a pair of antagonistic regions within each of which simple areal summation occurs, and a pair of antagonistic regions with more complex properties. It has recently been suggested that the retinal ganglion cells in the frog termed "convex edge detectors" by Lettvin and colleagues (17) have receptive fields with an excitatory center and an inhibitory surround (7). To judge from the accounts of Lettvin and co-workers it seems likely that if the fields in question have a center-surround organization it is only in some highly complex sense. They seem to be quite different from retinal ganglion cells or geniculate cells in the cat, and indeed they may have a complexity approaching that of hypercomplex cells in areas 18 and 19.

The properties of a hypercomplex cell are most easily explained by supposing that the afferents to the cell are complex, and that some synapses are excitatory and others inhibitory. It is only necessary to assume that the excitatory input is a complex cell (or perhaps more than one) with a receptive field identical in position and arrangement to the excitatory or activating part of the hypercomplex field, and that inhibitory inputs originate from complex cells with fields in the territory of the antagonistic flanks. This general scheme is illustrated in Fig. 38. The simplest case, that of a cell with its field stopped at only one end, is given in Fig. 38*A;* the cell could be the one illustrated in Figs. 8 through 11. Only two afferent cells are shown, an excitatory and an inhibitory, but there might be many of each type. In Fig. 38, *B* and *C,* two possible arrangements are suggested to account for the properties of a double-stopped hypercomplex cell (see Figs. 16 through 20, and 27). Figure 38*B* requires two inhibitory cells, or sets of cells, both complex, with their fields covering the two flanking areas. In an alternative scheme (Fig. 38*C*), the hypercomplex cell receives an excitatory input from a complex cell whose field covers the activating center, as before, and an inhibitory input from a single complex cell with a field having the same size and position as the entire hypercomplex field, both center and flanks. This arrangement could only work efficiently if the inhibitory afferent gave a good response to a long slit, but little or no response to a stimulus confined to the activating area. This was true for the complex cell (large spikes) of Fig. 27, which responded well to a large slit, but not to a small one. Except for the difference in ocular dominance, one might imagine that the two simultaneously recorded cells in Fig. 27 were interconnected, the complex cell sending inhibitory connections to the hypercomplex one.

In the schemes just proposed, the highly specific properties of hypercomplex cells in 18 and 19 seem to demand highly specific sets of connections from lower order cells. Compelling evidence to support the schemes is given by the functional architecture of visual II and III. As we have shown, these areas, like visual I, are subdivided into columns each containing complex and hypercomplex cells with identical receptive-field orientations

and a certain variation in receptive-field position—in short, the very cells that the physiology predicted should be interconnected. It is known from Golgi preparations of the cortex that cells within a region having the size and shape of a column would in fact be richly interconnected. As in area 17, then, the morphological anatomy, the functional architecture, and the single-cell physiology all seem to be completely consistent. The columns of areas 18 and 19, like those of 17, may be considered as functional units of cortex, there being many interconnections between cells of one column, far fewer between cells of adjacent columns. The main purpose of the aggregation of cells into columns is presumably an enormously efficient reduction in the lengths of these connections.

Hypercomplex Cells of Higher Order

An even higher degree of complexity, and still another example of a correlation between response properties and functional architecture, is provided by the cells in area 19 that responded to two orthogonal stimulus orientations. The simplest mechanism for the dual receptive-field orientation would involve convergence upon the cell of two sets of afferent hypercomplex cells having their receptive-field orientations 90° apart. Cells with dual orientation seemed to occur within columns that also contained complex and lower order hypercomplex cells, some having one receptive-field orientation, others an orientation at right angles to the first. It seems, in fact, that here again the very cells that the physiological experiments suggest are interconnected are aggregated in columns. Perhaps it should be stressed, however, that our notions about these higher order cells and the columns containing them are tentative, based as they are on a very few cells (11 in all), in only three penetrations. Experiments with more cells and penetrations may help to settle a number of questions, especially the relation, within visual area III, between these columns and ones in which a single orientation is represented.

A second quite different type of higher order transformation was seen in several cells. The cell recorded in Figs. 23 and 24 responded best to a double-stopped edge with a sharply defined orientation and length (Fig. 24). This was no ordinary hypercomplex cell, however, since there was no division of its field into excitatory and inhibitory areas, and since it responded to movement over an area many times the width of the optimum stimulus (Fig. 23), so that the hypercomplex properties were, in a sense, generalized in the direction of the receptive-field orientation. (A similar generalization was probably also present, though to a lesser extent, in the higher order hypercomplex field of Figs. 21 and 22.) Such behavior could obviously be explained by imaging a convergence of many lower order hypercomplex cells onto a cell of higher order, the afferent cells differing only with respect to the exact positions of the boundaries between centers and flanks. This convergence could occur in the same columns in which the lower order hypercomplex properties were elaborated.

The phenomenon of progressive attenuation of responses shown by this cell (Fig. 26) is one that we have seen from time to time in all three visual areas. Here it was clearly not a question of progressive unresponsiveness of the cell itself, since the responses came back as soon as the stimulus was introduced in a new part of the receptive field. Presumably the failure was somewhere along one particular pathway leading to the cell. Lettvin *et al.* (18) have found cells with somewhat similar behavior in the frog tectum.

Transformations in the Three Visual Areas

We have already referred, in the first part of this DISCUSSION, to the relative structural uniformity of the cerebral cortex. It seems astonishing that neural aggregations so similar in organization can be concerned with functions so diverse as vision, audition, somatic sensation, and motor movements. It becomes important to learn whether the anatomical similarity of the different cortical areas reflects common functional features. For this reason it seems worth while to compare the different transformations that occur in visual areas I, II, and III.

In the striate cortex one can distinguish two successive processes of convergence, each involving many excitatory afferents. The convergence of incoming geniculate fibers onto a simple cell is apparently such that the cell responds maximally only when most of the excitatory afferents are simultaneously activated. A spot is a feeble stimulus, but a slit may be a powerful one; if the cell has connections with the two eyes, a maximal response occurs only when the eyes are stimulated together.

The result of the process is an enormous increase in specificity, each cell requiring a particular stimulus position, shape, and orientation, and preferably stimulation of both retinas. This increased specialization is attained by an immense increase in the number of cells, and through multiple branching of the afferent fibers. At the next stage, from simple to complex cells in the striate cortex, the convergence is again excitatory, but with the difference that for activation of the complex cell only a small proportion of the afferents need be activated at any one time. For example, a slit becomes effective wherever it is shone within the receptive field, and, for reasons not clear, two parallel slits shone in the same receptive field seldom give a more powerful response than either by itself. On the other hand, sequential activation of the afferents by movement of a line across the field is generally a very powerful stimulus, perhaps partly because none of the antecedent cells has time to adapt. The transformation from simple receptive field to complex involves a generalization of one of the qualities of the stimulus, namely its orientation.

In 18 and 19 a still different mode of convergence takes place, apparently one in which excitatory and inhibitory influences come together on one cell. Here the result is again to increase stimulus specificity, rather than to generalize. The hypercomplex cell does not necessarily respond to a properly oriented line crossing the receptive field; it accepts only a line that is appropriately terminated. A line covering the entire field presumably activates two processes that mutually cancel to an amazingly precise degree. This powerful mechanism for enhancing stimulus specificity has already been encountered in two different contexts in the mammalian visual system. In the retina, the geniculate, and the striate cortex, it is used to discriminate against diffuse light in favor of patterned stimulation; in the monkey retina it is used to enhance specificity of the response to certain monochromatic wavelengths at the expense of others and of white light. Analogous mechanisms involving inhibition are known to occur in the somatosensory and auditory systems.

The next step, shown in the example of Figs. 23 and 24, and seen so far only in a few penetrations in area 19, seems again to be one of convergence of excitatory afferents. For the higher order hypercomplex cell to respond, the line must now be properly oriented (sometimes with two possible orientations 90° apart) and limited in its extent, as before, but it need not necessarily be accurately specified as to position. Still more generalization has taken place, this time along a direction parallel to the receptive-field orientation, i.e., at right angles to the direction of generalization in the transformation from simple cells to complex. Here again the convergence must be such that one only need activate small sets of antecedent hypercomplex cells in order to activate the higher order cell. The transformation is thus analogous to that between simple and complex cells in the striate cortex. Indeed, there is an analogy between simple cells and lower order hypercomplex cells, with their centers and flanks and high specificity, and also between complex and higher order hypercomplex cells, in each of which generalization has taken place.

Though these transformations show certain similarities in their details they also exhibit a considerable variety, and there seems to be no doubt that impressive differences exist in the details of connections between one cortical area and the next. These differences are undoubtedly related to the cytoarchitectural distinctions between the various areas. The common features are perhaps more fundamental—the occurrence of one or more intricate transformations between incoming and outgoing messages, taking place within a system of more or less independent columns with little lateral dissemination of information, and the possibility of explaining the transformations by simple, relatively well-known neural mechanisms like the nerve impulse, excitatory and inhibitory synapses, convergence, and so on, with the strong indication that the connections are not random, but highly specified.

The highly structured and specific nature of these connections raises the question of their origin, and in particular whether they are developmentally determined, or depend for their evolution on visual experience after birth. For connections up to and including the striate cortex it is clear that the development is largely innate, since kittens shortly after birth and prior to any visual experience show virtually the same response specificity as is found in the adult (15). In some respects this seems quite natural, since at these levels in the visual pathway one is still dealing with what are undoubtedly building blocks of perception, elements that would hardly be expected to differ from individual to individual with experience (except for pathological early experience such as results from sensory deprivation (30)). If this reasoning is valid for the striate cortex, it is probably also valid for 18 and 19; one would expect to find the connections innately determined there too. The experiments have not yet been done.

Columnar Organization of the Cortex

The most conspicuous property common to the three visual regions is to be found not in the details of the transformations that occur there, but in the columnar organization. Although Lorente de Nó (19) had emphasized the richness of the radial connections and the relative paucity of horizontal connections in the cortex, Mountcastle (21) was the first to show that one area of cortex, the somatosensory, was organized in discrete columnar regions, and to enunciate the principle that the column was the elementary unit of organization. This notion was based on the anatomically known richness of connections between cells in a column, and the assumption that neighboring columns, containing cells that subserved entirely different sensory submodalities, were functionally independent. A demonstration of columnar organization in the primary visual cortex (13, 14) showed that this plan was not unique to the somatosensory system. In the striate cortex, furthermore, the subdivision into columns depended on more subtle criteria: not on the submodality of the afferents, but rather on the connections within the columns. The present study shows that the columnar organization is not confined to sensory receiving areas, but holds also for certain higher visual areas. Thus all four cortical areas in which functional architecture has been examined show a columnar organization; it would be surprising if other cortical areas were not similarly subdivided. It is perhaps worth noting that functional parcellations of gray matter nuclei have been found outside the cortex, for example by Poggio and Mountcastle (24) in the ventrobasal complex of the thalamus. These subdivisions, like columns in the somatosensory cortex, are defined by differences in submodality from one cell aggregate to the next. The lateral geniculate body provides an extreme example of an especially coarse aggregation of cells within an otherwise functionally uniform mass of gray matter: in the monkey the small-cell and large-cell portions of the geniculate are each parcellated into layers according to eye dominance. Perhaps it is a rule, in the central nervous system, for sets of cells that are interconnected to be grouped together, and separated from other similar groups with which they have few or no connections.

The most interesting aspect of columnar organization, in the visual system at any rate, is the clear role that it appears to play in function. The concept of the column as a functional unit becomes more vivid when the transformations occurring within it are known, and it is realized that the segregated cells are just those that must be interconnected to explain the transformations. Far from being a mere aggregation of cells with common characteristics, the column emerges as a dynamic unit of function.

In the visual areas the columnar system can probably be looked on as a solution to the problem of dealing with three independent variables—two to specify a position on the retina, and the third for receptive-field orientation—in a structure, the cortex, that is in a sense two-dimensional. If there were four variables one might expect there to be two columnar systems, superimposed, as it were; this in fact appears to be the case in the monkey striate cortex where cortical subdivisions depending on ocular dominance are superimposed on the receptive-field orientation columns (unpublished).

So far nothing has been said of the horizontal cortical subdivisions into layers, divisions that are anatomically far more obvious than the vertical cytoarchitectonic subdivisions. In area 17 there are strong hints of physiological differences among layers (13), in that the fourth-layer cells seem to be almost exclusively simple. In 18 and 19 the results are even less clear. Part of the reason for our ignorance about the significance of layering is that in the cat the boundaries between layers are not always easy to find accurately in Nissl-stained sections. Moreover, most layers contain a variety of cell types, so that one cannot expect physiological properties of cells in one layer to be uniform. Finally, it is technically difficult to localize a particular cell along a given electrode track. For these reasons we have deferred a study of this aspect of the physiology, with the hope that the problem may

be more easily undertaken in the monkey, where the layering is more clean-cut.

Implications for Perception

It remains to discuss the possible implications of this work for an understanding of perception. This can be approached by asking what cells in a given area are responding to any particular part of an image. In the striate area cells respond to the contours of a form: most cells whose receptive fields lie entirely inside the homogeneous part of an image are uninfluenced, since for them the stimulus is in effect diffuse. A portion of the boundary of a figure will activate that population of complex cells whose receptive fields are not only crossed by the boundary but also oriented in the direction of the boundary. A segment of a curve will activate a complex cell best if the tangent to the curve does not greatly change its direction within the receptive field. The impression of the homogeneous interior of a figure as bright or dark is presumably derived from the activity of cells whose fields cover the boundaries, and from the lack of any signals from cells whose fields are entirely within.

Hypercomplex cells are still more selective. From these cells continuous straight boundaries, or boundaries that curve to a negligible degree within the confines of a receptive field, evoke no response. There must be discontinuities such as interruptions of a line or changes in direction. A simple image like a square activates only hypercomplex cells whose fields include the vertices, and then only if the receptive-field orientations are appropriate. Awareness of a straight edge may thus be derived from signals in hypercomplex cells activated by the ends of the edge, plus the failure of other hypercomplex cells to signal other directional changes in the edge. If perception of an entire line can arise solely from information on changes in direction one may have an explanation for the "completion" phenomenon, in which patients with an occipital lobe lesion perceive a line as uninterrupted even though it crosses the blind part of the visual field.

The hypercomplex cell can, in a sense, serve to measure curvature; the smaller the activating part of the field, the smaller the optimal radius of curvature would be. To term such cells "curvature detectors" seems unwise, however, since the term neglects the importance of the orientation of the stimulus, and does not capture the essential importance of a line stimulus to one region and the absence of a line stimulus to an adjacent, antagonistic region. Similar objections would apply to terms like "corner unit." The word "hypercomplex," while ugly and unwieldy, and perhaps also unwise in view of the possibility of finding even more complex cells, is at least relatively neutral.

Finally, it should perhaps be stressed that a proper understanding of the part played by any cell in a sensory system must depend not simply upon a description of the cell's responses to sensory stimuli, but also on a knowledge of how the information it conveys is made use of at higher levels. Just as one can better grasp the meaning of cells in the retina or geniculate, with their on-center or off-center fields, by knowing that such cells converge on the more specific cells of area 17, so an understanding of hypercomplex cells will be incomplete until we have a description of the cells they converge upon. How far such analysis can be carried is anyone's guess, but it is clear that the transformations occurring in these three cortical areas go only a short way toward accounting for the perception of shapes encountered in everyday life.

SUMMARY

In 1941 Talbot and Marshall (27) mapped the cat's visual cortex by recording slow potentials evoked by small-spot stimulation of the retina. In each hemisphere they found two separate but adjacent projections of the contralateral field of vision, which they termed visual areas I and II. In recordings from single cells we have confirmed these findings and have found a third systematic projection (visual III) of the contralateral visual field bordering on and lateral to visual area II. In crossing visual areas I, II, and III from medial to lateral, the corresponding receptive-field areas in the contralateral visual field moved progressively into the vertical meridian, then out into the periphery of the visual field, and finally back into the vertical meridian. On correlating the areas so mapped with microscopic anatomy as seen in Nissl- and myelin-stained sections, we conclude that the three visual areas are identical to areas 17, 18, and 19, as defined in the cat by Otsuka and Hassler (23).

In experiments using silver-degeneration (Nauta) techniques, cells in area 17 (visual I) pro-

jected both to 18 and 19 bilaterally, suggesting that visual messages are transmitted from visual I to visual II and III for further processing.

Cells in visual areas II and III, like those in visual I, responded best to line stimuli such as slits, edges, and dark bars; for optimum response the orientation of the stimulus was critical. The great majority of cells in visual II and half of the cells in visual III were "complex," in the sense that we have used this term in visual I. Other cells, which we term "lower order hypercomplex," formed 5–10% of the cells in visual II and about half of those in visual III. Finally, a few cells in visual III with even more elaborate response properties were termed "higher order hypercomplex."

A lower order hypercomplex cell, like a complex one, responded either to a slit, an edge, or a dark bar, but the length of the stimulus had to be limited ("stopped") in one or both directions. The adequate stimulus was thus a critically oriented line stimulus falling within a given region of retina (the "activating" region), provided a similarly oriented line did not fall over an adjacent ("antagonistic") region. For a cell that responded to an edge limited at one end only, a powerful stimulus was thus a right-angle corner formed by two edges, one of which fell across the activating region in the optimum orientation, while the other fell on the boundary between the activating and the antagonistic regions. A lower order hypercomplex cell thus behaved as though it received inputs from two complex cells (or sets of cells), one excitatory to the cell, with a receptive field occupying the activating portion, and one inhibitory to the cell, having its field in the antagonistic portion.

Higher order hypercomplex cells, of which only 11 were studied, resembled lower order hypercomplex cells in requiring that a line stimulus be limited in length at one or both ends. The higher order cells, however, differed in responding to the line in either of two orientations 90° apart, and the point where the terminus of the line or edge fell within the receptive field was not necessarily critical. These hypercomplex cells behaved as though they had their input from a large number of lower order hypercomplex cells.

Visual areas II and III were both organized in columns which appeared to extend from surface to white matter, within which there were both complex and hypercomplex cells, all with the same receptive-field orientation, but differing in the precise position and arrangement of receptive fields. In visual II and III a single column thus contained hypercomplex cells and also the complex cells that on physiological grounds one would predict projected to the hypercomplex cells. In addition, in visual III there were columns in which some cells had one receptive-field orientation, others had an orientation at 90° to the first, and still others, higher order hypercomplex cells, responded to both these orientations. Again the cells that seem to be interconnected on physiological grounds are apparently all contained within a single column.

In visual II, as in visual I, some groups of columns were arranged in a highly ordered fashion: as one moved across the cortical surface, the orientation of the underlying columns changed in small regular steps. In other regions the shifts in orientation between neighboring columns appeared to be random in direction and variable in size, sometimes small but sometimes approaching 90°.

The majority of cells of visual II and III were driven from both eyes. A cell that was binocularly driven had fields in corresponding parts of the two retinas, which were, as far as one could tell, identical in their arrangements. Ocular dominance varied from cell to cell, ranging from cells that were driven only from the contralateral eye, through those driven equally well by the two eyes, to those driven exclusively by the ipsilateral eye. The distribution of cells according to relative ocular dominance was remarkably similar in the three visual areas, and in visual III the distribution of hypercomplex cells was similar to that of complex cells. Thus the partial functional separation of cells according to ocular dominance seems to be maintained as far centrally as area 19.

ACKNOWLEDGMENT

We express our thanks to Jane Chen and Janet Tobie for their technical assistance.

References

1. Clare, M. H. and Bishop, G. H. Responses from an association area secondarily activated from optic cortex. *J. Neurophysiol.*, 1954, *17:* 271–277.
2. Cowey, A. Projection of the retina on to striate and prestriate cortex in the squirrel monkey, *Saimiri sciureus. J. Neurophysiol.*, 1964, *27:* 366–393.
3. Curtis, H. J. Intercortical connections of corpus callosum as indicated by evoked potentials. *J. Neurophysiol.*, 1940, *3:* 407–413.
4. Davies, P. W. Chamber for microelectrode studies in the cerebral cortex. *Science*, 1956, *124:* 179–180.
5. Doty, R. W. Potentials evoked in cat cerebral cortex by diffuse and by punctiform photic stimuli. *J. Neurophysiol.*, 1958, *21:* 437–464.
6. Garol, H. W. Cortical origin and distribution of corpus callosum and anterior commissure in the cat. III. *J. Neuropath. Exp. Neurol.*, 1942, *1:* 422–429.
7. Gaze, R. M. and Jacobson, M. 'Convexity detectors' in the frog's visual system. *J. Physiol.*, 1963, *169:* 1P–3P.
8. Hubel, D. H. Tungsten microelectrode for recording from single units. *Science*, 1957, *125:* 549–550.
9. Hubel, D. H. Single unit activity in lateral geniculate body and optic tract of unrestrained cats. *J. Physiol.*, 1960, *150:* 91–104.
10. Hubel, D. H. and Wiesel, T. N. Receptive fields of single neurones in the cat's striate cortex. *J. Physiol.*, 1959, *148:* 574–591.
11. Hubel, D. H. and Wiesel, T. N. Receptive fields of optic nerve fibres in the spider monkey. *J. Physiol.*, 1960, *154:* 572–580.
12. Hubel, D. H. and Wiesel, T. N. Integrative action in the cat's lateral geniculate body. *J. Physiol.*, 1961, *155:* 385–398.
13. Hubel, D. H. and Wiesel, T. N. Receptive fields, binocular interaction and functional architecture in the cat's visual cortex. *J. Physiol.*, 1962, *160:* 106–154.
14. Hubel, D. H. and Wiesel, T. N. Shape and arrangement of columns in cat's striate cortex. *J. Physiol.*, 1963, *165:* 559–568.
15. Hubel, D. H. and Wiesel, T. N. Receptive fields of cells in striate cortex of very young, visually inexperienced kittens. *J. Neurophysiol.*, 1963, *26:* 994–1002.
16. Kuffler, S. W. Discharge patterns and functional organization of mammalian retina. *J. Neurophysiol.*, 1953, *16:* 37–68.
17. Lettvin, J. Y., Maturana, H. R., McCulloch, W. S., and Pitts, W. H. What the frog's eye tells the frog's brain. *Proc. Inst. Radio Engrs.*, 1959, *47:* 1940–1951.
18. Lettvin, J. Y., Maturana, H. R., Pitts, W. H., and McCulloch, W. S. Two remarks on the visual system of the frog. In: *Sensory Communication*, edited by W. A. Rosenblith. Cambridge, Mass. and New York, M.I.T. Press and Wiley, 1961, pp. 757–776.
19. Lorente de Nó, R. Cerebral cortex: Architecture, intracortical connections, motor projections. In: *Physiology of the Nervous System* (2nd ed.), edited by J. F. Fulton. Cambridge, England, Oxford Univ. Press, 1943, pp. 274–301.
20. Minkowski, M. Experimentelle Untersuchungen über die Beziehungen der Gross-hirnrinde und der Netzhaut zu den primären optischen Zentren, besonders zum Corpus geniculatum externum. *Arb. Hirnanat. Inst. Zürich*, 1913, *7:* 259–362.
21. Mountcastle, V. B. Modality and topographic properties of single neurons of cat's somatic sensory cortex. *J. Neurophysiol.*, 1957, *20:* 408–434.
22. Nauta, W. J. H. and Gygax, P. A. Silver impregnation of degenerating axons in the central nervous system: A modified technique. *Stain Tech.*, 1954, *29:* 91–93.
23. Otsuka, R. and Hassler, R. Über Aufbau und Gliederung der corticalen Sehsphäre bei der Katze. *Arch. Psychiat. Nervenkr.* 1962, *203:* 212–234.
24. Poggio, G. F. and Mountcastle, V. B. The functional properties of ventrobasal thalamic neurons studied in unanesthetized monkeys. *J. Neurophysiol.*, 1963, *26:* 775–806.
25. Polley, E. H. and Dirkes, J. M. The visual cortical (geniculocortical) area of the cat brain and its projections. *Anat. Rec.*, 1963, *145:* 345.

26. Polyak, S. An experimental study of the association, callosal, and projection fibers of the cerebral cortex of the cat. *J. comp. Neurol.,* 1927, *44:* 197–258.

27. Talbot, S. A. and Marshall, W. H. Physiological studies on neural mechanisms of visual localization and discrimination. *Amer. J. Ophthal.,* 1941, *24:* 1255–1263.

28. Thompson, J. M., Woolsey, C. N., and Talbot, S. A. Visual areas I and II of cerebral cortex of rabbit. *J. Neurophysiol.,* 1950, *13:* 277–288.

29. Vastola, E. F. A direct pathway from lateral geniculate body to association cortex. *J. Neurophysiol.,* 1961, *24:* 469–487.

30. Wiesel, T. N. and Hubel, D. H. Single-cell responses in striate cortex of kittens deprived of vision in one eye. *J. Neurophysiol.,* 1963, *26:* 1003–1017.

31. Winkler, C. and Potter, A. *An Anatomical Guide to Experimental Researches on the Cat's Brain.* Amsterdam, W. Versluys, 1914.

32. Woolsey, C. N. Organization of somatic sensory and motor areas of the cerebral cortex. In: *Biological and Biochemical Bases of Behavior,* edited by H. F. Harlow and C. N. Woolsey. Madison, Wis., Univ. Wisconsin Press, 1958, pp. 63–81.

AFTERWORD

When this paper was written, the quest of finding a progressive increase in complexity of behavior of cells as one went centrally along the visual path seemed to be panning out. Finding hypercomplex cells in 18, and even higher-order hypercomplex cells in 19, seemed to give ample evidence for a path in which form analysis became increasingly elaborate. Cells could be thought of as forming a hierarchy, with ones of progressively higher complexity housed in successive areas. Just as 17 contained simple and complex cells, so 18 contained complex and hypercomplex cells, and 19 contained ordinary hypercomplex cells and ones of higher order. Presumably one had only to forge ahead to find more areas, and more elaborate and sophisticated physiology.

One of the most exciting moments in these experiments was when, proceeding laterally across the cat's cortex, in penetration after penetration, we suddenly realized that the fields were moving back in toward the vertical midline, and had become decidedly smaller—indicating a third visual area lateral to V-2. Just as exciting was our first realization that some cells in this new area failed utterly to respond to long slits, indicating that we had stumbled on cells of a new cell type. We called them *hypercomplex*. We thought at first that these cells were confined to visual 3—they were so common there that we could hardly miss them—but we went back to visual area 2 to be sure we hadn't missed them there—and we had. Before writing the paper we should have returned to 17 and checked there, but we were too negligent or lazy. In his thesis work in cats, our graduate student, Charles Gilbert, found clear end-stopping (as hypercomplexity came to be called), in simple cells of layer 4, and complex cells of layers 1 and 2 (*J Physiol*, 1977; 268:391–421).

A need to revise some of our ideas came around 1968 when Geoffrey Henry and Bogdan Dreher, in Australia, discovered cat cortical cells that resembled our simple cells except that they did not respond to long lines. In these cells one had to imagine six receptive-field subregions, not three, as in ordinary simple fields. A slit of light of limited length might produce an on-response, but a longer slit would produce no response, as though three zones were arranged along a line, giving "off", "on", and "off" responses, each region flanked on either side by antagonistic areas. Henry agreed, by and large, with our description of the hypercomplex cells of our '1965' paper, but considered them to result from the convergence of many of these more complicated simple cells, just as ordinary complex cells resulted from the convergence of many ordinary simple cells. These cells came to us as a surprise, and at first we were sceptical. But subsequently we saw clear examples of them in cats, and we had to agree with Henry and Dreher. The term *hypercomplex,* besides being cumbersome, seemed no longer appropriate. The simple cells we had described would have to assume a sibling relationship to these more complicated simple cells (or *end-stopped simple cells,* as they came to be called) and ordinary complex and end-stopped complex cells would then be first cousins. "End-stopped" was in any case more descriptive and neutral than "hypercomplex".

There nevertheless seemed to be no question that cells differed in degree of complexity; a hierarchy clearly existed, and the details had to be filled out. In macaque monkeys we have not recorded anything like the simple end-stopped cells of Henry and Dreher, and if we were only concerned with primates we could probably forget the matter and continue using *hypercomplex.*

In a hypercomplex cell, one had to think of receptive fields as extending beyond the region from which explicit responses could be evoked. It was not clear, and is still not clear, why no explicit opposing responses are obtained from end-stopped cells when the outlying antagonistic areas are stimulated alone: even spontaneous activity, when present in these anesthetized animals, was unaffected when the outlying areas were stimulated by themselves. We were not totally surprised at our failure to get responses to stimulating these end regions, because we had seen analogous examples even at the retinal ganglion cell and geniculate cell levels. In the geniculate, especially in cells close to the fovea, it is generally difficult to obtain responses to annuli unless one illuminates the field center with a steady light. In these cases it is not that the inhibition is weak: it is strong enough to abolish the center responses completely, as one finds on comparing responses to small spots with responses to large ones. It seems that the inhibition has to work, as it were, through the center. One can probably dream up a mechanism that would explain this, perhaps one involving presynaptic inhibition.

What seemed important to us, in this paper, was showing that the outlying antagonistic areas of these cells were themselves complex. To bring out the antagonism one had to stimulate the outlying area with lines in the same orientation as the optimal orientation for the activating area. This was our justification for the circuits shown in Fig. 38, for which evidence was found some years later by Charles Gilbert. He was the first to describe long, narrow complex fields in layer 6 of cat cortex (*J. Physiol,* 1977, 268: 391–421) which seemed tailor-made to fulfil the role of the cell proposed in Figure 38C. (Bolz & Gilbert *Nature* 1986, 320: 362–365)

We have often been asked how we can be sure that the behavior we ascribe to our cells is not determined by the stimuli we use. How can we know that some other, even more complex, behavior would not be brought out by stimuli we haven't had the imagination to try? Of course that is a problem, as our early failure to see hypercomplex cells illustrates. But we have generally used as wide a range of stimuli as we could dream up. We varied our stimuli as much as our imaginations would permit; indeed, our very sloppiness in devising stimuli must have added to the variety. That is doubtless why eventually we caught on to hypercomplex cells (or why we missed them in the beginning). It is worth emphasizing that our use of lines was not a preconception that lines were some magical concept in form analysis. The notion that orientation-selective cells are "line detectors" seems to us a seriously mistaken one. What most cortical cells are concerned with is surely orientation or, what amounts to the same thing, a responsiveness to oriented short line segments. Strictly speaking, to represent a straight line, a cell should receive convergent input from many such short-line-segment cells, with their fields arranged in collinear fashion; specialization for curved lines would require convergence of many cells with appropriately positioned receptive fields, with progressively differing orientations, and preferably end-stopped. Perhaps future work will reveal such cells.

It is tempting to speculate about what end-stopped cells are for. They certainly respond well to interruptions in lines, and to curves. One can perhaps go further: to detect, or represent, a straight line it should be sufficient to localize the terminations of the line and show that no change in orientation has taken place between the terminations. Similarly, to represent the interior, diffusely lit, part of any form such as a square or circle it should logically be enough to establish the boundaries separating the outside from the inside, and show the absence of any intensity changes in the interior. To a student who has trouble accepting such ideas—that in the case of a brightly lit circle the perceptual apparatus need not react to the innards of the circle, but attend only to the borders—we simply answer that any engineer interested in building a machine to process forms in the most efficient way would probably do it just this way. Any requirement that the nervous system should "fill in" a form—for a square, the interior, or for a line, the region between the ends—thus would seem unnecessary.

We recognize that form perception may *not* be done this way. For lines, we have plenty of ordinary complex cells to take care of the parts between the terminations. For a circle or a square, cells that respond to diffuse light will be activated by the interior, and though such activation is usually weak, we only have to suppose that weak activation of many cells could define the form. The point here is that lines or squares or circles do not logically have to be "filled in", that the edges and terminals are logically sufficient to define the line or form.

Meanwhile, we do not know how long straight lines or curves are handled by the brain, any more than we know what happens when we see triangles, boats, or faces. All we can do is to plod along from one stage in the path to another, asking what kinds of stimuli make cells fire. Our attitude, perhaps a mistaken one, is that it is best to proceed without prejudices as to how things work, and let the chips fall where they may. Until we happened on orientation selectivity, no one to our knowledge had even remotely suggested that visual information might in the early stages be processed in that way.

Much of our research over our 25-year partnership can be described as a massive fishing trip, an expression commonly used by study sections to disparage bad grant requests. Our research was seldom "hypothesis driven", to use another term (this one always implying approval). So be it: our research was by and large a huge fishing trip and was seldom hypothesis-driven— unless by "hypothesis" one means the idea that the brain works in a way that can be understood. But the lack of a hypothesis need not necessarily prevent one from catching big fish.

Our reluctance to speculate on how perception works may dismay, even irritate, some readers. It is a matter of scientific style, and our style has been to observe with as little prejudice as possible, and let the theoreticians do the speculating. We have felt that there is at present no way out of the eternal problems of how different submodalities of vision get together—the binding question, how one imagines a red hat is mediated or, in the extreme, whether "grandmother cells" exist. We have preferred to plod on and record from cells farther and farther downstream and hope that the questions will be answered or will melt away as meaningless or ill-posed.

We were puzzled by finding so little that was new or intriguing in visual 2. Besides the hypercomplex cells (which in the end turned out not to be a new property of visual 2 or 3), and besides the marked increase in the sizes of receptive fields (which was not all that exciting) there seemed to be little to justify the existence of visual 2 as a separate area. Visual 2 thus seems very different in cats and primates. To be sure, the topographic maps of the visual fields are similar, that of V-2 being a cruder mirror-image of V-1, in both cats and primates. But in the cat, V-2 receives a strong input from the lateral geniculate body, whereas primate V-2 receives little or none. And in the cat it fails to show the stripes that are so prominent in macaques and squirrel monkeys. It is as if the process of differentiation of V-2 has been carried further in primates.

In the cat, the farthest we got in the direction of increasing complexity was in the area we called *19* or *visual 3*. There the cells we called *higher-order hypercomplex* were of several types, the most interesting of which responded to short lines regardless of where in the receptive field they were placed, but failed to respond to long lines. (Such cells were later described by Palmer and Rosenquist in cat striate cortex [*Brain Research,* 1974; 67: 27–42] and by Charles Gilbert [*J. Physiol.,* 1977; 268: 391–421], and were termed *special complex*). They had the same relationship to ordinary end-stopped cells as complex cells had to simple cells. In the early 1980s in macaque monkeys, Margaret Livingstone and I found cells in the thin dark stripes of V-2 that responded to small spots of light regardless of where they were positioned in a large receptive field, but failed to respond to larger spots that filled the field. They showed the same relationship to Kufflerian on- or off-center cells as complex cells showed to simple. We gave to this process the ungainly term *complexification (Nature,* 1985, 315:325–327). We were struck by these analogies in transformations at the different steps in the hierarchies. The analogy between simple-to-complex and lower-to-higher-order hypercomplex was too prominent to ignore, as was the analogy between geniculate-to-simple and complex-to-hypercomplex. Some kinds of circuits seem to occur repeatedly in the cortex, serving analogous purposes but in very different contexts—a little like positive or negative feedback in electronics. We began to wonder just how general such circuits are—whether comparable transformations occur in the auditory or somatosensory cortex, or in the hippocampus or the frontal lobes.

Today (to come back to earth), research in vision at levels central to the retina is done mainly in primates. The cat has lost its place as the most studied mammal in central nervous system (CNS) neurophysiology, for several reasons. First, its cost has been artificially driven up through the efforts of animal rights groups, so much so that cats, while still far less expensive than macaque monkeys, are very far from cheap. (Ironically, cats are plentiful. Strays are picked up every day in large numbers and taken to "shelters", where they are killed. But in most states in the United States of America these cats cannot be obtained for research from shelters because of animal-rights activity.) Second, the trend today is away from research in acutely prepared animals, in favor of work in awake behaving animals, and cats are totally unsuited to vision research in which training is required. Unfortunately, monkeys are so expensive today that to kill one just to obtain the anatomy after each acute experiment, as we did decades ago, is out of the question. The result, sadly, is a marked trend away from experiments in which one can combine physiology with experimental anatomy.

Pressing forward along the cortical visual path has not continued to meet with spectacular success in unearthing cells that respond to more and more complex spatial configurations. An exception seems to be the face-recognition cells in the inferotemporal cortex first discovered by Charles Gross, and subsequently confirmed in many ways—by replication of the original results and by clinical observation coupled with magnetic resonance imaging (MRI). We still have little knowledge of the intermediate steps involved in building up such cells.

Chapter 12 • Survey of the Monkey Lateral Geniculate Body—A Foray into Color •

FOREWORD

In this survey of the lateral geniculate, our original intent was not particularly to study color. We mainly wanted to learn whether geniculate cells in monkeys had orientation selectivity or movement direction selectivity or any of the other properties we had found in the monkey cortex—or whether they were more like retinal ganglion cells, in having circularly symmetric receptive fields. We wanted to be certain that the properties we were finding in the monkey cortex were ascribable to cortical circuits, and not just a passive handing-on of properties arising in the geniculate. Our motives were the same as those for looking at the cat geniculate. What we found, in both species, was that the orientation selectivity and so on must be elaborated in the cortex, rather than at prior levels.

But as soon as we got started we found that the monkey geniculate is loaded with cells with specific color properties. This paper consequently represents the first effort in mammalian visual neurophysiology to examine the color sensitivities of the different spatial subdivisions of receptive fields.

Mammalian color neurophysiology had gotten off to a terrible start. Ragnar Granit had the misfortune to choose the cat for physiological studies of color, a poor choice of species, given the cat's poor color capabilities. Only with heroic effort was it possible, by behavioral methods, to demonstrate a cat's ability to discriminate color. Nancy Mello and Neil Peterson finally accomplished the feat in 1964 (*J Neurophysiol* 27:323–333), as did Sechzer and Brown that same year (*Science* 144:427–429). It took a long search for our colleagues Nigel Daw and Alan Pearlman to demonstrate color coding convincingly in a few rare cells in the C-layers of the cat lateral geniculate (*J Physiol* 1970, 211:125–137). To Granit's work on retinal ganglion cells in the cat we owe terms such as *modulators* and *dominators,* which to the two of us and to Stephen Kuffler were complete mysteries. Students must have been bewildered by these terms, but for years no one was brave enough to express their mystification aloud. So every graduate student's studies of color physiology began with Granit and puzzlement. We were no exceptions, but we had the benefit of Steve's complete disdain for authority, and he made no bones about his inability to understand Granit on any subject. A milestone came in 1960 with Giles Brindley's book on vision (*The Physiology of the Retina and Visual Pathway*, 1960, London, Edward Arnold). Here Brindley makes it clear that he has really no idea what "modulators" are supposed to be. To us that came as a great relief.

Work by deValois, in 1958, had clearly shown color coding in monkey geniculate cells, with excitation to one set of wavelengths and inhibition to others (De Valois, Smith, Kitai, and Karoly, *Science* 127:238–239). A similar result had been obtained in fish by Svaetichin, in 1956 (*Acta Physiol Scand* 39, suppl. 134:17–46), in records that he attributed to receptors but were probably horizontal cells. DeValois's stimuli were diffuse, so that the contributions of different parts of the receptive fields were confounded. As we were to learn, the color properties of center and surround are often strikingly different.

For years, a large part of everyone's fascination by the lateral geniculate had been its subdivision into clearly defined layers. The significance of the layering had excited much speculation—for example, Le Gros Clark's notion (1941, 1942) that each of the three pairs of layers might be related to one of the three cone receptor types. The results of DeValois failed to bear out the Le Gros Clark prediction, but rather suggested that the cells in the dorsal pair of layers gave on responses; the middle pair, on and off responses; and the ventral pair, off responses. But again, the use of diffuse light tended to confuse the picture and, ironically, in the present (1966) paper we show that ventral layer cells are usually on-center but with the off-surround dominating the center when diffuse light is used.

In our cat geniculate study of 1961, we had had the excitement of learning an important way in which the geniculate transforms information coming in from the eye. There the power of the receptive-field surround to antagonize the effects of the center is greatly increased. The prepotentials, which we showed were produced by retinal ganglion cell axons, had made it possible to compare directly the firing of geniculate cells with that of retinal ganglion cells. We had hoped to make this same comparison in the monkey geniculate but failed to. We did not see the prepotentials, perhaps because monkey geniculate cells are much smaller than cat geniculate cells, with correspondingly smaller impulse amplitudes. We still do not know whether the monkey geniculate carries out this function, though our guess would be that it does.

The main precedent for our color studies was work done in the goldfish, in papers that appeared beginning in 1960, by Wagner, MacNichol, and Wolbarsht (*J Gen Physiol,* 43:45–62) and subsequently, in various permutations of those names. They led the way in emphasizing the need to look at wavelength sensitivities as a means of learning the cone inputs, not of the entire receptive field lumped together, but of its different parts taken separately. (Strictly speaking, in fish the receptive-field center and surround components overlap, and one has to use "on" and "off" responses to separate them. In monkeys, overlap surely exists, especially in type 2 cells; in type 1 cells the small size of the field centers makes the overlap less important.) At a meeting around 1960, Myron Wolbarsht said to me: "The trouble with you guys is that you don't know what a receptive field is". We, who regarded ourselves as authorities in that domain, were annoyed—though we should not have been, given Wolbarsht's well-known brashness. We had the sense to take his remarks seriously, and the present paper reflects the influence of the goldfish work, more than any other set of contemporary studies.

We have another reason to forgive Wolbarsht: he made a completely unrelated contribution to our progress in science by letting us in on an important technical secret. In the early 1960s we had been plagued by electrical interference from a nearby hospital paging system (probably the Peter Bent Brigham's), and had even given up trying to do recording in one of our few available rooms, which we finally made into a tearoom. TV interference, that bane of the modern neurophysiologist, was seldom a problem in our labs, probably because of the thick marble medieval-castle-like walls of Harvard Medical School, and we had never had to install the expensive shielded cages that are so common in our field. But the paging transmitting antenna was directly in line with one of our windows. Wolbarsht had a trick: he simply placed, in series, two small resistors, right at the input of his preamplifier. This simple R-C circuit made use of stray capacitance to ground to bypass the high-frequency FM and TV stuff. We installed the two resistors and were never again bothered by paging or background music, and for four decades all of our input stages have been graced with Myron's filters. That more than made up for his cheekiness, and saved us a fortune in copper sheetmetal shielding.

Spatial and Chromatic Interactions in the Lateral Geniculate Body of the Rhesus Monkey[1]

TORSTEN N. WIESEL AND DAVID H. HUBEL • *Neurophysiology Laboratory, Department of Pharmacology, Harvard Medical School, Boston, Massachusetts*

The receptors and nerve cells that make up the visual pathway must convey and interpret information on both the form and the color of retinal images. In higher mammals little is known about the degree to which nerve cells are specialized for handling these types of information. In a visual stimulus the importance of spatial attributes, and especially of dark-light contours, first became obvi-

Received for publication March 9, 1966.

From *J. Neurophysiol.* (1966) 29, 1115–1156

[1]This work was supported in part by Research Grants NB-05554-02, NB-15304-06, NB-02260-06, and NB-02253-06 from the National Institutes of Health, and in part by Research Grant AF-AFOSR-410-62 from the U.S. Air Force.

ous with the discovery by Hartline (20) of lateral inhibition in the *Limulus,* a type of study that was extended to mammals when Kuffler (28) demonstrated that the receptive fields of retinal ganglion cells in the cat are subdivided into a center and an opponent surround. The opponent principle, in which spatially separated excitatory and inhibitory regions are pitted against each other, has now been observed for retinal ganglion cells in the frog (1), the lizard (9), the rabbit (3), the rat (4), the ground squirrel (33), and the monkey (24). Similar effects have been seen in the lateral geniculate body and visual cortex in the cat (23, 25, 26), and also recently at these levels in the monkey.

In 1958 De Valois and his collaborators (15) observed geniculate cells in the macaque monkey that were excited by one set of wavelengths and inhibited by another, making it apparent that in higher mammals the spectral composition of the stimulus was also an important variable. Similar opponent-color effects have since been described in the primate at the level of the retinal ganglion cell (24), and in the visual cortex (34). In the cat the absence or rarity of opponent-color mechanisms (19, 36) may be related to an inferior ability to discriminate color (31, 32, 40); indeed since Svaetichin's (41) original observation of opponent-color responses in the fish retina (S-potentials), similar response patterns have been seen only in animals thought to have good color vision.

Given the existence of two opponent mechanisms in the monkey visual system, one for the spatial variable and the other for color, it is natural to ask whether these occupy the same channels, or are confined to separate groups of cells. In the goldfish it is clear from the work of Wagner, MacNichol, and Wolbarsht (43, 45) that opponent-color and opponent-spatial effects can be found in common retinal ganglion cells. In the monkey, with its great visual capacity, similar mechanisms are to be expected, perhaps in more developed form. The rhesus monkey was chosen for the work to be described because behaviorally its vision seems to be very similar to that of man(10). In this species, moreover, absorption spectra of the three cone types are possibly identical to those of man, with maxima at about 445, 535, and 570 mμ. (5, 30). Any knowledge of the receptor properties obviously makes it easier to interpret responses to color at more central levels of the nervous system.

The purpose of the present study was to examine in detail how cells respond to variations in stimulus size, shape, and wavelength. By working in various states of light and dark adaptation we also tried to learn something about the connections of rods and cones with single fourth-order cells. The decision to record from the geniculate was made because of the obvious interest in learning how cells function at an early stage of the visual pathway, especially the stage that forms the input to the striate cortex. We also hoped to learn more about the significance of the layering in this puzzling structure.

Some of the findings of the present paper have already been described in preliminary notes (27, 47).

METHODS

Sixteen monkeys were used, ranging in age from 1 to 3 years. Animals were anesthetized with intraperitoneal sodium Pentothal (35 mg/kg.), and additional doses of the drug were given at half-hour intervals. The head was held rigidly in a Horsley-Clarke stereotaxic apparatus (42). The eyes were immobilized with a continuous infusion of succinylcholine (20–40 mg/kg. per hour). For complete immobilization it was often necessary to give additional intramuscular injections of gallamine triethiodide (10 mg/hour). Pupils were dilated with 1% homatropine. Contact lenses were fitted to the corneas after measuring corneal curvature with a keratometer (Bausch & Lomb, type 71-21-35). Focus was checked at a distance of 1.5 m. (the distance from the eyes to the projection screen) with a slit retinoscope, and any necessary correction was made with supplementary lenses mounted in front of the animal's eyes. With a properly fitted contact lens, correction by more than ±1.0 diopters was seldom necessary.

For most work the animal faced a large white screen at a distance of 1.5 m. When receptive-field centers were smaller than about 10 min. of arc, the screen was moved back to a distance of 5 m., and the eyes refocused. The projected positions of the foveas and the optic discs of each eye were marked out on the screen by an opthalmoscopic projection method (24, 42), which with our present instrument was accurate to within about 1/2°.

For work in the light-adapted state the screen was lit diffusely with a tungsten lamp at a distance of about 5 m. This background measured about 1.0 log cd/m², and the light impinging on the screen was bright enough so that fine print could easily be read and objects appeared normally colored. The spectral energy content of the background light is discussed below.

Stimuli consisted of spots of white light or monochromatic light projected onto the screen with a modified slide projector containing a 500-W. tungsten bulb. Stimulus durations of about 1 sec. were produced by a crude mechanical shutter. Monochromatic light was obtained by placing interference filters (Baird Atomic, B-1, half-bandwidth 7 mμ.) directly in front of the projection lens, which was far enough from the screen that the rays could be regarded as practically parallel. Sixteen filters gave wavelengths about 20 mμ. apart over the visible range (400–700 mμ.). Spots at the highest intensities available showed up brightly against the high mesopic background, at all but the longest and shortest wavelengths.

To calibrate the stimulator it was necessary to have a sensitive photometer whose spectral sensitivity was known. We used a Photovolt model 520M (Photovolt Corp., New York City) with a photomultiplier tube type IP28 (RCA). The spectral-sensitivity curve of the individual tube was supplied by the manufacturer, and this was checked independently by comparing the set of photomultiplier readings for beams of monochromatic light at different wavelengths with readings made on a thermopile (Kipp and Zonen: Delft, Holland, model E-20). The light from the stimulator, having passed through the optical system consisting of slide projector, neutral density wedge, and an interference filter, was directed into the calibrated photometer. With the wedge at some constant setting, readings were made on the photometer for each interference filter, and these were converted into relative energy units and then into quanta. This set of numbers furnished corrections which, when added to the wedge reading, gave the relative energy of any monochromatic beam of light.

The system was calibrated for several projection lamps that had been in use for various periods, and no significant differences were found in the spectral energy content. Although the absorption spectrum of the glass part of the neutral density wedge was taken care of in the over-all calibration, the emulsion was not, since this differed in density for different settings. We therefore recalibrated the stimulator at wedge settings 2 log units apart. From 440 mμ. to 680 mμ. the curves were similar in shape to within 0.02 log units, for our purposes a negligible error. The interference filters together with their blocking filters were calibrated in a Beckman spectrophotometer to check bandwidth and center frequency. It was fortunate that these precautions were taken, since a number of filters were unacceptable and had to be replaced. The whiteness of the screen was examined by comparing readings made directly from the projector (as described above) with readings made upon light reflected from the screen. The reflectivity was constant to within 0.05 log units from 440 mμ. to 660 mμ.

The background lamp was run at less than its rated voltage, and was slightly yellow in appearance. To obtain a measure of its spectral energy content, photometer readings were made with the different interference filters interposed, and the results compared with those obtained when a standard lamp (U.S. Bureau of Standards, color temperature 2,854°K) was used as source. The two curves of energy versus wavelength when placed so as to cross at 540 mμ. deviated so that the background had a spectral content 0.14 log units below that of the standard lamp at 440 mμ., and 0.17 log units above it at 640 mμ.; deviations were proportionately less at intermediate wavelengths. The background was used at a fixed intensity for all measurements to be described, except in the studies of chromatic and dark adaptation, and in studies specifically designed to test the effects of varying background intensity and color temperature.

The animal's eyes were dark adapted by turning out the background light and waiting 1/4 to 1 hour before making further measurements. For chromatic adaptation the white background light was left on, and the monochromatic light from a second identical stimulator was directed so as to fill most of the screen. This light was intensely colored, and the areas of screen lit by it contrasted vividly with the parts lit only with the white light. The white background was kept on in order to keep the retinas light adapted, something that was especially important for chromatic adaptation at long wavelengths. The 1 sec. duration spot was superimposed upon both of these diffuse, steady adapting lights. In several cells we examined the effects of confining the monochromatic adapting light to the center or the surround of the receptive field.

Threshold stimulus intensities were determined by listening for a change in maintained firing while stimulating once every 5 sec., gradually raising or lowering the wedge setting to find the weakest intensity at which some change could be heard. For "on" responses the change took the form of an increase in firing rate while the light was on; for "off" responses it was either the burst of impulses on turning off the light or the suppression of firing while the stimulus was on, whichever was detected first. This procedure has the obvious disadvantage that auditory thresholds may vary with the listener, and may depend upon whether the response is excitatory or inhibitory and upon the amount of maintained activity. The method nevertheless usually gave results reproducible to within 0.1–0.2 log units, and had the advantages of convenience and speed, important in a survey the object of which was to make a variety of studies on each cell and to sample many cells. Many of the irregularities in the curves were probably due to the problems of threshold determinations, and, while more accurate curves would doubtless have been obtained by suitable averaging techniques, we do not feel that this would have changed any of our main conclusions.

Methods of recording have been described in detail elsewhere (21, 23). Tungsten microelectrodes were introduced through a closed chamber. The electrode was protected by a 19-gauge needle, which was stereotaxically inserted vertically until the tip came to rest 2 mm. above the lateral geniculate; the electrode was then advanced by a hydraulic driver. All recordings were extracellular. Criteria for distinguishing cells from fibers have been discussed elsewhere (22). One or two lesions were made in each track (21) and Nissl-stained sections of the formalin-fixed, celloidin-embedded brain were used to reconstruct the tracks. No cells were included in the study unless the track and lesions were histologically identified.

Procedure. When a single cell was identified the eyes were stimulated separately with white light (or with monochromatic light if white was ineffective), and the eye that did not drive the cell was then covered. With the white background light turned on the receptive field was found and the field-center size roughly estimated. Spectral sensitivities were determined by measuring the thresholds for monochromatic light at different wavelengths, first for small (center-size) spots and then for large. Log sensitivity (the negative of log threshold) was then plotted against wavelength. The spectral-sensitivity curves were used as a guide in making the choice of background wavelengths for chromatic adaptation and stimulus wavelength in plotting area-sensitivity curves. Finally, the measurements were remade in the dark-adapted state.

Note on anatomical terminology. The six layers of the lateral geniculate are conventionally numbered from ventral to dorsal, the most dorsal layer being the sixth. This system has the disadvantage that it can be confused with a second system, seldom if ever used today, in which the layers are numbered in the opposite direction. A second difficulty is that of remembering which layers receive input from the contralateral eye and which from the ipsilateral. In the present paper we introduce an alternative system of labeling the layers. The four dorsal, histologically identical small-cell layers we label "D," numbering them D_1 to D_4 from dorsal to ventral. The two ventral (large-cell) layers are labeled "V," and numbered from ventral to dorsal. The six layers in order of penetration from above by an electrode are therefore D_1, D_2, D_3, D_4, V_2, V_1. Reversing the numbering for the ventral layers makes the odd-numbered layers receive input from the contralateral eye, and the even-numbered layers from the ipsilateral. Separate numbering of the dorsal and ventral layers is consistent with the relative histological and physiological uniformity within each set, and the marked differences between them.

RESULTS

Eighteen penetrations were made in 16 monkeys, and 244 units were examined in enough detail to permit their categorization. Spectral sensitivities were determined in 49 of these cells for both large and small spots, and 25 of the 49 were also examined in the dark-adapted state. Physiologically the monkey geniculate turns out to be more complex than that of the cat, the difference being related mainly to a large variety of responses to colored light. In the 4 dorsal layers one can distinguish 3 main cell groups, which we designate type I, type II, and type III. Each of these contains several subgroups. In the ventral layers there are at least 2 major groups. Receptive fields of all of the cells had 1 common feature, that of circular symmetry, and the great majority (though not all) showed a concentric center-surround arrangement. No directional asymmetries were seen with stationary or moving stimuli, and no cells showed the types of complex behavior seen in the cat and monkey cortex. In these respects the geniculates of cat and monkey seem to be similar.

In the following paragraphs we first describe the properties of dorsal layer cells, considering the behavior of the three main groups, first in the light-adapted state and then in the dark-adapted state. Next, we discuss the organization of the four dorsal layers, considering the distribution of different cell types within the layers and the size of receptive fields. Finally, we describe the cells of the two ventral layers.

DORSAL LAYERS

Type I Cells: Center-Surround Fields and Opponent-Color Responses

Two hundred thirteen cells were recorded in the four dorsal layers. Of these, 164, or 77%, were classed as type I (see Table 1). A cell was placed in this group if it had a receptive field with an antagonistic center-surround arrangement and if the center and surround had different spectral sensitivities. These properties may best be illustrated by an example.

Figure 1 shows the responses of a type I cell situated in the most dorsal layer (D_1). A white spot illuminating the center of the field gave a brisk on-

Table 1. 213 cells recorded from the dorsal layers

| Layer | TYPE I | | | | | TYPE II | TYPE III | | Totals |
	Red, on-center	Red, off-center	Green, on-center	Green, off-center	Blue, on-center		On-center	Off-center	
D_1	39 (45%)	11 (13%)	12 (14%)	2 (2%)	2 (2%)	4 (5%)	11 (13%)	6 (7%)	87
D_2	19 (37%)	8 (16%)	9 (18)%	5 (10%)		5 (10%)	2 (4%)	3 (6%)	51
D_3	10 (23%)	13 (30%)	6 (14%)	4 (9%)	1 (2%)	3 (7%)	1 (2%)	5 (12%)	43
D_4	7 (22%)	6 (19%)	8 (25%)	2 (6%)		3 (9%)	0	6 (19%)	32
Totals	75 (35%)	38 (18%)	35 (16%)	13 (6%)	3 (1%)	15 (7%)	14 (7%)	20 (9%)	
		164 (77%)				15 (7%)	34 (16%)		213

response (lower left record, Fig. 1); a white spot covering the entire receptive field gave no response.[2] A small red spot made by placing a 620-mμ. interference filter in front of the stimulator evoked a vigorous on-response. A large spot of the same intensity produced a similar response, neither weaker nor stronger. This suggested that the center was sensitive to light of long wavelength but that the periphery was not, since including it had no effect upon the response. A blue spot of center size evoked no consistent change in the irregular background discharges, whereas a large blue spot suppressed the maintained firing and evoked a brisk off-discharge. Thus within the receptive field only the surround was sensitive to short wavelengths.

In summary, the receptive field as examined by these rough tests appeared to have an excitatory center and an inhibitory periphery, with the center differentially sensitive to long wavelengths and the

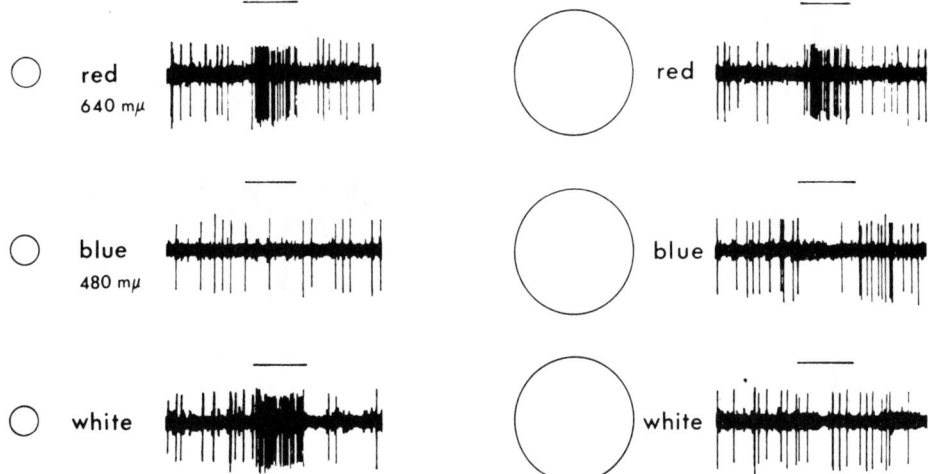

Fig. 1. *Responses of a dorsal-layer geniculate cell to white and monochromatic light. Top line, red, 640 mμ.; middle line, blue, 480 mμ.; bottom line, white. Left: illumination of field center with 1/2° spot. Right: illumination of whole receptive field. Colored spots were produced by placing an interference filter in the beam of white light. They therefore contain far less energy than the white stimuli. Light-adapted state. Field center 19° from the fovea, 6° below the horizontal meridian. Recorded from layer D_1. Further studies of this cell are illustrated in Figs. 2–4.*

[2]So far, these responses are typical for an on-center geniculate cell in the cat. However, using monochromatic light it became clear that the situation was more complex.

surround to short wavelengths. The responses to white light, seen in the lower records of Fig. 1, can now be understood as the resultant of the effects of long and short wavelengths. On the other hand, the responses to diffuse light, shown to the right in the figure, suggest immediately that the cell was specialized to register color stimuli, and was not particularly interested in diffuse white light.

Measurements were made in this cell to determine spectral sensitivities of the center and surround, separately and together, and to establish more accurately the spatial distributions of the two systems. Here, as in every cell in which measurements were made, our first step was to determine sensitivities at different wavelengths, first for a center-size spot and then for a large one. This relatively simple procedure gave enough information to categorize the cell. In Fig. 2 sensitivities are shown for center-size spots with interrupted lines and for large spots with continuous lines; crosses designate on-responses and triangles off-responses. The peak sensitivity of the center system (interrupted lines) was at about 580 mμ. At long wave-

lengths the small-spot and large-spot curves almost coincided, reflecting the insensitivity of the periphery to red. As wavelength was progressively shortened, the influence of the inhibitory surround became more and more powerful. Thus between 560 and 600 mμ., sensitivities to large spots fell below those to small ones, indicating that over this range there was peripheral suppression. At 540 mμ., the neutral point, the two effects balanced and a large spot gave no response at any available intensity. At still shorter wavelengths the surround dominated the center and large spots evoked off-responses. This inhibitory limb of the curve for large spots might well have been displayed below the wavelength axis, but the use of a log sensitivity scale made this awkward. It will be noted that at 480 mμ. and 460 mμ. a bright center-size spot evoked an on-response. The small blue spot used in Fig. 1 was evidently below threshold for a response.

To determine the spectral sensitivity of the receptive-field periphery alone, the most direct method would be to use an annulus. Technically this was difficult because of the small center size, and we therefore studied the opposing systems separately by chromatic adaptation of the entire receptive field. With the white background still on to avoid dark adaptation, the screen was flooded with diffuse light at 640 mμ., a wavelength to which presumably only the center system was sensitive (Fig. 2). With this background the spectral sensitivity to large monochromatic spots, measured as before by observing the cell's transient response, is given by the curve labeled 640 in Fig. 3. Off-responses were now evoked from 460 mμ. to 580 mμ., and the peak response, though not well defined, was somewhere around 540 mμ. The effect of the adapting light in suppressing the center system was the same whether it was confined to the center or covered the entire receptive field, and in fact it now made no difference whether the stimulus was an annulus covering all but the center system, or a large spot. This curve was therefore taken to represent the spectral sensitivity of the surround. By using an adapting light at 460 mμ. the effectiveness of the surround region was differentially reduced, and under this condition the sensitivities to diffuse light (dotted line, labeled 460) were about the same as those obtained with a small spot, shown in Fig. 2. The mechanism underlying these differ-

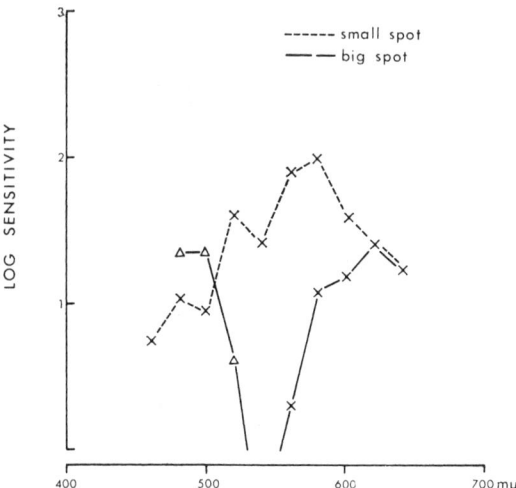

Fig. 2. Spectral sensitivity of the red on-center geniculate cell of Fig. 1. Relative sensitivities obtained by determining log reciprocal thresholds. Crosses = on-responses; triangles = off-responses. No response to 540 mμ. at any available intensity. Light-adapted state; stimuli are superimposed on a 1 cd/m² steady diffuse white background. (In this and other similar curves, points corresponding to "no response" are either omitted or plotted as circles slightly below zero on the log sensitivity scale.)

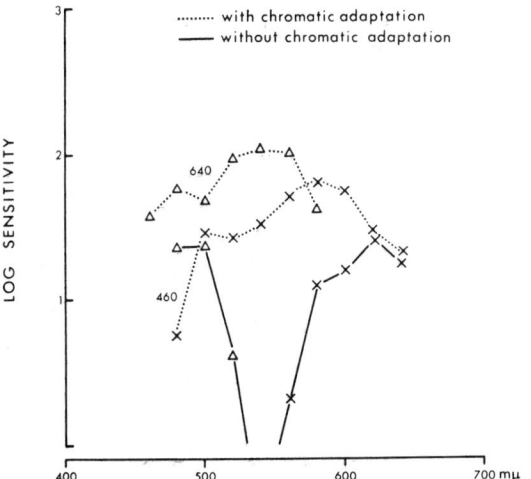

Fig. 3. *Effects of chromatic adaptation on responses to diffuse light. Same cell as in Figs. 1 and 2. Continuous lines, reproduced from Fig. 2, show responses to large spots against the constant 1 cd/m² white background. A steady monochromatic diffuse 640-mμ. light was now added to the white background, and with large spot stimulation the sensitivities are given by the dotted curve marked 640. All responses from 460 mμ. to 580 mμ. were inhibitory (triangles). Similar chromatic adaptation with light at 460 mμ. resulted in the second dotted curve marked 460. All responses were now "on" (crosses), from 480 mμ. to 620 mμ., and the curve was roughly the same as that for center-size spots, shown in Fig. 2.*

ential adaptation effects is taken up in the DISCUS-SION.

To measure the size of the receptive-field center, thresholds were determined for different spot sizes, first using red light at 640 mμ. and then green at 520 mμ. The area-sensitivity curve for the center system was made using a white background light. Because of the overlap of the two systems at short wavelengths, the field periphery was measured using, in addition to the white background, a steady diffuse adapting light at 640 mμ. These values for stimulating and adapting wavelengths were chosen using information given in Fig. 3. The two area-sensitivity curves are shown in Fig. 4. Sensitivity to red light increased from 1/8°, the smallest spot to evoke a response at any available intensity, to 1/2°, where it leveled off; 1/2° was therefore taken as the field-center size. The peripheral response to 520-mμ. light was first seen at 1°, and the curve leveled off at about 6°, which was taken

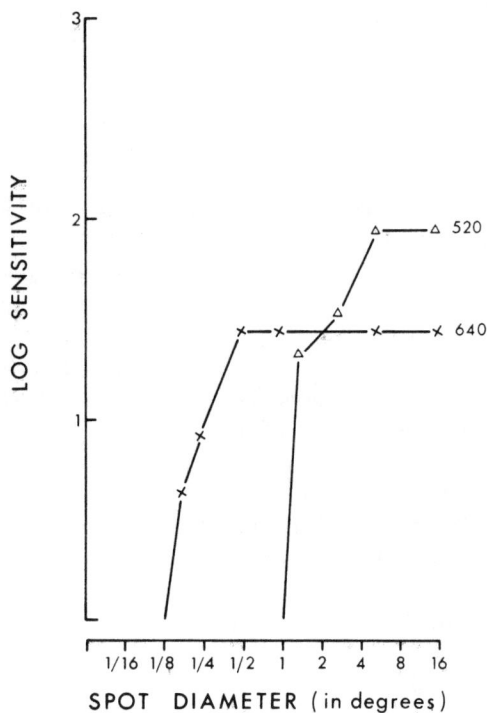

Fig. 4. *Area-sensitivity curves for two wavelengths of monochromatic light. Same red on-center cell as in Figs. 1–3. Sensitivities were first determined for various sizes of spots at 640 mμ., against the usual white background. On-responses indicated by crosses. With 520-mμ., spots and a steady background of 640-mμ. diffuse light added to the white, off-responses were evoked (triangles). Inhbiitory effects with short wavelengths were seen only for spots 1° and over, and the effect leveled off at about 6°. Because of the difference in backgrounds the sensitivities of the two systems cannot be compared in this figure.*

to be the total field diameter. (Because of the differences in background light, the relative sensitivities of center and surround cannot be compared using these two curves.)

To sum up, the receptive field consisted of a 1/2° excitatory center with a spectral sensitivity peak in the high 500s, and a peripheral inhibitory zone 6° in outer diameter with maximum sensitivity in the mid-500s. Given three sets of cones with peak absorption spectra at about, 445, 535, and 570 mμ. (5, 30), the results at once suggest that the geniculate cell received excitatory input from the red-sensitive cones in the field center, and inhibitory input from green-sensitive cones in the periphery.

This cell seems identical to the "red-green" type already described by De Valois and co-workers (12) in the monkey lateral geniculate body. De Valois was not concerned with spatial aspects of stimulation, but using chromatic adaptation and diffuse light stimulation he found that the two opponent systems had peak spectral sensitivities around 540 and 580 mμ.

As discussed below, it seems most likely that only red- and green-sensitive cones provided the input to this cell, but it is conceivable that the field periphery received contributions from the blue-sensitive cones also. Evidence that this cell received input from rods as well as cones is presented below, in the section on dark adaptation.

Subgroups within Type I

The cell just described belonged to a subgroup which we term "red-on center, green off-surround." This was by far the commonest subgroup, there being 75 examples of a total of 213 dorsal-layer cells (35%). Assuming the existence of both on-center and off-center fields, and given three cone types, there are obviously many possible subgroups within type I. Besides the red no-center cell just described, we have seen four other varieties, several of which are described in the following paragraphs (see also Table 1).

Thirty-eight cells (18% of 213) had fields of the "red off-center, green on-surround" type, an arrangement that was, in a sense, the reverse of that found in the cell just described. An example of one of these is given below in the section on dark adaptation. "Green on-center, red off-surround" was a combination that occurred in 35 of the 213 cells recorded in the dorsal layers (16%). Figure 5 shows spectral-sensitivity curves for a cell of this type; they are similar to the curves of Fig. 2, the two sets being roughly mirror images of one another. A "green off-center, red on-surround" combination was found for 13 cells (roughly 6%). Thus many examples were seen of the four possible red-green combinations. On the other hand, there were only three clear examples of type I cells that received a blue cone contribution. The cell of Fig. 6 had a field with a blue-sensitive on-center and a green-sensitive off-surround, the two opponent systems having spectral-sensitivity peaks at about 450 mμ. and 540 mμ. No examples were seen of cells receiv-

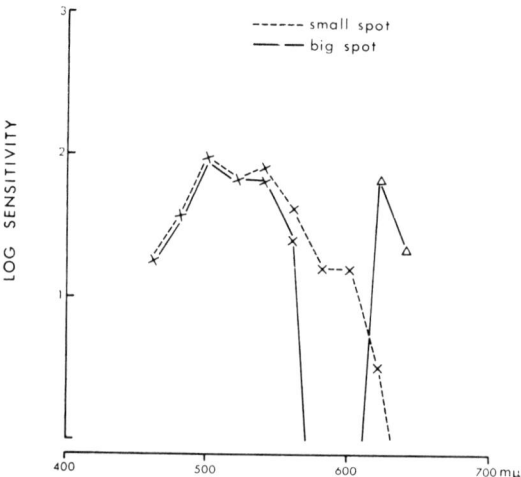

Fig. 5. Spectral sensitivities for small spots and large spots, in a "green on-center, red off-surround" cell recorded from layer D$_2$. Field center 10–12 min. in diameter, situated 10° from the fovea.

ing opponent inputs from blue- and red-sensitive cones.

To identify a particular cell as a member of one or another subgroup it was not necessary to make detailed measurements of the type just described. In order to classify enough cells to study the distribution of the different subtypes in the geniculate, some quick means of identification was necessary. Using white spots we usually first established the center-surround arrangement and the field-center position and size; then with monochromatic light peripheral suppression was compared at different wavelengths, and the neutral point determined. This gave enough information to identify the cell group. Detailed measurements, like those described above, were made in about one-fifth of the cells.

The balance between the center and surround systems varied from cell to cell, as reflected in the position of the neutral point and in the type of response, "on" versus "off," to white light. A cell-to-cell variation in the balance between opponent systems was far more prominent in type I cells than in type II.

The neutral point of the individual type I cell varied also to some extent with the intensity and spectral composition of the "white" background light. To estimate roughly the importance of color

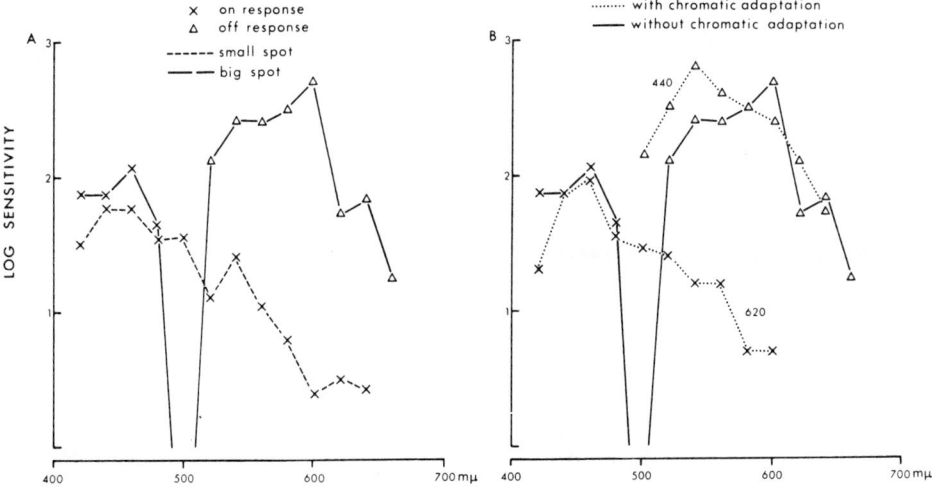

Fig. 6. Spectral sensitivities of a type I "blue on-center, green off-surround" cell recorded in layer D₂. Field center 1/2° in diameter, situated 9° from the fovea. Left: *spectral sensitivities for small-spot and large-spot stimulation.* Right: *effect of chromatic adaptation at 620 mμ. and 440 mμ. upon the responses to large spots. Conventions as in Figs. 2–5.*

balance we compared the neutral points of several type I cells before and after filtering the background light through Wratten 85 or 80B color-balance filters (Eastman Kodak Co., Rochester, N.Y.). These filters made the background distinctly yellowish or bluish, and yet changed the neutral point in either direction by less than about 10 mμ. Varying the intensity of the background with neutral density filters likewise tended to influence the neutral point, usually in a direction predictable from the response to diffuse white light.

Type II Cells: Opponent-Color Responses; no Center-Surround Arrangement

Type II cells were in many respects the most remarkable of the dorsal layer cells. Like those of type I they showed opponent-color responses, but their fields differed in having no trace of any center-surround arrangement. Only eight examples were seen and studied well enough to allow positive identification, suggesting that they are rather rare.

Responses of a typical type II cell are illustrated in Fig. 7. The receptive field occupied a region 1/2° in diameter, situated about 1° from the fovea. Within this area, on-responses were evoked by a 580-mμ. spot regardless of its exact size or position. As shown in the upper row of Fig. 7, large spots evoked more vigorous responses than small ones. A blue spot at 480 mμ. suppressed firing throughout the field, and again the effect was more marked the larger the spot (middle row). White light, containing much more energy than either of the monochromatic stimuli, evoked no obvious response regardless of the size or shape of the spot. The simplest interpretation of these findings is that the cell received input from two populations of cones, one excitatory and the other inhibitory, and that these two sets of receptors were distributed in an almost identical way throughout the circular 1/2° region.

Figure 8 gives the spectral sensitivities of a type II cell whose behavior was similar to that of the cell just described, but with responses of opposite sign, "on" to short wavelengths and "off" to long. Neither white light nor a 500-mμ. monochromatic light gave any obvious responses, again regardless of shape, position, or intensity. The interrupted lines refer to spots slightly smaller than the 1/2° field, and continuous lines correspond to

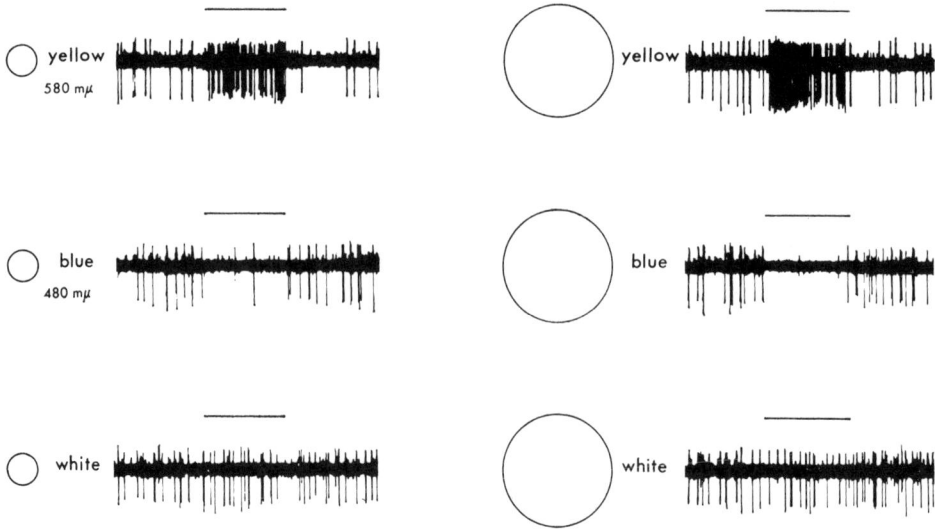

Fig. 7. Responses of a type II "blue-off, green-on" cell. Top line, yellow, *580 mμ.; middle line,* blue, *480 mμ.; lower line,* white. *Small spots, 3/8° in diameter; large spots, 6° in diameter. Cell located in layer D₂, at the posterior tip of the lateral geniculate. Field 1/2° in diameter, about 1° from the fovea.*

10° spots. The two curves were similar in shape and virtually parallel, the increased sensitivity to the larger spots reflecting spatial summation within the receptive field. The neutral point was at 500 mμ. for all spot sizes and shapes. These curves were thus quite different from the corresponding ones for type I cells (Figs. 2, 5, 6A), where the neutral point could be shifted from one end of the spectrum to the other by changing the region of the field that was stimulated.

The most direct evidence that the two opponent systems converging upon this cell had the

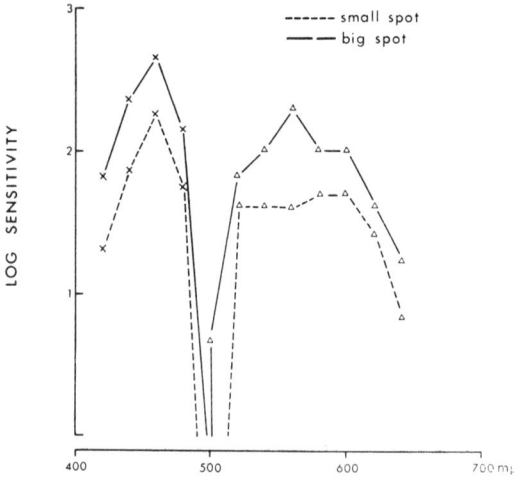

Fig. 8. Spectral sensitivities of a type II "blue-on, green-off" cell from layer D₂. Field 1/2° in diameter, 9° from fovea. Small spots were about 0.4° in diameter, large spots 10°.

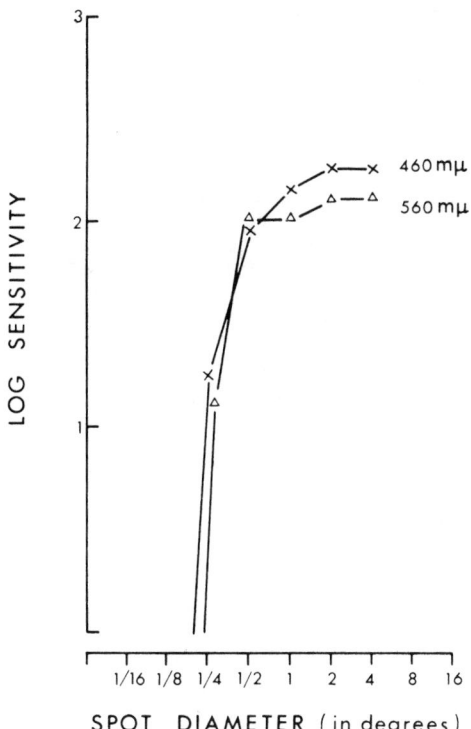

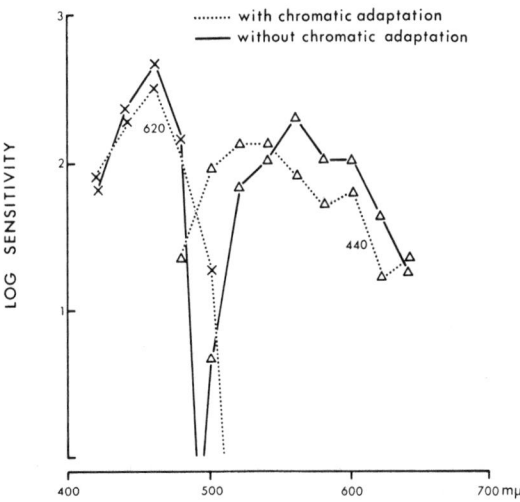

Fig. 10. *Effects of chromatic adaptation on large-spot responses of the cell of Figs. 8 and 9. Adapting lights at 620 mμ. and 440 mμ.*

Fig. 9. *Area-sensitivity curves for the cell of Fig. 8, for light at 460 mμ. (on-responses) and 560 mμ. (off-responses). Background in both cases white, 1 cd/m².*

same spatial distributions came from a comparison of area-sensitivity curves. Figure 9 shows two curves, one for on-responses using spots at 460 mμ., the other for off-responses to spots at 560 mμ. The curves were almost identical, indicating that the two systems were balanced throughout the field. On comparing area-sensitivity curves of type I cells (Fig. 4) with those of type II (Fig. 9), the difference in arrangement of receptive fields is obvious at a glance.

Chromatic adaptation was used in an attempt to obtain the spectral sensitivities of the two systems. Figure 10 shows the results of adapting *1)* with light at 440 mμ. and *2)* with light at 620 mμ. The two resulting curves (dotted) have their peaks at about 460 mμ. and 530 mμ., suggesting that the excitatory input was from blue-sensitive cones and the inhibitory input was from the green. That the two opponent systems had overlapping spectral sensitivities was confirmed by adapting with light

at 500 mμ., i.e., light that was precisely at the neutral wavelength and evoked no response at any available intensity (cf. Fig. 8) Flooding the screen with this light, on top of the white background, produced a uniform suppression in sensitivity at all wavelengths, shown by the curves of Fig. 11.

The eight most thoroughly studied type II cells had properties practically identical to those of the two just described. All had neutral points at 500 mμ., with spectral sensitivities suggesting opponent inputs from both blue and green cones. In all these examples the spatial distributions of the opponent systems seemed to be identical. Besides these cells there was a group of seven that had neutral points at 600 mμ., and whose spectral sensitivities suggested opponent inputs from red and green cones. These cells were not thoroughly studied, and it is not clear whether any of them were truly type II cells, i.e., whether they had opponent systems with identical spatial distributions. The results we did obtain suggested that the two components of the receptive field had spatial distributions that overlapped but were not identical. The over-all size of the regions occupied by the opponent systems seemed to differ slightly, with the suggestion that one component (the excitatory or the inhibitory) prevailed in the center and the other toward the periphery. The arrangement may thus

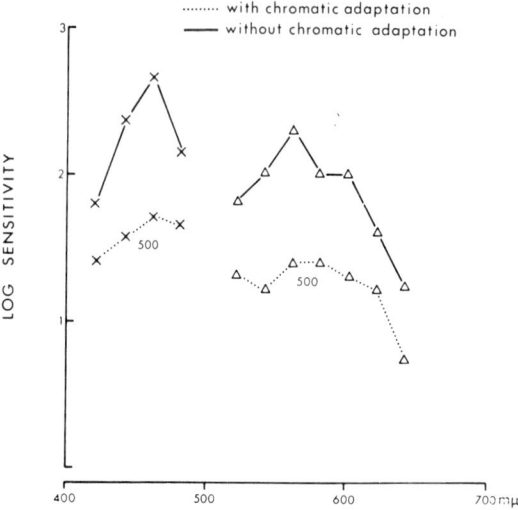

Fig. 11. Effects of chromatic adaptation with light at 500 mμ., the neutral wavelength, in the cell of Figs. 8–10. Though producing no response by itself, the adapting light lowered the sensitivity of the cell to stimulation at other wavelengths.

be similar to that described by Wolbarsht, Wagner, and MacNichol (49) for some goldfish retinal ganglion cells. These cells are for the time being classed as type II in Table 1.

Type III Cells: no Opponent-Color Mechanism

Of 213 cells recorded in the dorsal layers, 34, or 16%, were classed as type III cells. These were defined as cells showing no opponent-color responses. Receptive fields were subdivided into center and concentric surround, some centers being excitatory and others inhibitory. In most cells there was moderate or marked peripheral suppression, with little or no response to diffuse light, but in some the effect of the periphery was small or even negligible. For all cells, however, the peripheral suppression was the same at all wavelengths.

Figure 12 shows some results from a typical type III on-center cell. In Fig. 12A spectral sensitivities are given for the on-responses evoked by a 1° center spot (crosses), and off-responses from a 1°–8° annulus covering all of the receptive field except the center area (triangles). The two curves are nearly parallel, showing that there was little or no

difference in the spectral sensitivities of the two opposing systems. This would mean, as a corollary, that peripheral suppression should be just as pronounced at all wavelengths, and this was directly demonstrated by further measurements. Figure 12B shows area-sensitivity curves made at two different wavelengths, 540 mμ. and 620 mμ. For each wavelength the sensitivity increased (spatial summation) for spots up to about 1°, the diameter of the field center. Sensitivity then decreased progressively (peripheral suppression) up to 5° or 6°, where it leveled off, indicating the outer boundary of the field. The shapes of the two curves are almost identical. This result is to be contrasted with that obtained for a type I cell in Fig. 4, in which entirely different area-sensitivity curves were obtained at two different wavelengths, and with that for a type II cell shown in Fig. 6 in which the curves were identical, but the responses were of opposite sign. Behavior of this type III cell in the dark-adapted state is discussed below.

It is probably easiest to understand the behavior of a type III cell by supposing that it receives an excitatory input from cones in one part of the receptive field (center or surround) and inhibitory input from the remainder, and that in these two sets of cones the relative representations of the three cone types are the same. From cell to cell the relative contributions of the three cone types doubtless differ, since the spectral-sensitivity curves of different cells have different peaks. This has long been known to be so for retinal ganglion cells in the cat (19), which resemble type III cells in most respects. Type III cells are probably the same as the nonopponent broad-band cells described in the rhesus monkey by DeValois (11). Further evidence that more than one cone type supplies these cells has been obtained by chromatic adaptation studies (Fig. 20B).

To sum up the properties of these dorsal-layer cells, there seem to be three rather sharply defined types: type I with center-surround receptive fields, in which center and opposing surround have different spectral sensitivities; type II with two opposing systems having different spectral sensitivities and identical spatial distributions; and type III with opponent center and surround systems having the same spectral sensitivity. In addition, a few cells seem to have properties somewhere between

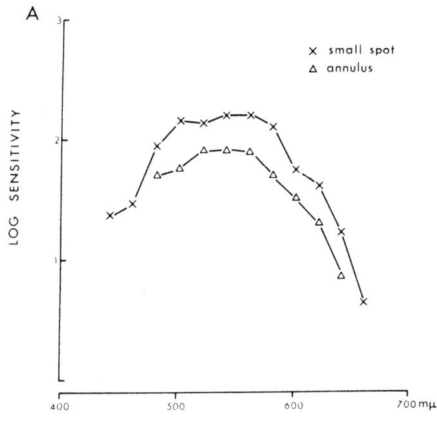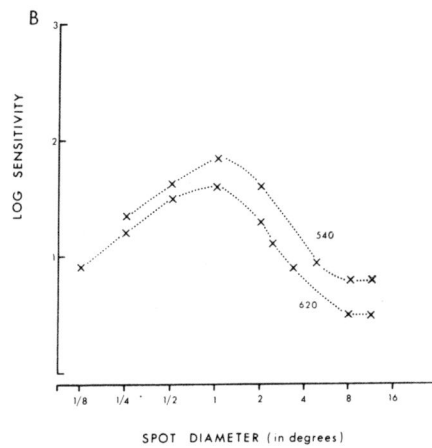

Fig. 12. Type III cell with an on-center 1° in diameter, located 25° from fovea. Recorded from layer D₁. A: spectral sensitivities to small spots 1° in diameter, and annuli with inner diameter 1°, outer diameter 8°. Light-adapted state. B: area-sensitivity curves at two wavelengths, 540 mμ. and 620 mμ.

those of type I and type II, but these have not been thoroughly studied.

Cells of all three types had the interesting property that on-off responses were rare. This is in marked contrast to retinal ganglion cells and geniculate cells in the cat (26, 28) and to retinal ganglion cells of the goldfish (48), where on-off responses are often seen when opponent systems are simultaneously stimulated. The absence of on-off responses in the monkey presumably indicates that the on-system and the off-system have similar time courses, excitation in one always being opposed by inhibition in the other.

Dark Adaptation

We were naturally interested in learning whether all types of geniculate cells were connected to both rods and cones, or whether some were connected to rods and others to cones. Twenty-five cells were therefore observed and categorized first in the light-adapted state and then after dark adapting the eyes for 15–20 min.

Type I Cells. Not all cells in this group were affected in the same way by dark adaptation. An example of one pattern of adaptation is given in Fig. 13. The cell was a typical red on-center, green off-surround, similar to the cell of Figs. 1–4 (which, in fact, reacted to dark adaptation in the same way). After 15 min. dark adaptation the cell's

sensitivity increased by about 4 log units, as shown in Fig. 13 by the interrupted curve. With diffuse light, on-responses were now obtained throughout the spectrum, with peak sensitivity at about 500 mμ. Our own thresholds for perceiving the spot with dark-adapted eyes agreed to within a few tenths of a log unit with those obtained for the cell. Moreover, for all wavelengths below about 620 mμ. the spot appeared colorless at threshold intensities and for the first few log units above threshold.

We conclude that this cell received input from rods as well as from cones. Thresholds were the same in the dark-adapted state for a center-size spot and for diffuse light, indicating that any rod contribution from the surround was not detectable at levels of intensity that were capable of stimulating the cell from the field center. Unfortunately the periphery of the field was not tested at suprathreshold scotopic levels, so that we do not know whether the cell made connections with rods in the field periphery.

The shift in response patterns between the two states of adaptation took place very quickly, this being especially obvious when the change in background reversed the response type from "on" to "off" and vice versa. Thus for the cell of Fig. 13, diffuse light at 500 mμ. gave off-responses with the background turned on, and on-responses with the background off. Here the response type reversed with a delay too short to be detected on rough test-

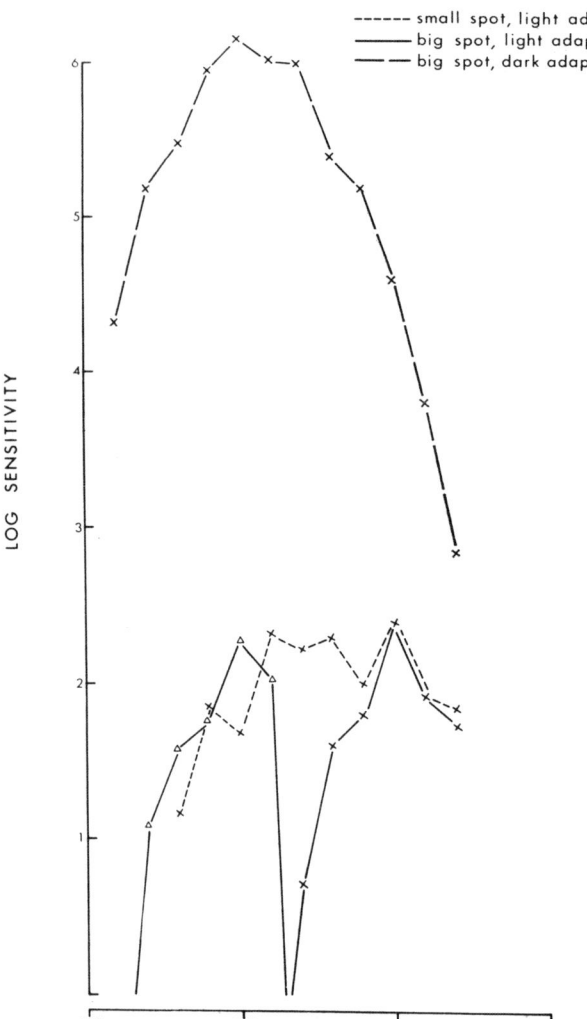

------- small spot, light adapte
——— big spot, light adapted
— — big spot, dark adapted

Fig. 13. Dark-adaptation effects in a type I red on-center cell in layer D₄. Field center 1/2° in diameter, situated 19° from the fovea. Lower curves show spectral sensitivities to small and large spots in the usual way (cf. Figs. 2, 5, and 6), with a 1 cd/m² white background light. Eliminating practically all the background for 15 min. produced the marked increase in sensitivity and shift in the maximum on-response sensitivity toward the short wavelengths shown for big spots by the upper curve. All responses were now "on" in type. Note that for wavelengths below 520 mμ., responses to large spots were "off" in light adaptation, "on" in dark adaptation. As far as one could tell the change occurred immediately upon switching the background light on or off.

ing, but certainly no more than a few seconds. It should be emphasized that the background in the light-adapted state was probably not intense enough to produce much bleaching of rod pigments; with a high photopic background the rods would undoubtedly have taken several minutes to reassert themselves.

Four of the 17 type I cells examined in the dark-adapted state had input from rods, showing similar increases in sensitivity and a Purkinje shift. In all four the response evoked from the center in dark adaptation ("on" or "off") corresponded to the center-type response in light adaptation. There was no obvious change in field-center size with dark adaptation, and stimuli that were threshold for the center seemed to have no influence on the periphery.

The remaining 13 type I cells showed neither a Purkinje shift nor any comparable increase in sensitivity on dark adaptation. The red off-center cell of Fig. 14 is an example. Spectral-sensitivity curves for small spots and for diffuse light were typical for red off-center cells. The diffuse-light curves are plotted in Fig. 14A in the light-adapted state and after 15 min. of dark adaptation. Each opponent system increased in sensitivity by roughly 1 log unit, and there was little difference in the cells' behavior, with peripheral suppression occurring at intermediate wavelengths as before. The thresholds of our own dark-adapted eyes were

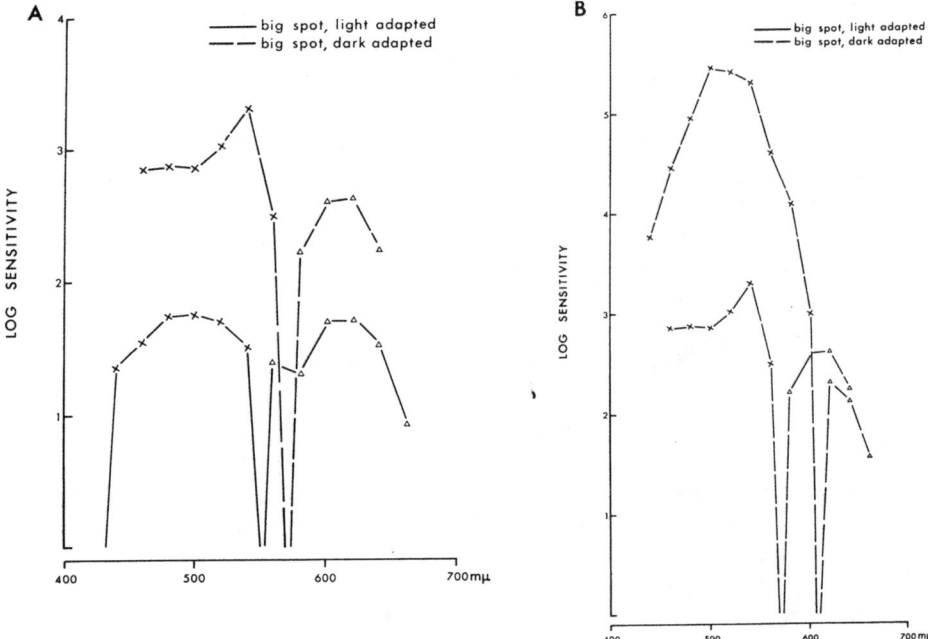

Fig. 14. *Effects of dark adaptation in a type I cell with a red sensitive off-center 3 1/2° from the fovea. Recorded from layer D₂. Center size was 1/4° and the whole field was about 4° in diameter. A: spectral sensitivities for large spots before and after dark adaptation. Both systems increased in sensitivity, but only by about 1 log unit. B: comparison of dark-adaptation effects in the cell of A with that of a simultaneously recorded green on-center, red off-surround cell. Though studied under identical conditions, one cell has sensitivity some 2 log units greater than the other.*

several log units lower than those of the cell, and it was interesting to observe that the cell began reacting to the stimuli at about the intensities at which the spot first appeared colored.

While making the determinations on this cell we noticed a second, simultaneously recorded unit of lower spike amplitude, which turned out to have a much lower threshold, one close, in fact, to that of our own dark-adapted eyes. A spectral-sensitivity curve of this cell was made for comparison, and is shown in Fig. 14B. Thresholds were as much as 2 log units lower than those of the first cell, with peak sensitivity at about 520 mμ. This type I cell was a green on-center. It seems clear from this that cells with only cone input can exist side by side in the geniculate with cells having both rod and cone connections.

To sum up these results, some geniculate type I cells have connections with rods and cones, as manifested by about a 4 log unit increase in sensitivity, a disappearance of opponent-color effects at scotopic stimulus levels, and a shift in peak spectral

sensitivity to the low 500s. Others show none of these changes and appear to make connections with cones only, even though having their fields outside of the fovea, where rods are abundant. The relative frequency of cells with and without rod input is not at all clear, but presumably it varies with position of receptive fields in the visual field, so that a thorough study would require a generous sampling from different parts of the geniculate.

TYPE II CELLS. Two type II cells were examined with the eyes dark adapted. In both there was an increase ins ensitivity of about 0.5–1 log unit for both systems, with no change in neutral point, suggesting a lack of any rod input. (It is worth noting that once again changing the white background light produced some change in sensitivity, even though white light, like the 500-mμ. light, evoked no response itself.)

TYPE III CELLS. Of the four dorsal-layer type III cells tested, two showed only a slight increase in sensitivity with no Purkinje shift, suggesting that they lacked connections with rods. The other two cells increased markedly in sensitivity and showed a clear shift in spectral sensitivity. One of these, an on-center cell, was studied in some detail. The results for the light-adapted state have already been given in Fig. 12. There it was shown that center and surround had practically identical spectral sensitivities and that peripheral suppression was the same at two widely separated wavelengths. When the eyes were dark adapted the threshold fell by over 2 log units (Fig. 15). At stimulus intensities just above threshold a large spot gave a weaker response than a small spot, indicating that rods fed into the cell from both center and surround, in opponent fashion. For a center-size spot the spectral sensitivity, shown by dotted lines in Fig. 15A, had a peak in the low 500s, being displaced to the short end of the spectrum compared with the light-adapted curve. Stimulation of the surround alone failed to evoke any response. If,

however, a just-suprathreshold white spot was directed on the center and left there, monochromatic stimuli now evoked clear peripheral responses in the form of suppression of firing with off-discharges. Thresholds for these responses at different wavelengths are shown in the upper, interrupted curve of Fig. 15B. Again there was a marked threshold decrease with a clear Purkinje shift giving further evidence that rods from the periphery of the field were connected to the cell.

On comparing the area-sensitivity curves for light and dark adaptation in Fig. 16, it appears that the field-center size remained about the same in the two states, yet to our surprise the contribution of the periphery was not evident, there being no decline in sensitivity for large spots. Stimuli that were just suprathreshold, on the other hand, evoked much stronger responses from the center than from the whole receptive field, indicating that the surround made an important contribution, and that its threshold was in fact not much higher than

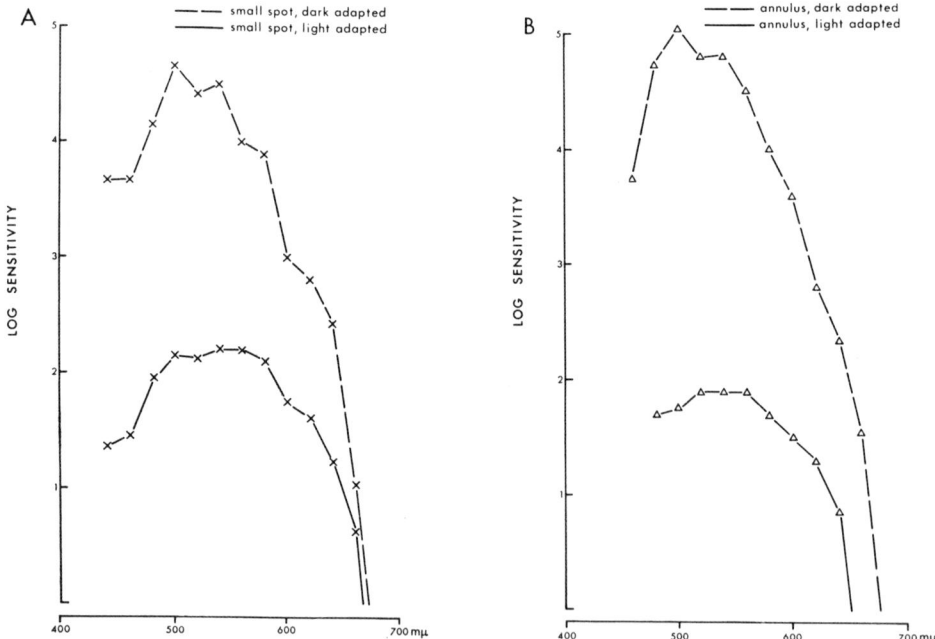

Fig. 15. Effects of dark adaptation in the cell of Fig. 12. A: on-responses to 1° spots. B: off-responses to an annulus, inner and outer diameters 1° and 6°, respectively. A suprathreshold 1° white spot was directed steadily on the field center during these measurements, so that thresholds are not strictly comparable with those of A.

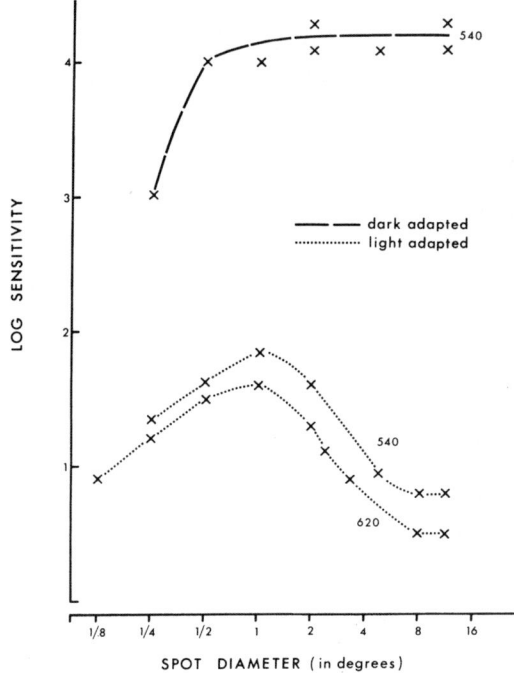

Fig. 16. *Area-sensitivity curves for the cell of Figs. 12 and 15. Lower curves, light-adapted state for spots at 540 mμ. and 620 mμ. (redrawn from Fig. 12B). Upper curve, dark-adapted state.*

that of the center. Once more it was as if some activation of the center was necessary before the peripheral effect could manifest itself.

In summary, of four type III cells tested in dark adaptation, two had rod input from both center and surround and two appeared to lack rod input.

Distribution of Cell Types in the Dorsal Layers

TOPOGRAPHICAL CONSIDERATIONS. It is well known from the anatomical work of Clark and Penman (7) and Polyak (38) that the contralateral half-visual fields are mapped in an orderly way upon the six geniculate layers. The six maps are in register, with layers D_1, D_3, and V_1 connected to the contralateral eye and D_2, D_4 and V_2 to the ipsilateral (see METHODS for discussion of terminology). While no attempt was made at a complete or detailed mapping in the present experiments, our results are in good agreement with the anatomy. The topographical representation is clearly a precise one: the receptive fields were small and restricted, and for simultaneously or successively recorded cells they either overlapped or were close together. As the electrode advanced through a layer in a radial direction there was no over-all drift in receptive-field positions of successively recorded cells, only a slight variation in position, even in long sequences. In very oblique penetrations there was always a steady drift in receptive-field positions, superimposed, as in the cortex (26), upon a small, apparently random staggering in field position. Figure 17 indicates the parts of the visual field explored. Each dot represents the average position of the receptive fields observed in a given penetration. The positions of these dots taken together reflect the parts of the lateral geniculate studied. Eleven of the 19 penetrations were made in areas serving retinal regions within 10° of the fovea. No recordings were clearly established as having been made in the area representing the fovea, but a few cells had fields that were at most within a degree or two of the center.

A fairly typical track reconstruction is shown in Fig. 18, an example chosen partly because it illustrates the danger of relying heavily on shifts from one eye to the other in estimating the electrode position with respect to the different layers.

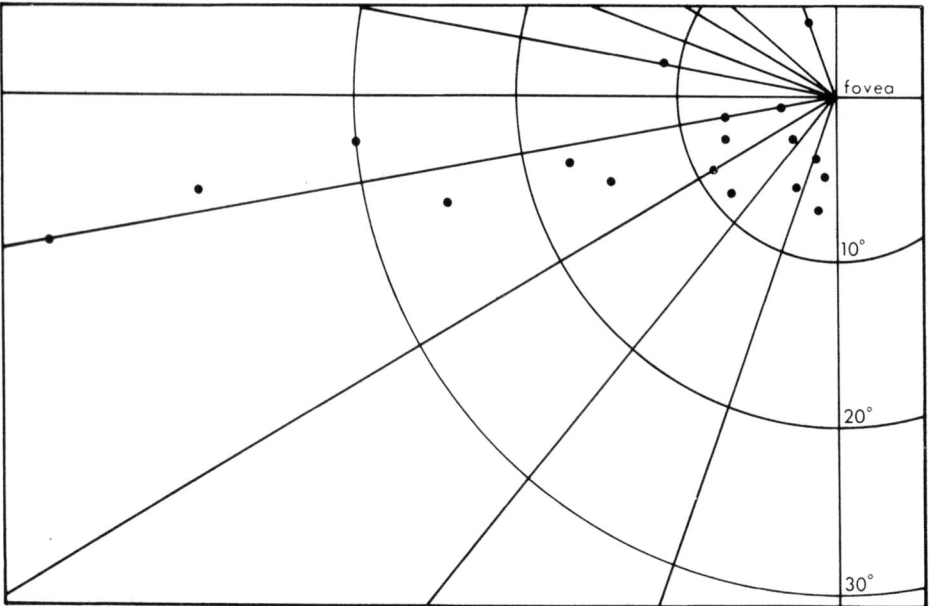

Fig. 17. Regions of visual fields explored in 18 penetrations of the lateral geniculate. Each dot represents the average visual-field position of the receptive fields in a single penetration. Most penetrations were normal to the geniculate layering, so that there was little variation in the positions of the individual receptive fields.

In this experiment one might have concluded from the eye shifts that the penetration terminated in V_1, the most ventral layer, instead of layer D_3. In fact, had the penetration continued in the same direction through the interlocking folds it would have passed through D_2 three times instead of once, and would never have reached the ventral layers.

DISTRIBUTION OF CELL TYPES IN THE DORSAL LAYERS. It was obviously important to learn whether the various cell types were evenly distributed throughout the four dorsal layers. The results are summarized in Table 1. The sampling of cells was largest for layer D_1 and progressively smaller for each of the other layers, because many penetrations were discontinued before the deeper layers were reached. To allow for this, the number of cells in a particular layer is given also as a per cent of the total number of cells in that layer, so that in comparing the different layers it is the percentages that are important.

Table 1 shows that all major cell types were represented in both pairs of dorsal layers, indicating a lack of any rigid separation of functional groups. There was some unevenness in the distribution of red on-center cells, these being almost twice as common in the dorsal two layers as in the middle two. On the other hand, the red off-center cells were about twice as common in the middle layers. We are nevertheless hesitant to accept what appears at first glance to be a statistically significant result for reasons having to do with the distribution of cells within each layer. Within a given layer there was no obvious systematic segregation of the different cell types, yet as the electrode advanced from cell to cell there were frequent sequences in which one subtype occurred two to six times in a row. As might be expected, this was most often seen with red on-center cells, for these were the most common. Clearly even a slight tendency toward grouping makes one cautious about interpreting the relatively small samples represented by Table 1. Meanwhile one can sum up the table by saying that *1*) no group of cells is confined to any layer or pair of layers; *2*) red on-center cells, red off-center cells, green on-center cells, and green off-center cells are all represented in all four layers; and *3*) the two dorsal layers are perhaps richer than

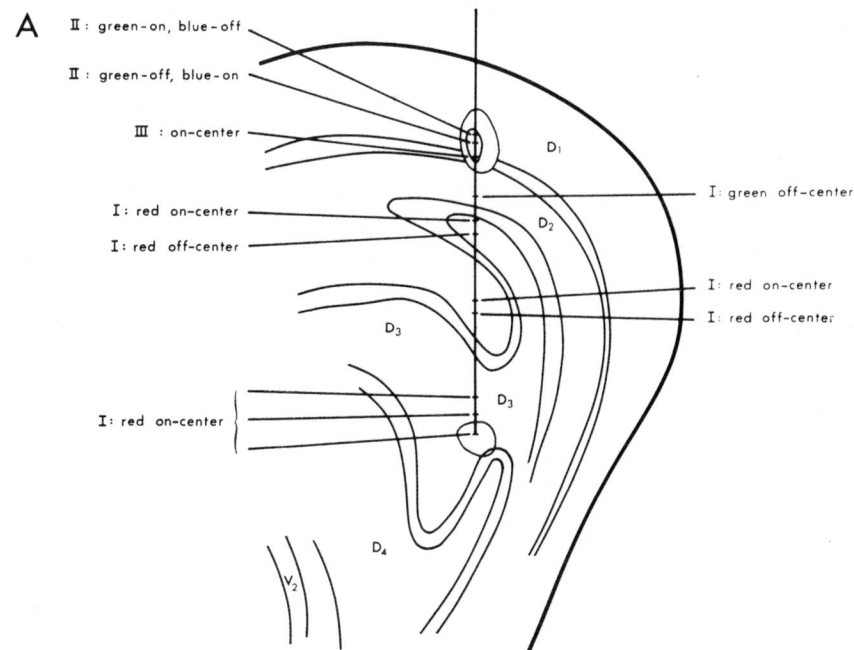

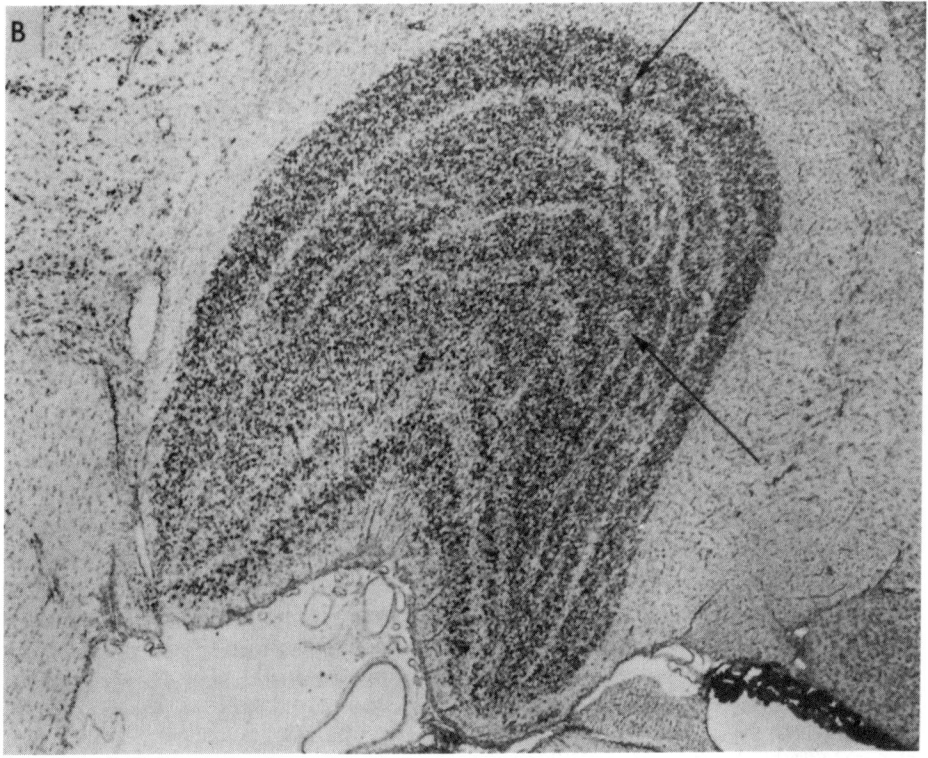

Fig. 18. A: *reconstruction of an electrode track through right lateral geniculate. Coronal section. Electrode track is shown entering layer D_1 and ending in layer D_3; lesions made near the beginning of the penetration and at the end are outlined as irregular ovals. Short lines intersecting the electrode track show the positions of cells studied during the penetration. Labels indicate, by their position to left or right of figure, whether cells were recorded from contralateral or ipsilateral eye. Distance from entry of track into geniculate to end of track was about 1.5 mm. B: one of the Nissl sections from which the track was reconstructed, showing lesions (arrows) and first part of electrode track (outlined by inflammatory reaction).*

the middle two in red on-center cells and poorer in red off-center cells.

SIZES OF RECEPTIVE-FIELD CENTERS. Cell centers ranged in diameter from 2 min. of arc up to about 1°. Distributions of type I cells according to field-center size are given in Fig. 19, with separate histograms for on-center (left) and off-center (middle). On comparing the two histograms, it can be seen that, though the size ranges overlapped, on-centers tended to be smaller than off-centers, and in fact all of the very small field centers (1/32° to 1/16°) were "on" in type. This agrees with our previous observations in spider monkey optic nerve (24). The relative proportions of red-center and green-center cells (shaded versus unshaded) were about the same for all center sizes. Fields of type III cells (Fig. 19, right) tended to be larger than those

of type I, though again the size ranges overlapped. For both type I and type III cells there was a loose correlation between field-center size and distance from fovea. The smallest centers, 1/32° to 1/16°, were all within 10° of the fovea. Type II fields ranged in size from 1/4° to 1°, and were found as close as 2° from the fovea and as far out as 12°.

VENTRAL LAYERS

Thirty-one cells were recorded from the ventral layers. The sampling was relatively small because many penetrations either did not reach the ventral layers or missed them entirely (Fig. 18), and because the ventral layers are relatively thin. Cells in these layers fell into two main groups: those of the first resembled type III cells in the dorsal layers; cells in the second group were different from any

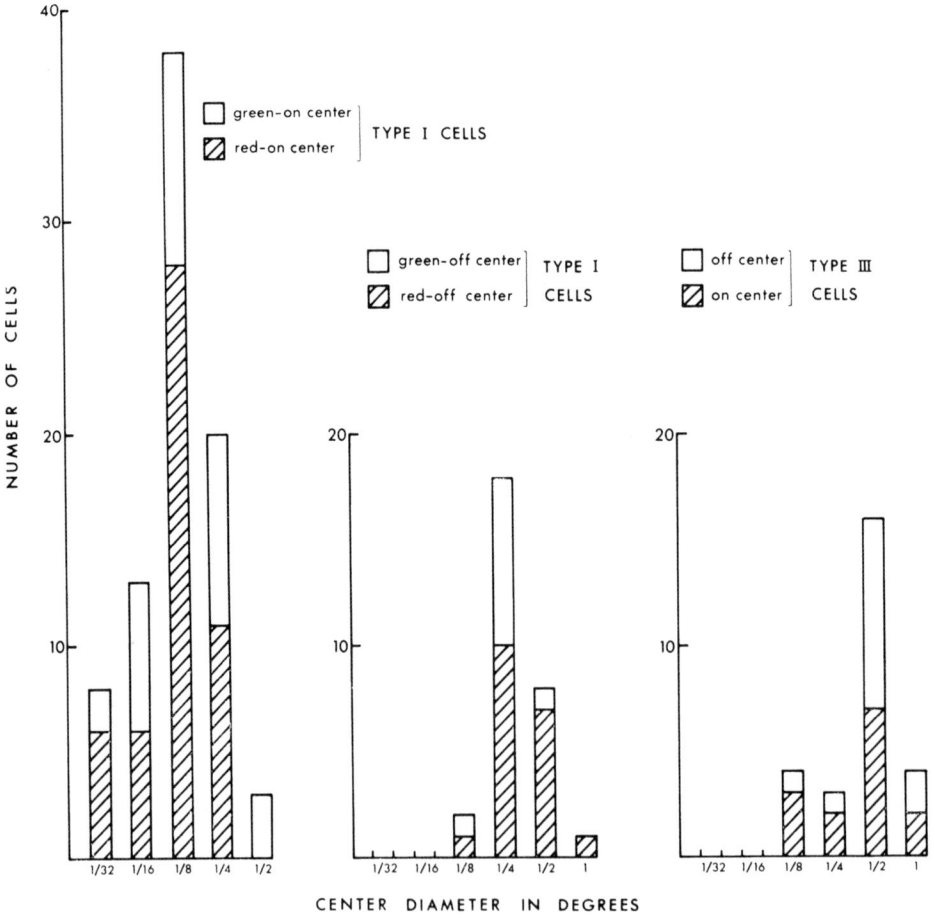

Fig. 19. Distribution of geniculate cells with respect to size of field centers. Left and middle histograms: type I cells. Right: type III cells.

seen in the dorsal layers, and are termed type IV cells.

Ventral-Layer Type III Cells

As with dorsal-layer type III cells, both on-centers (7 cells) and off-centers (14 cells) were seen. By definition, a cell in this group responded in the same way ("on" versus "off") to a spot of a given size or shape for all effective wavelengths, and showed the same degree of peripheral suppression over the entire spectrum. Most cells were unresponsive, or virtually so, to diffuse light, peripheral suppression being practically complete for white light and all wavelengths of monochromatic light, and at all available intensities.

An off-center type III cells was examined to learn whether more than one cone type contributed to the receptive field. To estimate center and surround dimensions, sensitivity (reciprocal threshold) was plotted against spot size for white stimuli in the light-adapted state (Fig. 20A). Peripheral suppression was complete at 6–8° spot diameter, sensitivity falling by over 3 log units from the maximum at 1/2°. Next, spectral sensitivity was determined for spots just under center size

(Fig. 20B). After adapting the field center with light at 640 mμ., threshold measurements were repeated for stimuli at 480, 520, and 620 mμ. The effect of the steady adapting light, shown by the arrows, was to reduce sensitivity at all three wavelengths, but more for the long than the short. This result is just what one would expect if the cell received contributions from more than one type of cone in the field center, in a nonopponent system.

Dark adaptation was not done for any ventral-layer type III cells, so that we have no information about the possible contribution of rods to these cells. The fields were found as close as 3° from the fovea and as far out as 12°. Center diameters ranged from 1/8° to 1/2°. Sampling was too small to allow any comparison of field-center sizes in ventral as opposed to dorsal layers.

Type IV Cells

Type IV cells, of which 10 were studied in detail, were quite unlike anything seen in the dorsal layers, or in the cat retina or geniculate. A typical example is illustrated in Fig. 21A. As with every cell in this group the receptive field was concentric in type, with an excitatory center and an inhibitory

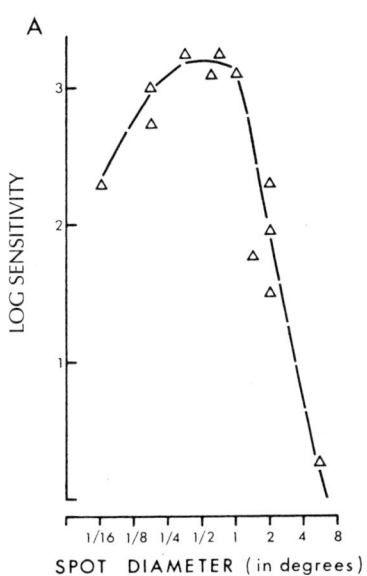
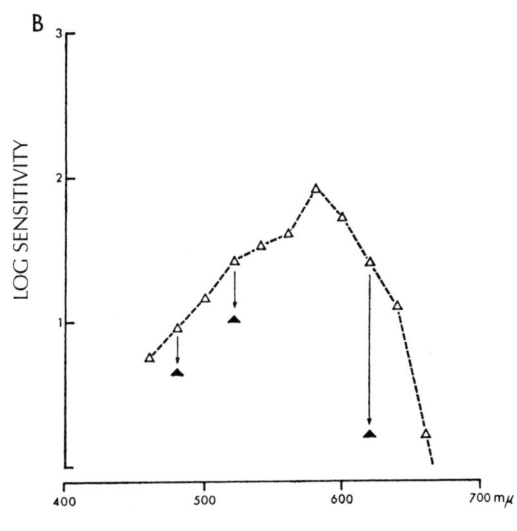

Fig. 20. Off-center type III cell recorded in light-adapted state from layer V₂. Field center 6° from fovea. A: area-sensitivity curve for white light stimuli, showing field-center size to be about 1/2°, and overall field at least 6–8° in diameter. B: spectral sensitivity plotted for 3/8° spots. Empty triangles, off-responses with the usual white background. Filled triangles, three measurements made in the presence of 640-mμ. diffuse steady background. Decline in sensitivity is greater for long wavelengths than for short, suggesting that more than one type of cone had a nonopponent connection with the cell.

surround. There was active maintained firing. Small spots evoked on-discharges with sensitivities shown by the rather broad upper (interrupted) curve. These responses were poorly sustained, lasting for a few seconds or less. To large spots the responses were most unusual: at short and medium wavelengths (violet through yellow) there was no effect at any intensity, i.e., peripheral suppression was complete. In the red, however, the influence of the surround actually predominated over that of the center, and the maintained activity was suppressed by large spots. The cessation of firing, unlike the center response, was well maintained, usually lasting as long as the light was left on. The effect required relatively high intensities, especially for complete suppression of firing. There was summation over a tremendous area, in some cases with clear differences in the effects of a 20° and a 25° spot. White light acted like red, producing a sustained suppression of firing with no marked off-discharge but, rather, a simple resumption of the maintained firing.

Cells of this type seemed to be plentiful. One of the common signs that the electrode had entered the ventral layers was the nearly complete suppression of unresolved background activity by diffuse light, especially diffuse red light, in contrast to the general activation of the background by small spots. These are the only cells we have seen in which surround prevailed over center with white

light, or where there was this center-surround difference in temporal adaptation.

A few cells had properties somewhat different from those just described. For the cell of Fig. 21B the surround system seemed to be not only richer than the center in red cone concentration, but also poorer in green or green plus blue. At wavelengths up to the mid-500s the surround had no discernible influence, while at wavelengths beyond 580 mμ. the sustained surround effect dominated and was apparent even at relatively low stimulus intensities. Diffuse white light was ineffective or evoked a weak on-response. It is thus clear that opponent-color cells occur in the ventral layers, though they seem rare. Too few have been seen to justify their classification as type I cells, or as a separate group.

Two type IV cells were studied after dark adaptation. One of these was the cell of Fig. 21A. In both there was an increase in sensitivity of about 1 log unit for all responses, with no obvious change in any of the qualitative behavior just described. Sensitivities were many log units below that of our own dark-adapted eyes. These two cells thus seemed not to have any significant rod input.

DISCUSSION

In this study the object was to learn how information on form and color of a stimulus is handled at

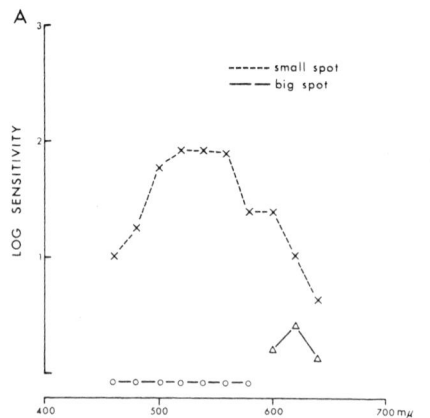
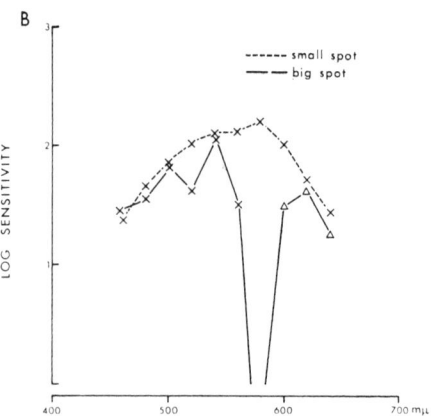

Fig. 21. A: *typical type IV cell, with brief on-responses to small spot stimulation, sustained suppression of maintained firing to large spots, but only at long wavelengths. At wavelengths up to 600 mμ. no response could be evoked with large spots. Field center 1/2° in diameter, situated 11° from fovea. Recorded from layer V₂. B: type IV cell with no obvious peripheral suppression at short wavelengths, but otherwise similar in properties to the cell illustrated in A. Field center 1/4°, 12° from fovea. Layer V₁.*

an early stage in the central nervous system. Given two opponent processes in the monkey, a chromatic and a spatial, it seemed important to learn whether these existed in independent pathways or were combined in common cells. The answer seems to be that both things occur: some cells are mainly concerned with form, others mainly with color, while the majority handle both variables at the same time. In the case of color, as originally shown by De Valois (10, 11), a cell may be excited by one group of cones and inhibited by another group with a different spectral sensitivity, so that white light covering a large retinal area and stimulating both groups of cones may evoke little or no response. For the spatial variable the receptors may excite or inhibit a cell, depending on retinal position, with the result that diffuse light has little effect regardless of wavelength (24). In any given cell one or both of these mechanisms may be found. Both opponent mechanisms seem aimed at increasing the specialization of single cells, in the direction of color as opposed to white, or spatial contrast as opposed to diffuse light. Thus the existence of inhibitory mechanisms leads to the surprising result that the optimum response of a cell in the visual pathway is not obtained by stimulation of all of the receptors—in general that is the least efficient stimulus. For the cell to respond optimally a particular set of receptors must be activated, the set varying from one cell to the next. The function of a structure like the geniculate can thus be studied by asking how the receptors are categorized into set and subsets by the different cells.

The findings can be summed up by saying that in the light-adapted state practically all cells are influenced by two antagonistic sets of connections, one excitatory and the other inhibitory. Depending upon the details of these connections, three main cell types can be distinguished. For type III cells the opponent inputs take origin from two groups of receptors that are spatially separated into center and surround. A given cell is generally supplied by cones of more than one type, and the relative proportions of the three cone types are the same for center and surround, though from cell to cell they undoubtedly differ. This is shown diagrammatically in Fig. 22*A* for a type III on-center cell; here a cell is considered to receive excitatory input from cones in the field center, with the red-, blue-, and green-sensitive cones represented in the

ratio of 1:1:1, and inhibitory input from peripherally located cones in the same ratio. (For simplicity, intervening synaptic stages are omitted, as are the rods.) Type III cells presumably represent an elementary step in form analysis, registering not simply the general level of illumination but rather comparing light that falls on one retinal region with that falling on the immediate surround. This is done to a large extent irrespective of wavelength. For these cells unevenness of illumination is a powerful stimulus, and diffuse light tends to be inadequate.

For type II cells the scheme is just the converse: opponent sets of receptors of different spectral sensitivities are distributed in identical fashion throughout the same retinal area. The cell of Fig. 22*B* receives excitatory input from green-sensitive cones over the entire receptive field, and inhibitory input from blue cones throughout the same region; over all parts of the receptive field the proportion of excitatory to inhibitory cones is constant. Thus these cells react mainly to unevenness of spectral energy distribution, and diffuse light is as good a stimulus as an optimally placed spot.

For type I cells, finally, the two sets of receptors are not only spatially segregated but also have different spectral sensitivities. The red on-center cell of Fig. 22*C* is supplied by the red-sensitive cones from the field center, and the green-sensitive cones from the periphery. The properties of the other two cell types are thus combined in the type I cell, which deals with black-white images in the same way as the type III cell does, but for diffuse light or parts of images lacking spatial intensity gradients has all of the wavelength-discriminating ability of the type II cell. In sum, diffuse light is to the type III cell what white light is to the type II, and what diffuse white light is to the type I.

The schemes proposed in Fig. 22 must be considered tentative, with several details still unsettled. The first of these concerns the relative contribution of the three cone types. While the simplest assumption consistent with the experimental evidence is that each opponent-color cell receives input from two of the cones, it is often difficult to be sure that the third cone does not also contribute. Cells that we regard as receiving opponent inputs from red and green cones could, for instance, receive contributions from the blue-sensitive cones along with the green. The result would be to

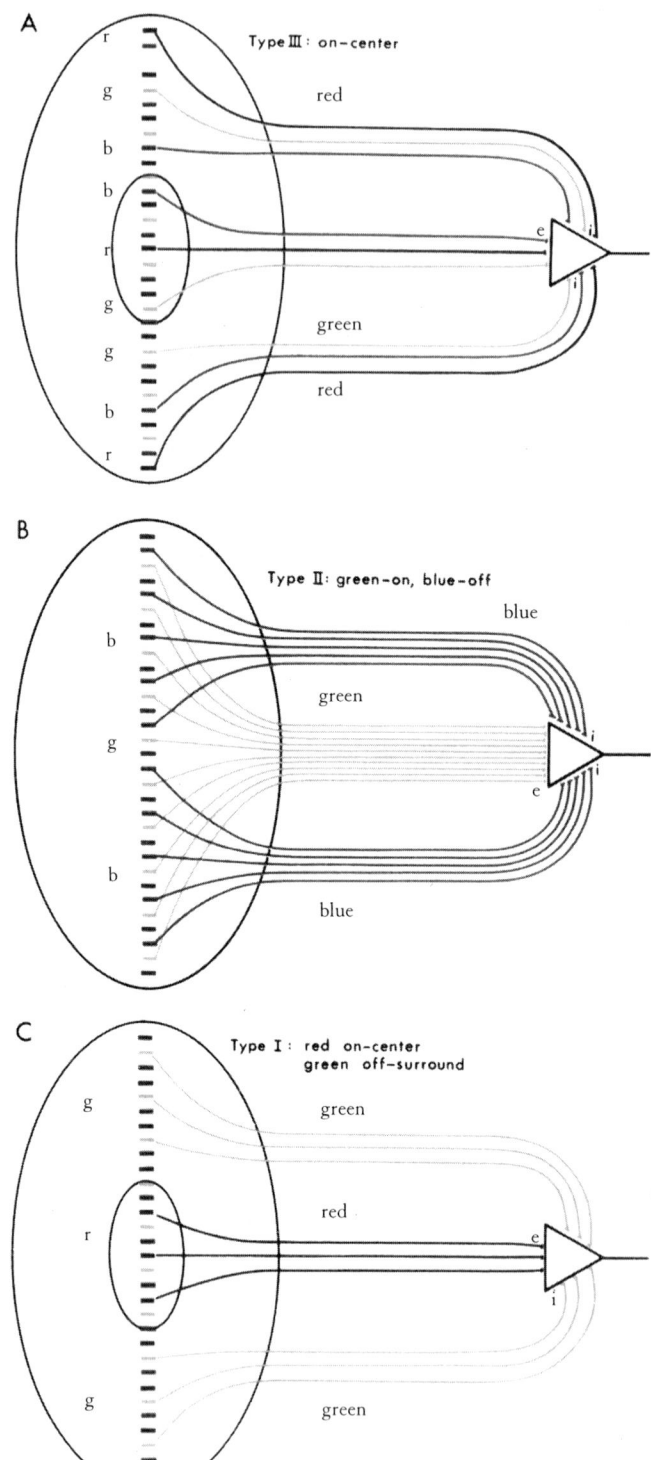

A Type Ⅲ: on-center

red

green

red

r
g
b
b
r
g
g
b
r

e i

B Type Ⅱ: green-on, blue-off

blue

green

blue

b

g

b

i
e
i

C Type Ⅰ: red on-center
green off-surround

green

red

green

g

r

g

e
i

Fig. 22. Three types of cones are illustrated by letters 'r', 'g' and 'b'. A: proposed contribution of cones to a type III on-center cell. Three types of cones are illustrated by colors and, for simplicity, receptors are shown only along a line through the field center. Cones project to the cell, via intervening synapses which are not shown, and activation of those in the center of the receptive field leads to excitation of the cell (e), those in the periphery to inhibition (i). The three cone types from the center are arbitrarily shown as being present in the ratio of 1:1:1, and this ratio is the same for the periphery. B: schematic representation of a type II cell, receiving excitatory input from green-sensitive cones and inhibitory input from the blue. The relative contributions of the two afferent cone types are the same in all parts of the receptive field. C: representation of a type I cell receiving excitatory input from red-sensitive cones in the field center and inhibitory input from green-sensitive cones in the periphery. Note that in these figures "i" is used simply to imply that light falling on the cone leads to an increased tendency toward cessation of firing of the cell. This could depend on an inhibitory synapse at any stage in the path from receptor to geniculate cell, and need not imply active inhibition at the geniculate cell itself.

broaden the spectral sensitivity of the short-wave-length system and displace the peak even further to the short-wavelength end of the spectrum. Since, in fact, the spectral sensitivity of the short-wave-length system in these cells generally has its peak in the mid-500s, falling off markedly by the mid-400s, the contribution of the blue cones must at most be a minor one. But if the ratio of green cones to blue in the input to the short-wavelength system were the same as it is in the local cone population the contribution of the blue cones would be hard to detect, for even outside the fovea there are probably far fewer blue cones than green ones.

The situation is different in the case of the blue-versus-green opponent cells (a few type I cells and most of the type II). Here the problem is to tell whether or not the red cones as well as the green contribute to the long-wavelength system, and in what proportion. This is not easy, since the two cones have extensively overlapping spectral sensitivities. Thus whether the green cones make up the entire contribution to the long system, or just half of it, will determine whether the spectral-sensitivity peak is at 540 mμ. or 560 mμ., a subtle difference for techniques as coarse as those used in this study.

Finally, there is the possibility of opponent-color cells having one system fed by green cones and the other by red cones plus blue cones. The result would be two neutral points, a cell being excited at intermediate wavelengths and inhibited at the long and short ends of the spectrum, or the reverse. So far we have not seen any cells of this type, though they should be easy to recognize. De Valois and Jones (13), recording also from the macaque geniculate, have reported finding such cells, but the results may not necessarily have to be interpreted in terms of three cone inputs, since with the eyes dark adapted a contribution from rods would seem possible. For example, a "red off-center, green on-surround" cell with inhibitory rod input, a type we have seen, might well masquerade as a "purple-off, green-on" cell if examined only in the scotopic state.

A second qualification to the interpretations implied by Fig. 22 concerns the arrangement of the receptive field of type I cells. The problem can best be approached by comparing our results in the monkey geniculate with a similar study made in the goldfish retina by Wagner, MacNichol, and Wolbarsht (43–45, 48, 49). The comparison reveals some striking similarities but also certain differences in the details of receptive-field organization. In the goldfish some cells showed no opponent-color effects, but had center-surround receptive fields of the type described by Kuffler (28) (type III in the present study). Other cells showed opponent-color responses, but in these the opponent systems overlapped instead of being distributed on the retina in a center-surround manner. The two systems had sensitivities that were maximal in the field center, but tapered off toward the periphery at different rates so that the effects of one predominated in the center and those of the other in the surround.

One might ask whether in the monkey the fields of type I cells are not also organized as two partially overlapping opponent systems with different spatial distributions. Experimentally, it is difficult to obtain a clear answer to this. As a rule the size of receptive-field centers of type I cells is very small relative to the size of the whole field, so that a spot of center-size placed anywhere in the periphery evokes no response at any wavelength or intensity. On the other hand, a small spot in the center evokes only center-type responses regardless of wavelength. Thus if the opposing system is activated at all from the center, its effects are apparently outweighed. In the goldfish, on-off responses indicate that opposing systems are being simultaneously activated, but in the monkey these mixed responses do not occur—either one system is dominant and completely submerges the other or the two mutually cancel and no response is seen. In any case, a distinction between overlapping and non-overlapping arrangements seems of theoretical rather than practical importance in the monkey, given the small size of field centers relative to the total field size. The scheme suggested in Fig. 22 seems to us the simplest consistent with the results. If, as seems likely on anatomical grounds, there are ganglion cells in or near the fovea whose field centers are supplied by single cones, then the receptive-field periphery of such cells must obviously be annular. Type II cells have overlapping opponent systems, but with the important difference that the sensitivities of the two systems have the same spatial distribution. No such cells have been reported in the goldfish. Possibly the model proposed by Wolbarsht *et al.* (49) might apply in the monkey to the relatively rare red-green opponent cell that seems to combine features of the type I and type II cells (see RESULTS section, under *Type II cells*).

Here a comment may be made on the organization of center-surround fields of types I and III. The descriptions in this and other papers may give the impression that the center and surround of a concentric receptive field are roughly equal and opposite in their influence on a cell. This is not strictly so. Peripheral responses are often difficult to evoke with annular stimuli alone, especially in the lateral geniculate of the cat and monkey. This has also been noted for retinal ganglion cells in the rabbit (3). Nevertheless it is clear that the periphery is highly effective, since a large spot evokes a weaker response (excitatory or inhibitory) than a small one, and often evokes none at all. In cells of the cat geniculate diffuse light has on the average less effect than it does at the retinal ganglion cell level (25), reflecting an increase in the potency of the receptive-field periphery; yet, compared with retinal cells, geniculate cells respond especially grudgingly to annuli. This is true both for on-center and off-center cells. Apparently the more potent the surround is in suppressing the center effects the more difficult it is to obtain a response from the surround alone. One can, however, always obtain a response from the periphery by first shining a spot steadily on the center and then turning on and off the annulus—it was necessary, for example, to use this device to obtain a spectral-sensitivity curve for the field surround in the dark-adapted type III on-center cell of Fig. 15B. The reciprocal phenomenon does not seem to occur, in that a center stimulus is not made more effective by shining a steady annulus in the periphery. It is as though the surround system could only exert its effects provided the center system was also activated. As indicated below, this peculiarity may help explain the difficulty in demonstrating peripheral effects at threshold in the dark-adapted state. The point to be emphasized is that the center and surround of concentric receptive fields seem to function in quite different ways, the effects of the surround working as it were, through the center.

CHROMATIC ADAPTATION. The importance of neural mechanisms in light and dark adaptation is well recognized and has most recently been emphasized by Rushton (39) and Dowling (16); they found, by very different methods, that within a wide range of intensities the amounts of pigment actually bleached were too small to account for the observed large changes in sensitivity. In the present experiments the rapid recovery from the rather moderate intensities of adapting lights likewise suggests that neural mechanisms are important: the effects of chromatic adaptation on opponent responses subside within seconds of the time the adapting light is turned off, rather than after several minutes as one would expect if it were solely a matter of pigment bleaching and regeneration. It is thus likely that chromatic adaptation involves a change in the stimulus-response relationship in one opponent system without any equivalent change in the other, the effect presumably occurring at some point prior to the convergence of the two systems. In the cat it is well known that the response to an intermittent white stimulus of constant intensity declines as the white background is turned up. Presumably in the monkey the decline in sensitivity with chromatic adaptation is similar in nature but the effect is selective, being confined to one of the opponent systems.

These remarks apply to chromatic adaptation of the type employed in our experiments, in which the intermittent stimulus is superimposed upon a steady adapting light. Obviously the mechanisms would be quite different if the adapting light were first turned out and then the stimulus applied. We have avoided this method because of the complications involved in stimulating during the transient off-effects following the change in background.

DARK ADAPTATION. That rods and cones may converge on single retinal ganglion cells in the cat was shown first by Granit (19) and later confirmed by Barlow, FitzHugh, and Kuffler (2). In the monkey similar conclusions have been reached by Gouras (18). From the results of De Valois (10, 15) in the rhesus geniculate it seems clear that some lateral geniculate cells receive input from rods and cones, and others from cones only. Our findings confirm those of De Valois, and further show that cells with fields clearly outside of the rod-free fovea may receive input from rods and cones, or from cones only. Indeed, to our surprise, the majority of cells recorded from the 10° parafoveal region received no rod input. We have seen no examples of cells with connections to rods but not to cones. As shown in Fig. 14*B,* two cells can exist side by side, one with a powerful rod input and the other with none. This, then, is still another example of the striking specificity of connections seen already in the geniculate in other contexts.

In the present work we were particularly interested in the receptive-field organization of cells that receive both rod and cone input. In the type I cell the receptive fields in the dark-adapted and light-adapted states had about the same center size, and in all cells the center responses were the same (on versus off) in the two states. The question of whether the receptive-field periphery supplies rods as well as cones in type I cells is still not answered, and while it is true that at threshold no effects were seen from the periphery, this was also the case in the type III cell of Fig. 15*B,* which turned out to have a clear input from rods in the periphery.

It seems that some type III cells receive rod contributions and others do not. In the one well-studied cell the rods from the center were excitatory and those from the surround inhibitory, and the same was true for the cones, so that there was no basic difference in the field arrangement in the two states. Only at threshold did the surround fail to manifest itself (Fig. 16), perhaps, as discussed above, because of the necessity for having some center activation for the surround to work upon.

The dark-adaptation effects in type III cells are in some ways similar to those obtained in the cat by Barlow, FitzHugh, and Kuffler (2). They found that rods project onto single retinal ganglion cells, producing excitatory effects from the center and inhibitory effects from the surround, or the reverse. After some hours of adaptation the surround effects were no longer detectable, not only from area-threshold measurements but also on comparing small and large spots as much as several log units above threshold. In these cells both center and surround increased in sensitivity as the rods became effective in dark adaptation, but ultimately the center sensitivity considerably exceeded that of the periphery. As shown in Fig. 15, no such center-periphery differences were seen in the monkey. This suggests a possible difference in dark-adaptation mechanisms in the two species, which would not be surprising since the cat is a nocturnal animal.

Just as with chromatic adaptation, the change in spectral sensitivity occurred within a second or less of the time that the background light was turned off. This would surely not have been so had our background been a high photopic one. The quickness of the change, from responses dictated primarily if not entirely by cones to responses due to rods, suggests that neural mechanisms were chiefly involved.

DISTRIBUTION OF CELL TYPES IN THE LATERAL GENICULATE BODY. The significance of the layering in the geniculate has puzzled anatomists and neurophysiologists for many years, and a number of theories have been proposed, notably those of Clark (6) and Walls (46). In the present study one of our main objectives was to learn whether cells as categorized by receptive-field organization differed from layer to layer. It was no surprise to find the biggest disparity between the four dorsal layers and the two ventral, given the glaring histological dissimilarities in the two sets of layers. Distributions of cell types were entirely different, there being no typical type I or type II cells in the ventral layers, and no type IV cells in the dorsal. Among the four dorsal layers the only difference, besides the obvious one related to ipsilateral and contralateral eyes, was in the distribution of the type I subgroups, the red on-centers being somewhat more common in the dorsal two layers than in the middle two, and the red off-centers somewhat less common. Both groups were nevertheless clearly represented in both pairs of layers. The lack of any fundamental differences in response properties of cells in these four layers once more fits well with the lack of any distinguishing histological features.

Our results are to some extent inconsistent with those of De Valois and co-workers (14), who concluded that cells are segregated into three groups by response type, with on-responses occurring in the two most dorsal layers (D_1 and D_2 in our terminology), on- and off-responses in the middle two, and off-responses (with inhibition during the stimulus) in the ventral layers. With respect to the ventral layers our findings actually are not in disagreement, since practically all of the cells we have observed were either unresponsive to diffuse light or, in the case of type IV, were inhibited. Nevertheless, type IV cells are, ironically, on-center in type, having a periphery that dominates in diffuse light, and type III contains both on-center and off-center, so that it would be misleading to continue speaking of the ventral layer cells as "off" or "inhibitory."

The middle pair of layers was shown by De Valois *et al.* (14) to contain predominantly opponent-color cells, giving on-responses or off-responses to diffuse light depending on wavelength. Our results confirm this. On the other hand, the dorsal pair of layers was initially described as containing on-cells, which constituted at first "the overwhelming majority" (14) and later 75% (13) of the cells. These cells were originally thought to be narrow band "modulators" of five types, but subsequently, as a result of using chromatic adaptation, they were found to have opponent-color properties (12). Our results show that the majority of dorsal-layer cells are opponent color in type and tend to suggest that there are more on-center cells than off-center in these two layers, though off-center cells are certainly quite common.

Anatomically and physiologically, the significance of the layering of the lateral geniculate body continues to be obscure. Anatomically, one would like to learn more about the afferent supply and the efferent projections of the different layers: whether, for example, ventral-layer and dorsal-layer cells receive projections from separate classes of retinal ganglion cells, and whether the axons of the dorsal layers have cortical terminations different from those of ventral layers. The present physiological study, like that of De Valois and collaborators (13), fails to bear out either the trichromatic theory of Clark (6) or the photopic-scotopic theory of Walls (46). What one can say in summary is that in the dorsal four layers the cells are predominantly of the opponent-color type, at least for the part of the geniculate representing parafoveal parts of the retina, whereas in the ventral two layers the importance of color seems to be reduced.

SIZES OF RECEPTIVE FIELDS. The smallest field centers measured in the present work were of the order of 2 min. of arc, which would correspond to about 10 μ. on the retina. These receptive fields were all type I, suggesting that the center was supplied by one type of cone only. The intercenter distance between cones is 2.0–2.5 μ. in the central part of the human fovea and, to judge from Østerberg's drawings, it is probably several times larger 1° from the center of the fovea (35, 37, 38). The smallest field centers were thus supplied by a few cones at the most, and possibly some were made up of one cone only, though more careful measurements

would be necessary to establish that. No area-threshold measurements were made on these cells so the exact size of field centers and surrounds are not known, but it is clear that the peripheries were orders of magnitude larger than the centers.

FUNCTIONS OF THE LATERAL GENICULATE. It should be emphasized that the present study tells us little about the part the lateral geniculate plays in vision. The electron microscope leaves no doubt that something more than a one-to-one relationship exists between optic fibers and geniculate cells (8), and it would be most interesting to know what physiological interactions these complex connections subserve. We have no reason to think that the classes of cells we have described for the geniculate do not also exist in the optic nerve, since opponent-color responses have been described in the spider monkey optic nerve (24), and several fibers which we recorded from the optic tract in the present work were not obviously different in their properties from geniculate type I cells. It is true that in the spider monkey optic nerve opponent-color cells were not nearly as common as in the rhesus geniculate, but this was probably related to the species difference and to the large area of visual fields explored in the spider monkey rather than to any difference between retina and geniculate. The exact function of the monkey geniculate is probably more subtle. In the cat there are clear differences between responses of geniculate cells and those of retinal ganglion cells, one contribution of the geniculate being a more precise adjustment of the balance between field center and surround, with decreased effectiveness of diffuse light (25). Similar kinds of interactions may well occur in the monkey but, if so, a different type of study will probably be required to reveal them.

There are, finally, some obvious correlations between the responses observed in the geniculate and perceptual phenomena. Given a cell whose receptive field is organized in center-surround fashion, and supposing, for simplicity, that diffuse light is ineffective, illuminating the field center with a white spot of a particular intensity can produce excitation or inhibition depending on whether the surround is simultaneously illuminated with a brighter or dimmer white light. There is a compelling parallel between these responses and one's impression of the spot as "white" or "black," and it is hard to think that the two events are not in some way related. Type I and type III cells are of course equally capable of mediating these black-white sensations. In the case of color there is a similar parallel between the virtual ineffectiveness of diffuse white light in opponent-color cells of type I or II, and the addition of complementary colors to produce the sensation "white." This involves the assumption that a necessary condition for a white sensation is a failure of an opponent-color cell to respond. Here the type II cells would seem to play the more important part, since in these the responses depend predominantly on stimulus wavelength and to a much smaller extent on stimulus geometry.

One is naturally inclined to ask whether a similar parallel can be made between spatial color-induction effects or the spatial-color effects described by Land (29) and the behavior of the type I cell. Surprisingly, it turns out that type I cells are of no direct help. The responses to a centered red spot are not enhanced by simultaneously shining green in the surround, since for type I cell this amounts to the same thing as using diffuse white light. For color contrast in this situation one would seem to require something like a red on-center green on-surround, a field type we have not so far seen. On the other hand, as already indicated, the type I cell is as good a candidate as the type III for the mediation of black-white contrast mechanisms. It may be that color contrast effects are not dealt with at a retinal or geniculate level at all, but only in the cortex. This would be consistent with the finding that Land's effects can occur when the two images are presented binocularly (17), which suggests that the necessary machinery is present in the cortex— though of course it does not rule out its existence at lower levels as well.

SUMMARY

In the visual system of primates, mechanisms exist for the analysis of both spatial and chromatic qualities of a retinal image. The present study was designed to examine these processes at the lateral geniculate level in the rhesus monkey. Extracellular recordings were made from 224 cells while stimulating the retina with spots of light of various sizes and wavelengths, and in various states of light and dark adaptation.

In the four dorsal (small cell) layers three types of cells were distinguished. Type I cells were by far the most common. In the light-adapted state they had concentrically arranged receptive fields which were divided into an excitatory or inhibitory center and an opponent surround, the center and surround having different spectral sensitivities. With diffuse light stimuli they showed opponent-color responses, giving on-responses to one set of wavelengths, off-responses to another set, and no response at some intermediate wavelength—the "neutral point." Chromatic-adaptation studies suggested that the cell had connections with one of the three types of cones in the field center, and another in the surround. Five varieties were seen, in order of frequency: *1)* red on-center, green off-surround; *2)* red off-center, green on-surround; *3)* green on-center, red off-surround; *4)* green off-center, red on-surround; and *5)* blue on-center, green off-surround. All type I cells behaved in the same way to white light, showing the usual center-surround arrangement seen in the retina or geniculate in the cat. On-off responses were rare or absent.

Type II cells made up a small minority of the dorsal-layer cells. They lacked any center-surround receptive-field arrangement, but gave opponent-color responses over all regions of the receptive field and had a 500-mμ. neutral point that was independent of stimulus geometry. These cells behaved as though they received opponent inputs from two sets of cones with identical distributions over the retina. Two types were seen: green-on, blue-off, and green-off, blue-on. A few cells seemed to have opponent connections with green and red cones. Here the two cone types were distributed throughout overlapping regions, but one set of cones seemed to predominate in the field center and the other in the surround.

Type III cells had concentrically arranged on-center or off-center receptive fields, the center and surround having identical spectral sensitivities. A large spot evoked a weaker response than a small one regardless of wavelength. These cells probably received input from cones of several types, the proportions of the three types being the same for the field center as for the surround.

A number of cells with fields outside the fovea were studied also in the dark-adapted state. Some type I cells behaved as though they had no connections with rods, while others showed clear evidence for rod input, giving a 4 log unit increase in sensitivity with a shift in the peak sensitivity to a point near 500–520 mμ. Opponent-color effects were no longer seen, and center-type responses occurred over the entire spectrum except at high stimulus intensities in the red. At threshold levels of intensity these responses were evoked from the field center only, so that whether they receive input from rods in the field periphery is still uncertain. Two type II cells examined in dark adaptation showed no evidence for rod connections. Of four type III cells two lacked a rod input, and the other two had rods feeding in from center and surround, forming opponent systems just as in the light-adapted state; for these cells scotopic thresholds were practically the same for center and surround.

All of the cell types were seen in both pairs of dorsal layers, and there were no differences in distribution of cell types in these four layers except for a suggestion that red on-center cells were more common in the two dorsal layers than in the two middle, and red off-center cells less common. Field-center sizes were generally smaller for type I cells than for type III, and among type I cells on-centers tended to be smaller than off-centers. Field centers were smaller the closer they were to the fovea, the smallest being 2 min. of arc in diameter, for fields 1° or 2° from the fovea; the largest were around 1°. Fields of type II cells ranged in diameter from 1/4° to 1°.

Ventral-layer cells were of two kinds. The first seemed similar to type III as described above. The second, termed type IV, had concentrically arranged on-center fields with a very large off-surround whose spectral sensitivity was displaced to the red with respect to the center. With red light, and generally also with white, the receptive-field periphery prevailed over the center, so that diffuse light produced a well-maintained suppression of the background firing.

In summary, a wide variety of cell types are present in the monkey geniculate. Some are concerned mainly with spatial variables, others with color, but most are able to handle both variables. Some have connections both with rods and cones and others with cones only.

ACKNOWLEDGMENTS

We express our thanks to Jane Chen, for histological work, and to Janet Tobie Wiitanen and John Tuckerman for their technical assistance.

References

1. Barlow, H. B. Summation and inhibition in the frog's retina. *J. Physiol.,* 1953, *119:* 69–88.
2. Barlow, H. B., FitzHugh, R, and Kuffler, S. W. Change of organization in the receptive fields of the cat's retina during dark adaptation. *J. Physiol.,* 1957, *137:* 338–354.
3. Barlow, H. B., Hill, R. M., and Levick, W. R. Retinal ganglion cells responding selectively to direction and speed of image motion in the rabbit. *J. Physiol.,* 1964, *173:* 377–407.
4. Brown, J. E. and Rojas, A. J. Rat retinal ganglion cells: receptive field organization and maintained activity. *J. Neurophysiol.,* 1965, *28:* 1073–1090.
5. Brown, P. K. and Wald, G. Visual pigments in single rods and cones of human retina. *Science,* 1964, *144:* 45–52.
6. Clark, W. E. L. Anatomaicl basis of colour vision. *Nature, Lond.,* 1940, *146:* 558–559.
7. Clark, W. E. L. and Penman, G. G. The projection of the retina in the lateral geniculate body. *Proc. roy. Soc., Ser. B.* 1934, *114:* 291–313.
8. Colonnier, M. and Guillery, R. W. Synaptic organization in the lateral geniculate nucleus of the monkey. *Z. Zellforsch.,* 1964, *62:* 333–355.
9. DeJours, S. F. *Receptive Fields of Optic Tract Fibers in Lizards (Sceloporus SPP)* (Doctoral dissertation). Cambridge, Mass., Harvard Univ., 1965.
10. De Valois, R. L. Color vision mechanisms in the monkey. *J. gen. Physiol.,* 1960, *43*(6), Part II: 115–128.
11. De Valois, R. L. Behavioral and electrophysiological studies of primate vision. In: *Contributions to Sensory Physiology,* edited by W. D. Neff. New York, Academic, 1965, vol. I, pp. 137–178.
12. De Valois, R. L., Jacobs, G. H., and Jones, A. E. Responses of signle cells in primate red-green color vision system. *Optik,* 1963 *20:* 87–98.
13. De Valois, R. L. and Jones, A. E. Single-cell analysis of the organization of the primate color-vision system. In: *The Visual System: Neurophysiology and Psychophysics,* edited by R. Jung and H. Kornhuber. Springer, Berlin, 1961, 178–191.
14. De Valois, R. L., Smith, C. J., Karoly, A. J., and Kitai, S. T. Electrical responses of primate visual system: I. Different layers of macaque lateral geniculate nucleus. *J. comp. Physiol. Psychol.,* 1958, *51:* 662–668.
15. De Valois, R. L., Smith, C. J., Kitai, S. T., and Karoly, A. J. Response of single cells in monkey lateral geniculate nucleus to monochromatic light. *Science,* 1958, *127:* 238–239.
16. Dowling, J. E. Neural and photochemical mechanisms of visual adaptation in the rat. *J. gen. Physiol.,* 1963, *46:* 1287–1301.
17. Geschwind, N. and Segal, J. R. Colors of all hues from binocular mixing of two colors. *Science,* 1960, *131:* 608.
18. Gouras, P. Primate retina: duplex function of dark-adapted ganglion cells. *Science,* 1965, *147:* 1593–1594.
19. Granit, R. *Sensory Mechanisms of the Retina.* London, Oxford Univ. Press, 1947.
20. Hartline, H. K. Inhibition of activity of visual receptors by illuminating nearby retinal areas in the *Limulus* eye. *Fed. Proc.* 1949, *8:* 69.
21. Hubel, D. H. Single unit activity in striate cortex of unrestrained cats. *J. Physiol.,* 1959, *147:* 226–238.
22. Hubel, D. H. Single unit activity in lateral geniculate body and optic tract of unrestrained cats. *J. Physiol.,* 1960, *150:* 91–104.
23. Hubel, D. H. and Wiesel, T. N. Receptive fields of single neurones in the cat's striate cortex. *J. Physiol.,* 1959, *148:* 574–591.
24. Hubel, D. H. and Wiesel, T. N. Receptive fields of optic nerve fibers in the spider monkey. *J. Physiol.,* 1960, *154:* 572–580.

25. Hubel, D. H. and Wiesel, T. N. Integrative action in the cat's lateral geniculate body. *J. Physiol.,* 1961, *155:* 385–398.

26. Hubel, D. H. and Wiesel, T. N. Receptive fields, binocular interaction and functional architecture in the cat's visual cortex. *J. Physiol.,* 1962, *160:* 106–154.

27. Hubel, D. H. and Wiesel, T. N. Responses of monkey geniculate cells to monochromatic and white spots of light. *Physiologist,* 1964, *7:* 162.

28. Kuffler, S. W. Discharge patterns and functional organization of mammalian retina. *J. Neurophysiol.,* 1953, *16:* 37–68.

29. Land, E. H. Color vision and the natural image. Parts I and II. *Proc. nat. Acad. Sci., Wash.,* 1959, *45:* 115–129, 636–644.

30. Marks, W. B., Dobelle, W. H., and MacNichol, E. F. Jr., Visual pigments of single primate cones. *Science,* 1964, *143:* 1181–1182.

31. Mello, N. K. and Peterson, N. J. Behavioral evidence for color discrimination in cat. *J. Neurophysiol.,* 1964, *27:* 323–333.

32. Meyer, D. R. and Anderson, R. A. Color discrimination in cats. In: *Color Vision* (Ciba Foundation Symposium). Boston, Little, Brown, 1965, pp. 325–339.

33. Michael, C. R. *Receptive Fields of Simple Optic Nerve Fibers in the Ground Squirrel* (Doctoral dissertation). Cambridge, Mass., Harvard Univ., 1965.

34. Motokawa, K., Taira, N., and Okuda, J. Spectral responses of single units in the primate visual cortex. *Tohoku J. exp. Med.,* 1962, *78:* 320–337.

35. O'Brien, B. Vision and resolution in the central retina. *J. opt. Soc. Amer.,* 1951, *41:* 882–894.

36. Okuda, J., Taira, N., and Motokawa, K. Spectral response curves of postgeniculate neurons in the cat. *Tohoku J. exp. Med.,* 1962, *78:* 147–157.

37. Österberg, G. Topography of the layer of rods and cones in the human retina. *Acta ophthal., Kbh.,* 1935, Suppl. 6.

38. Polyak, S. *The Vertebrate Visual System.* Chicago, Univ. Chicago Press, 1957.

39. Rushton, W. A. H. Increment threshold and dark adaptation. *J. opt. Soc. Amer.,* 1963, *53:* 104–109.

40. Sechser, J. A. and Brown, J. L. Color discrimmination in the cat. *Science,* 1964, *144:* 427–429.

41. Svaetichin, G. II. Spectral response curves from single cones. *Acta physiol. scand.,* 1956, *39,* Suppl. 134: 19–46.

42. Talbot, S. A. and Marshall, W. H. Physiological studies on neural mechanisms of visual localization and discrimination. *Amer. J. Ophtal.,* 1941, *24:* 1255–1263.

43. Wagner, H. G., MacNichol, E. F., Jr., and Wolbarsht, M. L. Opponent color responses in retinal ganglion cells. *Science,* 1960, *131:* 1314.

44. Wagner, H. G., MacNichol, E. F., Jr., and Wolbarsht, M. L. The response properties of single ganglion cells in the gold fish retina. *J. gen. Physiol.,* 1960, *43,* Part II: 45–62.

45. Wagner, H. G., MacNichol, E. F., Jr., and Wolbarsht, M. L. Functional basis for "on"-center and "off"-center receptive fields in the retina. *J. opt. Soc. Amer.,* 1963, *53:* 66–70.

46. Walls, G. L. The lateral geniculate nucleus and visual histophysiology. *Univ. Calif. Publ. Physiol.,* 1953, *9:* 1–100.

47. Wiesel, T. N. and Hubel, D. H. Receptive fields of monkey geniculate cells in the dark adapted state, *Physiologist,* 1964, *7:* 287.

48. Wolbarsht, M. L., Wagner, H. G., and MacNichol, E. F., Jr. The origin of "on" and "off" responses of retinal ganglion cells. In: *The Visual System: Neurophysiology and Psychophysics,* edited by R. Jung and H. Kornhuber. Springer, Berlin, 1961, pp. 163–170.

49. Wolbarsht, M. L., Wagner, H. G., and MacNichol, E. F., Jr. Receptive fields of retinal ganglion cells: extent and spectral sensitivity. In: *The Visual System: Neurophysiology and Psychophysics,* edited by R. Jung and H. Kornhuber. Springer, Berlin, 1961, pp. 170–175.

AFTERWORD

In tackling the monkey lateral geniculate, we got into color studies whether we wanted to or not. Little did we know what kind of hornet's nest we were invading. Scientists who study color do not comprise a pure culture of contentious or surly people, but the atmosphere in the field is hardly what one would call calm. When provoked, some of our best and warmest color-vision friends can rise up in intense wrath at public meetings, as William Rushton once did at a seminar at Harvard conducted by George Wald. I forget exactly what provoked William, but the audience, largely of undergraduate students, must have been perplexed at the heat generated in these two titanic figures in science by such a seemingly pacific topic. As we left the auditorium and proceeded to the elevators, William said to me, "David, I feel terrible. I do not know what can possibly have come over me to make such an outburst". An early reaction to this monkey-color paper came when William visited us shortly after its publication. As he walked into our tearoom, he launched forth with a heated denouncement of our failure to attribute the early determinations of the three cone spectral sensitivities to him, rather than to the quintet of Wald, Brown, Dobelle, MacNichol, and Marks. We had admired those people because they were the first to make such measurements in single receptors, but Rushton was certainly right. His work not only had the priority, but was celebrated for its ingenuity and elegance. We felt terrible and heartily apologized. He accepted our apologies and at once became his usual friendly self—and the matter was never again mentioned. But our omission was inexcusable and we still feel guilty.

A few years later I visited a group of visual scientists at Tallahassee, Florida, where William Rushton was doing a sabbatical. He greeted me warmly, saying, "David, I know neither of us wants to sit here talking about dry science. Let's go outside to the swimming pool, where there are far more interesting things to look at than slides and posters". William died in 1980. He was brilliant, warm, with a wonderful sense of humor, and we miss him sorely.

In the mid-1960s our methods were far cruder and less flexible than those available today. We had no computers, and because of the bizarre action spectra of video-monitor phosphors no one had thought of using color-TV techniques to generate stimuli. Reverse correlation methods for mapping receptive fields were far in the future, as were cone-isolation techniques. We mapped our receptive fields by generating white or monochromatic stimuli with an optic bench whose main components were a slide projector, a shutter, and a set of interference filters. To evaluate responses the ideal method would have been to measure light intensities required to evoke responses of criterion magnitudes for different wavelengths. We would have plotted responses against stimulus intensities and extrapolated back to zero response, but we lacked the equipment and the electronics engineer to build it. So we decided to use thresholds as our "criterion response magnitudes", and to do that by ear. Anyone who tries that soon learns that it is not easy. That is the reason for the alpine profiles of many of our threshold-versus-wavelength curves.

It almost immediately became apparent that the dorsal four geniculate layers contain a mixture of cells, which we designated types 1, 2, and 3. We began by calling them A, B, and C, but changed over to 1, 2, and 3 when Richard Jung objected that A–C would make for confusion with his labels for cat cortical cells. Ironically, it turned out that his types B, C, D, and E were, after all, almost certainly geniculate axons.

Type 1 cells (opponent-color center-surround) are still the subject of some disagreements. The field centers are clearly supplied by a single cone type. The main question concerns the makeup of the receptive-field surrounds—whether these are supplied by a single cone type, as we had thought (or two, in the case of blue center yellow (red & green) surround cells) or all three, and therefore "broadband". The argument goes back and forth, with participants ranging from retinal anatomists, predominantly Peter Sterling, our erstwhile postdoc—and physiologists. We still find our main evidence, comparing responses to small and large spots at short and long wavelengths, simple and compelling. Present-day techniques (cone isolation, reverse correlation) should help settle the question.

As we point out in the paper, it may well be that the centers and surrounds of type 1 cells interpenetrate, so that one might, if one had mathematical leanings, describe the fields as "difference-of-Gaussians". For the goldfish cells of Wolbarsht et al. this was easy to establish, because in goldfish the time courses of the on and off systems are not perfectly complimentary, and stimulating both together produces on-off responses. That makes it relatively easy to map separately the two opponent systems, using "on" responses to assess excitation and "off" responses to assess inhibition. In macaques the time courses of the two opponent systems are apparently well enough matched so that their effects cancel, and instead of on-off responses one sees little or no response. Mapping the separate overlapping components then becomes difficult. Still, there seems little doubt that the two opposing systems overlap. The question seems somewhat academic given the tiny size of the field centers. We are, perhaps pedantically, unhappy with the term "difference-of-Gaussians", which we suspect represents wishful or wistful thinking by mathematically oriented biologists. To call any bell curve "Gaussian" seems to us like the solecism of using the word "ellipse" to refer to any oval.

We found broadband cells (**type 3**) fairly common in the dorsal four laminae. Peter Schiller once flatly declared to me that all dorsal-layer cells are type 1, and Margaret Livingstone has tended to agree with him, in thinking that all parvocellular cells are color-coded. Modern methods, again, should easily resolve this.

We had, looking back, amazingly few examples of **type 2** cells. More examples are sadly needed. These were cells in which the two opponent systems (red vs. green, or yellow vs. blue) overlapped extensively or completely. We now think that they—at least the yellow-blue ones—are confined mainly to the narrow interlaminar leaflets, the thin and thinly populated layers between the principal six geniculate layers. That would help explain the relative rarity of type 2 cells in our penetrations. For the yellow-blue cells (called "blue vs. green" in the paper), the almost perfect superimposition of the area-threshold curves obtained with short and middle wavelengths (shown in Fig. 9) convinced us of the complete overlap of the two opponent systems. For our red-green type 2 cells, the overlap of the two systems was usually incomplete, one of the two components exceeding the other in diameter. Nevertheless, these cells seemed quite unlike type 1 cells, whose centers were far smaller, and whose surrounds were larger. The dimensions of the type 2 receptive-field regions seemed to fit better with our acuity for color than was true for the type 1 cells. Our present guess is that these are the cells that feed into the double-opponent cells of cortical V-1.

Type 4 cells, the commonest in the magnocellular layers, are in some ways the most interesting and puzzling of all the geniculate cells. Outside of our paper, one has to search the literature for any inkling of the special peculiarities of these cells: the clear color opponency present in the receptive-field surrounds; the extremely sustained quality of the surround responses; the very transient quality of the responses from the broadband field centers; the dominance, in the case of the sustained response components, of the surround over the center when longwave light is used. From one magnocellular cell to the next these cells show a stereotyped behavior. When an electrode enters the ventral layers, the effect of bathing the projection screen with red light is to produce utter and sustained silence from all the cells within recording range, whereas with diffuse white light the suppressive effect is much weaker, or entirely lacking. We found this to be the easiest way of knowing that an electrode has passed from the parvocellular layers to the magnocellular. Adding short or middle wavelength light to the red in the surround immediately brings back the activity, demonstrating vividly the color opponency in the surround. Nevertheless, magnocellular geniculate cells are still widely regarded as not color coded, and as giving transient responses.

Strangely, we have seen no reflection of any of this type 4 behavior in cells in layer 4C alpha of cortical V-1, even though that layer receives its geniculate input exclusively from magnocellular cells.

We wonder what function these prominent and bizarre cells serve. Why the importance of red? Why the very sustained quality of the surround responses, compared to the brief responses to centre stimuli? Above all, why has their strange behavior largely been ignored? Perhaps part of the reason for the neglect is the extensive and exclusive use, in many of the studies that followed ours, of sinewave grating stimuli, which seems far from ideal if one wants to study receptive field centers and surrounds separately. Given the concentric organization of the centers and surrounds of geniculate fields, to use gratings in working out the cells' properties seems to us a mistake; one might even say, perverse.

To return to **type 1** cells, we ask what part they can be playing in primate color vision. That they are color coded in any ordinary sense is undeniable. The opposite-type responses ("on" vs. "off") to diffuse light at different ends of the spectrum and their failure to respond to diffuse white light is prima facie evidence for color coding. Yet there are reasons to be sceptical about their role in color vision. First, as already mentioned, the small size of their field centers seems to match our acuity for luminance, but to be a poor match for our relatively coarser acuity for color, to which the larger size of type 2 fields seems a better fit. Second, to explain color contrast or color constancy would seem to require receptive fields with a center fed by one cone type and a surround fed by a different one, but both should be excitatory, or both inhibitory, surely not one of each. A cell with a red-on center and green-off surround is the very thing one does *not* want for red-green color contrast: rather, one expects a red-on center and green-*on* surround. The closest thing to this is found in the blobs of monkey V-1 cortex, in the double-opponent cells. Thus the candidate for red-green contrast would be a cell with red-on green-off center and red-off green-on surround. Such cells were originally described in the goldfish retina by Nigel Daw (*J Physiol* 1968, 197:567–592), by us in our 1968 monkey cortex paper, by Charles Michael in squirrel geniculate (*J Neurophysiol* 1973, 36:536–550) and monkey striate cortex (*J Neurophysiol* 1978, 41:572–588), by Margaret Livingstone and Hubel in cortical blobs (*J Neurosci* 1984, 4:309–356) and by Bevil Conway in striate cortex (*Journal of Neuroscience,* 2001, 21(8): 2768–2783). How double-opponent cells are built up from simpler antecedents is still not known. It would seem easiest to imagine that they are derived from type 2 cells, rather than from type 1, in which the field centers seem too small and the surround suppression is of the wrong sign.

Another reason to doubt that type 1 parvocellular cells play an important part in color vision comes from studying cells in the upper layers of striate cortex (V-1). The massively preponderant inputs to these cortical cells, the parvocellular geniculate cells, are type 1. We might therefore have expected upper-layer cortical cells to be overwhelmingly color coded, but we quickly found that they are not. We wondered if combining the effects of the various subtypes of type 1 cells might have led to the loss, through pooling, of the color information. To test whether a cell is totally color-blind, one can stimulate with a slit of one color moving against a background of another, and vary the relative intensities of the two. If a cell is totally color blind, at some pair of relative intensities the cell should fail to respond. Work by Gouras and Kruger (*J Neurophysiol* 1979, 42:850–860) and confirmed by Hubel and Margaret Livingstone (*J Neurosci* 1990, 10(7), 223–2237) showed that about half of the cortical cells responded to slits of one color against a background of another, at all relative intensities. Hence for these cells the color information is not lost, even though they show no overt opponency. For example, they respond well to white light, whereas opponent-color cells do not. Such cells could be useful in defeating camouflage, but it seems unlikely that they play a major part in color recognition.

Though we delight in our color vision and sympathize with those that lack it, clearly our vision depends mainly for its success on luminance differences. That is something the upper-layer cortical cells handle very well, doubtless because geniculate parvocellular cells when studied with white light likewise do very well. For the fovea the case is clear: there, a cell whose field center is fed by a single cone has to be fed by some kind of cone, and we see black-white well enough with our foveas.

Given that most of the receptors in our retinas are rods, it seemed important to ask whether the geniculate cells we studied received any rod input. For a time we avoided the question because it is tiresome to work in the dark—one has to grope, and we tended to fall asleep. Moreover we had thought that to test each of our cells for rod inputs we would have to turn out the lights and wait for at least a half hour. We used ourselves to assess whether at any given moment we and the monkey were dark-adapted or not: we turned down the background light, made a green stimulus spot progressively fainter, and waited until it disappeared when we looked right at it, and reappeared and became grey when we looked away. To our surprise that usually happened after five to 10 minutes, provided the room was not dazzlingly bright to begin with. So we found we could test every cell for rod inputs fairly quickly, without waiting for complete dark adaptation.

Our first effort to study dark adaptation was exciting and a cause of some hilarity (at least on our part). To avoid the scattering of light from our powerful tripod-supported Leitz slide projector, we had draped a large black cloth over the entire rig. On that occasion Dr. Otto Krayer, our chairman, paid us a rare visit—we don't remember his reason. Just as he entered the room the entire cloth burst into flames. Dr. Krayer must have wondered what kinds of postdocs Steve had imported to his department. He was, as usual, kind, but obviously did not think the whole thing was very funny.

In our small sample of dark-adapted cells we showed that both magnocellular and parvocellular cells can receive rod inputs, though not all do. All the cells we recorded received cone inputs. For cells that do receive rod inputs, it was always the case that if the centre was "on" in photopic conditions, it was also "on" in dark adaptation, and the same for off-center cells. Contrary to the impression given by Barlow, Fitzhugh, and Kuffler in their study of dark adaptation in cats in 1957 (*J Physiol* 137:327–337), we found that all the type 1 cells that we examined in scotopic conditions showed clear rod input to the surrounds. We saw no obvious change in field center size when the eye was dark-adapted. Our overall impression, from measurements of thresholds of dark-adapted cells, was that a cell either received abundant rod input (i.e., had a very low threshold, matching our own behavioral thresholds) in dim light, or it failed to show any rod input. If center sizes are the same in scotopic and photopic conditions, how can one account for our lowered acuity in dim light? We suspect that outside the fovea it is the cells with smaller field centers that receive no rod input. One obviously needs a survey of different parts of the lateral geniculate to correlate receptive field size with distance from the fovea (eccentricity).

One lesson from this paper seems to be that if we had wished to make a lasting impact on a field, we should have extended the work, pushing it further, using newer and more powerful methods to build on what we had already done, and correcting any errors along the way. As usual in research, one has to make choices. I doubt if today we would trade our work on visual deprivation and columnar organization for a more thorough account of geniculate cells. And perhaps we chose wisely after all, given the primitive nature of the equipment available to us in the mid-1960s.

Chapter 13 • Recording Fibers in the Cat Corpus Callosum •

FOREWORD

This paper represents a slight deviation from our receptive-field research in normal animals. We had found it hard to imagine what part the corpus callosum might play in vision. It had long been thought to link homologous parts of the two hemispheres, with little idea of how, exactly, that might be useful. For the prefrontal areas, about which so little was known in terms of function, it was impossible to think about the problem at all. For the somatosensory cortex or the visual cortex one could ask some more clearly defined questions. It would make no sense, it seemed to us, to link regions of cortex subserving the two thumbs or the two feet, or two mirror-symmetric regions of the peripheral left and right visual fields. It was not until we learned that callosal connections in the visual system linked cortical regions subserving the midline that the structure began to make any sense.

Rarely, humans are born without a corpus callosum. Occasionally it is necessary to sever the corpus callosum surgically, either to prevent the spread of epileptic seizures from one hemisphere to the other, or to allow the surgeon to reach deeply buried brain or pituitary tumors. In such cases little or nothing had been found in the way of neurological deficits. The first experimental demonstration of major deficits from callosal sectioning came from the work in cats by Ronald Myers, in Roger Sperry's laboratory (*J Comp Physiol Psychol* 1955, 48:470–473). Ronald showed that a task learned by one hemisphere failed to transfer to the other side. The findings were striking, and provided vivid examples of the necessity, in brain research, of designing ingenious behavioral tests, rather than simply noting the absence of obvious defects. Roger Sperry, J. Bogen, and M. S. Gazzaniga extended Myers' work to humans (Gazzaniga et al., *Brain* 1965, 88:221–236; Gazzaniga and Sperry *Brain* 1967, 90:131–148), taking advantage of the relative ease of doing behavioral work in humans, and making use of human attributes such as speech, whose function is largely lodged in the left hemisphere. As an example of such tests, one could show an object to a person's (or animal's) left visual field, and consequently the right visual cortex, and ask the subject to grasp it with the right hand, which would require the information to get over to the left motor cortex. Such a problem proved easy for a normal person or animal, but impossible after the corpus callosum had been cut.

In the case of vision it was not hard to think of reasons for linking the two hemispheres. Our schemes for the elaboration of simple and complex cells in striate cortex pointed to abundant, very local, short, lateral connections, linking neighboring cells whose receptive fields were overlapping or adjacent. So it was natural to think that cells whose receptive fields came close to the midline of the visual fields or straddled them should be similarly interconnected. Some such cells would be in one hemisphere of the brain and some in the opposite hemisphere; and many connections would therefore have to cross from one hemisphere to the other. (Presumably delays, caused by the distance to be traversed, could be made up for simply by adding myelin to the axons.) Work by Choudhury, Whitteridge, and Wilson in cats also pointed strongly to this idea (*Quarterly J Exp Physiol* 1965, 50:214–219). Having cut the optic chiasm in the midsagittal plane, so that the left eye was connected to the left hemisphere and the right eye to the right hemisphere, they stimulated the left eye, and observed responses from *both* cortical hemispheres. The only way to get from the left eye to the right hemisphere then had to be via the corpus callosum. We decided to test these ideas directly by looking for receptive-field overlap of cells near the 17-18 border, and by recording directly from the corpus callosum.

Cortical and Callosal Connections Concerned with the Vertical Meridian of Visual Fields in the Cat[1]

DAVID H. HUBEL AND TORSTEN N. WIESEL • *Department of Physiology, Harvard Medical School, Boston,*
Massachusetts

In higher mammals the left half of the visual field is represented in the right visual cortex, and the right half in the left cortex. The fact that our visual fields appear uniform, with no obvious interruption along the vertical midline, would seem to call for connections linking the two hemispheres. The present paper deals with the physiological properties of some of these connections.

In the cat the vertical midline of the visual field has its primary representation in and close to the poorly defined boundary between areas 17 and 18 (7, 10). Each half-visual field is represented in

From *J. Neurophysiol. (1967), 30*, 1561–1573

Received for publication March 20, 1967.

[1]This work was supported by Research Grants NM-02260-08 and NB-05554-03 from the National Institutes of Health.

both 17 and 18 in mirror fashion, so that as one proceeds away from the 17-18 boundary in either direction, medially along 17 or laterally along 18, the corresponding region of visual fields moves outward from the vertical meridian into the contralateral visual field. Recent anatomical evidence indicates that the part of area 17 adjacent to the 17-18 boundary sends callosal projections to the other hemisphere, ending in 18 near the 17-18 boundary (2, 7, 8) and possibly also in the adjacent part of 17 (8). Thus the parts of 17 and 18 having to do with the vertical midline of the visual fields are apparently connected on the two sides by the corpus callosum. In contrast, the more medial parts of 17, representing the peripheral parts of the visual fields, seem not to be reciprocally interconnected, and indeed one would hardly expect that cells concerned with a particular part of the left visual field should be connected specifically to cells concerned with the corresponding region in the right field.

These anatomical findings have lately been confirmed in the elegant physiological experiments of Choudhury, Whitteridge, and Wilson (1). They showed that with one optic tract cut, responses to light could be evoked in the ipsilateral hemisphere only near the 17-18 border, and only when the stimulus was applied near the vertical meridian. The responses were abolished either by cooling the corresponding region in the contralateral hemisphere or by cooling or cutting the posterior corpus callosum.

Several lines of evidence thus indicate that fibers in the corpus callosum originating in the most lateral part of 17 and projecting to 18 on the other side have special functions involving the vertical midline of the visual field. If this is so, then some cells in 18 near the 17-18 boundary ought to have receptive fields that straddle the vertical midline. Experimentally this is difficult to verify directly, since in the cat the exact position of the vertical midline is not easy to establish. Our first objective was to circumvent the difficulty by making simultaneous recordings from visual areas in the two hemispheres, looking for possible overlap between receptive fields of cells on the two sides. Any overlap would of course mean that at least one of the two receptive fields extended across the vertical meridian. A second objective was to record fibers directly from the corpus callosum, examine their responses to visual stimulation, and see to

what extent they are preoccupied with the vertical midline.

METHODS

The experimental preparation was similar to that used in our previous work (4–6). The cat was anesthetized with intraperitoneal thiopental, the head held in a Horsley-Clarke stereotaxic apparatus, the eyes paralyzed with intravenous succinylcholine and held open facing a white tangent screen at a distance of 1.5 m. Pupils were dilated with homatropine, and the corneas protected with contact lenses. The focus of images on the screen was determined with a slit retinoscope, and if necessary adjusted by interposing spherical lenses. Positions on the screen corresponding to the area centralis and optic disc of each eye were determined by using an ophthalmoscope (4), and the points were remeasured every hour or so, or whenever there was suspicion that the eyes had moved. Stimuli consisted of black or white lines or edges projected against a diffuse white background (6).

Cortical recordings were made with two independently positioned tungsten electrodes connected to separate recording channels. The electrodes were introduced through small holes in the skull and dura 1–2 mm to either side of the midline at the same Horsley-Clarke level. The corpus callosum was explored between planes A2 and A6 with a single electrode inserted stereotaxically 1–2 mm to the left or right of the midline. In all penetrations electrolytic lesions were made to identify the electrode tracks by passing 1–5 μa for 5–10 sec (4).

RESULTS

Simultaneous Recordings from the Two Hemispheres

An exploration was first made of the cortical representation of the vertical midline of the visual field, looking especially in 17 and 18 for any possible overlap between the two half fields across the midline. Five such experiments were done. In each of these, two electrodes were placed initially in roughly corresponding parts of the postlateral gyrus, close to the region representing the area centralis (Horsley-Clarke frontal plane −2 to +1). Receptive-field positions were mapped for several cells in each hemisphere, and if necessary one electrode was moved forward or back until the fields were at about the same horizontal level.

In the experiment of Fig. 1*A* one penetration was made on the left side and three on the right.

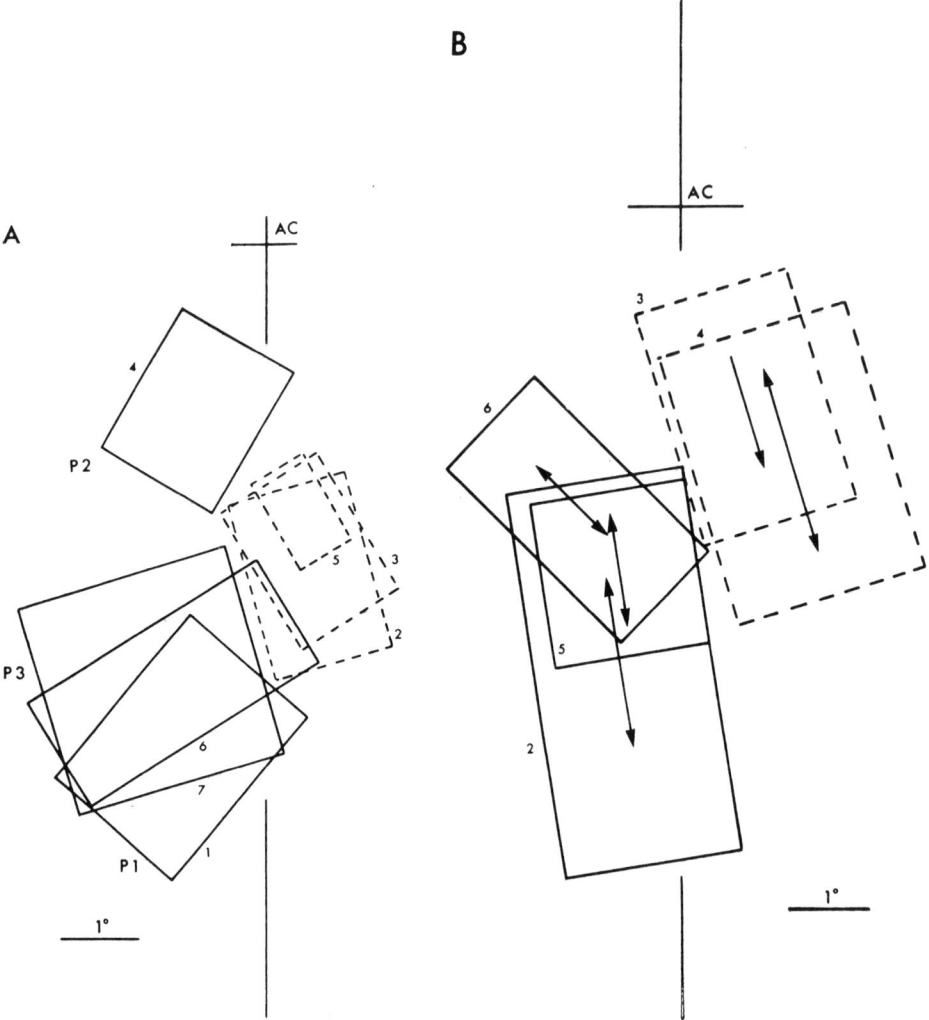

Fig. 1. Receptive fields of cells plotted in simultaneous recordings from the two hemispheres. Fields outlined by interrupted lines correspond to cells in the left hemisphere; continuous lines, right hemisphere. AC = area centralis. A: one penetration was made in the left hemisphere (L) and three (P1–P3) in the right (R), at different anteroposterior levels. All penetrations were in 17, close to the 17-18 border. Simultaneous recordings were made of units 1 (R) and 2 (L); then 4 (R) and 2 (L); then 4 (R) and 5 (L); and finally 6 and 7 (R) together with 5 (L). In none of these simultaneous recordings was there any trace of overlap. B: a similar experiment in which the left electrode was in 17 and the right in the transition zone between 17 and 18. Unit 2 recorded simultaneously with 3 and then with 4; unit 4 recorded simultaneously with 5 and then 6.

Both electrodes were in area 17, close to the 17-18 border. Some fields of simultaneously recorded cells touched, but in no case was there a common region of visual field within which a stimulus excited cells in both hemispheres simultaneously. Cells 2 and 6, whose fields might seem to overlap, were studied some time apart, and it is possible that small eye movements may have occurred in the interval. Because of the imprecision in estimating the exact center of gaze, the vertical meridian in all these figures is only a rough estimate, to the nearest degree or so.

Two other experiments also failed to show a convincing overlap across the midline. In one of these, both electrodes again were in 17; in the other (Fig. 1*B*), one electrode was in 17 and one in the transitional region between 17 and 18.

In two of the five experiments there was clear overlap between fields of cells on the two sides. In the first animal one electrode was in 17 and the other in 18. In the second experiment, illustrated in Fig. 2, both electrodes were in the 17-18 transitional zone. The field maps of Fig. 2 were obtained by first advancing one electrode and then the other, making a number of simultaneous recordings. In Fig. 2*A* the two maps correspond to two sets of simultaneously recorded cells. In the upper set cells 1 and 2 were studied together, then 3 and 2, and then 3 and 4, one electrode always being kept in place while the other was advanced, to be sure that the eyes had not moved in the meanwhile. Similarly for the lower set, cell 9 was recorded from the left hemisphere together with units 10 and 11 on the right; then the left electrode was advanced and cell 12 was observed together with 10 and 11. In both these sets the stimulus could be moved strictly within the region of overlap while the responses of the two cells were observed.

The fields of all 22 cells recorded in this experiment are shown superimposed in Fig. 2*B*. Eleven cells were recorded from the right hemisphere (continuous lines) and 11 from the left (interrupted lines). By always having a cell under observation in one hemisphere or the other we could be certain that there were no eye movements of more than about 1/4°. As usual in studies of visual cortex, the total visual-field area occupied by the overlapping receptive fields of a group of cells in a small region of cortex was two to four times that of an average receptive field in the group. The two groups of receptive fields from the two hemispheres themselves overlapped over about 1/3 of their total area.

CORRESPONDENCE OF RECEPTIVE-FIELD POSITION IN BINOCULARLY DRIVEN CELLS. The following observations have little direct bearing upon the problem of midline overlap of receptive fields, but were made incidentally while recording from pairs of cells simultaneously with two electrodes. The two receptive fields of a binocularly driven cell are known to occupy corresponding positions in the two retinas, at least to within a degree or so (6). Obviously, any slight departures from correspon-

dence from one cell to the next would be of great interest, especially if one found a variation in the horizontal direction and not in the vertical, for this would suggest that some cells were specialized to respond to images of objects in front of or behind some surface of reference determined by the degree of convergence of the two eyes. Whether a cell's two receptive fields always correspond precisely in position has been hard to judge, because the position of the area centralis cannot be accurately determined by ophthalmic inspection. Moreover, the relative positions of the receptive fields in the two eyes as one proceeds from cell to cell often seem to vary slightly, but it is difficult to evaluate this apparent variation because of occasional small eye movements. The problem of eye movements can be overcome in double recordings by keeping one binocularly driven cell under observation at all times and noting any change of position of either of the projected receptive fields.

In the experiment of Fig. 3, recordings were made from area 17 on the two sides. Here the receptive fields are shown just as they were mapped on the projection screen. With the eyes paralyzed the two visual axes were crossed, and the fields in the right eye were to the left of those in the left eye. For each pair of cells one then asked whether the relative positions of the receptive fields in the two eyes were the same. In all of the eight simultaneous recordings the positions matched to within about 1/2°. Moreover, the directions of the deviations were more or less random, with no particular tendency for horizontal variation.

It is hard to say whether or not these variations represent departures from true correspondence, given the difficulties in comparing the two receptive-field positions precisely. For example, if one eye is strongly dominant the field in the weaker eye generally appears smaller than its counterpart in the dominant eye, since the more peripheral parts of a field often exert progressively weaker effects on the cell. Thus the possible error in determining the positions of such large fields could be of the order of 1/2°. Judging from human experience, a horizontal variation in receptive-field correspondence of up to about 1-2° would be required if such a mechanism were to be linked to binocular depth perception, but in this and other experiments one can be reasonably sure that there were no variations this great, and certainly no pref-

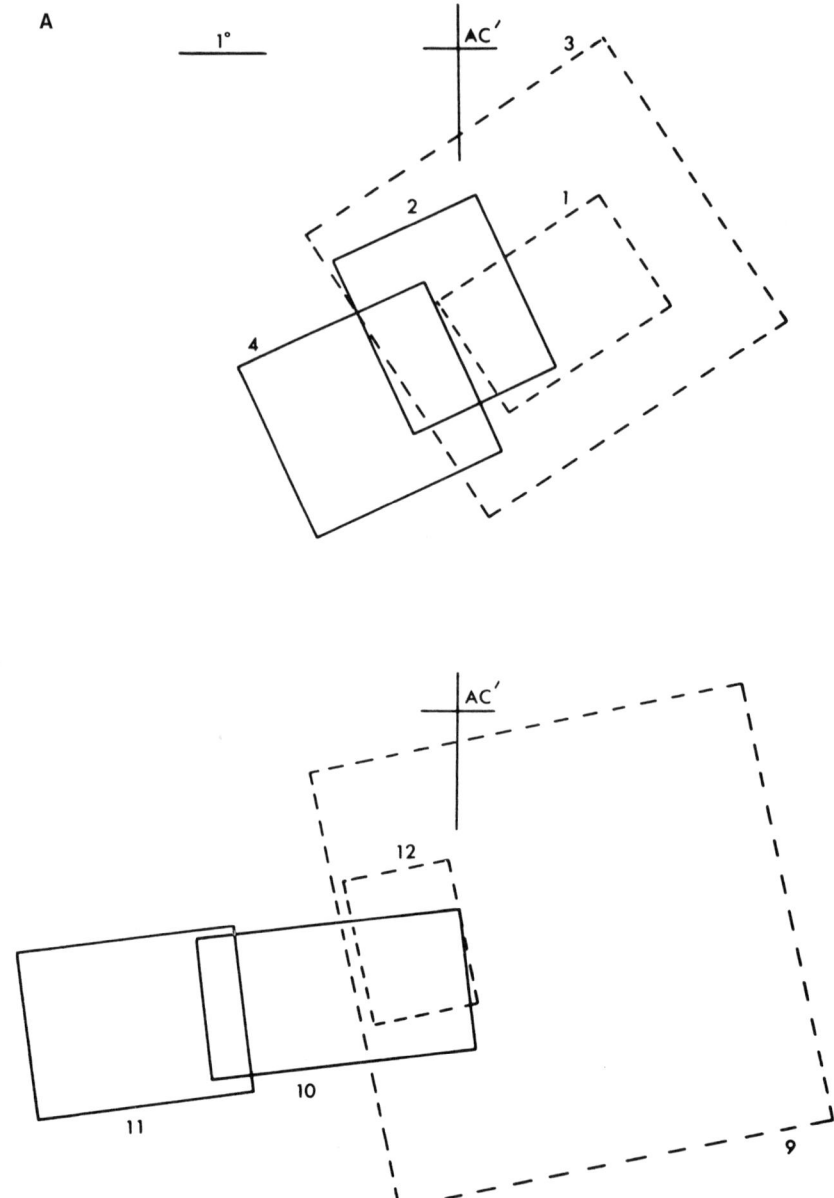

Fig. 2. A: fields of cells recorded with two electrodes in the 17-18 transition zone on the two sides, showing over-lap across the midline. Upper sequence: simultaneous recordings made of cells 1 and 2, 2 and 3, 3 and 4. Lower sequence: 9, 10, and 11 recorded simultaneously; then 10, 11 and 12. B (opposite page): same experiment, all fields from the two penetrations shown superimposed. Fields of cells from the right hemisphere are outlined by continuous lines; from left hemisphere, by interrupted lines.

(continued)

erential horizontal variations. The possibility remains that there are regional specializations within 17 or 18, with variation in relative field positions in some areas and not in others. This might partly explain the apparent discrepancy between our results and those of Bishop and Pettigrew, and of Pettigrew and Barlow; in a more extensive study of binocular correspondence of cortical cells in the

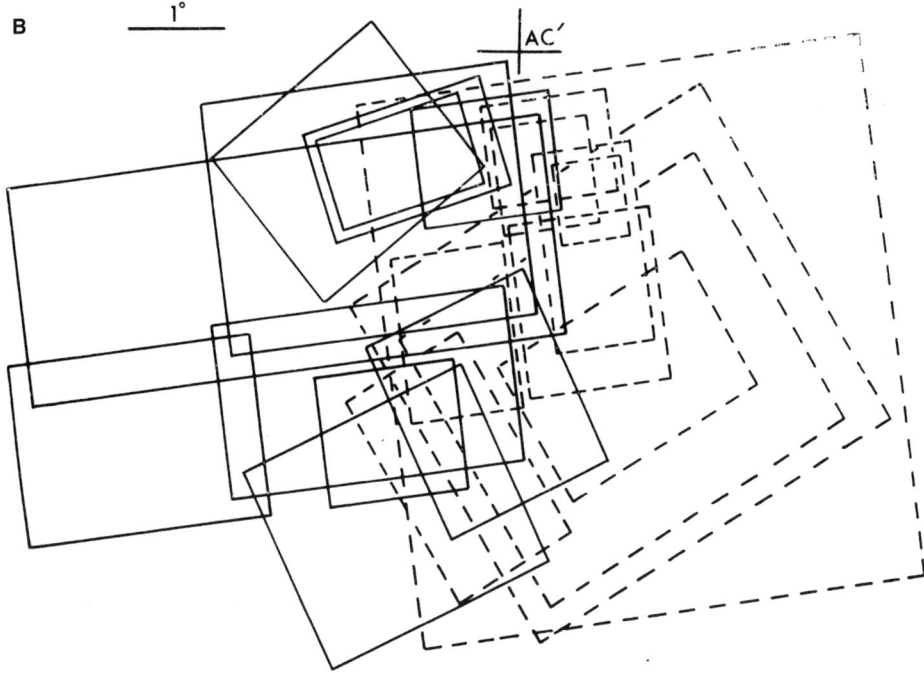

Fig. 2 (continued)

cat these workers found considerable variation in relative field positions in the two eyes, both horizontal and vertical (unpublished).

Recordings from Corpus Callosum

In three experiments, seven successful penetrations were made in the corpus callosum, at Horsley-Clarke levels ranging from A2 to A6. Spikes typical of large myelinated fibers (3) were observed immediately after the electrode entered the corpus callosum, and with one or two exceptions the discharges were easily driven by visual stimulation, suggesting that this part of the callosum is strongly preoccupied with vision. In each penetration, from 2 to 8 fibers were recorded, and in all, 34 responsive fibers were studied. Just as in cortical recordings, diffuse light was without obvious effect, but by exploring with a narrow slit of light (occasionally an edge or dark line) and constantly varying its orientation, responses were soon obtained and the receptive-field position and orientation established.

For 15 fibers an attempt was made to find out whether the field was simple or more complex. Of the 34 neurons, 7 had simple fields, with clear sub-division into excitatory and inhibitory areas; 7 were clearly complex and 1 was hypercomplex. The rest were not studied long enough for categorization. Fibers with simple fields presumably had their origin in area 17, while those with complex and hypercomplex fields could have originated from 17, 18, or 19.

For our present purposes the most interesting characteristic of these cells was the distribution of their receptive fields. Of 34 fibers, all but 2 or 3 had fields that came up to within a degree or so of the vertical meridian or overlapped it, and only 1 cell (no. 17, penetration *E*, Fig. 5) had a field more than 4° from the midline. Figures 4 and 5 summarize the receptive-field positions for the cells of all 7 penetrations. About half of the fields were in or very near the area centralis, and most of the others were scattered above and below it along the vertical meridian. Some indication of a crude topographic organization may be seen in Fig. 5, the cells of a given penetration tending to be mostly in the area centralis (penetration *B*), or all in the inferior fields of vision (penetration *C* and *E*), or the superior (penetration *A*). It was shown histologically that all of these penetrations passed through the

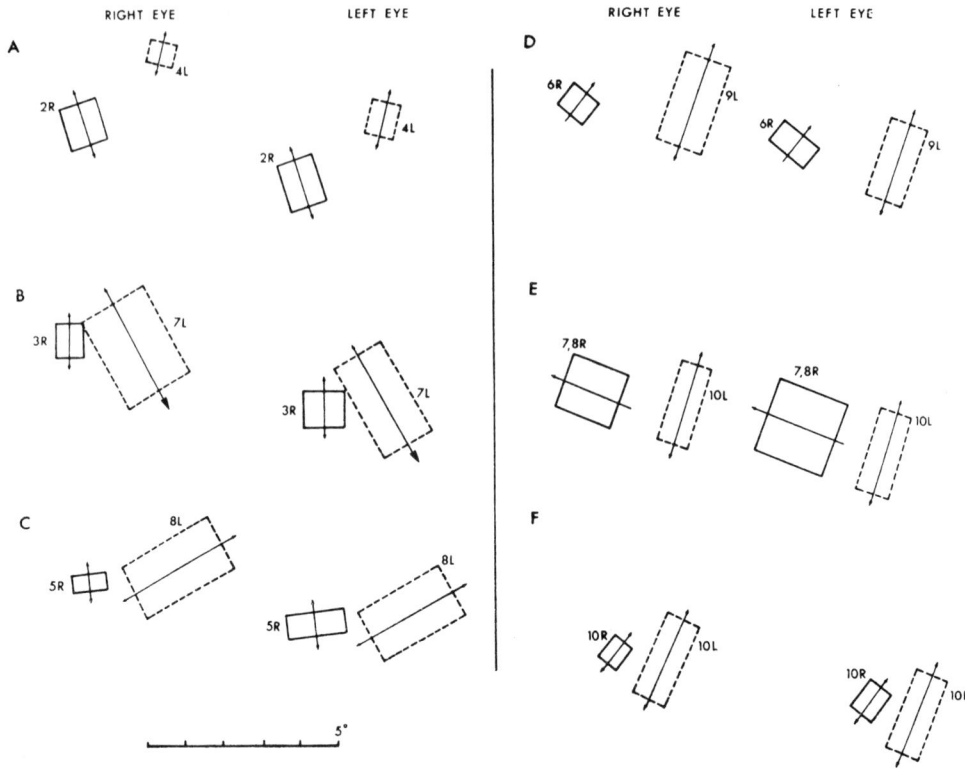

Fig. 3. Penetrations were made in the two hemispheres (area 17) at the same time, and a number of simultaneous recordings made of cells on the two sides. For each recording the object was to compare the relative positions of the two fields as mapped in one eye with the relative positions of the corresponding fields in the other eye. Fields are shown just as they were mapped on the screen, the left member of each pair corresponding to a cell in the right hemisphere, and conversely. The two visual axes were crossed, so that in each section (A–F) the fields in the right eye appear to the left, those from the left eye, to the right.

corpus callosum, as illustrated in Fig. 6 for one of the penetrations of Fig. 4 (cells 8–13).

All of the fibers in the corpus callosum were binocularly driven, but just as in cortical recordings there was wide variation in the relative influence of the two eyes, from fibers strongly dominated by the left eye, through equal influence, to strong right-eye dominance. As usual, the fields in the two eyes had otherwise identical characteristics, including field position, size, and orientation.

DISCUSSION

From the present results it seems clear that close to the 17-18 border in the cat cortex there is a bilateral representation of the vertical meridian of the visual field. Stated in terms of single cells, there are in this 17-18 border region cells whose receptive fields are not confined to the contralateral half of the visual field, but spill over into the ipsilateral half. The question immediately arises as to the connections responsible for this encroachment on the ipsilateral field. An indication that callosal connections are involved comes from the experiments in which Choudhury et al. (1) cooled the contralateral cortex or the corpus callosum, or cut the callosum while recording from the cortex on the side of the cut optic tract. Their conclusion receives support from our observations that the fibers in the posterior callosum are largely concerned with the midline.

At first glance the fact that the midline region of the visual fields is bilaterally represented in the cat cortex might seem to bear on the well-known but controversial question of macular sparing following total occipital lobe removal in man. Obviously, however, any bilateral representation which

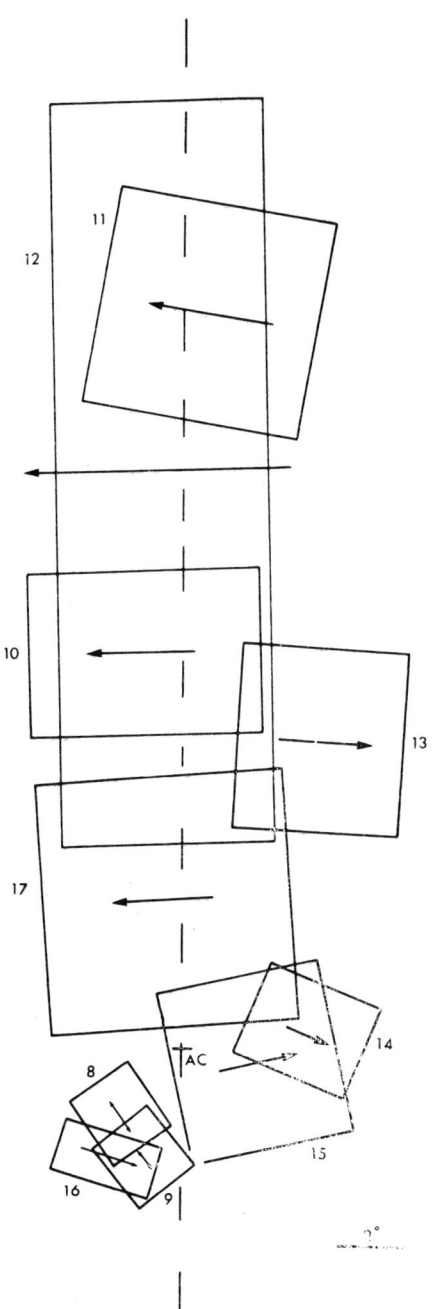

Fig. 4. Receptive-field positions of 10 cells recorded from the corpus callosum in 2 penetrations. Histology from the second electrode track (units 8–13) is illustrated in Fig. 6.

depends on projections from visual areas in the contralateral hemisphere could play no part in macular sparing attending the removal of these visual areas.

One should perhaps point out that the optic tract and lateral geniculate probably receive some ipsilateral input, and indeed it would be strange if geniculate cells with field centers along the vertical meridian were not just as plentiful as any others. These cells would have to have input from the ipsilateral half of the visual field to take care of a part of their field centers and about half of the field peripheries. The retrograde-degeneration studies of Stone (9) indeed indicate that the ganglion cell populations projecting to the two optic tracts overlap along the midline by about 0.9°.

Our results, as well as those of Choudhury et al. (1), fit well with anatomical studies which indicate that area 17 on one side projects to contralateral 18 and 19 and to the lateral bank of the suprasylvian gyrus (Clare and Bishop area; 7). We have recently found from Nauta silver-degeneration studies that 18 also has rich connections with 18 on the opposite side, but probably sends little or nothing to contralateral 17. These commissural connections by themselves would make one expect some overlap in receptive field position of cells in the two hemispheres, and indicate that one such region should be the part of 18 near the 17-18 border. The present experiments with two electrodes were too few in number to allow one to say conclusively that the region of overlap is entirely in 18. Moreover, the frequent difficulty in being certain of the exact position of the 17-18 border makes it hard to be sure that the most medial strip of 17 is not also involved. This problem is likely to be less serious in the monkey, where the 17-18 border is far more precise. Taken together, the results of Choudhury et al. (1), the two experiments described here, and the anatomical studies (2, 7, 8) all indicate that a special set of connections exists for dealing with the midline representation of the visual fields. These fibers might be expected to serve the same functions as intracortical fibers linking cells with receptive fields clustered in other, more outlying parts of the visual fields. The kinds of connections required can be reasonably inferred from what is known about the single-cell physiology of 17, 18, and 19. A complex cell in 18 which overlaps the midline could, for example, receive input from simple cells, some directly from nearby 17 in the same hemi-

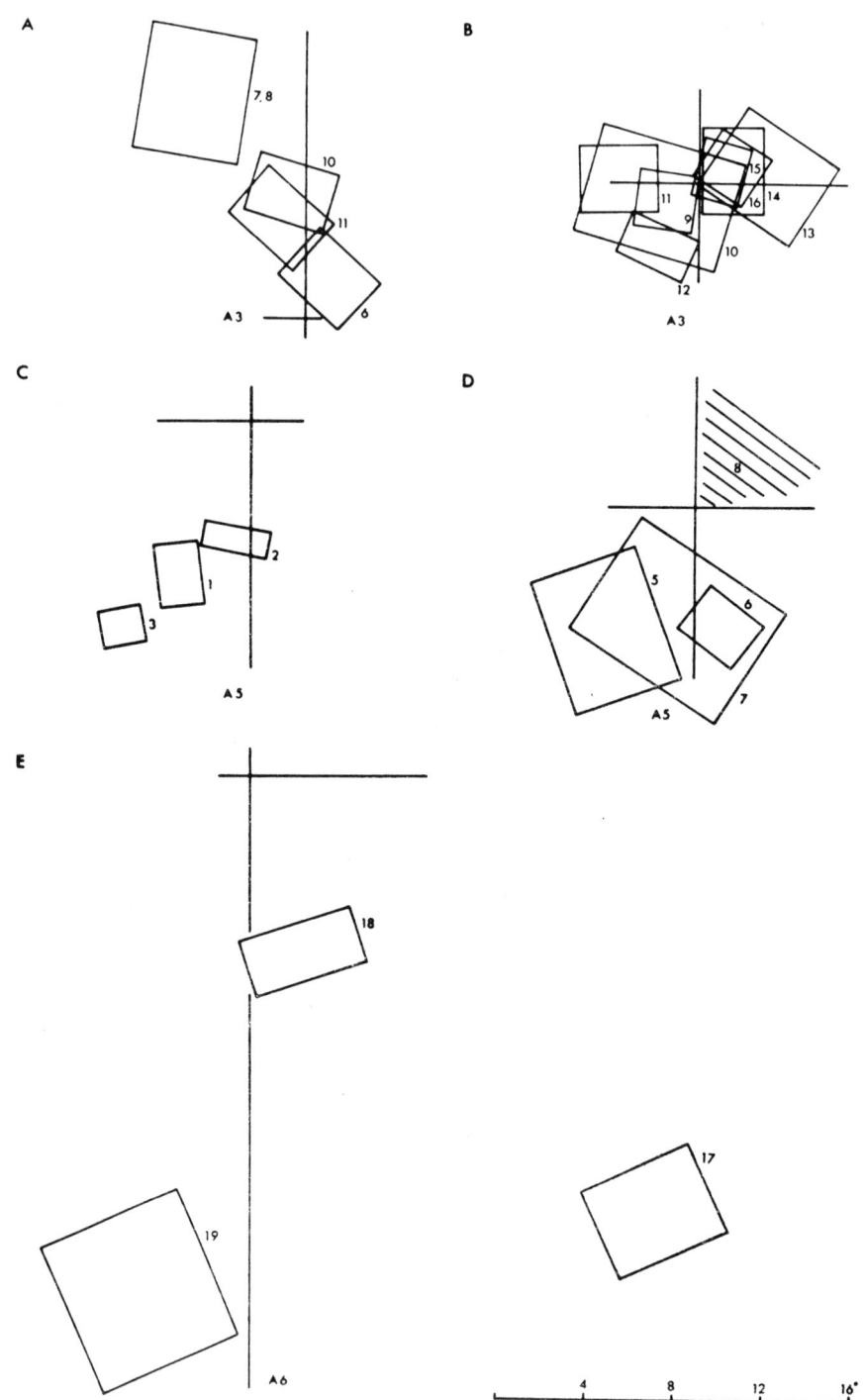

Fig. 5. Receptive-field positions of cells recorded in five penetrations in the corpus callosum. Penetration A is from one experiment, B–E from a different one. In each diagram the intersection of vertical and horizontal lines indicates the area centralis, to within a degree or so. (Field 8 of penetration D occupied the entire upper right quadrant.) The anterior-posterior position of the electrode in Horsley-Clarke coordinates is indicated for each penetration.

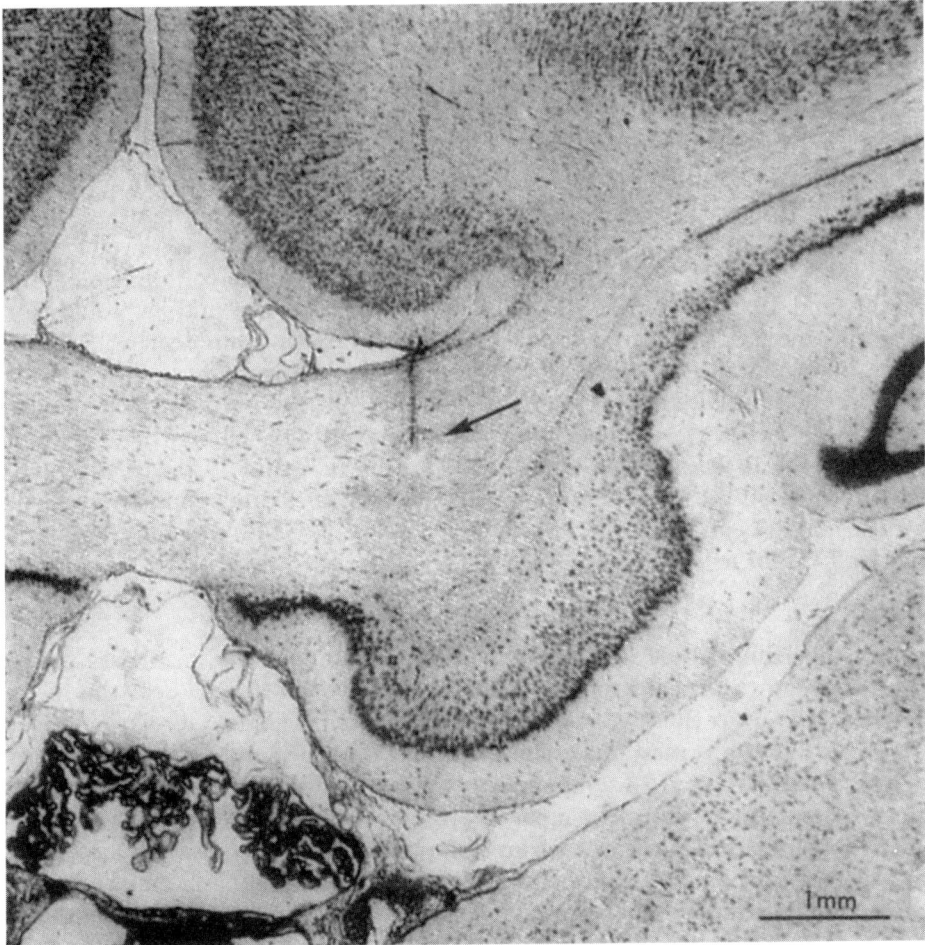

Fig. 6. Coronal section through corpus callosum at Horsley-Clarke level A5, showing microelectrode track and terminal lesion (arrow) for the penetration in which cells 8–13 of Fig. 4 were recorded. Cresyl violet stain.

sphere, and some from the opposite hemisphere via the corpus callosum. For this reason it seems interesting that the corpus callosum contains clear examples of fibers with simple receptive fields, which are not found, as far as is known, in area 18. From the fact that 17 projects to contralateral 19 on the two sides, one may similarly infer analogous connections for the elaboration in 19 of hypercomplex receptive fields which straddle the two half-visual fields.

SUMMARY

By recording single cells simultaneously in opposite hemispheres in the cat it was shown that the receptive fields of some cortical cells near the 17-18 boundary overlap the vertical midline of the visual fields. Overlapping was found only in the transitional zone between 17 and 18, and the adjacent part of 18. These areas are known anatomically to be interconnected, and to receive connections from the most lateral part of area 17.

Of 34 single fibers recorded from the posterior corpus callosum, all but 1 or 2 could be driven by visual stimulation, and of these all but 1 had receptive fields that overlapped the vertical midline or came up to within a degree or less of it. About half of the receptive fields were clustered around the area centralis; the rest were scattered widely above and below the horizontal meridian.

Seven cells had "simple" properties, the others being complex or hypercomplex.

These results suggest that certain fibers in the corpus callosum link cells whose fields are close together but lie on opposite sides of the vertical meridian or straddle it. These fibers would therefore seem to serve the same functions as intracortical fibers linking cells with receptive fields clustered in more outlying parts of the visual fields.

ACKNOWLEDGMENT

We express our thanks to Jane Chen and Janet Wiitanen for their invaluable technical assistance.

ADDENDUM

Since this paper was submitted, Gazzaniga, Berlucchi, and Rizzolatti have published a preliminary report on single-unit recordings in cat corpus callosum (*Federation Proc.* 26: 1864, 1967). Their main findings are in agreement with those reported here.

References

1. Choudhury, B. P., Whitteridge, D., and Wilson, M. E. The function of the callosal connections of the visual cortex. *Quart. J. Exptl. Physiol.* 50: 214–219, 1965.
2. Ebner, F. F. and Myers, R. E. Distribution of corpus callosum and anterior commissure in cat and raccoon. *J. Comp. Neurol.* 124: 353–366, 1965.
3. Hubel, D. H. Single unit activity in lateral geniculate body and optic tract of unrestrained cats. *J. Physiol., London* 150: 91–104, 1960.
4. Hubel, D. H. and Wiesel, T. N. Receptive fields of single neurones in the cat's striate cortex. *J. Physiol., London* 148: 574–591, 1959.
5. Hubel, D. H. and Wiesel, T. N. Integrative action in the cat's lateral geniculate body. *J. Physiol., London* 155: 385–398, 1961.
6. Hubel, D. H. and Wiesel, T. N. Receptive fields, binocular interaction and functional architecture in the cat's visual cortex. *J. Physiol., London* 160: 106–154, 1962.
7. Hubel, D. H. and Wiesel, T. N. Receptive fields and functional architecture in two nonstriate visual areas (18 and 19) of the cat. *J. Neurophysiol.* 28: 229–289, 1965.
8. Polley, E. H. and Dirkes, J. M. The visual cortical (geniculocortical) area of cat brain and its projections. *Anat. Record* 145: 345, 1963.
9. Stone, J. The naso-temporal division of the cat's retina. *J. Comp. Neurol.* 126: 585–599, 1966.
10. Talbot, S. A. and Marshall, W. H. Physiological studies on neural mechanisms of visual localization and discrimination. *Am. J. Ophthalmol.* 24: 1255–1263, 1941.

AFTERWORD

The results were as we had expected. When we put two electrodes into opposite hemispheres, at or near the 17-18 borders on the two sides, the two receptive fields that we mapped often overlapped. In the corpus callosum, the receptive fields of the crossing fibers were almost always close to the vertical midline or straddled it. This indicated that, for cells subserving the vertical midline of the visual fields, the callosum carries out the same functions that the connections between neighboring cells carry out, away from the midline. Its purpose is at least partly to deal with the awkward and artificial circumstance of having a cortical representation that is split along the midline.

We would have liked to know the exact origin and destination of the fibers in the callosum: did they come from, and go to, 17 or 18 (V-1 or V-2)? Here we had the problem of the vagueness, in the cat, of this 17-18 border region. In primates it is histologically as sharp as a knife, but in cats it is not well defined, and consequently, over a millimeter or so of its extent, one cannot be sure which of the two areas, 17 or 18, one is looking at, or recording from. This border region is the representation of the vertical midline, and is the region that the callosum interconnects. Because of the poor definition of the border in cats, the question of whether it is 17 or 18 that sends or receives callosal fibers becomes hard to answer. One even wonders if there *is* a border in any well-defined sense. In primates the geniculate projects only to 17, not to 18, so that the border is at the place were the geniculo-cortical projections leave off. In cats the geniculate projects strongly to both areas, so that criterion is not available. Thus V-2 seems to be different in the two species, and less well differentiated in the cat.

In the early 1970s, Carla Shatz, one of our first graduate students, made a careful examination of physiology and anatomical connections of corpus callosum in normal cats and in Siamese cats. She examined the connections by making injections of horseradish peroxidase into the 17-18 border region on one hemisphere, after identifying the border region by showing that cells recorded from the injection pipette had their fields along the midine. In normal cats she found that the incoming labelled fibers in the opposite hemisphere were indeed confined to the 17-border regions, in clear confirmation of the physiological results. We describe her results in Siamese cats in Chapter 23

A most ingenious illustration of corpus callosum function came from an experiment done by Giovanni Berlucchi and Giacomo Rizzolatti in Pisa in 1968 (*Science,* 159:308–310). They transected the optic chiasm midsagittally, as Choudhury, Whitteridge, and Wilson had done, and recorded from cortical cells close to the 17-18 border looking for cells that could be driven from both eyes. The binocular cells they observed were just what one might have predicted: for each cell the receptive field spanned the vertical midline, and the part in the left visual field was driven from the right eye and the part in the right field was driven from the left eye. The two half receptive fields joined perfectly across the midline, and the optimum orientation was the same in the two halves. That nicely confirms one's ideas about corpus callosum function, and tells us how specific the connections can be.

Knowledge of callosal connections and function was later used by David Van Essen and Semir Zeki in their mapping of primate prestriate visual areas (J Physiol 1978, 277:193–226). They reasoned that any of the visual areas on one side of the occipital lobe would be likely to contain a map of half of the field of vision, bounded by the vertical midline, and that these midline representations in the two hemispheres would be likely to be joined by the corpus callosum. So they transected the callosum and looked for degenerating terminals in the cortex with the Nauta method. They found multiple areas of degenerated terminals, and deduced that each such area must be a representation of the vertical midline, and probably part of a distinct prestriate region. That method, coupled with the mapping of responses to visual stimuli, helped make it possible to tease apart and map the many visual areas that lay beyond the striate cortex, a task that was beyond our patience and fortitude.

Chapter 14 • Recordings in Monkey Striate Cortex, 1968 •

FOREWORD

Between our 1962 cat-area-17 paper and this monkey striate-cortex paper is a lapse of six years. That may seem strange given that we began working in monkey cortex, in parallel with the cat work, while we were still at Johns Hopkins, in 1959. But the monkey cortex was far more intricate, like a Rolls Royce compared with a Model-T Ford, and the work went more slowly. We regarded these animals as precious and wanted to begin by covering as much ground as possible in cats.

Another reason for the delay in publishing our results in the monkey striate cortex was the near-absence of competitors, which made us feel less pressure to publish small bits of work as we went along. In this complicated field we thought that we would have a better chance of getting things right if we took our time. That luxury hardly exists today, given the competition for grants, for publication, and for jobs and promotions. In 1968 we did not feel that we lacked time for lunch with colleagues or afternoon tea. Overpopulation in science can have sad consequences, as we see when, in a new field such as olfaction, one breakthrough leads to the piling in of competitors from all sides, and priority for discoveries can be determined by days or weeks, not years. For us that would have taken away much of the fun. We were lucky.

Today it would be far harder to do a project like this one. Monkeys are so much more expensive, and regulations as to their use so much more onerous, that recording from one monkey each week and then sectioning the brain for the anatomy would be almost out of the question. One is forced to use awake-behaving techniques, with the obvious advantage that one monkey can be recorded from for months or years, and that anesthetics can be avoided. Also a recording session can begin at 10:00 A.M. and end at 3:00 in the afternoon, allowing one to get home for dinner, in contrast to our acute experiments, which typically started at 8:30 A.M. and went on to the next day, to the dismay of our wives. But awake-behaving methods have the grave

shortcoming of being far less compatible with the anatomical studies that are necessary to identify electrode placements.

Our work had come to rely increasingly on combining the neurophysiology and anatomy. We routinely examined the brains of all the monkeys that we recorded from to determine the exact location of our recording electrodes, using electrolytic lesions to mark each electrode track in several places. To get maximum information from every monkey, in an unrelated set of studies, we would also usually make a geniculate or cortical lesion (for Nauta degeneration studies, see below) or tracer injections (of horseradish peroxidase or a radioactive amino acid), five days or so before the recording. The time interval between the injections or lesions and the final recording allowed the axons from the damaged cells to degenerate or the injected label to be transported. In alert monkey research there is little hope, when the animal is finally killed, of recognizing particular electrode tracks among 50 or more others, or of recovering lesions months after they are made. Acute experiments such as the ones we did every week have become much less common, and progress in working out functional architecture of the different cortical areas has consequently been slow or nonexistent.

Magnetic resonance imaging techniques (MRI) may allow us to overcome some of these problems. Richard Born has shown in rats that electrode tip positions marked by depositing iron from stainless steel electrodes can be recovered after many months, and the iron deposits show up beautifully in the images. It seems almost certain that such a method will be used extensively in monkeys. MRI has a resolution that is far from what one gets with conventional histology, so identifying recording sites in terms of cortical layers or blobs may still be out of reach.

To someone reading this paper today, the nomenclature we used for labelling the cortical layers will surely be a source of confusion. Any logical system of labelling layers must rely at least partly on knowing the sites of termination of the inputs to the cortex and the destinations of fibers leaving the different layers. In 1968 we knew neither. We adopted a compromise between the various nomenclatures that had been based on the cytoarchitectonics of Brodmann, von Bonin, and Lorente de Nó. In subsequent papers we used a slightly different terminology, because we finally learned much more about where the fibers coming in from the different geniculate layers terminated in the cortex. What made this possible was the use of our tungsten electrodes to make lesions (as already mentioned), in geniculate layers that we identified by recording, coupled with Nauta staining of the fibers that degenerated as a result of the lesions (1972). Later we came more and more to inject radioactive tracers, whose transport we could follow with autoradiography. Finally we made increasing use of stains for cytochrome oxidase, which gave a much sharper definition of layer 4, and incidentally the blobs in area 17. (All this will be described in subsequent papers in this book.) The Golgi studies of Jennifer Lund have made for a more logical modern terminology for numbering and lettering these layers, on which most neurobiologists have come to agree.

The following paragraph compares the terminology used in our 1968 paper with today's terminology, and is meant to help anyone particularly interested in the history of the subject, or the details. For everyone else the table that follows will sum things up. The main thing to realize is that layer terminologies differ from author to author and from one time to the next.

In present-day terminology (and do skip this paragraph unless you are very zealous) we call layer 4A the *upper tier* of parvocellular geniculate terminations. This is roughly the deepest part of what in the present (1968) paper we call *layer III*. What is now called *4C-alpha* is the site of termination of magnocellular inputs and what we call *4C-beta* is the termination of the bulk of the parvocellular inputs. Together these comprise what in 1968 we called *layer 4B*. What we then called *4A* is more or less congruent with the classical line of Gennari, which was formerly thought to be the site of geniculate terminals, but was found in our Nauta studies to be free of them. We will have more to say about the physiology of the layers in the afterword to this paper, and when we come to the papers on geniculo-cortical connections.

Comparison of layer designations in the 1968 paper with more modern terminology.

Today	1968 Paper	Nissl	Connections (partial list)
1	1	sparse	
2,3	2,3 minus deepest part	dense	from 4C beta
4A	deepest part of 2,3	dense	from parvo genic
4B (Gennari)	4A	sparse	from 4C alpha & beta
4C alpha & beta	4B	dense	from mgno & par genic
5	5	sparse	
6	6	dense	from lgb and upper layers of 17, to m & p genic

Receptive Fields and Functional Architecture of Monkey Striate Cortex

D. H. HUBEL AND T. N. WIESEL • *Department of Physiology, Harvard Medical School, Boston, Mass., U.S.A.*

SUMMARY

1. The striate cortex was studied in lightly anaesthetized macaque and spider monkeys by recording extracellularly from single units and stimulating the retinas with spots or patterns of light. Most cells can be categorized as simple, complex, or hypercomplex, with response properties very similar to those previously described

From *J. Physiol.* (1968), **195**, 215–243
Received 6 October 1967.

in the cat. On the average, however, receptive fields are smaller, and there is a greater sensitivity to changes in stimulus orientation. A small proportion of the cells are colour coded.

2. Evidence is presented for at least two independent systems of columns extending vertically from surface to white matter. Columns of the first type contain cells with common receptive-field orientations. They are similar to the orientation columns described in the cat, but are probably smaller in cross-sectional area. In the second system cells are aggregated into columns according to eye preference. The ocular dominance columns are larger than the orientation columns, and the two sets of boundaries seem to be independent.

3. There is a tendency for cells to be grouped according to symmetry of responses to movement; in some regions the cells respond equally well to the two opposite directions of movement of a line, but other regions contain a mixture of cells favouring one direction and cells favouring the other.

4. A horizontal organization corresponding to the cortical layering can also be discerned. The upper layers (II and the upper two-thirds of III) contain complex and hypercomplex cells, but simple cells are virtually absent. The cells are mostly binocularly driven. Simple cells are found deep in layer III, and in IV A and IV B. In layer IV B they form a large proportion of the population, whereas complex cells are rare. In layers IV A and IV B one finds units lacking orientation specificity; it is not clear whether these are cell bodies or axons of geniculate cells. In layer IV most cells are driven by one eye only; this layer consists of a mosaic with cells of some regions responding to one eye only, those of other regions responding to the other eye. Layers V and VI contain mostly complex and hypercomplex cells, binocularly driven.

5. The cortex is seen as a system organized vertically and horizontally in entirely different ways. In the vertical system (in which cells lying along a vertical line in the cortex have common features) stimulus dimensions such as retinal position, line orientation, ocular dominance, and perhaps directionality of movement, are mapped in sets of superimposed but independent mosaics. The horizontal system segregates cells in layers by hierarchical orders, the lowest orders (simple cells monocularly driven) located in and near layer IV, the higher orders in the upper and lower layers.

INTRODUCTION

Over the past ten years we have studied the sequential processing of visual information in the cat by examining the responses of single cells at various points along the visual pathway. In extending this work it seemed natural to turn to the monkey, an animal that comes close to man in its visual capabilities, especially its high acuity and well developed colour vision. In contrast with the cat, moreover, most primates have a visual pathway that is further differentiated, with a rod-free fovea, a six-layered geniculate, and a striate cortex that lends itself well to studies of functional architecture, being conspicuously laminated and well demarcated from neighbouring cortical areas.

In this paper we present the results of a series of recordings from the monkey striate cortex. The study may be regarded as a continuation of previous work on the monkey optic nerve (Hubel & Wiesel, 1960) and lateral geniculate body (Wiesel & Hubel, 1966). The early experiments were done in the cortex of the spider monkey (*Ateles*), but the rhesus (*Macaca mulatta*) was used in all of the more recent work.

METHODS

Six spider monkeys and sixteen macaques were used. Details of stimulating and recording procedures have been published elsewhere (Hubel & Wiesel, 1962; Wiesel & Hubel, 1966). Animals, 2–3 kg in weight, were anaesthetized with thiopental sodium, and light anaesthesia was maintained throughout the experiment. Since intravenous succinylcholine alone was often insufficient to prevent all eye movements, gallamine triethiodide (2–3 mg/kg) was also usually given intramuscularly at half-hour intervals.

When only one or two penetrations were planned in a single animal, a small hole was drilled in the skull, the dura incised keeping the arachnoid intact, and the electrode introduced through a hollow 19-gauge stainless-steel needle, which was cemented into the hole to make a closed chamber. In a few experiments designed to explore a wider area of cortex a modified Davies chamber was cemented to the skull (Hubel & Wiesel, 1963). Microelectrodes were sharpened tungsten wire insulated with a clear vinyl lacquer (Hubel, 1957).

To help reconstruct the electrode tracks, one or several lesions were made in each penetration by passing direct current through the electrode (Hubel, 1959). In the monkey cortex 2μA for 2 sec (electrode negative) was usually sufficient. All brains were fixed in formalin, photographed, embedded in celloidin, sectioned serially at 20 μ, and stained for Nissl substance with cresyl violet.

RESULTS

Part I. Receptive Field Types

This study is based upon recordings of 150 cells in seven penetrations in six spider monkeys, and 272 cells in twenty-five penetrations in sixteen macaque monkeys. Most of the penetrations were made in cortical regions subserving the 0–4° parafoveal region; a few passed through buried cortical folds subserving the mid or far periphery, and in two laterally placed penetrations the fields were in the fovea. The approximate recording sites in the sixteen rhesus experiments are shown for a representative brain in Text-fig. 1.

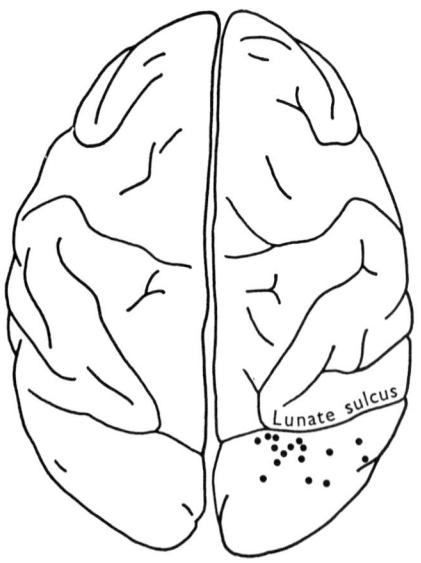

Fig. 1. Recording sites for the sixteen rhesus experiments. Diagram of monkey brain viewed from above; anterior is up. Many of the dots represent several closely spaced penetrations in a single monkey. Several deep penetrations went into buried folds of striate and non-striate cortex.

We begin by describing the various types of receptive fields that can be distinguished in the monkey striate cortex, emphasizing especially any differences between monkey and cat. Implicit in these descriptions is the possibly over-simplified concept of a hierarchical system dependent on anatomical wiring, in which geniculate cells with concentric fields converge on simple cortical cells, simple cells in turn converge upon complex cells, and complex on hypercomplex. The evidence for such connexions (Hubel & Wiesel, 1962, 1965a) is derived from the properties of the fields themselves, and also from the functional architecture of the cortex.

SIMPLE CELLS. As in the cat, these cells are defined as having receptive fields with spatially distinct 'on' and 'off' areas separated by parallel straight lines (Hubel & Wiesel, 1959). Twenty-five of the 272 cells studied in rhesus were definitely established as simple, and a similar proportion was seen in the spider monkey. This small number almost certainly does not reflect the actual proportion of simple cells in striate cortex, since judging from spike size and difficulties in isolation these cells are mostly small. Moreover, some penetrations stopped short of the layers where simple cells are most populous. In a typical penetration through the full cortical thickness, when the electrode was fine enough to isolate cells easily, three or four out of thirty or so cells could be expected to be simple. An example of such a penetration is described in detail in the next section.

Even in this small sampling, we found representatives of all of the 'simple' receptive field subtypes described in the cat (Hubel & Wiesel, 1962, Fig. 2). The commonest simple fields were those with long narrow 'on'-centres sandwiched between two more extensive 'off' regions, and those with an 'on' and an 'off' region lying side by side, but a few examples of each of the other types were also seen. Knowing the exact configuration of a field made it possible to predict the optimum stimulus: its size, shape, orientation, and position on the retina. As described below, and in contrast with what we found in the cat, most simple cells were driven by one eye only. Six of the twenty-five cells showed opponent-colour properties, suggesting that the proportion of colour coded cells may be higher in simple cells than in complex.

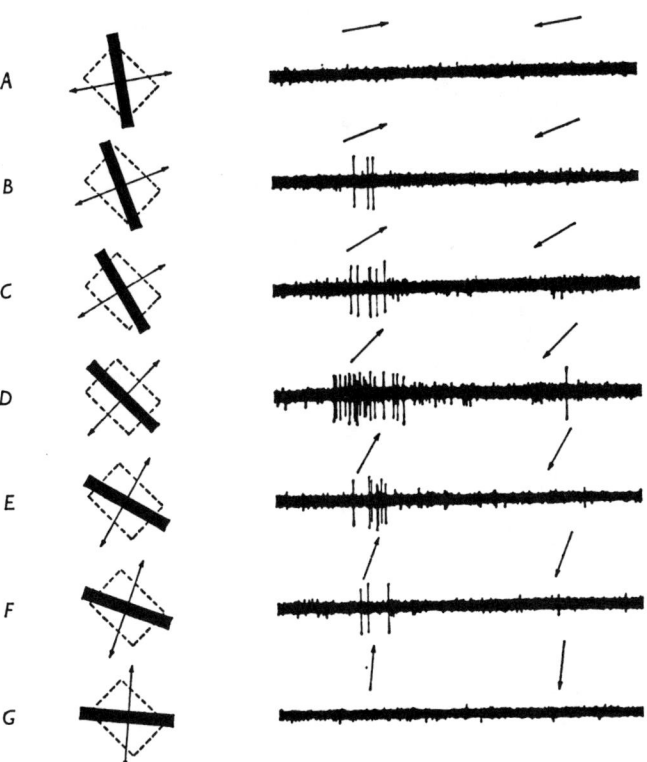

Fig. 2. *Responses of a complex cell in right striate cortex (layer IV A) to various orientations of a moving black bar. Receptive field in the left eye indicated by the interrupted rectangles; it was approximately ⅜ × ⅜° in size, and was situated 4° below and to the left of the point of fixation. Ocular-dominance group 4. Duration of each record, 2 sec. Background intensity 1·3 log_{10} cd/m², dark bars 0·0 log cd/m².*

COMPLEX CELLS. Complex cells are the commonest of all types, making up 177 of the 272 cells in the rhesus. The properties of these cells were similar to those we have described for the cat (Hubel & Wiesel, 1962). By definition, there was no separation of receptive fields into excitatory and inhibitory parts. As for simple cells, a line stimulus (slit, dark bar, or edge) in a particular orientation evoked optimum responses, and as the orientation was varied the responses fell off, usually failing long before an angle 90° to the optimum was reached. Prolonging the line in either direction did not reduce the response. But whereas for the simple cell the position of the stimulus was crucial, in the complex a response was evoked on shining the correctly oriented line on any part of the field, or by moving the line over the field. As in the cat, about half of the cells showed highly asymmetrical responses to diametrically opposite directions of movement, while the rest showed little or no directional preference. Even when responses were highly asymmetrical, the less effective direction of movement usually evoked some minimal response (see Text-fig. 2), but

there were a few examples in which the maintained activity was actually suppressed.

Individual complex cells differed markedly in their relative responsiveness to slits, edges, or dark bars. The majority responded very much better to one than to the other two, but some reacted briskly to two of them, and a few to all three. For a cell that was sensitive to slits, but not to edges, the responses increased as slit width was increased up to some optimal value, and then they fell off sharply; the optimum width was always a small fraction of the width of the whole field. For complex cells that responded best to edges, some reacted to one configuration and also to its mirror image, while others responded only to one edge configuration. In the first type a broad slit or dark bar usually gave more vigorous responses than an edge, as though it combined the advantages of the two types of edge. On narrowing the stimulus down to a width that might be close to the optimum for the usual slit or dark-bar complex cell, the response usually failed. Presumably the two types of cells are connected to simple cells in entirely different ways.

A complex cell that responded best to a moving dark bar is illustrated in Text-fig. 2. Here the optimally oriented stimulus (Text-fig. 2 D) gave very different responses to the two different directions of movement, with a minimal, inconstant discharge to movement down and to the left. The rate of decline of this cell's responses as the stimulus orientation deviated from the optimum was fairly typical; while the decline varied to some extent from cell to cell (see below), it was generally steeper in the monkey than in the cat. Most field orientations could be specified to within 5–10°, as compared to 10–15° in the cat.

HYPERCOMPLEX CELLS. Fifty-three of the 272 cells recorded from the rhesus were lower-order hypercomplex. For these, extending the line (slit, edge or dark bar) beyond the activating part of the receptive field in one or both directions caused a marked fall-off in the response, and there was usually no response at all if the line was made long enough. The proportion of hypercomplex cells occurring here may well be higher than our figures suggest, since in the early monkey experiments we did not know that such cells existed and did not systematically vary the lengths of the stimuli. We have recently found hypercomplex cells in the cat striate cortex, but they seem to be less common than in the monkey.

Responses of a typical hypercomplex cell are shown in Text-fig. 3. The more or less square central activating region, indicated by interrupted lines, was flanked by a weak antagonistic region above and by a stronger one below, so that to evoke a consistent response a line (edge or bar) had to be terminated within the rectangle or at its borders (Text-fig. 3A–D). When it extended beyond them, as in Text-fig. 3 E–G, the response was reduced or obliterated. Another example is shown in Text-fig. 4; here the most powerful stimulus was an obliquely oriented slit moving in either direction across the region marked by broken lines. Lengthening the stimulus in both directions again greatly reduced the response, though this time the suppression was not complete.

No higher-order hypercomplex cells were seen in monkey striate cortex (Hubel & Wiesel, 1965a).

SIZES OF RECEPTIVE FIELDS. For comparable regions of the visual field, simple receptive fields in the monkey were on the average much smaller than in the cat. At 1–4° from the centre of gaze, for example, fields ranged from ¼ × ¼° up to ½ × ¾°, as against about ½ × ½° up to about 4 × 4° for the cat. Complex and hypercomplex fields in the monkey were likewise smaller than in the cat, perhaps about one quarter the size in linear dimensions. They tended to be somewhat larger than simple fields, perhaps 1½ to 2 times as big, in linear dimensions.

In the two experiments made in the region representing the fovea one or two simple fields were less than ¼ × ¼°, but their exact boundaries were not determined. Surprisingly, the range of sizes of complex and hypercomplex fields was not very different from that seen a few degrees further out. As we have discussed elsewhere (Hubel & Wiesel, 1962), acuity is probably not closely related to over-all receptive field dimensions, but rather to the widths of optimally shaped stimuli.

UNITS LACKING ORIENTATION SPECIFICITY. In layer IV we usually recorded monocularly driven units whose receptive fields were similar to those of geniculate cells. The spikes of these units were small and negative, being quite different from the typical spikes of myelinated fibres seen in optic tract and radiations, and corpus callosum (Hubel, 1959; Hubel & Wiesel, 1967). The field properties and localization of these IVth layer units makes one suspect that they are axons or axon-terminals of geniculate cells, but they could be cortical cells, and it will probably be necessary to stimulate electrically the subcortical optic radiations to settle the question. Some units with concentric receptive fields had more complex responses to coloured stimuli than anything we saw in the lateral geniculate; these are discussed below.

CELLS WITH SPECIFIC COLOUR RESPONSES. In the rhesus lateral geniculate body the majority of the dorsal-layer cells have opponent-colour properties, light exciting them at some wave-lengths, inhibiting them at others, diffuse white light evoking little or no response (De Valois, Jacobs & Jones, 1963; Wiesel & Hubel, 1966). For cortical cells, we expected that with this input there might be a similar emphasis on wave-length discrimination. Motokawa, Taira & Okuda (1962) have in fact described opponent colour cells in monkey cortex. It was surprising to us, however, that the great

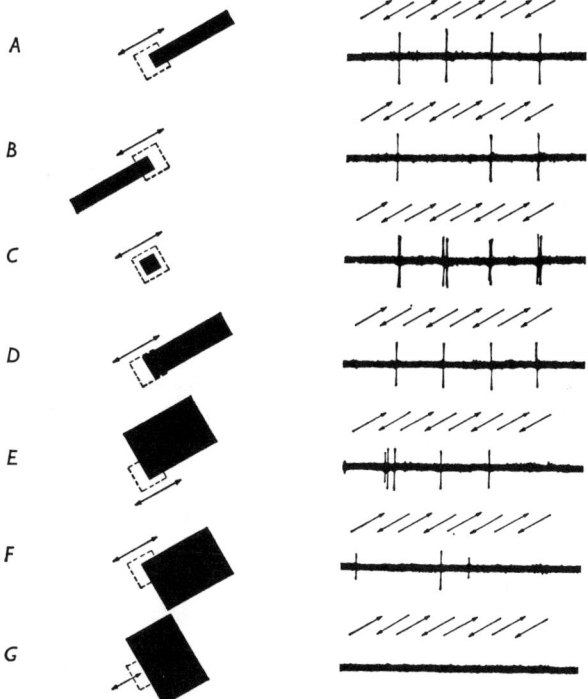

Fig. 3. Responses of a hypercomplex cell from layer III of monkey striate cortex. (This was cell 9 in Text-figs. 7 and 8). 'Activating' portion of receptive field (⅜ × ⅜°) is outlined by interrupted lines. Stimulus of this region by a moving edge activates cell (A–D). Below this region, and to some extent above it, are regions appropriate stimulation of which suppresses the response to an edge (E–G). Duration of each record 5 sec. Stimulus intensities as in Text-fig. 2.

majority of cells could discriminate precisely the orientation or direction of movement of a stimulus, but had no marked selectivity regarding wavelength. There were interesting and striking exceptions to this, which are described below, but on the whole the colour responses seen in area 17 have been disappointing: for a high proportion of cells the response to a given stimulus shape was qualitatively the same—firing being increased or firing being suppressed—regardless of wave-length, and the optimum stimulus shape was independent of

wave-length. Even in the two penetrations in the region representing fovea most cells seemed to be relatively unconcerned with colour, though here the proportion of cells with colour specific responses seemed higher than it was 2–4° from the fovea.

Of the twenty-five simple cells recorded in rhesus, six had more specific colour-coded behaviour, the excitatory and inhibitory parts of the receptive field differing in spectral sensitivity in the manner of geniculate Type I cells (Wiesel & Hubel,

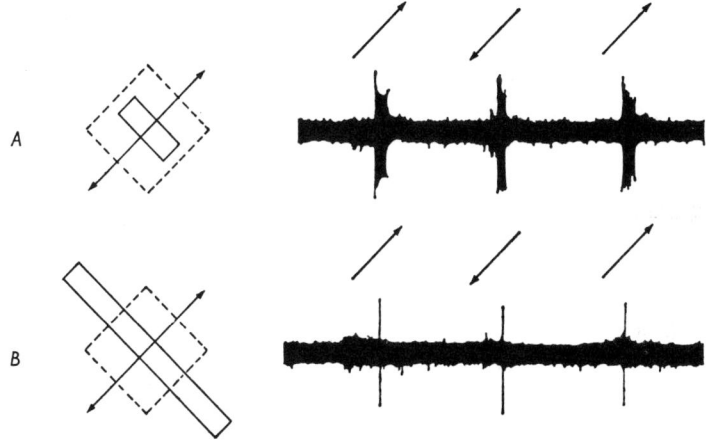

Fig. 4. Hypercomplex cell recorded from right striate cortex, layer II. A: stimulus of left eye by moving slit within activating region (¼ × ⅜°); B: similar stimulation with slit extending beyond activating region. Background, log 0.0 cd/m²; stimulus, log 1.3 cd/m². Duration of each record 10 sec.

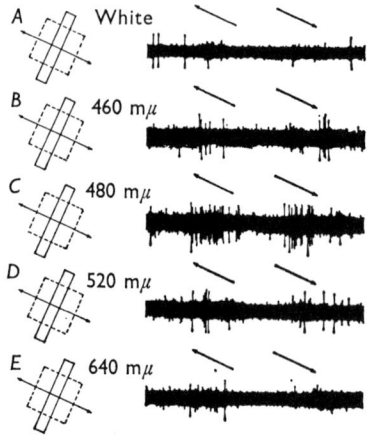

Fig. 5. Complex cell with colour coded properties recorded in layer II of striate cortex. Responses to movement of optimally oriented slits of white light and monochromatic light at various wave-lengths. Monochromatic light made by interposing interference filters in a beam of white light: stimulus energies are greatest for A, and progressively less for E, D, C and B. None of the responses was improved by lowering the intensity. Size of receptive field ½ × ½°. Ocular dominance group 1. Background and white stimulus intensities as in Text-fig. 4. Time for each record 5 sec.

1966). All six fields were similar in organization, with a long narrow excitatory region with highest sensitivity to long wave-lengths, flanked on either side by more extensive inhibitory regions with relatively greater blue-green sensitivity. These cells behaved as though they received input from a set of Type I red on-centre, green off- surround geniculate cells, the commonest variety found in the dorsal geniculate layers. Certain features of two of the cells were not so easily explained, however: one responded well to a properly positioned red slit but not at all well to a white slit; another failed to respond to diffuse white light, as expected, but also

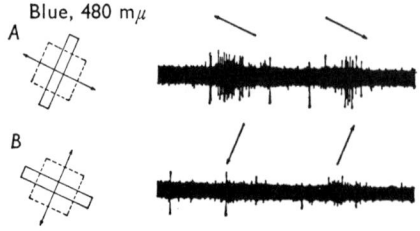

Fig. 6. Same cell as Text-fig. 5. Responses to two orthogonal stimulus orientations at 480 mμ.

responded poorly to diffuse red. Obviously it will be necessary to sample many more cells of this type, and to study them more thoroughly.

COMPLEX AND HYPERCOMPLEX CELLS WITH COLOUR SELECTIVITY. Of the 177 complex cells examined in rhesus, only twelve (about 7%) were identified as having clear colour specificity. Not all cells were studied with monochromatic stimuli, but enough were to be reasonably sure that colour coded cells are a small minority, probably not more than 10% for regions 2–4° from the fovea. Four cells gave responses to coloured stimuli that were qualitatively similar to their responses to white stimuli, but only over an unusually restricted band of wavelengths. A cell might respond actively in the blue-violet (or the red), but not to light at the other end of the spectrum.

Six cells showed still more specific reactions to coloured stimuli. They responded actively to a properly oriented slit at some wave-lengths but not others, and gave little or no response to a similarly oriented white slit at any intensity. An example is illustrated in Text-figs. 5 and 6. This cell had typical complex properties, favouring up-and-left movement of a 1 o'clock oriented slit and showing no response to a slit oriented at right angles to this. The only stimuli that evoked brisk responses were blue ones, and it was striking that white slits produced by removing the interference filter from the light path were completely ineffective. The other five cells behaved in a similar way, but favoured long wave-lengths.

Three cells, finally, had opponent-colour properties like the ones just mentioned, favouring monochromatic slits over white, but also had hypercomplex characteristics, in that a long slit was distinctly less effective than one of limited length.

CELLS WITH CONCENTRIC FIELDS AND DUAL-OPPONENT SYSTEMS. Under this heading we group a very few cells with centre-surround receptive-field organization, but with more complex behaviour than anything we have seen in the geniculate. The fields appeared to be organized in centre-surround fashion. With centre-size spots the cells were excited by long wave-lengths and inhibited by short, with little response to white light. On the other hand a large spot was almost completely ineffective regardless of wave-length, suggesting that the surround was red-off green-on, i.e. the reverse of the centre. It was as if two Type III (non opponent-colour) geniculate fields, an on-centre with maximum sensitivity in the red, and an off-centre with maximum sensitivity in the blue-green, had been superimposed. Since these cells were influenced from one eye only it is possible that they were axons of geniculate cells. We saw nothing this complicated in the rhesus geniculate, but our sampling there was small enough so that a relatively rare type could easily have been missed. Ganglion cells with somewhat similar fields have been described recently by Daw (1967) in the retina of the goldfish. In the units described above, however, the situation seems somewhat simpler, there being a single boundary between centre and surround instead of a separate boundary for each of the two opponent systems, as was found in the goldfish.

In summary, cells with interesting colour properties occur in the cortex but are in the minority, and, as in the geniculate, seem very diverse in type, with fields ranging in their spatial characteristics from non-oriented to hypercomplex. This survey is intended only to suggest the diversity; a satisfactory study will probably mean recording from thousands, rather than hundreds, of cortical cells.

Part II. Functional Architecture

A Representative Penetration Through Striate Cortex (Area 17)

As shown in Fig. 1, most of the penetrations through area 17 were made from the smooth exposed part of the occipital lobe a few millimetres behind the lunate sulcus, i.e. just behind the 17-18 border, which runs parallel to and just behind the sulcus. In all rhesus experiments the brain was sectioned in the parasagittal plane, which has the advantage of intersecting the lunate sulcus and the 17-18 boundary at right angles. The convention of numbering the layers (Pl. 1) combines that of von Bonin (1942) for layers I–IV, and that of Lorente de Nó (1943) and Brodmann (1909) for V and VI. In this system each layer can be identified easily in a Nissl preparation, except for the poorly defined II–III boundary, which we place arbitrarily between the upper ⅓ and the lower ⅔ of the cell-rich layer making up II and III. The pale layer beneath III is termed IV A, and the alternating cell-rich, pale, and cell-rich layers are termed IV B, V, and VI.

In the penetration to be described, three small lesions 50–70 μ in diameter were made at roughly ½ mm intervals, to help estimate shrinkage during fixation and embedding, and to increase the accuracy of estimating positions of the cells encountered (Text-fig. 7; Pl. 1). Except for cells tagged specifically by lesions, or cells very close to lesions, estimations made by this method are nevertheless only approximate. Sometimes, for example, the position of a superficial lesion corresponded poorly with depths calculated from two or more deeper lesions, possibly because of uneven shrinkage, or possibly due to dimpling of the cortex in the first part of some penetrations. The security with which one can assign a cell to a particular layer thus varies widely from cell to cell even in the same penetration, and statistics are difficult to compile. Specific questions can, nevertheless, often be answered with some certainty by placing lesions near cells of a particular type in penetration after penetration (see Text-Figs. 11 and 12 below). The penetration of Text-figs. 7 and 8 was exploratory, and lesions were not placed according to any particular plan.

In Text-figs. 7 and 8 the first nine cells were situated in layers II and III, lesion 1 marking the position of unit 9. Six of the nine cells were complex and, as in the cat, some showed highly asymmetrical responses to diametrically opposite directions of movement (cells 1 and 2), while the others showed no such directional preference. Cell 9 of this penetration was lower-order hypercomplex, and has already been illustrated in Text-fig. 3.

In layer IV A four complex cells were recorded, 10 and 11 responding best to dark bars, 12 and 13 to slits.

In IV B the fields of four successively recorded cells were simple in type. The second of these (unit 15) was marked by lesion 2. In three of the simple cells (14, 16, and 17) the long narrow excitatory region was most sensitive to light of long wavelengths, with hardly any responses in the green and blue, whereas the inhibitory flanks were most sensitive in the greens and blues with little response to red. It was as if these cells had received input only from a group of red on-centre green off-surround geniculate cells. In contrast to these opponent-colour cells, unit 15, whose field was similar geometrically, seemed identical to the usual simple cell in cat cortex, with no hint of opponent colour properties.

The remaining cells in this penetration were complex. The only one with remarkable colour

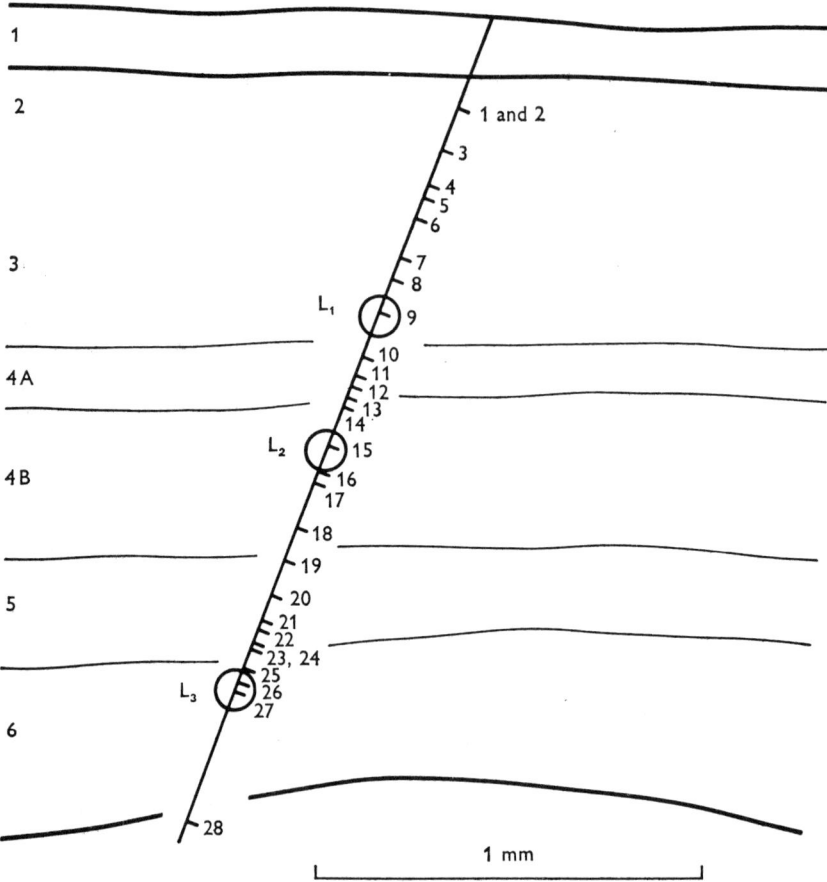

Fig. 7. Positions of twenty-eight units recorded in a single penetration through rhesus striate cortex. Positions of three lesions (L₁–L₃) are indicated by circles (see also Pl. 1 and Text-fig. 8).

features was No. 20, which lacked any opponent colour properties but favoured short wave-lengths strongly, as though it had its entire input from blue-sensitive cones.

The sequence of receptive field orientations seen in this penetration was less regular than in most, but as usual there were runs of cells in which the fields all had identical orientation, for example, cells 10, 11; 12–14; 16–18. At the beginning of the penetration, the sequence of cells 1–8 is of particular interest as an example of several small shifts of field orientation all in the same direction (see below).

Many of the cells in this penetration were driven from both eyes. Cells 1–17 were dominated by the left (contralateral) eye, except for No. 11, which favoured the right eye slightly; from 18 to 27 all cells favoured the right eye. The tendency for

neighbouring cells to favour the same eye was thus very pronounced, more so than is usual in the cat (Hubel & Wiesel, 1962).

This penetration illustrates several architectural features of the striate cortex which will be taken up in more detail in the remainder of the paper: (1) a tendency to aggregation of certain physiological cell types according to anatomical layering; (2) an aggregation of cells according to receptive field orientation; and (3) an independent clustering of cells according to eye dominance.

Vertical Organization

Given a set of properties of a cell, such as receptive-field position or orientation, eye preference, presence or absence of symmetry of responses to opposite directions of movement, colour coding, and so on, one can examine neighbouring cells to see

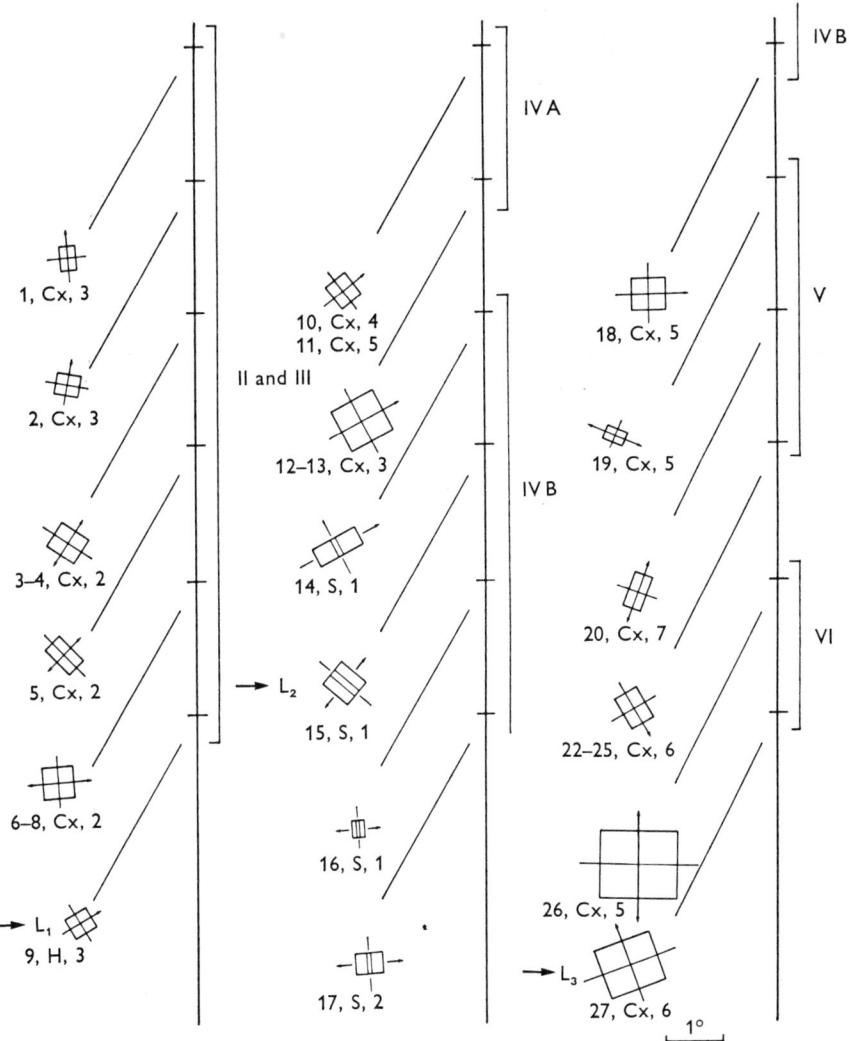

Fig. 8. Receptive-field diagrams for units recorded in the penetration of Text-fig. 7. Approximate positions and shapes of each field, referred to the fovea, are indicated by rectangles. Foveas are indicated separately for each field by the short horizontal lines intersecting the three long vertical lines. Responses to a moving line are shown for every field by arrows; a single arrowhead indicates strong directional preference. Square brackets refer to cortical layers. For each field the first number is the unit number; S, Cx and H mean simple, complex and hypercomplex; the last number refers to ocular-dominance groups. Cells of group 1 were driven only by the contralateral eye; for cells of group 2 there was marked dominance of the contralateral eye; for group 3, slight dominance. For cells in group 4 there was no obvious difference between the two eyes. In group 5 the ipsilateral eye dominated slightly; in group 6 markedly, and in group 7 the cells were driven only by the ipsilateral eye.

whether or not they share certain of these properties. If, for example, the same value of a stimulus variable is optimal for all cells in a small region, it can be asked whether that value changes steadily or in discrete steps as one progresses through the cortex. Where the steps are discrete one can try to discover the shape and extent of the regions.

In the visual cortex a number of variables remain unchanged, or at least show no systematic trend, in penetrations extending vertically from surface to white matter. The most fundamental are the two position co-ordinates by which the retinal surface is mapped on to the cortex. This mapping is continuous. Besides this, in the monkey striate cortex, as in that of the cat, each small area dealing with a particular part of the retina is subdivided by sets of vertical partitions into several independent systems of discrete cell aggregations. One of these systems is defined by receptive-field orientation, another by ocular dominance. It seems very likely that these aggregations are columnar, with walls parallel to the vertically running fibre bundles and perpendicular to the layering pattern. The evidence for this is chiefly that sequences of cells with common physiological characteristics tend to be long in penetrations that are perpendicular or almost perpendicular to the cortical surface, and short in oblique penetrations. In the cat the most direct evidence that aggregations were columnar in shape came from multiple closely spaced parallel penetrations in which a lesion was made at each change of receptive field orientation (Hubel & Wiesel, 1963). This type of experiment was not done in the monkey, but we have no reason to think that the results would be different.

Retinotopic Representation. Neighbouring cells in area 17 invariably have receptive fields in roughly the same part of the retina, and movement along the cortex corresponds to movement along the retina according to the well known retinotopic representation. We have not tried to make a detailed topographic mapping, but in a limited exploration of the dorsal convexity and ten or so additional penetrations through the buried calcarine fissure, our results agree well with Talbot & Marshall's early survey of the convexity (1941), and the subsequent extensive mapping by Daniel & Whitteridge (1961). This detailed topographic representation does not hold at a microscopic level. As in the cat (Hubel & Wiesel, 1962), the fields of successively recorded cells in a perpendicular track are not precisely superimposed: instead there is an irregular variation in field position from cell to cell, small enough so that the fields overlap, and large enough so that, in a perpendicular penetration with fifteen or twenty fields superimposed, the area covered is about 2–4 times that of the average receptive field. In a long oblique penetration one finds some drift in field position corresponding to the gross topography, but when the component of movement along the surface is only a millimetre or so, for the part of the cortex subserving regions of retina within about 5° of the fovea, the drift is considerably less than the

random staggering, and is obscured by it. In the peripheral retina the topographic representation becomes coarser, but to compensate for this the receptive fields become larger, and the situation is therefore similar.

This topographic representation does not by itself constitute a columnar system even though the retinal position co-ordinates remain virtually constant in a penetration perpendicular to the cortical surface. The term 'column' as first used by Mountcastle (1957) and as it is used here, refers to a discrete aggregation of cells, each aggregation being separated from its neighbours by vertical walls that intersect the surface (or a given layer) in a mosaic. In the retinotopic projection the representation is continuous; there are no sudden jumps as the surface is traversed. It is upon this continuous topographic map that the column-systems described below are engrafted.

Receptive-Field Orientation. Sequences of cells with identical receptive-field orientations can be seen in Text-figs. 8, 10, 11, and 12. The sequences tended to be shorter than in the cat, and penetrations in which the same orientation was maintained from surface to white matter were somewhat less common, occurring only when the track was normal to the cortical surface or almost so. An example can be seen in Fig. 12, penetration 1. Some idea of the cross-sectional size of a column can be obtained by projecting the distance spanned by a single sequence on to the cortical surface. This projected distance was seldom more than about ¼ mm, and most sequences were considerably shorter, an average being more like 0.1–0.2 mm (see Text-fig. 10).

Ordered Orientation Columns. In several experiments in the cat certain regions of the striate cortex seemed to be highly organized, with changes in orientation from column to column taking place in small regular progressive steps, all in the same direction, either clockwise or counterclockwise. Hints of such organization were seen in many penetrations in the monkey, but the sequences tended to be short. For example, in the first six cells of Text-fig. 7, five orientations are represented, each shifted about 20° clockwise compared with the previous. Following such a sequence there was often a shift of orientation in

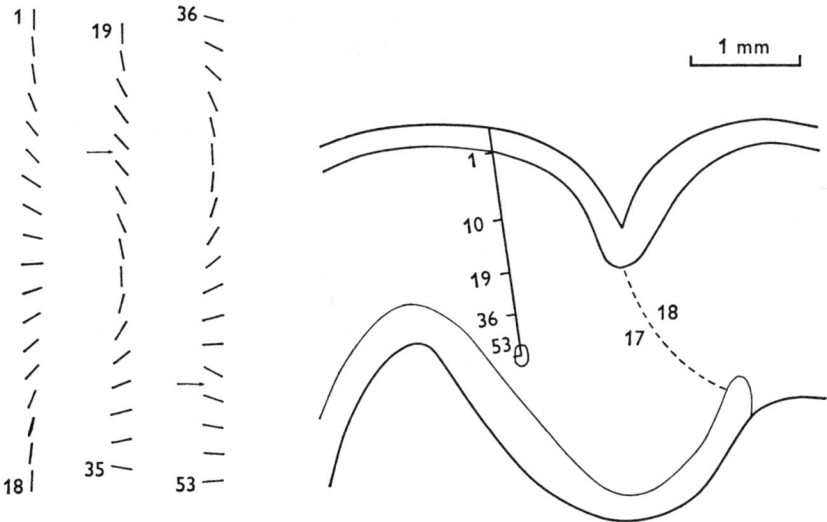

Fig. 9. Reconstruction of a penetration through striate cortex about 1 mm from 17–18 border, near occipital pole of spider monkey. To the left of the figure the lines indicate orientations of columns traversed; each line represents one or several units recorded against a rich unresolved background activity. Arrows indicate reversal of directions of shifts in orientation. Histological section through first part of this penetration is shown in Pl. 2.

the reverse direction, perhaps followed by a resumption of the sequence for a few more steps and then another similar interruption. Large shifts, of 45–90°, while not rare, were less common than small ones.

By far the most impressive example of orderly sequences was seen in one experiment in the spider monkey, illustrated in Text-fig. 9. The penetration entered area 17 very close to the 17–18 border, at an angle of about 30° to the normal. Fields of the first cells were oriented almost vertically. Subsequent cells and unresolved unit activity showed regular small shifts in orientation, consistently in a counter-clockwise direction, so that at a depth of about 1 mm, after eighteen shifts, the orientation had revolved through 180° and was again vertical. The progression continued in a counter-clockwise direction for another 45°, and then, at the point marked by the first arrow, the direction of shifts suddenly reversed. Now fifteen clockwise changes in orientation took place in the next 180°, followed by another ten clockwise shifts through almost another 180°. Finally, near the end, the process seemed to be reversing itself again, with counter-clockwise shifts beginning at the second arrow. There were, in all, 52 shifts in orientation, the smallest being about 6° and the largest around 20°,

and in the course of the penetration each orientation was represented about 4 times. The field positions of the final cells were in exactly the same place as those of the first, indicating that the distance traversed in a direction parallel to the surface had been too small to produce a measurable shift in receptive field position.

In this penetration the average shift was about 13°, associated with an average electrode movement of 40 μ, or, given the obliquity of 30°, a movement parallel to the cortical surface of 20 μ. From the higher-power photomicrograph of the cortex in the area of this penetration, shown in Pl. 2, 20 μ seems to be the order of magnitude of the widths of the vertical pallisades of cells in this area. The vertically orientated striations may thus represent the actual columns of cells, at least in this experiment, and the columns must have close to the minimum possible width, since the pallisades are only one or a very few cells wide. From this degree of orderliness and the probability that a similar order would have held for any direction of horizontal movement across the cortical surface, it seems likely that columns have the form of parallel sheets rather than pillars. In the cat this sort of geometry was also suggested in one surface-mapping experiment (Hubel & Wiesel, 1963, Text-fig. 4 and Pl. 2).

OCULAR DOMINANCE. In the monkey there was a marked tendency for successively recorded cells to have the same eye-preference (Text-figs. 8, 10, 11 and 12). Neighbouring cells did not necessarily fall into the same ocular-dominance group, but they usually favoured the same eye. Since there were several vertical penetrations from surface to white matter in which there was no change in eye preference, it is likely that the aggregations of cells are columnar. It is also evident that these regions of common eye-preference have nothing to do with orientation columns, the two systems apparently having entirely independent borders. Of the two types of columns, those associated with eye dominance seem to be larger, often including several orientation columns.

Aggregation of cells according to ocular dominance was first established in the cat striate cortex (Hubel & Wiesel, 1962; 1965b), but in the cat the organization was less clear cut, since, besides regions in which all cells had similar eye preference, there were regions of mixed allegiance, in which cells of all ocular-dominance groups, including group 4, were mingled. (For definitions of ocular-dominance groups see legend of Fig. 8.) These mixed regions tended to obscure the parcellation into columns in the cat (Hubel & Wiesel, 1962, p. 140), and indeed it was not until the columns had been accentuated by raising cats with strabismus that we became fully convinced of their existence (Hubel & Wiesel, 1965b). In the monkey the parcellation is far more obvious: the columns are possibly larger, mixed columns are racer if they exist at all, and cells of dominance groups 1, 2, 6 and 7 make up a larger proportion of the population.

DIRECTION OF MOVEMENT. As noted above, the monkey striate cortex resembles that of the cat in that complex cells tend to respond actively to a moving stimulus, with great cell-to-cell variation in directional selectivity—some firing actively to diametrically opposed directions, others responding to one direction and hardly at all to the other, and still others with various degrees of intermediate directional asymmetry. There is some intermixing between these groups, in that two simultaneously recorded cells are often driven by opposite directions of movement (Hubel, 1958). In the present series there nevertheless appeared to be some grouping of cells according to the presence or absence of directional preference. In most penetrations there were sequences, sometimes long ones, in which all cells showed strong directional preference, followed by sequences in which the cells all responded well to both directions of movement. This is seen in Text-fig. 10, which illustrates a penetration cutting across a gyrus in the spider monkey. Cells 1–5, 13–20, 23–27, 30–33, were all bidirectional, whereas those of sequence 6–12 were unidirectional. There may thus be another independent, perhaps columnar system of cortical subdivisions, this one dependent on symmetric vs. asymmetric responses to movement.

Finally, there was some indication of a grouping of cells according to their preference for stimulus form—slits, edges, or dark bars. Colour coded cells similarly often came in clusters. The shape of the aggregations for these systems is not clear: they could be nests or columns.

Horizontal Organization

The most conspicuous anatomical feature of the striate cortex is its rich layering—indeed it was so named for that reason. From the outset it has been clear that there are differences from layer to layer in the physiological properties of cells in area 17. These differences are more prominent than in the cat, just as the histological differences in layers are more prominent. In five experiments done specifically to investigate the layering differences, fourteen penetrations were made, six through the full cortical thickness and eight to the 4th layer. Two experiments, to be discussed in more detail below, are illustrated in Text-figs. 11 and 12, and the results from all rhesus experiments are tabulated in the histograms of Text-figs. 13 and 14.

RECEPTIVE FIELD ORGANIZATION. In the second layer and upper part of the third almost all of the cells were complex or hypercomplex, and as a rule the optimum stimulus orientation was precisely defined. We found no simple cells in layer II, and in III they occurred only in the deepest parts, close to IV. On entering this border zone and crossing into upper IV the first simple cells appeared, hypercomplex cells were no longer seen, and in complex cells the orientation specificity began to relax, with brisk responses over a wider range of orientations to either side of the optimum, but still no response at 90° to the optimum.

Usually in IV A, but sometimes only on entering IV B, a sudden change took place in the unresolved background activity: it became more prominent, higher in pitch, and lost all trace of orientation preference. Text-figure 11 and Pl. 3 illustrate an experiment done expressly to determine the depth at which the background lost its orientation specificity. In each penetration this point was marked by a lesion, shown as a filled circle. All lesions were in IV A or near the IV A–IV B border. A similar experiment, with the same outcome, is illustrated in Text-fig. 12. Here the points of appearance of non-oriented background are shown to the left of each penetration by open circles.

Throughout IV B there was a mixture of simple cells and units which lacked orientation specificity. This was the layer with the fewest complex units and the most non-oriented ones (Text-fig. 13). In V and VI the background again became selectively responsive to specifically oriented lines, and

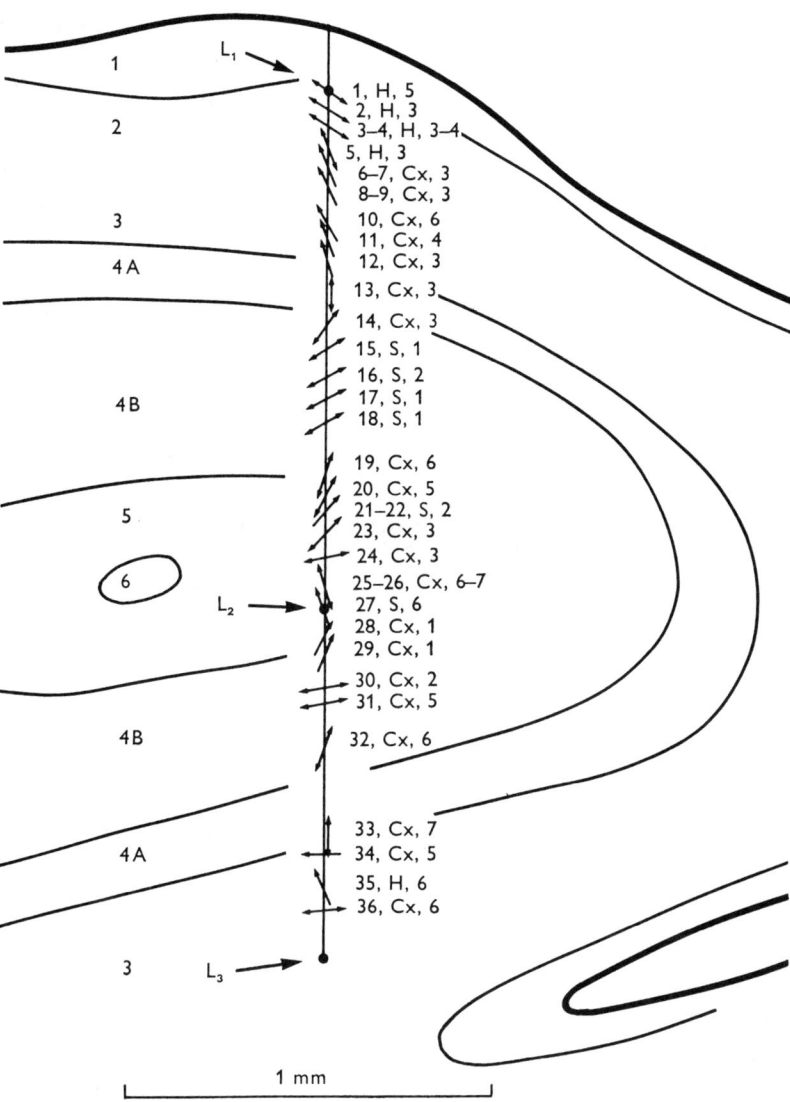

Fig. 10. Reconstruction of an oblique penetration through striate cortex of spider monkey. This experiment indicates laminar grouping of cells according to complexity, and aggregation according to orientation, directionality of movement, and ocular-dominance. As in Text-fig. 8, 19 Cx 6 means 'Unit 19, complex, ocular-dominance group 6'.

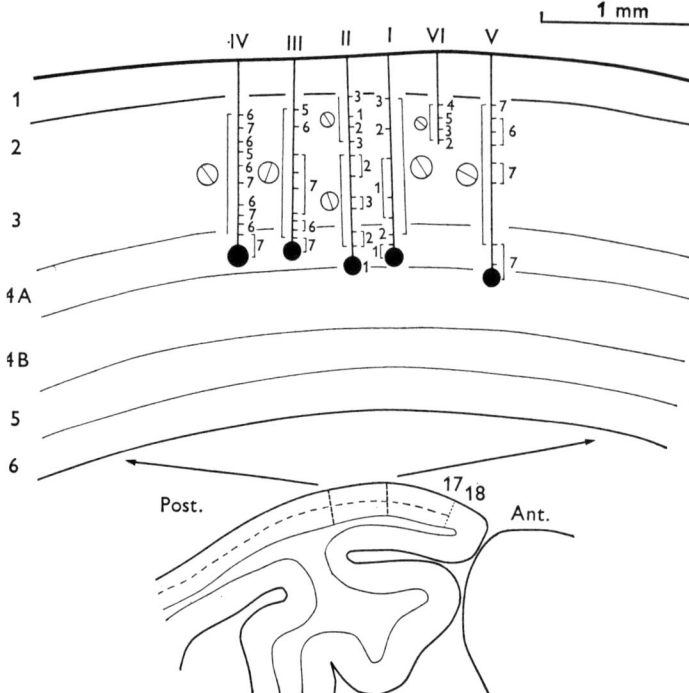

Fig. 11. Six closely spaced parallel penetrations through rhesus striate cortex made to determine the layer in which background and some units lacked orientation specificity, and in which most cells were driven by one eye exclusively. Lesion made in these regions are indicated by black circles. Lines within the open circles indicate optimum stimulus orientation. Numbers to right of each penetration refer to ocular dominance group of each isolated unit.

the units were mainly complex, with some hyper-complex ones intermixed.

Some of these laminar differences in field types are illustrated also in Text-fig. 10.

BINOCULAR INTERACTION. One marked difference between layers was related to binocular interaction. This is illustrated in the histograms of Text-fig. 14, and in Text-figs. 11 and 12. At the beginning of a typical penetration one eye or the other was consistently dominant, and through layer II and most or all of III one encountered a mixture of cells in groups 2 and 3 with a few from group 1, or else a mixture of 5 and 6 with an occasional group 7. At some stage, usually in upper IV, but occasionally as deep as the border of IV A and IV B, the eye that had been non-dominant would drop out completely, and through the remainder of layer IV cell after cell would be in group 1 instead of 2 or 3, or group 7 instead of 5 or 6. This was just the point at which the background became poorly oriented (i.e. the regions marked by lesions in Text-figs. 11 and 12). Simple cells recorded here were almost always groups 1 or 7, but a few exceptions were seen in groups 2 and 6 and there was a single group 4 simple cell. In penetrations that extended through

most of the cortical thickness, binocularly driven units remained scarce as layer IV was traversed, but reappeared abruptly in layer V, and persisted throughout V and VI.

Finally, ocular-dominance differed markedly with cell type (Text-fig. 14). This is not surprising since both ocular dominance and cell type tended to vary from layer to layer. There was an increase in binocular interaction in going from simple to complex and from complex to hypercomplex, with groups 1 and 7 becoming rarer, and the intermediate groups more common. But in general cells driven equally by the two eyes were less common in the monkey than in the cat, most monkey cells falling in groups 1, 2, 6 and 7. The ocular-dominance distribution of cells in the cat is closer to that of monkey area 18, than to monkey 17 (unpublished). These results suggest that in monkey striate cortex impulses from the two eyes probably converge not so much on the simple cell, as occurs in the cat, but chiefly on the complex cell.

DISCUSSION

From this and previous studies it is clear that any small region of the striate cortex analyses some

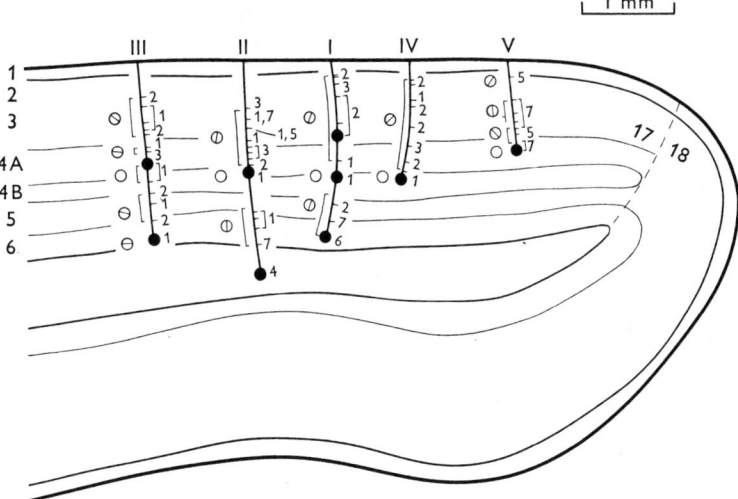

Fig. 12. *Five close-spaced penetrations in rhesus area 17. Open circles indicate a lack of background orientation specificity; other conventions as in Text-fig. 11.*

small part of the visual field in terms of the direction of light-dark contours (in particular, the tangent to the contour lines), a detection of movement of the contours, a registration of the type of contour (light against dark, edge, and the like), and, at the hypercomplex level, a detection of any change in direction (curvature) of the contours. At any one time only a small proportion of cells are likely to be influenced (activated or suppressed), since contours of inappropriate orientation and diffuse light have little or no effect on a cell.

Hypercomplex cells, which we had thought occurred only in 18 and 19 in the cat, turn out to be fairly common in 17, both in cat and monkey. Presumably in early studies their presence was not detected because they gave no response to a line that was too long, or perhaps they were classed as complex when they responded well to a line that happened to be the correct length. For these cells the proportion responding to a given contour must be extremely small, since even an appropriately oriented line is ineffective if it maintains that orientation over too great a distance.

The elaboration of simple cortical fields from geniculate concentric fields, complex from simple, and hypercomplex from complex is probably the prime function of the striate cortex—unless there are still other as yet unidentified cells there. One need not assume, of course, that the output consists entirely of the axons of hypercomplex cells, the

other types being merely interposed as links between input and output. We know, for example, that in the cat the posterior corpus callosum contains axons of all three cell types (Hubel & Wiesel, 1967).

A second function of the striate cortex concerns the convergence upon single cells of input from the two eyes. At the geniculate level any binocular interaction must be relatively subtle, since no one has yet mapped out receptive fields in the two eyes for a single geniculate cell, as can be done routinely for cortical cells. In the cortex stimulation of both eyes in corresponding parts of the receptive fields usually gives a greater response than stimulation of either eye alon. In the monkey as in the cat, this convergence takes a special form in which the influence of the two eyes is combined in varying proportions in different cells. Indeed, in the monkey the process of amalgamation of the two inputs is further delayed, so that interaction is minimal for simple cells, distinctly more for complex, and possibly still more for hypercomplex.

Given that contour analysis and binocular convergence are two prime functions of striate cortex, the parallel and independent manner in which the processes are carried out by this structure is worth noting. For both functions columns are the units of organization. In a given 'eye-preference' column one eye is emphasized, in the next the other eye. In a superimposed but quite independent sys-

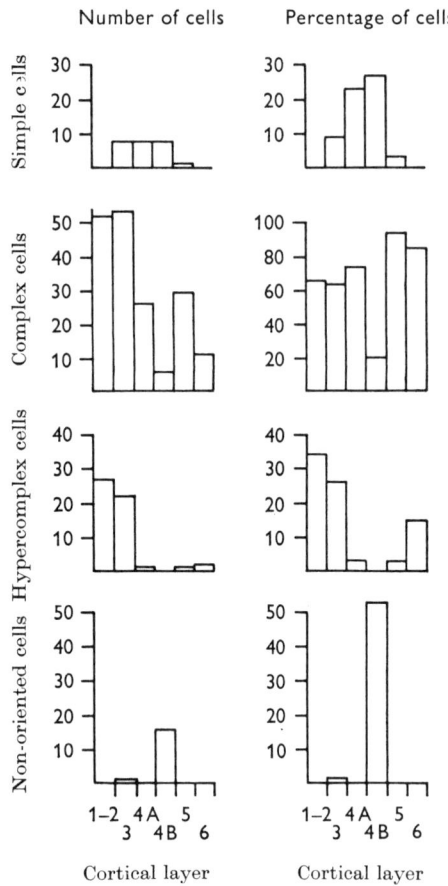

Fig. 13. Histograms of 272 cortical cells showing numbers of the different cell categories, in each layer. Only the cells from rhesus monkeys are included. In the right-hand set of histograms, cells are expressed as a percentage of the total number in a given layer.

tem, one 'orientation' column subserves one orientation, another column a different one. In both types of column the contour analysis and binocular convergence occur in a vertically interconnected system of layers, with the earliest stages in IV B, the latest ones in II and III, and probably also in V and VI. Thus IV B is made up chiefly of simple cells and units (possibly afferent fibres) that show no orientation preference, and these are almost all monocularly driven, whereas in II and III one finds complex and hypercomplex cells, mostly binocularly driven. This difference by layers in complexity of responses and in binocular interaction is entirely consistent with the Golgi type anatomy of Cajal (1911) and Lorente de Nó (1943), since in

terms of connexions cells of layer IV are closest to the input, and the upper and lower layers are furthest away. It is hardly surprising that physiologically the populations of individual layers are not pure, in view of the mixture of morphological cell types in each layer, and the presence of axons passing up and down from other layers. In the cat the layering is less distinct, and the tendency for each layer to contain a mixture of cell types seems to be greater—in any case the physiological evidence for segregation of different cell types in different layers, while suggestive in the cat (Hubel & Wiesel, 1962), was not nearly as clear as in the monkey. The present demonstration of a clear difference in function between cells in different cortical layers is, of course, only a first step toward the goal of correlating histologically defined cell types with function.

The form taken by the two systems of columns deserves some comment. The existence of regions in which orientation columns are highly ordered continues to be baffling, for if there are two kinds of striate cortex, one ordered and the other not, the anatomy gives no hint of this. There is a suggestion that the narrow orderly columns may sometimes correspond to the radial fascicles seen microscopically, but these are seen everywhere in 17, and the ordered regions seem not to be present everywhere. Where columns are ordered, it seems likely that they are very long narrow slabs, perhaps not straight, but swirling, if one can judge from the reversals in shifts seen in Text-fig. 9. It is possible that these ordered regions may be more common than we realize, for their detection depends on rather ideal recording conditions in which the electrode moves forward steadily rather than in jumps, and records activity at all times. The possible purpose served by such an ordered system of columns has been discussed elsewhere (Hubel & Wiesel, 1963).

In view of the recent work of Campbell & Kulikowski (1966) showing a difference in ability of humans to discriminate between horizontal or vertical lines and oblique lines, we have looked for any differences in the occurrence of horizontally and vertically oriented fields as opposed to oblique fields, but have seen none, in cat or in monkey. The problem is presumably one of comparing the frequency or size of the various orientation columns, and our series is doubtless too small to permit this, especially if one wishes to detect a difference of a

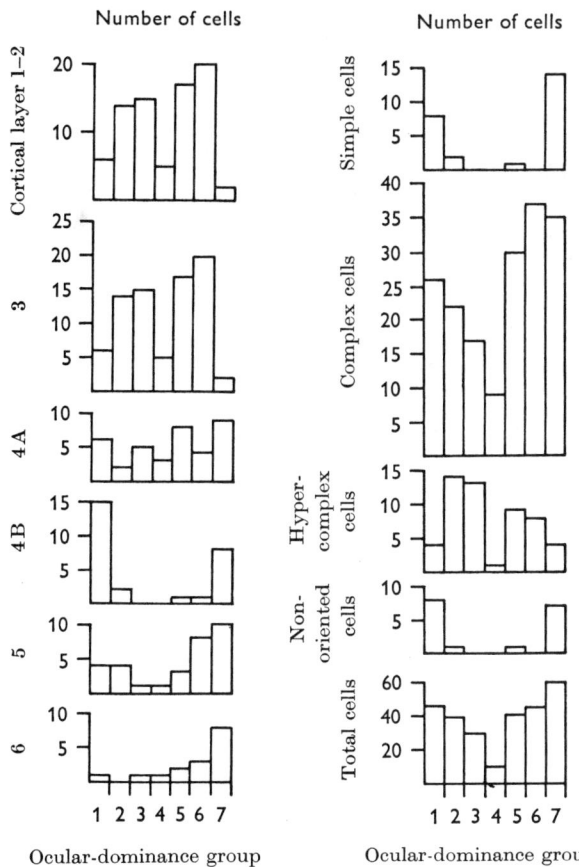

Fig. 14. Left: Distribution of 272 rhesus cells among the various layers according to ocular-dominance group. Right: Distribution of 272 cells among the different cell-classes, according to ocular-dominance group.

few per cent. At least it is clear that horizontal and vertical orientations are not many times more common than others.

In the binocular columnar system the columns seem to be coarser, and take a special form. At the level of layer IV B there is a mosaic of alternating left-eye and right-eye representation, each apparently almost pure. This presumably simply reflects the tendency for afferents to the cortex to be grouped (Hubel & Wiesel, 1965*b*), as is so for the columns of the somatosensory cortex described by Mountcastle (1957). As the visual input is transmitted over several stages to the more complex cells in the upper and lower layers, there must be progressively more intermixing between the eyes, presumably by interconnexions that run obliquely. The columns nevertheless remain discrete, with almost all cells in one column favouring one eye, though no longer dominated completely by it. There do not seem to be regions of mixed dominance, as one finds

in the cat. For the binocular columns the physiological evidence thus indicates that there is some interchange between one column and its immediate neighbours, minimal in layer IV, but increasing in the superficial and deep layers. (By definition two adjacent binocular columns must favour opposite eyes.) This is in sharp contrast to the orientation columns, since for these there is no evidence to suggest any cross talk between one column and its immediately adjoining neighbours. There is of course no reason why an orientation column should not have rich connexions with another column of identical field orientation even though the two may be separated by as many as 15–18 different columns. Indeed, if eye-preference columns are interconnected, and if one eye-preference column does contain many orientation columns, then the interconnexions must be highly specific, one orientation column being connected to another some distance away. These suggestions depend of course on rather indirect inferences from physiological experiments, but they may have some value in indicating certain patterns of connexions to look for with morphological techniques.

If there are indications that the orientation columns take the form of parallel pillars, or, in more ordered areas, parallel slabs, we have no hints at all about the shape of the eye-preference columns. They differ from the orientation columns in being of just two types, instead of more than a dozen, and the two should be about equally prominent, given the lack of any marked dominance of one eye or other in the cortex as a whole. One would therefore expect a patchwork of alternating columns like a checker board, or a confluent matrix of one type with pillars of the other type embedded within it, or a series of parallel slabs. These possibilities are mentioned here because the term 'column' itself implies a series of pillar-like structures, which is probably the least likely form in this case.

The columnar system seems to represent a method by which many areas of cortex—somatosensory (Mountcastle, 1957) visual, including 17, 18 and 19, and perhaps motor (Asanuma & Sakata, 1967)—deal with multi-dimensional problems using a two-dimensional surface. In the visual system the two co-ordinates of the visual field are mapped on the two surface co-ordinates; other variables, notably line orientation, eye dominance, possibly movement directionality, are handled by subdividing this surface into overlapping mosaics which are independent, just as the picture of a jigsaw puzzle is independent of the borders separating the pieces. With two such mosaics known and a third suspected, it will not be surprising if more are found in the future.

To conclude, it is easy to draw up a large list of gaps still to be filled in our understanding of this structure. To mention only a few, the binocular interaction we have described tells us nothing about mechanisms for handling stereoscopic depth perception. Bishop's group in Sydney and Barlow's in California have evidence for horizontal non-correspondence of some cells in cat area 17, and the relation of these to the binocular mechanisms described here for the monkey will be most interesting. Our knowledge of cortical colour mechanisms is still very sketchy. Anatomically one is just beginning to understand the layering of the cortex, and some features, such as the significance of layers

I, V and VI are still a complete mystery. At a synaptic level the correlation of structure with physiology, as is now being done in the retina (Dowling & Boycott, 1966), is still lacking in the cortex. The part, if any, that area 17 plays in attention mechanisms in conscious animals is completely obscure. But despite the large areas still unexplored, in broad outline the function of area 17 is probably now relatively well understood. One knows roughly how the output differs from the input, and it is possible to make guesses that can be tested concerning the circuits that underly these transformations. Knowing what image is falling on the retina at any given moment, one can predict with some confidence what most types of cells will be doing.

Specialized as the cells of 17 are, compared with rods and cones, they must, nevertheless, still represent a very elementary stage in the handling of complex forms, occupied as they are with a relatively simple region-by-region analysis of retinal contours. How this information is used at later stages in the visual path is far from clear, and represents one of the most tantalizing problems for the future.

We thank Janet Wiitanen for her excellent technical assistance. This work was supported by N.I.H. Research Grants, Nos. 5 RO 1 NB 02260 and 5 RO 1 NB 05554.

References

Asanuma, H. & Sakata, H. (1967). Functional organization of a cortical efferent system examined with focal depth stimulation in cats. *J. Neurophysiol.* **30**, 35–54.

Brodmann, K. (1909). *Vergleichende Lokalisationslehre der Grosshirnrinde.* Leipzig: J. A. Barth.

Cajal, S. Ramon Y (1911). *Histologie du système nerveux de l'homme et des vertébrés,* vol. 2. Paris: Maloine.

Campbell, F. W. & Kulikowski, J. J. (1966). Orientational selectivity of the human visual system. *J. Physiol.* **187**, 437–445.

Daniel, P. M. & Whitteridge, D. (1961). The representation of the visual field on the cerebral cortex in monkeys. *J. Physiol.* **159**, 203–221.

Daw, N. W. (1967). Color coded units in the goldfish retina. Ph.D. Thesis, Johns Hopkins University, Baltimore.

De Valois, R. L., Jacobs, G. H. & Jones, A. E. (1963). Responses of single cells in primate red-green color vision system. *Optik* **20**, 87–98.

Dowling, J. E. & Boycott, B. B. (1966). Organization of the primate retina: electron microscopy. *Proc. R. Soc.* B **166**, 80–111.

Hubel, D. H. (1957). Tungsten microelectrode for recording from single units. *Science, N.Y.* **125**, 549–550.

Hubel, D. H. (1958). Cortical unit responses to visual stimuli in nonanesthetized cats. *Am. J. Ophthal.* **46**, 110–121.

Hubel, D. H. (1959). Single unit activity in striate cortex of unrestrained cats. *J. Physiol.* **147**, 226–238.

Hubel, D. H. & Wiesel, T. N. (1959). Receptive fields of single neurones in the cat's striate cortex. *J. Physiol.* **148**, 574–591.

Hubel, D. H. & Wiesel, T. N. (1960). Receptive fields of optic nerve fibres in the spider monkey. *J. Physiol.* **154**, 572–580.

Hubel, D. H. & Wiesel, T. N. (1962). Receptive fields, binocular interaction and functional architecture in the cat's visual cortex. *J. Physiol.* **160**, 106–154.

Hubel, D. H. & Wiesel, T. N. (1963). Shape and arrangement of columns in cat's striate cortex. *J. Physiol.* **165**, 559–568.

Hubel, D. H. & Wiesel, T. N. (1965a). Receptive fields and functional architecture in two non-striate visual areas (18 and 19) of the cat. *J. Neurophysiol.* **28**, 229–289.

Hubel, D. H. & Wiesel, T. N. (1965b). Binocular interaction in striate cortex of kittens reared with artificial squint. *J. Neurophysiol.* **28**, 1041–1059.

Hubel, D. H. & Wiesel, T. N. (1967). Cortical and callosal connections concerned with the vertical meridian of visual fields in the cat. *J. Neurophysiol.* (In the Press.)

Lorente de Nó, R. (1943). Cerebral cortex: architecture, intra-cortical connections, motor projections. In *Physiology of the Nervous System,* ed. Fulton, J. F., 2nd edn., pp. 274–301. New York: Oxford University Press.

Motokawa, K., Taira, N. & Okuda, J. (1962). Spectral responses of single units in the primate visual cortex. *Tohoku J. exp. Med.* **78**, 320–337.

Mountcastle, V. B. (1957). Modality and topographic properties of single neurons in cat's somatic sensory cortex. *J. Neurophysiol.* **20**, 408–434.

Talbot, S. A. & Marshall, W. H. (1941). Physiological studies on neural mechanisms of visual localization and discrimination. *Am. J. Ophthal.* **24**, 1255–1263.

von Bonin, G. (1942). The striate area of primates. *J. comp. Neurol.* **77**, 405–429.

Wiesel, T. N. & Hubel, D. H. (1966). Spatial and chromatic interactions in the lateral geniculate body of the rhesus monkey. *J. Neurophysiol.* **29**, 1115–1156.

AFTERWORD

This paper represents a first attempt to survey physiologically the monkey striate cortex. Since 1968 our knowledge has greatly expanded with regard to of the properties of the cells in the different layers. End-stopping has been discovered to be present in monkey striate cortex, the geometry of the two main types of columns (orientation and ocular dominance) has been determined, and more of the color properties have been worked out. It was not until around 1980 that the blobs were discovered, together with their relation to the double opponent cells that were so briefly mentioned in the 1968 paper. There have been some disagreements as to the existence of blobs and the existence of double opponent cells in V-1. Fortunately, the case for the latter has now been well established through the combined use, by Bevil Conway, of reverse correlation receptive-field mapping and cone-isolation techniques.

Columns

Our missing the blobs in all the early years of exploring the monkey striate cortex has long been a puzzle to us, and probably also the the rest of the world of cortical neurophysiology. When, around 1980, blobs were first drawn to our attention by Margaret Wong Riley, who sent us slides of cytochrome-oxidase stained transverse sections, we were mystified, did not know what to make of them, and tried to forget them. We thought they probably had something to do with ocular dominance columns (as indeed was so), but it was only on seeing tangential sections that we realized that they could not be dominance columns and must be something quite new. Then a graduate student, Jonathan Horton, and I reconstructed tangential electrode tracks through upper-layer monkey striate cortex, stained for cytochrome oxidase, and found that the blobs coincided with regions of center-surround non-oriented cells. That we missed these structures for so long must at least partly be related to our custom of making vertical penetrations through the cortex. On examining old protocols it seems clear that

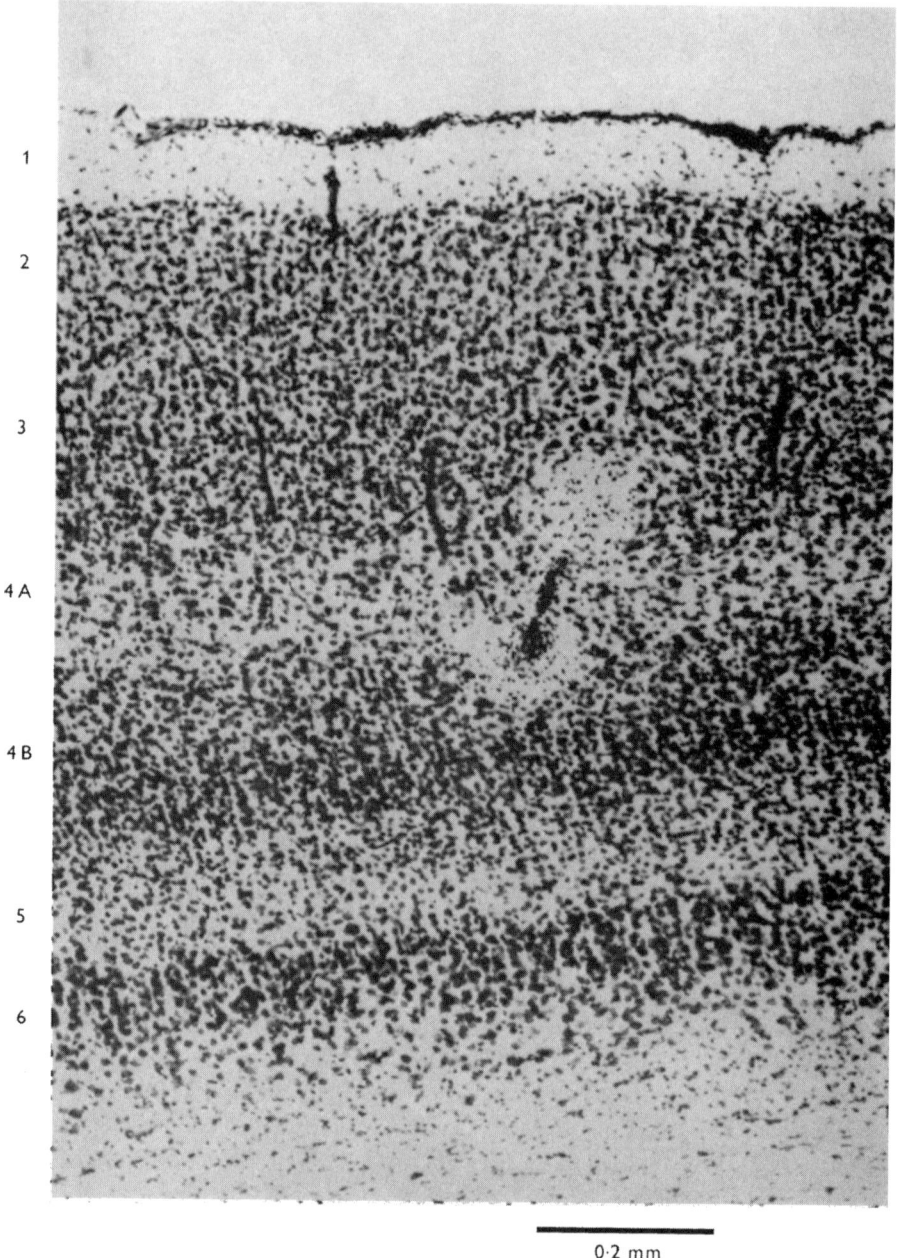

0·2 mm

Plate 1. Nissl-stained section corresponding to the experiment of Text-figs. 7 and 8, showing part of penetration and two lesions. Layers are indicated to left.

we had gone through blobs at times but attributed the lack of orientation selectivity to local damage. Today the evidence for blobs—their identification with lack of orientation selectivity and color selectivity—has been confirmed in many laboratories, but still some prominent workers have failed to find them. Neurophysiology is surely not the easiest of fields!

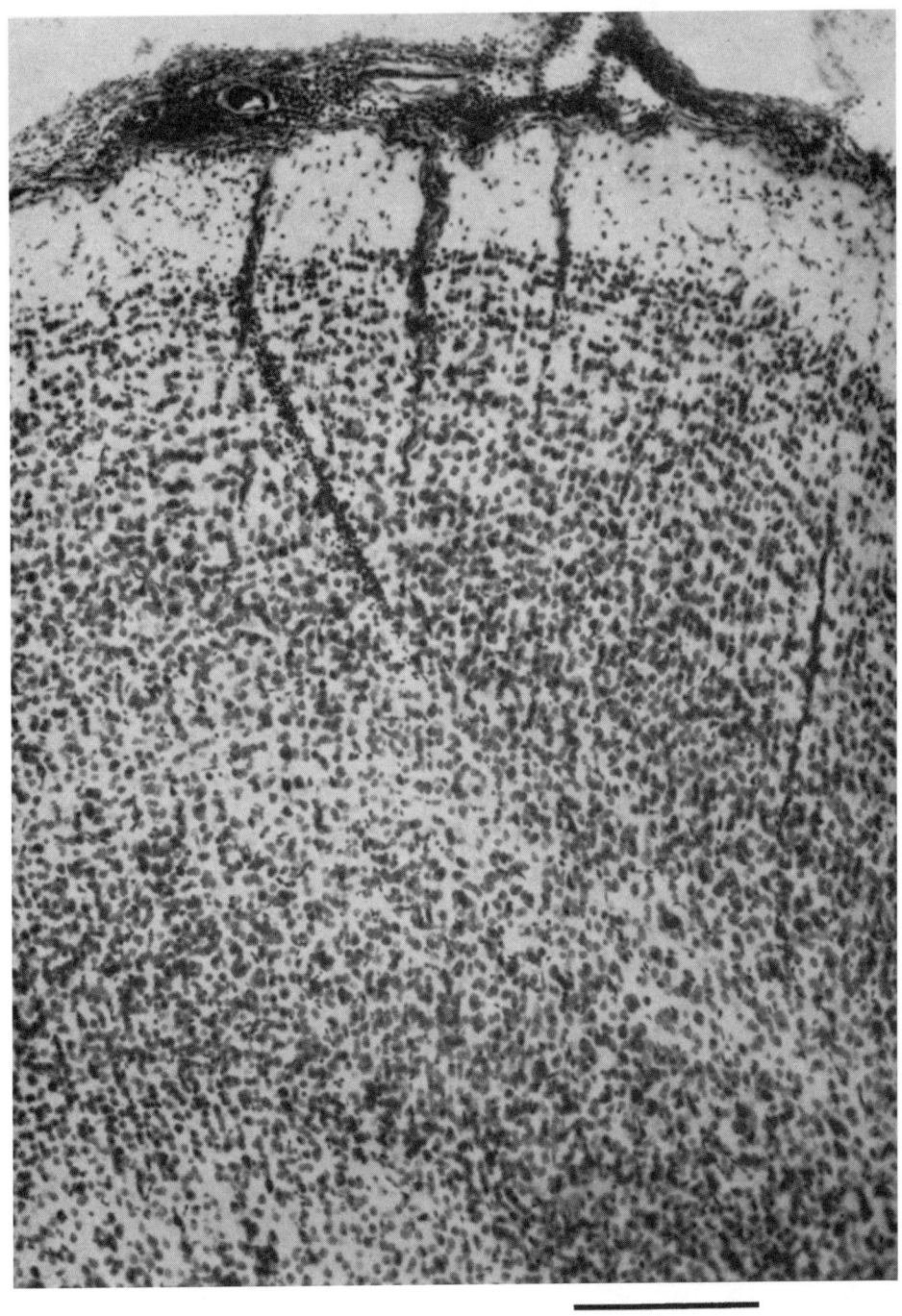

0·2 mm

Plate 2. Nissl-stained section through the electrode track of Text-fig. 9, showing first part of the track outlined by inflammatory reaction.

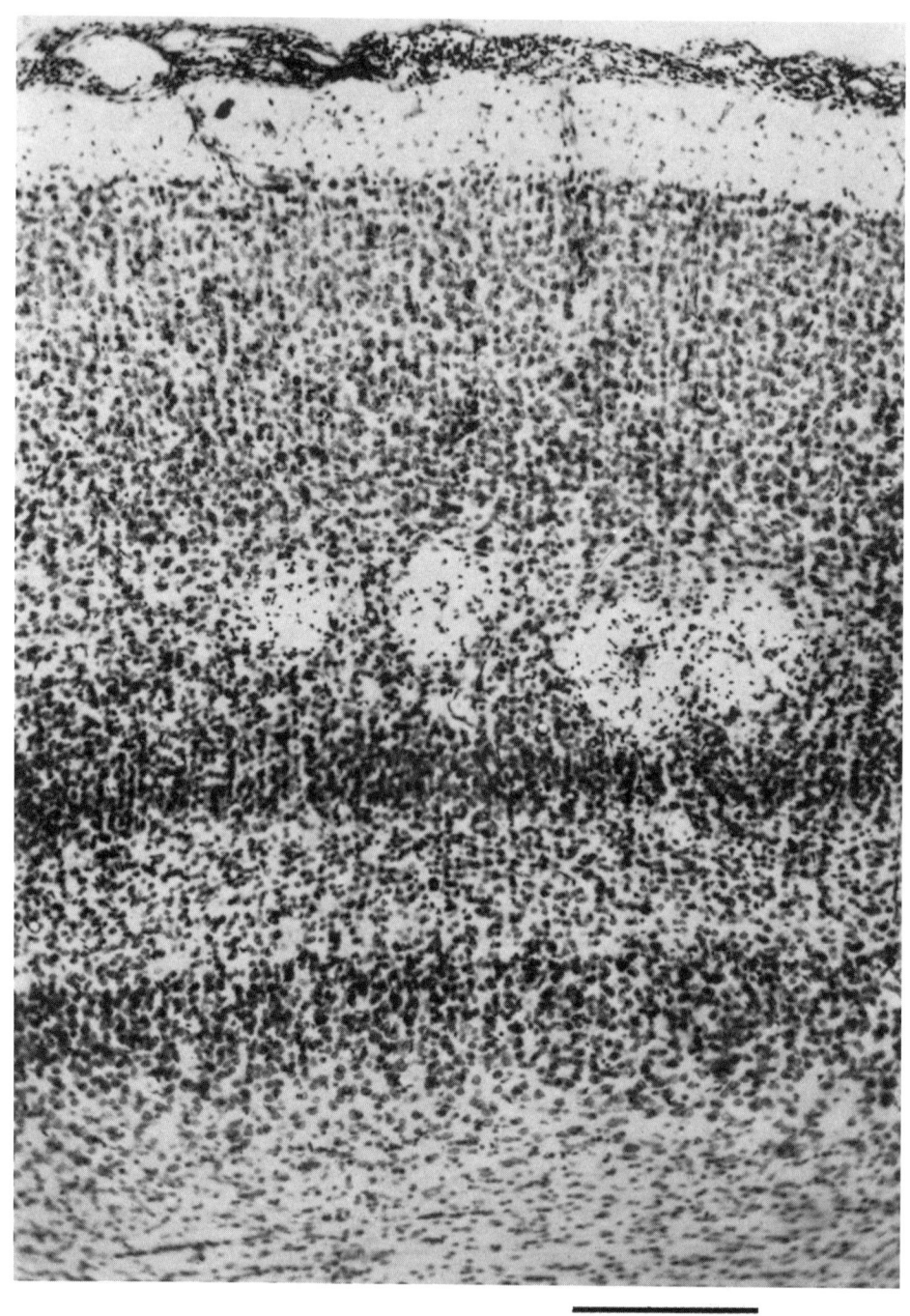

0·2 mm

Plate 3. Nissl section showing four of the five lesions of Text-fig. 11.

Ocular dominance columns, described in this paper in detail for the first time, were much easier to study in macaques than in cats, because they are so much better defined. In cats we only became convinced of their existence when we brought up kittens with artificial squint, which leads to a marked sharpening of their borders. In macaques there is much less mixing of inputs from the two eyes near the borders of columns, so that the transitions, as an electrode advances parallel to the surface, are far more abrupt. The abruptness is especially marked in layer 4C, in which the cells are monocular. Our physiological studies, in both cats and macaques, were done before we began to apply the anatomical methods that put ocular dominance columns on a firmer footing. Those studies are described in the next few papers.

In 1968 we were puzzled by how rarely we saw regions of highly ordered orientation shifts. We had the one overwhelming example of Figure 9 of the present paper, in a spider monkey named George. That memorable recording session lasted five hours, during which neither of us budged from our seats. We had previously seen a few examples that were less compelling, and in most penetrations we had seen little trace of such order. The reasons are now clear, and we have abundant physiological evidence that order is the rule, and breaks in the order are the exception. It is much easier to see the regularity if one makes very oblique microelectrode penetrations, and it is easiest if one uses electrodes that not too selective, so that one can see and hear a continuous background of undifferentiated activity as the electrode is advanced, in addition to a succession of occasional well isolated cells. Very selective electrodes give nice big well-isolated impulse deflections, but size and isolation are not so important when looking at properties that are shared by neighboring cells, such as optimum orientation. To struggle to obtain large isolated units is important for impressing visitors but can be carried too far. Perhaps our gravest early mistake in looking for order was in not realizing how useful it is to plot orientation against position along the cortex. Very selective electrodes record cells only here and there, and only by plotting the points does one realize that they usually fall along a straight-line trajectory. We did this plotting for George, our monkey of Figure 9, though in that case it was hardly necessary because the electrode happened to be relatively unselective. (Since 1985, with the advent of optical mapping, the evidence for order has become still more compelling.)

Our disdain of quantification and graph plotting had some advantages, including the freeing up of time, but on some occasions it could be a hindrance!

Layering

Cell properties in relation to layering presented some of the most difficult problems. In this paper we have almost nothing to say about the deeper layers, 5 and 6, partly because so many of our penetrations left off before we ever got that deep. We could have plunged in and started observing cells halfway down, but being human we always found it hard to forge ahead when we were recording nice big juicy cells. We could have doggedly kept on to the white matter, but we needed sleep, and never worked in relays or carried experiments over to the next day. It is not just that we were lazy: it was important to be sure of recovering the anatomy, and we hated to take chances on the animal dying before we could perfuse it.

We still have little to say about properties of cells in the very thin geniculate-recipient layer 4A (to use modern terminology). In 1968 we had no idea of this layer's existence, which only became clear as a result of our 1972 study of geniculate afferents using the Nauta method, and our subsequent autoradiographic studies. (Recent recordings by Chatterjee and Callaway, made in V-1 of monkeys in which mucimol was used to inactivate the cells, have shown that geniculate blue-yellow afferent fibers end in layer 4A and deep 3, whereas red-green afferents end only in deeper layers. [*Nature*, in press]). Layer 4B, now known to be the layer to which cells in the upper part of 4C project (layer 4C-alpha) and hence a continuation of the magnocellular path, seems to contain mainly complex cells, many of which are highly selective to movement direction, and many of which are sharply selective for binocular disparity.

In monkeys one of the biggest surprises was the center-surround organization of a large proportion of cells in layer 4. In cats, units with center-surround fields had been common, but we convinced ourselves these were geniculate afferent fibers. In the macaque things were more difficult. In 1968 we had no idea that the upper and lower halves of 4C received inputs from the magno and parvo geniculate subdivisions—that first became clear when we began our anatomical work around 1972 (see below). The units recorded from the deeper half of layer 4C were tiny and the spike shape was hard to assess. And unlike records from cats, in which the background unresolved activity is always orientation-selective, records from deep layer 4 of macaques (4C-beta) showed no hint of orientation selectivity. It was a surprise to learn that monkeys differed so markedly from cats, in having an interpolated stage of cortical cells lacking orientation selectivity. Gradually the consistent lack of any hint of orientation selectivity in layer 4C-beta convinced us of this extra stage, but at the time of the paper we were still undecided.

Though it is fairly clear that the units we recorded from 4C-beta were cells, and not afferent fibers, amazingly little is known even today about them. We do not know to what extent they resemble or differ from the parvocellular geniculate cells that feed this layer. They have concentric center-surround fields and the centers are tiny, but we do not know how many are type 1 or type 2 or 3. At present both parvocellular geniculate cells and cells of cortical 4C-beta are suffering from neglect.

We had a hard time learning the properties of cells in the upper half of layer 4c (4c alpha), probably because we were using Nissl stained sections to reconstruct our electrode tracks, and we now know that in Nissl material the border between this layer and 4b is not well defined. The border is more sharply defined in a cytochrome oxidase stain, and we have learned that it coincides with the upper margin of the projection of the magnocellular geniculate cells. This has made it far easier to relate track reconstructions to layers, and in subsequent anatomically controlled recordings, Margaret Livingstone and I found that this uppermost half of 4c contains a mixture of center-surround cells and well-oriented simple cells (*J Neurosci* 1984, 4:309–356). All this suggests that the magnocellular stream of macaques may be in some ways homologous with the geniculo-cortical projection in cats, in which the path proceeds directly from geniculate center-surround cells to cortical orientation selective simple cells, without having a second center-surround stage interposed—as one finds in the monkey parvocellular stream. If so, we wonder what, in the cat, corresponds to the monkey parvocellular system

We have, strangely, seen little suggestion of similarities between cells in 4c-alpha and the geniculate magnocellular cells that feed them, with their peculiar color properties and sustained surround responses.

Examples of simple cells in monkey striate cortex have been clear and plentiful, but the clearest examples we have seen have been in layer 4B. The prevailing evidence had until recently indicated that 4B received its main input from 4C-alpha, and must therefore be part of the magnocellular stream. Yet results by Sawatari and Callaway (*Nature* 1996, 380:442–446) suggest that some cells in layer 4B receive a substantial parvocellular input. In the parvocellular stream we would have expected to find simple cells in the deep part of layer 3, since it is here that cells of 4C-beta had been thought mainly to project. Simple cells of layer 4B need to be re-examined physiologically for signs of parvocellular input, such as color opponency.

Color

In the upper cortical layers, in addition to the massively preponderant group of cells that lack overt color coding, we have two major types of *overtly* color-coded cells, that respond best to specific sets of wavelengths, and often do not respond to white light. First, we have the orientation-selective color selective cells. In their orientation selectivity these relatively rare cells resemble the much more common non-color-coded complex or hypercomplex (end-stopped) cells, with their high spatial precision. They show marked color selectivity, responding selectively to a single group of wavelengths—long, middle, or short—and often give little or no response to white light. Most of the examples we have seen (perhaps 10 to 20 over 30 years or so) have preferred red slits, rather than green or blue.

Second, in this paper we identified double opponent cells for the first time in mammals, following their discovery by Nigel Daw in the goldfish retina. This foreshadowed results that were obtained in our separate laboratories, in cytochrome oxidase blobs, which is where these double opponent cells are lodged (Livingstone and Hubel, *J Neurosci* 1984, 4:309–356; Ts'o and Gilbert, *J Neurosci* 1988, 8(5):1712–1727). Blobs also contain center-surround cells that lack color coding but resemble double-opponent cells in having rather large on or off centers. The evidence that these cells (color coded and otherwise) are in blobs is direct and anatomical, consisting of identifying, with electrolytic lesions, the electrode-tip positions where the cells are recorded, and demonstrating, in adjacent sections stained for cytochrome oxidase, that the lesions are in blobs. In the past few years Bevil Conway, a postdoctoral fellow in our labs, has used cone-isolation stimuli to screen for over one hundred red-green double opponent cells in awake-behaving monkey V-1 (*J Neurosci* 2001, 21(8):2768–2783). In these awake, alert animals, direct anatomical evidence that these cells are in blobs is lacking, but the association seems highly likely given that the cells tend to occur in short sequences. Double-opponent cells would seem to form the most likely basis, at the level of V-1, for color contrast, color constancy, and the related color phenomena described by Edwin Land.

Recent failures by some workers to find double-opponent cells in macaque V-1 is hard to explain—Kandel, Schwartz, and Jessel's textbook (*Principles of Natural Science*, 4th edition, 2000, Chap. 29) makes no mention of double opponency. It is important to examine any cells with poor orientation selectivity with stationary colored-spot stimuli, and it is helpful to screen for cells using small-spot cone-isolation stimuli.

Like our efforts in the monkey lateral geniculate, the cortical recordings leave us with the feeling that there is still much to do if we are ever to get a complete picture of the physiology of striate cortex. And this may be a good place to admit that the account, in this book, of the progress that has been made in mammalian CNS vision neurobiology is necessarily very far from complete, and to apologize to the many workers whose contributions have been omitted. Had we tried to be complete, the book would never have been finished, and if finished would have cost an order of magnitude more money. And we would have had to be real scholars!

Chapter 15 • Another Visual Representation, the Cat Clare-Bishop Area •

FOREWORD

This was not one of our favorite papers, perhaps unjustly. We were naturally curious to record from a region that had long been known to be part of the cat visual path—in fact, since 1943, when Marshall, Talbot, and Ades discovered that it responded with slow waves to electrical stimulation of the optic nerve. There followed, in 1954, a study by George Bishop and Margaret Clare that showed that this area responded also to stimulation of the 17–18 region. We recorded from it because we hoped to find evidence for still more elaborate processing, beyond the hypercomplex cells we had seen in area 19. In that we were disappointed. We found no new interesting properties to distinguish the area from 17, 18, or 19—indeed, the only major difference we saw was in the very large receptive field size. To us it was simply a boring, if puzzling, area.

Visual Area of the Lateral Suprasylvian Gyrus (Clare-Bishop Area) of the Cat

DAVID H. HUBEL AND TORSTEN N. WIESEL • *Department of Neurobiology, Harvard Medical School, 25 Shattuck Street, Boston, Massachusetts*

SUMMARY

On anatomical and physiological grounds a zone of cat cortex deep in the medial bank of the suprasylvian sulcus (the Clare—Bishop area) is known to receive strong visual projections both from the lateral geniculate body and area 17. We have mapped receptive fields of single cells in this area in eight cats.

From *J. Physiol.* (1969), **202**, *pp.* 251–260
Received 16 December 1968.

Active responses to visual stimuli were found over most of the medial bank of the suprasylvian sulcus extending to the depths and over to the lowest part of the lateral bank. The area is clearly topographically arranged. The first responsive cells, recorded over the lateral convexity and 2–3 mm down the medial bank, had receptive fields in the far periphery of the contralateral visual fields. The receptive fields tended to be large, but showed considerable variation in size and scatter in their positions. As the electrode advanced down the bank, fields of successively recorded cells gradually tended to move inwards, so that in the depths of the sulcus the inner borders of many of the fields reached the vertical mid line. Here the fields were smaller, though they still varied very much in size.

Receptive fields were larger than in 17, 18, or 19, but otherwise were not obviously different from the complex and lower-order hypercomplex fields in those areas. No simple fields, or concentric fields of the retino-geniculate type, were seen. Cells with common receptive-field orientation were grouped together, but whether or not the grouping occurs in columns was not established.

Most cells were driven independently by the two eyes. Fields in the two eyes seemed to be identical in organization. Cells dominated by the contralateral eye were much more common than ipsilaterally dominated ones, but when cells with parafoveal and peripheral fields were considered separately, the asymmetry was seen to apply mainly to cells with peripheral fields.

INTRODUCTION

In 1943, Marshall, Talbot & Ades, while recording the responses of cat cortex to visual stimulation, observed evoked activity in a region close to the suprasylvian sulcus, some distance from the classical visual receiving areas. They could not abolish the response by making lesions in the lateral gyrus, and concluded that the area received projections from the lateral geniculate body or structures close to the geniculate. Over a decade later Clare & Bishop (1954) narrowed the responsive zone down to a strip of cortex deep within the suprasylvian sulcus, lying along its medial lip (Fig. 1). The responses were evoked by stimulating either the optic nerve or the lateral gyrus of the cortex (presumably areas 17 and 18 of Otsuka & Hassler (1962)).

Over the past few years anatomical studies have also implicated this same suprasylvian region as part of the visual system. Nauta methods have demonstrated projections to it from the lateral geniculate body (Glickstein, King, Miller & Berkley, 1967; Wilson & Cragg, 1967); from area 17 of either side (Hubel & Wiesel, 1965; Wilson, 1968); and from areas 18 and 19 of either side (Wilson, 1968). Removal of cortex lateral to areas 17, 18 and 19 gives by itself minimal retrograde degeneration in the lateral geniculate body (Sprague, 1966); to produce complete degeneration one must destroy these more lateral areas as well as 17, 18 and 19 (Garey & Powell, 1967). There is thus anatomical and physiological evidence for projections to the

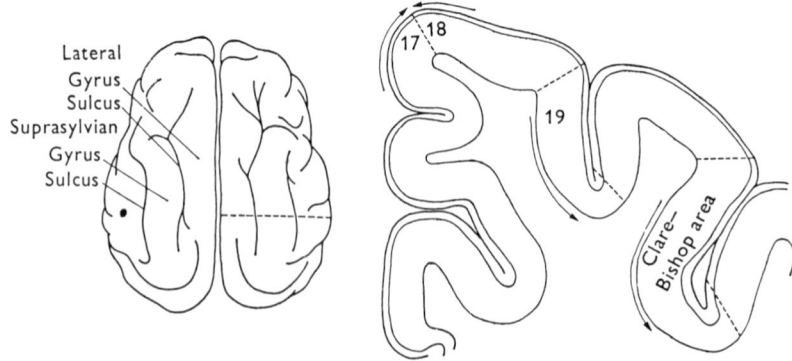

Fig. 1. Diagram of cat brain, as seen from above (anterior is up) and in coronal section, defining topographical terms used in this paper. For each of four topographically organized regions, arrows are directed from peripheral representation towards mid line representation.

lateral suprasylvian region from the lateral geniculate body and from 17, 18, and 19.

By studying responses of single cells to restricted spots and patterns of light, we have recently identified three distinct cortical visual areas in the cat (visual areas I, II, and III), and found them to be identical with architectonically defined areas 17, 18 and 19 of Otsuka & Hassler (1962). It seemed natural to extend this work by exploring the suprasylvian region, and the present paper represents a beginning in this direction. Cells in the area are easily influenced by visual stimuli, and their receptive fields are in many ways similar to those in 17, 18, and 19. The region is topographically ordered. We have seen little evidence that the analysis of form is carried further in this region, and so far its physiological significance remains a puzzle.

METHODS

Methods for stimulating and recording have been described in previous papers (Hubel & Wiesel, 1962, 1965), and will only be summarized here. A cat was anaesthetized with intraperitoneal thiopental, given intravenous succinylcholine to paralyse the eye muscles, and artificially respirated. Light anaesthesia was maintained throughout the experiment. The animal was placed in a stereotaxic head holder, and the eyes fitted with contact lenses to obtain a focus upon a screen at a distance of 1.5 m. Stimuli consisted of stationary and moving patterns of light projected against a diffuse photopic background. A tungsten micro-electrode was advanced hydraulically in a closed-chamber system, and several electrolytic lesions were made in each penetration. For track reconstruction all brains were fixed in formalin, embedded in celloidin, sectioned at 25 μ, and stained with cresyl violet.

Experiments were done in eight adult cats. The micro-electrode was inserted into the lateral part of the suprasylvian gyrus, at about Horsley—Clark level A4 to A6, and lowered along the medial bank of the suprasylvian sulcus. The regions explored consisted of the medial bank to the depths of the sulcus, and part way round to include the lowest part of the lateral bank.

RESULTS

Brisk activity was seen in response to visual stimulation either on first entering the suprasylvian gyrus or after descending about one-third of the way along its lateral bank (Fig. 1). As in 17, 18, and 19, diffuse light gave virtually no responses, but line stimuli (slits, dark bars, and edges) were very

effective over restricted regions. For optimum response the stimulus orientation was also critical, varying from cell to cell, and a moving stimulus was usually much more effective than a stationary one. About two thirds of the cells were 'complex', and the remainder 'hypercomplex' (Hubel & Wiesel, 1965). No 'simple' cells were seen. Hypercomplex cells were almost all of lower order. There was little suggestion that the kinds of form analysis occurring in 19 or even in 17 are carried further in the Clare—Bishop region.

Perhaps the main distinguishing feature of this area was the large size, and the great variation in size, of the receptive fields. On the average the fields even exceeded those of 18 in the territory they occupied, often taking up most of a visual-field quadrant. A second, less conspicuous difference concerned the responses to moving lines. As in 17, 18, and 19, the best responses were obtained to optimally oriented lines swept across the receptive field, and the responses were either about equal, for movements in the two diametrically opposite directions, or were very unequal. In the Clare—Bishop area cells strongly preferring one direction over the opposite were about three times as numerous as those showing no preference, in contrast to the more nearly equal representation of the two groups in 17, 18, and 19. To give an extreme example, in one penetration, described below (Fig. 3), only three out of thirty-two cells responded equally well to an optimally oriented slit moved in the two opposite directions.

Simultaneously recorded cells always had the same receptive-field orientation, and this was also usually true of successively recorded cells (see Fig. 3, below). Moreover, the orientation that was most effective for a given cell was also most effective for any unresolved activity audible in the background. There thus seems little doubt that cells of common receptive field orientation are grouped, as they are in 17, 18, and 19. We still lack compelling evidence that the groupings are in the form of columns, evidence such as comparisons between normal and tangential penetrations, lesions at points of transition in orientation in multiple parallel penetrations, or surface maps. Nevertheless, a columnar system seems a very likely possibility.

OCULAR DOMINANCE. Most cells were driven independently from the two eyes. As in areas 17–19 there were no obvious differences in the field struc-

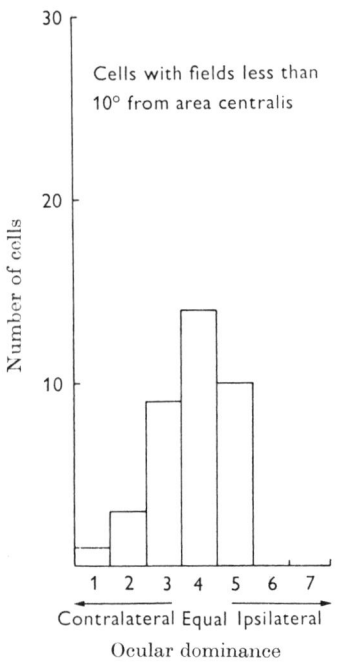

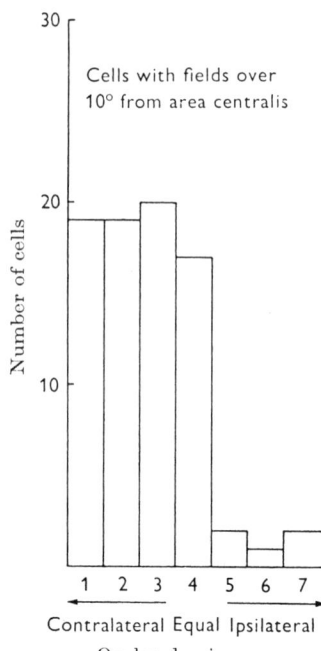

Fig. 2. Histograms showing distribution of cells according to ocular dominance. Cells with field centres within 10° of the area centralis are plotted separately from those with more peripheral fields. Cells of group 1 were driven only by the contralateral eye; for cells of group 2 there was marked dominance of the contralateral eye, for group 3, slight dominance. For cells in group 4 there was no obvious difference between the two eyes. In group 5 the ipsilateral eye dominated slightly, in group 6, markedly; and in group 7 the cells were driven only by the ipsilateral eye.

ture of a single cell in the two eyes, either in orientation, position, or optimal stimulus (Hubel & Wiesel, 1962, 1965). No thorough search was made for horizontal disparity in field positions. As in other areas, the ocular dominance varied from cell to cell. The relative abundance of cells in the different ocular dominance groups varied depending on the position of the fields, and hence in the region of the suprasylvian gyrus from which recordings were made. Figure 2*A* shows the ocular dominance distribution for cells having fields within 10° of the area centralis. This histogram resembles those previously obtained for cells in 17, 18, and 19 (Hubel & Wiesel, 1965) most of which likewise had centrally located fields, for reasons having to do with sampling. Cells whose field centres were further out than 10° tended strongly to favour the contralateral eye, as shown by the histogram of Fig. 2*B*. The surprisingly large number of group 1 cells (those responding only to the contralateral eye) would be even larger if it included cells whose fields were in the extreme periphery of the visual field, beyond the region of overlap of the two eyes.

Topography, Field Size, and Scatter. All the experiments showed a clear but rather crude topographic representation of the contralateral field of vision. Two typical examples are shown in Figs. 3 and 4. In the experiment of Fig. 3 the first responsive cells were found at point *a* (Fig. 3*A*). Fields of the twelve cells recorded between *a* and *b* were scattered over a region below the horizontal meridian, extending out 20–50 from the vertical mid line. These fields are shown diagrammatically superimposed in Fig. 3*B*. As the electrode advanced, the fields tended to be situated closer and closer to the mid line, so that by mid-penetration, between points *b* and *c* (Fig. 3*C*), they were centred some 10–15° out, and in the deepest part of the penetration, between *c* and *d* (Fig. 3*D*), they had moved in to within a few degrees of the vertical mid line. A graph summarizing the inward trend of field centres with electrode depth is given in Fig. 3*A*.

In the second example, illustrated in Fig. 4, responsive cells were recorded from the outset of the penetration. In this Figure the horizontal lines represent the horizontal extent of each field, and the short vertical marks indicate either the geometric centre or the region from which strongest responses were evoked. The first cells had fields that reached beyond 70° from the mid line. Again the inward trend with increasing depth was clear, though over any small segment of the penetration

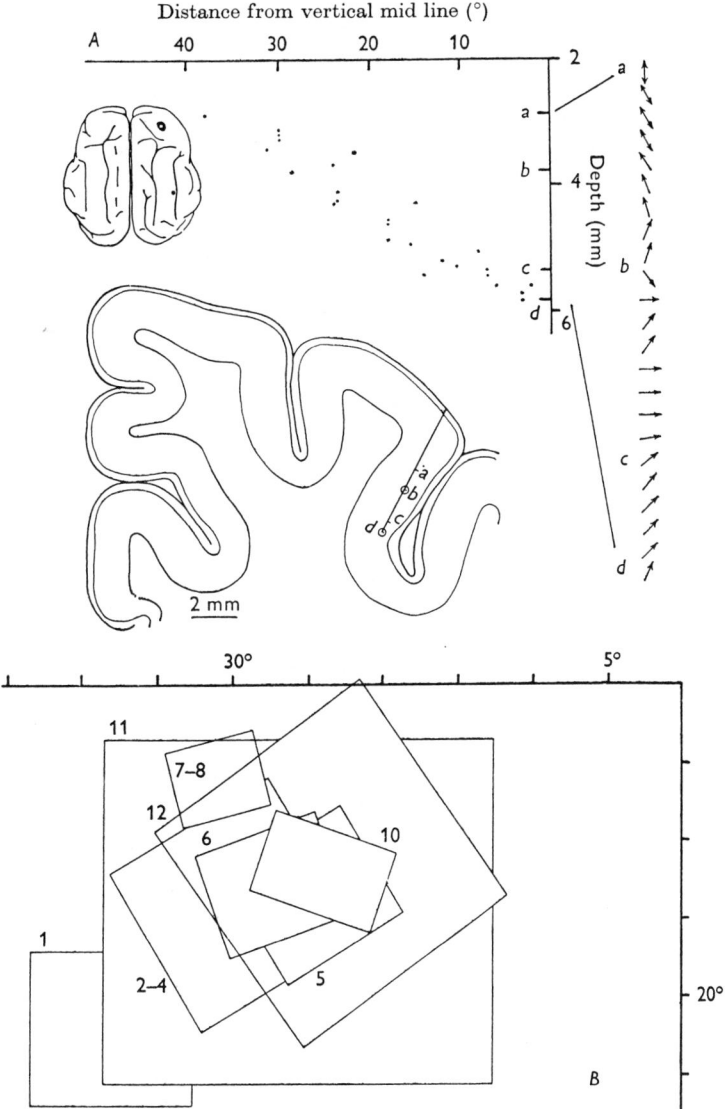

Fig. 3. *Reconstruction of a penetration through most of the lateral bank of the suprasylvian gyrus. Point of entry is marked by a dot in inset of Fig. 3A. Lesions indicated by circles were made at* b *and* d. *First responsive cells were recorded at point* a, *at a depth of about 3 mm; here fields were 30–40° out in the contralateral periphery, below the horizontal meridian. Fields of cells recorded between* a *and* b *are illustrated in Fig. 3B, those recorded between* b *and* c *in 3C, and between* c *and* d *in 3D. The dotted lines in Fig. 3C and 3D represent the area taken in by receptive fields of the preceding diagrams. In the upper right part of Fig. 3A positions of field centres are plotted against electrode depth. Receptive field orientations are indicated to the right of the graph. (continued)*

it tended to be masked by the large variation in field size and the scatter in position, up-and-down as well as mediolateral. Just as was seen in 17, 18, and 19, the scatter in field-centre position was roughly the same as the size of the largest fields.

All experiments gave similar results, with fields in the upper part of the bank far in the periphery, and those deep in the sulcus close to the mid line. At the antero-posterior levels explored, most fields were centred below the horizontal

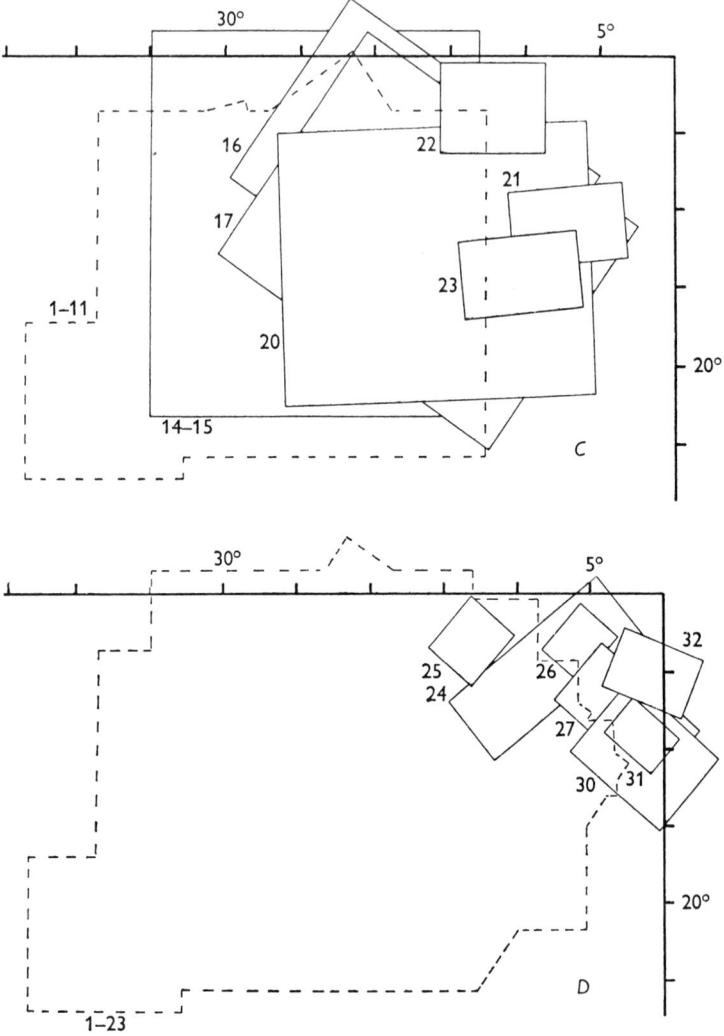

Fig. 3. (continued)

meridian: presumably the superior visual fields are represented more posteriorly in the cortex, just as they are in 17, 18, and 19, but this was not investigated.

On the average, fields close to the area centralis were much smaller than those in the periphery. This was seen in most experiments, and is well shown in Fig. 3B, C, and D. The tendency was less obvious in the experiment of Fig. 4, which was exceptional in this respect.

Many of the fields bordered on the vertical mid line, some of them extending into the ipsilateral field for several degrees. This overlap across the mid line presumably reflects the input the area receives from area 17 of the opposite hemisphere, and, hence, ultimately, from the ipsilateral visual field. A similar overlap has been seen in recordings from 18 (Hubel & Wiesel, 1967).

DISCUSSION

When one compares this lateral suprasylvian area with areas 17, 18, and 19, the similarities are far more marked than the differences. The preference for precisely oriented lines, especially lines moving through the visual field, the presence of asymmet-

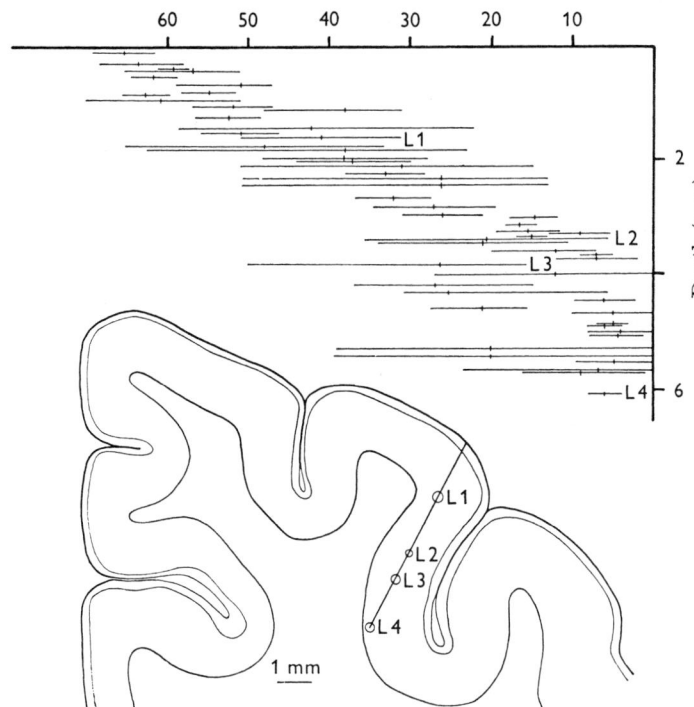

Fig. 4. Reconstruction of a penetration in the lateral bank of the suprasylvian gyrus. Circles (L1–L4) represent four electrolytic lesions made along the electrode trajectory. In the graph the horizontal lines show the mediolateral extent of the receptive fields, and the short vertical lines indicate either the geometrical centre or the area from which responses were maximal.

ric responses to the two opposite directions of movement of an optimally oriented line, and the topographic representation with staggering in field position, all are common to all four cortical regions. So far, receptive fields in the Clare-Bishop area seem roughly similar to those in the other three areas, except that there are no simple cells of the type seen in 17, and fewer higher-order hypercomplex cells than in 19, if indeed there are any at all.

The main differences between this area and the other three lie in the enormous size of many of the fields, the variability in size, and the correspondingly large scatter in field positions. In the coarseness of representation implied by the large fields and wide scatter this area exceeds 18, just as 18 exceeds 17 and 19. It is as though many of the same processes were taking place in the Clare-Bishop area and in 18, in parallel fashion, but with different degrees of refinement.

A paper recently published by Sterling & Wickelgren (1968) gives a description of cells in the cat optic tectum, studied by methods similar to the ones used here. The authors showed that although tectal cells resemble cortical cells in many respects they are also in many respects different, particularly

in not responding specifically to lines, in being relatively insensitive to orientation of contours, and in strongly preferring movement away from the mid line of the visual fields. The Clare-Bishop area thus seems much more akin to the other cortical areas than to the tectum. One reason for emphasizing the contrast between the tectum on the one hand and 18 or the Clare-Bishop area on the other concerns the dual projections that each of these receives: the tectum from the optic nerve and the 17, 18, 19 complex; 18 and the Clare-Bishop area from the geniculate and from 17, 18, and 19. In the optic tectum Wickelgren & Sterling (1968) showed that the more complex properties, e.g. the preferred direction of movement and much of the binocular convergence, disappear when the 17–19 complex is ablated; how the optic nerve contributes to the responses of the normal tectum is still not clear. For the Clare-Bishop area we found in one experiment that the responses similarly disappear on removal of 17, 18, and 19, but retrograde degeneration in the geniculate makes this result difficult to interpret. Thus, the question of the relative contributions of 17, 18 and 19 and the geniculate to the suprasylvian visual area still remains to be answered.

We are left, finally, with the puzzling prospect of an area for which we can, in our present state of knowledge, assign no obvious function. The main object of this study was to verify the existence of a region separate from the classical areas and strongly concerned with vision, to determine at least some properties of the cells, and to establish roughly the topographic organization, if any. A better understanding of its function, however, will require much more work on the receptive fields, and especially, perhaps, a comparison of the properties of cells in different layers. Some idea of where this region projects would also be useful.

We wish to thank Janet Wiitanen for her excellent technical assistance. This work was supported by N.I.H. Research Grants, nos. 5 RO 1 NB 02260 and 5 RO 1 NB 05554.

References

Clare, M. H. & Bishop, G. H. (1954). Responses from an association area secondarily activated from optic cortex. *J. Neurophysiol.* **17**, 271–277.

Garey, L. J. & Powell, T. P. S. (1967). The projection of the lateral geniculate nucleus upon the cortex in the cat. *Proc. R. Soc.* B **169**, 107–126.

Glickstein, M., King, R. A., Miller, J. & Berkley, M. (1967). Cortical projections from the dorsal lateral geniculate nucleus of cats. *J. comp. Neurol.* **130**, 55–76.

Hubel, D. H. & Wiesel, T. N. (1962). Receptive fields, binocular interaction and functional architecture in the cat's visual cortex. *J. Physiol.* **160**, 106–154.

Hubel, D. H. & Wiesel, T. N. (1965). Receptive fields and functional architecture in two nonstriate visual areas (18 and 19) of the cat. *J. Neurophysiol.* **28**, 229–289.

Hubel, D. H. & Wiesel, T. N. (1967). Cortical and callosal connections concerned with the vertical meridian of visual fields in the cat. *J. Neurophysiol.* **30**, 1561–1573.

Marshall, W. H., Talbot, S. A. & Ades, H. W. (1943). Cortical response of the anesthetized cat to gross photic and electrical afferent stimulation. *J. Neurophysiol.* **6**, 1–15.

Otsuka, R. & Hassler, R. (1962). Über Aufbau und Gliederung der corticalen Sehsphäre bei der Katze. *Arch. Psychiat. NervKrankh.* **203**, 212–234.

Sterling, P. & Wickelgren, B. G. (1968). Visual receptive fields in the superior colliculus of the cat. *J. Neurophysiol.* **32**, 1–15.

Sprague, J. M. (1966). Visual, acoustic and somesthetic deficits in the cat after cortical and midbrain lesions. In *The Thalamus*, ed. Purpura, D. P. & Yahr, M. D. New York: Columbia University Press.

Wickelgren, B. G. & Sterling, P. (1968). Influence of visual cortex on receptive fields in cat superior colliculus. *J. Neurophysiol.* **32**, 16–23.

Wilson, M. E. (1968). Cortico-cortical connexions of the cat visual areas. *J. Anat.* **102**, 375–386.

Wilson, M. E. & Cragg, B. G. (1967). Projections from the lateral geniculate nucleus in the cat and monkey. *J. Anat.* **101**, 677–692.

AFTERWORD

A careful rereading of the paper shows that we made one casual observation, ignored by ourselves and everyone else, that turned out to hold the key to much subsequent work in the cat and especially the monkey. Most of the cells were directionally selective, like the cell I had seen so many years before, waving my hands in front of my awake-behaving cats. Such cells are common enough in cat areas 17 and 18, where they are mixed in with the somewhat more prevalent non-direction-selective cells, and where, furthermore, cells responding to one direction are mixed with ones responding to the diametrically opposite direction, as was the case with the two hand-waving cells. In the Clare-Bishop area we had a strong suggestion of grouping of cells favoring a given direction of movement, such as left-to-right, perhaps into columns. We should have picked up on this, given the absence, in striate cortex, of columnar groupings of cells with common directional preference.

We not only did not follow up this result, but when we came to record from prestriate cortex of macaques we happened upon a region in the anterior lunate sulcus with very similar properties. The fields were again huge and again, to us, boring. We again failed to notice that such a large proportion of the cells were direction-selective, though it is obvious when we look back at the protocols. We recorded about 200 cells, but found the results so similar to those of the Clare-Bishop area that we abandoned the project and did not even write up the results. We had other priorities: we had no idea what the area was, and we were lazy and not very bright. This region of monkey cortex, now called MT or V-5, was one of the first prestriate areas to be mapped out and to be examined physiologically, by Allman and Kaas in a New World monkey, the owl monkey (in the middle temporal gyrus, or MT) (*Brain Research* 1971, 31:85–105), by Zeki in owl monkeys (*J Physiol* 1980, 207:239–248) and in macaques by Van Essen, Maunsell, and Bixby (*J Comp Neurol* 1981, 199:293–326). It is an important component of the dorsal visual stream of Mishkin and *Ungerleider*. It is now known to be organized in columns: one set defined by movement directionality rather than orientation (Albright, Desimone and Gross, 1984, *J. Neurophysiol.*, 51: 16–31; Born, 2000, *J. Neurophysiol.*, 84: 2658–2669), and a second set whose cells are sensitive to binocular disparity (De Angelis & Newsome, 1999, *J. Neurophysiol.* 19: 1938–1451).

The Clare-Bishop area has subsequently been mapped topographically, and christened "PMLS", perhaps because eponyms are regarded in some circles as unscientific.

Chapter 16 • Encoding of Binocular Depth in a Cortical Area in the Monkey •

FOREWORD

Like the recordings from MT just discussed, this represents another of our early forays into the prestriate monkey cortex, and again, not an entirely successful one. Like the MT work, the study has a curious and contorted history. We began looking at binocular interactions by following in the footsteps of the two groups already expert in stereopsis: Barlow, Blakemore, and Pettigrew, and Bishop, Nikara, and Pettigrew, in various arrangements of those names. They had the brilliant idea to put an adjustable prism in front of one eye to vary the relative directions of gaze, in order to look for cells that were tuned selectively for near or far objects or for objects at the fixation distance. The work of the two groups was in cats, and we had no success in reproducing it. The cat seemed to us an unfortunate choice for such work: eye movements are hard to control and monitor, and the cat lacks a rod-free fovea, having instead what is called the *area centralis,* which is in some ways equivalent to the primate fovea but is much larger and has poorly defined borders. This lack of a well-defined fovea made it difficult to line up the eyes precisely for studies of stereopsis.

We adapted their idea of using a prism in our work in the monkey, in which we explored a cortical gyrus buried deep in the lunate sulcus, just ahead of the primary visual cortex. We happened by chance upon this area, which was full of cells very responsive to visual stimuli, especially to stimuli of the two eyes. We soon realized that these cells were highly selective for the exact setting of the prism, and we established that some cells responded when the prism was set for near objects, others for far objects, and others for the distance on which the animal was fixated. For still others, about half, the settings were not critical. It was almost always the case that the cells that responded best for some critical prism setting, and therefore preferred some precisely determined stimulus distance, gave little or no response to stimulation of separate eyes. This was quite different from most of the cells we had studied in V-1, where binocular cells were common but responded well to stimulation through either eye alone. There was a marked tendency for cells

that responded to similar prism settings to be grouped, presumably into columns, for near, far, and zero disparities.

Cells Sensitive to Binocular Depth in Area 18 of the Macaque Monkey Cortex

D. H. HUBEL AND T. N. WIESEL • *Department of Neurobiology, Harvard Medical School, 25 Shattuck Street, Boston, Massachusetts*

Barlow, Blakemore and Pettigrew[1], and Nikara, Bishop and Pettigrew[2], have described a group of cells in the cat visual cortex that respond selectively to horizontally disparate stimulation of the two retinas. It seems very likely that such cells play an important part in stereoscopic depth perception. We wished to determine whether similar cells were present in the monkey cortex, especially in view of E. W. Bough's behavioural demonstration of stereoscopic depth perception in the monkey (*Nature*, 1970, 225: 42–44).

In fifteen macaque monkeys we have examined binocular interaction in 547 cells of area 18, a topographically ordered region anterior to area 17 (the striate cortex). Parallel anatomical studies show that there is an ordered projection from area 17 to area 18 on the same side; there is no evidence for any direct input to 18 from the lateral geniculate body[3,4].

Recordings were made simultaneously from an extracellular electrode in each hemisphere[5]. The main recording electrode was inserted into area 18, either in the posterior bank of the lunate sulcus or in the annectant gyrus, which is buried in the lunate sulcus. An adjustable prism in front of the left eye allowed the relative directions of gaze of the two eyes to be varied. Eye movements were almost completely prevented by the use of intravenous curare and gallamine[2]. The second electrode monitored the eye positions and detected any

residual movements. A binocular unit was recorded in area 17 and kept, if possible, for the duration of the experiment. The receptive fields in the two eyes were mapped on a projection screen 1.5 m away. The field positions were checked each time a new unit was studied with the main recording electrode; eye movements could thus be detected and corrected for immediately.

About half (57 per cent) of the cells in area 18 react to simultaneous stimulation of the two eyes in a manner similar to that of complex and hypercomplex cells of area 17 (ref. 6). We term these "ordinary cells of area 18". Most ordinary cells respond actively to either eye stimulated by itself, and the responses of the two separate eyes are usually about equal. Receptive fields of these cells are in anatomically corresponding parts of the two retinas. There is often moderate summation when the two eyes are stimulated together, and the relatve positioning of stimuli within the two fields is generally not critical for a cell to show maximum response.

Forty-three per cent of cells in 18 show more specialized properties. We term these "binocular depth cells". There are several distinct types of binocular depth cells; we describe here only the most common. In these, stimulation of either eye separately gives no response or only weak responses, whereas appropriate stimulation of the two eyes together results in very brisk responses. Some of these cells respond best with the two eyes

From *Nature*, Vol. 225, No. 5227, 41–42, *January* 3, 1970.
Received November 4, 1969.

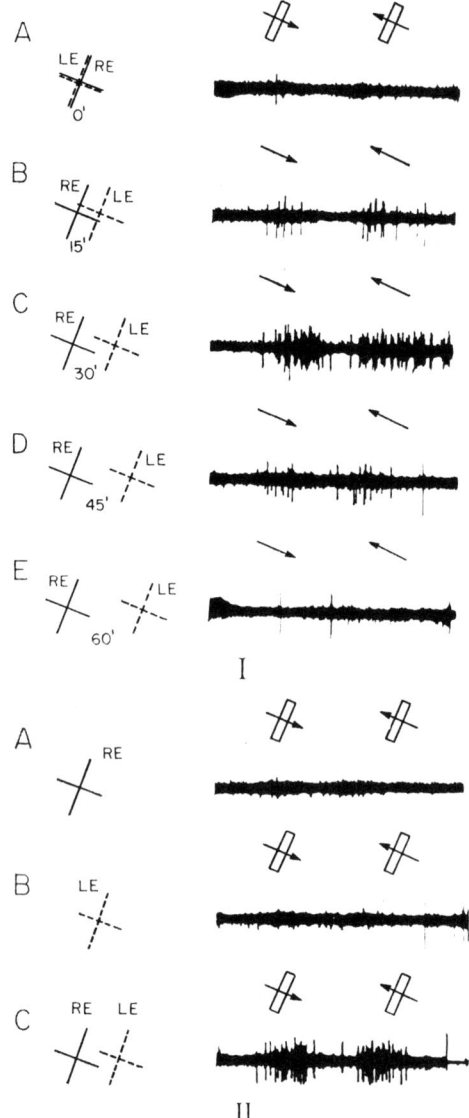

lined up so that exactly corresponding retinal regions are stimulated simultaneously; in others there is a disparity in the positions of the two receptive fields. The displacement of the field in one eye, relative to the field in the other, is usually at right angles to the receptive field orientation. Vertically oriented fields are thus horizontally displaced, whereas with oblique fields there is a vertical component to the disparity as well. In binocular stimulation, when the position of one eye (or the prism setting) is varied along a line at right angles to the orientation of the optimal stimulus (the receptive field orientation), the response rises from zero or some low value to a maximum and then falls off over a range that is usually very small compared with the dimensions of the receptive field. Variation in position along a line parallel to the orientation of the optimal stimulus gives a much more gradual rise and fall in response. Because of this, the responses of cells with obliquely oriented fields also peak sharply when the prism displacement is purely horizontal (Fig. 1). Binocular depth cells with receptive fields oriented within 15° of the horizontal are much less common than one would expect in a random distribution, and their responses have not yet been adequately analysed.

The frequency with which one encounters binocular depth cells varies in a systematic way in area 18. Just in front of the 17-18 border and 10–15 mm lateral to the midsagittal plane (representing the vertical midline, 3°–4° below the fovea), most cells are "ordinary"; many of these have fields straddling the vertical midline. As one proceeds forwards and down into the lunate sulcus, and then up over the buried annectant gyrus, the retinal representation moves out from the midline. At the same time, the proportion of binocular depth cells increases to more than 50 per cent. As an electrode traverses the cortex, sequences of cells that are all ordinary, or all of the binocular depth type, are recorded; neighbouring binocular depth cells often

Fig. 1. Responses of a cell recorded from area 18 in right hemisphere 12 mm lateral to the midline, on the anterior lip of the lunate sulcus about 3 mm in front of the 17-18 boundary. Cell was in layer 6. It responded best to a slit 1° long and ⅛° wide, oriented 20° clockwise from the vertical. The receptive field was approximately 1° by 0·75° in size, and in the right eye was situated 1·75° below and 1° to the left of the fovea. In the left eye it was displaced, relative to this, 0·5° to the right and slightly downwards. I: Both eyes stimulated together in anatomically corresponding regions (A). In B–E, position of stimulus to left eye was horizontally displaced to the right on the screen in steps of 15 min of arc. Maximum responses were obtained with a displacement of 30 min. (Displacement was produced by shifting direction of gaze of left eye to the left, with a prism.) Duration of each sweep was

Fig. 1. (continued)

4 s. II A, Right eye, stimulated alone; B, left eye, stimulated alone; C, both eyes, stimulus to left eye shifted 30 min to the right. Projection screen was 1·5 m away from the monkey. With eyes fixed on the screen, maximum response to a long object moved in front of the animal occurred when the object was 0·5 m in front of the screen. For eyes fixed at infinity this would be equivalent to a stimulus about 3 m from the animal.

have the same horizontal disparity, though varying in orientation. This suggests an organization in which cells representing a given stereoscopic depth relative to the surface of fixation are grouped together, and segregated from cells that are not particularly concerned with depth. These groupings may have the form of columns that extend from surface to white matter. There is probably also an independent system of columns containing areas of similar receptive field orientation as is found in area 17 (ref. 6). Sequences of cells with the same receptive field orientation are rather brief, suggesting that the orientation columns are very narrow compared with the depth columns.

We have also studied hundreds of cells in area 17, but have found no convincing examples of binocular depth cells. In this respect the monkey seems to differ from the cat[1,2]. Possible differences between binocular depth cells in cat area 17 and monkey area 18 are the failure of most depth cells in the monkey to respond to stimulation of either eye alone, and the linking, in the monkey, of vertical disparity to receptive field orientation.

Area 18 in the monkey seems, therefore, to have at least two independent functions, that of linking the two visual half fields across the vertical midline (as in the cat[5,7]), and the elaboration of stereoscopic depth mechanisms. The parts of 18 near the vertical meridian representation have both functions, whereas more peripheral areas probably lack the first.

We thank Janet Wiitanen for technical assistance. This work was supported in part by US National Institutes of Health research grants and in part by the Bell Telephone Research Laboratories, Inc.

References

1. Barlow, H. B., Blakemore, C., and Pettigrew, J. D., *J. Physiol.*, **193**, 327 (1967).
2. Nikara, T., Bishop, P. O., and Pettigrew, J. D., *Expt. Brain Res.*, **6**, 353 (1968).
3. Wilson, M. E., and Cragg, B. G., *J. Anat.*, **101**, 677 (1967).
4. Hubel, D. H., and Wiesel, T. N., *Nature*, **221**, 747 (1969).
5. Hubel, D. H., and Wiesel, T. N., *J. Neurophysiol.*, **30**, 1561 (1967).
6. Hubel, D. H., and Wiesel, T. N., *J. Physiol.*, **195**, 215 (1968).
7. Choudhury, B. P., Whitteridge, D., and Wilson, M. E., *Quart. J. Exp. Physiol.*, **50**, 214 (1965).

AFTERWORD

In modern terminology this area was probably what is known as the V-3/V-3A complex, and not 18 or visual area 2 as we thought at the time. This was long before the mapping out of primate visual regions beyond area 17, by Kaas and Allman in New World monkeys and by Zeki and Van Essen in macaques. At that time, anything north of the 17-18 borders was terra incognita. We hesitated to write a full-length paper when we did not even know for sure what area we were recording from, even though we had recorded from more than 600 cells and reconstructed 23 penetrations with the results tabulated and figures drawn, in what would have been a long paper even for us. Later Gian Poggio and Fisher had the insight to realize that the problem could best be addressed in awake behaving monkeys that could be trained to fixate to levels of accuracy of minutes of arc (*J Neurophysiol* 1977, 40:1392–1405). We wrote this short *Nature* paper on our results and abandoned our studies of stereopsis, returning to V-1 to learn more about topics such as columns.

Chapter 17 • Anatomy of the Geniculo-Cortical Pathway: The Nauta Method •

FOREWORD

The first phase of this work had been reported in a preliminary way in *Nature* three years before. The research gave us the rare satisfaction one experiences on thinking up an experiment that should work, and it turns out that it does work.

Our history with the Nauta method had its origin in the mid-1950s. I had met and become friends with Walle Nauta at Walter Reed, where he worked just down the hall. Neither Torsten nor I dreamed that one day we would make such extensive use of an anatomical method that was reputed to be forbiddingly difficult—we were, after all, not even trained anatomists. But one day, shortly after our move to Boston, James Sprague, a neuroanatomist and a good friend—and an established expert in the Nauta method—wrote from Philadelphia to tell us that his head technician, Jane Chen, had to move to Boston for personal reasons: was there any chance we could employ her? We thought it over and asked ourselves: Why not? We could probably think up uses for the Nauta silver-degeneration technique. It was the first of the new and powerful methods that were revolutionizing the field of neuroanatomy. It was the first reliable method for telling where any given group of cells in the central nervous system sent their axons. With Jane's help we could make lesions here and there in the brains of our cats and monkeys, wait a week for the axons of the killed cells to degenerate, and then do one of our usual recording experiments—which usually had nothing to do with the anatomy/lesion experiment. We would then section the brain to identify our electrode tracks, and also stain for degenerating fibers using the methods devised by Nauta, to find the terminals of the degenerating fibers that resulted from our lesion. In that way we could get extra mileage out of each of our experimental animals. We took a chance. Jane arrived, full of energy, and was soon turning out hundreds of beautiful slides. Our first lesions were made in cat striate cortex and allowed us to map some of the regions to which the striate cortex projected. Those results are included in our long paper on areas 18 and 19 of the cat.

We then had our exciting idea. We were already making tiny electrolytic lesions to identify our recording sites. Why not record from the monkey's lateral geniculate body, identify the layer our electrode tip was in by noting which eye produced the responses, make a lesion, wait the necessary days for fiber degeneration to occur, and use the Nauta method to reveal the degenerated projections to the cortex? That way we might hope to bring out anatomically the ocular dominance columns, whose existence we increasingly suspected, especially following our cat strabismus experiments in 1965 (see below). Perhaps we could confirm our suspicions that these were stripes rather than checkerboard-like patches. The Nauta method had recently been modified by Fink and Heimer to reveal degenerating nerve terminals rather than degenerating fibers, making the final destinations of the fibers easier to determine. (Degenerating fibers tend to obscure degenerating terminals.) The Fink-Heimer method had not been adapted for use in monkeys, but here again we were lucky. Jane Chen had to leave, but was replaced by Janet Tobie (later Wiitanen), who was a paragon of neatness and obsessive persistence. By varying concentrations of every possible reagent, she got the method to work beautifully in monkeys. We worried over two possible obstacles: a lesion would have to be very small for it to be confined to a single geniculate layer, but big enough to produce cortical degeneration that we could detect, over a wide enough cortical area to include at least several columns; second, we wondered if projections from one layer would not be contaminated by fibers passing up from deeper layers. Both problems proved surmountable, but at the start we had no assurance of success. At least the experiments were taking very little additional time, and no additional animals.

None of this work would ever have been approved by an Eye Institute study section. We had no experience in neuroanatomy, let alone the Nauta method, and no preliminary results. But the experiments cost us nothing over what we were paying for our usual experiments. And we had no assurance that the microlesion-plus-Nauta strategy would work.

We were lucky. In one of our first attempts the electrode passed obliquely along the most dorsal geniculate layer, and by listening to responses of unresolved cells we could make lesion after lesion as the electrode advanced, resulting in a nice long cigar-shaped area of destruction confined to the one layer. So it turned out that we could after all make rather large lesions. Our first glimpse of a cross-section through striate cortex (like that of Fig. 2) was one of those hugely satisfying treats when it is clear that everything has, after all, really worked. It took much labor to align, trace and reconstruct the sections, but the final picture of parallel stripes completely convinced us that the columns were in fact stripes. The fiber-of-passage problem solved itself by the obliquity of the trajectory that most fibers take after they leave their layer of origin.

But there was another pay off, probably just as important and completely unforeseen. Until then, no one knew which cortical layers received the geniculo-cortical inputs. It was widely assumed that the site of termination was the cell-sparse myelin-rich Line of Gennari, the component of layer 4 that gives the striatedness to the striate cortex on a freshly cut section. But our result showed quite unexpectedly that the Line of Gennari is virtually free of geniculate terminals. There had been one previous hint of this: Le Gros Clark and Sunderland had years before undercut the striate cortex and failed to see the loss of myelin that would be expected in this layer because of cutting the incoming geniculate fibres. (*J. Anat.,* 73: 563–574) For some reason their finding had been largely ignored.

When we first looked closely at the sections we could hardly believe our eyes. Instead of occupying the Gennari line, the terminals from the two geniculate subdivisions, the magnocellular and parvocellular, were distributed in quite distinct and separate sublayers just below the Gennari line. Endings from the parvocellular layers formed a dense thicket in the deep half of the cell-rich part of layer 4, and those from the magnocellular layers occupied the superficial half. From parvocellular geniculate we found a second thin layer lying just above the Gennari line in what we called the *upper tier.* The magnocellular and parvocellular sublayers of degeneration in layer 4C did not overlap at all. It took some Nissl counterstaining and careful comparisons to convince us of this palpable difference between the two inputs. In present day terminology of Jennifer Lund we say the magnocellular input is to 4C-alpha, and the parvocellular input to 4C-beta and 4A (*J. Comp. Neurol.* 147:455–496).

Laminar and Columnar Distribution of Geniculo-Cortical Fibers in the Macaque Monkey

DAVID H. HUBEL AND TORSTEN N. WIESEL • *Department of Neurobiology, Harvard Medical School, 25 Shattuck Street, Boston, Massachusetts*

ABSTRACT

Single cell recordings in monkey striate cortex have shown differences in response properties from one cell layer to the next and have also shown that the IVth layer, which receives most of its input from the geniculate, is subdivided into a mosaic of regions, some connected to the left eye, others to the right. In the present study small lesions were made in single layers or pairs of layers in the lateral geniculate body, and the striate cortex was later examined with a Fink-Heimer modification of the Nauta method. We hoped to correlate the laminar distribution of axon terminals in the cortex with functional differences between layers, and to demonstrate the IVth-layer mosaic anatomically.

After lesions in either of the two most dorsal (parvocellular) layers, terminal degeneration was found mainly in layer IVc, with a second minor input to a narrow band in the upper part of IVa. A very few degenerating fibers ascended to layer I. In contrast, lesions in either of the two ventral (mag-

From *the Journal of Comparative Neurology* Vol. 146, No. 4, December 1972.

nocellular) layers were followed by terminal degeneration confined, apparently, to IVb, or at times extending for a short distance into the upper part of IVc; no degeneration was seen in layer IVa or in layer I.

After a lesion confined to a single geniculate layer, a section through the corresponding region of striate cortex showed discrete areas or bands of degeneration in layer IV, usually 0.5–1.0 mm long, separated by interbands of about the same extent in which there was no terminal degeneration. When serial sections were reconstructed to obtain a face-on view of the layer-IV mosaic, it appeared as a series of regular, parallel, alternating degeneration-rich and degeneration-poor stripes. When a geniculate lesion involved both layer VI (the most dorsal, with input from the contralateral eye) and the part of layer V directly below (ipsilateral eye), the cortical degeneration, as expected, occupied a virtually continuous strip in layer IVc and the reconstructed face-on view of this layer showed a large confluent region of degeneration.

In some of the reconstructions the cortical stripes seemed highly regular; in others there was a variable amount of cross connection between stripes. The stripes varied in width from 0.25 to 0.50 mm, and width did not seem to correlate with region of retinal representation.

It is concluded that the long narrow stripes of alternating left-eye and right-eye input to layer IV are an anatomical counterpart of the physiologically observed ocular-dominance columns. Because of this segregation of inputs, cells of layer IV are almost invariably influenced by one eye only. A cell above or below layer IV will be dominated by the eye supplying the nearest IVth layer stripe, but will generally, though not always, receive a subsidiary input from the other eye, presumably by diagonal connections from the nearest stripes supplied by that eye.

A glance at a section through the cerebral cortex shows that it is subdivided into alternately cell sparse and cell rich horizontal layers. This subdivision is especially striking in the primary visual, or striate, cortex (area 17) of the monkey. By recording from single cells in this area it has been possible to demonstrate clear differences in responses to visual stimuli from the different layers. Not surprisingly, cells of layer IV, which is the site of termination of afferents from the lateral geniculate body, have the simplest properties and show the least intermingling of inputs from the two eyes. The more complex cell-types, for the most part binocularly driven, are found in layers above and below. In its structure layer IV is itself non-uniform, consisting of several distinct subdivisions; up to the time of the present study the exact distribution of the afferent endings within this layer was not known, though this is of obvious importance for an interpretation of the physiology.

Physiological studies have shown that the cortex is also parcelled by vertical partitions into at least two independent but overlapping systems of columns (Hubel and Wiesel, '68). In the first of these, cells with similar orientation preference are grouped together. In the second system, cells are grouped according to eye dominance, the cells of one column mostly favoring the left eye, those of the next the right. Layer IV, whose cells are strictly monocular, is thus divided into a mosaic of left-eye and right-eye patches. While it has long been known that cells deep to a given point on the cortical surface are richly interconnected, there has been no hint from the anatomy that the interconnected cells occur in discrete groupings.

The primary object of the present work was to demonstrate the ocular-dominance columns anatomically. We were anxious to have the satisfaction of actually seeing the mosaic whose existence the physiology suggested, and wanted especially to learn if it had the form of a checkerboard, or of islands of one type embedded in a matrix of the other type, or of alternating left-eye and right-eye stripes.

The following method of demonstrating the ocular-dominance columns occurred to us. A lesion in the lateral geniculate body leads to degeneration of thalamocortical axons and axon terminals that can then be selectively stained by silver-impregnation methods. The geniculate consists of six cell layers, each of which receives input from one eye only. If a lesion could be confined to a single geniculate layer there might be some hope of seeing the predicted patchy distribution of degenerating axon terminals entering the cortex. By using extracellular microelectrodes it should be possible to ascertain the position of the electrode tip by single-cell recording and then to make small lesions by passing current. Among silver-degeneration methods, the Fink-Heimer modification of the Nauta method seemed especially suitable, since it stains not only degenerating axons, but also what are almost certainly degenerating presynaptic terminals.

Such an experimental approach promised not only to outline the ocular-dominance columns, but also to show the exact distribution of the afferent terminals within layer IV of the cortex. It also opened the possibility of comparing the terminations of axons from the four dorsal geniculate layers with those from the two ventral layers, a matter of some interest because the two sets of layers differ both in their morphological appearance and their physiological properties (Wiesel and Hubel, '66). A preliminary account of some of this work has already been published (Hubel and Wiesel, '69).

METHODS

Eighteen monkeys were used, but not all lesions were suitably placed and for unknown reasons the staining was unsatisfactory in some animals. In all, 12 successful lesions were made, and complete reconstructions of the resulting intracortical fiber degeneration were made for eight of these. Survival times were 4–6 days.

The animal was anesthetized with thiopental and prepared for recording in the usual way (Hubel and Wiesel, '68), except that no neuromuscular blocking agent was used and intubation and artificial respiration were therefore not necessary. Tungsten microelectrodes with a shaft diameter of $125\,\mu$ were tapered to a tip of less than $1\,\mu$ over a distance of about 1 cm, and had an uninsulated tip length of $35\,\mu$. The electrode was inserted into the lateral geniculate body either vertically, through the folds of cortex and white matter directly above, or in the coronal plane at an angle of 45° to the vertical. It was usually possible to tell where the electrode tip was in relation to the layers by observing successive changes in the eye from which cells could be driven. On passing from the third to the second layer there was of course no change in the eye from which responses were evoked, but one could recognize the point of transition by the changes in response properties and receptive-field characteristics of single cells (Wiesel and Hubel, '66). By lowering and raising the electrode, the depths corresponding to the point of entering or leaving a given layer were determined. A large lesion or a series of lesions was then made between these points. When several lesions were made along a track they were spaced closely enough to produce a single long cigar-shaped lesion. This was an especially useful method when the electrode entered the lateral geniculate obliquely and advanced for some distance parallel to a single layer (fig. 8a).

Before the lesions were made the position of geniculate-cell receptive fields was noted on the projection screen, relative to the center of gaze. Because of eye movements it was usually possible to do this only to within a degree or so. From the receptive-field positions the site of the lesion in the geniculate could be estimated, and one could predict the region of striate cortex in which degenerating fibers would be found.

After perfusion-fixation with 10% formol-saline the cortex was cut in parasagittal serial frozen sections at 30 μ, and stained by a variant of the Nauta method (Nauta and Gygax, '54; Fink and Heimer, '67; Wiitanen, '69). The lateral geniculate body was sectioned in the coronal plane and alternate sections stained for Nissl substance or for degenerating fibers.

Degenerating fibers appeared, as in any Nauta preparation, as chains of black dots or black elongated particles about 2–4 μ in diameter that could usually be followed as long as the fiber remained in the plane of section. What we assumed were degenerating synaptic endings appeared as round dark-staining particles, also about 1–2 μ in diameter, peppered at random throughout sharply demarcated regions (see below) rather than in orderly chains. These dots could possibly be confused with background dust that is often found in these stains, but the dust, when it occurred, was much finer in consistency and was widely distributed throughout each section. The great majority of sections were fortunately almost totally free of this dust. It should be emphasized, however, that the main weakness of this method is the impossibility of knowing for certain whether any particular dot is a degenerating terminal: the recognition of endings must depend mainly on their grouping. In the present material the endings in layers IVa and IVc were so strikingly dense as to leave little doubt to their identification. On the other hand, it is not possible to say that there were no degenerated endings in the other layers. The proof that the large particles are presynaptic terminals will depend ultimately on electron microscopy. Similar particles in other material have in fact been so identified (Heimer and Peters, '68). While in the descriptions given below we shall refer to the particles as boutons, omitting quotation marks or qualifications, the absence of a rigorous identification should be borne in mind. An important feature of this modified Nauta stain is the ease with which (at least in the system in which we were working) the boutons were sharply distinguishable from degenerating fibers. The very feasibility of the present study depends on this distinction.

Fibers of Passage

A lesion in any but the most ventral geniculate layer will not only destroy cells, but also, presumably, geniculo-cortical fibers passing through the lesion site from the layers below. There was a risk that destruction of these fibers of passage might hopelessly contaminate the degeneration arising from destruction of cell bodies. As the geniculate axons leave a given layer, however, they tend to fan out, crossing the more dorsal layers not radially, along corresponding points in the successive retinotopic maps (lines of projection), but along the most direct route upwards and posteriorly. A lesion in a given layer might therefore be expected to lead to a dense and focal cortical projection due to cell-body destruction, and a more diffuse projection due to interruption of fibers of passage. The observed thalamo-cortical projections in fact took this form, with a main focus of dense degeneration occupying a restricted region a few millimeters in diameter, and a region of much lighter degeneration usually extending for many millimeters along the cortex, generally only on one side of the main focus and resembling the tail of a comet. In reconstructing lesions or determining the cortical laminar distribution of afferents, this sparse projection was ignored. As would be expected, lesions of the most ventral layer showed only the dense focus, with no comet tail.

Reconstructions

Once the region of cortical degeneration was found it was necessary to make a detailed reconstruction. Negative enlargements ($\times$ 33) were made directly from each slide, and the regions showing terminal degeneration, as seen by microscopic examination, were indicated on the print in ink. Small blood vessels and other features that appeared on the enlargement were used as a guide in positioning these marks (see Fig. 9). The regions of layer IVb or IVc showing degenerating terminals were then traced onto 1 mm lined tracing paper, using a new line for each successive section. Blood vessels were used in bringing successive sections into register. (Where the cortex was curved it was obviously necessary to straighten, in effect, layer IV; this was done by dividing it into a number of segments). The result was a face-on view of layer IV magnified 33 times. No attempt was made to correct for shrinkage, but comparisons of cortical thickness suggested that it did not differ grossly from one brain to the next. To assess the sites of termination of afferent fibers relative to the cortical layering, occasional sildes were counterstained with cresyl-violet.

RESULTS

Of the 12 lesions, seven were in the dorsal (parvocellular) part of the geniculate, and five were in the ventral (magnocellular) part. No lesions were made in dorsal layers 3 and 4 and, while it seems highly likely that these layers project in the same way as the upper two parvocellular layers, studies are now under way to verify this. The lesions were scattered widely through the geniculate, two being within a degree or two of the foveal representation, eight in the midperiphery, and two in areas representing the far periphery, 50–80° from the fovea. The position of each of the lesions is given in Table 1.

The occipital cortex, and cortex associated with the lunate and superior temporal sulci were examined. No degeneration was seen outside the striate cortex.

For the present paper we have adopted Brodmann's layering system for the striate cortex. A superficial inspection of the Nissl-stained Macaque area 17 (Fig. 1) shows it to be composed of three cell-sparse layers alternating with three cell-dense layers. In Brodmann's system the cell sparse layers are I, IVb and V; the cell dense layers are II, III and IVa (which appear as a single layer in the Macaque), IVc, and VI. In previous papers (Hubel and Wiesel, '68, '69) we saw no justification for separating layers III and IVa, since we did not realize that geniculate afferents reach the lower part of the uppermost cell-dense region (II, III, IVa). We therefore adopted von Bonin's layering system, which makes no distinction between III and IVa. The results of the present work show that some afferents indeed ascend further than was previously realized, ending in the lower portions of the upper cell-dense region. We have therefore reverted to Broadmann's system, calling this region IVa even though it cannot easily be distinguished from layer III in Nissl preparations.

Laminar Distribution of Afferent Fibers

Lesions of Dorsal (Parvocellular) Geniculate Layers The laminar distribution of degenerating afferents following a dorsal-layer geniculate lesion formed a highly consistent pattern in the seven monkeys. Figure 2, from monkey 12, shows the degenerating fibers and terminals in a section that was not counterstained. Degenerating fibers entered from the white matter with uniform density throughout the entire main focus, criss-cross-

Table 1

Monkey number	Layer of LGB lesion	RECEPTIVE-FIELD POSITIONS RELATIVE TO FOVEAL PROJECTION			Period of stripes	Figure number
		Vertical[1]	Horizontal	Total distance		
					mm	
8	Dorsal (6)	−2.5°	4.5°	5°	1.2	14
9	Dorsal (6)	8.5°	11°	13.5°		
11	Ventral (2)	4°	10°	10°		
12	Dorsal (6)	−9°	10°	14°	0.7	2, 3, 7–10
14	Dorsal (5, 6)	−8°	12°	14.5°	0.6	5, 11–13
15	Dorsal (5)	0°	0°	0°	0.8	15
16	Dorsal (6)	−10°	20°	22.5°	0.7	
19	Ventral (1, 2)	−30°	40°	50°		
33	Dorsal (3), Ventral (2)	2°	10°	10°		
36	Ventral (1)	6°	13°	14.5°	0.5	16
37	Ventral (1, 2)			40–90°		
41	Ventral (1)	−1°	2.5°	3°	0.5	6, 17

[1]Negative numbers indicate field positions below the foveal projection.

ing diagonally in all directions and apparently branching as they ascended through layers VI and V, but giving off no obvious terminal arborizations. In IVc fibers were also abundant, but they were probably slightly thinner at this level. Here, however, there was a sudden very dense aggregation of degenerating boutons, so dense that at first glance it tended to obscure the fibers. The position of these endings relative to the layering is shown in a Nissl-counterstained section in figure 3. The boutons appeared abruptly at the base of IVc (which in Nissl sections is sharply demarcated from layer V), and showed a uniform density over its lower two-thirds, becoming gradually less dense in the upper third, paralleling, more or less, the decline in cell density. There were very few boutons within the uppermost part of IVc, and none in IVb. Layers IVb and IVc showed considerable numbers of degenerating fibers, perhaps one-third the number that were seen in the deeper layers.

In layer IVa there was another horizontal band of degenerating boutons, thinner than the band in IVc (roughly 1/4 the thickness, or about 30 μ), and less dense (fig. 2). Counterstained sections (Fig. 3B) showed that this upper tier of degeneration was not situated immediately above layer IVb, i.e., not right at the base of the cell-dense II-III-IVa complex, but somewhat above this level.

Although Nissl and myelin stains showed no hint of a separate layering correlated with this upper tier of degeneration, the Fink-Heimer material often showed a faint but clear line precisely at this level, that appeared as a white band in the negative prints (Figs. 9, 12, arrows). The line was seen both within the focus of degeneration and well outside it, in the normal cortex, and so could not have been produced by degenerating fibers or endings. We do not know what is being stained to produce it.

Although Nissl stains of Macaque area 17 showed nothing that would correlate with this upper tier, favorable sections of *Ateles* striate cortex show a cell-sparse lamina in roughly the same region (Fig. 4). A similar lamination was noted by von Bonin in *Cercocebus* and *Cebus* monkeys ('42, Figs. 7, 8). It would be interesting to make geniculate lesions in the New-World monkeys in order to see how the upper tier, if there is one, correlates with the more elaborate layering pattern.

Above the upper tier of degeneration an occasional degenerating fiber was seen running vertically. In lesions that produced the densest degeneration (such as that in monkey 14) an occasional fiber ran all the way to layer I, and then turned, or divided in the form of a T, the branches running horizontally precisely in the middle of the first layer (Fig. 5). On an occasional section, two or

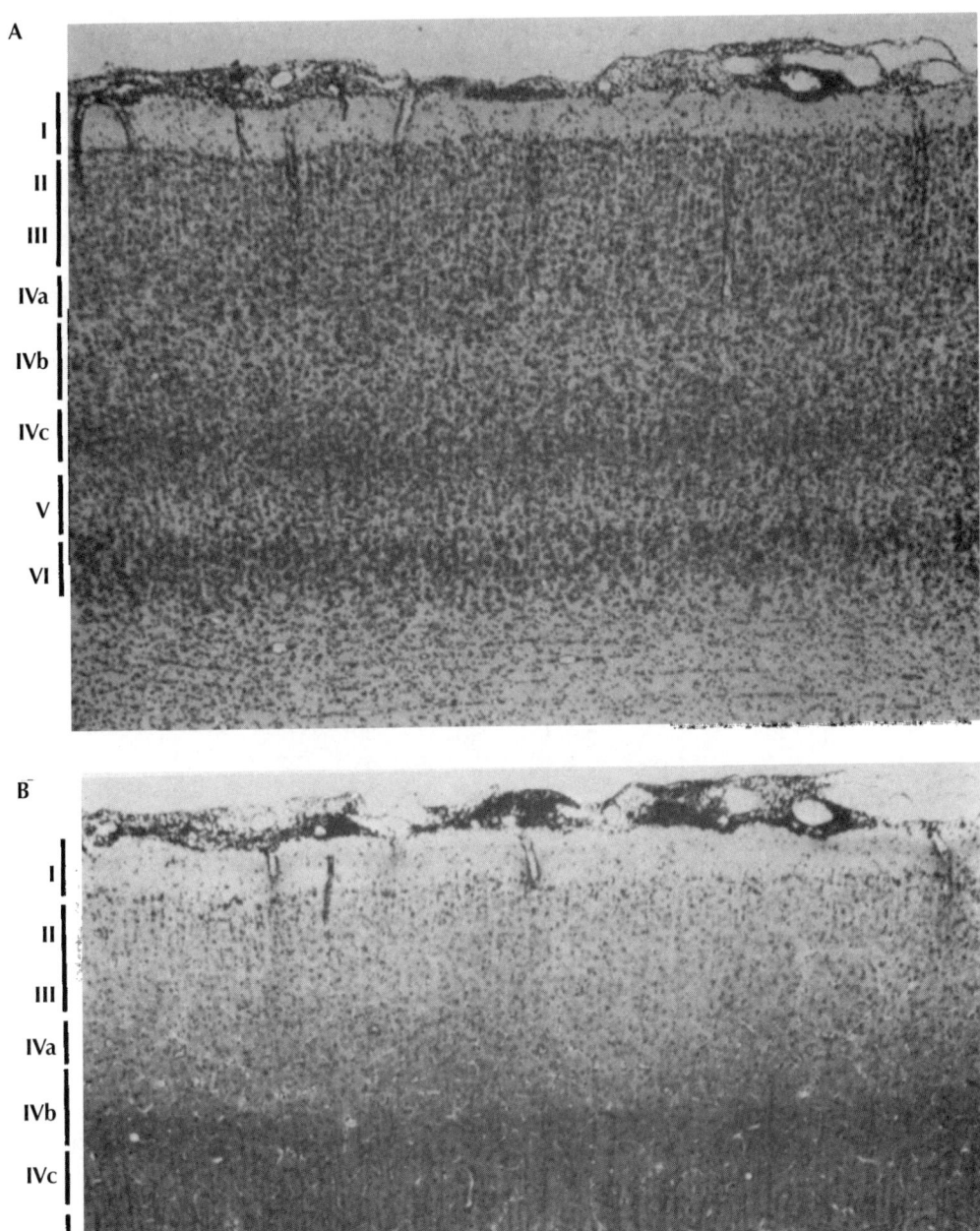

Fig. 1. Nissl- (cresyl-violet) (A) and myelin-(Loyez) (B) stained sections through striate cortex (area 17) of Macaque monkey to show the layering system used in this paper. The Nissl stain shows three cell-sparse regions, layers I, IVb and V, and three cell-dense regions, layers II, III and IVa collectively, layer IVc, and layer VI. The line of Gennari is roughly located in layer IVb.

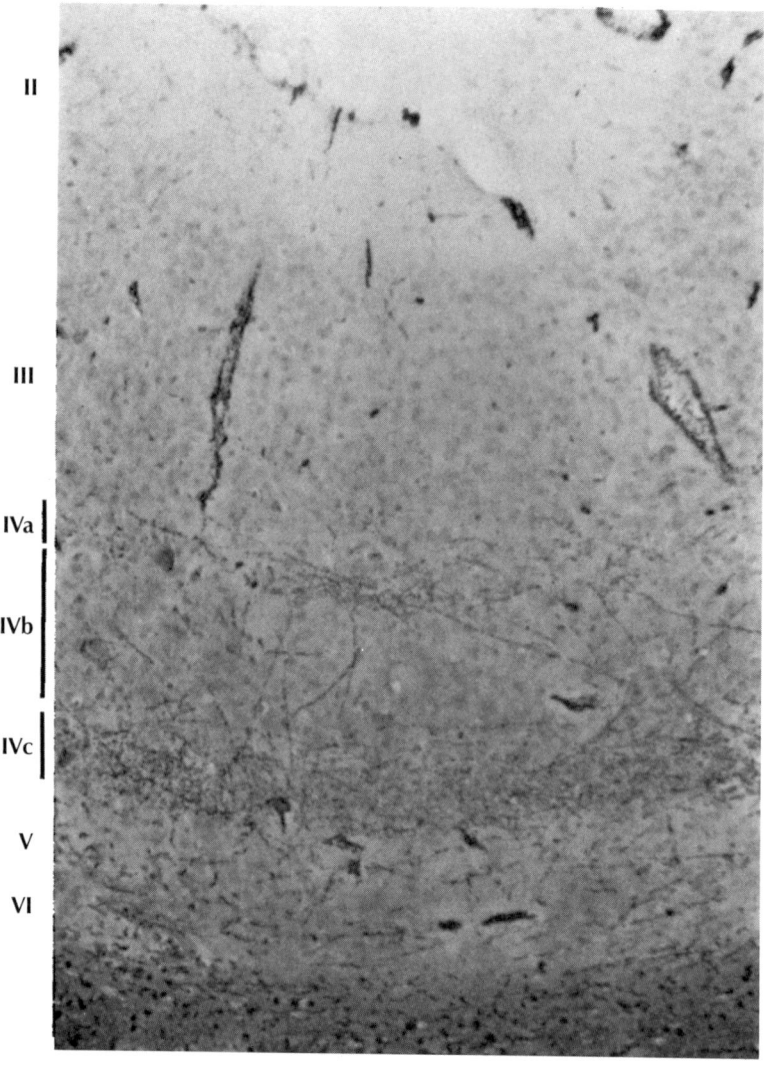

II

III

IVa

IVb

IVc

V

VI

0.2mm

Figs. 2A, 2B. Low and high power photographs of a Fink-Heimer stained section through the striate cortex of monkey 12 in which a microelectrode lesion had been made in LGB layer 6, four days prior to perfusion (see Table 1 and Figs. 3, 7–10). Degenerating fibers ascend diagonally through layers VI and V, and presumably branch extensively in IVc, which is densely loaded with boutons. A moderate number of fibers ascend further through layer IVb to IVa, where more boutons are seen. (continued)

three such horizontal fibers could be seen running closely spaced at this level for at least 0.5 mm before leaving the plane of section. At least one or two such fibers were seen on each section in monkey 14, undoubtedly because the lesion in this animal was relatively large. Very rarely, a vertical fiber on its way to layer I could be seen emitting a horizontal branch in layers II or III.

In summary, there appears to be a three-fold distribution of endings from the dorsal (parvocellular) layers of the lateral geniculate to area 17: a dense thicket of terminals in IVc, a second much

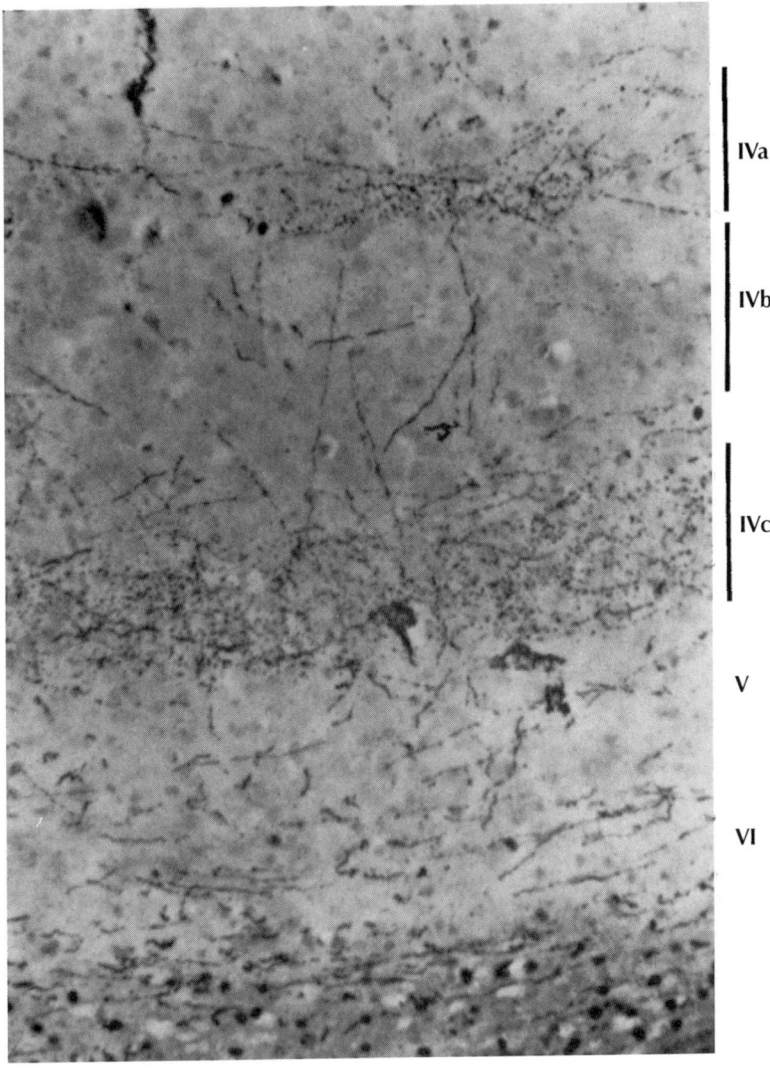

IVa

IVb

IVc

V

VI

<u>0.1mm</u>

Fig. 2B.

smaller but still substantial outcropping in IVa, and a third very sparse set of fibers running in the midthickness of layer I, whose terminals were not seen. One cannot, of course, rule out a scanty distribution of endings, or the presence of very fine endings, in layers II, III, V, or VI.

LESIONS OF VENTRAL (MAGNOCELLULAR) GENICU-LATE LAYERS A different distribution of degenerating endings was seen following lesions of the ventral layers. Figure 6 shows the results of a lesion in

the most ventral layer (cf. Fig. 17, monkey 41). As before, obliquely running fibers threaded their way up through layer VI and V but instead of producing a dense mass of boutons in IVc, they bypassed this layer in its lower portions. There was a dense layer of terminal particles in the deeper half of IVb, extending into IVc for a distance that varied from brain to brain. The very cell-dense part of IVc was either spared entirely or was occupied only in its upper one-third or one-half. Precise estimates of the regions involved are made difficult by the lack of

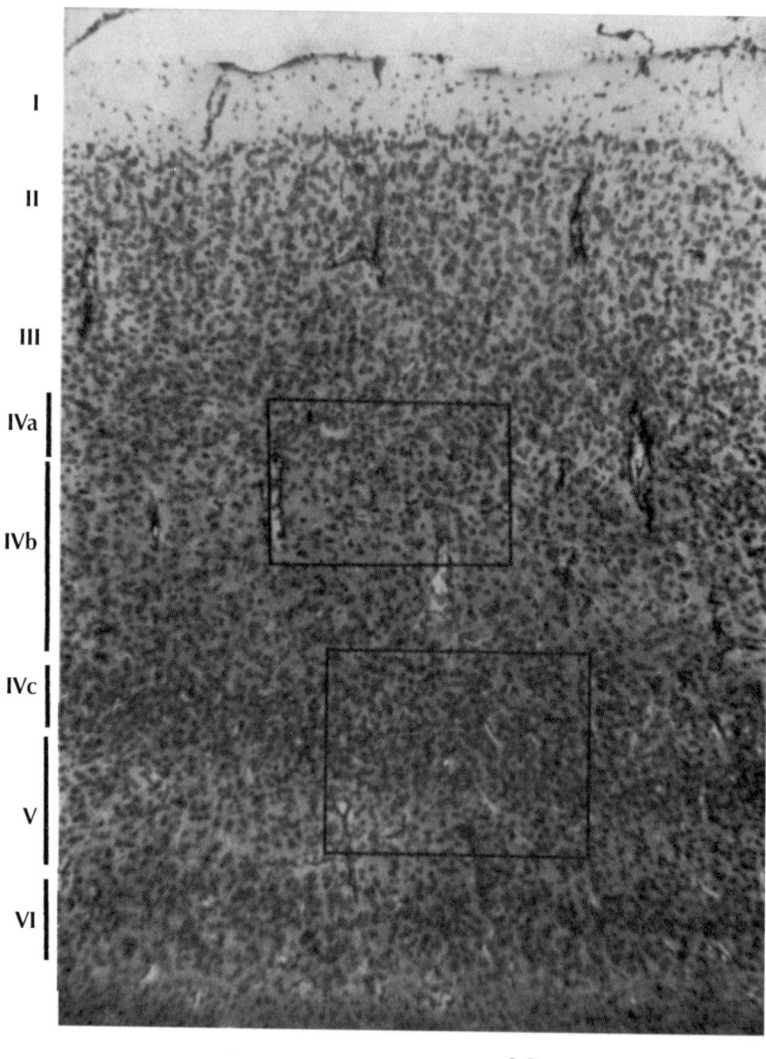

I

II

III

IVa

IVb

IVc

V

VI

0.2mm

Figs. 3A, 3B, 3C. Counterstained Fink-Heimer section showing relationship between distribution of degenerated boutons and the cytoarchitecture. A, low power, B and C, high power of enclosed areas. Same monkey as in Figure 2. (continued)

sharpness in the boundaries between these layers. What was clear, however, was that following every ventral-layer lesion the region occupied by the degenerating terminals was at a higher level than the degeneration following dorsal-layer lesions. Results from the two ventral-layer experiments in which the staining was of best quality suggest that in some monkeys the two sites of termination may not overlap at all (compare Figs. 3C, 6B).

Layers above IVb and IVc showed no degenerating fibers and no hint of terminals; there was thus no obvious upper tier of degeneration following ventral-layer lesions. The ventral layers of the geniculate are much thinner than the dorsal ones, and presumably as a consequence of this the cortical degeneration was considerably less dense than that following lesions in the dorsal layers. Since in the dorsal-layer lesions the upper tier of degenera-

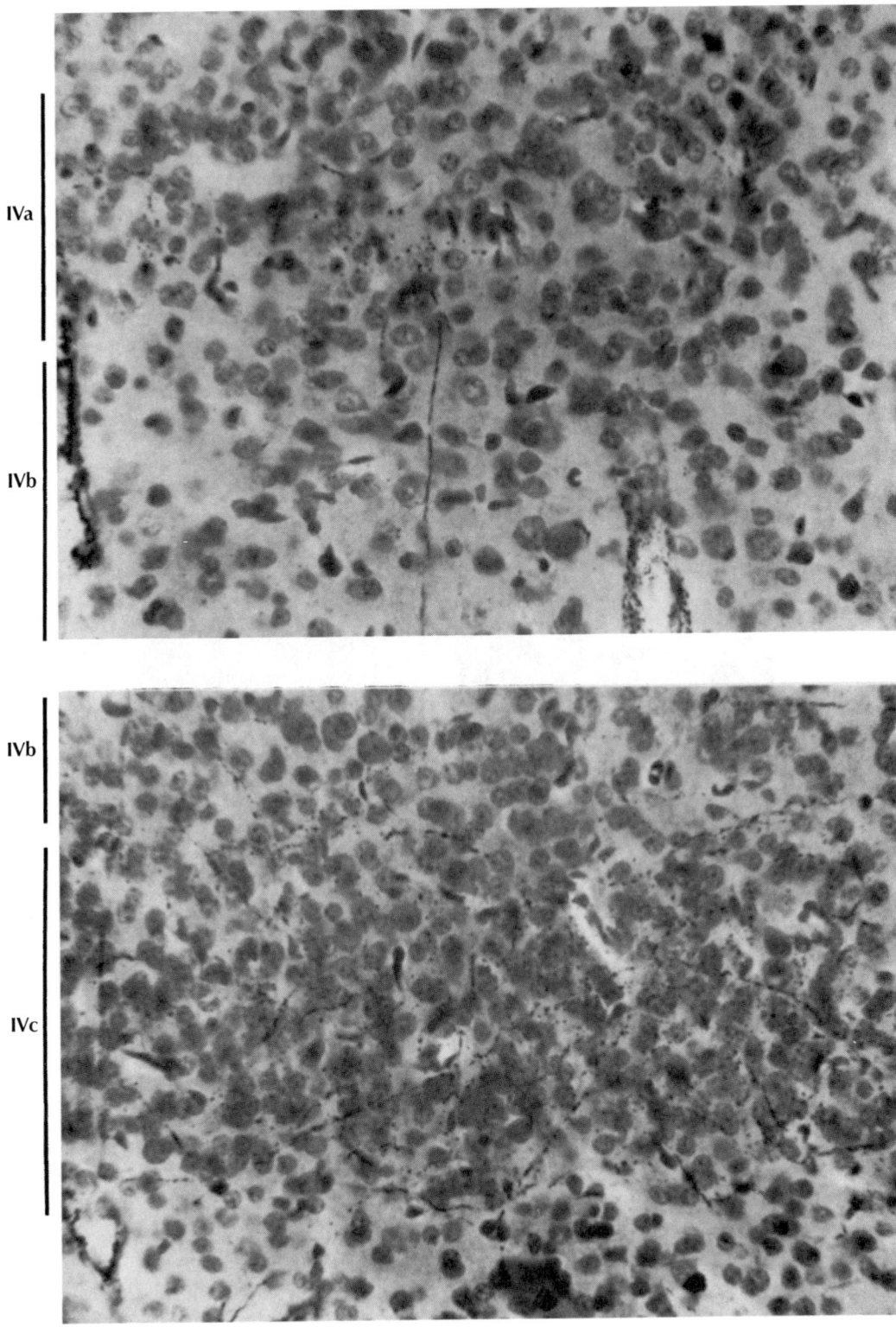

IVa

IVb

IVb

IVc

0.1mm

Figs. 3B, C.

297

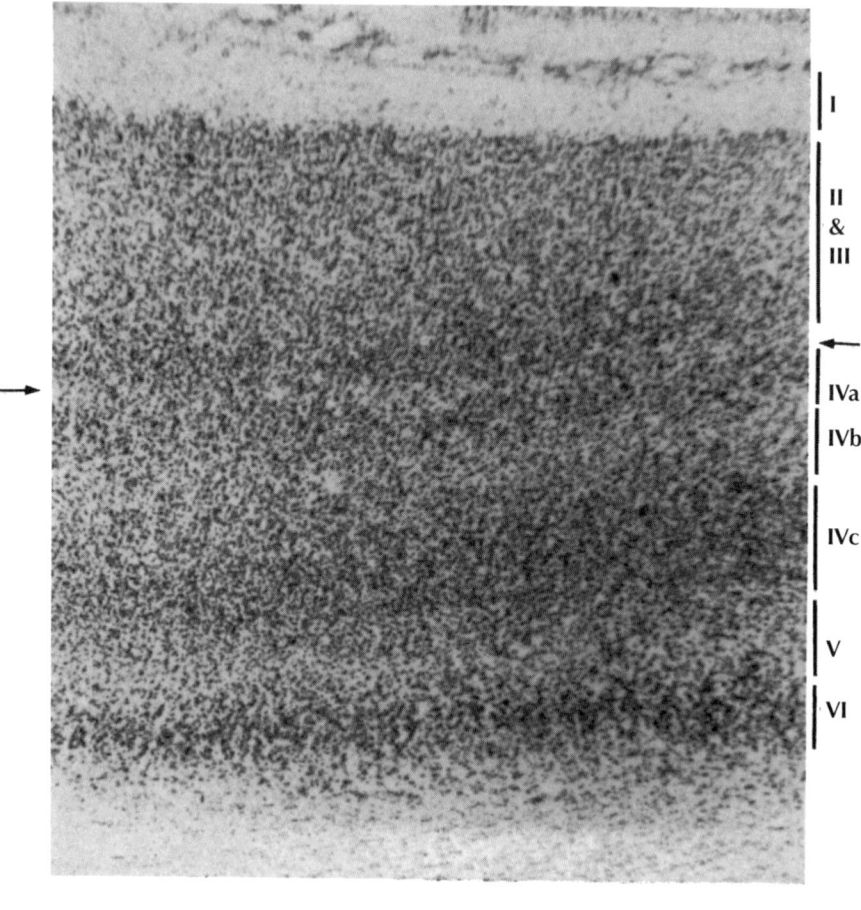

0.5mm

Figs. 4. Nissl-stained section through area 17 in spider monkey (Ateles), showing an additional narrow cell-sparse layer in what is tentatively assumed to be layer IVa (arrows), and which may be the site of an upper tier of terminations in this species.

tion was always more scanty than that observed in the lower tier, it is possible that an upper tier following ventral layer lesions was missed, being that much more sparse. The same problem exists, to an even greater degree, with respect to the possibility of degeneration in layer I. Subject to these reservations, however, one can say that terminals from ventral layers are probably confined to one major level.

Ocular-Dominance Columns

After geniculate lesions involving either the two most dorsal geniculate layers, as in monkey 14, or the two ventral layers, as in monkey 37, degenerating terminals occupied a continuous band or bands in the fourth layer, interrupted only at the end (see Fig. 12). A marked difference was seen in animals in which the lesion involved one layer only. Here the bands of degenerating terminals were interrupted at regular intervals by segments of equal extent that were, as far as one could tell, completely free of terminals. We call these regions "interbands." The borders of the bands, where the transition took place from a high concentration of terminals to few or none, were usually distinct (Fig. 7). We assume that this pattern of bands and interbands is the anatomical counterpart of the ocular-dominance system and represents regions of alternating left-eye and right-eye inputs to layer IV (Hubel and Wiesel, '68).

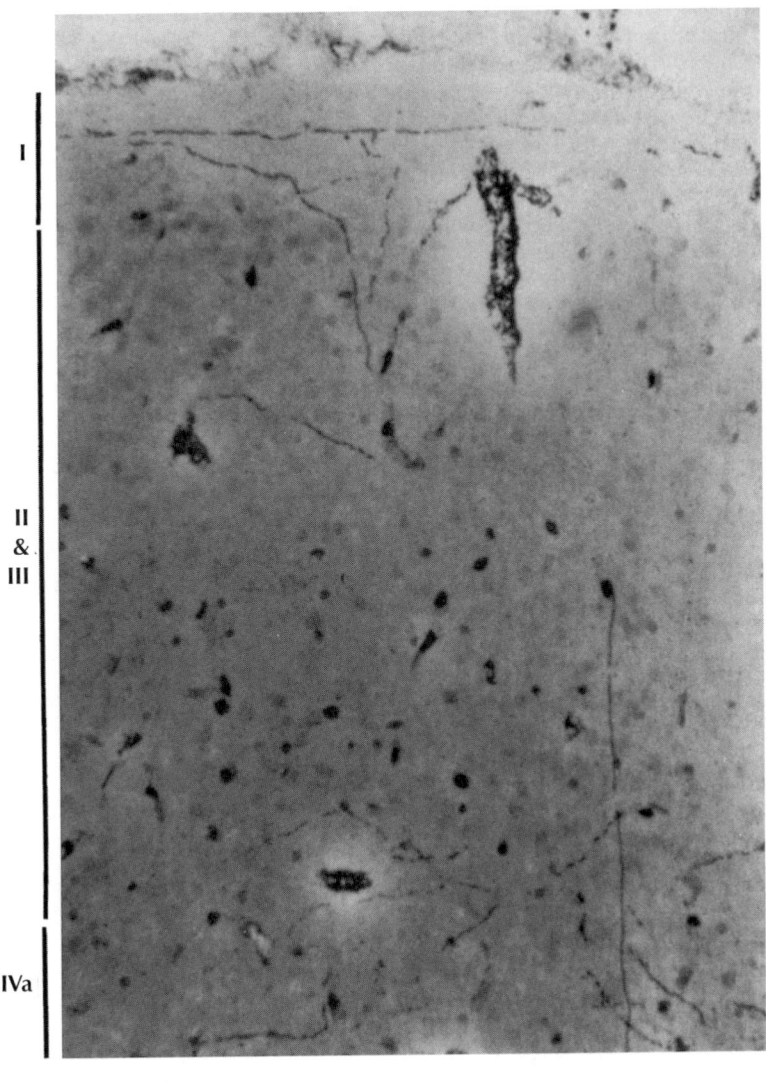

Figs. 5A, 5B. Two photomicrographs from upper part of cortex in monkey 14 (see also Figs. 11–13). One or two fibers ascend vertically through layers III and II, branch a few times in II and I and then run horizontally through the middle of layer I. Fink-Heimer stain.

In the smallest lesions, such as that made in monkey 8 (Fig. 14) a single cortical section showed only one or two patches of degeneration, whereas with longer lesions there were as many as 6–8 sets of bands and interbands (Figs. 8–10). Following a lesion of a dorsal layer, the band appeared as before in layers IVa and IVc. Here, as a rule, the bands and interbands lay in register one above the other, though this pattern was sometimes distorted when the cortex was markedly curved or was cut in a plane that was not perpendicular to the surface.

The degenerating fibers entering cortex from white matter did so rather uniformly and criss-crossing fibers were present throughout layers VI and V. It was as if a fiber only decided on its destination after entering the cortex, and took a diagonal course in the deeper layers in order to get to an appropriate band or interband in layer IV. In the

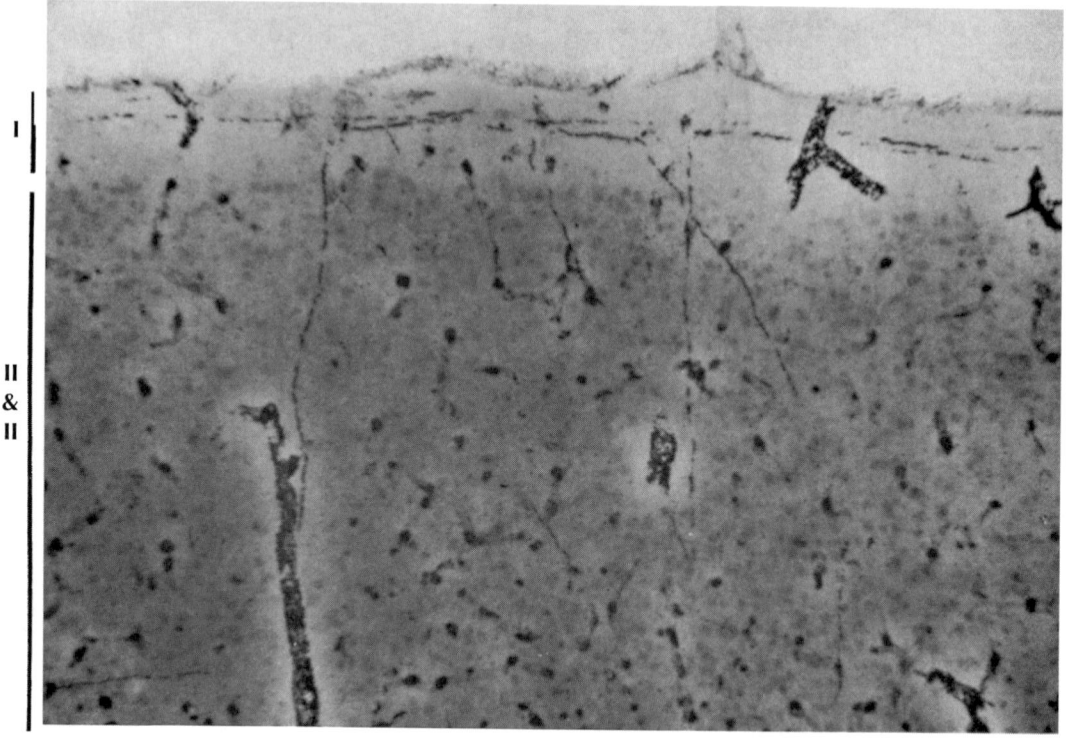

I

II
&
II

0.1mm

Fig. 5B.

interbands of layer IV there were many horizontally or diagonally running degenerating geniculate fibers, perhaps as many as in the bands themselves. These seemed frequently to be spanning the gap between one band and its neighbor, supplying branches and terminals in the bands but none at all in the interbands. Layer IVb, though having few or no terminals, nevertheless showed numbers of degenerating fibers, running mostly vertically or obliquely, in about the same numbers over the bands as over the interbands. It is perhaps worth emphasizing that degenerating fibers in a given layer were fairly uniform in their horizontal distribution, so that the conventional Nauta method, staining fibers but not terminals, would not necessarily have demonstrated the columnar organization.

Horizontal Distribution of Degeneration: Reconstruction of Columns from Serial Sections

The most extensive lesion confined to a single layer was seen in monkey 12 (Figs. 8, 9). Here the electrode entered layer 6 of the left lateral geniculate at

its medial aspect, and lesions were made over a distance of 1 mm. The initial receptive fields were located in the visual field 9° below the horizontal, and 10° from the vertical midline, and as the electrode advanced these moved out and down. As expected from the known topography, the resulting degeneration appeared in the anterior corner of the mushroom-like buried calcarine cortex, occupying a region of cortex measuring about 4 mm × 8 mm. Each section showed some six to eight bands of degeneration. In the final reconstruction (Fig. 10) the degeneration in layer IVc took the form of a series of more or less distinct parallel stripes, roughly 0.35 mm wide, separated by spaces of roughly the same width. The definition of the stripes is best on the right of the figure (anteriorly) and becomes progressively poorer towards the left of the map. This parallels the abrupt beginning of the degeneration anteriorly and a gradual tapering off posteriorly. In terms of topography, the point of entry of the electrode into the geniculate corresponds to the anterior boundary of the cortical degeneration. It is likely, therefore, that the lesion

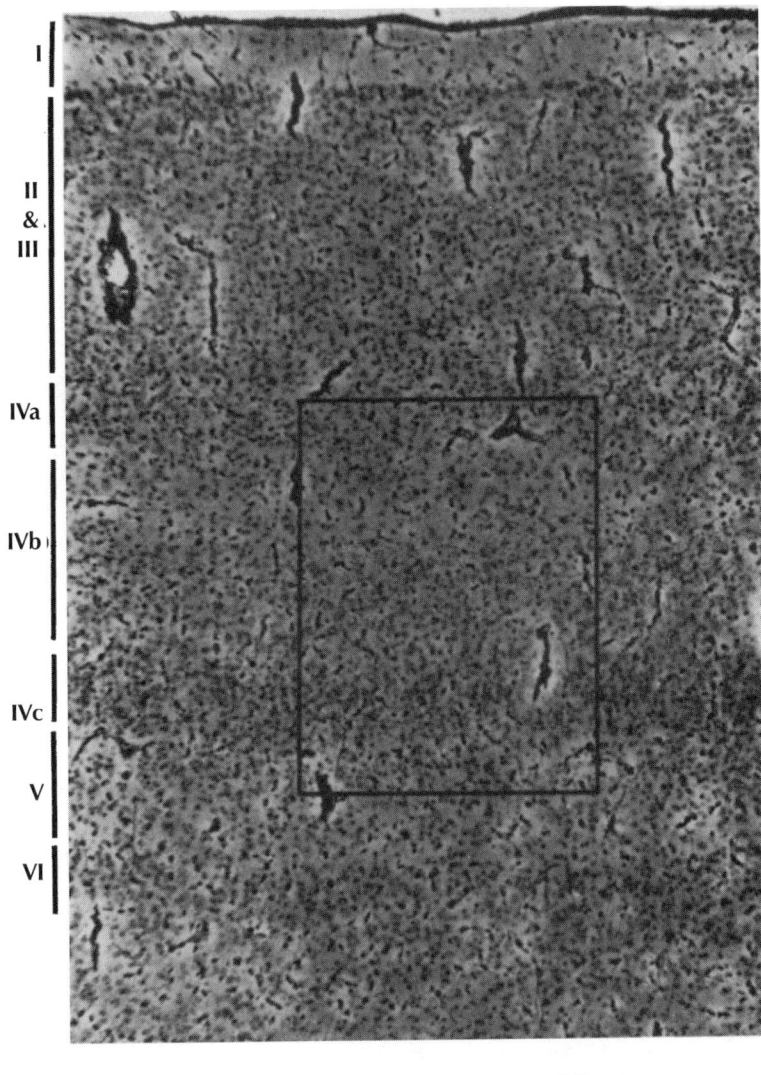

I
II & III
IVa
IVb
IVc
V
VI

0.2mm

Figs. 6A, 6B. Low and high-power photographs showing distribution of degenerating terminals following a ven-tral-layer geniculate lesion (layer 1) in monkey 41. Degenerating terminals are confined to cortical layer IVb in its deeper half, for the most part. Fink-Heimer counterstained section.

caught fibers of passage from deeper layers destined for the most posterior part of the degeneration area.

The stripes are not entirely independent, but in places are cross-linked to their neighbors. The original slides were rechecked carefully and it was verified that two neighboring stripes do at times coalesce, and that single stripes in places split to form two. The reciprocal situation, of a stripe being interrupted by coalescence of two interspaces

(representing the other eye) was not seen in this experiment but was very common in one of the others (monkey 41, Fig. 17).

If destruction confined to one geniculate layer, corresponding to one eye, gives stripes of cortical degeneration separated by equal blank spaces, the assumption is that the blank spaces represent the destination of fibers linked to the other eye. Since the maps from the contralateral half visual field in the different geniculate layers are in exact

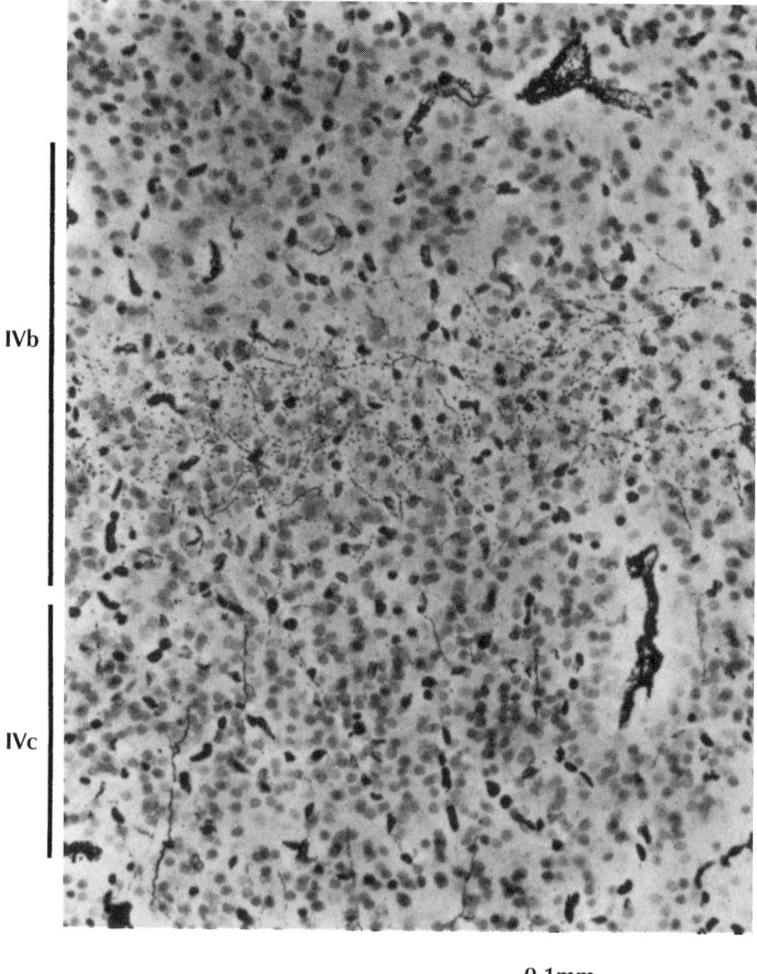

IVb

IVc

0.1mm

Fig. 6B.

register a lesion involving layer 6 and layer 5 directly beneath should give a continuous patch of degeneration, rather than a series of stripes. The lesion in monkey 14 (Figs. 11–13) was designed to test this. Here the electrode entered the geniculate in almost the same place as in the previous monkey (12), with the initial receptive fields situated about 8° below the horizontal and 12° out from the midline. This time the lesion was extended into layer 5, the final fields being 15° out and 19° down in the visual field. The cortical area showing terminal degeneration was found in almost exactly the same part of area 17, but now in most sections there was a long continuous strip of degeneration in layers IVc and IVa, interrupted only at the two ends. The reconstruction showed a dense elongated central

patch of degeneration, with a suggestion of stripes on both sides. We assume that the continuous band of degeneration reflects the destruction of geniculate cells lying in the two most dorsal layers along the same radial projection lines, and therefore representing the same region of visual field, whereas the stripes to the upper left and lower right in the figure arise because at the beginning of the lesion the sixth (most dorsal) layer was involved without corresponding involvement of the fifth, and similarly at the end, the fifth was injured without an involvement of the corresponding part of the sixth. Thus a stripe beginning in the upper left should continue into an interband in the lower right: unfortunately the method is not good enough, or the stripes themselves are not quite orderly

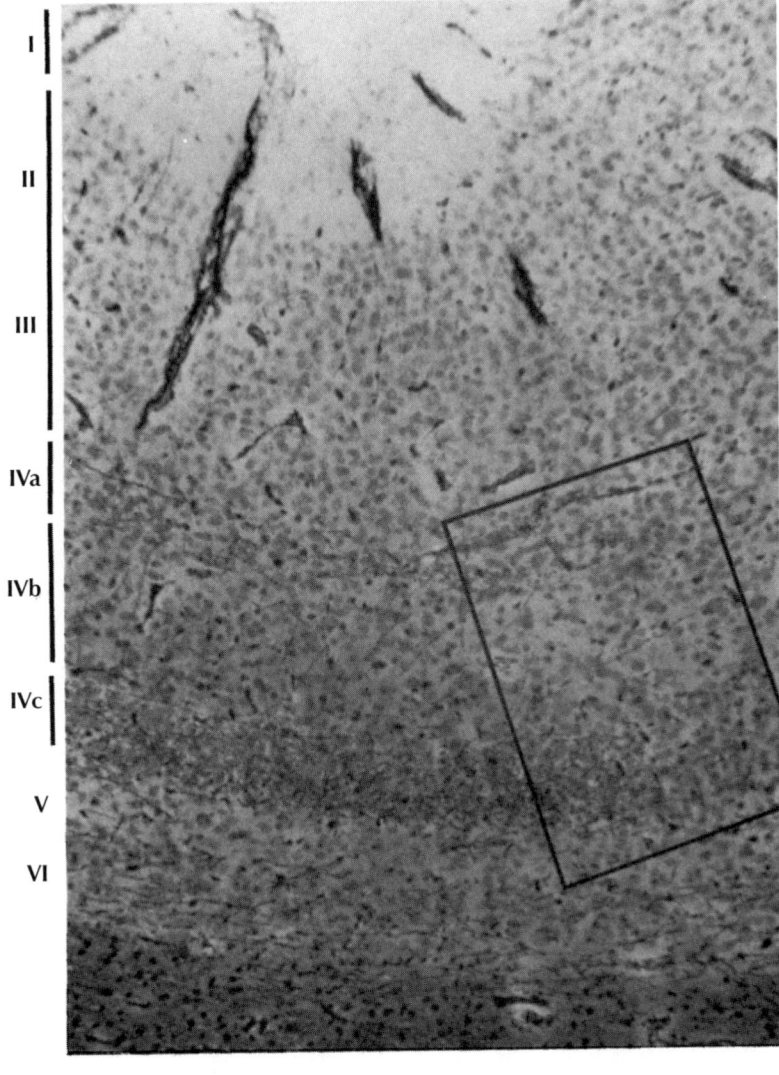

Figs. 7A, 7B. Terminal degeneration following lesion of a dorsal geniculate layer (layer 6) showing boundary between a band, to the left, and an interband, to the right. Note abruptness of the transition in both the upper and lower tiers of degeneration (layers IVa and IVc), the fact that the transition points lie roughly one above the other. Monkey 12. Fink-Heimer stain.

enough, for one to be sure of this, given the size of the dense overlapping region.

It may be worth noting that the direction of the stripes in the first experiment, and the direction suggested by the second, are almost identical. This raises the question of whether the stripes always have the same direction in a given part of the cortex, and whether they bear any constant relationship to the coordinates of the visual field, parallel-

ing the horizontal or vertical meridians, or lying along circles concentric about the fovea, for example. The material we have so far is too scanty and the lesions too widely spread through the visual fields to allow us to answer this.

The results from two other dorsal-layer lesions (monkeys 8, 15) are shown in figures 14 and 15. These were close to, and probably within, the foveal region.

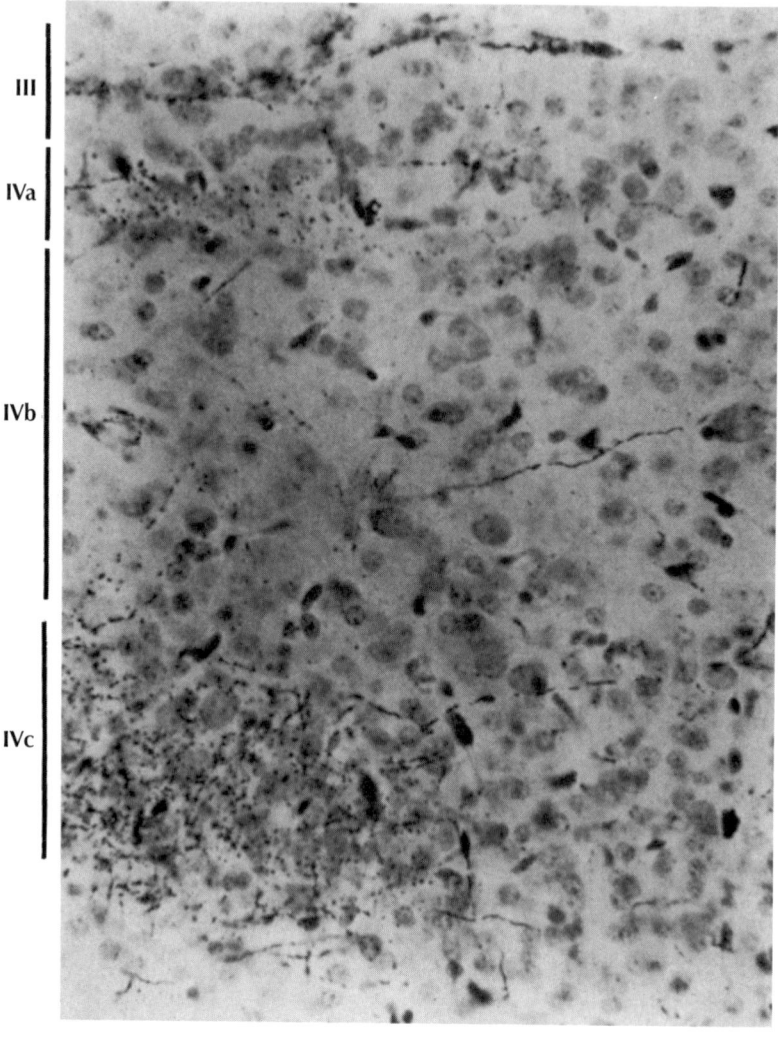

III

IVa

IVb

IVc

0.1mm

Fig. 7B.

Two ventral layer lesions are illustrated in Figures 16 and 17. The layer-1 lesion in monkey 36 (Fig. 16) was in the superior visual-field representation (lateral aspect of geniculate, posterior half of calcarine cortex). That of monkey 41 (Fig. 17) was also in the most ventral layer, in the region receiving input from an area 2–3° from the fovea, close to the horizontal meridian. The pattern in this monkey was again striped, in some sense, but here the tendency for interlacing and cross links was very marked, and was seen in both the areas of degeneration and in the spaces between.

We were interested in learning whether there was any obvious relationship between the widths of the bands of degeneration, i.e., the period of the alternating stripes, and the distance of the visual-field representation from the fovea. The magnification factor, or degrees of visual field per millimeter of cortex (Daniel and Whitteridge, '61) is well known to be related to distance from fovea, so that our question was the same as asking whether the stripe periodicity was constant in terms of millimeters along cortex, or in terms of degrees of visual field. The apparent period of stripes varied from

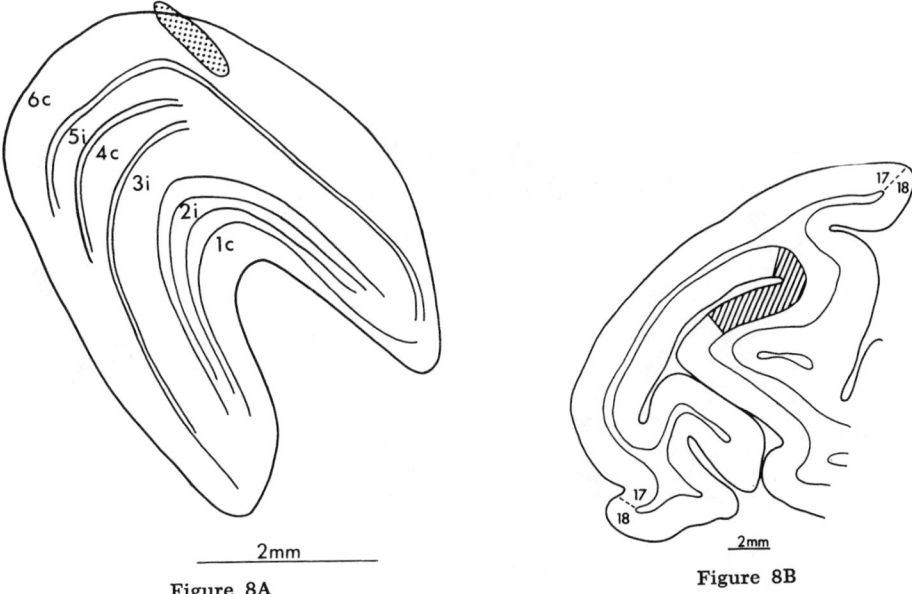

Figure 8A

Figure 8B

Fig. 8A. Tracing of left lateral geniculate body in monkey 12 to show the extent of the lesion in the most dorsal layer. Coronal section. Left is lateral. c, input from contralateral eye; i, input from ipsilateral eye.

Fig. 8B. Site of degeneration in left striate cortex of some monkey. Parasagittal section about 1 cm from midline, left is posterior. Shading indicates region with degenerating terminals.

about 0.5 mm for monkeys 36 and 41, up to 1.2 mm for lesion monkey 8. These measurements are taken from the frozen-section Nauta-degeneration slides, and have not been corrected for shrinkage. It is common experience that shrinkage may be substantial, up to 30% or more, in linear dimensions, and is far from constant from brain to brain or even in the same brain. Furthermore, the process of reconstruction may have led to distortions that could influence stripe width. But from the present material one can say that, at least in order of magnitude, the stripe periods were from 0.5 to 1.0 mm or slightly more, and that there was no obvious systematic variation in stripe width over the cortex, certainly none that would be comparable with the variation in magnification factor or in the size of cortical receptive fields. For example, Daniel and Whitteridge ('61, Fig. 4) found that in the fovea 1° is represented by about 6 mm of cortex, whereas about 15° from the fovea 1° occupies roughly 0.2–0.3 mm. If the stripe widths had varied by a factor of 20–30 this would surely have been detected in the present study.

DISCUSSION

The findings of this paper are of two different kinds, one having to do with the distribution in the striate cortex of terminals from the magnocellular and parvocellular geniculate layers, the other with the anatomical identification of the ocular-dominance columns and a description of their three-dimensional shape. The first of these represents a step towards understanding the wiring of the striate cortex, for clearly, not even a rudimentary description can exist if the site of terminations of the afferents is not known to the nearest layer, or if it is not appreciated that the two main subdivisions of the geniculate project to different cortical regions, or if, to take another example, a structure as conspicuous as the line of Gennari is erroneously (and despite the study of Clark and Sunderland, '39) thought to consist largely of afferent fibers. This is not to say that with the present study the input end of the wiring diagram of the striate cortex is by any means solved. Perhaps the most serious gap in our knowledge of area 17's morphology

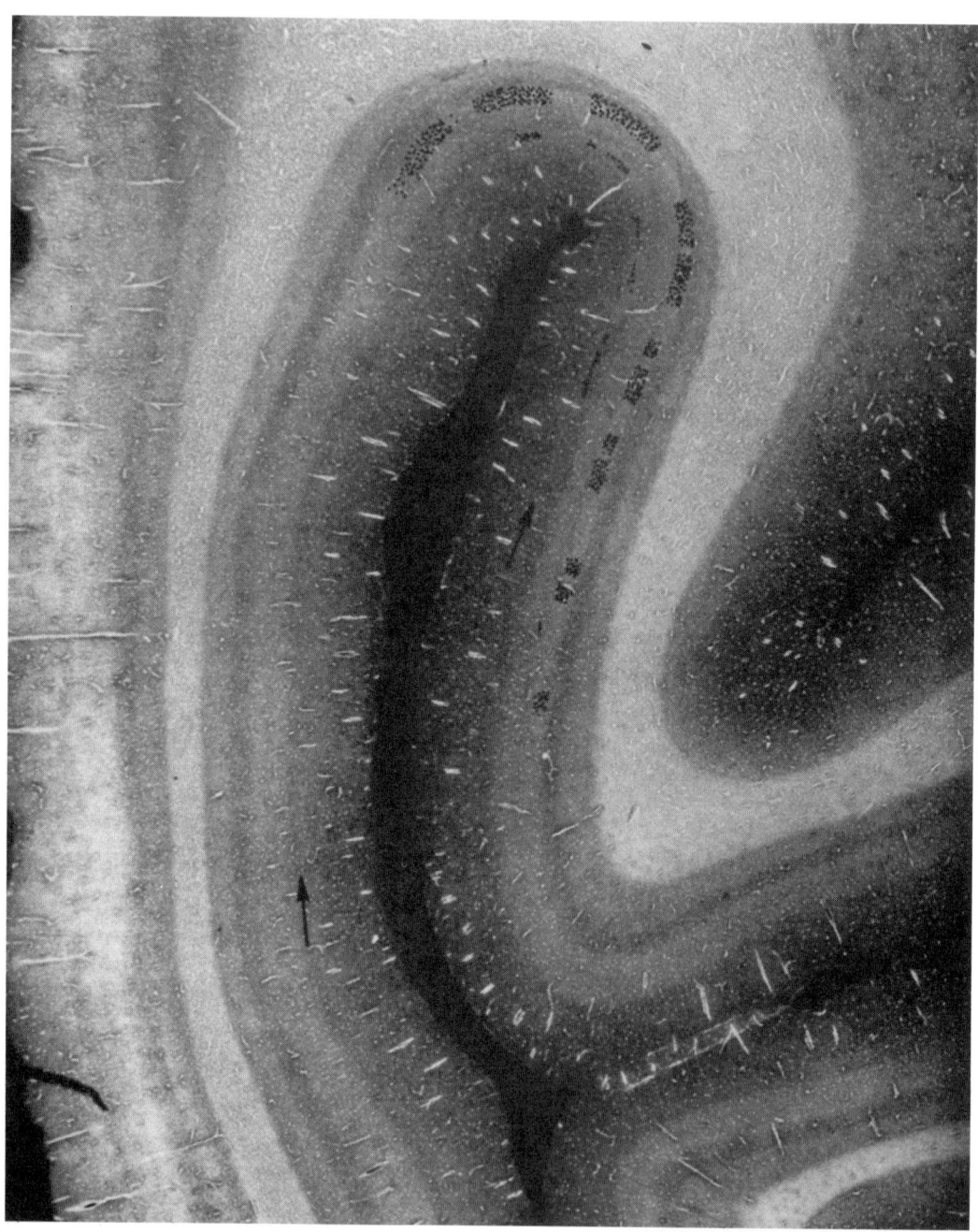

Fig. 9. Enlargement made directly from one parasagittal section through the occipital lobe in the region of degeneration in monkey 12 (Fig. 8). (Light areas are dark on the original slide.) The areas showing degeneration have been dotted in. A complete set of photographs such as this was used to make the reconstruction shown in Figure 10. Note the pale band at the same level as the upper tier of degeneration (arrows). Fink-Heimer stain.

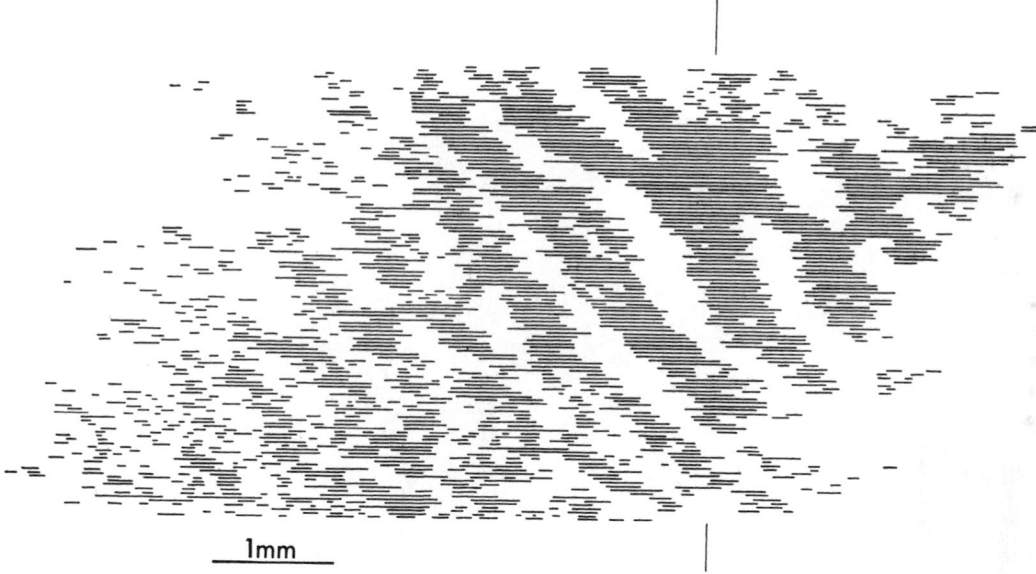

Fig. 10. Reconstruction of region showing terminal degeneration in layer IVc in monkey 12 (see Figs. 8, 9). The figure shows a face-on view of the flattened cortex at the level of layer IVc. Each horizontal line segment represents the degeneration in a single band of a single section such as that shown in Figure 9. Adjacent 30 μ-thick sections were plotted on 1 mm graph paper. Curved sections of gyrus were straightened graphically. Anterior is to the right, medial is up. The vertical lines represent the point of sharpest curvature of the gyrus (see Fig. 9).

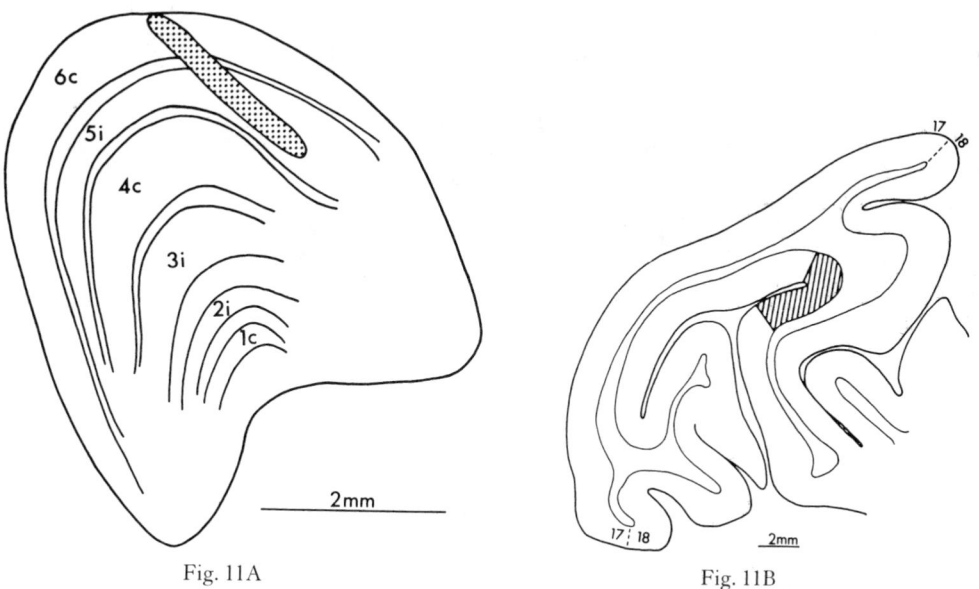

Fig. 11A   Fig. 11B

Fig. 11A. Tracing of left lateral geniculate body in monkey 14 to show the extent of the lesion in the two most dorsal layers. Coronal section, left is lateral. Fig. 11B. Site of degeneration in left striate cortex of same monkey in parasagittal section about 1 cm from midline. Left is posterior. Shading indicates region with degenerated terminals.

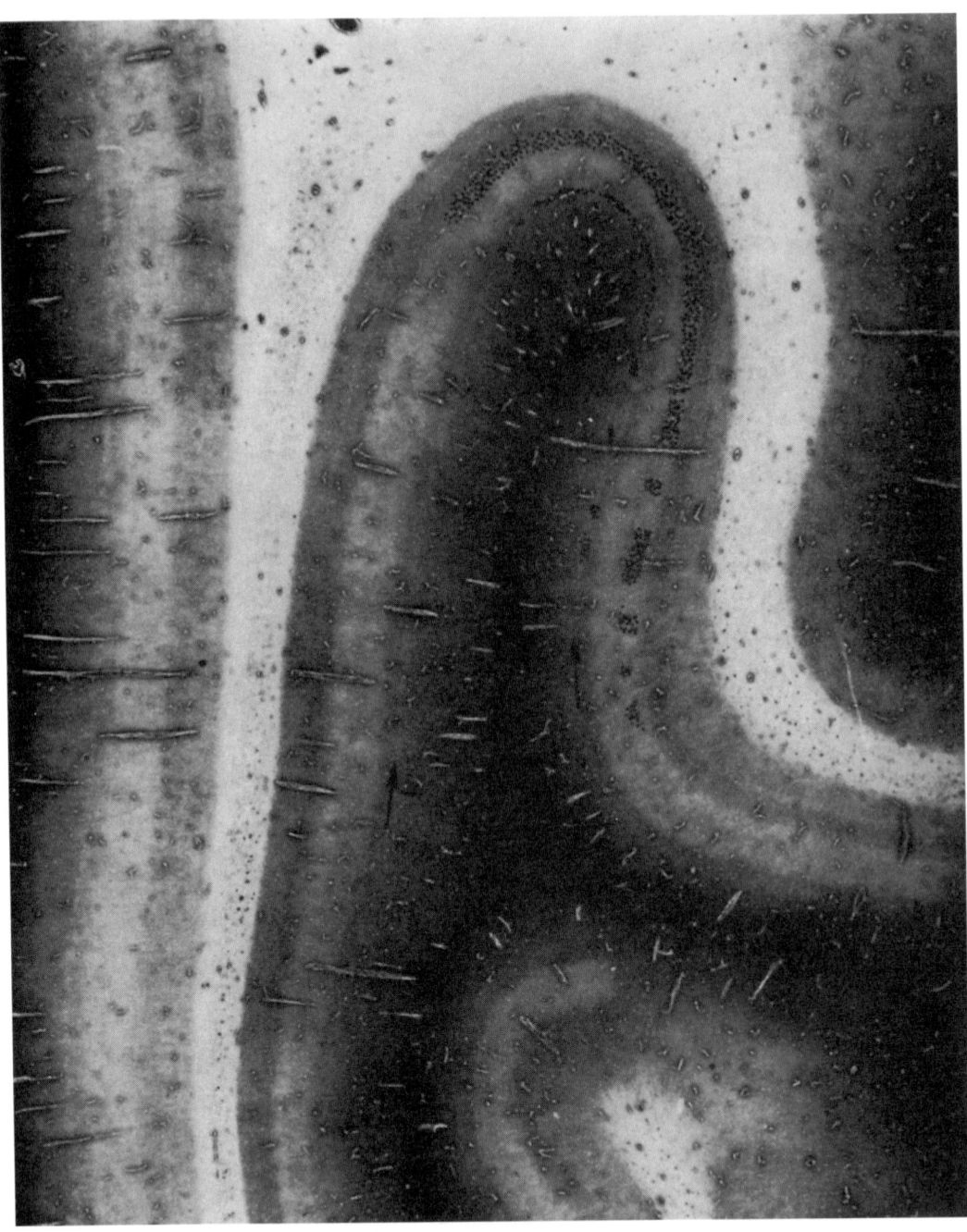

Fig. 12. Enlargement made directly from one parasagittal section through occipital lobe in the region of degeneration in monkey 14 (Fig. 11). The areas showing degeneration have been dotted in. A complete set of photographs was used to make the reconstruction shown in Figure 13. Note the pale band at the same level as the upper tier of degeneration (arrows). Fink-Heimer stain.

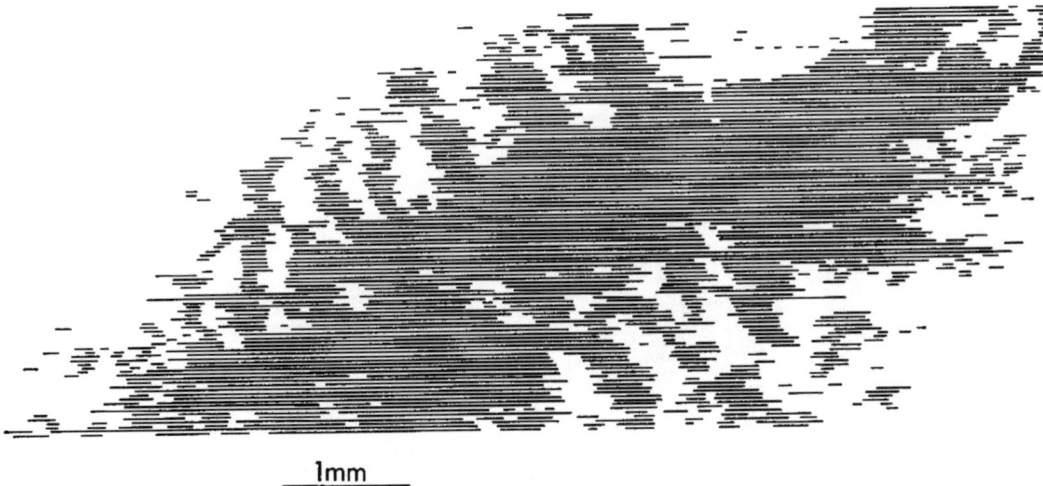

Fig. 13. *Reconstruction of region showing terminal degeneration in layer IVc in monkey 14 (see Figs. 11, 12). Other conventions as in Figure 10.*

concerns the class of cells upon which the afferents terminate—whether these are stellate or pyramidal cells. This question has been a somewhat vexed one (see Garey and Powell, '71), but recent Golgi studies in the monkey (Valverde, '71; Lund, in press) suggest that, after all, the stellate cells are probably the main targets of the input. Certainly, results of the present study, given the dense pack-

ing in layer IVc of an almost pure stellate-cell population, provide little encouragement to the idea that the afferents end primarily on pyramidal cells.

The finding that the dorsal geniculate layers project to two very distinct regions of layer IV (Hubel and Wiesel, '69) has been noted by Polley ('71) and confirmed by Garey and Powell ('71) both of whom used the Fink-Heimer method. Earlier

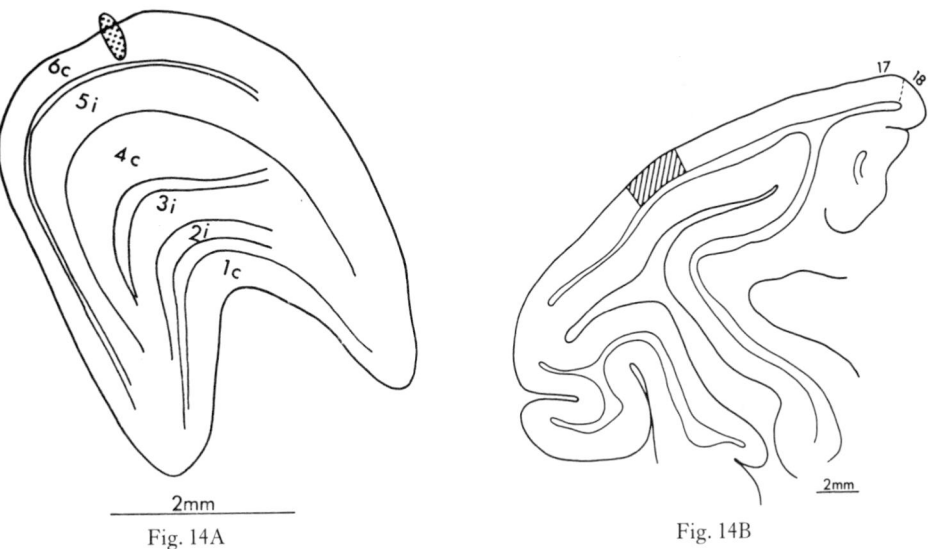

Fig. 14A

Fig. 14B

Fig. 14. *Monkey 8. (A) Tracing of left lateral geniculate body to show the extent of a lesion in the most dorsal layer. Coronal section. (B) Site of degeneration in left striate cortex. Parasagittal view about 1.5 cm from midline. (C) Reconstruction of region showing terminal degeneration in layer IVc. Conventions in Figure 10.*

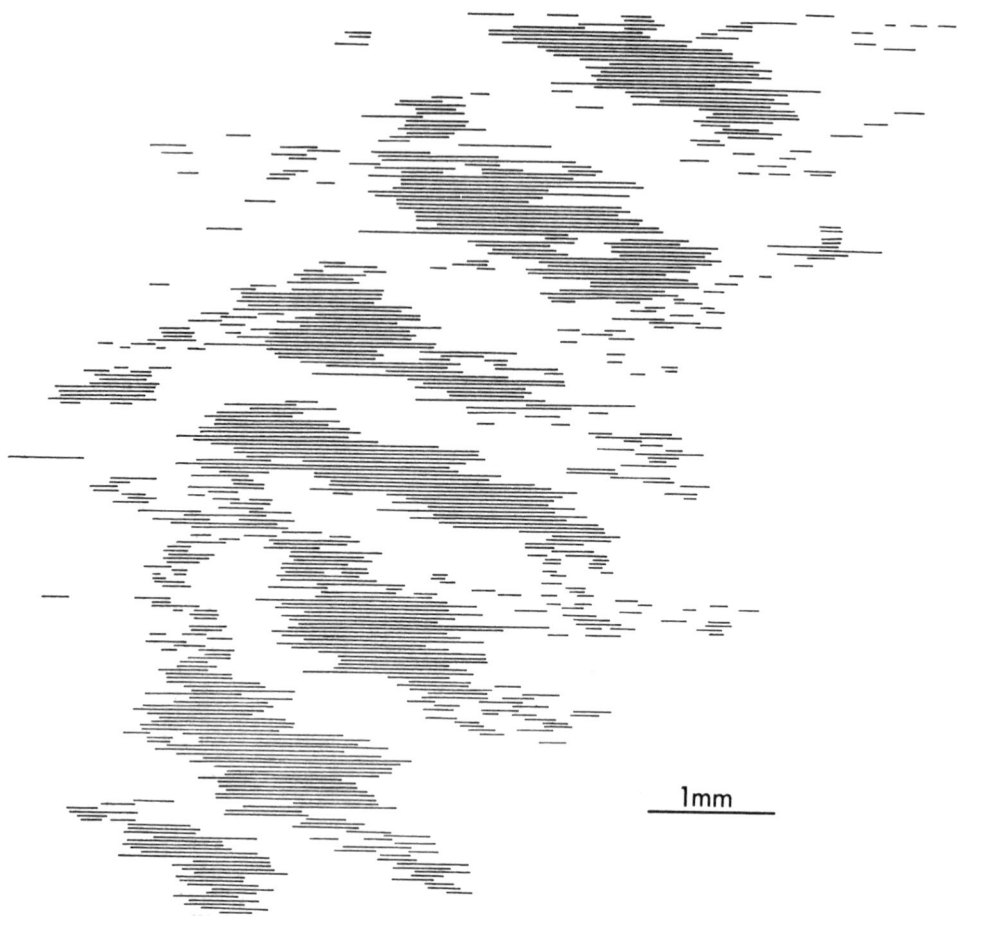

Fig. 14C.

studies (e.g., Wilson and Cragg, '67) already observed dense degeneration following geniculate lesions, extending superficially as far as layer III (perhaps what we have termed IVa) but the Nauta method did not make it possible to observe two distinct regions of termination. So far there is no hint of the physiological meaning of this two-tiered input. Our previous studies (Hubel and Wiesel, '68) showed the presence of simple cells and strictly monocular responses throughout layer IV. Given the present results, it would be worthwhile to study area 17 looking particularly at responses from the various subdivisions of layer IV. The fact that fibers from the dorsal and ventral layers of the geniculate terminate in different parts of layer IV is also difficult to interpret at present, but it is of potential interest since one knows that these two sets of geniculate layers have very different physiological properties (Wiesel and Hubel, '66). Thus ventral layer cells, on the whole, seem to have less of the color specificity and the variety of receptive-field types that are found in the dorsal group of layers. If one wishes to understand the reasons for the magno-parvo cellular duality in the geniculate, perhaps the best hope is to learn how the information transmitted by the two types of cells is used at higher levels. It thus comes as welcome news that the terminals are not immediately intermixed in the cortex, but are kept to a very large extent separate.

In recording from monkey visual cortex one of the most striking findings has been the vertical subdivisions into ocular-dominance columns. An anatomical demonstration of the corresponding

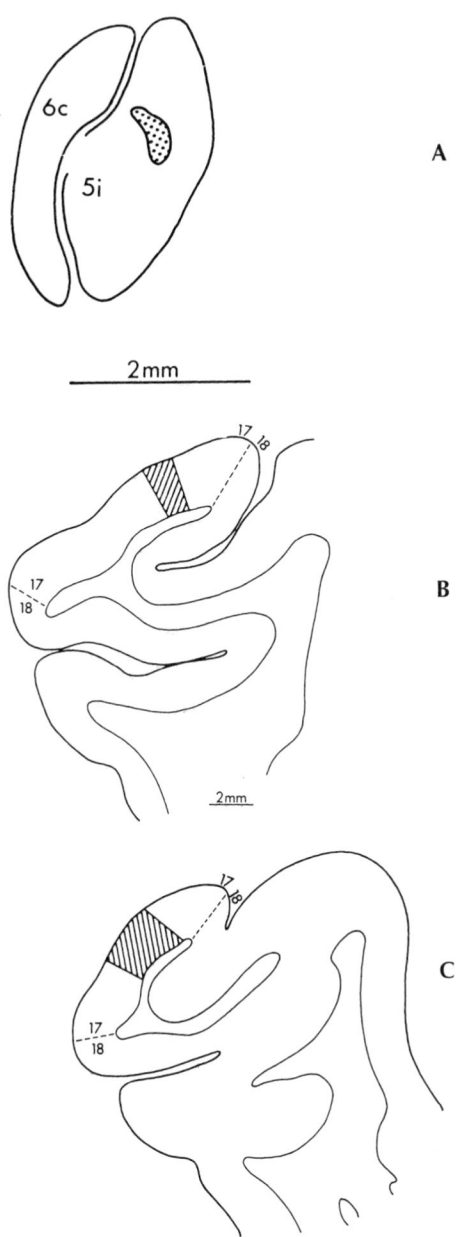

Fig. 15. Monkey 15. (A) Tracing of left lateral geniculate body to show extent of the lesion in layer 5. Coronal section which passes through geniculate in its most posterior part. (B and C) Two parasagittal section through left striate cortex, very far lateral. Foveal representation. C is a few millimeters lateral to B. (D) Reconstruction of region showing terminal degeneration in layer IVc. Conventions as in Figure 10.

IVth layer left-eye right-eye mosaic not only confirms this observation but also gives some idea of the geometry and degree of regularity of the mosaic. It turns out that the form is a highly regular one, consisting of alternating parallel stripes, with a variable amount of cross linking. The width of the stripes seems fairly constant at about 0.25–0.5 mm; any variation with position in the cortex was too little to detect, and in any case was certainly far less than the variation in magnification factor. The problem of constancy of stripe direction from animal to animal will be difficult to solve without doing many more experiments of this type. At present we are attempting to evolve a method that will show the stripe pattern over very wide areas of cortex in a single animal.

It is worth stressing that the IVth-layer mosaic brought out by these anatomical methods is only one manifestation of the system of ocular-dominance columns. Each column, as defined physiologically, extends from surface to white matter. In layer IV the cells almost always have fields that are concentrically arranged or simple, and they are almost always strictly monocular. (We have seen exactly one example of a binocularly driven simple cell in the monkey). In upper and lower layers most cells are binocularly influenced, but even here cells favoring a given eye are grouped together, and the grouping occurs in such a way that cells favoring, say, the left eye are directly above and below the IVth layer region monopolized by the left eye. The conclusion that the boundaries between neighboring columns are vertical is based on vertical and oblique microelectrode penetrations, but it receives anatomical support from the fact that the upper-tier patches in the present material are directly above and in register with the lower patches except occasionally in regions of high cortical curvature, where it is likely that the planes of section were oblique.

The surprising regularity of the ocular-dominance columns naturally makes one wonder if the orientation columns are similarly regular and long and narrow in cross section. There are some hints that they may be. Long oblique cortical penetrations (e.g., Hubel and Wiesel, '68, fig. 9) have sometimes, though not always, shown a marked regularity, with long sequences of small shifts in orientation all in the same direction clockwise or counter-clockwise. In 1968 we argued that this in

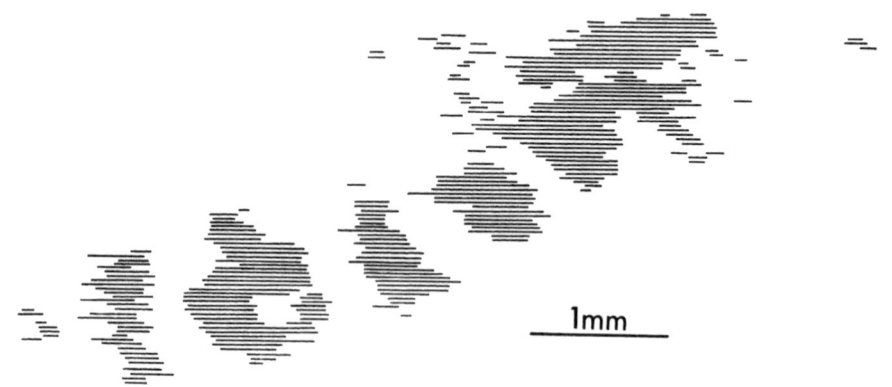

Fig. 15D.

itself suggested that the columns might be slab-like in shape. The evidence for this was indirect, though surface mappings had also pointed to the same conclusion (Hubel and Wiesel, '63, Fig. 4). The finding that the ocular-dominance columns are slabs would seem to strengthen the possibility that the orientation columns are also. If they are, it would be especially interesting to know whether in horizontal section the stripes are orthogonal to the ocular dominance stripes, or parallel, or have any fixed relationship. The answer to this may be important, for the input that a binocular complex cell, lying above or below layer IV, receives from two adjacent ocular-dominance columns must at the same time originate from the same orientation column—unless it comes from two similar orienta-tion columns and has to cross over all the interven-ing ones. The problem is obviously easily solved by having the two systems orthogonal to each other. A diagrammatic example of such an arrangement is given in Figure 18.

The two coexisting column systems are of course superimposed upon the two-coordinate mapping of the visual fields. It might reasonably be asked whether a complex cell receiving input from two neighboring ocular-dominance columns would not necessarily, as a consequence, receive its input from two disparate positions on the two reti-nas. The answer seems to be that the topographic representation does not hold over distances compa-rable to column widths; in an oblique penetration traversing a single column from one side to the other, no overall drift in receptive-field positions

can be discerned against the random variations (Hubel and Wiesel, '62). Even in a penetration that crossed 53 orientation columns (Hubel and Wiesel, '68) there was no detectable change in receptive-field position. The retinocortical mappings are decidedly not point-to-point, but are region-to-region.

In comparing the results of recordings from striate cortex in cat and monkey, one of the most conspicuous differences has been the sharpness of definition of the ocular-dominance columns. What was such a striking feature in the monkey was only barely detectable in the cat (Hubel and Wiesel, '62, '65). We have repeated the experiments described in the present paper in the cat, and, as might have been predicted from the physiology, find no obvi-ous suggestion of a right-eye left-eye mosaic in layer IV. In cats brought up from birth with stra-bismus (Hubel and Wiesel, '65) the relative num-bers of binocularly influenced cells drops sharply to about 20% and there is a concomitant strong ten-dency to grouping of cells according to eye domi-nance. Our hope was that a mosaic might be demonstrable in these animals by making laminar geniculate lesions, and studies with this objective are now under way, though the results so far have not been very encouraging.

In a previous paper (Hubel and Wiesel, '68) we have drawn attention to the similarity between ocular-dominance columns in the visual cortex, and the "skin" versus "deep" columns originally described by Mountcastle ('57) in the somatosen-sory cortex. Both are two-fold columnar systems,

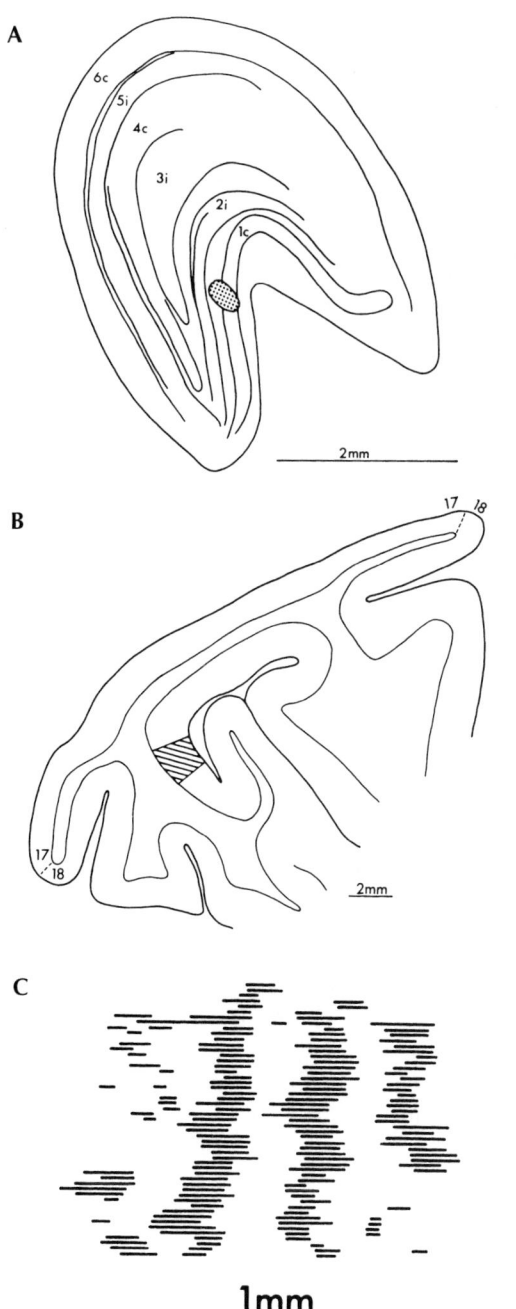

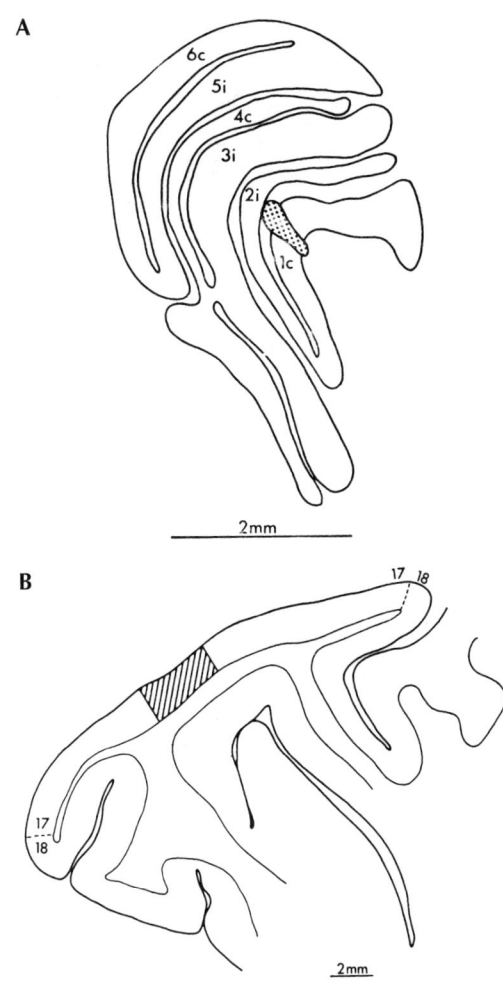

as opposed to the many-fold orientation columns in area 17; both depend on the distribution of input fibers rather than subsequent intracortical connections. It would be interesting if similar methods could be used to demonstrate the IVth layer mosaic in the somatosensory cortex. That this might be feasible is suggested by the observation of Poggio and Mountcastle ('63) that cells are aggregated in the thalamic ventrobasal complex according to their responsiveness to superficial versus deep

Fig. 16. Monkey 36. (A) Tracing of left lateral geniculate body from coronal section showing the extent of a lesion in the most ventral layer. (B) Site of degeneration in left striate cortex. Parasagittal section about 10 millimeters from midline. Shading indicates area of degeneration. (C) Reconstruction of region showing terminal degeneration in layer IVb. Conventions as in Figure 10.

Fig. 17. Monkey 41. (A) Tracing of left lateral geniculate body from coronal section showing the extent of a lesion in the most ventral layer. (B) Site of degeneration (indicated by shading) in left striate cortex. Parasagittal section about 15 mm from midline. Left is posterior. (C) Reconstruction of region showing terminal degeneration in layer IVb. Conventions as in Figure 10.

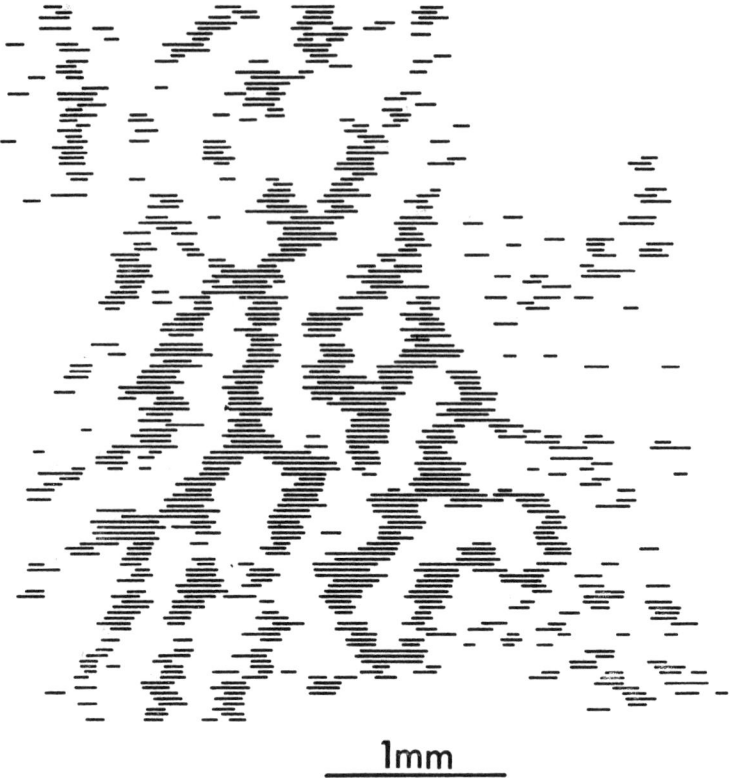

Fig. 17C.

stimuli. In a sense, these aggregations may be analogous to the geniculate layers.

It is worth noting that the elegant system of "barrels" described by Woolsey and Van der Loos ('70) in the mouse somatosensory cortex seems to represent a columnar system in which the IVth layer mosaic is visible by routine staining methods, especially if the cortex is sectioned tangentially. Here each column apparently represents a single whisker of the snout of the mouse, being a part of the two-dimensional cortical topography but nevertheless fulfilling the requirement of discreteness. This is the only case so far where a correlation of columns was observed anatomically before a physiological identification had been made. One wonders, of course, whether cells below and above the barrels represent the site of convergence from several neighboring whiskers.

Finally, the development of these highly regular column systems is worth considering. The ocular-dominance columns are evidently determined by the mode of ingrowth of the afferent fibers. The orientation columns, as we have argued before, must be determined by patternings of intracortical connections, perhaps at the first or second synapse. The orientation columns are probably present at birth (Hubel and Wiesel, '63); we have as yet done too few studies of infant monkeys to know whether ocular-dominance columns are also, but it seems very likely that they are. How such ordered systems can develop innately promises to be a challenging question for the future.

ACKNOWLEDGMENTS

We wish to think Julia Currie and Martha Egan for histological assistance, and Marian Carlson for help with the cortical reconstructions. Our special thanks to Janet Wiitanen for her invaluable assistance with the photomicrographs and in the preparation of the manuscript, to say nothing of her contribution to the staining method! This work was supported by NIH Research grants 5RO1 EY00605–13 and 5RO1 EY00606–08 and also grant 4916 from Bell Telephone.

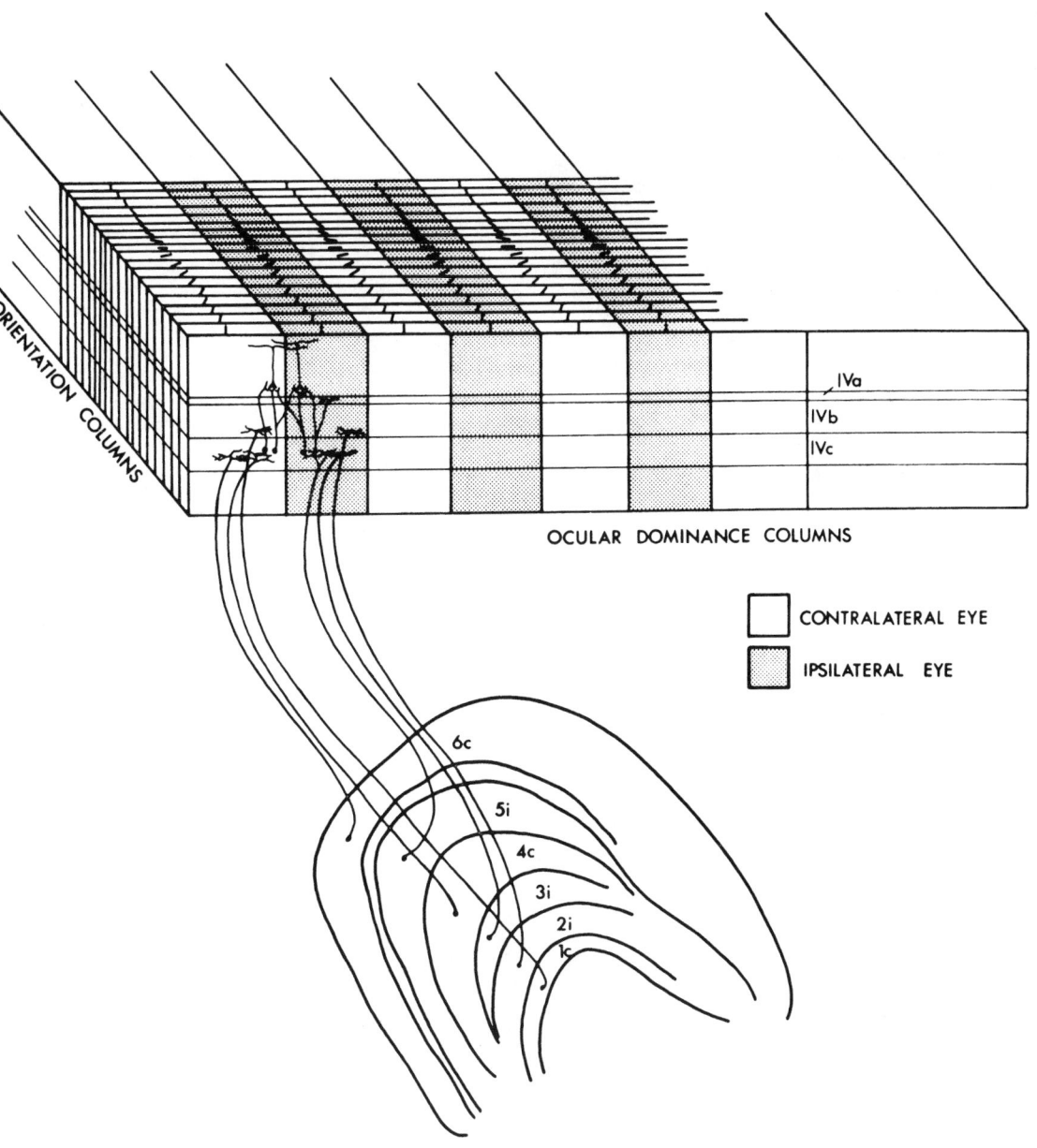

Fig. 18. Diagram showing a possible relationship between ocular-dominance columns and orientation columns assuming the orientation columns are also long narrow parallel slabs, and that their arrangement is very orderly. Note that the width of these orientation slabs is much less than that of the ocular-dominance columns. A complex cell in an upper layer is shown receiving input from two neighboring ocular-dominance columns, but from the same orientation column.

315

Literature Cited

Clark, W. E. Le Gros, and S. Sunderland 1939 Structural changes in the isolated visual cortex. J. Anat., *78:* 563–574.

Daniel, P. M., and D. Whitteridge 1961 The representation of the visual field on the cerebral cortex in monkeys. J. Physiol., *159:* 203–221.

Fink, R. P., and L. Heimer 1967 Two methods for selective silver impregnation of degenerating axons and their synaptic endings in the central nervous system. Brain Res., *4:* 367–374.

Garey, L. J., and T. P. S. Powell 1971 An experimental study of the termination of the lateral geniculo-cortical pathway in the cat and monkey. Proc. Roy. Soc. Lond. B., *179:* 41–63.

Heimer, L., and A. Peters 1968 An electron microscope study of a silver stain for degenerating boutons. Brain Res., *8:* 337–346.

Hubel, D. H., and T. N. Wiesel 1962 Receptive fields, binocular interaction and functional architecture in the cat's visual cortex. J. Physiol., *160:* 106–154.

——— 1963 Shape and arrangement of columns in cat's striate cortex. J. Physiol., *165:* 559–568.

——— 1965 Binocular interaction in striate cortex of kittens reared with artificial squint. J. Neurophysiol., *28:* 1041–1059.

——— 1968 Receptive fields and functional architecture of monkey striate cortex. J. Physiol., *195:* 215–243.

——— 1969 Anatomical demonstration of columns in the monkey striate cortex. Nature, *221:* 747–750.

Lund, J. S. 1972 Organization of neurons in the visual cortex, area 17, of the monkey (Macaca mulatta). J. Comp. Neur., in press.

Mountcastle, V. B. 1957 Modality and topographic properties of single neurons of cat's somatic sensory cortex. J. Neurophysiol., *20:* 408–434.

Nauta, W. J. H., and P. A. Gygax 1954 Silver impregnation of degenerating axons in the central nervous system: A modified technic. Stain Technol., *29:* 91–93.

Poggio, G. F., and V. B. Mountcastle 1963 The functional properties of ventrobasal thalamic neurons studied in unanesthetized monkeys. J. Neurophysiol., *26:* 775–806.

Polley, E. H. 1971 Intracortical distribution of lateral geniculate axons in cat and monkey. Anat. Rec., *169:* 404.

Valverde, F. 1971 Short axon neuronal subsystems in the visual cortex of the monkey. Intern. J. Neuroscience, *1:* 181–197.

von Bonin, G. 1942 The striate area of primates. J. Comp. Neur., *77:* 405–429.

Wiesel, T. N., and D. H. Hubel 1966 Spatial and chromatic interactions in the lateral geniculate body of the lateral geniculate body of the Rhesus monkey. J. Neurophysiol., *29:* 1115–1156.

Wiitanen, J. T. 1969 Selective silver impregnation of degenerating axons and axon terminals in the central nervous system of the monkey (Macaca mulatta). Brain Res., *14:* 546–548.

Wilson, M. E., and Cragg, B. G. 1967 Projections from the lateral geniculate nucleus in the cat and monkey. J. Anat., *101:* 677–692.

Woolsey, T. A., and H. Van der Loos 1970 The structural organization of layer IV in the somatosensory region (SI) of mouse cerebral cortex. Brain Res., *17:* 205–242.

AFTERWORD

This was the first indication that the magno and parvo subdivisions of the geniculate keep their separated identities at central levels in the visual path. How much further into the brain they maintain their separation—how much they overlap, if they do—is a major source of discussion among neurobiologists. Jennifer Lund has extended the story by showing with Golgi techniques that 4C-beta projects to the deepest part of layer 3, whereas the magno-affiliated 4C-alpha projects to 4B, roughly to the Line of Gennari. As mentioned in the afterthoughts to our 1968 monkey paper, it appears that 4B may receive substantial input from 4C-beta.

It was hugely gratifying to be invited to present these results at a meeting of the austere Cajal Club, at the anatomy meetings in Chicago in 1970, and to be treated like respected members of that august society. All thanks to Jim Sprague, Jane Chen, Janet Wiitanen, and of course Walle Nauta.

Chapter 18 • Ocular Dominance Columns Revealed by Autoradiography •

FOREWORD

In these experiments we used the relatively new (at least to us) method of axon transport of radioactive labels coupled with autoradiography, to reproduce and extend the experiments with the Nauta method. Autoradiography was just beginning to be used in neuroanatomy, and we had been looking for a chance to try it. The method consists of injecting a radioactive aminoacid into some part of the nervous system; the amino acid is incorporated into a protein that is taken up by the cells and, one hopes, transported by the cells' axons to their terminals, perhaps some distance away. One then sections the tissue and mounts it on slides that are covered by silver emulsion and developed just as a photographic negative is. The radioactivity will have produced a reduction of the silver compounds in the emulsion, so that the terminations of the labelled cells show up as black.

In 1971 Bernice Grafstein and R. Laureno, at the Cornell University Medical College (*Exp Neurol* 38, 44–57), reported a result that made us sit up. They injected a radioactive amino acid into the eye of a mouse, and found by autoradiography not only the expected transport to the superior colliculus and lateral geniculate, but also in small amounts to the primary visual cortex. That meant that the tracer had gone beyond the geniculate, somehow presumably crossing the synapse there—an unprecedented result. We thought of trying the same thing in a monkey but worried that the amounts that made it to the cortex might not be enough to detect. When we finally made the attempt, with a rather huge eye injection of tritiated fucose and proline, our pessimism seemed to be confirmed: we saw large amounts of tracer in the appropriate layers of the geniculate but no hint of silver grains in the striate cortex. In the spring of 1974 I visited the labs of the neuroanatomist Ray Guillery in Madison, Wisconsin, to give a seminar. Guillery was making much use of autoradiography of transported tracers and was routinely viewing his slides under dark-field illumination. Evidently everyone but a rank beginner knew that the scattering of light by silver grains in the photographic image was greatly enhanced when viewed under dark field. I made no mention of our experiment to Guillery, but within minutes of my return to Boston out came the slides—and there under dark field, were the columns in all their glory. Because the entire eye had been injected we could of course see the columns throughout the entire binocular part of the striate cortex, compare their sizes near the foveal representation and in the periphery, and compare the two temporal crescents—none of which could be done with the tiny local geniculate lesions in the Nauta experiments. On the other hand we obviously could not distinguish magnocellular and parvocellular projections, so each method had its own advantages.

This convinced us that travel can sometimes pay dividends, especially if one chooses carefully the people one visits.

Autoradiographic demonstration of ocular-dominance columns in the monkey striate cortex by means of transneuronal transport

T. N. WIESEL, D. H. HUBEL AND D. M. K. LAM • *Harvard Medical School, Department of Neurobiology,*

Boston, Mass. 02115 (U.S.A.)

In the past few years the technique of mapping pathways in the central nervous system by anterograde axoplasmic transport of radioactive molecules has come into wide use and is now an important supplement to Nauta degeneration methods[2,6,10,13]. Several investigators[1,3,7,9,12] have noted radioactive substances in the postsynaptic cells, which suggests that these cells take up labeled material released from the terminals[1,3,7]. Grafstein[4] was the first to explore the possibility of tracing a pathway beyond the terminals of the initially labeled cells, by examining also the projections of the recipient postsynaptic neurons. By radiochemical measurements and by autoradiography, it was shown that after injection of [³H] proline and [³H]fucose into one eye of a mouse the contralateral striate cortex was more heavily labeled than the ipsilateral, and that the label was concentrated in layer IV[5,14]

In the macaque monkey the geniculostriate pathway terminates in a very dense, highly localized manner, mainly in layer IV C. Furthermore, projections from the 2 eyes end in a characteristic alternating stripe-like pattern of ocular-dominance columns[8]. It occurred to us that if radioactive substances were transported transneuronally, injection of labeled material into one eye followed by autoradiography of the cortex might reveal the entire system of ocular-dominance columns.

For the autoradiographic study of transneuronal transport in the primate visual system, 50 µl of a saline solution containing L-[6-³H]fucose (2.5 mCi/ml, 13.4 Ci/mmole) and L-[³H]proline (7.5 mCi/ml, generally labeled, 6.8 Ci/mmole) was injected into the vitreous of the left eye of a 3 kg normal Rhesus macaque. This injection was repeated 5 times at 12 h intervals (total dose 3.0 mCi). The animal was perfused with 10% formalin 3 weeks after the initial injection. The lateral geniculate nucleus was cut into 20 µm frozen sections, and the striate cortex was embedded in paraffin and cut into 15 µm

From *Brain Research,* 79 (1974) 273–279

Accepted July 3rd, 1974.

sections. The sections were coated with Ilford K5 emulsion, left in the dark for 2–4 months and developed in Dektol. Sections were counter-stained with thionin.

In the lateral geniculate nucleus all layers receiving projections from the injected eye were strongly labeled (Fig. 1A and B). The other layers showed grain counts higher than background, perhaps partly because of fibers of passage from the retina, but also, probably, because of diffusion of radioactive material from recipient layers to adjacent ones.

In the striate cortex an accumulation of silver grains in layer IV was most easily visualized under dark-field illumination. A typical section is shown in Fig. 2. Deposition of granules can be seen in layer IV C and as a thin 'upper tier' in layer IV A. This distribution agrees well with that seen in Fink-Heimer stained material after a geniculate lesion[8]. An apparent difference between the two methods was a lack of any obvious concentration of radioactive material in layer I, which receives a very sparse input in Nauta stained material.

The accumulation of silver grains in layer IV

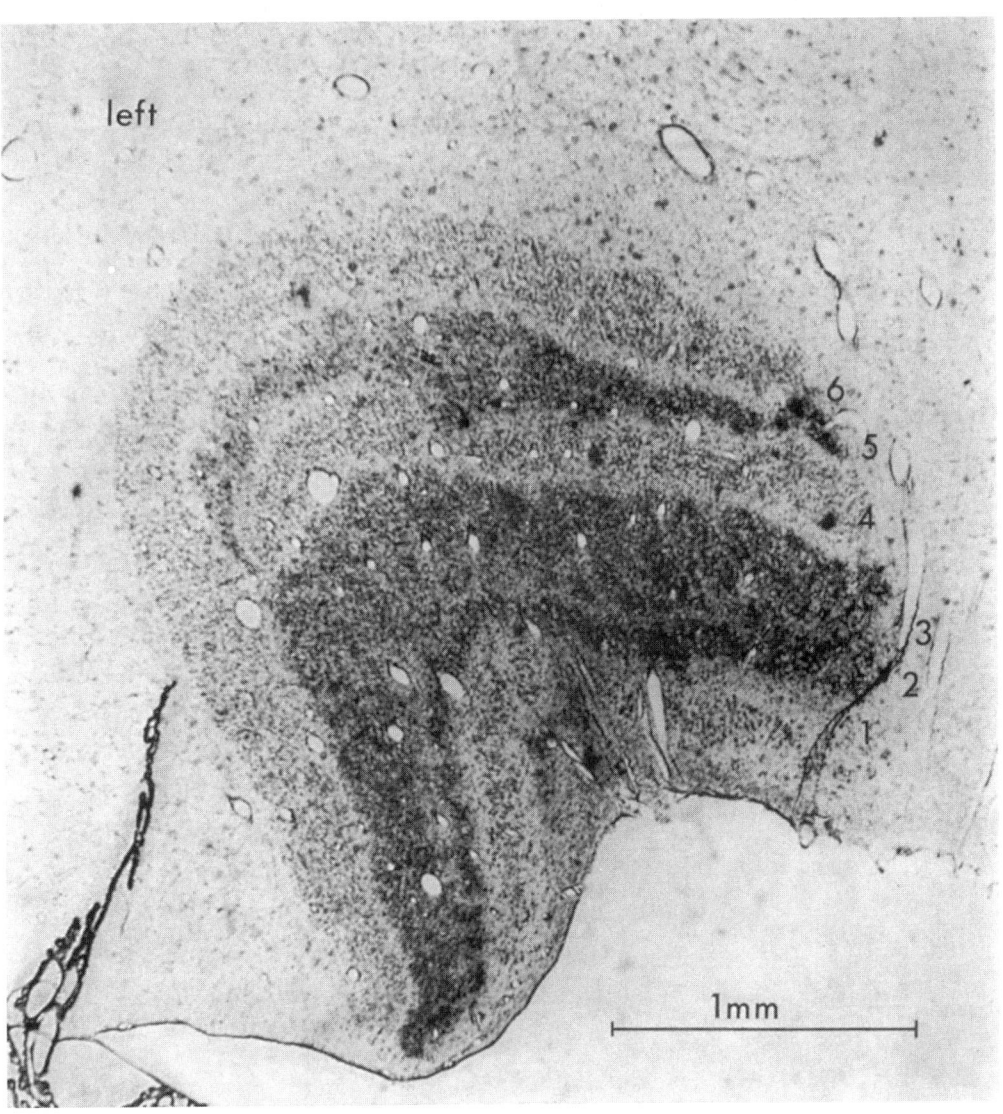

Fig. 1. Autoradiograph of left (A) and right (B) lateral geniculate bodies; coronal sections, Nissl counterstained, bright-field illumination. 1–6, the layers are numbered 1–6 from ventral to dorsal.

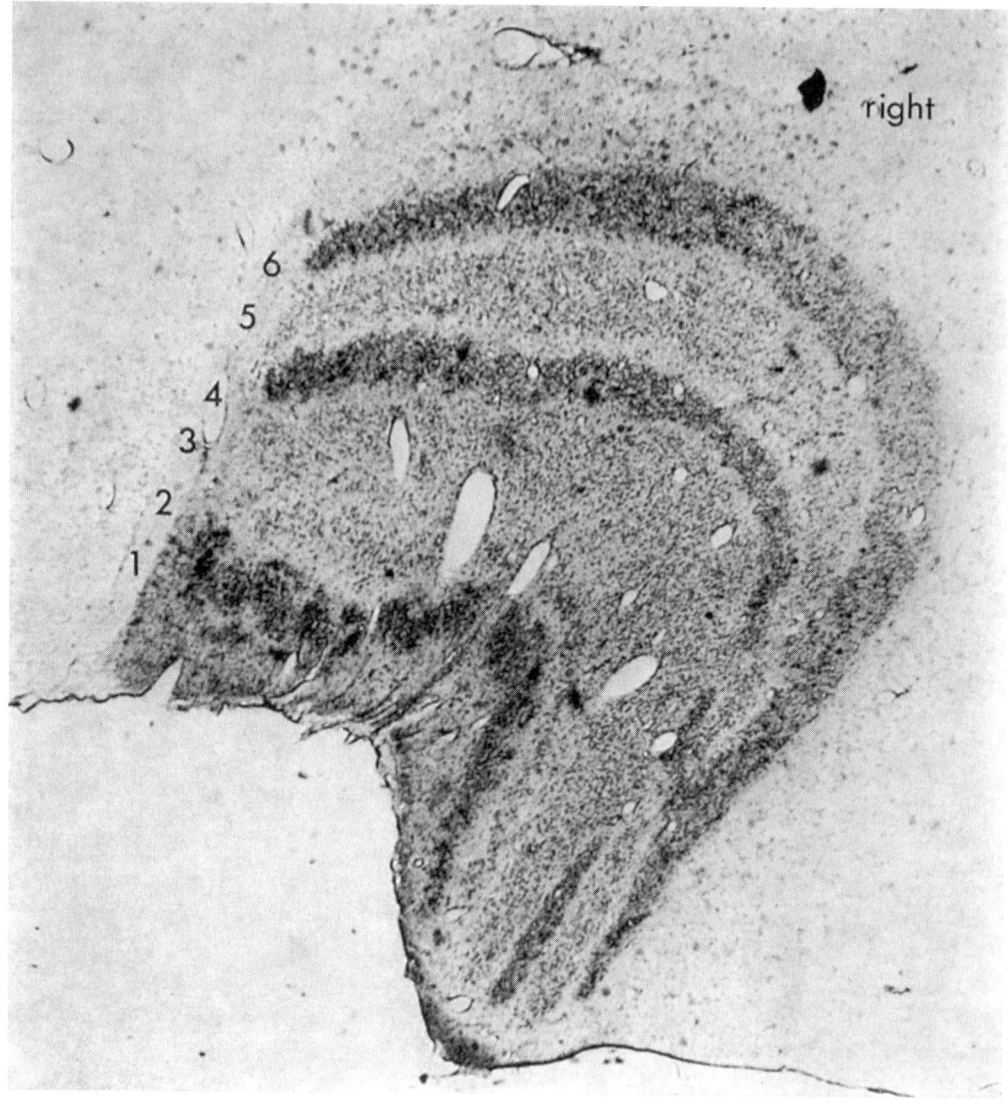

Fig. 1B.

was interrupted by conspicuous gaps in which the density of grains was considerably less, although it was higher than that of the background (Fig. 2). The widths of the dark and light bands were about equal, measuring 0.3–0.5 mm. Fig. 3 shows a montage reconstruction of a section through cortex in the calcarine fissure. The plane of section is almost tangential to the cortex, cutting through layer IV C and grazing layer V. The alternating bands of IV C thus form an oval surrounding layer V. In the upper part of the reconstruction 5 or 6 columns are cut tangentially and appear as parallel stripes. The

pattern revealed by Figs. 2 and 3 is identical to that seen with the Fink-Heimer modification of the Nauta method after a lesion confined to one layer of the lateral geniculate nucleus, and certainly represents the morphological equivalent of the physiologically defined ocular-dominance columns. In the monocular segment of the cortex, contralateral to the injected eye, there were, as expected, no gaps, but a continuous band of silver grains in the IVth layer (Fig. 4). No attempt was made to reconstruct the columns in the entire occipital lobe, since we have subsequently found a simpler method of

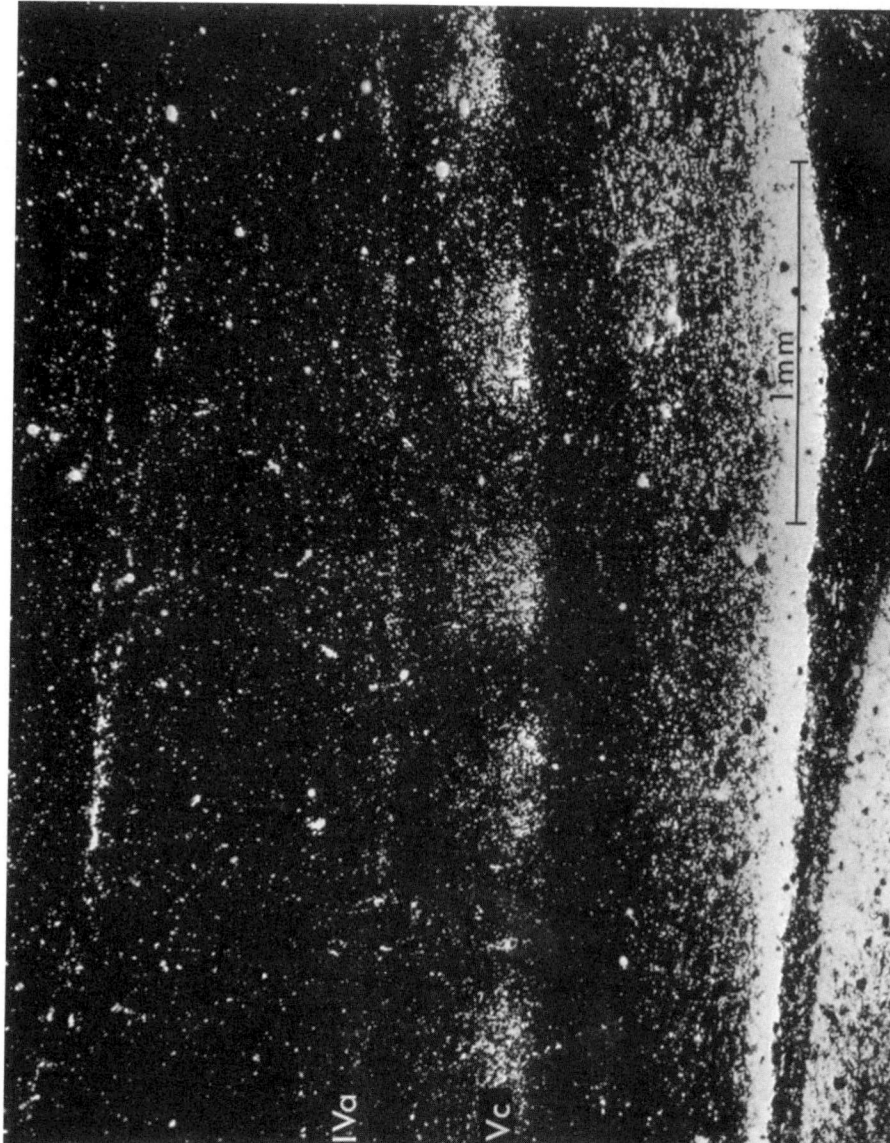

Fig. 2. Autoradiograph of a section through calcarine cortex (area 17), photographed under dark-field illumination. Bright bands of silver-granule accumulations appear in layer IV C at regular intervals, separated by gaps of equal width in which grains are fewer, although still more numerous than in the layers immediately above and below. Similar bands, much fainter and thinner, form an upper tier in layer IV A.

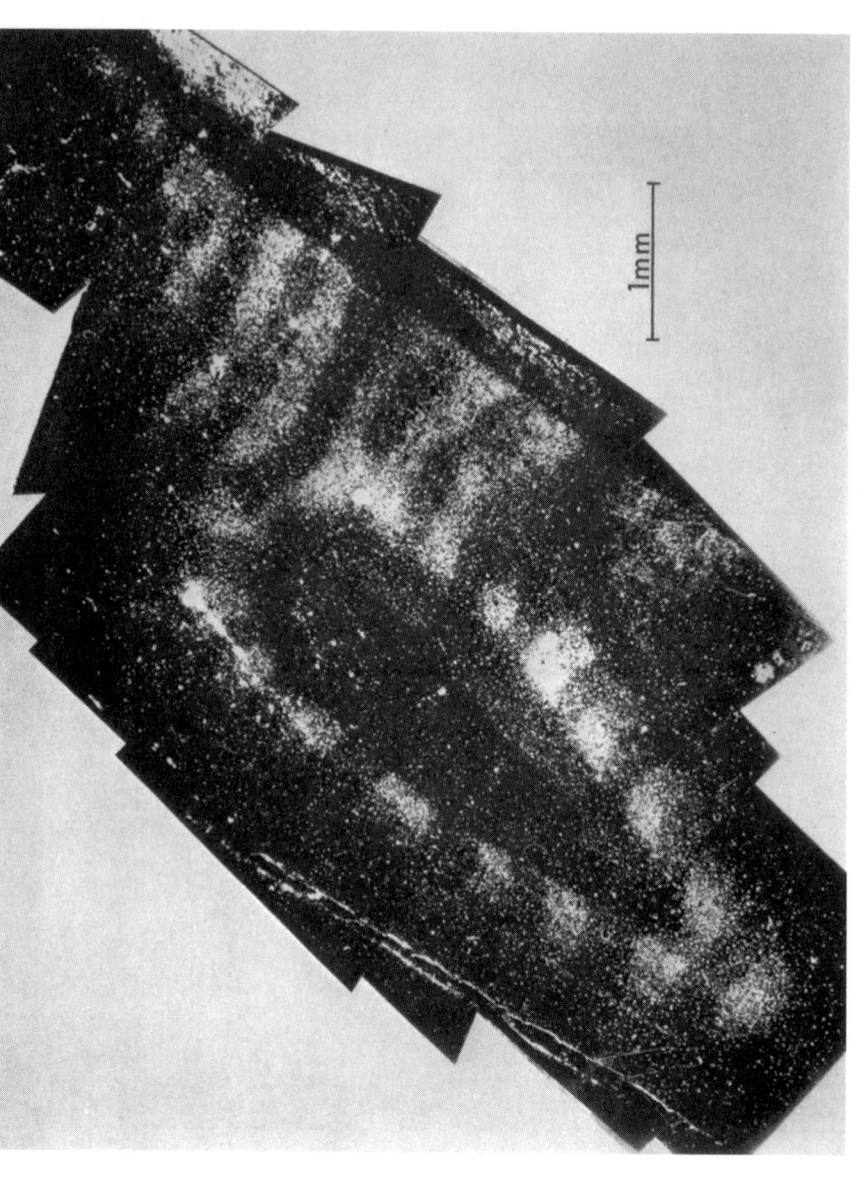

Fig. 3. Montage of a set of dark-field microphotographs from a section through calcarine cortex. The section passes almost tangentially through a dome-shaped region of cortex, cutting through layer IV to form an oval ring of alternating light and dark patches. The oval encloses a part of layer V which has been grazed by the plane of section. Above, 5–6 of the layer IV C patches are cut tangentially and form a set of parallel stripes. Two-thirds of the way from pia to layer IV C, one can see a suggestion of the thin layer IV A 'upper tier'. Below, the thin pial surface is visible; together with the pial surface of adjacent cortex it forms parallel lines like train tracks.

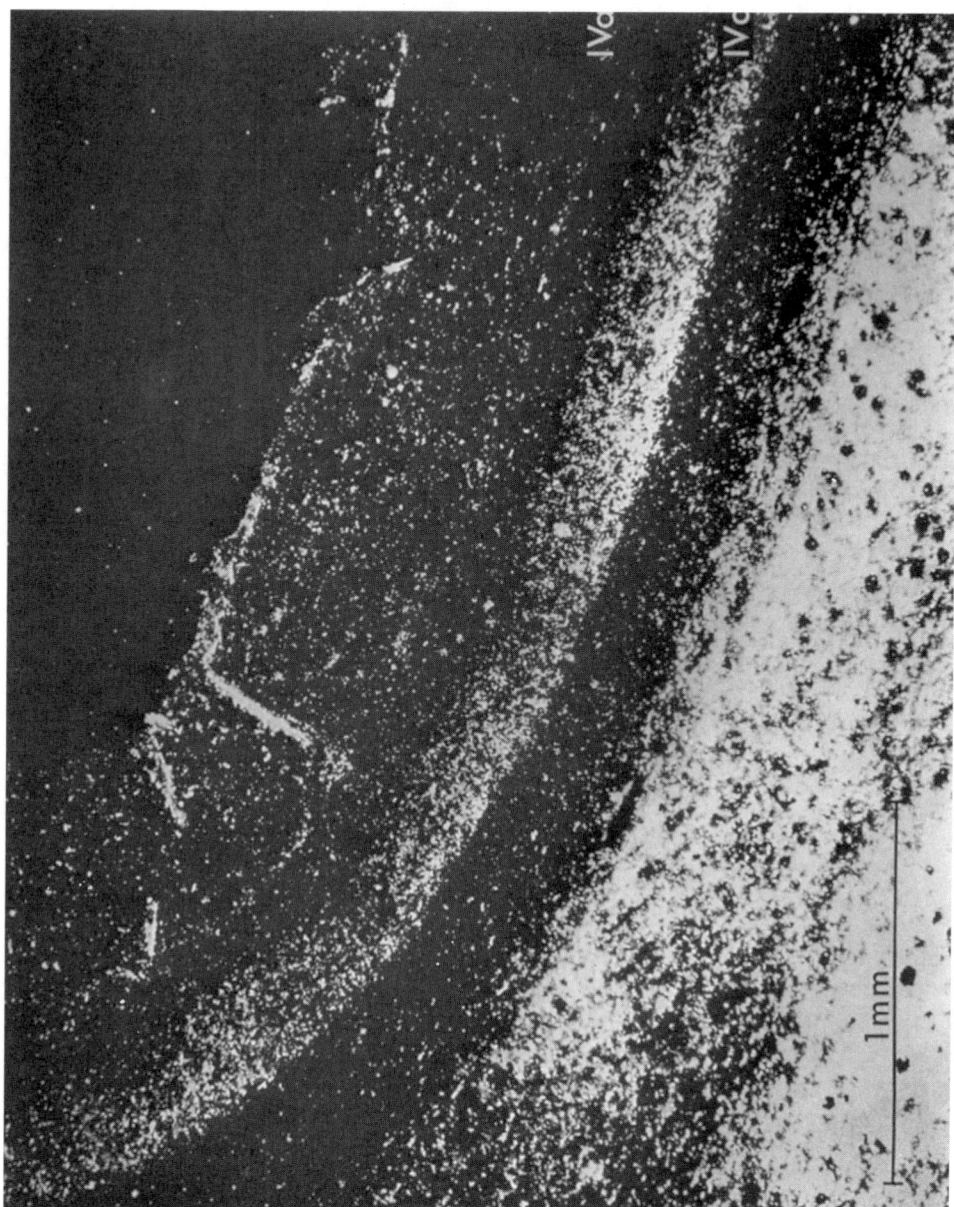

Fig. 4. Autoradiograph of a section through the stem of the calcarine cortex, photographed under dark-field illumination. Same section as in Fig. 2, but shows the temporal-crescent representation. Since the ipsilateral eye has no input to this region, the granules form a continuous band in layer IV C, with a sparse accumulation in IV A.

demonstrating ocular-dominance columns in normal material[11].

The presence of labeled material within the IVth-layer gaps may be due to fibers of passage from the geniculate layers representing the injected eye. It may also be the result of diffusion within the geniculate, from the 3 layers on each side receiving input from the injected eye, to their neighbors.

In summary, this study confirms Grafstein's original findings of transneuronal transport in the mammalian visual system and also provides an additional independent demonstration of the ocular-dominance columns in the striate cortex.

We wish to thank Sarah Kennedy for her technical assistance. The work was supported by NIH Grants 5ROIEYO 0605 and 5ROI EYO0606 and grants from the Rowland Foundation, Inc. and the Esther A. and Joseph Klingenstein Fund, Inc.

References

1. Alvarez, J., and Püschel, M., Transfer of material from efferent axons to sensory epithelium in the goldfish vestibular system, *Brain Research*, 37 (1972) 265–278.
2. Cowan, W. M., Gottlieb, D. I., Hendrickson, A. E., Price, J. L., and Woolsey, T. A., The autoradiographic demonstration of axonal connections in the central nervous system, *Brain Research*, 37 (1972) 21–51.
3. Droz, B., Koenig, H. L., and Di Giamberardino, L., Axonal migration of protein and glycoprotein to nerve endings. I. Radioautographic analysis of the renewal of protein in nerve endings of chicken ciliary ganglion after intracerebral injection of [^{3}H]lysine, *Brain Research*, 60 (1973) 93–127.
4. Grafstein, B., Transneuronal transfer of radioactivity in the central nervous system, *Science*, 172 (1971) 177–179.
5. Grafstein, B., and Laureno, R., Transport of radioactivity from eye to visual cortex in the mouse, *Exp. Neurol.*, 39 (1973) 44–57.
6. Hendrickson, A. E., Electron microscopic distribution of axoplasmic transport, *J. comp. Neurol.*, 144 (1972) 381–397.
7. Hendrickson, A., Electron microscopic radioautography: identification of origin of synaptic terminals in normal nervous tissue, *Science*, 165 (1969) 194–196.
8. Hubel, D. H., and Wiesel, T. N., Laminar and columnar distribution of geniculocortical fibers in the macaque monkey, *J. comp. Neurol.*, 146 (1972) 421–450.
9. Korr, I. M., Wilkinson, P. N., and Chornock, F. W., Axonal delivery of neuroplasmic components to muscle cells, *Science*, 155 (1967) 342–345.
10. Lasek, R., Joseph, B. S., and Whitlock, D. G., Evaluation of radioautographic neuroanatomical tracing method, *Brain Research*, 8 (1968) 319–336.
11. LeVay, S., Hubel, D. H., and Wiesel, T. N., The pattern of ocular dominance columns in macaque visual cortex revealed by a reduced silver stain, (1974), in preparation.
12. Miani, N., Transport of S-100 protein in mammalian nerve fibers and transneuronal signals, *Acta neuropath. (Berl.)*, 6, Suppl. V (1971) 104–108.
13. Moore, R. Y., and Lenn, N. J., A retinohypothalamic projection in the rat, *J. comp. Neurol.*, 146 (1972) 1–14.
14. Specht, S., and Grafstein, B., Accumulation of radioactive protein in mouse cerebral cortex after injection of ^{3}H-fucose into the eye, *Exp. Neurol.*, 41 (1973) 705–722.

AFTERWORD

We made much subsequent use of radioactive labels and autoradiography, in normal monkeys and in monkeys after various kinds of visual deprivation, and in a variety of other species including mouse and tree shrew, looking at both superior colliculus and cortex. We were most interested to find, in monkey superior colliculus, a marked clumping of projections especially from the ipsilateral eye, very reminiscent of cortical ocular dominance columns. That finding came at the same time as results by Ann Graybiel on work done in the cat, published in 1976 (*Brain Res* 114:318–327). It came some years before her remarkable discovery of clumps of several kinds in corpus striatum. Evidently columns, or structures analogous to columns, must be widespread in the central nervous system.

Chapter 19 • Regular Sequences of Orientation Shifts in Monkeys •

FOREWORD

This paper is concerned with the geometry of orientation columns—establishing that they are slabs perpendicular to the cortical surface, discussing whether the slabs are discrete or continuous, and the question of the orderliness of the sequences. Some of the topics were already addressed in the first, 1968 monkey cortex paper, and the purpose of this one was to enlarge on those topics in the light of what we had learned in the intervening six years. Lurking in the background is the fact that we still, at this stage, had no anatomical picture of the face-on geometry of the columns. In several discussions published separately, (e.g., Hubel, D. H., Wiesel, T. N., & LeVay, S., 1976 *Cold Spring Harbor on Quantitative Biology*, 40: 581–589) we illustrate the columns as though they were strictly parallel slabs, more or less orthogonal to the ocular dominance slabs, in what we came to call our "ice-cube model", but we had no evidence for this assumption: we simply took it as the simplest possibility. Indeed, the reversals and fractures suggested that the slabs could hardly be parallel planes. The subsequent discovery by Blasdel, with optical methods, of the complexity of the orientation columns as seen face-on, with the swirls and pinwheel formations, came to us as a complete surprise (see p. 352).

Sequence Regularity and Geometry of Orientation Columns in the Monkey Striate Cortex

DAVID H. HUBEL AND TORSTEN N. WIESEL • *Department of Neurobiology, Harvard Medical School, 25 Shattuck Street, Boston, Massachusetts*

ABSTRACT

The striate cortex of the macaque monkey is subdivided into two independent and overlapping systems of columns termed "orientation columns" and "ocular dominance columns." The present paper is concerned with the orientation columns, particularly their geometry and the relationship between successive columns. The arrangement of the columns is highly ordered; in the great majority of oblique or tangential microelectrode penetrations the preferred orientations of cells changed systematically with electrode position, in a clockwise or counterclockwise direction. Graphs of orientation vs. electrode track distance were virtually straight lines over distances of up to several millimeters; such orderly sequences were often terminated by sudden changes in the direction of orientation shifts, from clockwise to counterclockwise or back. The orientations at which these reversals occurred were quite unpredictable. Total rotations of 180–360° were frequently seen between reversals. In tangential or almost tangential penetrations orientation shifts occurred almost every time the electrode was moved forward, indicating that the columns were either not discrete or had a thickness of less than 25–50 μ, the smallest order of distance that our methods could resolve. In penetrations that were almost perpendicular to the surface, the graphs of orientation vs. track distance were relatively flatter, as expected if the surfaces of constant orientation are perpendicular to the cortical surface. Stepwise changes in orientation of about 10° could sometimes be seen in perpendicular penetrations, each orientation persisting through several clear advances of the electrode, suggesting a set of discrete columnar subdivisions. The possibility of some kind of continuous variation in orientation with horizontal distance along the cortex was not, however, completely ruled out. Occasionally a highly ordered sequence was broken by an abrupt large shift in orientation of up to 90°. Shifts in ocular dominance occurred roughly every 0.25–0.5 mm and were independent of orientation shifts. In multiple parallel penetrations spaced closer than about 250 μ the slopes of the orientation vs. track distance curves were almost the same; reconstruction of these penetrations indicated that the regions of constant orientation are parallel sheets. On crossing perpendicular to these sheets, a total orientation shift of 180° took place over a distance of 0.5–1.0 mm. Column thickness, size of shifts in orientation, and the rate of change of orientation with distance along the cortex seemed to be independent of eccentricity, at least between 2° and 15° from the fovea. A few penetrations made in area 17 of the cat and in area 18 of the monkey showed similar orderly sequences of receptive-field orientation shifts.

In the monkey striate cortex there exist two independent and overlapping systems of columns which we have termed "orientation columns" and "ocular-dominance columns" (Hubel and Wiesel, '68). The ocular-dominance columns are parallel sheets or slabs arranged perpendicular to the cortical surface subdividing it into a mosaic of alternating left-eye and right-eye stripes 0.25–0.5 mm in width (Hubel and Wiesel, '72). For the orientation columns the geometry is less clear, though we have had indications that they are slab shaped. The present paper is concerned in part with this question. The main subject, however, is the degree to which the orientation columns are ordered. As the cortex is explored with a tangentially or obliquely moving electrode, the sequence of ocular-dominance columns is obviously back and forth from one eye to the other, since there are by definition only two kinds of ocular-dominance columns. For the orientation columns one can distinguish something like 18–20 possible orientations, and it is not trivial to ask whether the electrode encounters a random or ordered sequence. We have previously had hints that the columns were highly ordered (Hubel and Wiesel, '63, '68) and the results to be described make it very clear that this order is the rule rather than the exception.

METHODS

The series consisted of nine macaque monkeys (rhesus and stumptail) one to three years of age, and one cat. Of the nine monkeys seven were normal, one had long-standing monocular blindness, and one had artificial strabismus from birth. The cat also had strabismus from birth. The total number of cells recorded in monkeys was 1410, in 45 penetrations.

Most penetrations were made from the convexity of the occipital lobe, 2 to 7 mm posterior to the 17–18 border and about 10–15 mm lateral to the midline. This corresponds to a region of visual field 4–10° below and out from the fovea. Four penetrations were made far lateral, in the cortical region representing the fovea, and two were made in the buried calcarine cortex, with fields 12° and 18° from the fovea. In one experiment five penetrations were made in area 18, in the posterior bank of the lunate sulcus about 10 mm from the mid-sagittal plane (Fig. 12). To help reconstruct the electrode tracks one or more electrolytic lesions were made in each penetration.

Methods for animal preparation, stimulation, and recording were generally those described in previous papers (Hubel and Wiesel, '68). Since it was important to record activity continuously as the electrode advanced, we made the tungsten electrodes slightly coarser than usual, with 25–35 μ of uncoated tip rather than 15–25 μ. With such electrodes many isolated units were still recorded in each penetration, but background activity was more plentiful, with fewer gaps during which no responses to stimulation could be heard on the audio monitor.

The electrode was advanced in steps of 25–50 μ, and at each advance the responses were checked for changes in optimal stimulus orientation. Steps smaller than 25 μ usually did not result in a change of optimal orientation or of electrical activity, either because the uncoated tip length was 25 μ or more, or because of the inevitable stickiness in the movement of the electrode relative to the tissue. Obviously these factors impose a lower limit on the size of the columns that can be resolved.

We stimulated routinely by sweeping a slit of white light of variable length and width across the receptive field in different orientations. When necessary we used dark bars or monochromatic slits. As the electrode advanced through the cortex each new optimal orientation for activating single cells or groups of cells was recorded as a line drawn on the receptive field chart (Fig. 1). The accuracy in estimating optimal orientations var-

ied from cell to cell, from roughly ±2–3° at best, to ±5–10° for less sharply tuned cells; in layer IV C most cells lack orientation specificity. Orientations were plotted against micrometer readings of electrode position, with a new point marked each time the orientation changed or each time any change in electrical activity made it clear that the electrode had advanced. To determine orientation we occasionally used a PDP-12 computer to produce a graph of average response vs. orientation, generating the slit electronically on a television screen. This method took much longer, and the usual minute-to-minute variations in responsiveness of the cells tended to make the curves broader and noisier. We concluded that for both speed and for precision it is hard to beat judgements based on the human ear. Certainly a curve such as the one in Figure 2 could not have been obtained with computer averaging methods before the authors reached the age of mandatory retirement.

For binocular cells in which the two eyes were equally effective or almost so (groups 3, 4, 5 . . . Hubel and Wiesel, '62), orientation was determined separately for the two eyes. For cells dominated strongly by one eye (groups 1, 2, 6, 7) only one point corresponding to the dominant eye was plotted. Open circles in the graphs represent contralateral eye, closed circles, ipsilateral. Thus an idea of the dominant eye and the degree of binocular interaction can be obtained from the graphs at a glance. When the orientations of a binocular cell consistently differed in the two eyes by a measurable amount (as in Fig. 6, for example), the discrepancy could be accounted for by a relative rotation of the paralyzed eyes in the equatorial plane.

After perfusion of the brain with 10% formol saline the occipital lobes were embedded in celloidin, cut in the parasagittal plane at 25 μ, and stained with cresyl violet. The angle of the electrode track was measured in the histological slides either with respect to the cortical surface and the layers or by taking the complement of the angle made with the radial fascicles. In estimating this angle an error is introduced by sectioning the brain in the parasagittal plane rather than in a plane perpendicular to the surface, but this was small in penetrations that were within 10–15 mm of the midline. Small errors in estimation of track angles were important only in nearly perpendicular penetrations, and then only in calculations involving estimates of the horizontal component of track distance. Numbers based on such calculations are omitted from Table 1.

RESULTS

Regularity of Orientation Columns

In this study the main finding was the high degree of order in the arrangement of orientation columns. For many years our only good example of this order was a single experiment in a spider monkey (Hubel and Wiesel, '68, Fig. 9), but since we began to use lower impedance electrodes and the plotting procedure described below we have seen a high degree of order in almost every penetration.

Figure 1A shows an example of a typical ordered sequence in a very oblique penetration in a normal monkey. The first cell or group of cells in the sequence (No. 96 in the experiment) strongly favored the right (ipsilateral) eye and had a 1 o'clock–7 o'clock receptive-field orientation. The next 14 (Nos. 97–110) were all strongly dominated by the right eye and had the orientations shown, each counterclockwise to the one before, with steps that were small and fairly uniform. At cell No. 111 the right eye suddenly became ineffective, and subsequently recorded cells were all strongly dominated by the left eye. The sequence, however, continued in a counterclockwise direction without interruption.

These results are shown graphically in Figure 1B. Orientations are plotted against electrode-track distance in millimeters. In plotting orientations, 0° is taken as vertical, angles clockwise up to 90° are designated as positive, counterclockwise to 89° as negative. The first cell in the sequence thus had an orientation of +32°. Track distances are taken directly from the micrometer advancer readings, with zero as the depth at which unit activity was first encountered.

The graph, like others obtained in this series, showed a high degree of regularity, and indeed a linearity, over long distances. Almost every 25–30 μ advance of the electrode was followed by a fairly constant small shift of about 10° in the optimal stimulus orientation. Since any particular orienta-

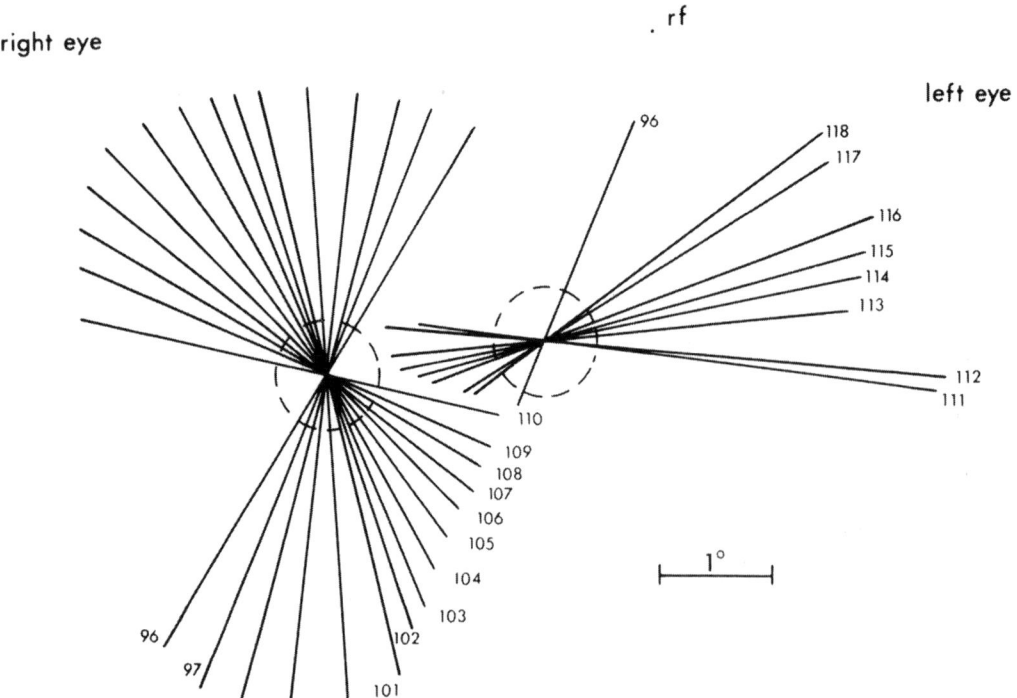

Fig. 1A. Normal 2–3 year-old monkey. Observations during an oblique microelectrode penetration through striate cortex. The drawing was made on a sheet of paper affixed to the tangent screen 146 cm from the monkey. The eyes converged slightly so that the visual axes crossed, with the left and right foveas ophthalmoscopically projected as shown (1 f and r f). The receptive fields of 22 cells or clusters of cells were distributed through the regions marked with interrupted circles, 3° below and 3° to the left of the foveas. The first cell in the sequence, No. 96 in the experiment, had an orientation 32° clockwise to the vertical, and was influenced from both eyes but more strongly from the right (ipsilateral). Cells 97–110 were likewise strongly dominated by the right eye; at No. 111 there was an abrupt switch to the left (contralateral) eye, which dominated for the rest of the sequence (same penetration as in Fig. 8,A,D). (Experiment No. 5).

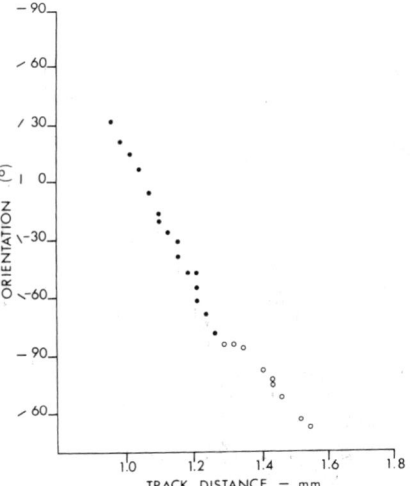

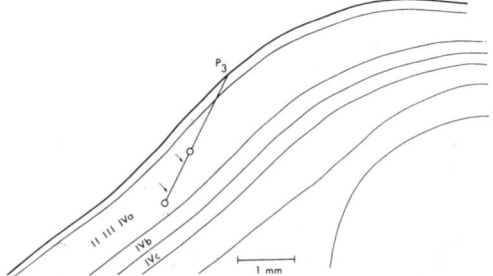

Fig. 1C. Reconstruction of the electrode track. Electrode entered the striate cortex 8 mm behind the lunate sulcus in the parasagittal plane, 10 mm to the right of the midline, intersecting the surface at 20°. The sequence described here was recorded between the two arrows. Circles represent electrolytic lesions. Anterior is to the right.

Fig. 1B. Graph of orientation vs. track distance for the sequence of Figure 1A. In plotting orientations, 0° is vertical, angles clockwise up to 90° are positive, counterclockwise to 89°, negative. Closed circles, ipsilateral (right) eye; open circles, contralateral (left) eye. Track distance is taken from micrometer advancer readings.

tion could be measured only to the nearest 2–5° it was at times hard to be sure that a shift had actually occurred, but once the slope of the curve had been established the orientation arrived at after several advances in 25–30 μ steps was predictable with surprising accuracy.

As pointed out in the method section, an advance of the electrode by a substantially smaller distance, such as 15–20 μ, often did not result in an orientation shift, but with such a small advance it was difficult to be sure the electrode had moved relative to the tissue. Since most 25–30 μ advances of the electrode did result in orientation shifts the regions of constant orientation were obviously that size or smaller. Thus the distances between observed shifts in orientation, or their horizontal components ("horizontal distance/shift" in Table 1), represent an upper bound to the thickness of the columns, and not necessarily the true values. This should be kept in mind in interpreting Figures for the distance between orientation shifts, or the number of degrees for each orientation shift, given in the present descriptions and in Table 1. The possibility that orientation may vary in some sense continuously with horizontal electrode movement is taken up in the discussion, but here it may be

well to point out that 25–30 μ is close to the dimensions of a cell body, so that the column widths are already close to the lower limit. As shown below, the distance an electrode traveled between shifts in orientation was large enough to be measurable in nearly perpendicular penetrations, but then the horizontal component of the distance became critically dependent on the angle between electrode and cortex, and could not be accurately estimated.

The part of the electrode track in which the sequence of Figure 1 occurred is shown between the arrows in the track reconstruction of Figure 1C. The sequence was part of a longer one described in Figure 8D. The span of 158° was covered in 22 shifts, giving a mean orientation shift of 7.2° ± 2.8° (S.D.), (Linear coefficient of correlation, 0.98). The 22 shifts in orientation took place over a distance of 0.59 mm, giving an average distance between shifts of 27 μ, or 25 μ in terms of distance parallel to the cortical surface. This is equivalent to 40 shifts/mm horizontal excursion. Since the radial column-like bands of cells seen in Nissl-stained transverse sections of striate cortex are separated by intervals of about this order of magnitude we thought it might be interesting to compare the sizes directly. Figure 1D shows a photomicrograph of the cortex with two lesions made before and after the sequence of 22 shifts; the part of the track in which the sequence occurred is indicated by arrows. (The track could only be seen with dark-field illumination.) The bands are not sharply defined and can be counted only very roughly, but

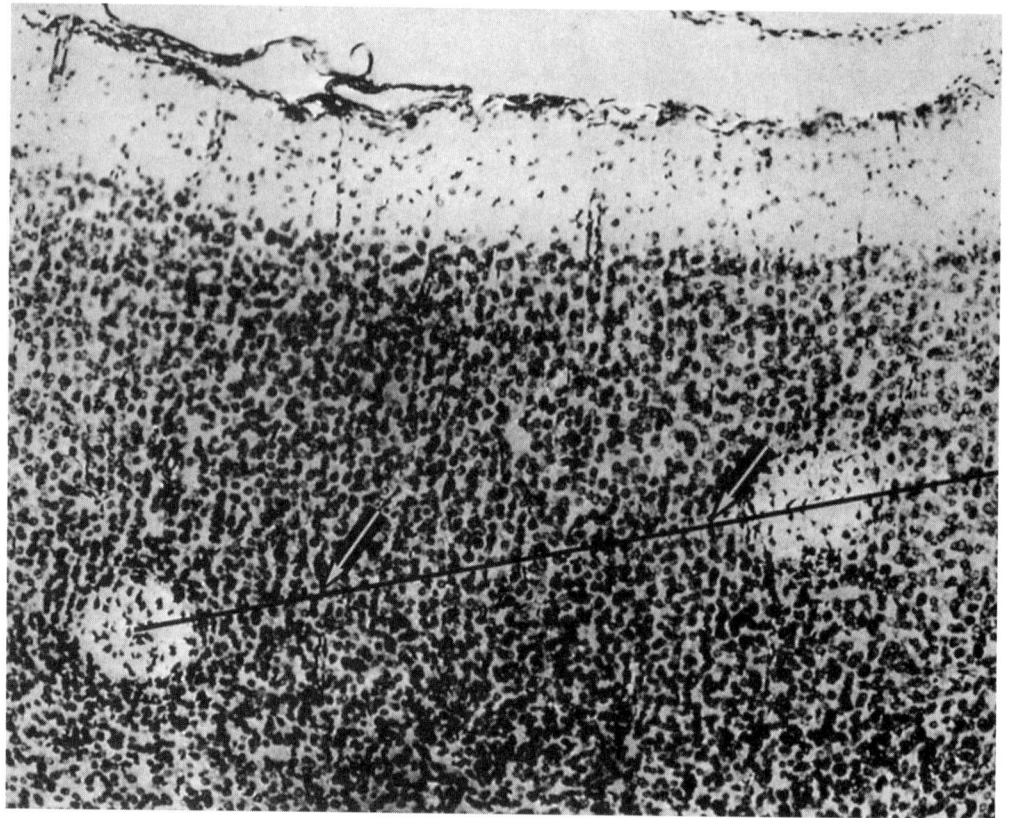

Fig. 1D. Photomicrograph of a Nissl-stained section through the two lesions and the electrode track. The track was visible only with dark-field illumination. The sequence of 22 orientation shifts occurred between the two arrows, within which space roughly 32 vertical bands of cells can be counted.

in this part of the track there appear to be about 32, or 54 bands/mm.

Reversals in the direction of rotation were seen in about half of the penetrations in the series. Several examples of such reversals are shown in Figure 2, a graph from a highly regular penetration in a normal macaque monkey. Here one long clockwise progression spanning 188° in 17 orientation shifts (average 11.1°/shift) was followed by an even longer counterclockwise rotation through 267° in 26 shifts (10.3°/shift). This in turn was followed by two shorter sequences. The total number of orientation shifts in the 2.2 mm track was 53, or 24 shifts/mm of horizontal excursion. The number of radial bands of cells counted along the electrode track was about 110, giving 50 bands/mm.

Throughout almost the entire penetration the ipsilateral eye (closed circles) was strongly dominant, though the contralateral eye was able to influ-

ence most of the cells. Towards the end of the penetration the dominance began to change, with a few cells influenced about equally from the two eyes, and by the very end the contralateral eye had become dominant. The relationship between orientation columns and ocular-dominance columns is considered below.

The regularity shown in these two examples was typical. Within any progressive sequence, clockwise or counterclockwise, the slope of the curve was generally fairly constant. The total rotation taking place before a reversal in direction of rotation was highly variable, but the majority of uninterrupted spans were over 100°, one-third exceeded 200°, and a few were over 300°. Many linear sequences were cut short, not because of a reversal in direction of rotation, but because the penetration was terminated or entered white matter or layer IV C (in which most cells have no ori-

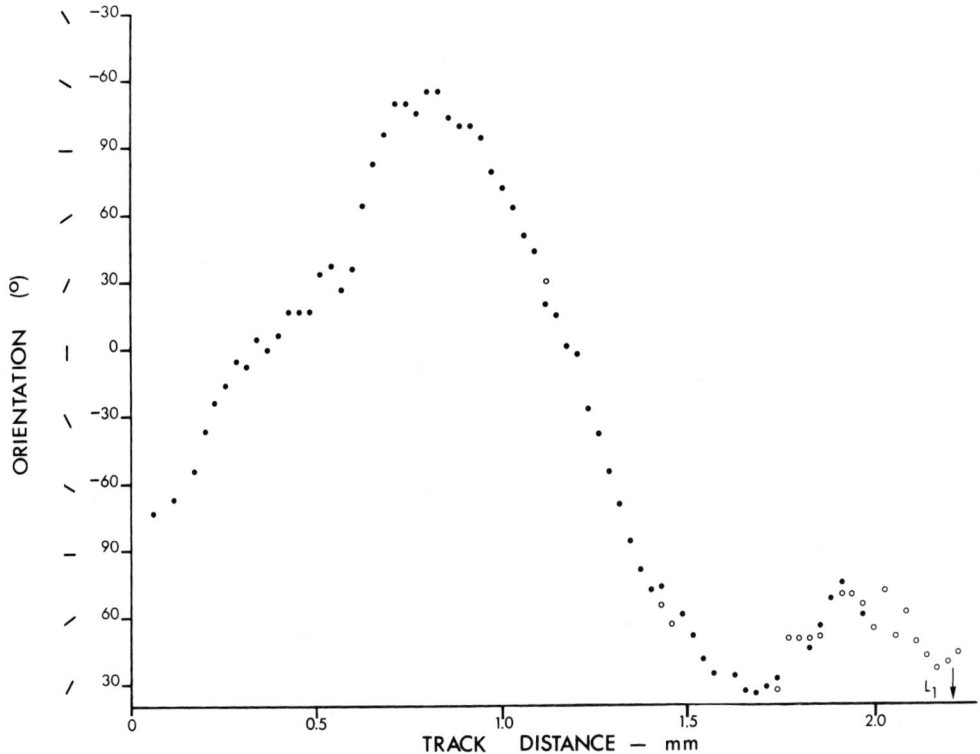

Fig. 2A. Graph of orientation vs. track distance for an oblique penetration through striate cortex in a normal monkey. Note the reversals in direction of orientation shifts, the first two of which bracket a long sequence spanning 267°. (Experiment No. 7.)

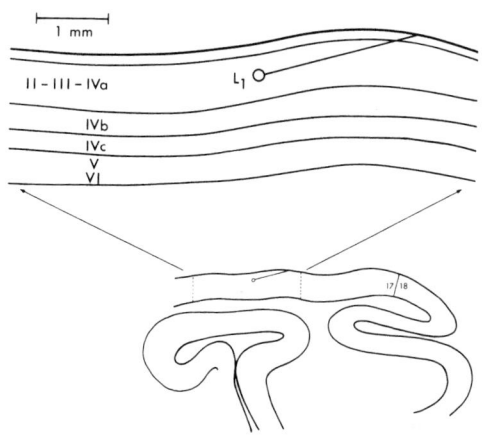

Fig. 2B. Reconstruction of the electrode track, which entered the striate cortex 10 mm behind the lunate sulcus and 10 mm to the right of the midline, making an angle of 7° with the surface. Section is parasagittal. One lesion was made at the end of the 2.2 mm penetration. Receptive fields were 1° below and 7.5° to the left of the fovea.

entation specificity). The angles at which reversals occurred were quite unpredictable, there being no tendency for any particular orientations, such as vertical or horizontal, to be favored as points of reversal.

Though most of the sequences were regular, isolated large jumps in orientation did occur. Some of these may simply have reflected a sudden movement forward of the electrode after sticking relative to the tissue, but others were certainly genuine. An example of a pair of breaks in the order of a sequence is shown in Figure 3 from a penetration described further in another context below (Fig. 8C). Here the orientation had been systematically changing in a counterclockwise direction when suddenly there was a 70° counterclockwise jump, followed by a short regular clockwise sequence and then a second counterclockwise jump of 105°. The previous counterclockwise sequence was finally resumed with the same slope, just as though it had

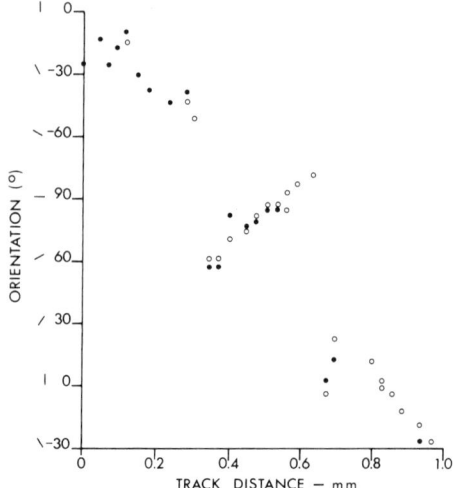

Fig. 3. Graph of orientation vs. track distance for a sequence that showed two clear breaks in regularity (Experiment No. 5, penetration 2; see Fig. 8C).

never been interrupted. At this point the electrode was pulled back slowly and then readvanced, whereupon the entire sequence was reproduced, making it almost certain that the jumps were not in some way related to uneven electrode movements.

Effects of Varying the Direction of a Penetration through the Cortex

For reasons taken up in the discussion the prevalence of regularity in the sequences makes it likely that the columns have the form, not of pillars, as the word "column" implies, but of parallel slabs. Further evidence for this will be presented below. Here we discuss the variation in slope of graphs of orientation vs. track distance as the direction of the electrode through a given set of orientation slabs is varied.

Most penetrations that were parallel or almost parallel to the cortical surface gave relatively steep curves of orientation vs. track distance, with slopes ranging from 100°/mm to 400°/mm. The absence of flatter curves may seem surprising, since there is no obvious reason why tangential penetrations should not meet the slabs at all possible angles, from 0° to 90°, with equal likelihood. As pointed out in the discussion, however, it is not the angle itself that is important in determining the slopes of the curves, but the sine of the angle, so that with randomly distributed angles between electrode and slabs it is expected that the slopes of the curves should be skewed towards large values, i.e., most curves

should be relatively steep. It would have been interesting to test this directly by making several tangential penetrations through some small region of cortex in various directions, but for the present the idea was abandoned because of the difficulties in finding a suitable plane of sectioning for histological reconstruction. The results of making multiple parallel penetrations are taken up below.

In tangential penetrations individual shifts in orientation tend to be obscured in orientation-vs.-distance curves because of limitations in resolution along the distance axis. On the other hand a penetration that is deliberately made almost normal to the surface should intersect the columns at a very small angle and pass through relatively few of them; the curve should be relatively flat, and individual shifts should be further apart and consequently more easily seen.

The two penetrations of Figure 4 were made about 1.5° from the foveal representation of the right hemisphere in a normal monkey. In penetration 3 (Fig. 4B), which was almost normal to the surface, the slope of most of the curve was −54°/mm, the flattest of the entire series. Steps were conspicuous, occurring about every 120 μ. In contrast, penetration 4 (Fig. 4C), which made an angle of 46° to the surface, had a slope of 273°/mm and the orientation changed with each 25–30 μ advance of the electrode, i.e., too frequently for individual steps to be resolved. The interruption in this penetration between 1.8 and 2.5 mm marks the passage of the electrode through layer IV C, where as usual there was no hint of any orientation specificity and responses were strictly monocular (Hubel and

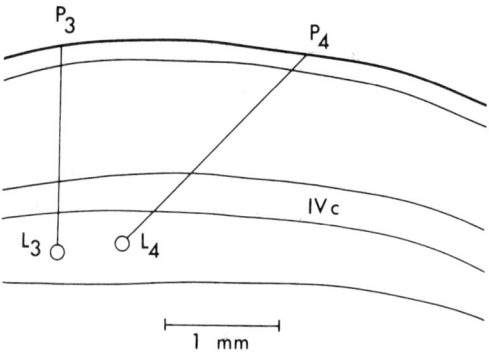

Fig. 4A. Reconstructions of two penetrations in the right striate cortex. P3 was almost normal to the surface, whereas P4 made an angle of 46° with it. Fields were 1° below and 1° to the left of the fovea. (Experiment No. 10.)

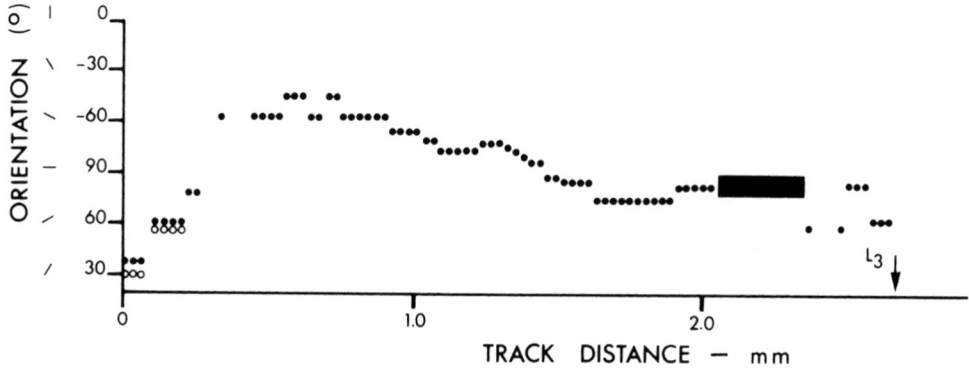

Fig. 4B. Graph of orientation vs. track distance for the perpendicular penetration P3. Slope −54°/mm, uncorrected for angle to surface. The filled dark bar represents activity in layer IV C, which was influenced exclusively from the ipsilateral eye and showed no orientation selectivity; the bar's placement along the orientation axis is arbitrary.

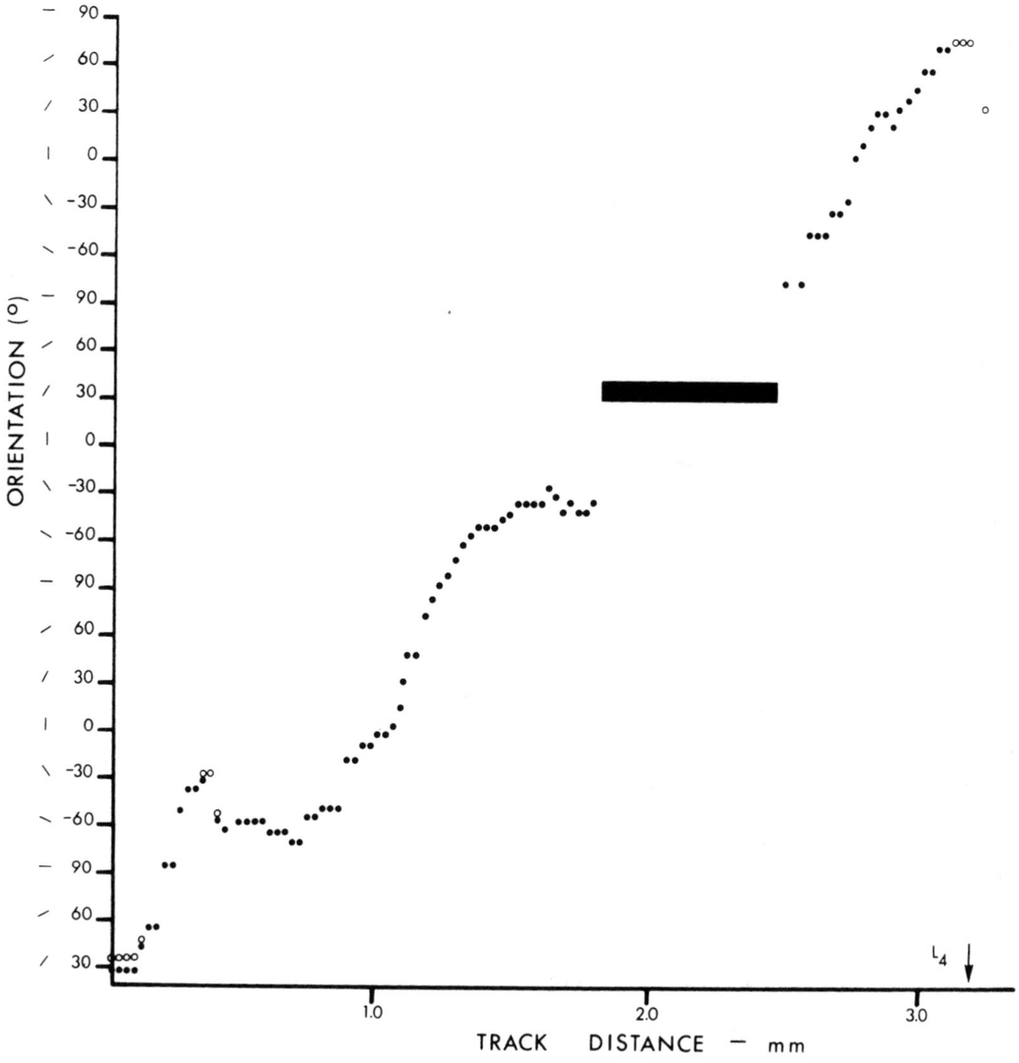

Fig. 4C. Orientation vs. track distance for the oblique penetration P4. Slope, 273°/mm, uncorrected.

Wiesel, '68). Following this interruption the curve showed about the same slope as before, and appeared to represent a simple continuation of the sequence. This is what is expected if the columns extend through the full thickness of cortex.

A second example comparing oblique and nearly perpendicular penetrations is shown in Figure 5. After crossing the outermost thickness of cortex and white matter beneath, the electrode entered the mushroom-shaped calcarine cortex, where it pierced one fold completely, at 82° to the surface, and finally entered the next fold at 51°. In the first of these calcarine folds the receptive fields were 12° from the fovea, in the second, 18°. Once again the more perpendicular traverse gave a relatively flat curve (–106°/mm), whereas for the oblique portion the curve was much steeper (283°/mm). (It is not clear why discrete steps did not occur in the first curve.)

A third comparison between perpendicular and oblique penetrations is shown below in Figure 13, for the cat.

That the three perpendicular penetrations in these examples gave very flat curves agrees with our previous experience (Hubel and Wiesel, '62, '68), and is in marked contrast with the relatively steep slopes observed for the straight segments of the curves in virtually every oblique or tangential penetration in the series.

Dimensions of Orientation Columns

A summary of the information obtained from all the penetrations of the series is given in Table 1. Our purpose here is chiefly to convey an overall impression of the degree of variability of the results. The mean value for the total orientation shift in 1 mm of tangential component of the electrode movement ("slope corrected") is 281°/mm. As already mentioned, the distribution of the slopes favored high values, with only one slope less than 100°/mm. The mean slope of 281°/mm, corresponds to 640 μ for a full sweep through 180°, a value that is likely to be a somewhat high estimate of the thickness of a full 180° complement of orientation slabs since, as mentioned above, we have no way of knowing in single penetrations the angle between the slabs and the horizontal component of the electrode tracks. The mean value for "horizontal distance/shift" of 43 μ is also probably a high estimate for slab width, partly for the same reason, and partly because it is likely that some orientation

shifts went unobserved. The same applies to the mean value for "angle/shift" of 11.9°, as an estimate of the angular shift between slabs.

A closer approach to the true values of these items can probably be obtained from the penetrations that gave the most frequent intervals, with the smallest shifts in angle. The sequence shown in Figure 1, for example, gives a mean value for "horizontal distance/shift" of 25 μ and a mean "angle/shift" of 7.2°; the comparable numbers from the second sequence of Figure 2 (experiment no. 7) are 31 μ and 10.3°. In the present study one objective was to obtain some rough estimate of column size. As a summary statement it seems reasonable to say that the columns are 25–50 μ wide and are arranged in sequences of 9–10° steps. Both of these figures are upper limits and obviously would be meaningless if orientation were a continuous function of horizontal distance, in the statistical sense discussed below (DISCUSSION). In either case, an array of columns subserving a full 180° has a total width of 0.5–1 mm.

Systematic shifts in orientation were seen in all layers of the cortex with the exception of layer 1, where no responses were generally seen, and IV C, in which responses were not orientation specific. There were otherwise no obvious differences from layer to layer in the shapes of the curves, the size of the orientation shifts, or slab thickness. Most of the recordings were made from layers II and III, however, and with such a limited survey one cannot rule out the existence of subtle differences between layers.

Variation of Columns Size with Eccentricity

Most of our experiments were done in cortical areas representing visual fields 5–10° from the foveal representation (Table 1), in order to form some idea of the range of variation of the columns in at least one region. One pair of penetrations, however, was made in the foveal representation (Fig. 4) and another went beyond the exposed surface of area 17 into the calcarine fissure where it intersected the cortex twice (Fig. 5), with receptive-field positions 12° and 18° from the fovea. As expected, in the fovea the fields and the random variation in field position ("scatter") were both very much smaller than what was found 5–10° out, and these in turn were smaller than the fields and scatter 12–18° out. In contrast, there was no indication

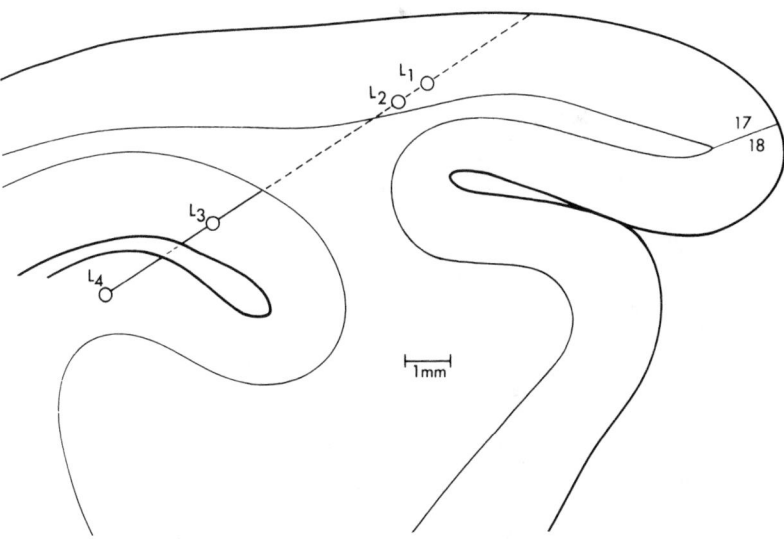

Fig. 5A. *Comparison of perpendicular and oblique penetrations. Reconstruction of a penetration that passed through two folds of striate cortex deep in the calcarine fissure. Field positions 12° and 18° from the fovea; parasagittal section, 10 mm to right of midline. Parts of track indicated by continuous line are plotted in Figure 5B. Electrode intersected the first calcarine fold at 82°, and the second at 51°. Monkey had an artificial strabismus from birth. (Experiment No. 3.)*

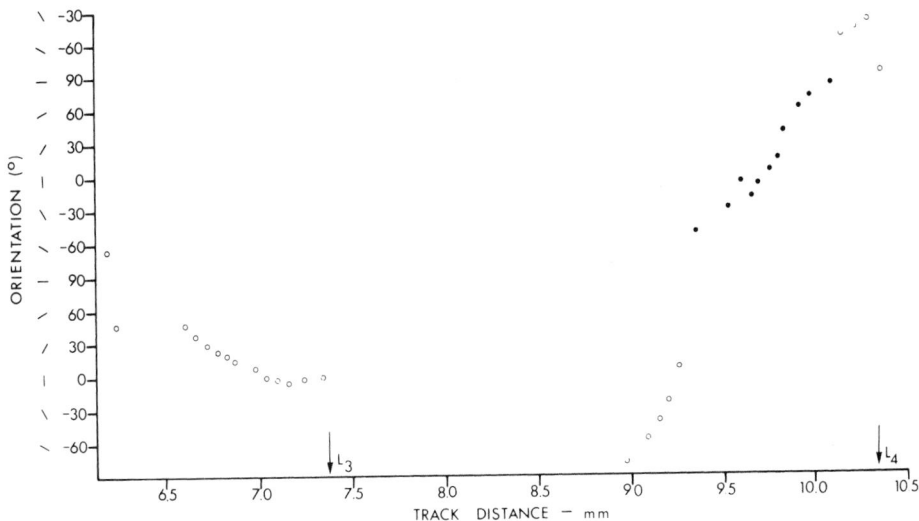

Fig. 5B. *Orientation vs. track distance, for the portion of penetration indicated by a continuous line, in Figure 5A. Open circles, contralateral eye; closed circles, ipsilateral eye. Slopes, −106°/mm, 283°/mm.*

that the column size varied with eccentricity: the slopes of the graphs of orientation vs. track length, the frequency of occurrence of shifts and their angular size, and the frequency of changes in ocular-dominance were all similar (Table 1).

To be certain that the columnar organization is uniform in all respects over the entire cortex would of course require a much more extensive survey. One can, however, be confident that there are no gross differences between center and

Table 1

Experiment No.	Penetration No.	Sequence No.[1]	Species and state	Horizontal[2] (degrees)	Vertical[3] (degrees)	Total[3] (degrees)	Span of sequence[5] (deg.)	Track length (mm.)	Angle (θ)[6] (deg.)	Horizontal track length[7] (mm.)	Slope uncorrected[8] (°/mm.)	Number of shifts	Angle/shift[10] (deg.)	Horizontal dist/shift[11] (μm)	Figure number
4	1	1	macaque normal	0	-3.5	3.5	130	1.01	40	0.77	-154	16	8.1	48	6
	2	2					159	0.50	31	0.43	-307	11	14.5	39	
	3	1					146	0.78	29	0.68	-177	13	11.2	52	
5	1	1	macaque normal	3	-3	4	215	0.84	25	0.76	-200	19	8.0	40	8B
		2					61	0.29	25	0.26	226	8	7.6	33	8B
	2	1					282	1.22	20	1.15	-218	31	9.1	37	3,8C
		1					42	0.28	20	0.26	154	7	6.0	37	3,8C
	3	1					323	1.27	20	1.19	-262	28	11.5	43	1,8D
6	1		macaque normal	3	-4.5	5.5	271	1.24	12	1.21	204	24	11.3	50	10
	2						204	0.59	31	0.51	363	14	14.6	36	10
	3						174	0.62	31	0.53	307	15	11.6	35	10
7	1	1	macaque normal	7.5	-1	7.5	188	0.73	7	0.72	263	17	11.1	42	2
	2	2					267	0.82	7	0.81	417	26	10.3	31	2
9	1	1	macaque normal			6	157	1.68	58	0.89	64	13	12.1	68	
	2	1					131	0.48	25	0.44	263	15	8.7	29	
		2					83	0.82	25	0.74	112	11	7.6	67	
	3	1					97	0.37	17	0.35	284	12	8.1	29	
		2					191	0.87	17	0.83	227	23	8.3	36	

Expt	Animal	fovea h²	fovea v³	dist⁴	θ⁶	H. track⁷	n shifts	slope⁸	slope/cos θ⁹	span/n¹⁰	track/n¹¹	seq. track	Fig.
10	macaque normal	−1	1.5		(90)	−54	9	—	1.07	—	—	59	4B
10	macaque normal				46	283	21	0.63	0.90	30	10.7	224	4C
10	macaque normal				46	263	13	0.59	0.85	45	11.7	152	4C
10	macaque normal				42	320	10	0.42	0.56	42	14.5	145	
3	macaque squint	−4.5	5	10.5	32	−244	—	0.46	0.54	—	—	107	5B
3	macaque squint	−4.5	5	10	(82)	−106	9	—	0.58	—	5.8	52	5B
3	macaque squint	−5.5	12		51	283	7	0.27	0.43	39	19.1	134	7B
3	macaque squint	−15	18		19	219	27	1.33	1.41	49	10.7	291	
3	macaque squint	−4.5	5		19	219	7	0.34	0.36	49	8.7	61	
3	macaque squint	−4.5	5		39	219	—	1.60	2.06	—	—	489	
2	macaque area 18	−4	4		67	142	11	0.41	1.1	37	13.5	149	12
2	macaque area 18				45	−194	9	0.64	0.9	70	19.4	175	12
2	macaque area 18				38	−139	9	0.50	0.64	55	9.9	89	
8	Cat				(90)	54	14	—	1.07	—	4.3	60	13b
8	Cat	2	2.25		3	−165	17	1.24	1.24	73	10.6	180	13c
Means¹²					43.26	222					11.91		
s.d.					11.5	83					3.4		

¹"Sequence" refers to a group of orientation shifts all in one direction. Figure 8D (expt. 5, penetration 3) contains one sequence; Figure 2 (expt. 7, penetration 1) contains two major and two (untabulated) minor sequences.

²Horizontal component of distance from fovea.

³Vertical component, positive values upward.

⁴Distance from fovea.

⁵Length of the sequence in degrees.

⁶Angle between electrode track and cortical surface (METHODS).

⁷Horizontal track length = track length × cos θ pene.

⁸Very roughly, this is given by span ÷ track length; usually computed from graphs: 177.2/tan (angle of curve to orientation axis).

⁹Uncorrected slope/cos θ.

¹⁰Span/(no. of shifts).

¹¹Horizontal track length/(no. of shifts).

¹²Means for all normal and abnormal macaque area 17 (all of Table 1 except Experiments 2 and 8).

periphery such as exist in magnification factor or receptive-field size. From the curve of Daniel and Whitteridge ('61, Fig. 4) the magnification factors corresponding to fovea and to points 7° and 15° from the fovea are roughly 6.3, 1.3 and 0.4 mm/°. Had the orientation columns differed in size in these proportions (16:3:1) it should have been evident. Our conclusion concerning the ocular-dominance columns (Hubel and Wiesel, '72), based on anatomical methods, was similar: there is no very striking change in the widths of the stripes with eccentricity.

Relationship between Ocular-Dominance and Orientation Columns

Physiological and anatomical studies in the macaque monkey indicate that the width of ocular-dominance columns is in the order of 0.25–0.5 mm (Hubel and Wiesel, '68, '72). In an average tangential penetration one should therefore expect to see many shifts in receptive-field orientation for each shift in eye dominance. The relation between the two types of column can be illustrated in several typical penetrations. In the example shown in Figure 6, from a normal monkey, cells in the first 0.5 mm of the penetration were driven almost exclusively from the ipsilateral eye. Then, for about 0.3 mm, the cells were roughly equally influenced from the two eyes. Finally, in the last 0.2 mm, the contralateral eye had complete control. All this time the orientation progressed steadily in a counterclockwise direction, at virtually the same rate for all parts of the penetration regardless of eye dominance.

In the strabismic animal the results were similar except that transitions from one eye to the other were abrupt, with, at most, only very short spans in which both eyes were represented. An example of this has already been seen in Figure 5, and another example from a different penetration in the same experiment (No. 3) is shown in Figure 7. The curve from the first part of this penetration, before entering layer IV, was the closest approach of any to a straight line (coefficient of linear correlation 0.996), and the line was again virtually uninterrupted by the transition from ipsilateral to contralateral eye. (The slight apparent shift in the curve is explained by a relative outward rotation of the eyes in the equatorial plane.) During the 2 mm long passage through layer IV C, marked by

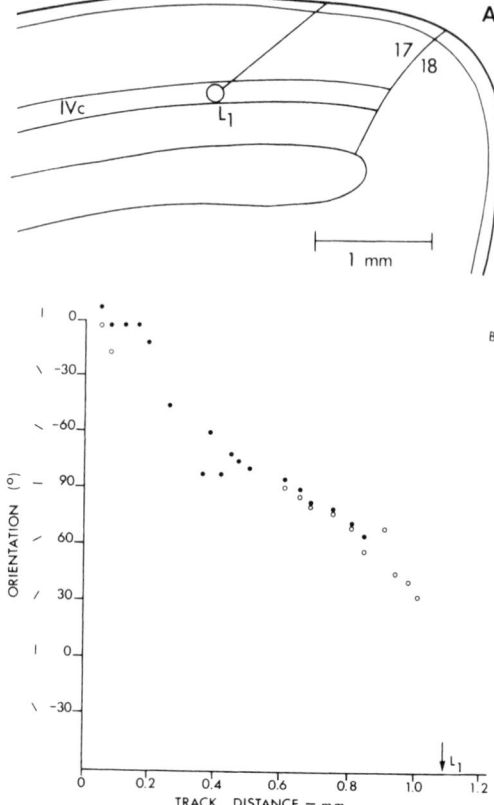

Fig. 6. Relation of orientation shifts to changes in ocular cominance, in crossing from one ocular-dominance column to another. Graph of orientation vs. track distance, for a penetration that entered striate cortex in the parasagittal plane 10 mm from the midline, making an angle of 40° to the surface. Normal monkey. Most of the first cells were strongly dominated by the ipsilateral eye (closed circles), but after the electrode passed through a region of mixed dominance between 0.6 and 0.9 mm, it entered a region of contralateral eye dominance (open circles). (Experiment No. 4.)

arrows in the reconstruction, there were three ocular-dominance shifts, and a final shift occurred in the traverse through layer V.

These results, in summary, indicate that sequences of orientation shifts are undisturbed by ocular dominance; to this extent the two column systems are certainly independent.

Reconstruction of Closely-Spaced Penetrations

It should be possible to test the idea that orientation columns are parallel slabs by making several paral-

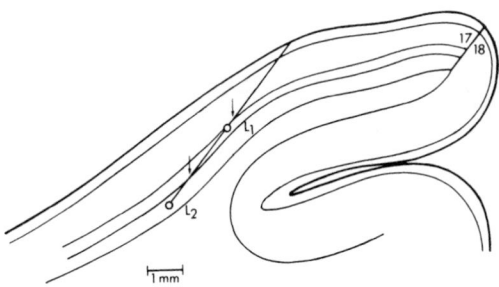

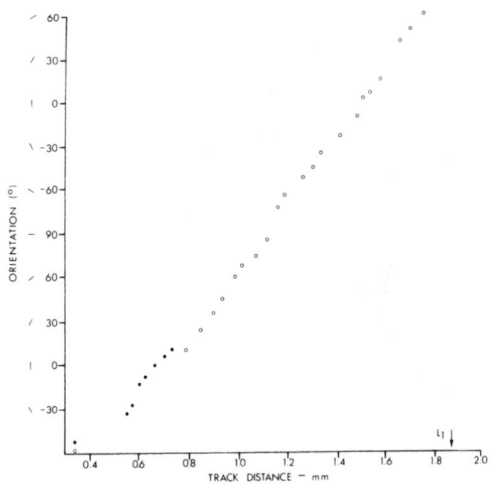

Fig. 7A. *Relation of orientation shifts to changes in ocular-dominance. Reconstruction of a penetration in the same monkey as in Figure 5 (strabismic), but at a slightly smaller angle to the surface (19°) and 200 μ lateral. Region of penetration in which responses lacked orientation specificity is marked with arrows. This coincides closely with layer IV C. (Experiment No. 3.)*

Fig. 7B. *Graph of orientation vs. track distance. Closed circles, ipsilateral eye; open circles, contralateral. The relative counterclockwise displacement of the graph at the point of transition from one eye to the other near the beginning of the penetration was caused by a relative extortion of the two eyes.*

lel penetrations through a small region of cortex, comparing receptive-field orientations of adjacent points. In practice this proved difficult. In our first attempt, two parallel penetrations were made 1 mm apart, and though both sequences were regular the rotation was clockwise in the first and counter-clockwise in the second. This result is perhaps not surprising, considering how abruptly a sequence can go from clockwise to counterclockwise or back in a single penetration, but if one is to understand the geometry of the columns a closer spacing of penetrations is clearly required.

Figure 8 illustrates the results of an experiment (No. 5) in which three penetrations were made 0.2 mm apart in a normal monkey. Three tracks intersected the surface of the cortex at angles of 25°, 20° and 20°. The pattern of shifts in each of the three penetrations was highly regular, and the slopes of the three graphs were reasonably similar, with values, corrected for inclination to the surface, of −221, −232, and −280°/mm. It is difficult to control the exact point of entry in a penetration that is close to tangential, and penetration 1 overlapped the other two for only about one-half of its length.

A reconstruction of these penetrations from the histology is shown in Figure 9. To the left in the figure the three penetrations are viewed from above, as though projected onto the plane of the cortical surface; in the right half of the figure they are viewed from the side as in Figure 8A. On comparing the receptive-field orientations in neighboring

tracks one can imagine the slab walls running in roughly the directions indicated by the thin continuous lines. These lines are drawn every 45° except in one place where they are spaced at 9° to give an indication of the probable upper limit of the column thickness. The lines representing the tracks are shown as continuous in regions of ipsilateral-eye domination, and interrupted where the contralateral eye dominated. While there is too little territory mapped to do more than suggest roughly the form of the ocular-dominance columns (dotted lines), one can at least get some idea of their size relative to that of the orientation columns.

The abrupt breaks in penetration 2 (Fig. 8C) have already been discussed above (Fig. 3). Curiously, just at the second discontinuity the cells responded to specifically oriented red slits but not to white stimuli of any kind. We have previously observed that color-coded cells in the monkey striate cortex tend to be aggregated in small groups (Hubel and Wiesel, '68), but whether or not these are columnar is not known. That such a group occurred here together with discontinuities in the main orientation sequence is interesting, and perhaps not entirely coincidental since it may be that groups of color-coded cells are interjected as sepa-

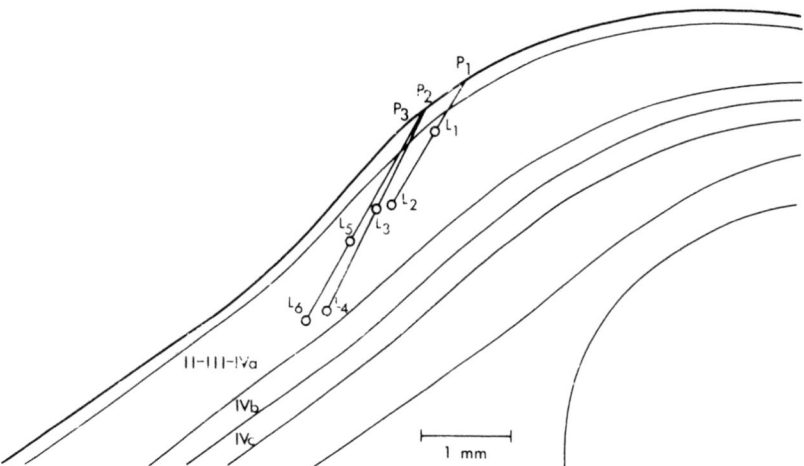

Fig. 8A. Reconstruction of three closely spaced penetrations ($P_1 - P_3$) in right striate cortex. Each penetration was in the parasagittal plane, with P_1 most medial, P_2 200 μ lateral to it, and P_3 200 μ lateral to P_2. In the reconstruction, the three are seen in profile, as though they were in the same parasagittal plane. All three penetrations were restricted to layers I–III. (Experiment No. 5)

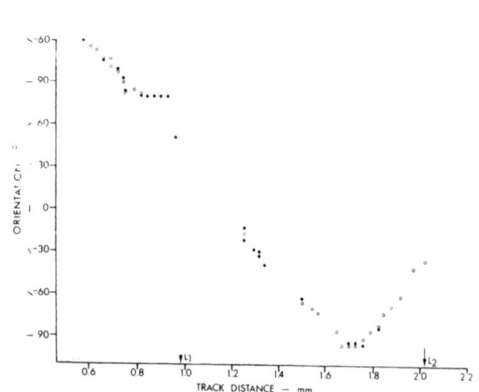

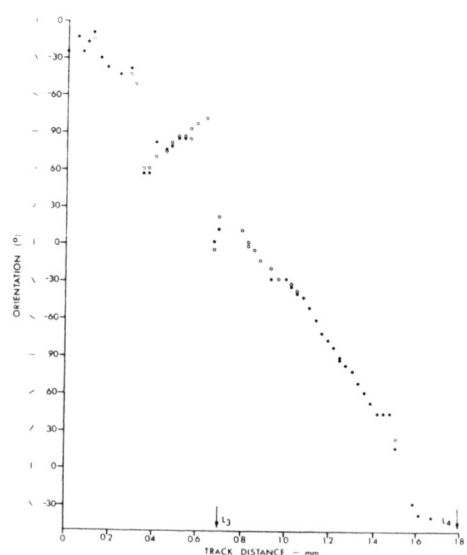

Fig. 8B. Orientation vs. track distance of P_1. The gap beginning at about 0.95 mm is caused by the first lesion (L_1). Activity at the outset was dominated by the left eye (contralateral, open circles), but the dominance soon switched to the ipsilateral eye, and finally it switched back again to the contralateral at 1.5 mm. Angle to surface, 25°. Slope of the first, descending, sequence, –200°/mm uncorrected, –221°/mm corrected, for the inclination of the electrode.

Fig. 8C. Graph for P_2, of orientation vs. track distance. Electrode inclination 20°; slope of the main sequence, uncorrected for inclination, –218°/mm; corrected, –232°/mm. For description of the breaks in the sequence at 0.3 mm and 0.6 mm, see text and Figure 3.

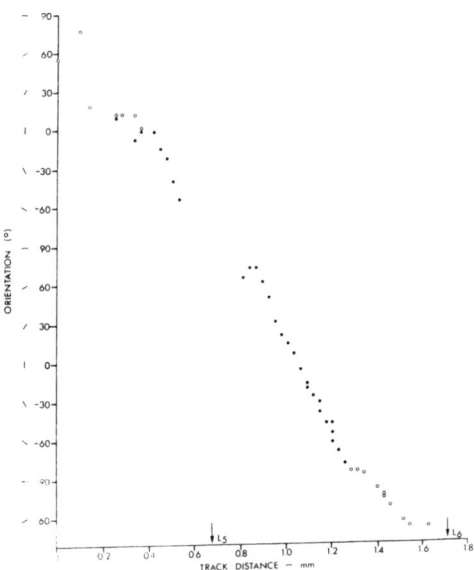

Fig. 8D. Orientation vs. track distance for P_3. Electrode inclination 20°. Slope −262°/mm uncorrected, −280°/mm corrected, for inclination.

rate islands with separate sequences of orientation, in an otherwise well-ordered matrix of columns. No color-coded cells or abrupt jumps were seen in the other two penetrations, but in the reconstruction the clockwise sequence of penetration 2 is physically very close to the similar clockwise progression at the end of penetration 1, and is probably related to it.

A second set of parallel penetrations in a normal monkey is illustrated in Figure 10 and reconstructed in Figure 11. Here the lateral spacing between penetrations was 0.1 mm; again one of the penetrations entered some distance beyond the others so that there was no overlap with them. The slopes of all three penetrations were again very similar, and the reconstruction of penetrations 2 and 3 are once more consistent with the idea that the columns are parallel slabs.

Area 18

In one monkey six penetrations were made in area 18 and 111 shifts in orientation were observed. One penetration in which 44 cells were recorded is illustrated in Figure 12. The animal had had one eye removed at birth for a different study, so that variation in ocular-dominance could obviously not be

examined. Although six penetrations are far from enough to allow any close comparisons between areas 17 and 18, it is clear that in area 18 orientation columns are present and are systematically arranged, with similar long sequences of orientation shifts broken occasionally by reversals. A similar orderliness in arrangement of orientation columns in area 18 was previously observed in the cat (Hubel and Wiesel, '65, Fig. 32). The fineness of orientational representation and the size of the columns seem not to differ very greatly in area 17 and 18.

Recordings from Cat

Four penetrations were made in the striate cortex of one cat. Systematic variations in orientation were seen in all four penetrations, two of which are described in Figure 13. Penetration 1 was almost perpendicular to the cortical surface, and penetration 4 in its latter part was almost parallel. As in the monkey, the slope of the graph of orientation vs. track distance was much less for the perpendicular penetration.

In comparing cat and monkey one major difference suggested by Figure 13 is in the size of the orientation columns. In the tangential penetration (P. 4, Fig. 13C) steps were evident, whereas in the monkey, as already mentioned, the steps were usually too small to be resolved by our methods except in nearly perpendicular penetrations. The horizontal distance/orientation shift for this penetration was 73 μ, compared with a mean of 43 μ in the monkey. The column thickness suggested by surface mapping techniques in our previous work in the cat was about 100 μ (Hubel and Wiesel, '63, Fig. 4).

The histological sections in the region of this tangential penetration were especially favorable for comparing numbers of radial bands of cells with the steps seen physiologically, since the point of entry into cortex from white matter was clearly marked by the track, and the end of the track by a lesion. We counted roughly 35 bands along this track (23 bands/mm, i.e., average width of band 43 μ) whereas the number of observed shifts was 17 (14/mm, average distance between shifts 73 μ). As in the monkey, the two seem to be about the same order of magnitude, the number of bands/mm again being somewhat larger than the number of shifts.

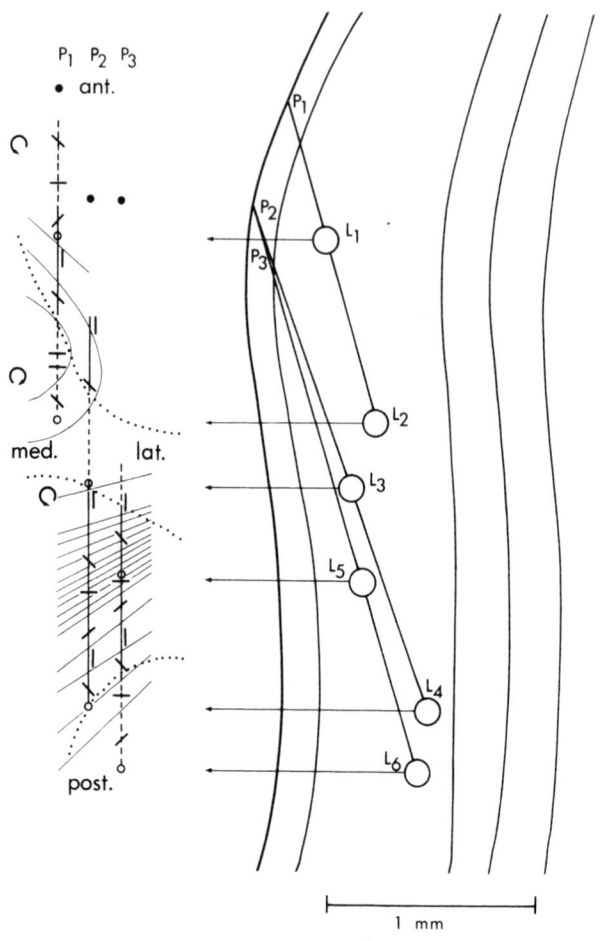

Fig. 9. Reconstruction of the three penetrations of Figure 8. To the right of the figure the tracks are seen from the side, as in Figure 8A. To the left, the three penetrations are seen as though the cortex were viewed from above. Each penetration is drawn as a vertical line, continuous for regions of contralateral-eye dominance, interrupted for ipsilateral. Black dots indicate points where the penetrations began: in P_3 no activity was recorded for roughly the first 1 mm. Dotted lines are intended to suggest boundaries between ocular-dominance columns. Continuous thin lines indicate boundaries of orientation columns, spaced at 45° except near L_5, where spacing is 9° to give a rough impression of the size of the individual orientation columns.

DISCUSSION

The Column Concept

The results of this paper indicate that orientation columns are highly ordered and probably have the form of parallel slabs. This seems to be true in the cat as well as in the monkey and in area 18 as well as in area 17. That stimulus orientation turned out to be so systematically related to position along the cortical surface was not entirely a surprise, since we had observed a compelling example of it before (Hubel and Wiesel, '68). Until the present study, however, with the use of lower impedance electrodes and the plotting of orientation against distance, we had not realized that the orderliness is the rule rather than the exception. Since such a highly patterned machinery must surely have some

important biological significance, it may be useful to think through once more the concept of the cortical column before discussing the implications of the orderliness.

The cortical column may generally be looked upon as arising from the necessity to portray more than two variables upon a two-dimensional surface. The two surface coordinates are used up by the topographic representation of the visual fields, and it is the engrafting upon this representation of two more variables in the form of receptive-field orientation and ocular dominance that leads to the two sets of subdivisions. It is important here to emphasize the hierarchy: the topographic projection is the primary one, and for each position in the visual field there is a machinery for each orientation and for each eye. How the topographic repre-

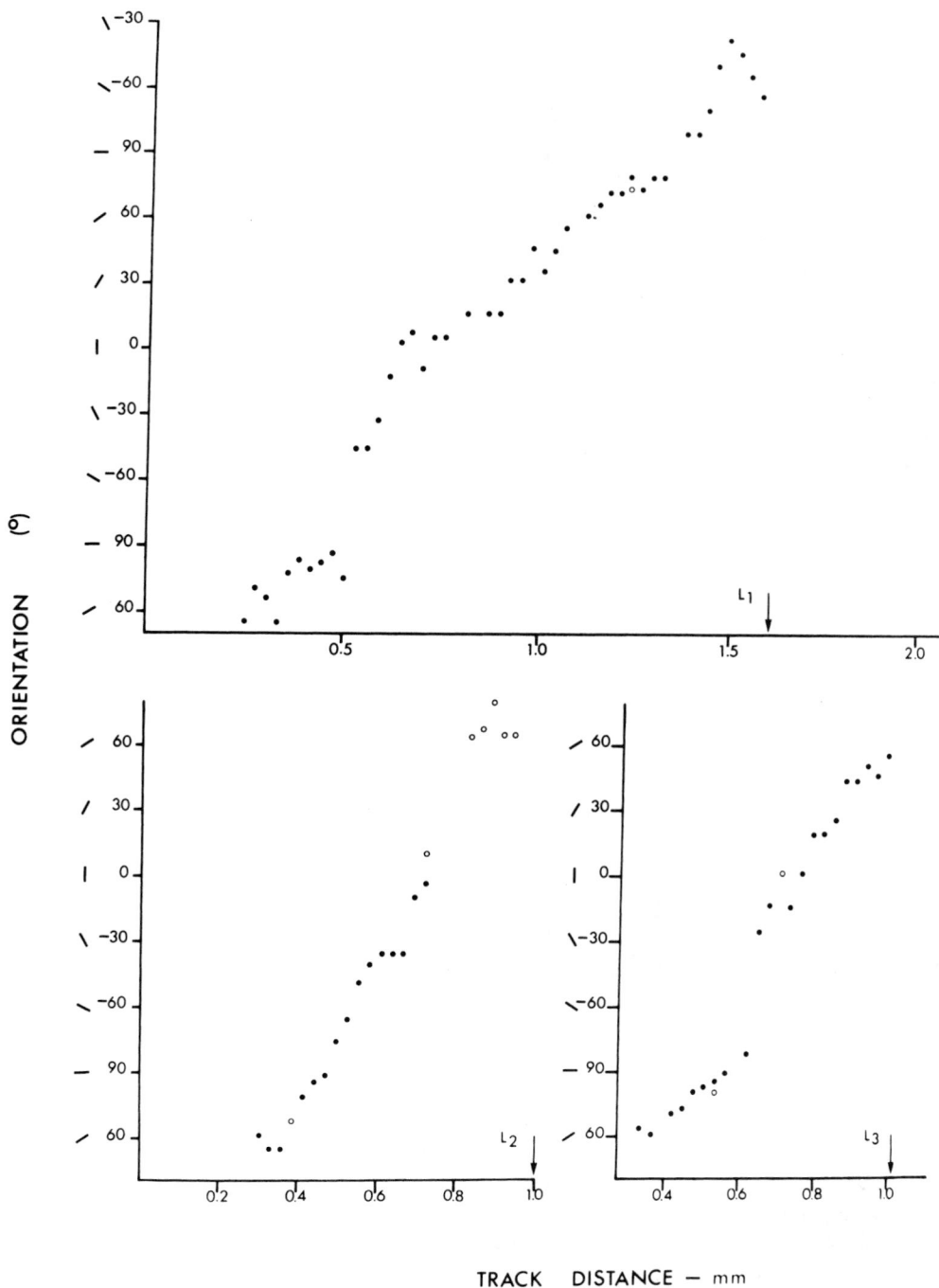

Fig. 10. Graphs of orientation vs. track distance for three parallel penetrations in parasagittal planes 100 μ apart. (The three reconstructions are seen in profile and plan views in Fig. 11.) Slopes, uncorrected and corrected for electrode inclination, P_1, 204, 208; P_2, 363, 424; P_3, 307, 358—all in °/mm. P_1 entered the cortex behind the other two, so that the total extent of cortex explored was about 2.2 mm, throughout which the trend of orientations was clockwise, going posteriorly. (Experiment No. 6.)

343

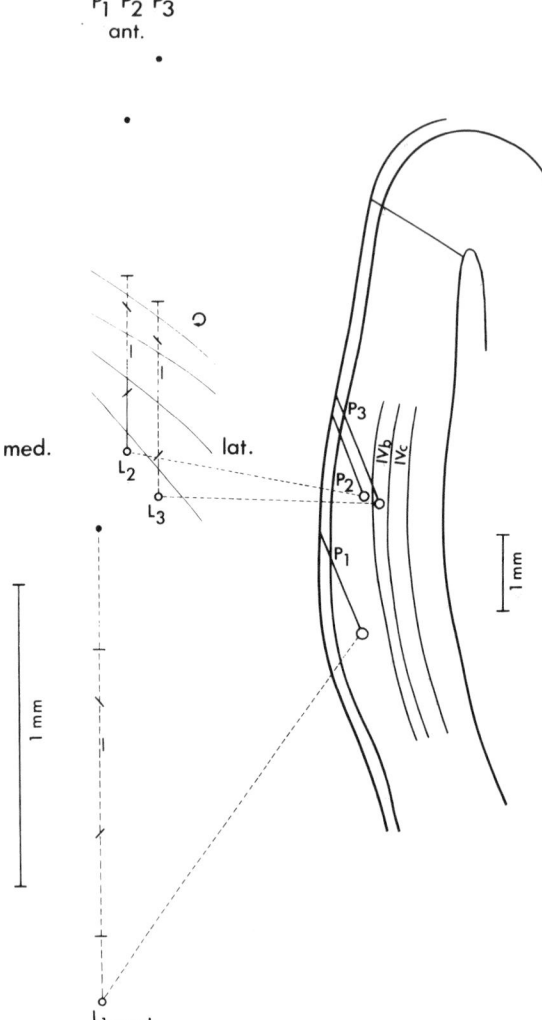

Fig. 11. Reconstruction of three parasagittal penetrations 100 μm apart, whose graphs of orientation vs. track distance appear in Figure 10. Side view is shown in the right part of the figure; surface view on the left. The large dots indicate points of entry of electrode into cortex; in P_2 and P_3 no responses were recorded for the first 0.5–0.75 mm.

sentation and the two columnar systems interrelate, in detail, is taken up in a later paper (Hubel and Wiesel, '74a).

That we speak of the cortex as a two-dimensional structure in this context is deliberate, for the three variables, visual-field position, orientation, and ocular dominance, all remain virtually constant during a perfectly perpendicular penetration. The cortical depth dimension is apparently concerned with other problems, such as the relative complexity of cells and their hierarchical order. For a columnar system, then, a prime criterion is that there be subdivisions extending vertically through the full cortical thickness, with walls perpendicular to the surface and to the layers. This is fulfilled by

the ocular-dominance columns, as we know from both anatomical and physiological evidence. For the orientation columns previous evidence (Hubel and Wiesel, '62, '63) has been reinforced, in the present paper, by comparing slopes of orientation-vs.-distance curves in perpendicular penetrations with those obtained in tangential or oblique ones.

The requirement that the walls of the columnar subdivisions be perpendicular to the surface and to the layers predicts a cylindrical shape (or a conical shape, if the cortical surface is curved). Since "cylinder" summons up visions of highball glasses, coins, or Greek pillars, the word "column" originally seemed a natural choice. In the somatosensory system, where the term was first used by Mountcas-

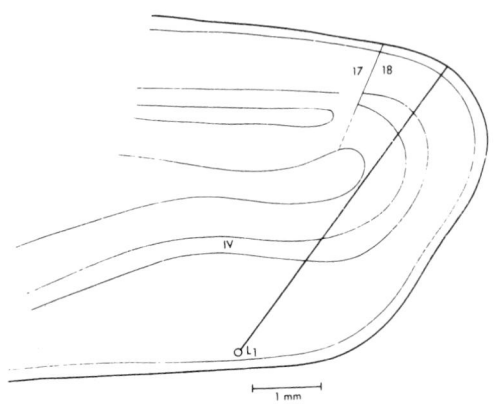

Fig. 12A. *Penetration in monkey area 18. Electrode entered the cortex in the parasagittal plane just anterior to the 17–18 border.*

tle ('57), the geometry is still unclear, but in the two column systems so far described for the visual cortex the cylinders seem to take the extreme form of a set of sheets, a shape that does not come to mind on hearing the word "column." We retain the term partly for historical reasons and partly because it has become associated, in cortical physiology, as much with the principle of grouping of cells with certain physiological similarities, as with any special shape.

Furthermore, before considering a change in terminology, it is well to note that even in the ocular-dominance system, where by anatomical methods we have obtained some inkling of the surface mosaic, the form seems to be one of stripes only to a first approximation: in some experiments the stripes seemed to subdivide and rejoin or to be crossconnected, occasionally to such an extent that the geometry resembled an interlacing kind of lattice rather than parallel plates (Hubel and Wiesel, '72, Fig. 17).

An additional requirement that has usually been insisted upon for a columnar system is that the subdivisions be discrete. This means that within a certain finite volume of cortex the variable concerned must remain constant. The ocular-dominance columns are certainly discrete, and hence properly named. With the orientation columns, on the other hand, the situation is less clear, especially in view of the present results. In tangential or oblique penetrations in the monkey any discrete steps were too small to be resolved, since every clear-cut advance of the electrode was accompanied by an orientation shift. The only exceptions to this were the relatively infrequent but nevertheless very clear large shifts such as the two illustrated in Figure 3; in cases like these there

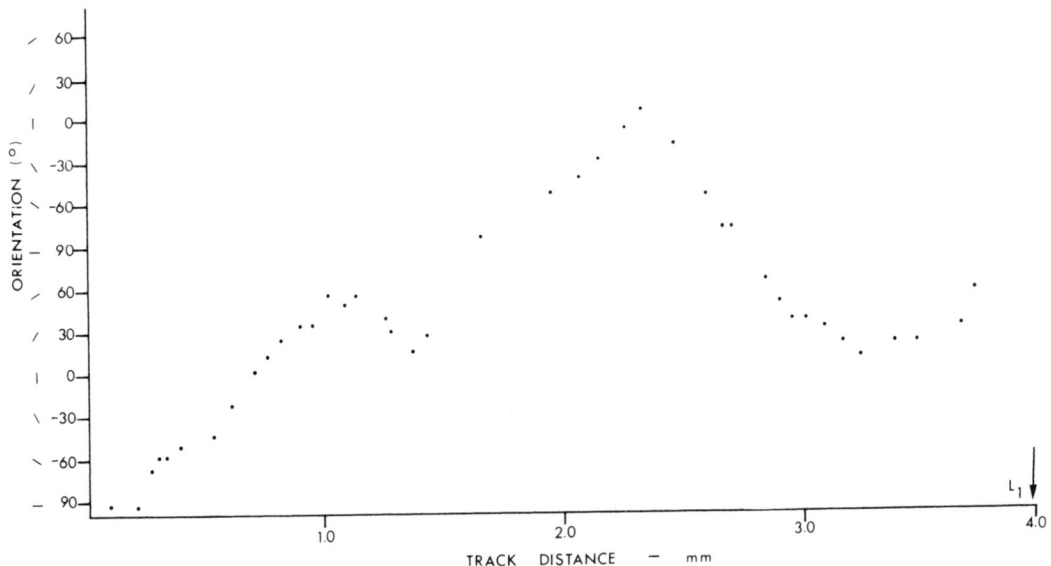

Fig. 12B. *The graph of orientation vs. track distance shows that orientation varied systematically with position. This animal, from a separate study, had had its right eye removed from birth, so that nothing can be said about eye dominance. (Experiment No. 2.)*

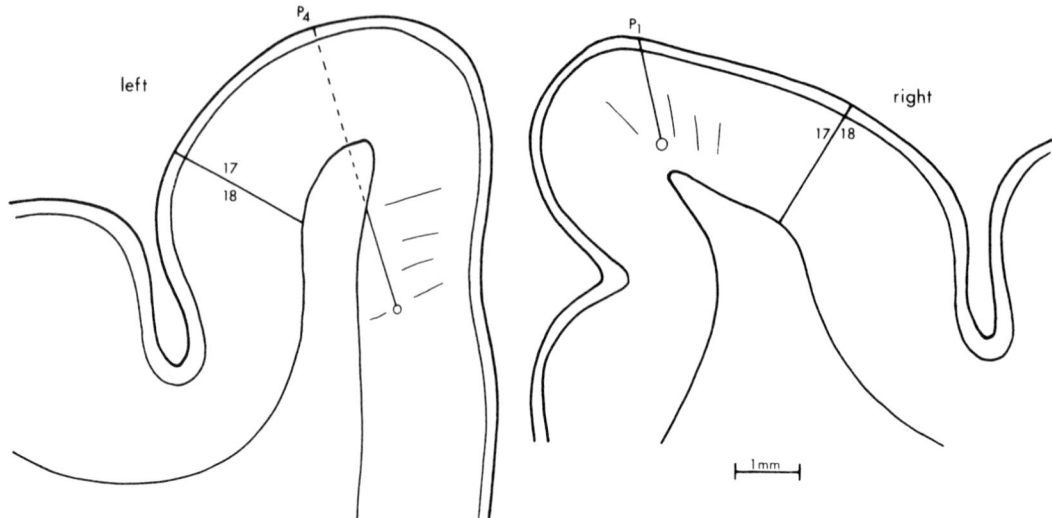

Fig. 13A. Cat striate cortex. Reconstruction, in the coronal plane, of two penetrations in the postlateral gyrus, roughly at Horsley-Clark P 2.0. Penetration in right hemisphere was virtually perpendicular to the layers throughout. On the left side the electrode passed through the dorsal thickness of grey matter, and then through white matter, finally re-entering the mesial segment of striate cortex, intersecting the radial fascicles at about 87°. (Experiment No. 8.)

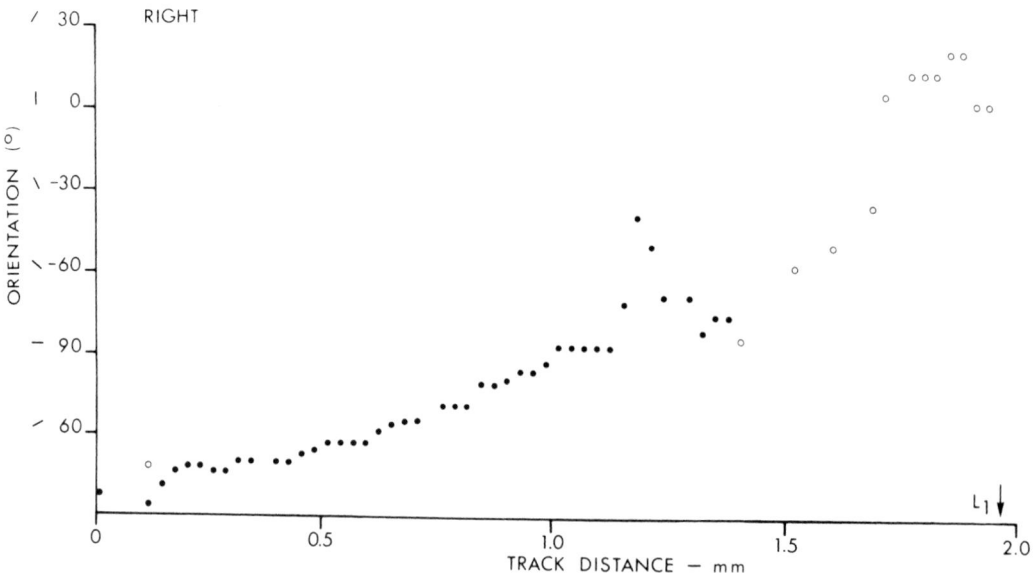

Fig. 13B. Graph of orientation vs. track distance for the perpendicular penetration in the right hemisphere. Slope, uncorrected, 54°/mm.

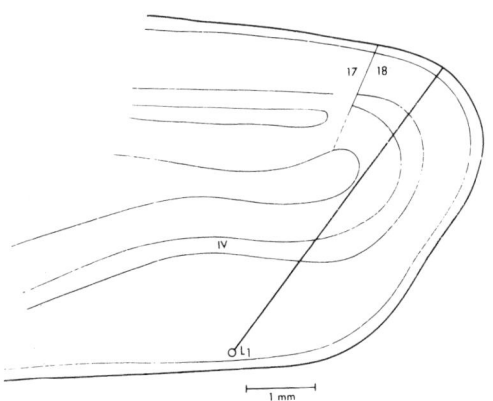

Fig. 12A. Penetration in monkey area 18. Electrode entered the cortex in the parasagittal plane just anterior to the 17–18 border.

tle ('57), the geometry is still unclear, but in the two column systems so far described for the visual cortex the cylinders seem to take the extreme form of a set of sheets, a shape that does not come to mind on hearing the word "column." We retain the term partly for historical reasons and partly because it has become associated, in cortical physiology, as much with the principle of grouping of cells with certain physiological similarities, as with any special shape.

Furthermore, before considering a change in terminology, it is well to note that even in the ocular-dominance system, where by anatomical methods we have obtained some inkling of the surface mosaic, the form seems to be one of stripes only to a first approximation: in some experiments the stripes seemed to subdivide and rejoin or to be crossconnected, occasionally to such an extent that the geometry resembled an interlacing kind of lattice rather than parallel plates (Hubel and Wiesel, '72, Fig. 17).

An additional requirement that has usually been insisted upon for a columnar system is that the subdivisions be discrete. This means that within a certain finite volume of cortex the variable concerned must remain constant. The ocular-dominance columns are certainly discrete, and hence properly named. With the orientation columns, on the other hand, the situation is less clear, especially in view of the present results. In tangential or oblique penetrations in the monkey any discrete steps were too small to be resolved, since every clear-cut advance of the electrode was accompanied by an orientation shift. The only exceptions to this were the relatively infrequent but nevertheless very clear large shifts such as the two illustrated in Figure 3; in cases like these there

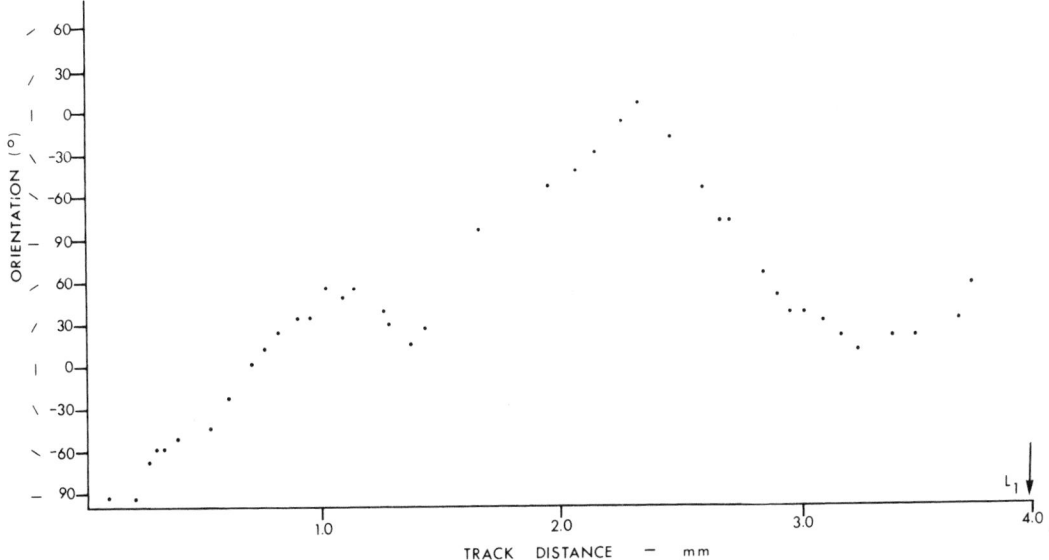

Fig. 12B. The graph of orientation vs. track distance shows that orientation varied systematically with position. This animal, from a separate study, had had its right eye removed from birth, so that nothing can be said about eye dominance. (Experiment No. 2.)

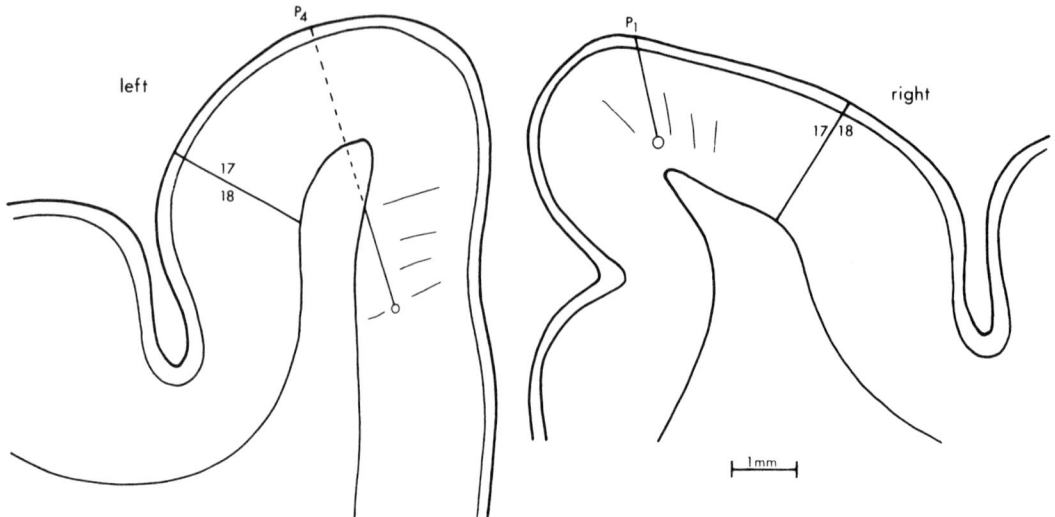

Fig. 13A. Cat striate cortex. Reconstruction, in the coronal plane, of two penetrations in the postlateral gyrus, roughly at Horsley-Clark P 2.0. Penetration in right hemisphere was virtually perpendicular to the layers throughout. On the left side the electrode passed through the dorsal thickness of grey matter, and then through white matter, finally re-entering the mesial segment of striate cortex, intersecting the radial fascicles at about 87°. (Experiment No. 8.)

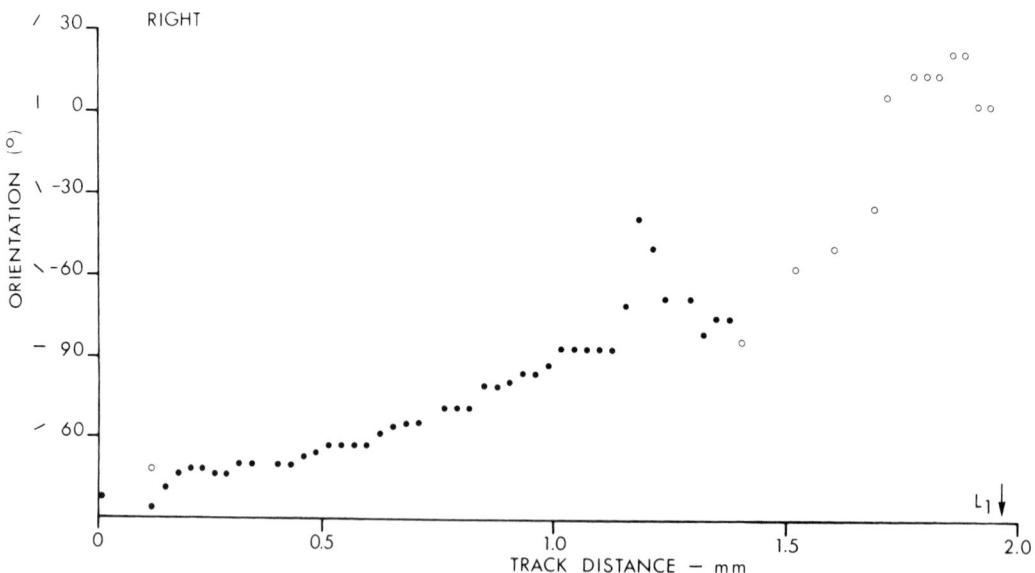

Fig. 13B. Graph of orientation vs. track distance for the perpendicular penetration in the right hemisphere. Slope, uncorrected, 54°/mm.

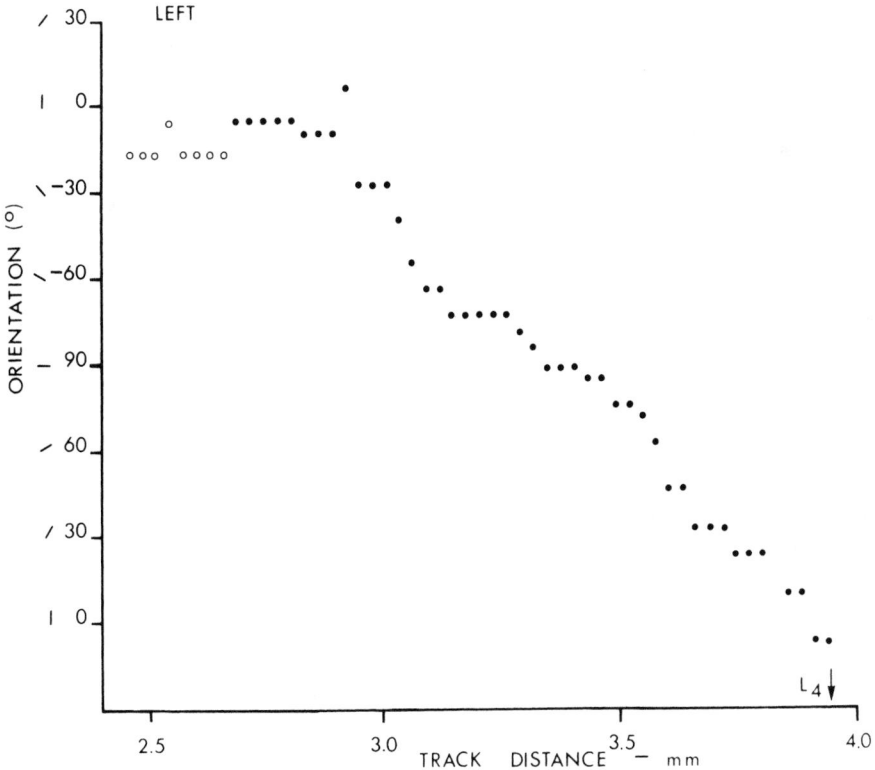

Fig. 13C. *Graph of orientation vs. track distance for the part of the penetration in the left hemisphere indicated by a continuous line. Slope, corrected for the 3° inclination, –165°/mm.*

can be no doubt that the change in orientation with movement parallel to the surface was abrupt and discrete. Otherwise the notion that the orientation shifts are discrete relies, in the monkey, upon a very few penetrations that were virtually perpendicular to the surface, in which the distance from slab to slab was presumably magnified, and in which the curves showed clear steps (Fig. 4B). In the cat cortex, where the columns are probably thicker, steps were apparent even in a penetration parallel to the surface (Fig. 13C), so that here the existence of discrete orientation columns seems reasonably clear.

Though it is conceivable that orientation may vary continuously with movement along the cortex, there are certain difficulties in the idea. Taken literally, it is contradicted by the fact that the cells which make up the cortex and from which one records are discrete entities. A kind of continuous variation might nevertheless be achieved if there were a small random variation in the orientations of neighboring cells, and if accompanying horizon-

tal movement through the cortex there were superimposed a steady drift or progression in the orientation. This would be analogous to the random variation or staggering in receptive-field positions of neighboring cells, upon which is superimposed a steady drift in receptive-field position with movement parallel to the surface. We did not, however, observe any such random variations in orientation, from one cell to the next. Variations comparable to those seen in receptive-field position would have produced jagged curves, not the smooth monotonic ones found in this study. Moreover the multiunit background activity showed an orientation preference that was generally the same as that of simultaneously recorded cells, and no less sharply tuned. There is thus no evidence to support the existence of a local random variation in orientation, but at present this possibility cannot be ruled out conclusively.

To recapitulate, the orientation slabs in the monkey, if discrete entities, are so thin that they

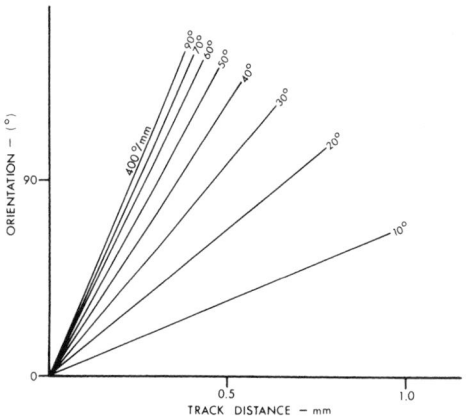

Fig. 14. Theoretical effects of varying the angle between a set of parallel orientation slabs and a tangential electrode, upon curves of orientation vs. track distance. The uppermost curve corresponds to a head-on 90° intersection of the electrode and the slabs; a slope of 400°/mm was arbitrarily selected for the example because the steepest experimental curves were in the range of 400–450°/mm. As the angle between the electrode and the slabs varies, the slope falls according to the sine of the angle, with little change up to about 40–50°, giving curves that are far from flat even at 20°. Thus if tangential penetrations intersect the slabs at random angles there should be a skew distribution of slopes, with a preponderance of steep curves. If the slabs are parallel but curved, reversals in direction of rotation from clockwise to counterclockwise or back should be abrupt.

cannot be clearly resolved in tangential penetrations, because of imprecision in measurements both of electrode distance and receptive-field orientation. The evidence favoring discrete entities comes from perpendicular penetrations, from the occasional abrupt discontinuities seen in tangential penetrations, and from results in the cat, where the columns are coarse enough to be resolved. The alternative notion, that substantial regions of visual cortex are organized with respect to the orientation variable in some kind of continuous manner, cannot be ruled out, though it seems rather less likely. Independent of which alternative is correct, the central concept of a subdivision of cortex into regions of common orientation specificity by surfaces arranged perpendicular to the cortical layers still holds. If the slabs are not discrete it obviously becomes incorrect to speak of steps of 9–10° or slabs 25–50 μ thick, but the notion of 180° being covered

in 0.5–1 mm movement normal to the surfaces is still valid.

If one accepts the notion that the orientation columns are discrete, with an interval of roughly 9–10°, does this mean that orientation over the entire 180° is quantized into 18–20 strictly defined groups in terms of angle? If, beginning at a certain point on the cortex, corresponding to a certain optimal stimulus orientation, one proceeds along the surface from orientation to orientation until a full cycle of 180° has taken place, will one have returned to precisely the same orientation, or will it be slightly different? At present we have no way of knowing the answer to this, and given the breadth of the tuning curves and the limitations in precision of measurement, it is not likely that an answer will be easily found. Intuitively the idea of strict quantization seems somewhat unattractive, since to develop such a system would probably be more difficult, with no obvious advantages over the fuzzier alternative.

To summarize: the column is usually defined as a discrete aggregate of cells whose shape is that of a sheet, or more generally a cylinder, with walls perpendicular to the surface. The physiological variable that defines a set of columns is represented by being engrafted upon a pre-existing two-dimensional mapping. Although field position in the cortex remains constant (aside from a random scatter) along the depth axis, this by itself does not result in a columnar system unless one is willing to see the concept of the column degraded, since there are no discrete aggregates, and since the topography itself forms the system upon which columns are engrafted. Similarly the projection-line system of topographic representation in the lateral geniculate body (Bishop et al., '62) should not be regarded as columnar. The mouse cortical whisker barrels are certainly discrete (Woolsey and Van der Loos, '70), but they constitute a topographic representation rather than being superimposed on one. Whether they should be considered columns seems a matter of taste and semantics. The orientation columns, finally, if discrete, certainly fall within the definition of the term column. If orientation varies continuously with distance there are again semantic difficulties—either one must broaden the definition of the column or decide that the system is not strictly columnar. In fact, however, the distinction may be somewhat academic, since if the columns are discrete their thickness is close to the size of a single cell body.

Geometry of Orientation Columns

Ever since our finding with silver-degeneration techniques that ocular-dominance columns are to a first approximation slab shaped, we have hoped to find a similar method for revealing the shape of the orientation columns. None has yet been forthcoming, though direct physiological evidence for a slab shape was obtained by making multiple superficial penetrations in the cat (Hubel and Wiesel, '63), and by reconstructions of parallel penetrations in the present study. To obtain a more exact idea of the shape of the slabs will require more studies using multiple penetrations but meanwhile we are given a much better insight into the geometry of the columns by the observation that their arrangement is highly regular. The slab shape, in fact, seems an inescapable consequence of the regularity. Suppose that whenever an electrode moves tangentially through the cortex it records either small regular orientation shifts or no shifts at all. Then a three-dimensional graph of orientation (as the Z-axis) against cortical position (X- and Y-axes) will give a smooth surface, or strictly speaking one terraced in 9–10° steps. Each of the curves of orientation vs. track distance simply represents the intersection of this surface with a plane perpendicular to the X-Y plane and passing through the electrode track. On such a surface the contour lines of constant orientation represent the column mosaic as it appears when the cortex is viewed face-on. These contour lines define the tops of the slabs. Thus without appealing to rigorous arguments involving topology or mathematical theories of continuity it seems intuitively obvious that the absence of breaks in regularity implies a set of slabs. These may be straight or curved depending on the shape of the surface in the three-dimensional graph.

If the columns indeed have the form of slabs, one may predict that in tangential penetrations some of the tracks should thread their way along the plane of the slabs, producing a flat or nearly flat graph of orientation vs. track distance just as was obtained with penetrations perpendicular to the surface. In this study most tangential penetrations gave relatively steep curves. Since most penetrations were made in the parasagittal plane, one wonders if the slab orientation is constant, from animal to animal, running perpendicular to the parasagittal plane, i.e., parallel to the 17–18 border behind the lunate sulcus. This seemed only a remote possibility until recently, with the finding that the ocular-dominance columns do in fact have a consistent pattern from animal to animal, intersecting the 17–18 border at right angles (LeVay et al., '75). As mentioned below, it is theoretically attractive to suppose that the two sets of slabs, if they have any constant relationship, intersect each other at right angles.

It turns out, however, from simple trigonometry, that a parameter such as the slope of these curves is very little affected by the angle of intersection of a horizontal track with the slabs, until that angle becomes very small. As an example (Fig. 14), suppose that an electrode intersecting the slabs at right angles were to give a curve of slope 400°/mm. How is the steepness of the curve affected for approaches different from 90°? The calculations show that the change in slope for angles up to about 50° is slight (the slope is 400 sin 50°, or 306°/mm), and even at 20° the curves are hardly what would be called flat (137°/mm). The same applies to variations in the angle between the electrode and the surface of the cortex, and indeed curves as flat as those of Figures 4B, 5B (first part) and 13B were obtained only in penetrations that were within a few degrees of perpendicular. Thus in tangential penetrations, at what are presumably random angles with respect to the slabs (since we do not have any idea of the slab orientations), the slopes cannot be expected to be distributed evenly between some maximum value, such as 400°/mm, and zero. In fact the slopes we obtained (Table 1) were not so distributed but were, as would be predicted, skewed markedly towards higher values.

One curious property of the orientation columns, illustrated in Figures 2A and 8B, is the reversal of the sequences from clockwise to counterclockwise and back between uninterrupted spans of the order of 270–360°. Only more ambitious mapping will help in understanding the origin of these reversals. Possibly the columns are virtually straight parallel slabs, and the order may simply reverse at irregular intervals. This would mean that the surface generated by plotting orientation against position on the cortical surface would be corrugated like the bellows of a camera. The abruptness of the reversals might seem to argue for this: the curves of orientation vs. track distance are not at all sinusoidal, but the sequences progress with remarkable linearity and reverse not by gradual flattening but fairly suddenly. A second possibility, however, is that the slabs, viewed from above, are not straight but form whorls, in which case the surface would consist of mountains and valleys. If that were so, a straight electrode track would constantly change its angle to the slabs, and would be expected at times to become tangential and then to reverse its direction through them. One might expect, on first thought, that this would give curves with gradually changing slopes, but as pointed out above the slopes of the graphs are not greatly affected until the approach becomes almost tangential. The result of this would be to increase the abruptness of the reversals. The information from reconstructions of parallel penetrations is so far too fragmentary to allow us to choose between these possibilities, but presumably more extensive mapping can settle the question.

The degree of order must be limited, for there seem to be regions that are more or less chaotic, and there are occasionally clear breaks between ordered regions, as if the slabs had been fractured or broken apart and other parallel arrays inserted in different directions. These intercalated slabs may conceivably represent some minor imperfections in development, or perhaps they have some special function, as suggested in connection with color by the experiment of Figure 8C. It seems likely that cells concerned with color are arranged in columns (Hubel and Wiesel, '68), and the relationship of these columns to the orientation slabs described in this paper should be very interesting.

The geometric relationship between ocular-dominance columns and orientation columns is still not clear, but the fact that when the electrode crosses from a left-eye to a right-eye region there is no noticeable disturbance in the sequence of orientation columns argues for a certain degree of independence between the two systems. It would be interesting to know whether the two sets of slabs are parallel or cut each other at right angles or have any consistent relationship. We have argued previously (Hubel and Wiesel, '72, p. 444) that it would put a great burden on the connections if the two column systems were parallel. A binocular cell with some particular receptive-field orientation must receive its input from two sets of monocular cells having the same receptive-field orientation; the two sets must, by definition, be located in separate ocular-dominance columns. Obviously it is most efficient if the binocular cell and the monocular cells supplying it are all housed in the same orientation column, for the alternative—the only one possible if the two column systems are parallel—is to have connections run from one orientation column through an entire array of intervening columns, stopping only when they reach the next column subserving the same orientation.

Histological Correlates

It is curious that in contrast to the horizontally-running layers, which are obvious at a glance, the boundaries between the vertical columnar subdivisions seem not to be evident by ordinary staining methods. The ocular-dominance columns are highly discrete, especially in layer IV C, yet to identify them histologically has required the use of specialized silver-degeneration techniques following laminar geniculate lesions, a method which depends on the fact that left-eye and right-eye columns differ because their inputs differ (Hubel and Wiesel, '72). Orientation columns are distinguished from each other by differences in intracortical connections, and consequently no analogous method is possible for their demonstration. It may be that the vertically running bands of cells are the slabs cut in transverse section: the measurements are consistent with this, for in the present series the horizontal distance between shifts was less than double the size of the bands in penetrations in which the two were compared. One would perhaps not expect better agreement, since some orientation shifts were probably missed, and the figures for distance between shifts were consequently probably overestimates. If the vertical bands of cells do indeed represent orientation slabs cut in cross section, tangential sections through the cortex might also be expected to reveal parallel lines of cells, straight or in whorls. In a few observations in the monkey we have so far seen nothing like this.

In this context the question discussed above of whether the orientation columns are discrete or merge continuously may be of some importance; if the variation is in some sense continuous one would hardly expect to find discrete anatomical subdivisions. Perhaps, indeed, the solution to this problem of discreteness vs. continuity should be sought using anatomical rather than physiological methods.

There is one puzzling apparent discrepancy between these physiological results and the morphology. The orientation-column (or slab) thickness is at most in the order of 25–50 μ, yet from sections of Golgi material most cells are known to have dendritic and axonal arborizations that extend, apparently in all directions, for distances of up to several millimeters. Perhaps the connections made by these processes have a selectivity not hinted at by the anatomy, for the physiological results predict strongly that different orientation columns should not be linked by important excitatory connections. Neighboring columns might, on the other hand, be linked by inhibitory connections subserving movement directional selectivity or the sharpening of response-vs.-orientation tuning curves. At present one can only say that, except for the cortical barrels seen in mice and related species (Woolsey and Van der Loos, '70), there is no example of a correlation between any of the columns yet described and the Nissl, Golgi or electron-microscopic anatomy.

The presence of highly ordered orientation sequences in area 18 deserves some comment. Area 18 in the monkey receives a powerful, systematic and orderly projection from 17 (Spatz et al. '70), but unlike area 18 in the cat it has not been shown to receive any direct input from the lateral geniculate body. For example, after small discrete lesions made in single dorsal or ventral layers of the geniculate we found no obvious Nauta degeneration in area 18, despite a careful search of the parts of 18 topographically corresponding to the lesion sites (Hubel and Wiesel, '72). Other inputs to area 18 in the monkey, for example from thalamus outside the geniculate, are at present conjectural. Thus the only well established direct visual input to 18 comes from 17. It therefore seems likely that a cell in 18 with high orientation specificity derives those properties from cells in 17 having the same orientation specificity and receives no important excitatory inputs from cells with different optimal orientations. By extension, cells within a given orientation column must receive most of their inputs from columns with identical orientations in 17. The fact that receptive fields in 18 are several times larger than those in 17 (Hubel and Wiesel, unpublished) suggests that several columns of like orientation

specificity in 17 may feed into one column in 18. In any case, the existence of two similar columnar systems in the two visual areas implies a specificity of 17-to-18 connections far transcending a mere region-to-region projection.

Biological Advantages of Ordered Orientation Columns

What advantage can such an ordered system of orientation columns be to the animal? We have suggested before that an economy of connections may result if columns subserving very similar orientations are close together. To build a simple receptive field from a set of geniculate afferents whose "on" or "off" field centers are arranged along a line calls for a specific set of convergent connections. By dropping a few geniculate inputs and adding a few, the orientation of the line can be changed slightly, but the inputs to the old line and the new will still be largely the same. On the other hand, two overlapping simple receptive fields with very different orientations would have far fewer afferents in common. Undoubtedly the wiring is made simpler and more efficient if cells with similar inputs are close together.

A second possible advantage is related to the suggestion by Blakemore and Tobin ('72) that orientation selectivity may be sharpened by a cell's receiving inhibitory inputs from cells with slightly different orientations, in a fashion analogous to the surround inhibition of receptive fields of retinal ganglion cells and geniculate cells. Again it would be an advantage, in terms of efficiency of wiring, if the interconnected cells could be kept close together. Psychophysical observations (Blakemore et al., '70) support the idea of mutual inhibition between neighboring orientation columns, but it is difficult to think of a direct way of testing this physiologically. Although Blakemore's experiments showing an inhibitory effect from a grid of lines moving outside the activating part of a cortical receptive field are suggestive, his results can also be explained by supposing that the cells he describes have hypercomplex properties.

As a third possibility, an orderly arrangement of columns may have advantages for development. Perhaps the order reflects a mechanism for guaranteeing that all orientations be represented once or only a few times in each part of the visual field, with no omissions and minimal redundancy. In this connection, the third paper in this series presents evidence that the entire ordered system is innately determined, and does not depend for its development on early experience (Hubel and Wiesel, '74b).

ACKNOWLEDGMENTS

We wish to thank Sandra Spinks, David Freeman and Claire Wang for technical assistance. The work was supported by NIH grants 5R01EY00605 and 5R01EY00606, and a grant from the Esther A. and Joseph Klingenstein Fund, Inc.

Literature Cited

Bishop, P. O., W. Kozak, W. R. Levick and G. J. Vakkur 1962 The determination of the projection of the visual field on to the lateral geniculate nucleus in the cat. J. Physiol., *163:* 503–539.

Blakemore, C., and E. A. Tobin 1972 Lateral inhibition between orientation detectors in the cat's visual cortex. Exp. Brain Res., *15:* 439–440.

Blakemore, C., R. H. S. Carpenter and M. A. Georgeson 1970 Lateral inhibition between orientation detectors in the human visual system. Nature, *228:* 37–39.

Daniel, P. M., and D. Whitteridge 1961 The representation of the visual field on the cerebral cortex in monkeys. J. Physiol., *159:* 203–221.

Hubel, D. H., and T. N. Wiesel 1962 Receptive fields, binocular interaction and functional architecture in the cat's visual cortex. J. Physiol., *160:* 106–154.

———— 1963 Shape and arrangement of columns in cat's striate cortex. J. Physiol., *165:* 559–568.

———— 1965 Receptive fields and functional architecture in two non-striate visual areas (18 and 19) of the cat. J. Neurophysiol., *28:* 229–289.

———— 1968 Receptive fields and functional architecture of monkey striate cortex. J. Physiol., *195:* 215–243.

———— 1972 Laminar and columnar distribution of geniculo-cortical fibers in the macaque monkey. J. Comp. Neur., *146:* 421–450.

———— 1974a Uniformity of monkey striate cortex: a parallel relationship between field size, scatter, and magnification factor. J. Comp. Neur., *158:* 295–306.

———— 1974b Ordered arrangement of orientation columns in monkeys lacking visual experience. J. Comp. Neur., *158:* 307–318.

LeVay, S., D. H. Hubel and T. N. Wiesel 1975 The pattern of ocular dominance columns in macaque visual cortex revealed by a reduced silver stain. J. Comp. Neur. (in press).

Mountcastle, V. B. 1957 Modality and topographic properties of single neurons of cat's somatic sensory cortex. J. Neurophysiol., *20:* 408–434.

Spatz, W. B., J. Tigges and M. Tigges 1970 Subcortical projections, cortical associations, and some intrinsic interlaminar connections of the striate cortex in the squirrel monkey (*Saimiri*). J. Comp. Neur., *140:* 155–173.

Woolsey, T. A., and H. Van der Loos 1970 The structural organization of layer IV in the somatosensory region (S1) of mouse cerebral cortex. Brain Res., *17:* 205–242.

AFTERWORD

What was lacking in the sequence-regularity study was a means of picturing the map of orientations face-on, for without that it was almost impossible to interpret the reversals and the breaks in the sequences of orientation versus electrode track distance. This came suddenly, like a thunderclap, in 1985 at a Society of Neuroscience meeting in a 10-minute paper presented by Gary Blasdel, a young investigator in the labs of Jenny Lund, then in Pittsburgh. Gary had the idea of using TV techniques to detect optical changes accompanying neural activity in the cortex, but was told it was not possible because of noise, weakness of signals, and so on. Urged on by Jenny he persisted, and succeeded, and here suddenly was the memorable map with color standing for orientation, with all the whorls that later came to be called pinwheels.

Gary's maps relied on the use of voltage-sensitive dyes, which had first been developed at Yale by Amiram Grinvald and Larry Cohen, in Larry's lab. The technique was further developed in Torsten's lab by Grinvald and Tobias Bonhoeffer, and has become one of the most important modern methods for cortical mapping. The voltage-sensitive dyes enhance the sensitivity of the technique, but are toxic to the cortex, so it was a step forward when Amiram Grinwald discovered that the dyes are not strictly necessary, and that what became known as *intrinsic signals* could supply the entire picture. This has made it possible to employ the method in human neuro-surgery.

I must hasten to add that the two authors of the present book are not in full agreement over the history of the development of these optical methods. In a scientific partnership that lasted 25 years and that goes back 40 years, it would be surprising if the two of us had not found one or two things to dis-agree on, and on this story I believe the two of us are in agreement—that we disagree!

The optical methods have gone a long way in explaining the reversals in direction of orientation shifts, but have perhaps been less successful in explaining the fractures. And I still have no clear idea of the exact relation-ship between the pinwheel centers, sometimes called *singularities,* and the centers of blobs. Recent work by Eric Schwartz suggests that the apparent offset in the positions of blobs as shown in cytochrome-oxidase stains, and pinwheel centers as revealed in the optical recordings, may be an artifact caused by the limitations in resolution of the optical method and by averag-ing vectors as opposed to scaler quantities. Probably the most important lim-itation has been the method's inability to map parts of the cortex that are hid-den from the brain surface by being buried in sulci. Surely future technical advances will overcome this limitation.

Chapter 20 • Cortical Modules and Magnification in Monkeys •

FOREWORD

This is one of our all-time favorite papers, occupying in our minds a place beside the 1959 and 1962 cortex papers. It resembles the 1962 cortex paper in deepening our understanding of this fascinating structure. It goes beyond description and attempts to get at the essence of what the cortex in general may be doing. It addresses the question of what determines the three-dimensional shape of any cortical area, and how any one area of cortex can be so uniform anatomically despite certain marked variations in function as the surface is traversed—in the case of area 17, variations especially in field size and magnification.

Our study stemmed from the discovery in the early 1960s, by Daniel and Whitteridge, (*J Physiol* 1961, 159:203–221), that the topological shape of the cortex—whether it is a plane or a sphere or something else—is dictated by its function. They were the first, to our knowledge, to point out that, in considering shape, what counted was the form taken by the cortical plate when the trivial crinkles are smoothed out. A paper crumpled before throwing it in the wastebasket is still basically a flat surface. In the case of the cortex, what one wants to know is the essential shape revealed when one goes inside the structure and blows gently. This is in effect what Daniel and Whitteridge did by using serial sections of cortex to model it in rubber, and discovering that its shape after unfolding was neither flat nor spherical, but rather like a pear. Given that the eye is necessarily spherical, as it has to be for optical reasons, one might have expected the cortex to have that shape too. But Daniel and Whitteridge showed that the pear shape could be exactly predicted from the variations in the retina-to-cortex magnification (a term they originated): the fact that the number of millimeters of cortex corresponding to a degree of visual field varies in a regular and consistent way with distance from the fovea (the eccentricity).

Around 1961 Whitteridge visited our group at Harvard and gave a seminar in which he demonstrated his India-rubber model and how it could easily be refolded to reproduce the shape it has in the skull, with calcarine fissure and all. At the time I thought it only mildly interesting, but slowly came to appreciate its profundity. It gradually dawned on us that any cortical region must have *some* basic (unfolded) shape and that the exact shape must be dictated by its function. So the somatosensory hand representation should be that of a distorted glove, perhaps with rips and splices, given the obvious awkwardness of having a region of cortex with anything like the shape of a glove.

The second realization that led to this paper came as a result of a visit I paid to Tübingen, where I presented our work on columns. Werner Reichardt was in the audience, and in the discussion he asked how the shifts in orientation, as one proceeded along the cortex, were related to positions of the receptive field in the visual field. If you got into a new region of visual field without having covered all the orientations, what then? We had taken it for granted that steady movement across the visual field, on moving along the cortex, would be slow enough that the visual fields would not be peppered with scotomata for specific orientations. I remember thinking that his question was rather silly. And once more, as weeks went by, it dawned on us that the question was profound. So we did experiments to correlate positions of receptive fields in the visual field, field size, and magnification—as one moved across the cortex. Was there a systematic relationship between the x-y cortical topography and receptive field size? Would examining it tell us anything interesting about the cortex in general?

The result was deeply satisfying in extending our ideas about how the retina can be so non-uniform; for example, there is a huge difference in layer thickness near the fovea and far out from it, whereas the visual cortex shows no comparable variations in thickness. The study also led to the concept of *modules,* small blocks of cortex each carrying out a set of functions with roughly the same machinery, for a given region of visual field. The term *module* seems not to be used in our papers. Where it originated, in the context of cortical function, is not clear to us, though I use it in the title of Chapter 6 in my book *Eye, Brain and Vision* (Scientific American Libras, Leslesz, New York, 1988), to refer to these blocks of cortex. The term *hypercolumn* designated all the columns of a given type (either ocular dominance or orientation) within a module. So within any one module, an ocular dominance hypercolumn would mean a left- plus a right-eye column; and an orientation hypercolumn would mean a set of columns subserving each orientation, once only. Some writers have used the term *hypercolumn* as roughly synonymous with *module,* to mean a complete set of columns of all kinds. That was not how we defined the word, but terminologies do tend to get degraded over time, and we should perhaps be tolerant.

Obviously, we are talking about these chunks of cortex not in a literal, but in an abstract sense, as it is arbitrary where one module begins and where it leaves off.

Uniformity of Monkey Striate Cortex: A Parallel Relationship between Field Size, Scatter, and Magnification Factor

DAVID H. HUBEL AND TORSTEN N. WIESEL • *Department of Neurobiology, Harvard Medical School, 25 Shattuck Street, Boston, Massachusetts 02115*

ABSTRACT

This paper is concerned with the relationship between orientation columns, ocular-dominance columns, the topographic mapping of visual fields onto cortex, and receptive-field size and scatter. Although the orientation columns are an order of magnitude smaller than the ocular-dominance columns, the horizontal distance corresponding to a complete cycle of orientation columns, representing a rotation through 180°, seems to be roughly the same size as a left-plus-right ocular dominance set, with a thickness of about 0.5–1 mm, independent of eccentricity at least out to 15°. We use the term *hypercolumn* to refer to a complete set of either type (180°, or left-plus-right eyes).

In the macaque monkey several penetrations were made at various eccentricities in various parts of the striate cortex subserving the fovea, parafovea and midperiphery. As observed many times previously, in any vertical penetration there was an apparently random scatter in receptive-field positions, which was of the same order of magnitude as the individual receptive fields in that part of the cortex; the field size and the scatter increased in parallel fashion with eccentricity. The movement through the visual field corresponding to a 1 mm horizontal movement along the cortex (the reciprocal of the magnification factor) also increased with eccentricity, in a manner that was strikingly parallel with the increase in receptive field size and scatter. In parts of the cortex representing retina, at least out to about 22° from the fovea, a movement along the cortical surface of about 1 mm was enough to displace the fields so that the new position they collectively occupied half overlapped the old. Such an overlap was thus produced by moving along the cortex a distance about equal to the thickness of a left-plus-right set of ocular-dominance columns, or a complete 180° array of orientation columns. It therefore seems that, independent of eccentricity, a 2 mm × 2 mm block of cortex contains by a comfortable margin the machinery needed to analyze a region of visual field roughly equal to the local field size plus scatter. A movement of 2–3 mm corresponds to a new visual field region and to several new sets of hypercolumns. The cortex thus seems remarkably uniform physiologically, just as it is anatomically.

As a recording electrode moves through the monkey striate cortex in a direction parallel to the surface, the position in the visual fields from which responses are evoked changes in a predictable manner, according to a systematic topographic map (Talbot and Marshall, '41; Daniel and Whitteridge, '61). Engrafted on this projection of the visual fields are two columnar systems, one subserving receptive-field orientation, the other, ocular dominance. In the preceding paper (Hubel and Wiesel, '74) we showed that changes in orientation with tangential movement occur in a highly systematic manner, in small, relatively constant steps of at

most about 10°. These orientation columns apparently have the form of parallel slabs, with a thickness of 25–50 μ or less. We had found in a previous study that the ocular-dominance columns are likewise slab shaped, with a thickness of 0.25–0.5 mm (Hubel and Wiesel, '72). Over the regions of cortex so far examined the dimensions of both column types are roughly constant, a result that is not unexpected given the relative histological uniformity of the striate cortex.

From a different standpoint, however, this relative constancy of column size over the cortex seemed surprising, since it is known that the num-

From *Journal of Comparative Neurology*, Vol. 158, No. 3, December 1, 1974.

ber of degrees of visual field corresponding to 1 mm movement along the cortex (the reciprocal of the magnification factor) is far from constant, being small for the foveal representation and larger—by a factor of about 35—for the periphery. Both receptive-field size and scatter in the field positions of neighboring cells are likewise small in the foveal region and large in the periphery. The present paper addresses itself to resolving this apparent inconsistency between a relatively constant histological appearance and column size, on the one hand, and a markedly inconstant magnification and field size, on the other. The crux of the problem turns out to lie in the exact relationship between field size, field scatter, and magnification, as position in the cortex (or in the visual field) is varied. Our conclusion is that the cortex is, after all, a remarkably uniform structure.

METHOD

Seven penetrations were made in two normal adult rhesus monkeys. In all, 125 cells were studied. Methods of recording and stimulating were generally the same as in previous studies (Hubel and Wiesel, '68, '74). Since in estimating field scatter and magnification it was important to determine the positions of receptive fields precisely, we used an eye-monitoring technique originally devised for measurements of retinal disparity (Hubel and Wiesel, '70). Cells were recorded in the usual way with an electrode in one hemisphere, and eye positions were monitored by recording from a single binocular cell for long periods with a second electrode placed in the opposite striate cortex; after recording from each new cell with the main recording electrode we quickly checked eye positions by switching the input stage to the reference electrode and re-mapping the receptive fields of the reference cell. Electrodes were selected to be fine enough to resolve single units easily, but coarse enough so that there was a reasonably high likelihood of dual-unit recordings.

RESULTS

In our previous work in cats ('62) we observed an apparently random variation in receptive-field position on recording from successive cells during a penetration perpendicular to the cortical surface.

The amount of variation in receptive-field position was such that the total visual-field area covered by the superimposed receptive fields in one penetration was several times the area occupied by a single field; most of the fields either overlapped or abutted each other. In a long tangential penetration, a gradual drift in field positions was superimposed on the random scatter, but electrode movements of a few tenths of a millimeter were far too small for this drift to be apparent. We concluded that there are limitations to the precision of the topographic map of visual fields on to cortex.

In the monkey we have had the strong impression that the organization is similar, but we wished to re-examine the problem in order to learn more about the relationship between receptive-field size and amount of scatter on the one hand, and topography on the other. The first step was to record from enough cells in a perpendicular penetration, in a particular region of monkey cortex, to form an idea of the range of receptive-field sizes and the amount of scatter. We monitored eye movements with a second electrode to be absolutely sure that the scatter was real (METHODS).

In the perpendicular penetration of Figure 1, the receptive-field positions of 14 consecutively recorded cells are superimposed. The penetration was made about 15 mm behind the lunate sulcus and 10 mm to the left of the midline, corresponding to a visual-field area 10° to the right of the fovea and 1–2° above it. The track ended in layer IV B, 1.3 mm from the surface. All cells were strongly dominated by the right (contralateral) eye. As expected, the fields overlapped extensively, and the total size of the region through which the fields were spread (about 4° × 4°) was several times the average size of the individual fields (about 1.3° × 1.3°). Two pairs of simultaneously recorded cells are indicated, one by heavy lines (13, 14) and the other by interrupted lines (15, 16). In both pairs the fields are certainly not superimposed and in fact hardly overlap, but instead come into contact along one border: such a degree of separation in the receptive fields of neighboring cells is not unusual, though it is more common to find some overlap. Simultaneous recordings such as these supply addi-

---

[1]*Note on magnification factor:* This term refers to millimeters of cortex corresponding to 1° of visual field (Daniel and Whitteridge, '61). The reciprocal of this index was found more useful in the present study. We designate it as "magnification^{-1}." "Eccentricity" refers to distance from fovea, in degrees.

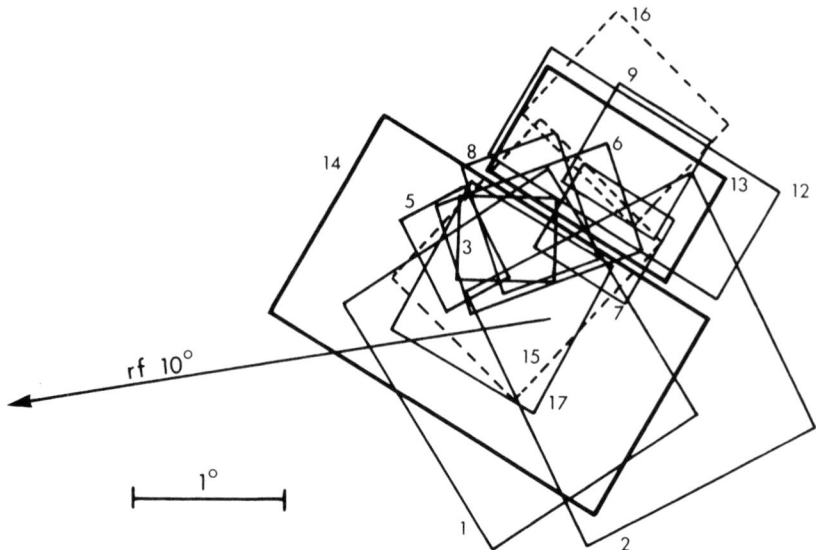

Fig. 1. Scatter of receptive fields in a perpendicular penetration. Receptive-field positions of 14 consecutively recorded cells from monkey striate cortex 10 mm to the left of the midline and 15 mm behind the lunate sulcus. The fields, mapped in the right eye, were 10° from the right fovea, just above the horizontal meridian. Fields 13 and 14 (heavy lines) are mapped for simultaneously recorded cells, as are fields 15 and 16 (interrupted lines). Eye positions are monitored with a reference electrode in the left striate cortex by repeatedly checking receptive-field positions of a binocular cell. The scatter, relative to the receptive-field size, is typical for area 17.

tional evidence that the scattering is real and not an artifact produced by eye movements. The relationship shown in this figure between overlap and scatter is typical of what we have seen in all perpendicular penetrations in striate cortex.

Our next step was to determine the number of degrees of visual field corresponding to a 1 mm horizontal movement along this part of the cortex, i.e., magnification^{-1}. To do this we inserted the electrode into the same cortical area but tilted it so as to penetrate in a posterior direction, making as acute an angle to the surface as feasible (30–35°). We first mapped the fields of whatever cells were within recording distance by stopping to stimulate and record each 20 μ for the first 100 μ. We then quickly advanced the electrode 900 μ. The whole procedure was repeated, mapping out four or five fields over the next 100 μ and advancing a further 900 μ. In this way a group of fields was plotted roughly every millimeter until after four groups (a distance of 3 mm) white matter was reached. The results are shown in Figure 2. Several shifts in eye dominance were seen, as expected for a movement of this length: cells were influenced first by the left eye only, next by both eyes with the right eye strongly dominant, then by the two eyes equally,

and finally once more by the left eye only. Thus the 3 mm penetration cut through at least three eye-dominance columns. At each advance of 1 mm there was a displacement of the mean field position upwards in the visual field, as expected from the known topography. Each displacement was roughly the amount required to produce a 50% overlap between the new territory over which the fields were scattered, and the old. Allowing for the electrode inclination (30°), the value of magnification^{-1} corresponding to this eccentricity of 10° was estimated to be 0.65°/mm.

A similar experiment was done in the same monkey for a region of the right striate cortex slightly further lateral and anterior, subserving a visual-field territory 7° from the fovea instead of 10°. From the results shown in Figure 3, allowing for electrode obliquity, it can be calculated that 1 mm represents about 0.5° in the visual field. As expected, both the receptive fields and the scatter were now smaller. Thus in both penetrations a 1 mm movement through the cortex produced a shift of receptive-field positions that was large enough to be obvious above the random staggering, but still small enough so that the two sets of fields overlapped.

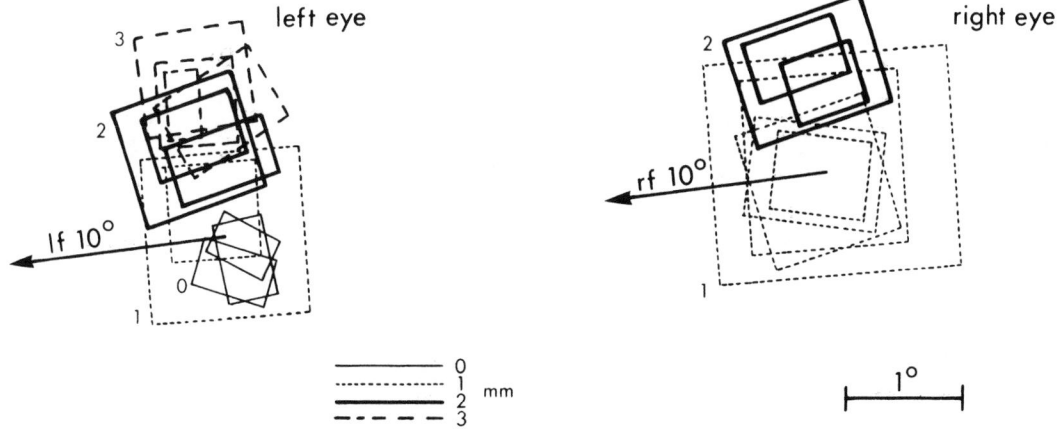

Fig. 2. *Relationship between receptive-field size-plus-scatter and magnification for an eccentricity of 10°. Same monkey as in figure 1, same region of cortex. In a penetration making an angle of 30° to the cortical surface, the fields of several cells were mapped in the first 0.1 mm and the electrode was advanced 900 µ. This procedure was repeated until white matter was reached. In this figure the first cluster of fields, marked "o," is drawn with thin continuous lines; the second, marked "I," with dots, and so on. Note the alternation of eyes as the electrode passed through successive ocular-dominance columns.*

The same procedure was repeated in two more monkeys, in regions with eccentricities of 1° and 4°. The diagram for 1° is shown in Figure 4. From the inset, which is the same diagram drawn to the scale of Figures 2 and 3, it can be seen that the fields and scatter are now much smaller, and so is the field displacement corresponding to each millimeter of movement. Magnification^{-1} was calculated to be 0.25°/mm.

For more peripheral penetrations a different strategy had to be adopted, since this part of the cortex is buried deep in the calcarine fissure and tangential penetrations are impractical. We therefore first made a long parasagittal penetration

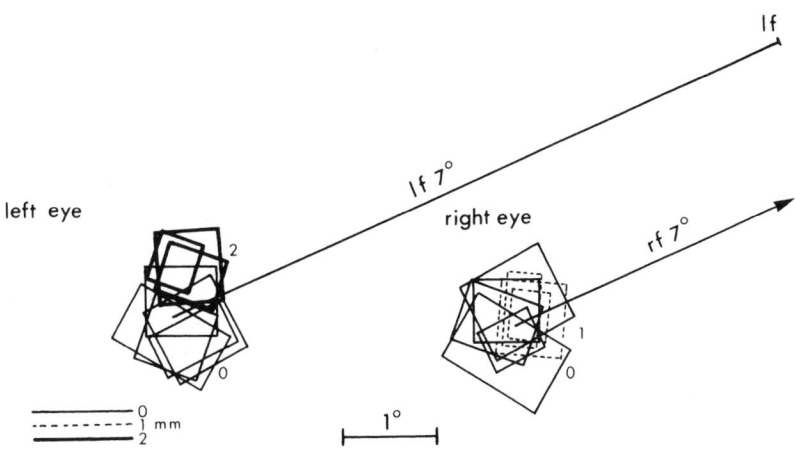

Fig. 3. *Relationship between field size-plus-scatter and magnification, for a 7° eccentricity. Same monkey as in Figures 1 and 2, right hemisphere. Angle between electrode track and surface of cortex, 30°. Scale is the same as in Figure 2. Note the decrease in field size and scatter and in the displacement in position with each 1 mm advance of the electrode.*

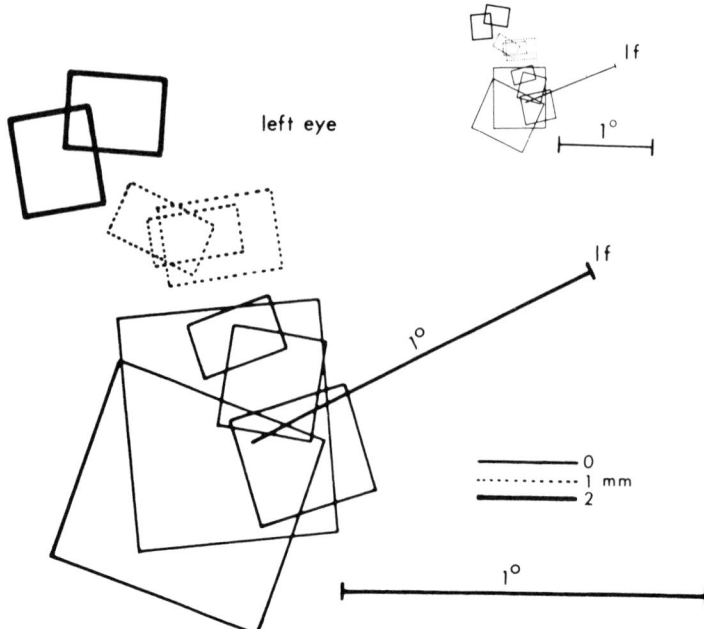

Fig. 4. Relationship between field size-plus-scatter and magnification, for a 1° eccentricity. Here the scale of the figure is about four times that of Figures 2 and 3, but the inset shows the same diagram reduced to match Figures 2 and 3. Different monkey from that of Figures 1–3. Angle of electrode to surface, 5°.

(same monkey as that of the 4° penetration) through the convexity (8.5°) and through two folds of the buried calcarine cortex (18° and 22°). A second penetration was then made parallel and 3 mm lateral to the first. The two tracks are reconstructed in Figure 5. As expected, the three field positions were now slightly displaced. Each time a thickness of cortex was traversed, four-six fields, on the average, were mapped. Thus for each of three field

positions the average field size could be determined, and magnification^{-1} obtained by dividing the field displacements by three.

The results of all seven determinations are shown in Figure 6A, in which we plot magnification^{-1} (open circles) and field size (crosses) against distance from fovea. As a measure of field size we took (length × width)$^{0.5}$. Given the smallness of the samples and the large variation in field size at each

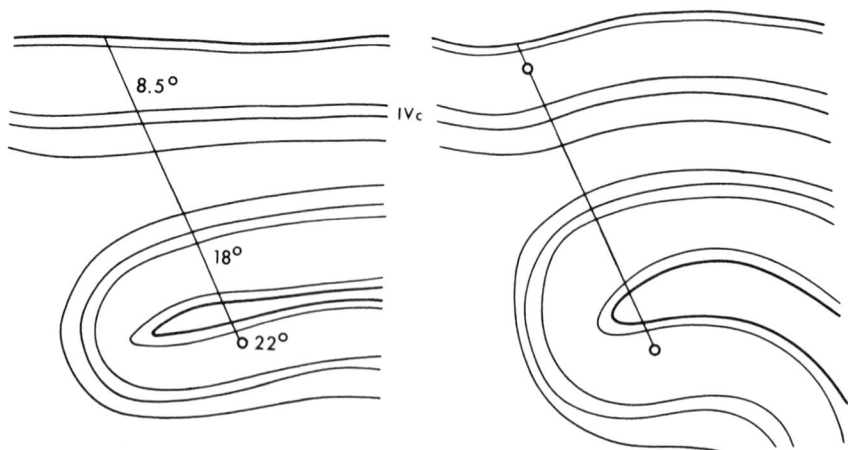

Fig. 5. Reconstruction of two electrode tracks, in two parasagittal planes 3 mm apart. Eccentricity for the surface traverse, 8.5°; for the two folds of the calcarine fissure, 18° and 22°. The results were used in plotting the 8.5°, 18° and 22° points in Figure 6A.

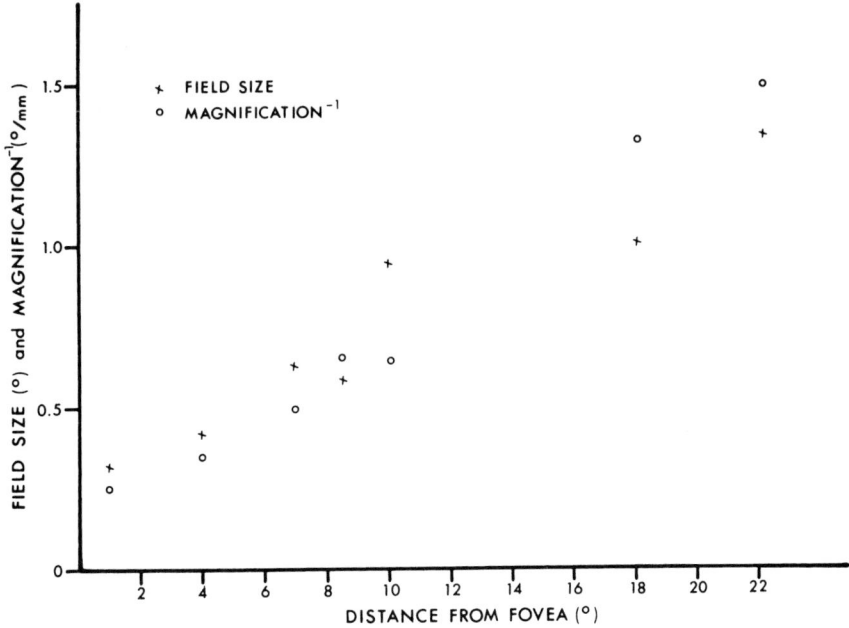

Fig. 6A. Graph of average field size (crosses) and magnification^{-1} (open circles) against eccentricity, for five cortical locations. Points for 4°, 8°, 18° and 22° were from one monkey; for 1°, from a second. Field size was determined by averaging the fields at each eccentricity, estimating size from (length × width)$^{0.5}$.

eccentricity (Figs. 1–4), it is perhaps surprising that the graph of field size vs. eccentricity is not more chaotic than it is. Cells in layer IV C, whose fields are very small, were excluded from the series, but in an exhaustive study of field size one would have to consider cells layer by layer. Despite this difficulty the graph confirms our expectation that field size and magnification^{-1} change with eccentricity in strikingly parallel fashion, at least as far peripheral as 22°.

Figures 2–4 suggest that magnification and receptive-field size are roughly proportional. In Figure 6B this is confirmed by plotting a graph of field size against magnification^{-1}, using information from the graph of Figure 6A.

Figure 7 sums up these results by showing a single cluster of fields from each of the 1°, 7° and 10° penetrations in relation to the fovea (f). For each pair of circles the two members are separated by a distance corresponding to a 1 mm movement along the cortex (i.e., by a distance equal to "magnification^{-1}") so that magnification and field size-plus-scatter can be compared directly. As eccentricity increases so does the distance between circles in each pair (magnification^{-1}), and parallel with this

there is a corresponding increase in the area taken up by each cluster of receptive fields.

DISCUSSION

Central to the concept of the cortical column is the idea of a group of cells with one common physiological characteristic, such as a particular value of some variable. The cells behave as though they shared certain connections among themselves, but not with cells of neighboring columns, and in this sense a single group of cells is looked upon as a more or less autonomous functional unit. If the variable has only two values, as is so for the somato-sensory columns described by Mountcastle ('57) or for the ocular-dominance columns, then on moving horizontally across the cortical surface the values of the variables must obviously simply alternate, from one eye to the other, for example. If the variable can have many values, as in the orientation columns, one can expect either an ordered sequence or a random one. In the preceding paper (Hubel and Wiesel, '74) the chief finding was that the orientation columns are arranged with great regularity, so that a probe moving along the cortex horizontally

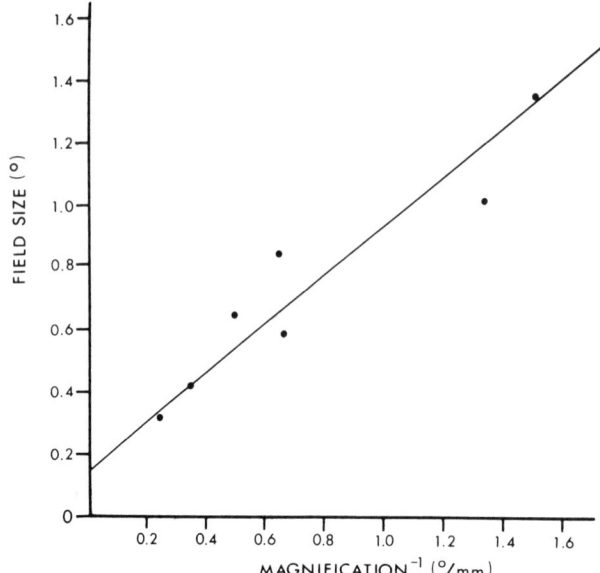

Fig. 6B. Graph of field size vs. magnification^{-1}, using the values from Figure 6A.

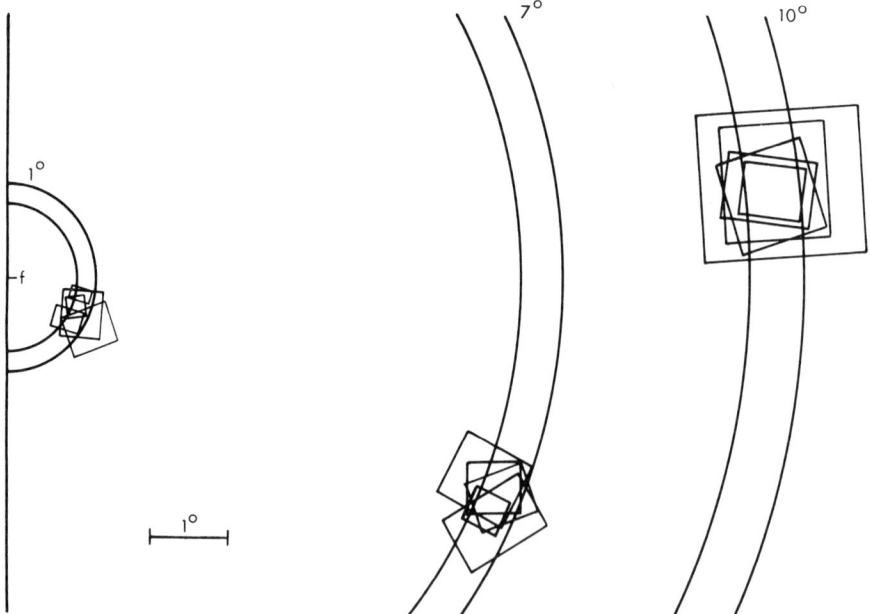

Fig. 7. Relation between field size-plus-scatter and magnification, for three different eccentricities, 1°, 7° and 10°. The diagram shows part of the right field of vision, with vertical meridian and fovea (f) represented on the extreme left. Three clusters of receptive fields are redrawn from Figures 2, 3 and 4; each represents the fields mapped in a 0.1 mm segment of penetration. (For economy of illustration, the 1° and 7° groups of fields, which were actually in the left visual field, have been mirror-reversed.) Each pair of concentric circles is drawn so that the difference in the two radii equals magnification^{-1} for that eccentricity.

may generally be expected to encounter all values of orientation (roughly 18–20) in regular sequence before any one value is repeated.

Given this result, it seems useful to extend the concept of the column, and consider a complete array of columns as a small machine that looks after all values of a given variable. For the orientation system this would be a full set of slabs subserving an entire 180° cycle, while for the ocular dominance system it would be a left-eye column plus a right-eye column. We may refer to such a group as a *hypercolumn.*

We had long been puzzled by the observation that ocular-dominance columns are 0.25–0.5 mm wide, and therefore an order of magnitude larger than the orientation columns. Only on seeing the orderliness of the orientation columns did we realize that there is a close similarity in *total* width between an array of orientation slabs that takes in all 180° of orientation, and a left-plus-right set of ocular-dominance columns. Both of these amount to something like 0.5–1 mm. That the two kinds of hypercolumns are of the same order of magnitude may not be purely coincidence, for the size itself must be of some importance. Suppose, for example, that orientation columns were so large that in going through a large angle, say 90°, the distance along the cortex corresponded to a considerable movement in the visual field. The result would be bizarre indeed: the animal would be sensitive to horizontal lines in one part of its visual field, to various obliques in others, and to verticals in still others. A similar problem would arise with respect to eye preference—the visual fields would be carved up into a mosaic of left-eye and right-eye areas, with each eye seeing only its own subdivisions. But it has been clear since our '62 paper that the precision of cortical representation holds only down to a certain size of cortical surface, and only down to a certain area of visual field. Cells in a given cortical region have finite sized receptive fields and a finite (and proportional) random variation in position; a certain constant distance along the cortex, amounting to 2–3 mm, must be traversed in order to obtain a shift in field position comparable to the size of the fields plus their scatter. Within such a distance one can have many subregions subserving different orientations of receptive fields, or subregions dominated first by one eye and then by the other, without getting into difficulties related to topography.

It is remarkable that this distance is about the same as the size of the hypercolumns—it would be more accurate to say that it is about double or triple, since roughly a 2–3 mm displacement is required to get out of one region of visual field and into an entirely new one, as compared with 0.5–1 mm for the widths of the hypercolumns. In a sense, then, a 2–3 mm region of cortex can be said to contain by a comfortable margin the machinery it needs to analyze the region of visual field that it subserves. It is probably significant that 2–3 mm is also roughly the horizontal distance over which cortical cells are interconnected (Fisken et al., '73).

The relationship seems to hold throughout the visual cortex, for everywhere the columns, and hence the hypercolumns, are probably about the same size and, at least over the region explored, the span of cortex corresponding to the local receptive-field size plus scatter seems to be constant. The receptive-field size plus associated scatter varies tremendously over the cortex, but so does the visual-field area corresponding to 1 mm of cortex. The degree to which these are matched is striking and surely no accident.

Thus the machinery may be roughly uniform over the whole striate cortex, the differences being in the inputs. A given region of cortex simply digests what is brought to it, and the process is the same everywhere. Certainly this general idea is not refuted by any striking histological non-uniformity over the visual cortex, from fovea to far periphery. If it is assumed that the number of optic-radiation fibers entering a square millimeter of cortex is roughly constant (Clark, '41) then differences from one region to the next must simply be related to the size of the geniculate receptive fields and their scatter.

Another example of this stereotyped processing of input can be seen on comparing striate cortex of normal and Siamese cats (Hubel and Wiesel, '71). The 17–18 border region in the ordinary cat subserves the visual-field midline, whereas in one type of Siamese cat the seemingly identical area, morphologically, serves a region 20° in the ipsilateral periphery, where the fields and scatter are much larger. Apparently this segment of cortex can carry out the same operation on the two widely differing sets of inputs. The capability is evidently an intrinsic property of the cortex, depending on genetically determined connections and not on postnatal experience, since the topography is the same in Siamese kittens whose eyes have been closed since birth.

This is not to deny the possibility of certain non-uniformities over the cortex—indeed regional differences are to be expected, given the relative preoccupation of the central visual fields with form and color, of the periphery with scotopic vision and movement, and the absence, in the far periphery, of binocular interaction. It would be surprising if careful studies even of such crude indices as cortical thickness failed to reveal differences between foveal and peripheral representations. The point here is that if differences in histology exist they are not so glaring as to be obvious at a glance and are certainly minor when one considers the 30–40 fold variation in magnification factor.

The tasks that a given region of cortex must fulfill are many and varied and include the machinery for establishing orientation specificity, directional selectivity, degree of complexity, selectivity to color, and binocular convergence, all for a particular region of visual field. It may be that there is a great developmental advantage in designing such a machinery once only, and repeating it over and over monotonously, like a crystal, for all parts of the visual field. The problem is to achieve the uniformity despite the great difference in detail of representation between central and peripheral visual fields.

How successfully the problem has been solved can be appreciated by comparing the relative uniformity of the cortex with the striking non-uniformity of the retina. The ganglion-cell layer of the monkey retina, for example, is some five cells deep near the fovea, whereas in the far periphery there are not enough cell bodies to make up one continuous layer (Van Buren, '63). For simple reasons of optics, the retina cannot adopt the strategy that the cortex employs; if the retinal surface must be spherical, the magnification factor has to be the same throughout, despite the difference in precision of representation between central and peripheral visual fields. Hence its histological non-uniformity. The cortex has no such arbitrary restrictions on surface shape. If the retina is mapped onto the cortex in such a way that magnification is at every point independent of direction and falls off with eccentricity, the resultant surface must be far from spherical. (If magnification is constant, the spheri-

cal retina obviously maps onto a sphere. If magnification falls off with eccentricity, one may imagine building up the cortical surface by beginning at the foveal projection and adding on successive circular rings having the foveal projection as a common center. The circumference of each ring is the product of the circumference of the corresponding retinal ring and the magnification, so that a variation in magnification will produce distortion of the sphere.) In 1962 Daniel and Whitteridge modelled the striate cortex in rubber and smoothed out the folds so as to examine the overall shape. As expected, the surface was far from spherical and was roughly what was predicted from a knowledge of the magnification factor at every eccentricity. The distortion in the shape of the cortical surface can be regarded as a consequence of the need to keep the histology uniform.

Despite this marked difference between retina and cortex in histological uniformity, similar principles probably prevail in the two structures. In the cortex, magnification changes with eccentricity, while cell density remains roughly constant: in the retina, magnification is constant but ganglion cell density (cells/unit area) varies. If the field size of cortical cells is matched to the magnification, we may reasonably ask if field sizes of retinal ganglion cells are matched to cell density. Just such an enquiry has been made in the cat retina by Fischer ('73), who measured field-center sizes at different eccentricities and correlated the results with ganglion cell densities as estimated by Stone ('65). With increasing eccentricity receptive-field center areas increase (Wiesel, '60), but ganglion-cell density declines, and Fischer found that the two vary inversely, the average number of ganglion cells in a receptive field center having a roughly constant value of about 35 throughout the retina. The two sets of results, in retina and cortex, are probably equivalent, for in the cortex the counterpart of the retinal receptive field under which Fischer estimates cell numbers is the cortical projection of the boundaries of an average cortical receptive field. The present study shows that the cortical area so enclosed is constant (in fact, it is the square of the slope of the graph of fig. 6B, i.e., 0.66 mm^2). If cell density in the cortex is roughly uniform the number of cells under this area will obviously be constant. It would be of great interest to make an analysis similar to Fischer's in the monkey retina and in the geniculate, for comparison with the present results in the cortex.

ACKNOWLEDGMENTS

We wish to thank Sandra Spinks, David Freeman and Claire Wang for technical assistance. The work was supported by NIH Grants 5ROI EYO 0605 and 5ROI EYO 0606, and a grant from the Esther A. and Joseph Klingenstein Fund, Inc.

Literature Cited

Clark, W. E. LeGros 1941 The laminar organization and cell content of the lateral geniculate body in the monkey. J. Anat., Lond., *75:* 419–433.

Daniel, P. M., and D. Whitteridge 1961 The representation of the visual field on the cerebral cortex in monkeys. J. Physiol., *159:* 203–221.

Fischer, B. 1973 Overlap of receptive field centers and representation of the visual field in the cat's optic tract. Vision Res., *13:* 2113–2120.

Fisken, R. A., L. J. Garey and T. P. S. Powell 1973 Patterns of degeneration after intrinsic lesions of the visual cortex (area 17) of the monkey. Brain Res., *53:* 208–213.

Hubel, D. H., and T. N. Wiesel 1962 Receptive fields, binocular interaction and functional architecture in the cat's visual cortex. J. Physiol., *160:* 106–154.

———— 1968 Receptive fields and functional architecture of monkey striate cortex. J. Physiol., *195:* 215–243.

———— 1970 Cells sensitive to binocular depth in area 18 of the macaque monkey cortex. Nature, *225:* 41–42.

———— 1971 Aberrant visual projections in the Siamese cat. J. Physiol., *218:* 33–62.

———— 1972 Laminar and columnar distribution of geniculo-cortical fibers in the macaque monkey. J. Comp. Neur., *146:* 421–450.

———— 1974 Sequence regularity and geometry of orientation columns in the monkey striate cortex. J. Comp. Neur., *158:* 267–294.

Mountcastle, V. B. 1957 Modality and topographic properties of single neurons of cat's somatic sensory cortex. J. Neurophysiol., *20:* 408–434.

Stone, J. 1965 A quantitative analysis of the distribution of ganglion cells in the cat's retina. J. Comp. Neur., *124:* 337–352.

Talbot, S. A., and W. H. Marshall 1941 Physiological studies on neural mechanisms of visual localization and discrimination. Am. J. Ophthal., *24:* 1255–1263.

Van Buren, J. M. 1963 The Retinal Ganglion Cell Layer. Charles C Thomas, Springfield, Ill.

Wiesel, T. N. 1960 Receptive fields of ganglion cells in the cat's retina. J. Physiol., *153:* 583–594.

AFTERWORD

To the Uniformity paper there has not been much reaction. It would seem to have impressed the world less than it did us. I find the students I teach have trouble absorbing its messages. And ultimately, what one finds attractive in scientific ideas is a matter of taste. I would not trade it for any of our other papers, except perhaps the 1962 cortical paper.

PART IV

DEPRIVATION AND DEVELOPMENT

Chapter 21 • The First Three Kitten Deprivation Papers •

FOREWORD

These three papers represent a major stream of studies that were done in parallel with the work in normal adult cats and monkeys. We made our first recording from a normal newborn kitten on June 22, 1961, about three years after the time we began our work in adult cats. By then we felt we had become familiar enough with the normal physiology of the adult visual cortex that we could begin to ask some questions about the development of the visual system, and about the effects of early visual deprivation.

Our motives for studying kittens were clearly tied to our clinical backgrounds. We wanted to know whether the response properties of the cells we had been studying in adults were innate or were developed in early life by some process analogous to learning. We wanted to learn whether we could alter the responses by modifying the animals' early experience, a question that had been raised and discussed by philosophers since the time of Descartes. Our experiments were undoubtedly influenced by the observations, described in detail by von Senden (*Space and Sight,* The Free Press, Glencoe, 1960), that children with congenital cataracts have substantial and often permanent visual deficits after removal of the cataracts. In animals, behavioral studies by Riesen had shown that dark rearing, or being raised in an environment devoid of contours, can similarly lead to severe visual impairments. It seemed important to establish whether these impairments were occurring in the eye or further downstream. Behavioral tests of vision are just one means of assessing the system, and we felt that our knowledge of cortical physiology might supply another useful index.

So we decided to sew closed the lids of one eye of a newborn kitten, wait for a few months, and then do a recording to see if anything interesting had happened. Parallel with that approach, we recorded from a series of normal kittens at various ages to see how the system developed. It turned out that after monocular deprivation the cortex was far from normal, and at that point it was natural to ask whether the abnormalities were a matter of a failure of the connections to develop postnatally, presumably the result of lack of experience, or were the results of a disuse-related deterioration of connections that were already present at birth. Whether we originally formulated these questions as clearly as this is hard to remember after so many years. We closed eyes to see what would happen, and if the cortical physiology of the deprived cats had been normal we would probably have dropped the project.

Our first recordings in young kittens were not without difficulties. The newborn animals simply died when we anesthetized them with a scaled-down dose of our usual anesthetic, thiopental (commonly known as pentothal). We soon found, to our surprise, that the local anesthetic we were using to suture the eyelids was, for kittens, not just an analgesic but also an excellent general anesthetic, and we did not need the thiopental at all. Immobilizing the head with its soft skull was impossible with our usual Horsley-Clarke stereotaxic head holder, so we cemented a cylindrical chamber to the skull and clamped the lid of the chamber to the head holder.

Our very first recording from a kitten began badly, with nothing but electrical artifacts during the first penetration. For penetration 2, our unedited typewritten records read:

> Even before contact with a new electrode the same damn crap. First unit rather close or 1 mm below the red line.[1] Syringe zeroed here. Unit 2: After an untold amount of buggaring around we get rid of the cathode follower[2] altogether, and thereby most of the artefact. At 0.488 we find a unit, contralaterally driven, i.e., by right eye this time, by a 10:00–4:00 slit moving downwards especially, slow movement, complex, T. thinks jibbery.[3] From ipsilateral eye we get nil.[4] [The experiment finally closes with the note]: We seem to have normal both simple and complex fields in a 3½ month old kitten and that really all we wanted to know. Since it soon midnight we quit. No lesion and no perfusion. N. B.: A. C. [area centralis, corresponding to primate fovea] not mapped out carefully in this experiment.

The coarseness, even obscenity of this description is useful in reminding us just how trying some of these experiments could be. Even with the patience of a couple of oysters we could end up yearning for the day to end, regardless of whether or not it was successful.

By September of 1961 we had obtained a rough idea of the physiology of normal kittens at the time of eye opening. Some cells showed virtually normal orientation selectivity and could be influenced from both eyes. In other cells, sluggish responses and poor orientation selectivity were hard to interpret, given the relative opacity of the media and, sometimes, the poor physical shape of the kittens, but there was no avoiding the conclusion that at least some cells had acquired their connections by mechanisms that must be innate.

---

[1] A line made with grease pencil on the plexiglas advancer to mark the piston's expected position at contact.

[2] Our input amplification stage, connected to the electrode.

[3] The term we used to describe a firing pattern in rapidly occurring high frequency bursts.

[4] There followed a succession of three cells, each well oriented, two of them clearly driven from both eyes.

Around the time of our first recordings from newborn kittens, we began our series of unilateral eye closures. These studies, too, had their difficulties, the main one being a tendency for a sutured eyelid to reopen after a few days to a week. A reclosure was then necessary, but a day or so of visual experience made the interpretation messy. We got better at the surgery, but for a time we had to contend with a mixture of clean experiments and a few that were contaminated by the intermittent periods of both eyes being open.

We wanted to have a rough idea of the deprived kittens' visual capabilities, so just before some of the recording sessions we opened the closed eye and fitted the normal eye with an opaque contact lens. No elaborate testing of vision was necessary. When we put the animal on a table it groped its way to the edge and tumbled onto a cushion we had placed on the floor. That is something that no self-respecting kitten would ever do. We took it as prima facie evidence that the animal was for all intents and purposes blind in the deprived eye.

When we looked at the histological sections from the monocularly deprived kittens, we were amazed at the pallor of cells in the geniculate layers supplied by the eye that had been closed. In a three-month closure the thinness and paleness of these layers was obvious even without the aid of a microscope. The phenomenon of *transneuronal degeneration*—shrinkage and pallor following transsection of the optic nerve—was of course well known, but it was not known that simple disuse would cause abnormalities that were almost as severe. On the other hand the visual cortex, when stained for Nissl substance, appeared normal. As more sophisticated anatomical methods became available to us, and as we got more familiar with the normal columnar architecture in normal adults, we applied the new methods to our deprivation-development studies and found that the cortical anatomy was anything but normal. So what started as a minor sideline gradually blossomed into a major effort—so much so that when in 1981 we shared the Nobel Prize we were cited for two pieces of work: the mainline physiology, and the deprivation-development work.

Only recently did it occur to us that we did deprivation studies for several years before applying for funds to support them. Cats and monkeys were cheap enough, and the prospect of writing another grant request repellent enough (even in those easy days) that we simply let the work we were doing in normal animals support the deprivation studies. Perhaps we were reluctant to publicize the deprivation work before our first papers came out. We knew (or soon learned) how easy it would be for competitors to charge in and begin closing eyes of monkeys, which was the next item on our list of things to do.

We submitted the first three deprivation papers in June 1963, and they came out that year. These were our first major papers that were not published in the British *Journal of Physiology*. We had no quarrel with that journal: the editors were wonderful to work with, and we were delighted with their handling of the illustrations. We only made the shift when it became clear that their policy of strict alphabetical order of authors was having an adverse effect on the one of us not blessed with a last name beginning with a letter close to A. Alphabetical order had the advantage of relieving authors of worries over priority, but one could not realistically expect deans to understand the ways of the British. The problem must have reached its ludicrous peak in the case of Edwin Furshpan and Taro Furukawa, who had to turn to the *Journal of Neurophysiology* to publish their Mauthner-cell work if Taro was to have any chance of being promoted on his return to Japan.

The order of these first three deprivation papers, while logical, had little to do with the order in which we did the work. We began with recordings from very young normal kittens and from of monocularly sutured kittens, more or less alternating the two. Only when it became clear that we had palpable deprivation effects in the cortex did we go back and look at geniculate responses. Of course the anatomical abnormalities we found in the geniculates made it doubly imperative to look at the geniculate physiology. But had we been real scientists we would probably have started by recording from the retina and then have continued inexorably downstream, to the geniculate and finally, if we lived long enough, the cortex, all in newborns, and only then have started sewing eyelids. Such an approach still seems to us to be soulless. As it is, the order in which we placed these first deprivation papers seems artificial, tending to promote false ideas about how the science was actually done.

Effects of Visual Deprivation on Morphology and Physiology of Cells in the Cat's Lateral Geniculate Body[1]

TORSTEN N. WIESEL AND DAVID H. HUBEL • *Neurophysiology Laboratory, Department of Pharmacology,*

Harvard Medical School, Boston, Massachusetts

INTRODUCTION

The importance of normal sensory stimulation in the development and maintenance of the nervous system is now generally recognized. In the visual system this problem has usually been approached by examining the effects of sensory deprivation on structure and behavior (see reviews by Hebb (12) and Riesen (28)). An obvious way of extending this work would be to examine electrophysiologically the functional effects of visual deprivation, but such experiments require some knowledge of normal function. During the last 10 years single-cell responses have been examined and receptive-field arrangements compared at several levels in the cat's visual pathway: in the retina (21), the lateral geniculate body (18), and the visual cortex (17, 19).

From *J. Neurophysiol.* 1963, *26*, 978–993.

Received for publication June 26, 1963.

[1]This work was supported in part by Research Grants GM-K3-15,304 (C2), B-2260 (C2), and B-2253-C2S1 from the Public Health Service, and in part by Research Grant AF-AFOSR-410-62 from the U.S. Air Force.

This information provides the necessary background for a study of the immature and the stimulus-deprived visual system.

The results of a physiological and anatomical study of the visual pathways in normal and visually deprived kittens will be presented in a series of three papers. In the present paper we describe single-unit recordings in the optic tract and lateral geniculate body of kittens in which one eye had been deprived of vision, and an anatomical examination of the visual pathways in these animals. The second paper (20) will describe single-unit recordings in the striate cortex of newborn kittens. The final paper (32) will deal with responses of cells in the visual cortex of visually deprived animals.

METHODS

Nine kittens and one adult cat were used in studying the morphological effects of 1–4 months of monocular visual deprivation. In two of the kittens recordings were made from the lateral geniculate body and the optic tract. In addition, three kittens were used in a study of the development of lateral geniculate cells. Table 1 summarizes the procedures carried out in the experimental animals.

Deprivation procedures. The most common method of deprivation was to suture together the lids of the right eye. Under local or general anesthesia the lid margins were trimmed and then sutured end to end. The reduction in intensity of a light beam passing through the eyelid, measured with a photoelectric cell, was found to vary between 4 and 5 log units, depending on fur color. The lid-sutured eyes were thus completely deprived of form stimulation, and also, to a large extent, of stimulation by diffuse light.

In two kittens a translucent plastic contact lens was placed over the right eye. This type of cover allowed more light to enter the eye but still excluded pattern stimulation. The technique was not wholly satisfactory because of a tendency to recurrent conjunctivitis. In a third kitten, to overcome this difficulty, the nictitating membrane was brought across the cornea of the right eye, and the edge of the membrane was trimmed and sutured to the abraded conjunctiva of the upper lid. These two types of covering were found by direct measurement to reduce retinal illumination by only about 1–2 log units.

Physiological methods. Single-unit recordings were made from the optic tract and lateral geniculate bodies in two kittens. Both animals were 3 months old and had had the right eyelid sutured before the time of normal eye-opening. The recordings were done under general anesthesia. Procedures for preparing the animals and details of methods for stimulating and recording have been described elsewhere (15, 18, 19). In both kittens, after separating the previously closed lids, we observed that the cornea was moist and clear; the fundus, including the optic disc, appeared normal, and the direct and consensual light reflexes were normally active.

Single units were recorded in the lateral geniculate body with tungsten microelectrodes (14), and electrode positions were marked by electrolytic lesions (15). Receptive fields were mapped by projecting small spots of white light on a wide screen which the animal faced from a distance of 1.5 m. The screen was lit diffusely by a moderately bright background light (–1 to +1 $\log_{10}$cd/m^2). Intensities of stimulus and background lights were adjusted so that the difference between the two did not exceed 2 log units.

Anatomical methods. After the acute experiments all animals were perfused with normal saline followed by 10% formalin. The eyes were also perfused separately with formalin according to a method described by Polyak (25). Brains and eyes were embedded in celloidin: the brains were serially sectioned at 26 μ and the sections stained with cresyl violet; the retina was sectioned at 10 μ and the sections stained alternately with hematoxylin and eosin and with cresyl violet.

Table 1. Experimental Animals

Procedure, Right Eye	No. of Animals	Age at Onset of Deprivation, weeks	Duration of Deprivation, weeks	Age at Time of Experiment, weeks
Lid closure	4	Just before normal eye opening	9–13	10–14
Lid closure	1	9	16	25
Lid closure	1	9	4	13
Lid closure	1	Adult	12	Adult
Plastic translucent occluder	2	Just before normal eye-opening	8–10	9–11
Occlusion with nictitating membrane	1	5	12	17

A quantitative method for measuring areas of the entire cell, the nucleus, and the nucleolus was adapted from the method of Matthews, Cowan, and Powell (23). Cell outlines were traced on 1-mm. graph paper after a linear magnification of 1,000. The number of square millimeters within a particular outline gave a direct measure of the projected area in square microns. Only cells showing a distinct nucleus and nucleolus were traced. Measurements in the two dorsal layers (A and A_1) did not give rise to any difficulties since these layers are clearly defined, relatively thick, and rich in cells. On the other hand, the ventral layer (B) was comparatively thin in coronal section. Here special care was taken to avoid the large intralaminar cells since they are considered by some to have binocular input (10). In the two dorsal layers cell density was estimated by counting the number of cells within a given area, using a Whipple net micrometer disc.

RESULTS

Single-Unit Recordings

Single units were studied in the lateral geniculate bodies of two kittens monocularly deprived of light and form by lid suture. The kittens were 3 months old and had had the right eyelids sutured together just before the time of normal eye-opening. Records were made from the left lateral geniculate body, and detailed receptive fields were mapped for 34 geniculate cells. Twenty of the cells were recorded in layers receiving input from the deprived eye, 19 in the dorsal layer (A) and one in the ventral layer (B); the remaining 14 were recorded in the middle layer (A_1), whose input was from the normal eye.

All cells, whether they received their input from the normal or from the deprived eye, had the usual concentric receptive-field arrangement consisting of an excitatory or inhibitory center and a peripheral region of the opposite type (18). With a few exceptions, which will be described below, the cells had field centers of normal size. They responded well to stimuli restricted to the field centers, and if the antagonistic periphery was included in the area stimulated by using large spots or diffuse light, there was a marked decrease in the response. From this it is clear that cells can have normal receptive-field arrangements in immature (3-month-old) kittens, and that patterned-light stimulation is not required for the development of the necessary connections.

Records were also made from seven optic-tract fibers, which were recognized by their firing pattern, response characteristics, and spike shape (16). Two of the fibers were activated from the normal eye and five from the stimulus-deprived eye. All fibers had normal concentric receptive-field arrangements, with "on" centers and "off" peripheries, or the reverse (21). The field centers were well defined and of normal size, and the units responded strongly when the centers alone were stimulated. The normality of the receptive fields of at least some retinal ganglion cells in these kittens is hardly surprising since, as already described, lateral geniculate cells with normal fields were found in the same animals.

In previous studies (18) we showed that geniculate cells were very similar to retinal ganglion cells in their receptive-field arrangements, the main difference being an increase in the peripheral suppression at the geniculate level. This difference was demonstrated directly in simultaneous recordings from a geniculate cell and its main excitatory afferent: the probability that the excitatory afferent would trigger the geniculate cell varied in such a way as to render diffuse light less effective at the geniculate level. In the present study simultaneous recordings were made of a geniculate cell and its main excitatory afferent on three occasions; in two of these the driving was from the normal eye and in the third it was from the deprived eye. In all three cases there was a clear increase in the peripheral suppression for the geniculate cells, indicating that the lateral geniculate body in a 3-month-old kitten, like that of the adult cat, is not merely a relay station, but modifies the input in an important way. Moreover, geniculate cells possess this power of modification even in animals that have not previously been exposed to patterned light.

Although the majority of the geniculate cells receiving input from the previously closed eye appeared normal, there were a few exceptions. Four cells, all in the dorsal (A) layer, were strikingly sluggish in their responses to light stimulation. These had field centers four to six times the diameter of neighboring cells—indeed, the centers were larger than any we have seen in the lateral geniculate body of the normal adult cat—and they showed less than normal peripheral suppression. Furthermore, in the two kittens in which recordings were made from the geniculate, the over-all activity seemed to be less in the visually deprived layers than in the normal ones; fewer units could be isolated, and the unresolved background activity was unusually sparse. Despite these signs of abnormal function, it was our general impression from these recordings that the geniculate physiology was relatively normal, a somewhat surprising finding in view of the striking anatomical changes to be described below.

Morphological Changes in the Lateral Geniculate Body Induced by Light and Form Deprivation

KITTENS MONOCULARLY DEPRIVED FROM BIRTH BY LID CLOSURE. In the two kittens described above and in two others also deprived for about 3 months the lateral geniculate bodies showed striking histological changes. In all four animals there was a profound atrophy in the geniculate layers receiving input from the covered eye. This is illustrated for one kitten in Fig. 1: coronal sections of the left lateral geniculate body, contralateral to the closed eye, show atrophy in the dorsal (A) and ventral (B) layers (Fig. 1A); in the right lateral geniculate body there is atrophy in the middle (A_1) layer (Fig. 1B). These changes were observed throughout the entire extent of the lateral geniculate bodies.

The abnormal layers stood out by virtue of several morphological changes (Figs. 1–3). Throughout their entire extent these layers were thinner than normal and appeared somewhat collapsed. The collapse was in part produced by a general reduction in cell size; a lack of Nissl substance gave most cells a pale, often ghost-like appearance, though a few normally stained, healthy-looking cells were interspersed among the mass of atrophic cells. Also contributing to the thinness of these layers was a reduction in the volume of the apparently homogeneous space between cell bodies, as a result of which the cells seemed to be more thickly packed. There was no obvious glial infiltration.

Cross-sectional areas of lateral-geniculate cell bodies, nuclei, and nucleoli were estimated for 50 cells in each layer. As shown in Table 2, cell bodies and nuclei were much smaller for layers receiving their input from the closed eye. Comparison of corresponding layers on the two sides showed a reduction of about 40% in mean cell area for the left dorsal (A) layer, and a similar reduction for the right middle (A_1) layer. The reduction in the left ventral

(B) layer was about 25%. These differences are highly significant ($P < 0.001$). Comparable shrinkages were found for the nuclei and nuceoli.

The distribution of cell areas in the different layers is shown in the histograms of Fig. 4. In the normal layers the variation in cell size was relatively large, ranging from about 180 to 600 μ. In contrast, in the layers receiving input from the light-deprived eye, cell areas ranged from 150 to 300 μ, reflecting a marked reduction in the number of large cells. In all three abnormal layers the proportion of cells with small areas was greatly increased. Values given here for upper limit and average cell areas in normal layers varied to some extent from one cat to the next, probably because of differences in details of fixation and histological processing. These variations emphasize the advantage of using monocular deprivation, since here the normal layers furnish the control in each animal. That cells in the "normal" layers were not hypertrophied was checked by measuring cell areas in a 3-month-old kitten raised with both eyes open.

The determination of cell areas, while useful in comparing the degree of atrophy produced by different schedules or types of deprivation (see below), did not seem to us as sensitive an index of abnormality as ordinary microscopic examination of the Nissl-stained sections. Histological changes in layers whose mean area was decreased by only 10% were obvious at a glance. This was probably because the measurements were based on only one criterion, the area, whereas in examining the slides one can to some extent unconsciously compare many features such as cell area, staining properties, cell density, and layer thickness, both in adjacent layers and in corresponding layers on the two sides.

Several other parts of the visual system were examined for anatomical changes. The normal and light-deprived retinas showed no gross morphological differences: there were no obvious differences in the thickness of the entire retinas or of the various layers, and the size and staining properties of retinal ganglion cells appeared normal. The two optic nerves, stained with osmium, appeared identical, as did the two superior colliculi and the striate cortex on the two sides. While more specialized histological methods might have shown abnormalities at various levels in the visual system, the most obvious changes undoubtedly occurred at the level of the lateral geniculate body.

Left LGB

A

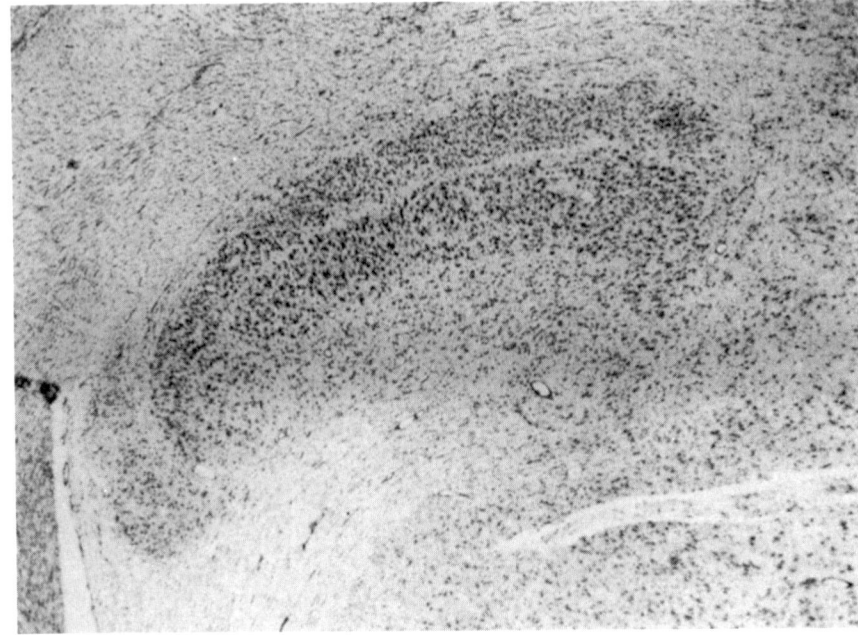

Right LGB

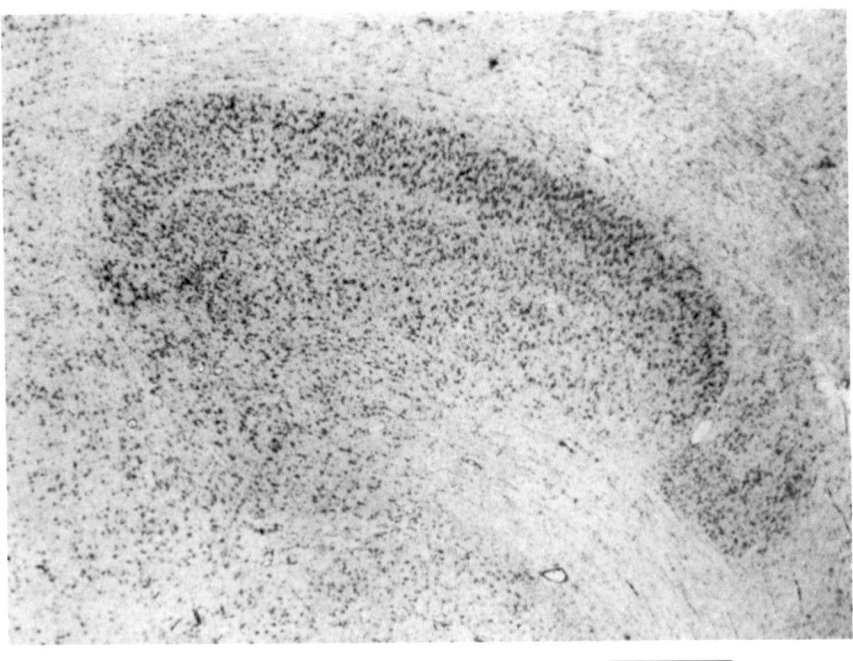

————— 1 mm

Fig. 1. Coronal sections through the lateral geniculate bodies of a kitten, aged 3½ months, whose right eye was closed by lid suture just before the time of normal eye-opening. Celloidin, cresyl violet. A: left lateral geniculate body (contralateral to the covered eye); B: right lateral geniculate body (ipsilateral to the covered eye).

Left   Right

A

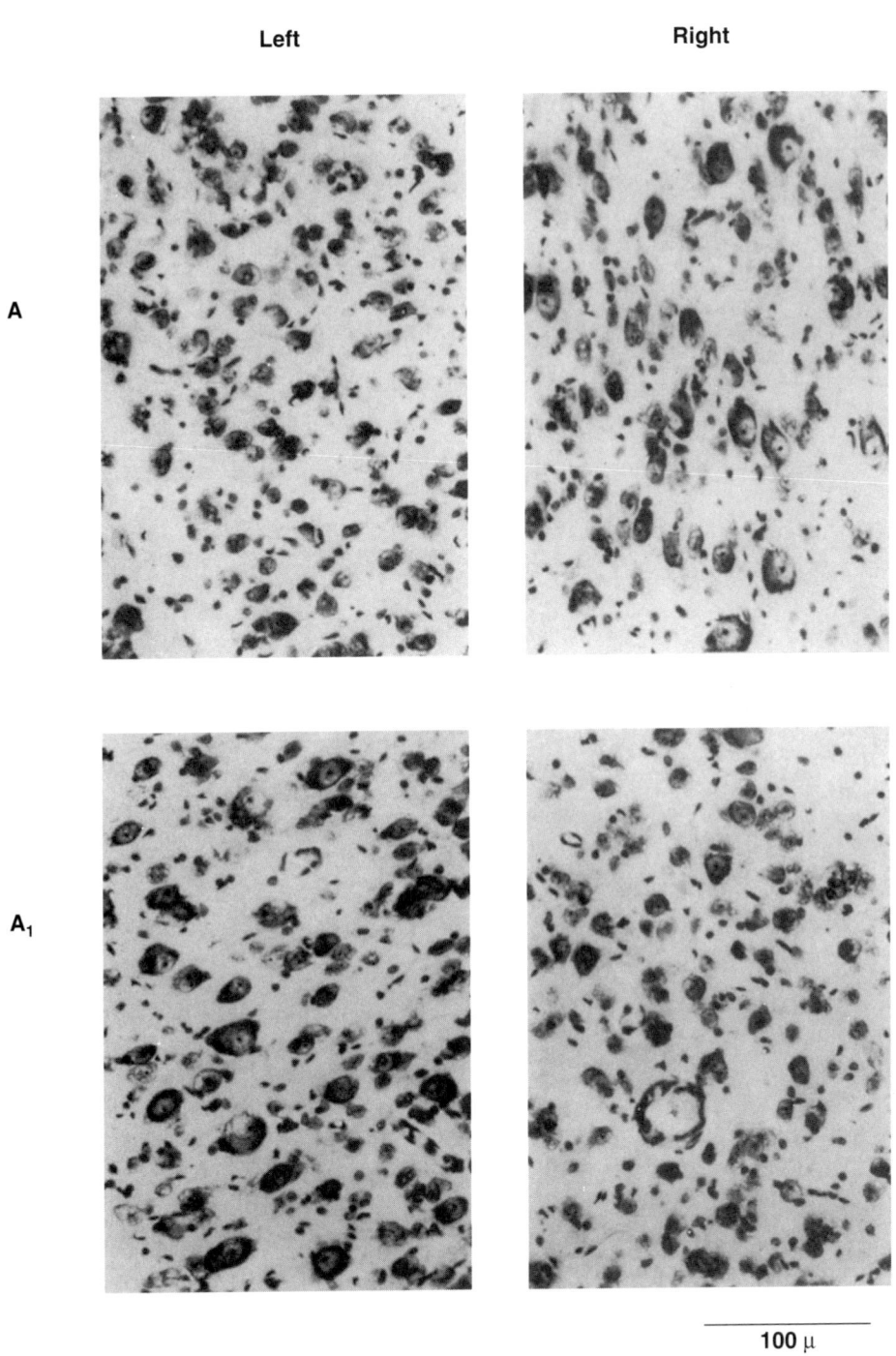

A₁

100 μ

Fig. 2. High-power photographs of dorsal and middle layers. Same sections as in Fig. 1.

Left　　　　　　　　　Right

A

A₁

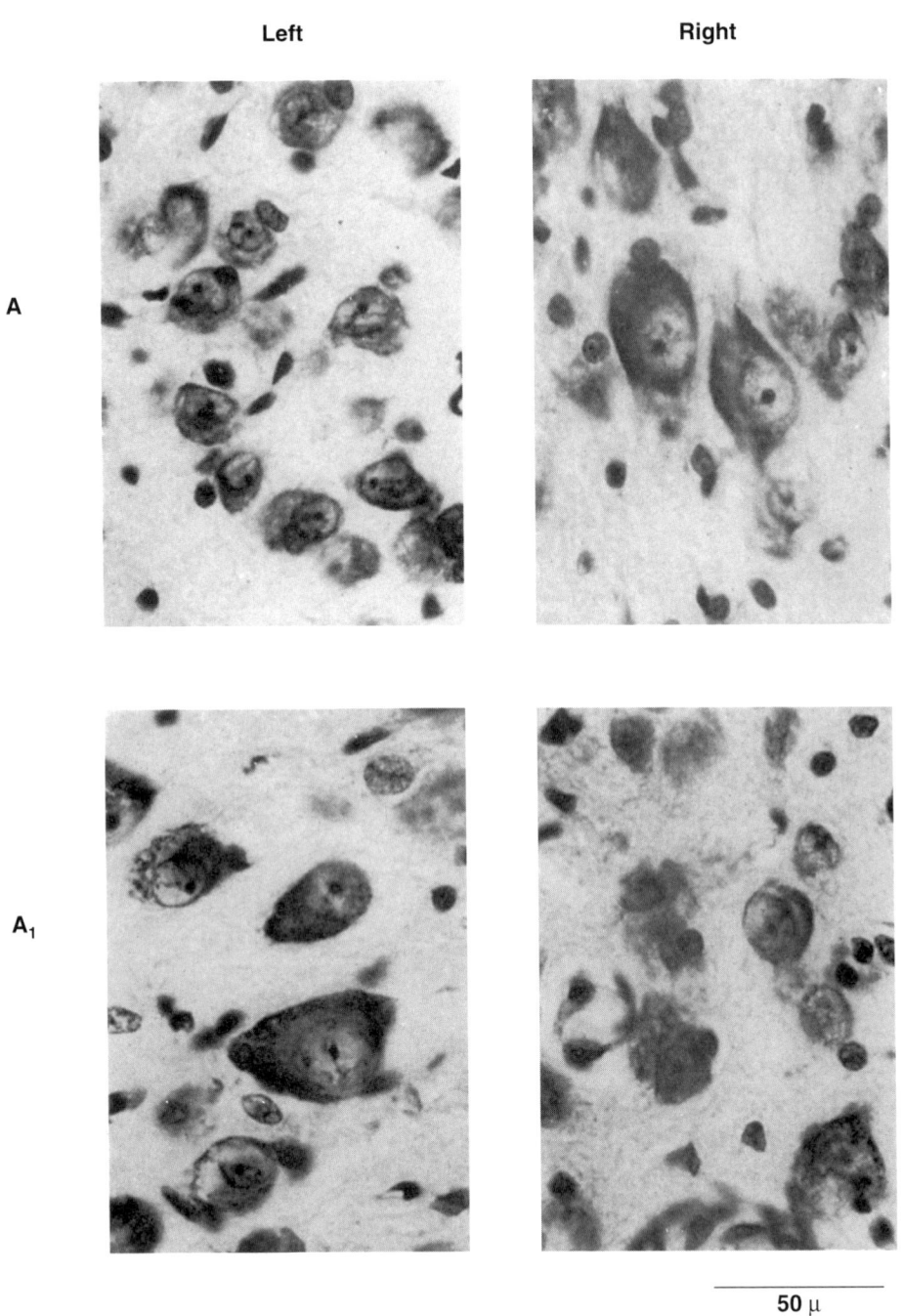

50 µ

Fig. 3. Same sections as in Figs. 1 and 2, but still higher magnification.

Table 2. Mean Areas ±SE of Mean) and Per Cent Shrinkage in Deprived Layers Relative to Corresponding Normal Layers

Layer	AREA OF CELLS			AREA OF NUCLEI		
	Left, μ^2	Right, μ^2	Shrinkage, %	Left, μ^2	Right, μ^2	Shrinkage, %
A	198 ± 7	365 ± 20	46*	88 ± 4	135 ± 7	35
A_1	340 ± 15	201 ± 6	41	136 ± 6	85 ± 4	38
B	236 ± 7	303 ± 14	22	106 ± 3	142 ± 5	25

All t values exceed 4.0 ($P < 0.001$).

*Sample calculation: $\dfrac{\text{difference of means}}{\text{mean of normal}} \times 100 = \dfrac{365 - 198}{365} \times 100 = 46\%$.

MONOCULAR LIGHT DEPRIVATION IN ANIMALS WITH PREVIOUS VISUAL EXPERIENCE. Monocular lid closure was performed in two kittens aged 2 months. In one of the kittens, deprived for 4 months, the lateral geniculate layers receiving input from the closed eye showed strong atrophic changes which were, however, less severe than those found in kittens deprived from birth. The other kitten had the right eye closed for only 1 month. In this animal the appropriate layers showed even less atrophy, although the changes were still very clear both on microscopic inspection and on measuring cell areas. Thus deprivation by lid closure caused atrophic geniculate changes in spite of the previous visual experience; furthermore, the changes could be observed after only 1 month of lid closure.

Finally, it seemed important to ask whether similar changes would occur in mature cats after similar periods of monocular light and form deprivation. Accordingly, the right eye was closed for 3 months in an adult cat. In this animal there was no difference between corresponding geniculate layers on the two sides: layers that received input from the closed eye were of normal thickness and contained cells normal in size and staining properties. Apparently there is an important difference between a growing kitten and an adult cat in susceptibility to these atrophic changes.

VISUAL DEPRIVATION WITH TRANSLUCENT COVERS. In the experiments described so far the kittens were visually deprived of form and also, to a large extent, of light. To assess the relative importance of form and light deprivation some experiments were done using translucent eye covers. In two kittens the cornea of the right eye was covered with a contact occluder made of translucent plastic. This was kept in place from the time of normal eye opening to an age of 2 months in one kitten, and 2½ months in the other. The occluder reduced retinal illumination by about 2 log units (compared to 4–5 log units in kittens with lid suture) and excluded all form vision. In both kittens the geniculate layers receiving input from the covered eye showed histologically obvious cell atrophy, with a reduction in cell area of 10–15% for the appropriate dorsal and middle layers. This may be compared with the reduction, following lid closure for a similar period, of 40%. The histological changes in the lateral geniculate body thus seemed to vary with the degree of diffuse light deprivation, strong light deprivation giving severe atrophy, moderate deprivation giving moderate atrophy.

In one of the experimental kittens morphological changes were completely absent. This kitten was raised in a normal environment for the first 5 weeks after birth and was then deprived for 3 months by suturing the nictitating membrane across the cornea. This procedure reduced retinal illumination by about 1 log unit and excluded form vision, but unlike translucent plastic occluders, it caused no infection or irritation of the conjunctiva. The lateral geniculate bodies of this kitten appeared quite normal: layers with input from the covered eye had the same thickness and the same mean cell areas as the corresponding layers with normal input. In the case of deprivation by lid suture, as described in a previous section, clear atrophy was found in kittens normally raised for 2 months and then deprived for as little as 1 month.

This again supports the conclusions of the last paragraph, that for the production of geniculate atrophy the amount of light deprivation is an important variable.

GROWTH OF GENICULATE CELLS DURING THE FIRST WEEKS AFTER BIRTH. A few experiments were done with the object of learning whether the geniculate cells of light-deprived kittens were small because of failure to grow at the normal rate or because of a decrease in size following previous growth. We therefore examined brains to determine geniculate cell size in visually naïve kittens at 1 day of age and at 8 days (i.e., before the time of normal eye-opening), and at 16 days in a kitten with plastic translucent contact occluders kept on both eyes from the eighth to the sixteenth day.

In the 1-day-old kitten the layering of the lateral geniculate body was poorly developed. The cells were densely packed and small, with a mean cell area for the dorsal layers of about 100 μ^2, as opposed to about 300 μ^2 in a normal 3-month-old kitten. In the 8-day-old kitten the layers were better differentiated: the cells were not so densely packed, and they had increased in size so that those of layers A and A_1 had reached a mean area of 170–180 μ^2, and those of layer B an area of 130 μ^2. At 16 days the mean cell areas for layers A and A_1 had further increased to about 200 μ^2, and for layers B to about 170 μ^2.

In summary, in newborn kittens geniculate cells are smaller than in the adult, and even smaller than cells in the atrophic layers of 3-month-old kittens deprived from birth. Moreover, even in the absence of patterned-light stimulation growth occurs, so that at 16 days the cells reached about the size of those in kittens deprived for 3 months. It would thus seem that under these conditions of deprivation cells continue to grow up to some time between the eighth and sixteenth days, and then remain stationary. It is conceivable that growth continues beyond this time, and that atrophy occurs subsequently; to rule this out would require more studies in animals deprived for intermediate periods. That visual deprivation can cause atrophy in the strict sense of a diminution in cell size was, of course, demonstrated in the experiments already described, in which light deprivation of 2-month old kittens was found to cause a clear decrease in cell area.

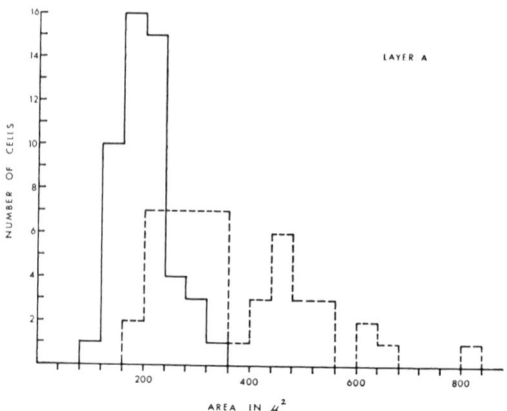

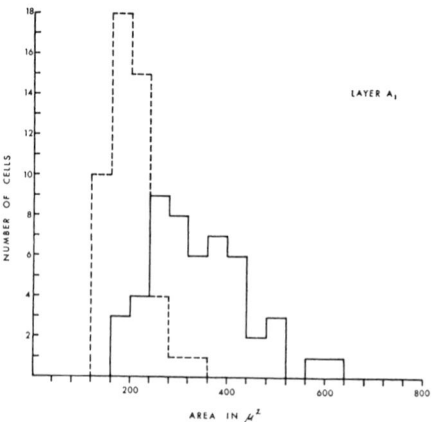

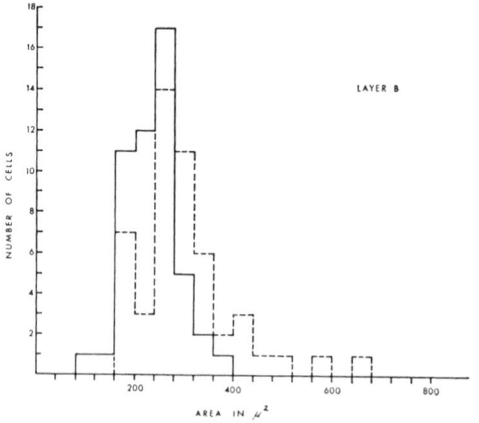

Fig. 4. Distribution by layers of cell areas in the two lateral geniculate bodies; kitten deprived by right eye-closure from the time of normal eye-opening to an age of 3½ months. Same kitten as in Figs. 1–3. Continuous lines, left lateral geniculate body; interrupted lines, right lateral geniculate body.

Table 2. Mean Areas ±SE of Mean) and Per Cent Shrinkage in Deprived Layers Relative to Corresponding Normal Layers

Layer	AREA OF CELLS			AREA OF NUCLEI		
	Left, μ^2	*Right, μ^2*	*Shrinkage, %*	*Left, μ^2*	*Right, μ^2*	*Shrinkage, %*
A	198 ± 7	365 ± 20	46*	88 ± 4	135 ± 7	35
A_1	340 ± 15	201 ± 6	41	136 ± 6	85 ± 4	38
B	236 ± 7	303 ± 14	22	106 ± 3	142 ± 5	25

All t values exceed 4.0 ($P < 0.001$).

*Sample calculation: $\dfrac{\text{difference of means}}{\text{mean of normal}} \times 100 = \dfrac{365 - 198}{365} \times 100 = 46\%$.

MONOCULAR LIGHT DEPRIVATION IN ANIMALS WITH PREVIOUS VISUAL EXPERIENCE. Monocular lid closure was performed in two kittens aged 2 months. In one of the kittens, deprived for 4 months, the lateral geniculate layers receiving input from the closed eye showed strong atrophic changes which were, however, less severe than those found in kittens deprived from birth. The other kitten had the right eye closed for only 1 month. In this animal the appropriate layers showed even less atrophy, although the changes were still very clear both on microscopic inspection and on measuring cell areas. Thus deprivation by lid closure caused atrophic geniculate changes in spite of the previous visual experience; furthermore, the changes could be observed after only 1 month of lid closure.

Finally, it seemed important to ask whether similar changes would occur in mature cats after similar periods of monocular light and form deprivation. Accordingly, the right eye was closed for 3 months in an adult cat. In this animal there was no difference between corresponding geniculate layers on the two sides: layers that received input from the closed eye were of normal thickness and contained cells normal in size and staining properties. Apparently there is an important difference between a growing kitten and an adult cat in susceptibility to these atrophic changes.

VISUAL DEPRIVATION WITH TRANSLUCENT COVERS. In the experiments described so far the kittens were visually deprived of form and also, to a large extent, of light. To assess the relative importance of form and light deprivation some experiments were done using translucent eye covers. In two kittens the cornea of the right eye was covered with a contact occluder made of translucent plastic. This was kept in place from the time of normal eye opening to an age of 2 months in one kitten, and 2½ months in the other. The occluder reduced retinal illumination by about 2 log units (compared to 4–5 log units in kittens with lid suture) and excluded all form vision. In both kittens the geniculate layers receiving input from the covered eye showed histologically obvious cell atrophy, with a reduction in cell area of 10–15% for the appropriate dorsal and middle layers. This may be compared with the reduction, following lid closure for a similar period, of 40%. The histological changes in the lateral geniculate body thus seemed to vary with the degree of diffuse light deprivation, strong light deprivation giving severe atrophy, moderate deprivation giving moderate atrophy.

In one of the experimental kittens morphological changes were completely absent. This kitten was raised in a normal environment for the first 5 weeks after birth and was then deprived for 3 months by suturing the nictitating membrane across the cornea. This procedure reduced retinal illumination by about 1 log unit and excluded form vision, but unlike translucent plastic occluders, it caused no infection or irritation of the conjunctiva. The lateral geniculate bodies of this kitten appeared quite normal: layers with input from the covered eye had the same thickness and the same mean cell areas as the corresponding layers with normal input. In the case of deprivation by lid suture, as described in a previous section, clear atrophy was found in kittens normally raised for 2 months and then deprived for as little as 1 month.

This again supports the conclusions of the last paragraph, that for the production of geniculate atrophy the amount of light deprivation is an important variable.

GROWTH OF GENICULATE CELLS DURING THE FIRST WEEKS AFTER BIRTH. A few experiments were done with the object of learning whether the geniculate cells of light-deprived kittens were small because of failure to grow at the normal rate or because of a decrease in size following previous growth. We therefore examined brains to determine geniculate cell size in visually naïve kittens at 1 day of age and at 8 days (i.e., before the time of normal eye-opening), and at 16 days in a kitten with plastic translucent contact occluders kept on both eyes from the eighth to the sixteenth day.

In the 1-day-old kitten the layering of the lateral geniculate body was poorly developed. The cells were densely packed and small, with a mean cell area for the dorsal layers of about 100 μ^2, as opposed to about 300 μ^2 in a normal 3-month-old kitten. In the 8-day-old kitten the layers were better differentiated: the cells were not so densely packed, and they had increased in size so that those of layers A and A_1 had reached a mean area of 170–180 μ^2, and those of layer B an area of 130 μ^2. At 16 days the mean cell areas for layers A and A_1 had further increased to about 200 μ^2, and for layers B to about 170 μ^2.

In summary, in newborn kittens geniculate cells are smaller than in the adult, and even smaller than cells in the atrophic layers of 3-month-old kittens deprived from birth. Moreover, even in the absence of patterned-light stimulation growth occurs, so that at 16 days the cells reached about the size of those in kittens deprived for 3 months. It would thus seem that under these conditions of deprivation cells continue to grow up to some time between the eighth and sixteenth days, and then remain stationary. It is conceivable that growth continues beyond this time, and that atrophy occurs subsequently; to rule this out would require more studies in animals deprived for intermediate periods. That visual deprivation can cause atrophy in the strict sense of a diminution in cell size was, of course, demonstrated in the experiments already described, in which light deprivation of 2-month old kittens was found to cause a clear decrease in cell area.

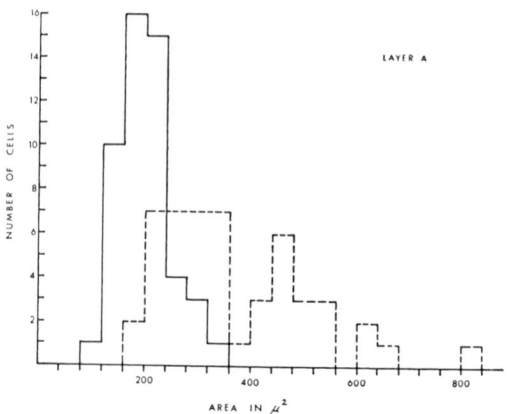

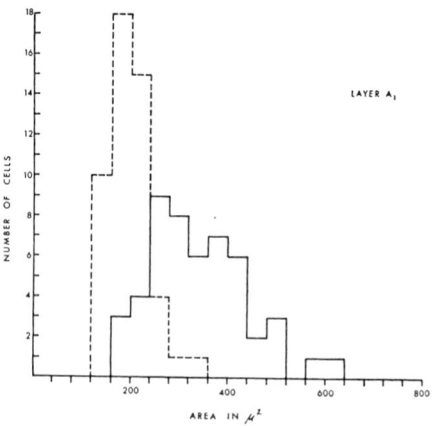

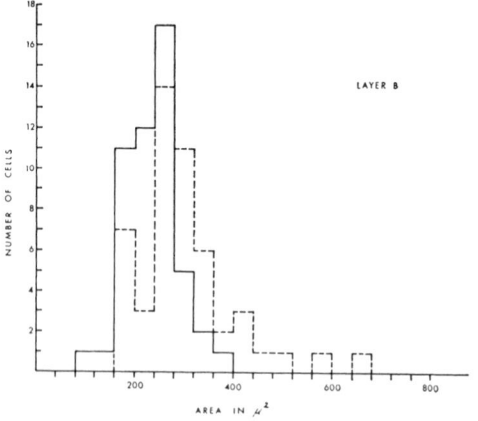

Fig. 4. Distribution by layers of cell areas in the two lateral geniculate bodies; kitten deprived by right eye-closure from the time of normal eye-opening to an age of 3½ months. Same kitten as in Figs. 1–3. Continuous lines, left lateral geniculate body; interrupted lines, right lateral geniculate body.

DISCUSSION

Our recordings from visually deprived kittens show that geniculate cells and optic-tract fibers can have normal receptive-field arrangements, indicating highly complex and functionally normal connections, even though the associated retinas have never been exposed to patterned-light stimulation. That this is also true for cells in the primary visual cortex will be shown in a subsequent paper (20). Consistent with these results are behavioral experiments in the rat by Lashley and Russel (22), Hebb (11), and Walk and Gibson (30), which show that at least in some mammals certain simple visual discriminations are not necessarily learned.

Such abnormalities as were found in lateral-geniculate receptive fields were minor but nonetheless interesting. The large center size seen in a few of the fields may be the result of some derangement in the lateral geniculate body, but it may also reflect a similar abnormality in the fields of incoming optic-nerve fibers. While no such abnormal optic-nerve fields were seen, the sampling was far too meager to rule out their existence. The apparent enlargement of some geniculate-field centers might seem to suggest some kind of proliferation of connections. It might also be accounted for by a diminution of input opposing the center response, from the transitional zone between field center and surround. Whatever the explanation, the observation suggests that sensory deprivation can lead to a distortion of function.

That there were at least some physiological abnormalities is not surprising in view of the marked atrophic changes observed in the lateral geniculate body of visually deprived kittens. The atrophy, present in all layers receiving input from the closed eye, was most pronounced in kittens deprived from birth, less marked in kittens deprived at later ages, and absent in the deprived adult cat. The exact age beyond which cat geniculate cells are no longer sensitive to light and form deprivation of several months duration was not determined. This age may represent the end of a critical period in the development of the nervous system, a period during which an animal is not only more sensitive to sensory deprivation, but also can more easily make new nervous connections, adapting itself to variations in sensory stimulation.

The marked anatomical changes in the lateral geniculate body were especially surprising since similar findings have not previously been reported. In 1889 von Gudden (9) introduced the method of depriving animals of visual stimulation by suturing the lids. Later Berger (1), using this technique in newborn kittens, could find no anatomical changes in the lateral geniculate body after 2½ months of binocular deprivation. Goodman (6) raised rabbits in darkness from birth to an age of 6 months, and Chow (3) kept immature monkeys (age not specified) in darkness for 8 months; no geniculate changes were found in either of these two studies. All of this work, then, has been unanimous in finding no geniculate abnormalities by conventional histological techniques. There may be several reasons for this discrepancy, besides the obvious one of species difference. In our study the deprivation was monocular, whereas all of those referred to above were binocular. The monocular technique tends to be more sensitive, since in each experiment the structures to be compared, deprived and nondeprived, appear in the same animal and on the same slide. But beyond this there is the possibility that in some way monocular deprivation may be very different from binocular: we might have found no atrophy had we closed over both eyes. Such a possibility is of course easy to test experimentally, and is now under study.

Apparently in kittens it is especially the lateral geniculate body that is sensitive to light deprivation, since similar atrophic changes could not be found in other parts of the visual system. In the retina, however, certain studies have demonstrated clear structural changes following light deprivation. An X-ray micrographic study of single retinal ganglion cells by Brattgård (2) showed marked reduction of cellular proteins in rabbits kept in darkness from birth to an age of 10 weeks; the same ganglion cells appeared normal when examined with ordinary histological techniques. Marked abnormalities, even complete disappearance of retinal ganglion cells, were first shown by Chow, Riesen, and Newell (4) in 2- to 3-year-old chimpanzees kept in darkness from birth. Less pronounced retinal changes have been reported in the cat (31, 27, 26).

The morphology of the deprived geniculate layers is strikingly similar to the transneuronal changes that occur some time after sectioning the optic nerve (24, 5, 23). In both conditions the abnormal layers are thin and contain small cells which lack Nissl substance. Comparing our results with those of Cook, Walker, and Barr (5), it appears that for similar periods of deprivation and deafferentation the amounts of cell atrophy were of the same order. Such a result might at first glance seem surprising, since the geniculate cells of light-deprived kittens, in contrast to the deafferented cells, may receive input from spontaneously active retinal ganglion cells (7, 21, 8); this input should, if anything, tend to limit the atrophy. The difference in age between the two types of preparation must, however, be taken into consideration: in the adult cat, in which optic-nerve section produces marked geniculate changes, visual deprivation was without discernible effect. Furthermore, transneuronal atrophy is known to be more pronounced and to develop faster in immature animals (13, 29), so that in a newborn kitten optic-nerve section might well produce a geniculate atrophy more severe than that which follows form and light deprivation. Preliminary studies indeed suggest that this is so (unpublished). In any case it is clear that such activity as does remain in optic-nerve fibers after prolonged deprivation is insufficient to maintain the cells in their normal healthy state.

We speak of the changes in deprived kittens as an "atrophy" because of the close histological resemblance to transneuronal atrophy found in adult cats, but it is important to realize that for the kittens one may be dealing at least in part with failure to grow rather than an atrophy in the strict sense. Ideally one would wish to compare two growth curves, one for normal cells, the other for visually deprived ones. In the present work we have shown that geniculate cells of newborn kittens are small by adult standards, and that they do increase in size even without benefit of visual stimulation. What is still not known is whether cells in the deprived cat grow to anything like a normal adult size and then atrophy, or whether they simply grow at a slower rate. In any case, in the normal kitten of about 2 months the geniculate cells are of about adult size, so that the changes observed when these kittens are then visually deprived can be termed an atrophy without any reservation.

From these experiments the exclusion of light seems to be an important factor in the development of atrophy in lateral geniculate cells, since the amount of atrophy varied with the amount of light deprivation, and, furthermore, a visually experi-enced kitten when subsequently light-deprived showed atrophy, whereas there was no atrophy in a comparable animal subjected to a similar period of form deprivation. These results are in line with the findings of Chow, Riesen, and Newell (4), that a few hours of diffuse light stimulation each day is enough to prevent degeneration of retinal ganglion cells in animals raised in darkness. It remains to be established whether geniculate atrophy can be caused by form deprivation alone, and also whether it can be caused by diffuse light deprivation without form deprivation.

SUMMARY

1. Kittens were subjected to deprivation of form and light in one eye, at various ages and for various periods. Deprivation was accomplished either by suturing the lids together or by placing a translucent contact occluder over the cornea.

2. In kittens with the lids of one eye sutured from birth for 3 months, most geniculate cells with input from the deprived eye had normal receptive fields, with an on-center and an off-periphery, or the reverse. The normal process by which the peripheral suppression demonstrable in retinal ganglion cells is increased at the geniculate level was observed. The over-all activity of cells in layers fed by the deprived eye was, however, diminished, and a few cells had sluggish responses and receptive fields with abnormally large centers.

3. Marked histological changes were present in layers fed by the deprived eye. Mean cell areas were decreased by about 40% for the dorsal and middle layers and 25% for the ventral layer, and nuclei and nucleoli were also shrunken. No obvious histological changes were found in the retinas, optic nerves, superior colliculi, or striate cortex.

4. Lid closure for comparable periods in 2-month-old, visually experienced kittens produced similar but less severe histological changes in the lateral geniculate bodies. No changes were seen in an adult cat visually deprived by lid suture of one eye for 3 months.

5. A translucent contact occluder placed over one eye from birth for 2 to 2½ months produced similar histological changes, but again these were less marked, with 10–15% reduction in

mean cell area, in the appropriate dorsal and middle layers. In one kitten a translucent occluder was placed over one eye at 5 weeks for a 3-month period; there was no atrophy of geniculate cells.

6. Geniculate cells measured in a newborn kitten are smaller than those in the adult, and are even smaller than cells in the atrophic layers of kittens deprived from birth by lid suture for 3 months, indicating that some growth of cells occurs subsequent to birth, in spite of visual deprivation.

ACKNOWLEDGMENT

We express our thanks to Jane Chen and Janet Tobie for their technical assistance.

References

1. Berger, H. Experimentell-anatomische Studien über die durch den Mangel optischer Reize veranlassten Entwicklungshemmungen im Occipitallappen des Hundes und der Katze. *Arch. Psychiat. Nervenkr.*, 1900, *33:* 521–567.

2. Brattgård, S.-O. The importance of adequate stimulation for the chemical composition of retinal ganglion cells during early postnatal development. *Acta radiol., Stockh.*, 1952, Suppl. *96:* 1–80.

3. Chow, K. L. Failure to demonstrate changes in the visual system of monkeys kept in darkness or in colored lights. *J. comp. Neurol.*, 1955, *102:* 597–606.

4. Chow, K. L., Riesen, A. H., and Newell, F. W. Degeneration of retinal ganglion cells in infant chimpanzees reared in darkness. *J. comp. Neurol.*, 1957, *107:* 27–42.

5. Cook, W. H., Walker, J. H., and Barr, M. L. A cytological study of transneuronal atrophy in the cat and rabbit. *J. comp. Neurol.*, 1951, *94:* 267–292.

6. Goodman, L. Effect of total absence of function on the optic system of rabbits. *Amer. J. Physiol.*, 1932, *100:* 46–63.

7. Granit, R. *Sensory Mechanisms of the Retina.* London, Oxford Univ. Press, 1947.

8. Granit, R. *Receptors and Sensory Perception.* New Haven, Yale Univ. Press, 1955.

9. Gudden, B. A. von. In: *Gesammelte und hinterlassene Abhandlungen,* edited by H. Grashey. Wiesbaden, Bergmann, 1889.

10. Hayhow, W. R. The cytoarchitecture of the lateral geniculate body in the cat in relation to the distribution of crossed and uncrossed optic fibers. *J. comp. Neurol.*, 1958, *110:* 1–64.

11. Hebb, D. O. The innate organization of visual activity: I. Perception of figures by rats raised in total darkness. *J. comp. Neurol.*, 1937, *51:* 101–126.

12. Hebb, D. O. *Organization of Behavior.* New York, Wiley, 1949.

13. Hess, A. Optic centers and pathways after eye removal in fetal guinea pigs. *J. comp. Neurol.*, 1958, *109:* 91–115.

14. Hubel, D. H. Tungsten microelectrode for recording from single units. *Science,* 1957, *125:* 549–550.

15. Hubel, D. H. Single unit activity in striate cortex of unrestrained cats. *J. Physiol.*, 1959, *147:* 226–238.

16. Hubel, D. H. Single unit activity in lateral geniculate body and optic tract of unrestrained cats. *J. Physiol.*, 1960, *150:* 91–104.

17. Hubel, D. H. and Wiesel, T. N. Receptive fields of single neurones in the cat's striate cortex. *J. Physiol.*, 1959, *148:* 574–591.

18. Hubel, D. H. and Wiesel, T. N. Integrative action in the cat's lateral geniculate body. *J. Physiol.*, 1961, *155:* 385–398.

19. Hubel, D. H. and Wiesel, T. N. Receptive fields, binocular interaction and functional architecture in the cat's visual cortex. *J. Physiol.*, 1962, *160:* 106–154.

20. Hubel, D. H. and Wiesel, T. N. Receptive fields of cells in striate cortex of very young, visually inexperienced kittens. *J. Neurophysiol.*, 1963, *26:* 994–1002.

21. Kuffler, S. W. Discharge patterns and functional organization of mammalian retina. *J. Neurophysiol.*, 1953, *16:* 37–68.

22. Lashley, K. S. and Russel, J. T. The mechanism of vision: XI. A preliminary test of innate organization. *J. genet. Psychol.*, 1934, *45:* 136–144.

23. Matthews, M. R., Cowan, W. M., and Powell, T. P. S. Transneuronal cell degeneration in the lateral geniculate nucleus of the Macaque monkey. *J. Anat., Lond.*, 1960, *94:* 145–169.

24. Minkowski, von M. Über den Verlauf, die Endigung und die zentrale Repräsentation von gekreuzten und ungekreuzten Sehnervenfasern bei einigen Säugetieren und beim Menschen. *Schweiz. Arch. Psychiat.*, 1920, *6:* 201–252.

25. Polyak, S. L. *The Retina.* Chicago, Univ. of Chicago Press, 1941.

26. Rasch, E., Swift, H., Riesen, A. H., and Chow, K. L. Altered structure and composition of retinal cells in dark-reared mammals. *Exp. Cell Res.* 1961, *25:* 348–363.

27. Riesen, A. H. Effects of stimulus deprivation on the development and atrophy of the visual sensory system. *Amer. J. Orthopsychiat.*, 1960, *30:* 23–36.

28. Riesen, A. H. Stimulation as a requirement for growth and function in behavioral development. In: *Functions of Varied Experience,* edited by D. W. Fiske and S. R. Maddi. Homewood, Ill., Dorsey Press, 1961, pp. 57–105.

29. Torvik, A. Transneuronal changes in the inferior olive and pontine nuclei in kittens. *J. Neuropath.*, 1956, *15:* 119–145.

30. Walk, R. D. and Gibson, E. J. A comparative and analytical study of visual depth perception. *Psychol. Mongr.*, 1961, *75:* 1–44.

31. Weiskrantz, L. Sensory deprivation and the cat's optic nervous system. *Nature, Lond.*, 1958, *181:* 1047–1050.

32. Wiesel, T. N. and Hubel, D. H. Single-cell responses in striate cortex of kittens deprived of vision in one eye. *J. Neurophysiol.*, 1963, *26:* 1003–1017.

Receptive Fields of Cells in Striate Cortex of Very Young, Visually Inexperienced Kittens[1]

DAVID H. HUBEL AND TORSTEN N. WIESEL • *Neurophysiology Laboratory, Department of Pharmacology, Harvard Medical School, Boston, Massachusetts*

INTRODUCTION

In a series of studies on the cat over the past 5 years we have recorded from single cells in the striate cortex and mapped receptive fields using patterned retinal stimulation. The results suggest that connections between geniculate and striate cortex, and between cortical cells, must be highly specific (5). Indeed, cells in the striate cortex respond in such a characteristic way that departures from the normal adult physiology should be easily recognizable.

In the present study we have made similar experiments in kittens ranging in age from 1–3 weeks. Our purpose was to learn the age at which cortical cells have normal, adult-type receptive fields, and to find out whether such fields exist even in animals that have had no patterned visual stimulation.

METHODS

Four kittens were included in this series. Three of these were from the same litter. The youngest was 8 days old at the time of the experiment, and had not yet opened its eyes. The second had both its eyes covered by translucent contact occluders at 9 days, at which time the eyes were just beginning to open; the experiment was done 1 week later, at 16 days of age. The third kitten had the right eye covered by a translucent occluder at 9 days, and the other eye was allowed to open normally; the experiment was done on the nineteenth day. The fourth kitten, from a different litter, was brought up normally and used in an experiment on the twentieth day, after 11 days of normal visual exposure. Thus two kittens had, at the time of the experiment, no patterned-light experience; the third had such experience in one eye only, and the fourth had normal visual stimulation in both eyes. Before the experi-

ments the two kittens that had been exposed to patterned light were beginning to show following movements of the eyes and visually guided behavior.

Procedures for stimulating and recording have for the most part been described in previous papers (4, 5). A few modifications were necessary for newborn and very young kittens. Since doses of barbiturate large enough to give surgical anesthesia were usually lethal, the kittens were first given a small dose of thiopental (15–20 mg/kg.), and just before surgery the appropriate regions of skin were infiltrated with local anesthetic (Xylocaine, 2%). A few minutes after injection of the local anesthetic the animal usually fell asleep and showed no sign of discomfort during the surgery or the experiment. From observations on these and other newborn kittens we have the impression that the Xylocaine has central effects as well as local ones. Since eye movements were not troublesome, no paralyzing agent was used, and artificial respiration was not necessary. The skull, too soft to be held by ear plugs, was supported by cementing it to a modified Davies chamber (2) which was then clamped securely. The electrode was introduced through a hole in the skull and dura a few millimeters wide. Tungsten microelectrodes were used for recording, and several electrolytic lesions in each track served to identify recording sites in histological sections. All brains were examined histologically.

Patterned stimuli were shone on a diffusely lit screen which the kittens faced from a distance of 1.5 m. Background light was about 1 c.d/m^2, and stimuli were generally 0.5–1.5 log units brighter. Identification of area centralis and optic discs by our usual projection method (4) was difficult because the cornea and media have a cloudy appearance and because the tapetum in cats does not develop fully until 3–4 weeks after birth (3). Receptive-field position could therefore not be determined accurately, though it was our rough impression that fields were within about 10° of the center of gaze.

From *J. Neurophysiol. 1963, 26,* 994–1002

Received for publication June 26, 1963.

[1]This work was supported in part by Research Grants GM-K3-15,304 (C2), B-2260 (C2), and B-2253-C2S1 from the Public Health Service, and in part by Research Grant AF-AFOSR-410-62 from the U.S. Air Force.

RESULTS

Cortical Activity and Responses in Kittens without Visual Experience

RESTING ACTIVITY AND RESPONSIVENESS. Seventeen single cells were recorded from the two visually naïve kittens, nine from the 8-day-old and eight from the 16-day-old. Perhaps the most marked difference between these experiments and our usual recordings from cortex in adult cats was in the maintained activity and responsiveness of the cells. With steady diffuse background illumination cells tended to be silent or to fire at a very low rate. Perhaps partly because of this paucity of maintained activity the number of cells studied in a penetration was unusually small, a few in each passage from surface to white matter as against 20–30 in an ordinary adult penetration. Cells were not only sluggish in their spontaneous activity but also responded grudgingly to the most effective patterned stimuli. This relative difficulty in eliciting responses reminded one of similar difficulties in driving cells in very deeply anesthetized adult cats (5, p. 122). Just as in deeply anesthetized adults, some cells did not respond at all to patterned stimuli unless the stimuli were moving.

Finally, cortical cells, especially in the 8-day-old kitten, showed a marked tendency to fatigue. To be sure of obtaining brisk responses one sometimes had to wait for as long as a minute between stimuli. While a tendency to such fatigability is occasionally found in cells of mature cats, it is far from the rule, and when the depressed responsiveness occurs, it does not last nearly so long. The fatigue would seem to be cortical, since similar effects were not seen in geniculate cells, and since in a binocularly influenced unit the intervals between effective stimuli could not be shortened by stimulating first one eye and then the other.

RECEPTIVE-FIELD CHARACTERISTICS. Except for this sluggishness, cortical cells of visually inexperienced kittens strongly resembled cells of mature cats in their responses to patterned stimuli. The cells responded poorly, and often not at all, to changes in diffuse retinal illumination. They responded best to straight-line stimuli (i.e., slits, dark bars, or edges), but only when these were appropriately oriented within the receptive fields, which averaged about 2–5° in diameter. The optimum orientation was found by moving the stimulus back and forth across the receptive field, adjusting the orientation between stimuli. In Fig. 1, a single-unit recording obtained from the 8-day-old kitten, a long narrow rectangle of light was moved back and forth across the receptive field as shown. Brief responses were consistently obtained when the slit was oriented in a 1 o'clock–7 o'clock direction (*A*) whereas there was no response when it was oriented at 90° to this (*B*). A similar kind of preference in stimulus orientation was common to all of the units isolated. Several of the cells, especially those in the 8-day-old kitten, gave responses over a range of stimulus orientations that was unusually wide by adult standards, yet even in these cells stimulating at an orientation of 90° to the optimum evoked no response at all. Moreover, the responses to moving an optimally oriented stimulus across the receptive field were not necessarily the same for the two diametrically opposite directions of movement (see Fig. 4). As in the adult cat, this kind of directional preference varied from cell to cell; some cells responded equally well to the two opposing directions of movement, while some responded well to one direction and not at all to the other.

The combination of sluggish responses and poor optics made it difficult to map receptive fields in a detailed way. Of those that could be mapped, however, some were clearly "simple" in type and others were "complex" (5).

BINOCULAR INTERACTION. The great majority of cells recorded from the two immature kittens (16 out of 17) could be influenced from each eye separately. Just as in adult cats (5), the receptive fields of these cells were situated in corresponding regions in the two eyes, and the two fields were, as far as one could tell, identical in arrangement, in degree of complexity and in orientation. Furthermore, the two eyes often differed in their relative ability to influence a given cell. We have again subdivided cells into seven groups according to the relative influence of the two eyes (see Fig. 2, legend). The distribution of cells among the groups is given in Table 1 and in the histogram of Fig. 2 (shaded portion). Comparison of this histogram with the corresponding one in the adult (9, Fig. 1) suggests that there is little or no difference in ocular-dominance distribution with age or visual experience.

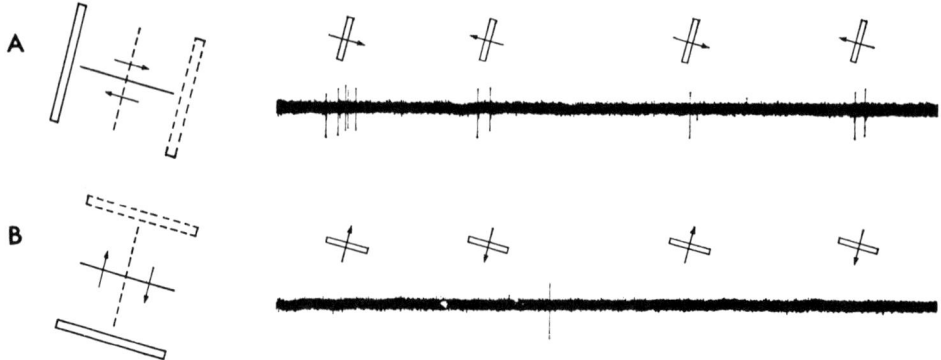

Fig. 1. Single-cell responses from cortex of an 8-day-old kitten with no previous visua experience. A rectangle of light 1° × 5° is moved back and forth across the receptive field in the contralateral eye. Unit binocularly activated, ocular-dominance group 3. Receptive-field sizes about 5° × 5°; fields situated in the central part of the contralateral visual field. A: stimulus oriented 12:30–6:30 (parallel to receptive-field axis). B: stimulus oriented 9:30–3:30 (at right angles to the optimal orientation). Rate of movement, 5°/sec. Time, 1 sec.

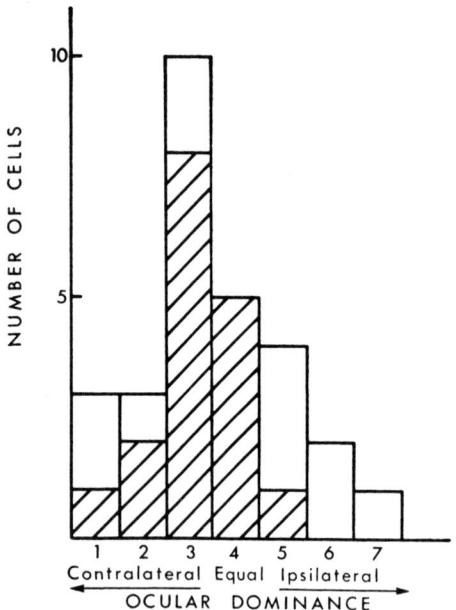

Fig. 2. Distribution of 28 cells among the seven ocular-dominance groups, defined as follows: cells of group 1 were driven only by the contralateral eye; for cells of group 2 there was marked dominance of the contralateral eye; for group 3, slight dominance. For cells in group 4 there was no obvious difference between the two eyes. In group 5 the ipsilateral eye dominated slightly, in group 6 markedly; and in group 7 the cells were driven only by the ipsilateral eye. The shaded portion refers to 17 cells recorded from two kittens with no prior visual experience (aged 8 and 16 days). The unshaded portion refers to cells recorded from the 20-day-old normal kitten.

FUNCTIONAL ARCHITECTURE. In penetrations perpendicular to the surface of the cortex and parallel to the radial fiber bundles there were long sequences of cells all having the same receptive-field orientation. In oblique penetrations more frequent shifts in orientation were seen. An oblique cortical penetration in the 16-day-old kitten is reconstructed in Fig. 3. Here there were three shifts in receptive-field orientation within a relatively short distance, and between each shift cells and unresolved background activity had the same field orientation. All of this is in good agreement with previous studies of the functional architecture of the visual cortex in adult cats (5), suggesting that the organization of cortex into columns of cells having common receptive-field orientations is already present in immature kittens that have never received patterned visual stimulation.

KITTENS WITH VISUAL EXPERIENCE

In their maintained activity, cortical cells of older, visually experienced kittens were much closer to normal. Most cells were active in the absence of patterned stimulation, so that isolation of single cells was much easier. Responses to restricted stimuli were brisker, and showed little of the fatigue that was so apparent in the 8-day-old kitten. As a rule the optimum stimulus was more precisely defined, especially the receptive-field orientation; in this respect these two kittens were closer to the

Table 1. Distribution of Cells Among the Ocular-Dominance Groups

Kitten	NUMBER OF CELLS IN EACH GROUP						
	1	2	3	4	5	6	7
8-day-old	1	2	3	3			
16-day-old			5	2	1		
19-day-old*	1	1	2	2	3	2	
20-day-old	2	1	2		3	2	1
Totals	4	4	12	7	7	4	1

*Not included in histogram of Fig. 2.

adult than they were to the 8- and 16-day-old visually naïve kittens. Both simple and complex types of fields were mapped, and reconstructions of electrode penetrations again tended to confirm the columnar organization of the cortex. In the responses to stimulation of the two eyes there were no obvious differences between the younger visually naïve kittens and the older experienced ones: the 11 cells recorded from the 20-day-old normal kitten varied greatly in ocular dominance, and are included in the histogram of Fig. 2, where they are represented by the unshaded portion.

The third, 19-day-old kitten was a useful control, since the right eye was covered from the time of normal eye-opening by a translucent occluder, and the left was allowed to remain uncovered. In the cortical recordings there was, on the whole, no obvious difference between the two eyes in their ability to influence cortical cells; the previously occluded eye was dominant about as often as the normal eye (see Table 1). In Fig. 4, a two-unit recording obtained from this kitten, a slit stimulus crossed the receptive field in three different orientations. The units responded well only to the second of these; to the first and third and to orientations still further from the optimum there was little or no response. The unit from which the smaller spikes were recorded gave hardly any responses to stimulation of the right eye (which had been covered), but responded well to the left. On the contrary, the cell giving the larger spikes strongly preferred the eye that had been occluded.

There was no tendency for cells dominated by the occluded eye to have less maintained activity or to respond less briskly and precisely than the other cells. We are therefore inclined to think that the

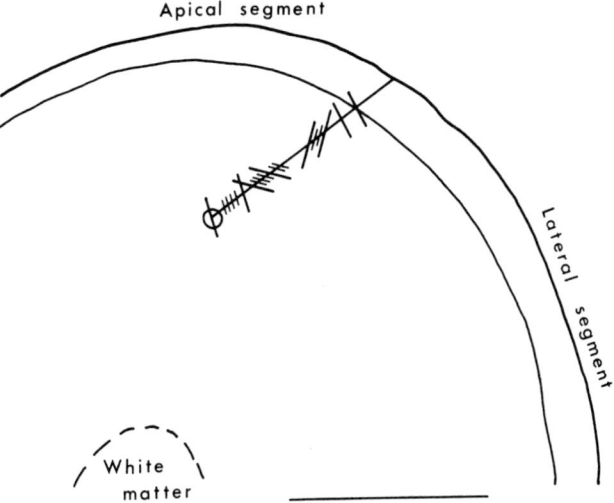

Fig. 3. Reconstruction of an oblique microelectrode penetration through the postlateral gyrus of a 16-day-old kitten without previous visual experience. Longer lines intersecting the electrode track represent single well-isolated cortical cells; directions of these lines represent receptive-field orientations, a line perpendicular to the track standing for a vertical orientation. Shorter lines show regions in which unresolved background activity was observed. At the end of a penetration an electrolytic lesion was made; this is indicated by the circle. Scale, 0.5 mm.

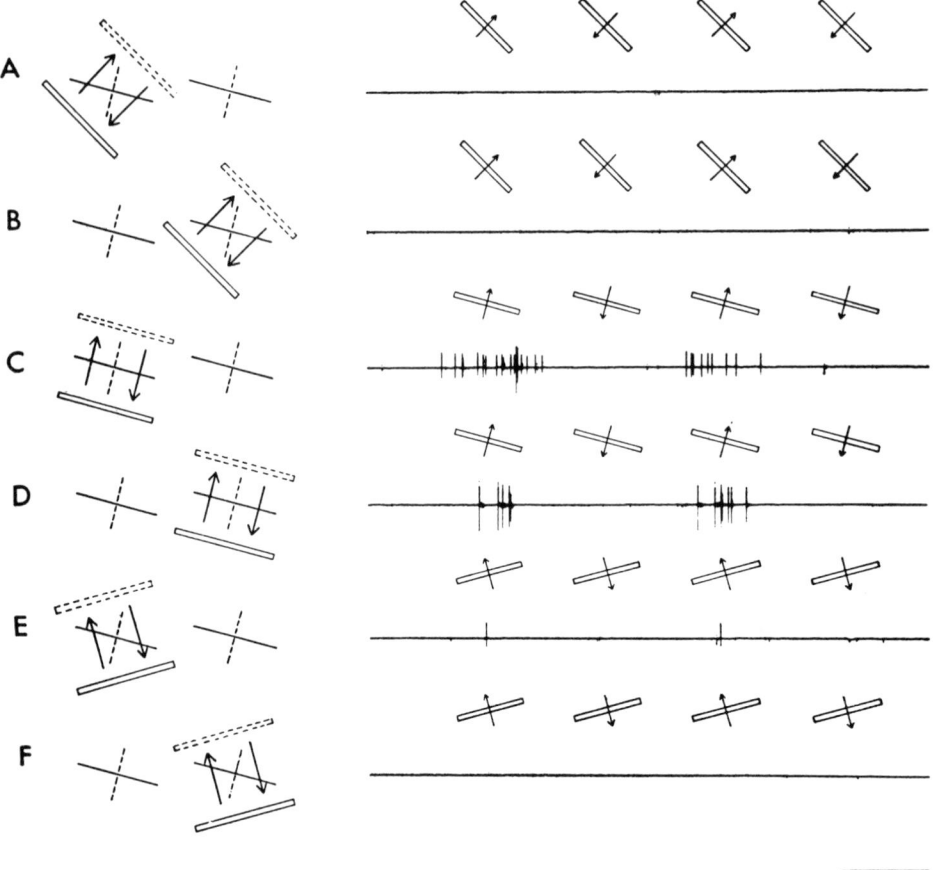

Fig. 4. Two-unit recording from a 19-day-old kitten whose right eye had been covered from the time of normal eye-opening by a translucent occluder. Each eye stimulated separately by a slit 0.5° × 0.4°, moved across the receptive field at a rate of about 1°/sec. Size of fields 2° × 4°. Time, 1 sec.

sluggishness of maintained activity and responses in the first two kittens was related to age rather than to visual experience. This is simply a tentative impression, since the difference in the two groups of kittens may be more related to differences in the animals' susceptibility to anesthesia than to a difference in properties of cortical cells, especially since we know that suppression of maintained activity and of responses is a characteristic effect of anesthesia in adult cats.

What can be concluded from this kitten is that even as late as 19 days of age a cell need not have had previous patterned stimulation from an eye in order to respond normally to it. This will be of some interest when the effects of longer periods of monocular deprivation are considered, as discussed in the accompanying paper (9).

DISCUSSION

The main result of this study has been to show that much of the richness of visual physiology in the cortex of the adult cat—the receptive-field organization, binocular interaction, and functional architecture—is present in very young kittens without visual experience. Our conclusion is that the neural connections subserving these functions must also be present, in large part, at or near the time of birth. This extends the work of the previous paper (8) in which we showed that visual experience was not necessary for the development of optic-nerve or geniculate receptive fields.

These findings were somewhat unexpected in view of behavioral observations in very young kittens. At birth a bright light evokes a lid reflex (10), as well as a sluggish pupillary response (1), suggesting that the visual system is to some extent functional. Nevertheless, kittens appear quite unable to use their eyes at the time of normal eye-opening, which usually occurs between the sixth and the tenth day. Avoidance of objects is seen at the very earliest around 14 days, while pursuit, following movements, and visual placing appear only at 20–25 days (10, 7). Visual acuity, measured by observing optokinetic nystagmus, increases rapidly from the second week and approaches adult levels by about the fourth week (7). To parallel this behavioral development in the first weeks we have in cortical cells only the increase in briskness of responses and extent of maintained activity—which may be related to differences in reaction or our experimental procedures rather than to real differences in the physiology—and the heightened precision of responses, especially to variations in stimulus orientation. This leads one to wonder whether the inability of young kittens to use their vision is related not so much to incomplete development of the visual pathway as to a lack of visuo-motor ability.

From the behavioral observations alone one might easily imagine that the improvement in visual skill during the first weeks after birth is closely paralleled by development in neural connections in the visual pathway. Such a concept has probably been reinforced by studies on the delay in development of visual ability produced by raising animals in darkness or in diffuse light (for reviews see ref. 6); it has been natural to assume that in the normal animal neural connections subserving vision are developed only if pattern stimuli fall on the retina. The present results make it clear that highly complex neural connections are possible without benefit of visual experience. In interpreting the results of visual deprivation, both the behavioral and the physiological, one must therefore consider the possibility that lack of stimulation may lead not simply to a failure in forming connections, but rather to the disruption of connections that were there from the start.

SUMMARY

Responses of single cells to visual stimuli were studied in the striate cortex of very young kittens. Two animals, aged 8 and 16 days, had had no previous exposure to patterned stimuli. Responses of cortical cells in these animals were strikingly similar to those of adult cats. Fields were simple or complex, with a clear receptive-field orientation. Cells with similar orientations appeared to be grouped in columnar regions. The majority of cells were driven by the two eyes, with patterns of binocular interaction that were similar to those in the adult. Compared with cells in the mature cat, those in young kittens responded somewhat more sluggishly to visual stimuli, and receptive-field orientations tended to be not quite so well defined.

In two other kittens, one monocularly deprived by translucent occluder from birth for 19 days, the other a normal 20-day-old, responses to patterned stimulation of either eye were entirely normal by adult standards.

It is concluded that many of the connections responsible for the highly organized behavior of cells in the striate cortex must be present at birth or within a few days of it. The development of these connections occurs even in the absence of patterned visual experience.

ACKNOWLEDGMENT

We express our thanks to Jane Chen and Janet Tobie for their technical assistance.

References

1. Abelsdorff, G. Bemerkungen über das Auge der neugeborenen Katze, im Besonderen die retinale Sehzellenschicht. *Arch. Augenheilk.*, 1905, *53*:257–262.
2. Davies, P. W. Chamber for microelectrode studies in the cerebral cortex. *Science*, 1956, *124*:179–180.
3. Hilbert, R. Ueber die nach der Geburt eintretenden entwickelungsgeschichtlichen Veränderrungen der brechenden Medien und des Augenhintergrundes der Katze. *v. Graefes Arch. Ophthal.*, 1884, *30*:245–250.
4. Hubel, D. H. and Wiesel, T. N. Receptive fields of optic nerve fibres in the spider monkey. *J. Physiol.*, 1960, *154*: 572–580.
5. Hubel, D. H. and Wiesel, T. N. Receptive fields, binocular interaction and functional architecture in the cat's visual cortex. *J. Physiol.*, 1962, *160*:106–154.
6. Riesen, A. H. Stimulation as a requirement for growth and function in behavioral development. In: *Functions of Varied Experience,* edited by D. W. Fiske and S. R. Maddi. Homewood, Ill., Dorsey Press, 1961, pp. 57–105.

7. Warkentin, J. and Smith, K. U. The development of visual acuity in the cat. *J. genet. Psychol.*, 1937, *50:*371–399.

8. Wiesel, T. N. and Hubel, D. H. Effects of visual deprivation on morphology and physiology of cells in the cat's lateral geniculate body. *J. Neurophysiol.*, 1963, *26:* 978–993.

9. Wiesel, T. N. and Hubel, D. H. Single-cell responses in striate cortex of kittens deprived of vision in one eye. *J. Neurophysiol.*, 1963, *26:*1003–1017.

10. Windle, W. F. Normal behavioral reactions of kittens correlated with the postnatal development of nerve-fiber density in the spinal gray matter. *J. comp. Neurol.*, 1930, *50:*479–503.

Single-Cell Responses in Striate Cortex of Kittens Deprived of Vision in One Eye[1]

TORSTEN N. WIESEL AND DAVID H. HUBEL • *Neurophysiology Laboratory, Department of Pharmacology, Harvard Medical School, Boston, Massachusetts*

INTRODUCTION

In the first paper of this series (11) we showed that in a kitten 2–3 months of monocular light and form deprivation can produce a marked atrophy of cells in the lateral geniculate body. The changes were confined to layers receiving projections from the deprived eye. Despite the atrophy, most of the cells recorded had normal receptive fields. The present paper extends this physiological study of monocularly deprived kittens to the next level in the visual pathway, the striate cortex. We wished to learn whether one could influence cortical cells from the deprived eye, and whether the receptive fields were normal.

At the cortical level any long-term effects of tampering with one eye might be expected to show up as a change in normal patterns of binocular interaction. It may therefore be useful to begin by summarizing some previous findings on binocular interaction in the normal cat. Approximately four-fifths of cells in the cat striate cortex are binocularly influenced. For any given cell the receptive fields mapped in the two eyes are similar in arrangement and occupy corresponding retinal positions. Although stimuli to corresponding retinal points thus produce qualitatively similar responses, the strengths of the responses from the two eyes are not necessarily equal: some cells respond best to the contralateral eye; others prefer the ipsilateral. Figure 1, reproduced from a previous study (7), shows the distribution of 223 cells according to eye-dominance. It will be seen from this histogram that on the whole the contralateral eye is decidedly the more influential. In the second paper of this series (9) we showed that very young kittens resembled adults in all of these respects. This was true even of animals with no previous patterned visual experience.

We have been particularly interested in learning whether the distribution of cells among the different ocular-dominance categories would be appreciably altered in recordings from monocularly deprived kittens. The histogram of Fig. 1 represents the lumped results of 45 penetrations, and cannot necessarily be used to predict the distribution of cells in a single penetration. To interpret the results of the present paper we need to know whether this distribution varies markedly from one penetration to the next. It might be much narrower and less constant from penetration to penetration if, for example, there were a strong tendency for cells with the same eye-preference to be

From *J. Neurophysiol.* 1963, *26,* 1003–1017.

Received for publication June 26, 1963.

[1]This work was supported in part by Research Grants GM-K3-15,304 (C2), B-2260 (C2), and B-2253-C2S1 from the Public Health Service, and in part by Research Grant AF-AFOSR-410-62 from the U.S. Air Force.

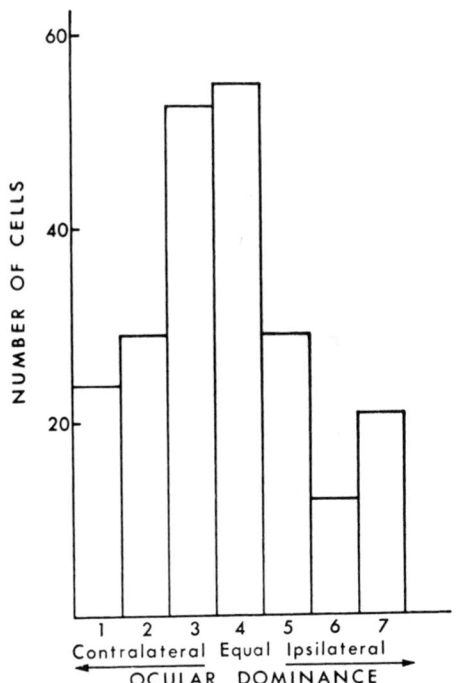

Fig. 1. *Ocular-dominance distribution of 223 cells recorded from striate cortex of adult cats in a series of 45 penetrations (7). Cells of group 1 were driven only by the contralateral eye; for cells of group 2 there was marked dominance of the contralateral eye, for group 3, slight dominance. For cells in group 4 there was no obvious difference between the two eyes. In group 5 the ipsilateral eye dominated slightly, in group 6, markedly; and in group 7 the cells were driven only by the ipsilateral eye.*

grouped together in the cortex. To have a better idea of the variation in distribution from penetration to penetration we have therefore taken 12 separate consecutive penetrations from the series used to construct Fig. 1, and plotted each of their ocular-dominance distributions separately (Fig. 2). It appears from these histograms that there is no very marked tendency for cells to be anatomically grouped by eye-preference: penetrations *2* and *4* represent the extremes in the two directions, of dominance by the ipsilateral eye (*2*) or the contralateral eye (*4*), and even in these two penetrations both eyes make a substantial contribution. In judging an individual penetration it is therefore probably reasonably safe to take the distribution of Fig. 1 as the normal, regarding as probably significant only departures much greater than those of penetrations *2* and *4*.

METHODS

Seven kittens and one adult cat were used. The animals were monocularly deprived either by lid closure or by a translucent eye cover (11). Closure of lids prevented form vision and reduced the level of diffuse retinal illumination by about 4–5 log units. The translucent occluders also prevented pattern stimulation, but reduced the diffuse illumination by only about 1–2 log units. Four of the kittens were deprived from the time of normal eye-opening; the others had some prior visual experience. Deprivation was for periods of 1–4 months. Before some experiments the lids of the closed eye were separated or the translucent eye cover was removed. The normal eye was then covered with an opaque contact occluder and the animal's visual behavior was observed.

Experimental procedures for preparing the animals and for stimulating and recording are given in previous papers (5, 6, 7, 11). Extracellular recordings were made with tungsten microelectrodes in the part of the lateral gyrus receiving projections from the retinal area centralis. In one animal electroretinograms and evoked cortical potentials were recorded, the electroretinograms with chlorided silver electrodes placed on the limbus of the upper outer quadrant of the cornea, the evoked potentials with similar electrodes placed on the dura over homologous points on the two lateral gyri (Horsley-Clarke frontal plane zero, 1 mm. from the midline); the indifferent electrode was the frame of the Horsley-Clarke head holder. Responses were evoked with a Grass photostimulator (model PS 2) set at maximum intensity and held 6 in. from the animal's eyes. The eyes were stimulated separately by covering each in turn with a patch of thick black rubber.

All brains were subsequently examined histologically in order to reconstruct electrode tracks marked by electrolytic lesions.

RESULTS

Behavioral Effects of Monocular Deprivation

Prior to some experiments in animals deprived from birth, the obstruction was removed from the right eye (by separating the lids or removing the translucent contact occluder), and an opaque occluder was placed over the normal left eye. Pupillary light reflexes were normal, and there was no nystagmus. No visual placing reactions could be obtained, though tactile placing was normal.

As an animal walked about investigating its surroundings the gait was broad-based and hesitant, and the head moved up and down in a pecu-

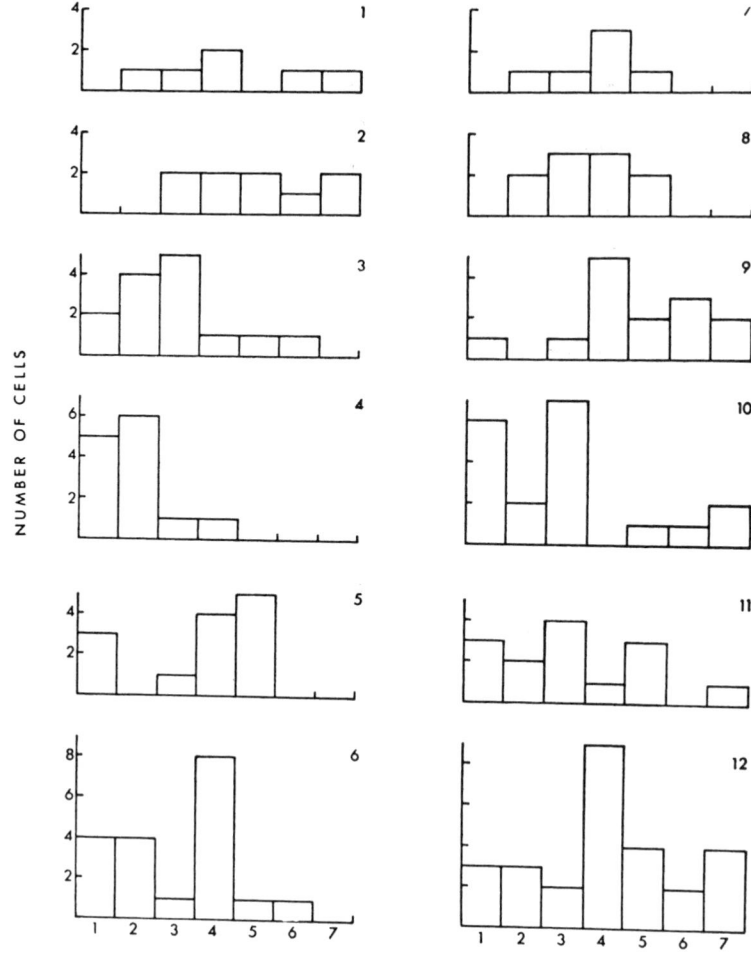

OCULAR DOMINANCE

Fig. 2. Ocular-dominance distribution of 12 separate consecutive penetrations from the same series as Fig. 1 (7).

liar nodding manner. The kittens bumped into large obstacles such as table legs, and even collided with walls, which they tended to follow using their whiskers as a guide. When put onto a table the animals walked off into the air, several times falling awkwardly onto the floor. When an object was moved before the eye there was no hint that it was perceived, and no attempt was made to follow it. As soon as the cover was taken off of the left eye the kitten would behave normally, jump gracefully from the table, skillfully avoiding objects in its way. We concluded that there was a profound, perhaps complete, impairment of vision in the deprived eye of these animals.

Physiological Findings in Kittens Deprived of Vision in one Eye from Birth

Of the 84 cortical cells recorded in kittens deprived from birth, 83 were completely uninfluenced by the deprived eye. The dominance of the normal eye in these cells was all the more striking since all but one of the five penetrations were made in the hemisphere contralateral to, and hence normally strongly favoring, the deprived eye (see Fig. 1).

The ocular-dominance histogram of a kitten whose right eye was sutured at 8 days for a 2½-month period is shown in Fig. 3. Of the 25 cells examined in a single penetration of the left striate cortex, 20 were driven exclusively by the normal

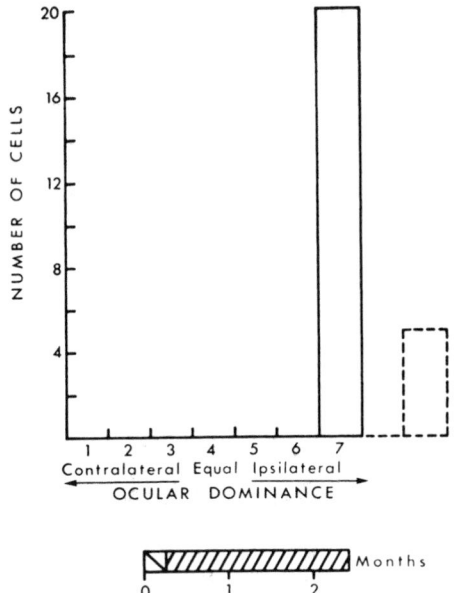

Fig. 3. Ocular-dominance distribution of 25 cells recorded in the visual cortex of a 2½-month-old kitten. Experimental procedures are indicated beneath; during the first week the eyes were not yet open; on the eighth day the lids of the right eye were sutured, and they remained closed until the time of the experiment (cross-hatched region). The left eye opened normally on the ninth day. Recordings were made from the left visual cortex, contralateral to the eye that had been closed. Five of the cells, represented by the interrupted column on the right, could not be driven from either eye. The remaining 20 were driven only from the normally exposed (left, or ipsilateral) eye, and were therefore classed as group 7.

(ipsilateral) eye, and none could be influenced from the deprived (contralateral) eye. The 5 remaining cells could not be driven from either eye, and would have gone unnoticed had it not been for their spontaneous activity. The presence in most of these penetrations of a small number of unresponsive cells is worth stressing, since in normal adult cats it has been possible to drive all cells with appropriate visual stimuli (7). The electrode track of this penetration, reconstructed from the histological slides, is shown in Fig. 4. The 20 cells whose receptive fields were mapped in the normal eye all responded to line stimuli, and each strongly favored one orientation and failed to respond to a slit, edge, or dark bar placed at right angles to the optimum. The receptive fields were arranged in

the usual "simple" or "complex" manner (in the sense that we have previously used these terms (7)) and varied in their orientation in a way consistent with a columnar arrangement. Unresolved background activity was present throughout the penetration, and, like the isolated units, it was strongly influenced by the normal eye but not at all by the deprived one.

In another 3-month-old kitten whose right eye had been closed from birth, penetrations were made in homologous regions in both hemispheres. The ocular-dominance histograms of these penetrations are shown in Fig. 5, and again illustrate a failure to drive any cell from the abnormal eye. Again there were several cells that could not be driven from either eye.

The one cell in the series that could be driven from the deprived eye was recorded from a third kitten, lid-sutured from birth to an age of 2½ months. This cell was unusual in having abnormal fields in both eyes. Unlike other cells in the same penetration, which were normal except for their unresponsiveness to stimulation of the deprived eye, this cell had no particular orientation-preference, and the responses were more sluggish than those of the other cells. The receptive fields were in roughly corresponding parts of the two retinas.

To try to evaluate the relative importance of form deprivation as against light deprivation we raised one kitten from birth to an age of 2 months with a translucent contact occluder over the right eye. This prevented patterned retinal stimulation and reduced the general retinal illumination by about 2 log units, as opposed to 4–5 for the sutured lids. The ocular-dominance distribution of 26 cells recorded from the left hemisphere (contralateral to the occluded eye) is shown in Fig. 6. Just as in the lid-suture experiments, all cells were driven exclusively from the normal (left) eye, except for three which could not be driven at all. The cells that could be driven had normal receptive fields. From the electrode track reconstruction shown in Fig. 7, the electrode is seen to have traversed three columns, both shifts in orientation being small, discrete, and anticlockwise. Such orderly sequences have been seen in penetrations in adult cats (8), and support our impression that in parts of the striate cortex the columns are arranged in an orderly manner. As in the first two kittens there was continuous unresolved activity throughout the pene-

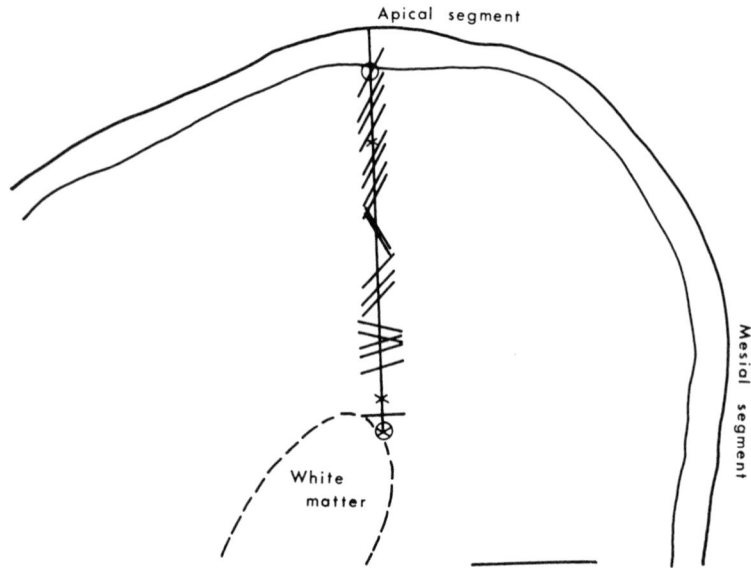

Fig. 4. Reconstruction of a microelectrode penetration through the postlateral gyrus of the left hemisphere. This 2½-month-old kitten had its right eye covered from birth by lid suture. Lines intersecting the electrode track represent cortical cells; directions of these lines indicate the receptive-field orientations. Crosses indicate cortical cells uninfluenced by light stimulation. Simultaneous recordings from two units, which occurred three times in this penetration, are each indicated by only one line or cross. A lesion was made while recording from the first unit, and another at the end of the penetration: these are marked by small circles. The ocular-dominance distribution of units recorded in this penetration is shown in Fig. 3. All fields positioned 5–6° to the left of the area centralis, slightly below the horizontal meridian. Scale, 0.5 mm.

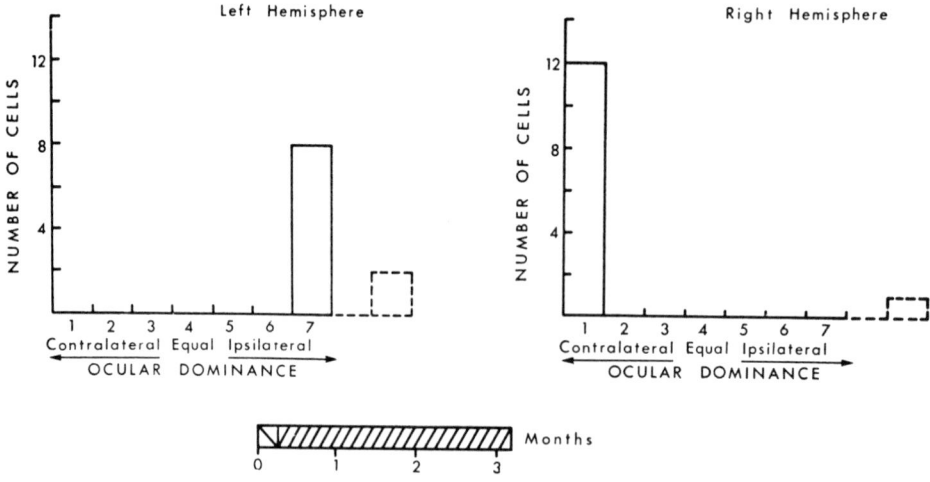

Fig. 5. Histograms showing ocular-dominance distribution of cells recorded in two penetrations, one in the left visual cortex and one in the right. A 3-month-old kitten with right eye closed by lid suture at 8 days (i.e., prior to normal eye-opening). Of a total of 23 cells, 3 were not influenced from either eye (interrupted lines). The remaining 20 could be driven only from the left (normally exposed) eye: 8 were recorded in the left hemisphere, and are therefore classed as group 7; 12 were recorded in the right hemisphere, and are classed as group 1.

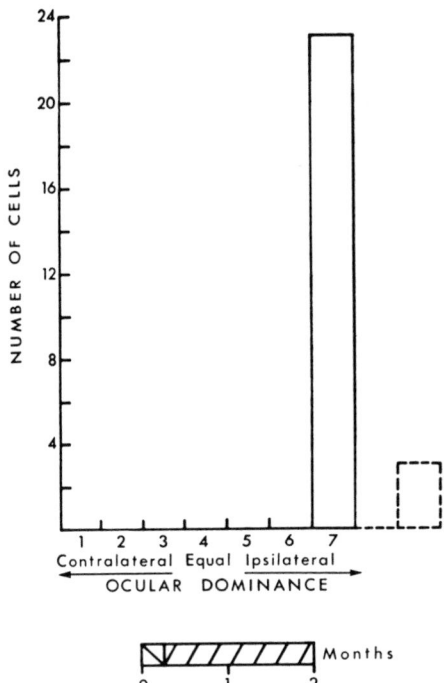

Fig. 6. *Ocular-dominance distribution of 26 cells recorded in the visual cortex contralateral to the deprived eye. This 2-month-old kitten had had its right eye covered from the time of normal eye-opening by a translucent contact lens; the left eye was normally exposed. Twenty-three cells were driven by the normally exposed (left, or ipsilateral) eye, and were therefore assigned to ocular-dominance group 7. Three cells could not be activated by either eye (interrupted lines).*

tration, briskly responsive to stimuli of the left eye, but with no hint of a response from the right.

In order to have a gross over-all impression of the retinal and cortical activity in this kitten, bilateral electroretinograms and evoked potential recordings were made (Fig. 8). The corneal electroretinograms evoked from either eye by a brief flash showed the normal a- and b-waves (Fig. 8, *A* and *B*). Successive responses were almost identical, and with stimulation rates of 1/sec. There was no sign of fatigue. (The amplitude was, if anything, greater from the deprived eye, but this could easily be due to minor differences in stimulating conditions.) This is consistent with the findings of Zetterström (12), that the electroretinogram develops normally except for a somewhat delayed time course in kittens raised in darkness. On the other hand, cortical potentials evoked from the two eyes

were far from equal. This was true for either hemisphere (Fig. 8, *C–F*). Responses from the previously occluded eye showed an initial positive component, but the later negative wave, so prominent in responses from the normal eye, was almost completely lacking. Moreover, the latency to stimulation of the deprived eye was 35–40 msec., as opposed to 25–30 msec. from the normal eye. That any cortical wave was evoked from the deprived eye indicates that some impulses originating from the eye must be relayed to the cortex, a finding that is not surprising since normal geniculate receptive fields were found in these animals. The striking differences in the negative phase support the single-unit findings in indicating that form deprivation and perhaps also moderate light deprivation during the first 3 months after birth can cause marked changes in the normal physiology of the striate cortex.

Deprivation of Kittens with Previous Visual Experience

In the first paper of this series (11) we showed that the geniculate atrophy resulting from 2–3 months of visual deprivation is much less if the animal has had 1 or 2 months of normal visual exposure, and that in the adult cat no detectable atrophy results from 3 months of monocular lid closure. The effects of delayed deprivation on the responses of cortical cells closely paralleled these anatomical findings. Figure 9 shows the ocular-dominance histograms from a kitten deprived by lid closure at the age of 9 weeks, for a period of 4 months. For both hemispheres the eye that had not been occluded was again abnormally dominant. Particularly abnormal was the large number of cells driven exclusively by the normal eye. Now, however, some cells (11 of the 34) could be driven also by the deprived eye, and while the deprived eye was dominant in only 3 of these, it clearly exerted far more influence than the deprived eyes of kittens operated on at birth. The responses of all cells seemed normal, and, in contrast to experiments done in kittens deprived from birth, there were no cells that could not be driven.

A second kitten was light-deprived by lid closure at the age of 2 months for a period of only 1 month. The ocular-dominance distribution of a penetration contralateral to the deprived eye was clearly abnormal (Fig. 10), though it was less so

Apical segment

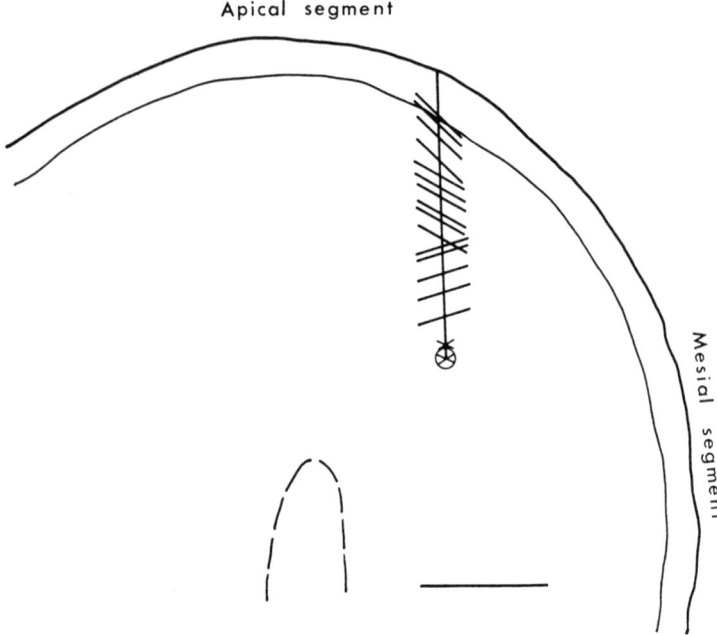

Mesial segment

Fig. 7. Reconstruction of a micro-electrode penetration through the left postlateral gyrus; ocular-dominance distribution of this penetration is given in Fig. 6. Conventions as in Fig. 4. Of the 17 recordings indicated, 8 were single-unit and 9 were 2-unit. Scale, 0.5 mm.

than that of the previous kitten. Again, all cells were responsive to patterned-light stimulation and had normal receptive fields.

In one kitten the nictitating membrane was sewn across the right eye at 5 weeks, for a 3-month period. It will be recalled that this animal showed no geniculate atrophy (11). Nevertheless the ocular-dominance distribution was clearly abnormal (Fig. 11), suggesting that a decrease in effectiveness of the deprived eye in driving cortical cells is not necessarily of geniculate origin. Once again, the ocular-dominance distribution of cortical cells was less distorted than that of a kitten deprived by a translucent occluder from birth, for an even shorter time (Fig. 6)

Finally, a single penetration made in the left hemisphere of an adult cat whose right eyelids had been sewn for 3 months was completely normal. Here again it will be recalled that the lateral geniculate bodies were histologically normal (11). The ocular-dominance distribution of 26 cells (Fig. 12) shows the usual over-all dominance of the contralateral eye—in this cat the eye that had been deprived. A few months of monocular lid closure was thus not enough to cause any obvious change

in cortical function; whether a longer period would have is not known.

DISCUSSION

The results of the present paper show that in kittens monocular deprivation of light and form from birth can produce both behavioral blindness in the deprived eye and a failure of cortical cells to respond to that eye. These findings must be viewed in the light of those reported in the preceding paper (9), that the specific responses seen in cortical cells of normal adult cats are present also in newborn and very young visually inexperienced kittens. We conclude that monocular deprivation produces physiological defects in a system that was once capable of functioning.

In view of the anatomical findings described in the first paper of this series (11), the results of the present study may at first seem paradoxical: that deprivation by lid closure from birth should produce in the geniculate marked atrophy of cells with only mild physiological effects, and in the cortex just the reverse, no obvious anatomical changes but profound physiological deficits. The reasons for

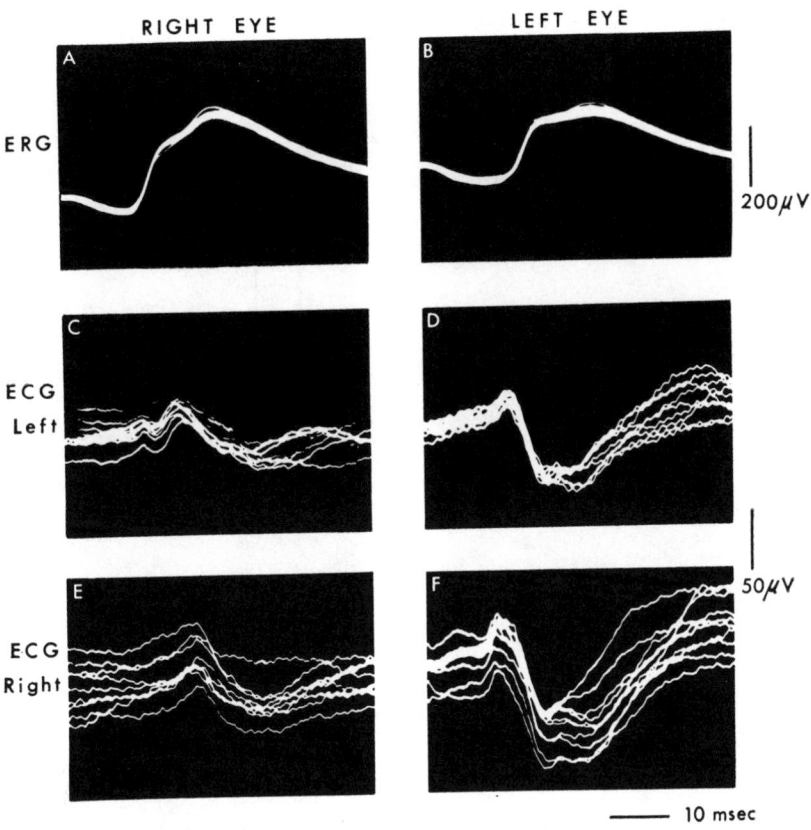

Fig. 8. *Corneal electroretinograms and cortical evoked potentials (ECGs) in a 2-month-old kitten whose right eye had been covered by a translucent contact lens from the time of normal eye-opening (same kitten as in Figs. 6 and 7). A, C, E: stimulation of right (previously occluded) eye. B, D, F: stimulation of left (normal) eye. A, B: electroretinograms. C, D: cortical evoked potentials, left hemisphere. E, F: cortical evoked potentials, right hemisphere. Positive deflections upward.*

the differences in morphological effects in the two structures are easy to imagine. Each geniculate cell receives visual input almost exclusively from one eye, and the cells receiving afferents from a given eye are aggregated in separate layers, so that any anatomical change is easy to see, the more so since it tends to contrast with the normality of the adjacent layers. The majority of cortical cells, on the other hand, have a binocular input (7), and the relatively few cells that are fed exclusively from one eye are intermixed with the others. One would therefore not expect a selective atrophy of the monocularly driven cells to stand out histologically.

It remains to account for the striking unresponsiveness of cortical cells to stimulation of the deprived eye, compared with the relative normality of geniculate responses and receptive fields. The cortical impairment was just as marked after dep-

rivation with a translucent occluder as with lid closure an especially surprising result since in the lateral geniculate the amount of light deprivation seemed to be important in determining the degree of anatomical change (11). These differences between geniculate and cortical cells can perhaps be best understood if we recall that in the normal cat cortical cells are much less responsive than geniculate cells to diffuse light (5, 6). Any light reaching the retina would thus help to keep geniculate cells active. On the other hand, most cortical cells would be practically uninfluenced regardless of the type of occlusion, and over a long period they might become unable to respond even to patterned stimulation of the deprived eye.

In discussing morphological changes in the lateral geniculate following visual deprivation (11), we pointed out that the maintained activity persist-

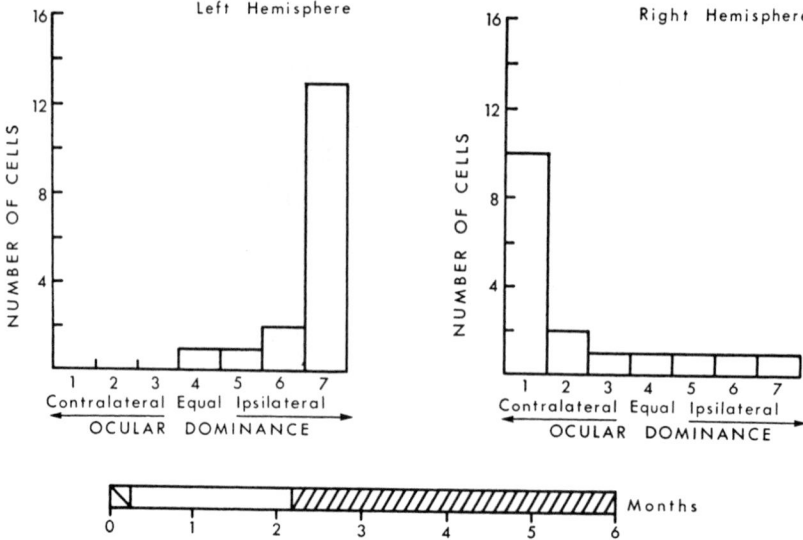

Fig. 9. Histograms of ocular-dominance distribution of 34 cells recorded in two penetrations, one in the left visual cortex and one in the right. Kitten whose right eye was closed by lid suture at 9 weeks, for a period of 4 months. Seventeen cells recorded from each hemisphere. All cells were influenced by patterned-light stimulation.

ing in the retina under these conditions of lid suture or translucent occlusion is insufficient to prevent the atrophy. The same obviously applies to the present cortical recordings: the functional pathway up to the cortex was evidently not maintained by whatever activity persisted in the lateral geniculate body.

Though we have no direct way of knowing the exact site of the abnormality responsible for cortical unresponsiveness, the main defect must be central to the lateral geniculate body, since geniculate cells respond well to stimulation of the deprived eye. Nevertheless these geniculate impulses have no apparent effect on cortical cells, even though the cortical cells fire perfectly well to stimulation of the normal eye. This suggests that the abnormality is in the region of the synapse between the axon terminals of geniculate cells (those receiving input from the deprived eye) and the cortical cells on which these terminals end.

Though the most abnormal feature in the physiological studies was the ocular-dominance distribution, there was another consistent difference from normal penetrations: in every experiment in kittens deprived from birth there were a few cells that could not be driven from either eye. This probably cannot be explained by the immaturity of the kittens, since in a previous study of even

younger animals all of the cells could be driven by appropriate stimuli (9). A more likely explanation is that the unresponsive cells were connected exclusively with the covered eye—at least the proportion of nondriven cells was about what one would

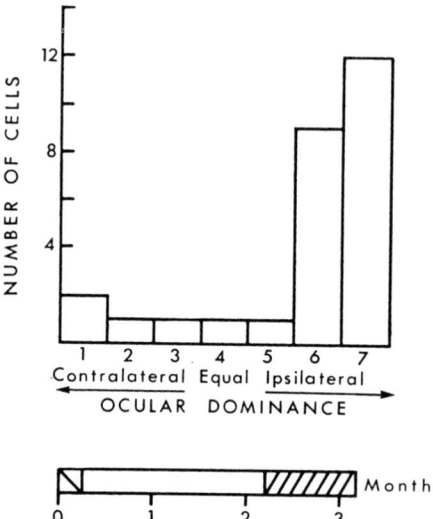

Fig. 10. Ocular-dominance histogram from a kitten whose right eye was closed by lid suture at the age of 9 weeks, for 1 month. Twenty-one cells were recorded from the left visual cortex. All cells were influenced by patterned-light stimulation.

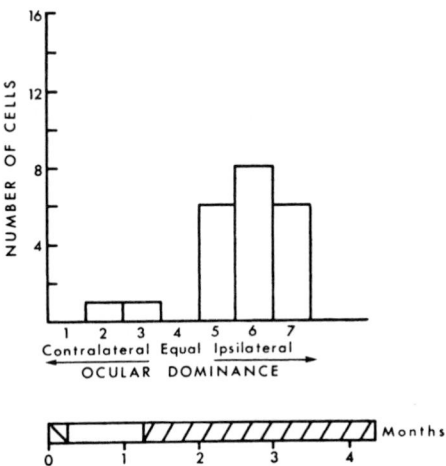

Fig. 11. *Ocular-dominance histogram of 22 cells recorded from the left visual cortex; kitten with nictitating membrane sutured across the right eye at an age of 5 weeks, for 3 months. The left (ipsilateral, normal) eye dominated markedly, and all cells were influenced by patterned-light stimulation.*

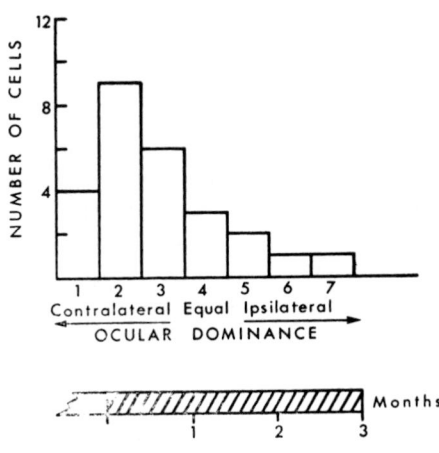

Fig. 12. *Ocular-dominance distribution of 26 cells recorded in the left visual cortex of an adult cat whose right eye had been covered by lid suture for a period of 3 months. As in the normal cat, the contralateral eye—in this case the deprived eye—dominated.*

expect on that assumption. Had it not been for their maintained activity these cells would probably have gone undetected, and one wonders if the maintained firing does not reflect some other, nonvisual input.

While the site of the physiological defect may be within the cortex, as suggested above, it would probably be wrong to assume that abnormalities at the geniculate level did not also contribute to the unresponsiveness of the cortical cells. Many of the geniculate cells were atrophic; in recordings from the geniculate there was an over-all decrease in activity in the layers connected with the deprived eye, and a few fields seemed abnormal (11). The cortical evoked responses to a flash made it clear that impulses in at least some geniculate fibers associated with the deprived eye reached the cortex of both hemispheres, but the marked increase in latency suggests that this input may have been abnormal. Thus it is probable that defects at several levels, from retina to primary visual cortex, contributed to the observed physiological abnormalities. At present we have no direct way of assessing their relative importance.

The behavior of our monocularly deprived kittens, under conditions in which they could use only the deprived eye, suggested the presence of gross visual deficits. This confirms the binocular-deprivation studies of other observers in several different mammalian species (2, 4, 10, 3). In monocularly deprived animals the visual pathway beyond the point of convergence of impulses from the two eyes was presumably intact, since cortical cells were actively driven from the normal eye, and since the animals were able to see with that eye. This suggests that also in bilaterally deprived animals the defect may not necessarily be at a far central level: e.g., the defect need not be in visually guided motor function, or the result of some emotional disturbance. There may indeed be such defects, but our results make it likely that abnormalities exist at a more peripheral level as well.

In interpreting the blindness resulting from raising animals in darkness it has generally been assumed that some of the neural connections necessary for vision are not present at birth, and that their development depends on visual experience early in life. Our results suggest the alternative possibility, that certain connections are intact at birth and become defective through disuse. One must, however, make one reservation: deprivation of one eye may be quite different in its morphological and physiological effects from binocular dark-raising. Conceivably if one eye is not stimulated, the fate of its projections in the central visual pathway may partly depend on whether or not the other eye is stimulated. This question of a possible competition between the eyes can only be settled experimentally, by studying animals that have been binocularly deprived of vision. For example, Baxter (1), comparing records from the visual cortex of normal and dark-raised kittens, could find no striking difference in the size or shape of the evoked potentials in the two groups. This finding contrasts sharply with the difference we saw in cortical potentials evoked from the normal, as opposed to the deprived eye (Fig. 8), and it remains to be learned whether or not the discrepancy reflects a difference in the two types of preparation.

The susceptibility of very young kittens to a few months of visual deprivation apparently does not extend to older animals, since there is a detectable lessening of effects when deprivation is begun at 2 months, and an absence of behavioral or physiological effects in adults. This is a clear demonstration of a pronounced difference between kittens and adults in susceptibility to deprivation, a difference one might have expected from the profound visual defects observed after removal of congenital cataracts in man, as opposed to the absence of blindness on removal of cataracts acquired later in life.

SUMMARY

1. Single-unit recordings were made from striate cortex of kittens in which one eye had been deprived of vision either from birth or subsequently, and for various periods of time.
2. Kittens deprived from birth for 2–3 months showed profoundly defective vision in the deprived eye. Visual placing and following reactions were absent, and there was no hint of any ability to perceive form. Pupillary light reflexes were nevertheless normal.
3. In kittens deprived from birth, either by suturing the lids of one eye or by covering the cornea with a translucent contact occluder, the great majority of cortical cells were actively driven from the normal eye, with normal receptive fields. On the other hand, only 1 cell out of 84 was at all influenced by the deprived eye, and in that cell the receptive fields in the two eyes were abnormal. A few cells could not be driven from either eye.
4. In one 2-month-old kitten monocularly deprived with a translucent contact occluder, the corneal electroretinograms were normal in the two eyes. On flashing a light in the previously occluded eye the slow-wave potentials evoked in the visual cortex of the two hemispheres were highly abnormal, compared with responses from the normal eye.
5. One to two months of normal visual experience prior to monocular deprivation by lid suture or with a translucent occluder reduced the severity of the physiological defect, even though the ability of the deprived eye to influence cortical cells was still well below normal. On the other hand, 3 months of deprivation by lid closure in an adult cat produced no detectable physiological abnormality.
6. We conclude that monocular deprivation in kittens can lead to un-responsiveness of cortical cells to stimulation of the deprived eye, and that the defect is most severe in animals deprived from bith. The relative normality of responses in newborn kittens (9) suggests that the physiological defect in the deprived kittens represents a disruption of connections that were present at birth.

ACKNOWLEDGMENT

We express our thanks to Jane Chen and Janet Tobie for their technical assistance.

References

1. Baxter, B. L. *An Electrophysiological Study of the Effects of Sensory Deprivation* Doctoral dissertation (unpublished). University of Chicago, 1959.
2. Berger, H. Experimentell-anatomische Studien über die durch den Mangel optischer Reize veranlassten Entwicklungshemmungen im Occipitallappen des Hundes und der Katze. *Arch. Psychiat. Nervenkr.*, 1900, *33:* 521–567.
3. Chow, K. L. and Nissen, H. W. Interocular transfer of learning in visually naïve and experienced infant chimpanzees. *J. comp. Physiol. Psychol.*, 1955, *48:* 229–237.
4. Goodman, L. Effect of total absence of function on the optic system of rabbits. *Amer. J. Physiol.*, 1932, *100:* 46–63.
5. Hubel, D. H. Single unit activity in striate cortex of unrestrained cats. *J. Physiol.*, 1959, *147:* 226–238.
6. Hubel, D. H. and Wiesel, T. N. Receptive fields of single neurones in the cat's striate cortex. *J. Physiol.*, 1959, *148:* 574–591.
7. Hubel, D. H. and Wiesel, T. N. Receptive fields, binocular interaction and functional architecture in the cat's visual cortex. *J. Physiol,* 1962, *160:* 106–154.
8. Hubel, D. H. and Wiesel, T. N. Shape and arrangement of columns in cat's striate cortex. *J. Physiol.*, 1963, *165:* 559–568.

9. Hubel, D. H. and Wiesel, T. N. Receptive fields of cells in striate cortex of very young, visually inexperienced kittens. *J. Neurophysiol.,* 1963, *26:* 994–1002.

10. Riesen, A. H., Kurke, M. I., and Mellinger, J. C. Interocular transfer of habits learned monocularly in visually naïve and visually experienced cats. *J. comp. Physiol. Psychol.,* 1953, *46:* 166–172.

11. Wiesel, T. N. and Hubel, D. H. Effects of visual deprivation on morphology and physiology of cells in the cat's lateral geniculate body. *J. Neurophysiol.,* 1963, *26:* 978–993.

12. Zetterström, B. The effect of light on the appearance and development of the electroretinogram in newborn kittens. *Acta physiol. scand.,* 1955, *35:* 272–279.

AFTERWORD

If one were to sum up the main message of the first of these three papers, the stress would be on the relative normality of the geniculate physiology in the face of the marked abnormality of the anatomy. Part of the explanation of the apparent discrepancy could lie in the methods: for the anatomy one had the possibility of a direct comparison of neighboring layers, whereas it was harder in interpreting the physiology to compare sluggishness of responses and the sizes of the field centers. In retrospect, the relatively mild differences we saw in the physiology of the left-eye and right-eye layers were probably real. The final explanation for the anatomical shrinkage came much later, with Ray Guillery's discovery that the geniculate cell shrinkage was probably the result of paring down of the axonal terminals of these cells in the cortex, accompanying the shrinkage of the cortical ocular dominance columns. We shall come back to this topic when we discuss the relative roles, in deprivation, of disuse and eye competition.

The second paper gives evidence that some at least of the wiring of the cat visual system is present at birth. The responses of cortical cells in the newborn clearly had some of the specificity that we had seen in the adult cat visual cortex. Because of the frailty of the newborn kittens and the relative opacity of the ocular media in the first few weeks, we usually waited for a few weeks before testing, sewing both eyes closed just at the time of normal eye opening and hoping that in the few weeks that followed any deprivation effects would be minimal. What surprised us was the presence of *any* orientation selectivity in these kittens. In retrospect, if we had given more stress to the differences between normal kittens and normal adult cats (the broader orientation tuning curves and so on, in the kittens) we might have saved ourselves some of the controversy that came in the years that followed. We never doubted the importance of experience or learning in the development of neural connections—that would be tantamount to claiming that learning had nothing to do with neural connections—but what was new was our evidence for any innate connections. The newborn brain was (and perhaps still is) thought by some psychologists to be a tabula rasa on which postnatal experience writes its messages. In the 1960s, to claim otherwise could get one into political trouble. We felt that in this series of studies we had bolstered the arguments for both sides, for both nature and nature. One of our main discoveries was, after all, the importance of postnatal experience for the maintenance of cortical connections.

Much of the controversy that followed these results was settled by our subsequent deprivation studies in macaque monkeys, because the relative maturity of responses in the newborn is so much more evident. In newborn kittens the relative immaturity of visual capabilities made the state of the connections far harder to establish, and it was no wonder that others were more impressed by the lack of responsiveness than by the specificity that one had to struggle to detect.

In at least one respect we may have gone too far in interpreting our results. We thought that the connections responsible for the orientation selectivity, and so on, in the newborn, must necessarily be the result of genetic coding. Nevertheless, we were careful, at least in our mainline papers, not to make any such claims in public: our molecular-biological friends had stressed to us the unlikelihood of there being enough genes to code for even a small percentage of the connections that must be present in the newborn animal. It had not occurred to us, or presumably to anyone else, that prenatal retinal activity unrelated to the environment could play a part in promoting cortical connections. Today we know from work by Meister, Wong, Baylor, and Shatz (*Science* 1991, 252:939) that in the months prior to birth, waves of activity crisscross the retina and are accompanied by impulses in retinal ganglion cells. Although there is as yet no evidence that this activity is responsible for specificity of connections beyond the retina, we are no longer forced, by exclusion, to the notion that the richly detailed connections that must exist in the visual cortex must all be determined by purely genetic processes.

The results of this second paper on innate connections were important in our interpretation of the third paper, reporting the physiological results of eye closures. We were forced to recognize the possibility that the abnormalities were caused by some kind of withering of disused connections that had existed at birth, as opposed to a failure to develop them though lack of experience. This went against interpretations, expressed or implied, of all the dark-rearing work that had been done previously. We would not have denied the importance of experience in developing connections (one is after all not born knowing the alphabet), but suddenly one had to admit that deprivation might, at least in part, be a matter of failure through disuse.

What had probably not occurred to us was the possibility that something more than simple disuse might be involved. Only when we deprived both eyes of vision, and when we induced artificial squint—the subject of the next set of deprivation/development papers—were we forced to conclude that our cortical deprivation effects were more related to competition than to simple disuse. That of course left the geniculate anatomical defects, the pallor and shrinkage, unaccounted for, since geniculate cells are fed exclusively by one eye, with no chance of competition. Or so we thought—until the work of Guillery and his colleagues, to be described in the Afterwords to the next set of deprivation papers.

Finally, today we are so used to thinking of the visual cortex as housing two types of columns, one subserving orientation and the other, ocular dominance, that we tend to forget how long it took to recognize the existence of the ocular-dominance columns. In our 1962 magnum opus on normal cat

cortex, we do, somewhat reluctantly, admit to seeing hints of grouping of cells according to eye dominance, but only, as it were, to keep the possibility open. At the time of these three papers, ocular dominance columns were still only vaguely in our minds. Later, three kinds of evidence forced us to recognize ocular dominance columns: the strabismus experiments in the cat, which made them obvious; our studies of the normal adult macaque monkey cortex, in which they are better developed; and the use of transport labels after eye injection, done by us in monkeys and by Torsten, Carla Shatz, and Sivert Lindström in cats.

Chapter 22 • Second Group of Deprivation Papers •

FOREWORD

The next three deprivation papers (pp. 404–439), which came out in 1965, deal with the effects of binocular eye closure, artificial strabismus (cross-eye or wall-eye), and the recovery induced by eye reopening. Finally, in the fourth (1970) paper (pp. 440–452), we examined the time course of the critical period.

In our first deprivation studies we had obvious reasons for closing one eye rather than both. Interpretation of responses was easier (or so it seemed to us at the time) because we had the normal eye as a control, and the procedure was certainly kinder to the kittens. This approach seemed vindicated when, in the very first monocular eye-closure experiments, practically all the cells were monopolized by the normal eye, with only rare responses from the eye that had been sutured. Furthermore, it was hard enough, in the beginning, to suture one eye closed and keep it closed, without attempting a doubly difficult binocular suture. Finally, it would have been much harder to see the geniculate morphological changes had we closed both eyes and not had the built-in control that let us compare neighboring geniculate layers. Nevertheless, out of a stubborn sense of rigor, we finally decided to do a binocular suture, with every expectation that we would be unable to drive cells from either eye. The result came as a complete surprise and convinced us that while controls can seem a bore, they should not be avoided indefinitely. (Our graduate students know this very well—they even believe in controls—but we were trained to be clinicians, not scientists. One colleague, a scientist, nevertheless remarked that her definition of a fool was one who did the control before doing the experiment.) In any case, along with the results on strabismus, the binocular-closure result provided the first indications that the deprivation effects we had been seeing were not related just to disuse, but must involve competition between the two eyes. This first binocularly deprived animal showed such striking and convincing differences from what we had expected that we wrote the paper on the strength of that animal alone and sent it, along with the two companion papers, to Eric Kandel for his comments. He wrote back full of enthusiasm, but with the plea that, given the importance of the binocular closure result, would we please consider doing just a few more binocular animals. We decided he was right and reluctantly rolled up our sleeves and spent an extra month or so. The results were essentially the same. We are glad we took the extra time and feel indebted to Eric.

The strabismus experiments, like the eye closures, were motivated by our clinical backgrounds. The unilateral blindness that can result from the cross-eye or wall-eye state, also known as *lazy eye* or amblyopia ex anopsia, is one of the commonest forms of human blindness in the Western world. It seems fair to say that before these experiments no one had thought that the site of the abnormality could be anywhere but the eye itself. We had no idea what we would find, but our knowledge of the physiology of the visual path up to and including the primary visual cortex seemed to put us in a good position to ask. We took a litter of six newborn kittens and proceeded to cut the right medial rectus muscle in all of them, causing the eye to turn out. After about three months we tested vision behaviorally in one of the kittens by putting an opaque contact lens over first one eye and then the other one and watching the animal get around. To our dismay vision seemed normal in both eyes. What we had obviously produced was an alternating strabismus, the condition commonly seen in humans with divergent squint, in which vision remains normal in both eyes but the eyes take turns fixating, while the non-fixating eye diverges. There seemed little point in going any further with these kittens. We were saddled with a roomful of wall-eyed kittens and no expectation of learning anything from them.

We debated whether to do any recordings, but finally we tossed a coin and decided to go ahead and waste a day recording from one kitten. We were dumbfounded at the result. We encountered one monocular cell after the other, first a batch driven from only one eye, then a batch from only the other eye. We had to concede that we did indeed have a result. That week, for the first and only time, we did a crash program of three experiments, on Monday, Wednesday, and Friday, and wrapped up the entire squint project. The squint experiments were thus unlike the slow plodding of most of the deprivation work.

We obviously had to find out whether the squint result was a matter of not using the eyes together in the normal way, or not using them together at all. This motivated us to do the next series using alternating occlusion, in which we placed an opaque occluder over one eye one day and the other eye the next, over a period of several weeks. Again we were surprised by the clear and striking result, practically identical to the strabismus results. (We naturally worry about the implications of this result for the commonly employed treatment of human lazy eye by placing a patch over the normal eye. That procedure does indeed work, to the extent of improving the vision of the lazy eye, but can only impair any possible residual stereopsis. And stereopsis is presumably a large part of the reason we have two eyes.)

The artificial squint experiments provided an unexpected byproduct, a clear demonstration of ocular dominance columns in cats. We had detected some grouping of cells according to ocular dominance in our 1962 paper but were relatively unimpressed. In normal cats, contrary to what one finds in monkeys, the variations in eye dominance are gentle rather than abrupt. Strabismus apparently had the effect of sharpening the differences in ocular dominance, so that a cell that in early life only mildly favored one eye would come to favor it markedly or end up responding only to that eye. (Groups 2 and 3 cells would thus become group 1, and 5 and 6 become 7.) In the squint animals we saw striking sequences of cells, ten or twenty in a row, all monopolized by one eye, then another stream of cells monopolized by the other eye. We concluded that similar groupings according to eye preference must be present in normal cats, but that the squint had made them more obvious.

The cat recovery study, like the strabismus study, was motivated by clinical considerations. The slow and unsatisfactory recovery of children after removal of congenital cataracts had led us not to expect dramatic recovery when our cats' eyes were reopened after prolonged deprivations, and indeed we saw little. Obviously our use of reverse suturing—opening the lids of the deprived eye and closing the lids of the normal eye—was modelled on the use of eye patching in cases of human amblyopia, and it certainly encouraged the recovery from amblyopia. The results further strengthened our impression that we were dealing with competitive effects and not simply disuse. Our alternating-occlusion results, on the other hand, suggested that eye patching in humans should only lead to a further loss of the ability of the two eyes to act together, and should if anything lead to further impairment of stereopsis.

We still had to establish the critical period for eye closures. In the third paper of the first set, on the physiological results of deprivation, we had shown a diminished effect when the closure was delayed and absence of effects in an adult. It remained to narrow down the time course. This, the topic of the fourth paper in this series (pp. 440–452), was slow work—we thought of it as plotting a set of graphs in which we varied two parameters, the onset and the cessation of the deprivation, and required an experiment, and a kitten, for each point.

The concientious reader of this book will probably notice that the references to the second paper in this series, on strabismus (p. 430), are somewhat less generous than those that follow most of our papers. When we wrote the penultimate draft we noticed that all but one of the references were to ourselves. We looked at each other, and one of us asked, "Do we really need this one?" We agreed that generosity should have its limits, and removed it.

Comparison of the Effects of Unilateral and Bilateral Eye Closure on Cortical Unit Responses in Kittens[1]

TORSTEN N. WIESEL AND DAVID H. HUBEL • *Neurophysiology Laboratory, Department of Pharmacology,*

Harvard Medical School, Boston, Massachusetts

INTRODUCTION

In the normal cat or kitten about four-fifths of cells in the striate cortex can be driven by both eyes (3, 4). If, however, one eye of a newborn kitten is sewn shut and the visual cortex recorded from 3 months later, only a small fraction of cells can be driven from the deprived eye (8). In contrast, many cells in the lateral geniculate are driven normally from the deprived eye (7), suggesting that the abnormality occurs somewhere between geniculate cells and cortex. Since clear receptive-field orientations and directional preferences to movement are seen in cortical cells of newborn visually inexperienced kittens, the deprivation effects presumably represent some sort of disruption of innately determined connections, rather than a failure of postnatal development related to lack of experience.

In these experiments the use of monocular deprivation made it possible to compare adjacent geniculate layers, and also to compare the two eyes in their ability to influence cortical cells, so that each animal acted, in a sense, as its own control. The results led us to expect that depriving both eyes for similar periods would lead to an almost total unresponsiveness of cortical cells to stimulation of either eye. That should be so, provided the effects of depriving one eye were independent of whether or not the other eye was simultaneously deprived. It seemed worthwhile to test such an assumption, since any interdependence of the two pathways would be of considerable interest. We accordingly raised kittens with both eyes covered by lid suture, and recorded from the striate cortex when the animals had reached an age of 2½–4½ months.

METHODS

In 5 kittens the lids of both eyes were sutured together bilaterally 6–18 days after birth, just before normal eye opening or up to 8 days after (Table 1). Lid closure reduces retinal illumination by 4–5 log units (7), and undoubtedly prevents any form vision. One kitten was observed behaviorally at 3 months of age and was kept aside for physiological studies of recovery (9). Single-cell recordings were made in the other 4 kittens (no. 3–6) at 2½–4½ months of age. In all, 10 penetrations were made and 139 units studied.

In two additional kittens the lids of one eye were sutured before the time of normal eye opening. These animals (no. *1* and *2*) were recorded from at 8–10 weeks, and the results, together with those from three monocular closures previously reported (8), were compared with the results of the binocular closures.

The acute experiments were done under thiopental anesthesia, and succinylcholine was injected intravenously in order to paralyze the extraocular muscles. Tungsten micro-electrodes were used in a closed-chamber system (2, 3). Receptive fields were mapped by projecting small spots of white light upon a wide white tangent screen, which the animal faced from a distance of 1.5 m. A background light was set at low photopic or mesopic levels (-1 to $+1$ $\log_{10}$ cd/m^2), and the intensity of the stimulating light was 1–1.5 log units brighter than the background.

After the recordings the animals were perfused with normal saline followed by 10% formalin. The brains were embedded in celloidin, sectioned at 25 μ, and stained with cresyl violet. These histological sections were used for reconstruction of the electrode tracks and for a morphological study of the visual pathways. Methods of measuring the size of cells in the lateral geniculate are described in a previous paper (7).

RESULTS

MONOCULAR CLOSURES. In our first series of deprivation experiments (8) three kittens were deprived by monocular lid closure from birth to 2½ to 3 months. Recordings made at that time gave highly consistent results: in each of the 4 penetrations there were steady successions of cells responding to

From *J. Neurophysiol.* (1965) 28: 1029–1040

Received for publication December 23, 1964.

[1]This work was supported in part by Public Health Service Grants NB-02260-05 and NB 05554-01, and in part by U. S. Air Force Contracts AF-AFOSR-410-63A and AF 49(638)1443.

the eye that had been open, interrupted by an occasional cell that would not respond to either eye, against an almost continuous background of unresolved unitary activity responding briskly to the normal eye. With a single exception, all of the 85 cells recorded gave no response to the previously closed eye, and at no stage in any of the penetrations was the unresolved background responsive to that eye.

In the paper that follows (5) it is shown that normal cortical cells are to some extent segregated with respect to eye dominance. The possibility arose that after monocular deprivation any cells still influenced from the deprived eye might be aggregated into small isolated islands, and might therefore not be encountered in a small number of penetrations. We therefore made a more intensive search, recording from 115 more cells in 2 kittens deprived by monocular closure from birth to an age of 2–3 months. Five additional penetrations were made, the results of which are shown schematically in Fig. 1. Each electrode track is expanded so as to illustrate the relative depths at which cells were recorded. The position of each cell is represented by a short horizontal line placed in the appropriate vertical row according to ocular dominance group; positions of cells that could not be driven are shown in a separate row to the right of the others.

Two penetrations were made in the first of these kittens, and are illustrated to the left in Fig. 1. No cells were driven from the right (deprived) eye. Cells recorded from the left hemisphere, all driven from the left eye, were therefore classed as group 7; cells recorded from the right hemisphere were all group 1. These two penetrations were thus similar to almost all of those made in the previous monocular deprivation series.

Three penetrations, reconstructed to the right in Fig. 1, were made in kitten no. 2. Two of these turned out to contain a region in which successively recorded cells and unresolved background activity were driven from both eyes or from the deprived eye alone. Each region formed only a small portion of the whole penetration. In the third penetration cells were driven entirely by the normal eye, with one exception, a cell that was influenced by the deprived eye but strongly dominated by the normal eye.

Of the 12 cells that were driven by the deprived eye, all but 1 were abnormal in one way or another. Most of them responded in a vague, unpredictable manner, and most lacked a precise receptive-field orientation. Some showed an unusually pronounced decline in responsiveness after several seconds of repeated stimulation. Curiously, some cells were driven abnormally not only from the deprived eye but also from the eye that had been open all along. Similar abnormal cells were found after binocular deprivation, as described below, and after attempts to induce recovery (9).

Figure 2 shows the ocular-dominance histogram of all 199 cells recorded in monocular deprivation experiments. The 13 cells that were influenced from the deprived eye amounted to about 7% of the total. While this figure is larger than the original monocular deprivation experiments suggested, it is undoubtedly more reliable, and confirms our impression that the proportion of cells influenced from the deprived eye is small. The proportion driven normally must be very small indeed. Perhaps more important is the suggestion that such cells may be aggregated in small regions of cortex which together make up only a small fraction of the total volume.

BINOCULAR CLOSURE. From the monocular closures one might have expected to find large areas of cortex containing no responsive cells, and only small islands of tissue with cells responding in an aberrant way to one eye or both. Right from the outset, however, it was clear that we were not dealing with cortex in which most cells were unresponsive. Throughout the greater part of all nine penetrations in kittens no. 3–6, most cells not only responded to visual stimuli, but over half of the ones that responded did so normally.

The cortex of these animals was nevertheless by no means normal. Numerous sluggishly responding unpredictable cells with vaguely defined receptive field properties made the penetrations difficult and frustrating. Of 139 cells recorded, 45 (32%) were classed as abnormal, as opposed to 57 (41%) normal cells. Thirty-seven cells (27%) could not be driven by visual stimulation at all, and were recognized only by their maintained firing. The cortex may have contained unresponsive cells without maintained firing; they would not have been observed, in which case 27% would be too low. These results are for the 4 kittens taken together, but figures for the individual experiments

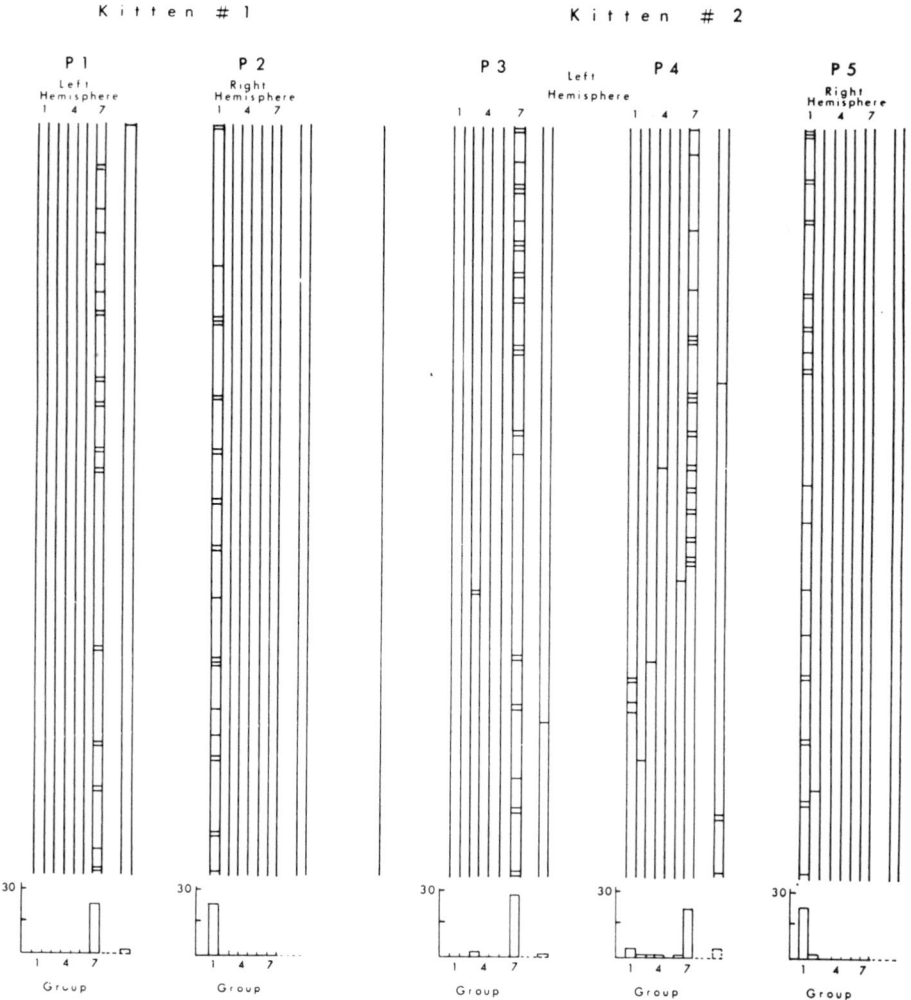

Fig. 1. Schematic reconstructions of five microelectrode penetrations in two kittens. Kitten 1 was 8 weeks old and kitten 2, 10 weeks; both had the right eye closed by lid suture at 8 days. Each penetration extended into cortical gray matter for about 1.5 mm. The penetrations are drawn so as to indicate relative positions of individual cells; each cell is represented by a short horizontal line placed in the appropriate vertical row according to ocular-dominance group. The separate row to the right of group 7 is for unresponsive cells. The total number of cells in each group is indicated in the histogram at the bottom. (For definitions of ocular-dominance groups see legend of Fig. 2.)

were in reasonable agreement (Table 1); the proportion of cells that could be driven, normally or abnormally, ranged from 67% for kitten no. *3* to 80% for no. *5.*

The normal cells showed all of the usual specific responses to properly oriented line stimuli. Some receptive fields were "simple" and others "complex," in the sense in which we have used these terms elsewhere (2, 3). Cells that responded abnormally had lost much of their specificity for

precisely oriented lines, reacting with uniform briskness over a wide range of angles, and often showing no orientation preference at all. Some of these cells were driven from both eyes, and gave abnormal responses to both. Like most normal cortical cells, the abnormal ones generally gave no responses to diffuse light. None had concentric center-surround fields of the type found in the lateral geniculate body or retina. Many showed a tendency to fire actively the first time a stimulus was

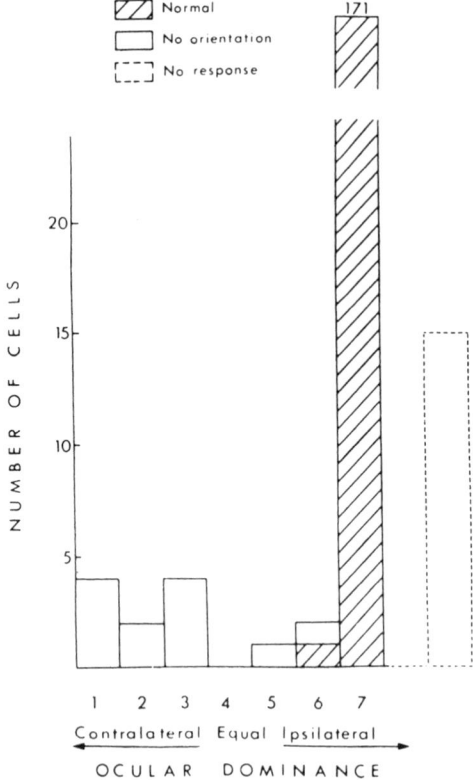

Fig. 2. Ocular-dominance distribution of 199 cells recorded in the visual cortex of 5 monocularly deprived kittens. The animals were 8–14 weeks old and all had the right eye closed by lid suture from the time of normal eye opening. Shading indicates cells that had the usual specific response properties to visual stimulation; absence of shading indicates cells that lacked the normal orientation specificity. Interrupted lines indicate cells that did not respond to either eye. Cells of group 1 were driven only by the contralateral eye; for cells of group 2 there was marked dominance of the contralateral eye; for group 3, slight dominance. For cells in group 4 there was no obvious difference between the two eyes. In group 5 the ipsilateral eye dominated slightly; in group 6, markedly, and in group 7 the cells were driven only by the ipsilateral eye.

introduced but with declining vigor as the stimulus was repeated. A period of 1/2 to 1 min. without stimuli was usually enough to revive a cell fully. We have observed this behavior in cells of normal adult cats in all three visual areas, but not as frequently or to as pronounced a degree.

The ocular-dominance distribution is shown for one binocularly deprived kitten (no. 3) in Fig. 3A, and for all four kittens in Fig. 3B. The major-ity of cells could be driven from both eyes. Normal and abnormal cells were present in all groups in Fig. 3B, though there was probably some decrease in the proportion of cells in groups 3–5 compared with the distribution in normal cats. The most conspicuous abnormality was seen in the large group of nonresponding cells, shown by the interrupted column to the right of each histogram. We have no evidence that unresponsive cells occur in the normal striate cortex (3, 4).

In Fig. 4 one of three penetrations made in kitten 4 is reconstructed in detail. To the right of the figure is a tracing of a coronal section through the right postlateral gyrus. To the left, the electrode track is expanded as in Fig. 1. Lines within the circles indicate by their tilt the receptive-field orientation. As in the normal animal, cells were aggregated according to receptive-field orientation. Within a single column, such as that formed by cells 1–10 and 13–16 and indicated by the large brackets, there were both normal cells and cells with nonoriented fields. Unresponsive cells were sometimes grouped together (cells 23–27), but were also frequently intermixed with more normal cells (12, 19, and 20). Finally, the figure illustrates a tendency for cells to be aggregated in the cortex according to the predominating eye. For example, cells 1–13 form a sequence in which the contralateral eye consistently dominated. As mentioned above, this grouping according to eye dominance is also found in normal cats, and is examined in more detail in the next paper (5).

HISTOLOGICAL OBSERVATIONS IN THE VISUAL PATHWAYS. Since the cortical physiology was so different from what might have been expected from the monocular closures, we were anxious to learn whether or not the geniculate histology would be consistent in the two studies. In monocular closures (7) there were marked abnormalities in the layers receiving input from the deprived eye, consisting of a change in staining characteristics of cells, a decrease in the volume of cell bodies and nuclei, and a loss of the clear unstained substance between cell nests. The changes were obvious at a glance, on comparing the normal and abnormal layers. The decrease in mean cross-sectional area of cell bodies amounted in the dorsal layers to 30–40%.

In animals with binocular closure there was surprisingly little to see on casual inspection. This

Table 1. *Effects of Bilateral Eye Closure on Cortical Cells*

	Kitten 3	Kitten 4	Kitten 5	Kitten 6	
Age at time of eye closure, days	18	18	6	6	
Age at time of recording, months	4½	4	2½	3	Totals (cells)
Number of penetrations	3	3	2	2	
Normal cells	14 (36%)	17 (46%)	15 (43%)	11 (39%)	57 (41%)
Abnormal but responsive cells	12 (31%)	10 (27%)	13 (37%)	10 (36%)	45 (32%)
Unresponsive cells	13 (33%)	10 (27%)	7 (20%)	7 (25%)	37 (27%)
Totals (cells)	39	37	35	28	139

is illustrated in the photomicrograph of Fig. 5*A*. The difference, however, was apparent rather than real. The changes were not obvious since abnormal cells did not stand out against normal ones on the same slide. Nevertheless, comparison with a normal geniculate as in Fig. 5*B,* or with normal layers in monocularly deprived kittens, showed that the same abnormalities were indeed present, and to an equal degree. In kitten 3 measurement of 200 cells in the two dorsal layers (A and A₁) showed a mean cross-sectional area of about 180 μ², compared with a normal value of about 300 μ². This represents a shrinkage of about 40%. The nucleus and nucleo-

lus likewise showed marked shrinkage. No obvious histological changes were seen on simple inspection of Nissl or myelin sections of retina, optic nerve, superior colliculus, or cortex.

Behavioral Effects. As the lid-sutured kittens grew up they adapted remarkably well to their blindness. They learned to move about adroitly in the large room where they were kept, and became so familiar with the objects in the room that a casual observer would hardly have guessed they could not see. Vision was tested in one kitten at 3½ months by observing its behavior after separating

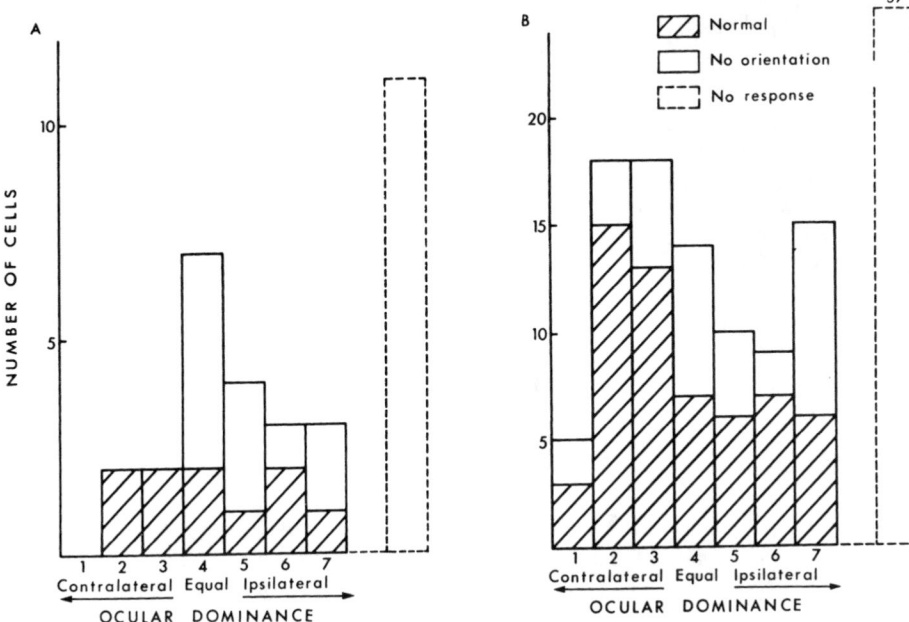

Fig. 3. A: *distribution of 32 cells according to eye preference, in a kitten (no. 3) raised for the first 3 months with both eyes sutured closed. One penetration was made in each hemisphere. B: ocular-dominance distribution of 126 cells recorded from the 4 binocularly deprived kittens (no. 3–6), in 10 penetrations.*

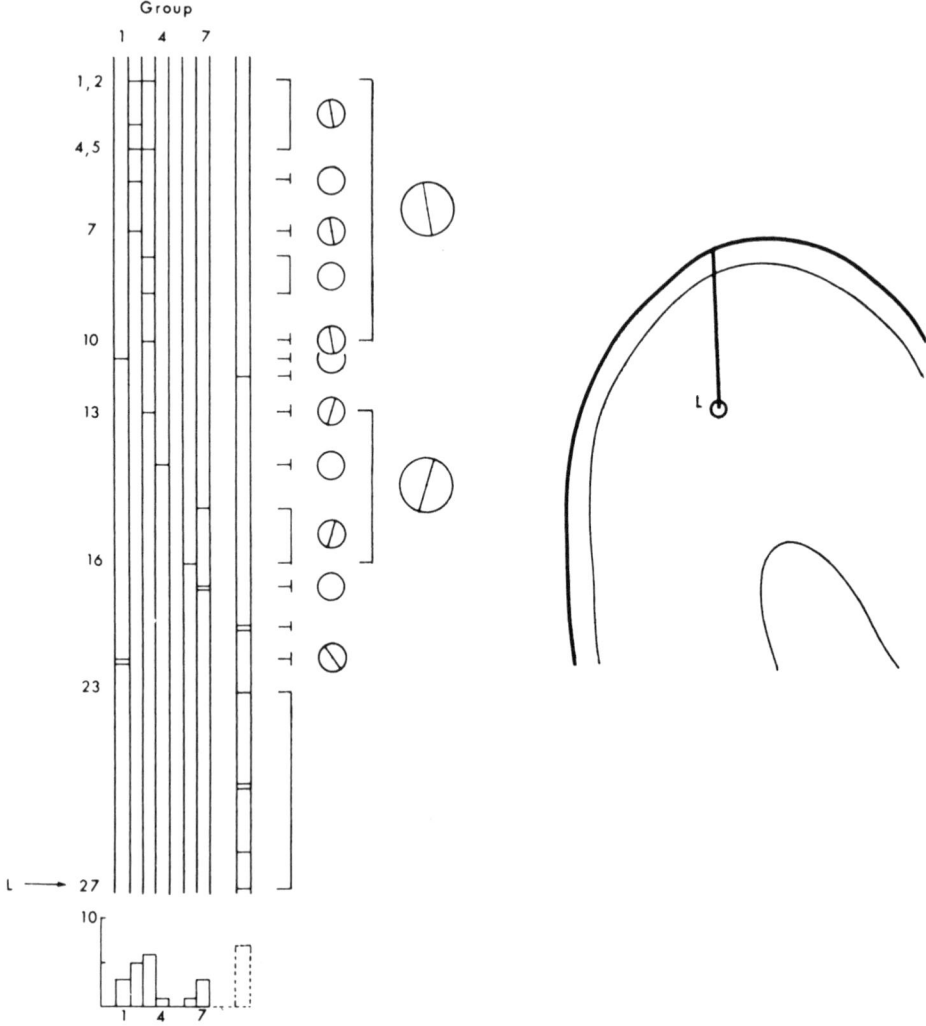

Fig. 4. Reconstruction of a penetration through the right postlateral gyrus in a kitten deprived by bilateral lid suture for the first 3 months. To the right is a tracing of a coronal section passing through the electrode track; an electrolytic lesion, made at the end of the penetration, is indicated by a circle. This track is expanded to the left of the figure. As in Fig. 1, cells are indicated by short horizontal lines placed in the appropriate vertical rows according to ocular-dominance group, and to the right of group 7 is a separate row for unresponsive cells. The total number of cells in each group is indicated by the histogram at the bottom. To the right of the reconstruction receptive-field orientations are indicated by the inclination of the lines inside circles; a circle without a line indicates absence of any clear receptive-field orientation (kitten no. 4).

the lids of one eye under a general anesthetic. The cornea and media appeared normal, the pupillary reflex was brisk, and there was no nystagmus. Tactile placing reactions were present, but there was no visual placing. As the kitten moved about the room there were no indications that visual cues were used; placed in an unfamiliar room, it frequently bumped into large obstacles in its path. We concluded from these crude behavioral observations that for practical purposes the animal was blind. The result is in agreement with behavioral studies on animals raised in darkness (6), and is similar to that obtained for the deprived eye in kittens raised with one eye covered (8).

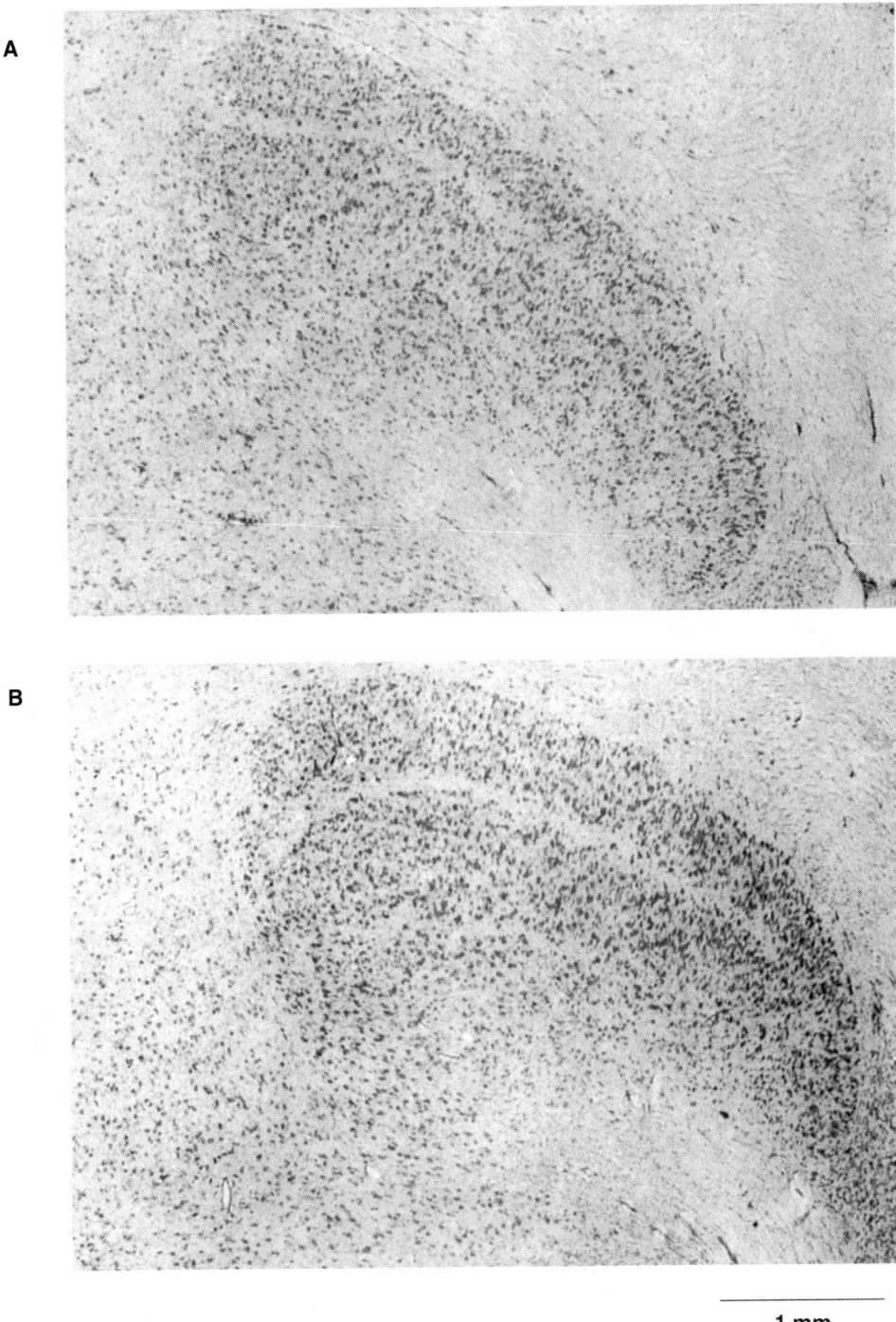

1 mm

Fig. 5. A: *coronal section through the right lateral geniculate body of a kitten (no. 3) in which both eyes were closed for the first 3 months of life. Celloidin, cresyl violet. Same animal as in Fig. 3A.* B: *coronal section through right lateral geniculate body of a normal 3-month-old kitten, for comparison with* A.

413

DISCUSSION

The experiments with binocular eye closure confirm the monocular results in showing that complete form deprivation with virtually complete exclusion of light can lead to marked morphological changes in the geniculate, and marked functional changes in the cortex. The surprising thing was not the extent of the physiological changes, but on the contrary the fact that they were not more severe. Penetration after penetration with little or no driving of cortical cells from the deprived eye in monocular closures had led us to expect little or no driving from either eye in the binocular experiments. In all nine penetrations it was as if the expected ill effects from closing one eye had been averted by closing the other. Taken together, the two sets of experiments seem to suggest that early in life the functional integrity of the pathway may depend not only on the amount of afferent impulse activity, but also on the interrelationships between the various sets of afferents. This suggestion receives support from the results of the next paper (5), which describes the cortical effects of interference with normal binocular interaction.

The mechanism of this apparent interaction between the two converging pathways is at present quite obscure. The site of the interaction is presumably the cortex, since the evidence so far available indicates that few cells in the geniculate receive input from the two eyes. Within the cortex the most important site for anatomical convergence of the two paths is probably the simple cells, for these seem to be the first cells in the path that can be driven by both eyes. The similarity of simple and complex cells in their ocular-dominance distribution suggests that no further binocular convergence takes place at the complex cell (3). No attempt was made in these experiments to distinguish simple and complex cells; to sample as many cells as possible we confined our efforts to mapping field position, size and orientation, and ocular dominance. If simple cells are the site of the interacting deprivation effects, it may be possible to learn more about underlying mechanisms by studying these cells separately.

Regardless of where the interaction takes place, it is almost as though the afferent paths were competing for control over the cell, so that a reduction in efficiency in one set of synapses permitted the other set to take over at the first set's expense.

This could simply be a matter of competition for space on the postsynaptic membrane, some synapses shrinking, others expanding to fill the space, and, as it were, pushing the first ones aside. If anything like that did occur one would expect that with monocular closure the effectiveness of the open eye would, on the whole, be enhanced. Unfortunately, it is difficult to establish such an improvement experimentally because of the great variation in briskness of responses from one cell to the next. A possible way of settling this and other questions would be to look in kittens for changes in responses of simple cortical cells over periods of many hours or a few days.

Our previous finding that visual experience is not necessary for the formation of specific connections at the striate level (4) is confirmed by the fact that in the bilaterally lid-sutured animals many cells were driven normally. We have no hint as to why some cells remained apparently normal while others became unresponsive and still others developed pathological responses. The presence of a high proportion of responsive cells in these experiments is consistent with Baxter's observation (1) of normal evoked responses in dark-reared cats.

It remains to comment on the relation between the physiological findings in these experiments and the behavioral defects. Monocular deprivation led to a marked decline in responsiveness of cortical cells to stimulation of the deprived eye, which agreed well with the marked blindness in that eye. Binocular deprivation produced a bilateral blindness even though there were plenty of responsive cells in the cortex, many of them apparently normal. The visual defects found in the two experiments may thus have different origins. The abnormalities in area 17 could by themselves account for the loss of vision following monocular occlusion. With binocular occlusion one may have to look for impairment at levels central to area 17 to explain the blindness we observed, and also that which follows dark rearing (6).

SUMMARY

If a kitten is raised from birth with one eye sutured closed, recordings from the visual cortex at 3 months show that very few cells can be driven from the deprived eye (8). As part of the present study these results were confirmed and extended in two kittens monocularly deprived for 8–10 weeks. In the 5 monocularly deprived kittens studied to date, 13 of 199 cells could be driven from the previously closed eye; all of these except 1 had abnormal receptive fields. Cells that responded to stimulation of the deprived eye tended to be aggregated into small regions of the cortex, so that over most penetrations no responses were seen from the deprived eye. From these results it was predicted that if animals were binocularly deprived for similar periods most of the striate cortex would be unresponsive to stimulation of either eye. To test this, the lids of both eyes were sutured together in 5 kittens shortly after the time of normal eye opening, and the animals raised in normal surroundings to an age of 2½–4½ months. Responses in single cells of the striate cortex were observed in 4 animals. Contrary to what had been expected, responsive cells were found throughout the greater part of all penetrations, and over half of these cells seemed perfectly normal. The cortex was nevertheless not normal in that many cells responded abnormally, and many were completely unresponsive. In the fifth kitten an eye was opened and vision tested. The pupillary response was normal but the animal from its behavior appeared to be blind.

Histologically the lateral geniculate body showed changes similar to those found after monocular deprivation, but they occurred throughout all layers bilaterally: the Nissl-stained cells appeared pale, cross-sectional areas of cell bodies were reduced by about 40%, and the pale substance between cell nests was greatly reduced in volume. There were no obvious changes in retinas or cortex.

It thus appears that at the cortical level the results of closing one eye depend upon whether the other eye is also closed. The damage produced by monocular closure may therefore not be caused simply by disuse, but may instead depend to a large extent on interaction of the two pathways.

ACKNOWLEDGMENT

We express our thanks to Jane Chen, Janet Tobie, and John Tuckerman, for their technical assistance.

References

1. Baxter, B. L. *An Electrophysiological Study of the Effects of Sensory Deprivation* (doctoral dissertation; unpublished). University of Chicago, 1959.
2. Hubel, D. H. Single unit activity in striate cortex of unrestrained cats. *J. Physiol.,* 1959, *147:* 226–238.
3. Hubel, D. H. and Wiesel, T. N. Receptive fields, binocular interaction and functional architecture in the cat's visual cortex. *J. Physiol.,* 1962, *160:* 106–154.
4. Hubel, D. H. and Wiesel, T. N. Receptive fields of cells in striate cortex of very young, visually inexperienced kittens. *J. Neurophysiol.,* 1963, *26:* 994–1002.
5. Hubel, D. H. and Wiesel, T. N. Binocular interaction in striate cortex of kittens reared with artificial squint. *J. Neurophysiol.,* 1965, *28:* 1041–1059.
6. Riesen, A. H. Stimulation as a requirement for growth and function in behavioral development. In: *Functions of Varied Experience,* edited by D. W. Fiske and S. R. Maddi. Homewood, Ill., Dorsey Press, 1961, pp. 57–105.
7. Wiesel, T. N. and Hubel, D. H. Effects of visual deprivation on morphology and physiology of cells in the cat's lateral geniculate body. *J. Neurophysiol.,* 1963, *26:* 978–993.
8. Wiesel, T. N. and Hubel, D. H. Single-cell responses in striate cortex of kittens deprived of vision in one eye. *J. Neurophysiol.,* 1963, *26:* 1003–1017.
9. Wiesel, T. N. and Hubel, D. H. Extent of recovery from the effects of visual deprivation in kittens. *J. Neurophysiol.,* 1965, *28:* 1060–1072.

Binocular Interaction in Striate Cortex of Kittens Reared with Artificial Squint[1]

DAVID H. HUBEL AND TORSTEN N. WIESEL • *Neurophysiology Laboratory, Department of Pharmacology,*

Harvard Medical School, Boston, Massachusetts

INTRODUCTION

Before a kitten opens its eyes, and long before the eyes are used in visual exploration, single cells of the primary visual cortex respond to natural stimulation with the same specificity as is found in the adult (5). This suggests that the anatomical connections between retina and striate cortex are for the most part innate. During the first 3 months of life the connections are highly susceptible to the effects of visual deprivation, to the extent that exclusion of all form and some light from one eye leads to a severe decline in the ability of that eye to influence cortical cells. Anatomical and physiological evidence suggests that the defect is chiefly, though not entirely, a cortical one (7–9).

The object of the present study was to influence cortical connections by some means less drastic than covering one or both eyes. We wished if possible to alter the input in such a way that there would be no question of effects on the visual pathway below the level of the striate cortex. A method was suggested by the well-known clinical observation that a child with a squint (strabismus or nonparallel visual axes) may suffer a deterioration of vision in one eye (amblyopia ex anopsia). Since the visual pathways from the two eyes are for practical purposes separate up to the level of the striate cortex, it is unlikely that in these children the defect is in the retina or geniculate. An artificial squint therefore seemed to provide a possible means of obtaining a cortical defect while sparing the retina and lateral geniculate body. Accordingly, we produced a divergent strabismus by cutting one of the extraocular muscles in each of four newborn kittens, with the plan of testing vision and recording

from single cortical cells after several months to a year.

When at length each eye was tested in these kittens by observing the animal's behavior with the other eye covered the results were disappointing: there was not the slightest suggestion of any defect in vision in either eye. This was not entirely unexpected, since with both eyes uncovered the animals had appeared to fix at times with one eye and at times with the other. At this stage there seemed to be little point in proceeding further, for there was no reason to doubt that the cortical recordings would be entirely normal—especially since we had not yet studied the kittens with binocular lid closure, and had no idea of the extent of interdependence of the two eyes in sustaining normal function (9). Nevertheless, we decided to record from the kittens before abandoning the project. The results from all four animals were to our surprise quite abnormal; they are presented in the first part of this paper, together with a related set of experiments on alternating monocular occlusion. An incidental finding in the course of these experiments prompted us to re-examine the problem of distribution of cortical cells by ocular dominance in the normal animal.

METHODS

Four kittens were operated upon at 8–10 days after birth, just at the time the eyes were beginning to open. Periorbital tissues on the right were infiltrated with a local anesthetic (Xylocaine, 2%), which was sufficient to produce general anesthesia for 10–15 min. (7). The right eyeball was retracted laterally and the conjunctiva cut at its medial scleral attachment. The medial rectus muscle

From *J. Neurophysiol.* 1965, 28: 1041–1059.

Received for publication December 23, 1964.

[1]This work was supported in part by Public Health Service Grants NB-02260-05 and NB-05554-01, and in part by U.S. Air Force Contracts AF-AFOSR-410-63A and AF-49(638)1443.

was caught with a blunt hook and cut. An asymmetry in the position of the two eyeballs was usually immediately obvious, and after recovery from anesthesia all four kittens had a marked divergent squint, with the sclera visible medial to the limbus. Except for some limitation in turning the eye inward there was no obvious reduction in movements of the right eye, which were as free and active as those of the normal one.

We recorded from three of the animals, no. *1,* no. *3,* and no, *4,* at 3 months of age, and no. *2* was studied at 1 year. Two kittens (no. *5* and no. *6*) were brought up from the time of normal eye opening with an opaque contact occluder covering one eye one day and the other eye the next. These animals were studied at 10 weeks. Two normal adult cats were recorded from as controls for the studies of distribution of cells by ocular dominance. Methods of stimulating and recording are described in other papers (1–4).

RESULTS

Strabismus

Cortical Penetrations. Seven penetrations were made in four kittens. The first kitten (no. *1*) was studied at 3 months of age. When it was anesthetized and paralyzed in the usual way the eyes diverged by 21°, as measured by the projected area centralis, instead of the normal 2–3°. We concluded that with the animal awake the eyes must have diverged by about 18°. In the remaining three animals the squints estimated in this way amounted to 29°, 12°, and 23°.

To begin with, the cortical activity seemed perfectly normal. The penetration were unusually rich, spikes from a new unit growing up to replace those of a declining one each time the electrode was advanced. The unitary discharges were seen against a background of almost continuous unresolved activity. Each cell was briskly responsive to one or the other eye and had the normal preference for a slit, edge, or dark bar in a particular orientation, which varied from one column to the next.

As more and more cells were studied it became obvious that the amount of binocular interaction was far less than normal. Most cells were driven by one eye only, some by the ipsilateral, others by the contralateral. Even more startling was the finding that there were regions of complete contralateral or ipsilateral dominance in which one eye drove cell after cell as well as the unresolved

background activity, with no trace of a response to stimulation of the other eye. As the electrode was advanced a region dominated by one eye would give way to a region dominated by the other. Mixed regions were also seen, containing cells driven from one eye and cells driven from the other, interspersed with an occasional cell driven from both eyes.

One of the two penetrations made in cat *2* is reconstructed in Fig. 1. To the left of the figure the long vertical lines separate the 7 ocular-dominance groups. The 61 cells are represented as short horizontal lines placed in the appropriate spaces at points corresponding to the electrode depths as interpolated from the two lesions, L' and L''. In this penetration, except for cells *7–9* and cell *13,* all of the first 33 cells were completely dominated by the contralateral eye. The electrode then entered a region of strong, almost exclusive ipsilateral dominance which extended to cell *46.* After a brief transitional phase (cells *47–50*), the electrode entered a third region, from *51* to the end, which showed complete contralateral domination.

Similar results were seen in the other six penetrations. In these, however, the regions of mixed dominance were more prominent. Figure 2 shows reconstructions of two penetrations made in cat *3,* at an age of 3 months. In the penetrations made in the left hemisphere (Fig. *2A*) an area of mixed dominance occurred between cells *22* and *28,* and another brief episode between cells *40* and *42.* The penetration in the left hemisphere (Fig. *2B*) showed even more extensive mixed zones. After an initial region of ipsilateral domination (cells *50–59*) the first mixed region extended from *60* to about *91.* There was then another ipsilaterally dominant area from about *91* to *106,* followed by a second mixed area. In the first mixed zone there were several examples of dual-unit recordings (indicated by dots) in which one cell was group 1 and the other group 7. Cell *64* in group 1 was recorded with *65* and *66,* both in group 7. In the single penetration made in cat *4* at 3 months (Fig. 3) the middle groups (no. *3–5*) were especially poorly represented. Here the mixed areas consisted almost entirely of cells of group 1 intermixed with cells of group 7 (cells *49–67;* cells *90–95*). It thus appears that in these kittens the cortex is subdivided into regions of three types, one containing contralaterally dominated cells, the second containing ipsilat-

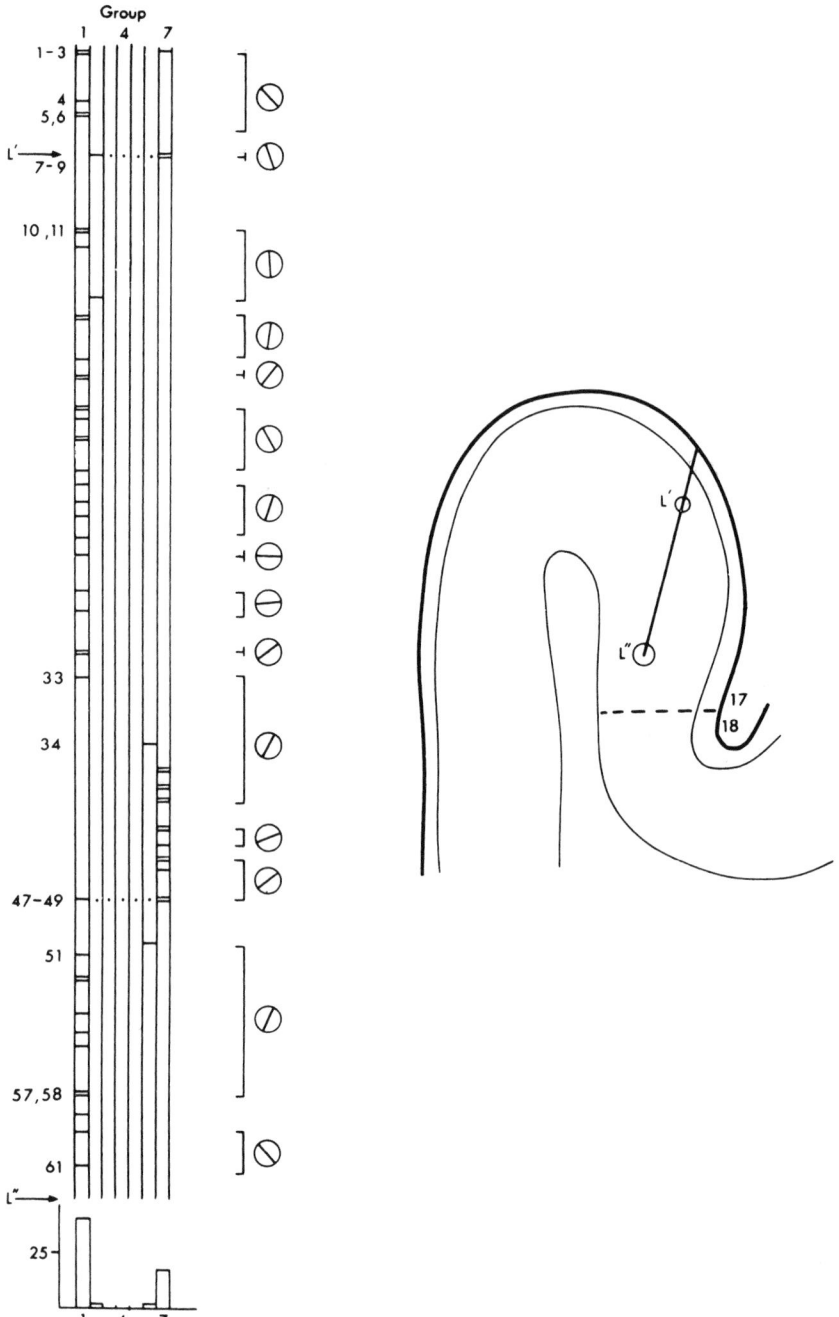

Fig. 1. Reconstruction of a penetration through right hemisphere of a 12-month-old cat with divergent strabismus from birth (cat 2). To the right is shown a coronal section through the right postlateral gyrus. The electrode track is shown passing through two electrolytic lesions, L' and L", indicated approximately to scale by circles. To the left of the figure the track is reconstructed, each cell being indicated by a short horizontal line placed in its appropriate ocular-dominance group. Two lines close together, or dots between pairs of lines, indicate two-unit recordings. Total numbers are shown for each group in the histogram below. Lines to the right within the circles indicate by their tilt the receptive-field orientations of the cells within the brackets. Note the strong tendency for cells of a particular ocular-dominance group to occur in sequence.

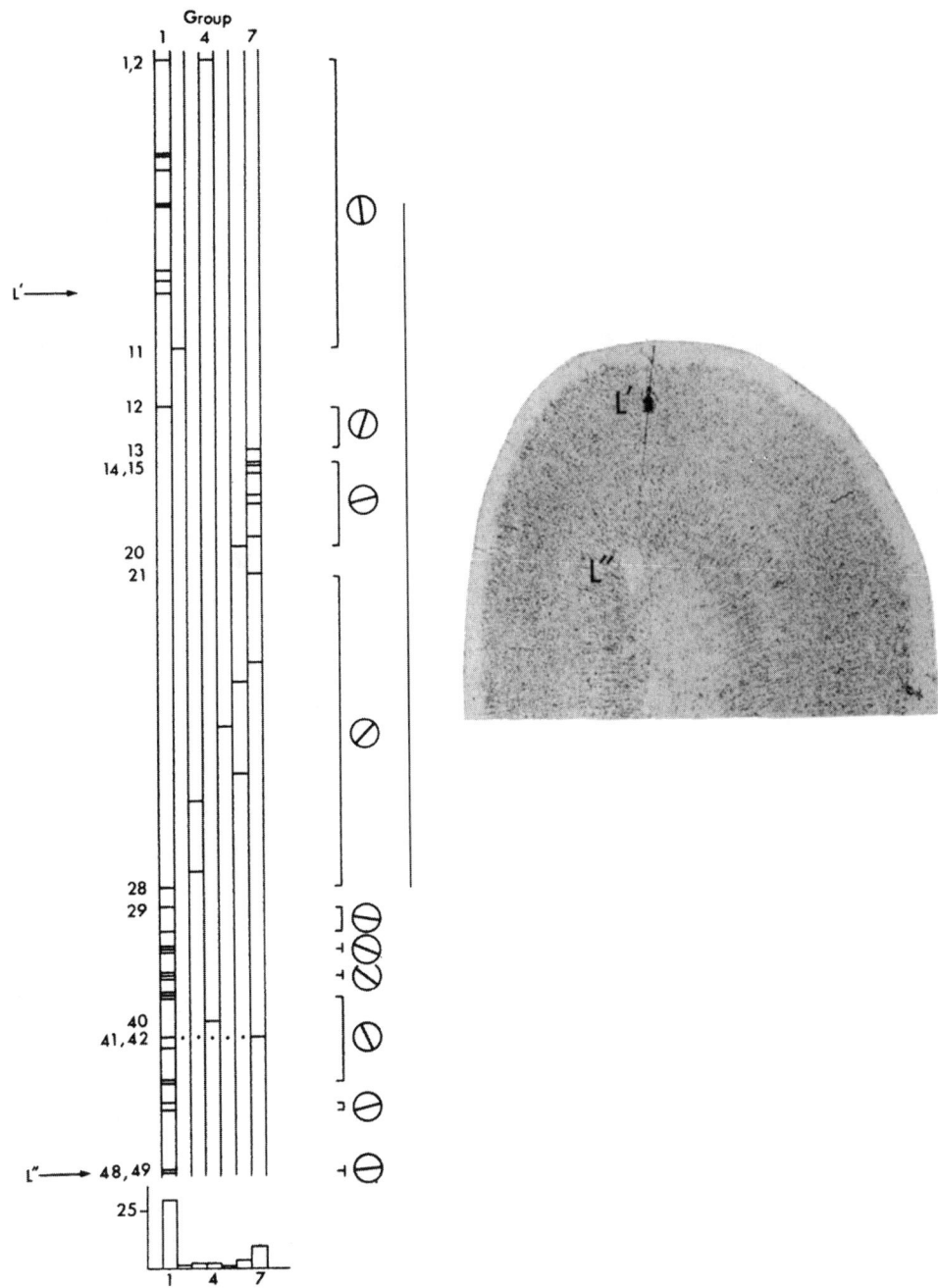

Fig. 2A. *Reconstruction of penetration through right hemisphere of cat 3, a 3-month-old animal with divergent strabismus from birth. To right of figure is a photomicrograph of a Nissl-stained coronal section through the post-lateral gyrus.*

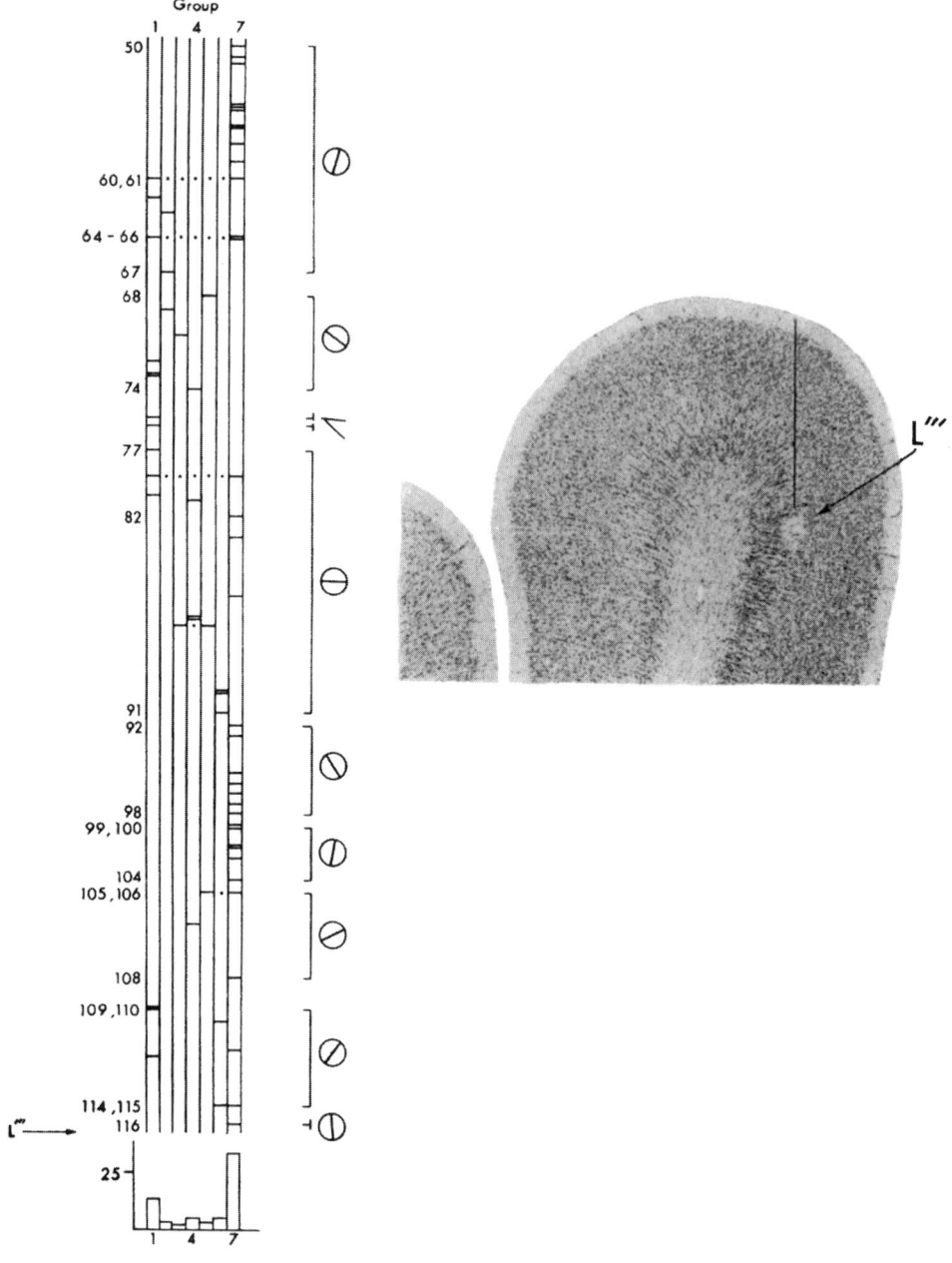

Fig. 2B. Reconstruction of penetration through left hemisphere of cat 3. Conventions as in Fig. 1.

erally dominated cells, and the third containing cells of both types as well as a few binocularly driven cells. As shown in a later section of this paper, the three types of region represent an exaggeration of regional variations in ocular dominance that occur in normal animals.

OCULAR-DOMINANCE DISTRIBUTION. The ocular-dominance distributions of cortical cells recorded in four of the penetrations in animals with strabismus are given in Figs. 1–3 below each track reconstruction. In all these penetrations the distributions were abnormal, with the extreme groups (no. 1 and

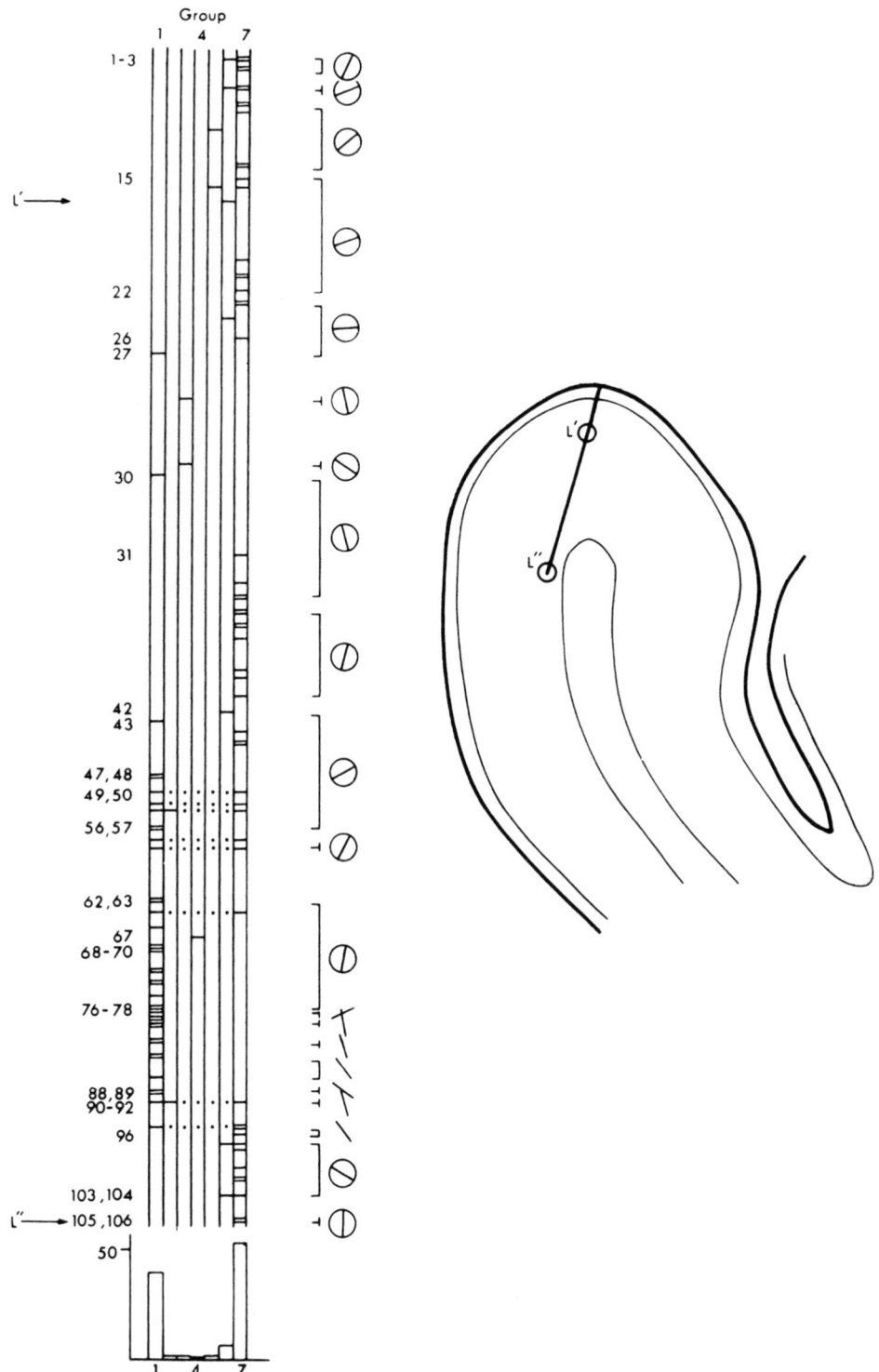

Fig. 3. Reconstruction of penetration in cat 4, through right hemisphere. Kitten, age 3 months, strabismus from 8 days. Conventions as in Fig. 1.

7) well represented and the inner ones (no. 3–5) poorly represented. To be sure of this result we recorded from many cells in each animal, 106 in one penetration in cat *4* (Fig. 3) and 116 in two penetrations in cat *3* (Fig. 2). In all seven penetrations deviations from normal were large, but there was some variation; the two least abnormal penetrations were seen in cat *1*, summarized in Fig. 4. Even in this experiment 50 of 81 cells, or roughly 60%, were driven from one eye only, compared with about 20% in the normal cat.

The distribution of the 384 cells from all four kittens is given in Fig. 5*B*. This histogram is to be compared with the distribution of 223 cells previously obtained in 17 penetrations in the normal adult, shown in Fig. 5*A*. Of the 384 cells recorded from animals with squint, 302, or 79%, were monocularly driven, as opposed to 20% in the normal.

That the difference represented by Fig. 5, *A* and *B*, has nothing to do with age differences is clear from a previous study in which normal kittens were found to have an ocular-dominance distribution similar to that of adult cats (ref. 5, Fig. 2). Finally, another measure of ocular-dominance distribution of an entirely different sort is described below and shown in Fig. 9*B*.

Anatomical findings. Histological sections of the lateral geniculate and the striate cortex showed

no sign of any abnormality. In one animal 50 cells from the dorsal layer of the geniculate (layer A) were measured on each side, and no significant difference was found between the two sides.

Ocular-Dominance Distribution in Kittens Raised with Alternating Monocular Occlusion

In the experiments just described, the strabismus kept the two eyes from working together without cutting down the input to either eye. It seemed worthwhile to ask whether a similar cortical defect would result if one were to stimulate the two eyes alternately, blocking light from entering one whenever the other was in use, and thus keeping the eyes from working together without introducing the possibility of antagonistic interaction between them. We therefore placed an opaque contact occluder over one eye one day, and the other eye the next, alternating eyes each day from the time of normal eye opening up to an age of 10 weeks. At that point the animals seemed to see perfectly well with either eye, and both eyes when uncovered moved together without obvious strabismus.

Three penetrations were made in these animals and are reconstructed in Fig. 6. The ocular-dominance histograms, shown below in the figure, are even more abnormal than those of the squint

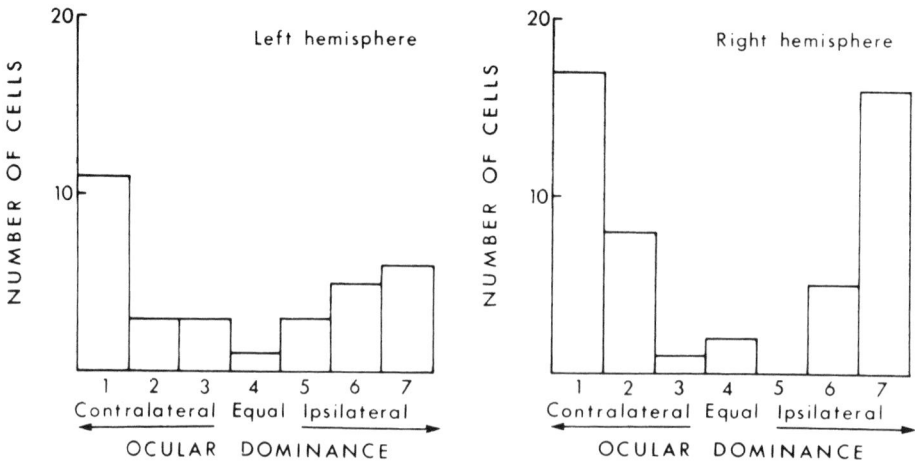

Fig. 4. Ocular-dominance distribution of 81 cells recorded in two penetrations, one in each hemisphere. Kitten 1, age 3 months, right medial rectus cut at 8 days. (Cells of group 1 were driven only by the contralateral eye; for cells of group 2 there was marked dominance of the contralateral eye, for group 3, slight dominance. For cells in group 4 there was no obvious difference between the two eyes. In group 5 the ipsilateral eye dominated slightly, in group 6, markedly; and in group 7 the cells were driven only by the ipsilateral eye.)

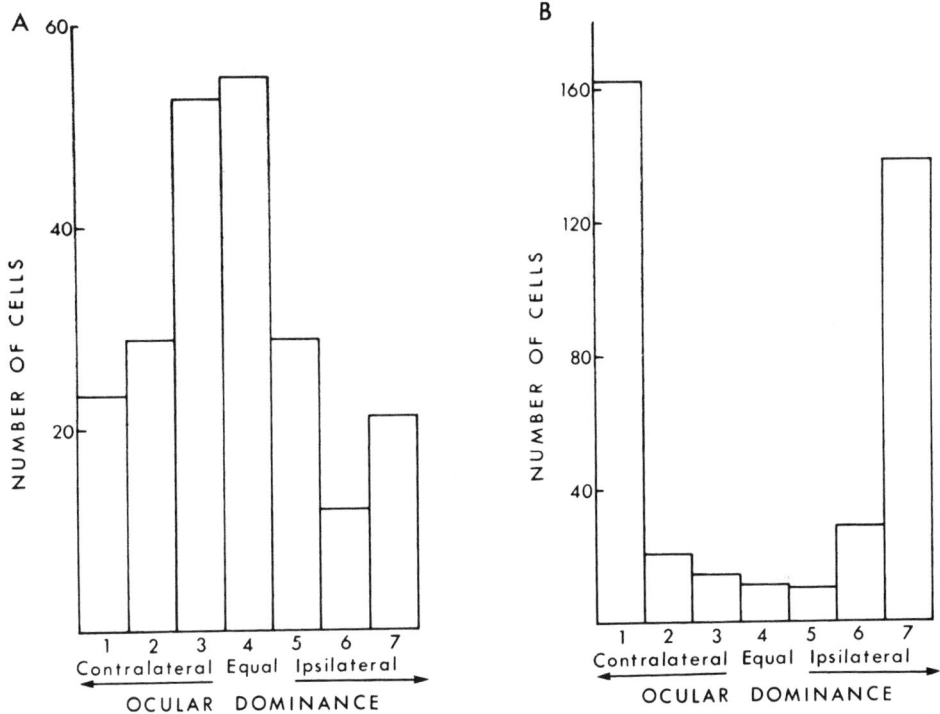

Fig. 5. A: *ocular dominance of 223 cells recorded from a series of normal adult cats (3).* B: *ocular dominance of 384 cells recorded from all four strabismus experiments.*

animals, with 176 of 194 cells (91%) driven by one eye only. The track reconstructions again show strong evidence for spatial aggregation of cells according to ocular dominance. We conclude that the results of the strabismus experiments do not depend on the fact that the two eyes were both open at the same time.

Spatial Distribution of Cells According to Ocular Dominance in Normal Cats

We were naturally interested in whether the division of striate cortex into areas according to ocular dominance was an abnormal state produced by squint, or alternating occlusion, or whether it also existed in the normal animal and was merely made more obvious by the exaggerated ocular dominance of the cells. Our previous studies of normal striate cortex had suggested that there was some tendency to aggregation of cells according to ocular dominance (ref. 3, p. 140 and Text-fig. 13). To help settle this problem we made four penetrations in two normal adult cats and reconstructed the results in Figs. 7 and 8. Here there indeed seemed to be a

subdivision of cortex according to eye dominance. In penetration 1 of Fig. 7, the first 13 cells favored the ipsilateral eye; this was followed by a small area of mixed dominance (cells *14–17*), and then the contralateral eye prevailed to the end (cell *25*). In penetration 2, the first few cells favored the ipsilateral eye and from then on there was a mixture. In Fig. 8, the penetration in the right hemisphere was first predominantly ipsilateral in emphasis, and at the end contralateral (cells *24–26*), cells *3* and *4* giving the only hint of intermixing in the early part. Penetration 2, made in the left hemisphere, was largely mixed.

This tendency for cortical cells in the normal cat to be segregated according to ocular dominance complicates the assessment of cortex as normal or abnormal in animals with strabismus. But while the ocular-dominance distributions for the individual penetrations in the squint and alternating monocular occlusions vary to some extent (Figs. 1–4; Fig. 6), the marked preponderance of cells in the two end groups (no. 1 and 7) is common to all of them. For the normal cat, on the other hand, an

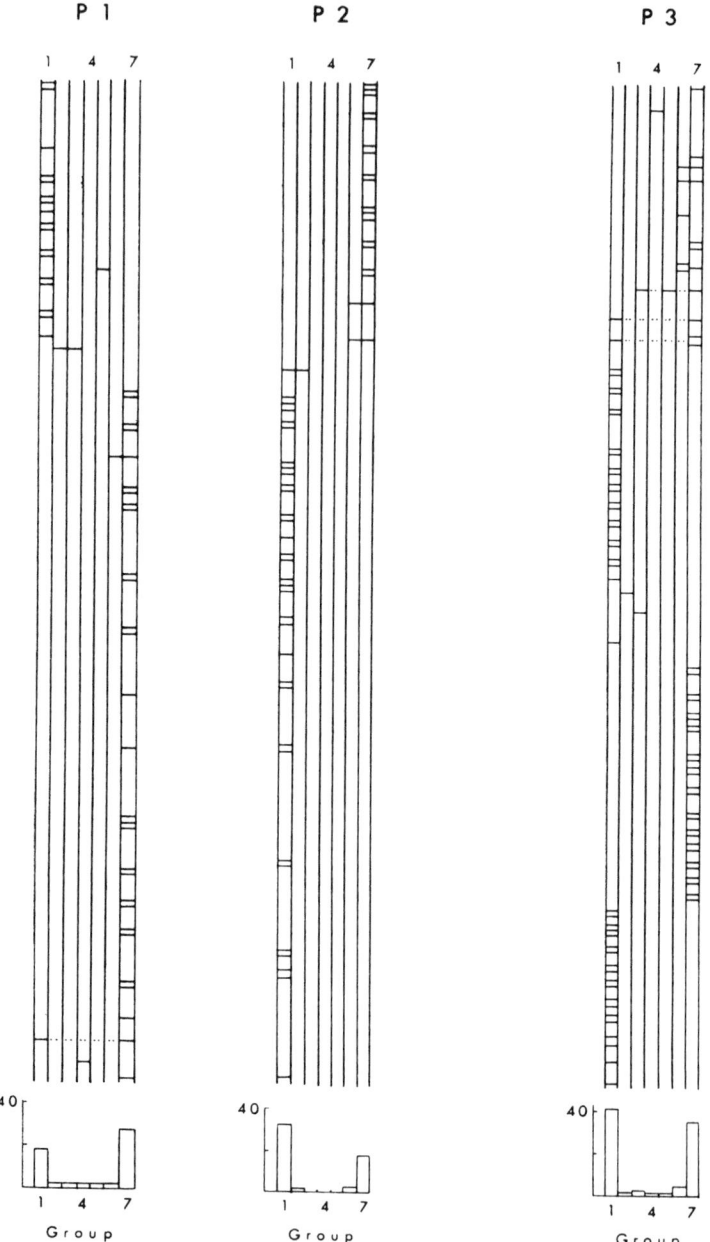

Fig. 6. Schematic reconstruction of three penetrations in the striate cortex of two 10-week-old kittens (no. 5 and no. 6) raised from the time of normal eye opening with an opaque contact occluder covering one eye one day, and the other eye the next. Each penetration extended into cortical gray matter for about 1.5 mm. Conventions as in Fig. 1.

idea of the variation from one penetration to the next can be obtained from the histograms of 12 individual penetrations, shown in a previous paper (ref. 8, Fig. 2) or from the histograms of the 4 normal penetrations in Figs. 7 and 8. None of these normal penetrations, and no others we have made,

have shown ocular-dominance distributions with anything like the shape of those from kittens with strabismus or alternating monocular occlusion.

In normal and abnormal animals the cortical subdivisions defined by ocular dominance seem to be quite independent of the columns defined by

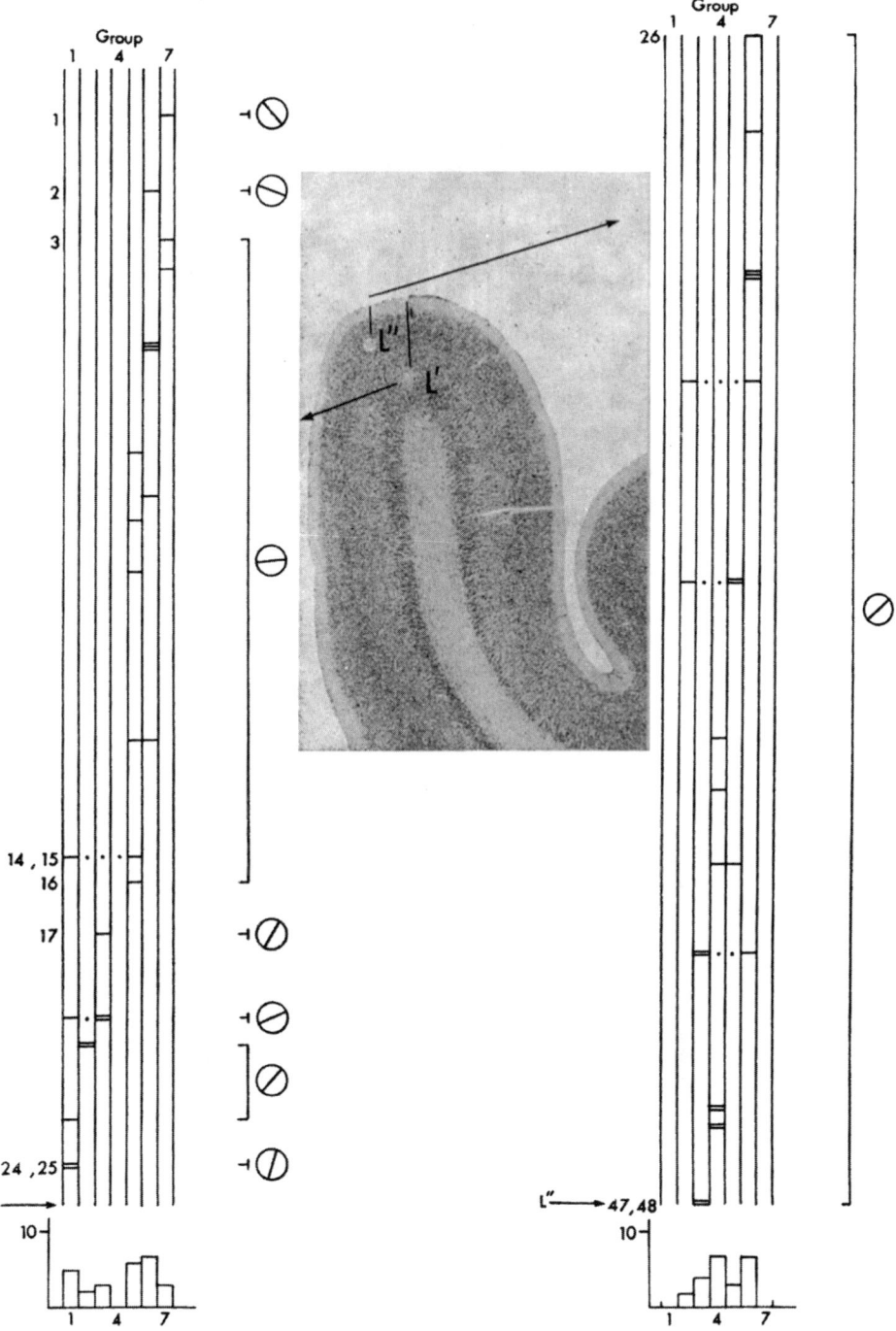

Fig. 7. Two penetrations in the right striate cortex (postlateral gyrus) of a normal adult cat. Conventions as in Fig. 1.

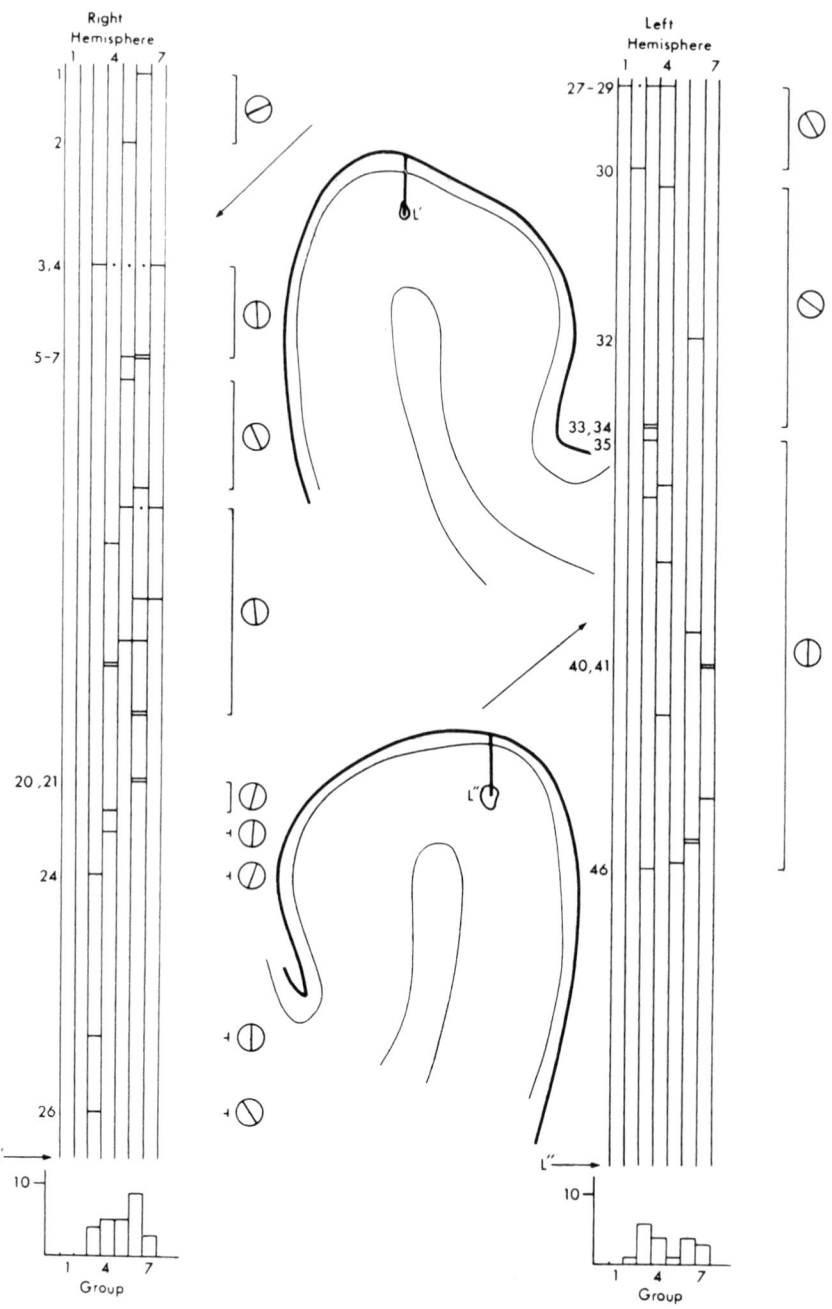

Fig. 8. One penetration in each hemisphere through striate cortex (post-lateral gyrus) of a normal adult cat. Conventions as in Fig. 1.

receptive-field orientation. Within an orientation column there may be more than one region defined by ocular dominance (Fig. 1, cells *33–40* and cells *50–58;* Fig. 2*A,* cells *21–28;* Fig. 2*B,* cells *77–99*) and, conversely, an ocular-dominance region may contain a large number of receptive-field orientation columns (see especially Figs. 1 and 3).

To study the interrelationship of the two kinds of aggregations we reexamined a series of experiments made originally for the purpose of mapping receptive-field orientation columns (4). Each experiment consisted of a number of superficial cortical penetrations. A typical map is redrawn in Fig. 9*A* (ref. 4, Text-fig. 3). The columnar regions of constant receptive-field orientation are roughly outlined as before by interrupted lines. Superimposed upon and cutting across these lines, the continuously drawn contours outline areas of marked ipsilateral eye dominance. Presumably, in an extensive enough mapping one might also out-

line regions of contralateral and mixed dominance, but in this experiment there were too few points and they were too far apart for comfort. The map does, however, reinforce the impression that the system of parcellation by ocular dominance is independent of, and cuts across, that of the orientation columns so that the same surface of cortex is simultaneously subdivided in two different ways.

The ocular-dominance distribution of cells in normal cat cortex has been estimated from a relatively small number of deep penetrations (3, 5, and 8). To obtain an entirely different measure of this distribution we tabulated the ocular dominance of the first units recorded, in all 167 superficial penetrations made in the mapping experiments (4). The resulting histogram, given in Fig. 9*B,* agrees reasonably well with those obtained from deep cortical penetrations (Fig. 5*A;* and ref. 5, Fig. 2).

We are still not absolutely clear about the shape and size of the regions of one-eye or mixed

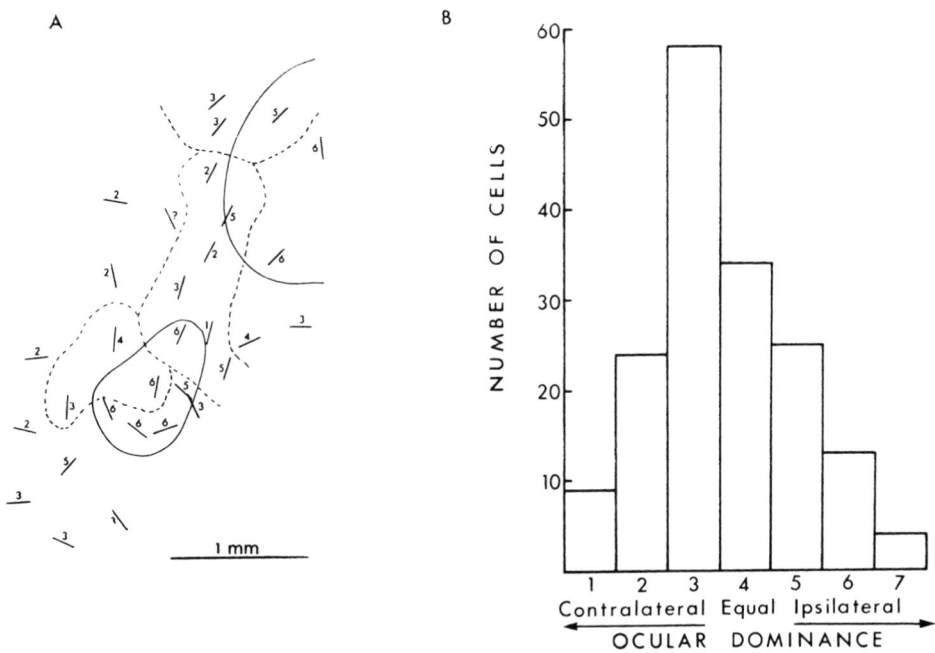

Fig. 9. A: *normal adult cat. Map showing receptive-field orientations and ocular dominance of first cells encountered near the surface, in 31 penetrations. The entire map covers a region of the right striate cortex measuring about 1 × 3 mm. Interrupted lines separate regions of relatively constant receptive-field orientation, partly outlining 3 columns. The numbers refer to ocular-dominance groups. Continuous lines separate areas of strong ipsilateral dominance from areas of mixed or contralateral dominance (redrawn from ref. 4, text-Fig. 3 and Plate 1).* B: *ocular-dominance distribution of the first units recorded in 167 superficial penetrations made in five normal adult cats.*

eye dominance. Penetrations like that of Fig. 1, together with the surface-mapping experiments described above, suggest that the regions may be large, extending along the cortex for some millimeters. Deep microelectrode penetrations (ref. 3, Text-fig. 13) indicate that they can, at least sometimes, extend from surface to white matter. Thus it seems likely that the regions are columnar, though evidence that the walls separating them are perpendicular to the cortical layers is still lacking.

The spatial segregation of cells by ocular dominance may have a relatively simple anatomical explanation. Geniculate axons as they enter the cortex may be grouped into small bundles, all of the fibers in a given bundle coming from the same geniculate layer and consequently all connected with the same eye. These fiber groups, entering the cortex and fanning out, could establish certain regions in which one or the other eye strongly dominated, and other regions of mixed dominance in which groups of the two types intermingled. The ocular dominance of a given cell in the cortex would then be determined by the relative regional concentration of the two types of axon.

DISCUSSION

The results presented here show that it is possible to produce abnormalities in neural functioning by alterations in sensory input that are relatively subtle, compared with light or form deprivation or cutting an afferent nerve. The neural abnormality was a severe decline in the number of cells that could be driven by both eyes in area 17 of the cortex. In the case of strabismus the sensory impairment was simply a misalignment of the two eyes; on the average, both retinas must have received the same sensory input. Thus it seems fairly certain that the squint produced no impairment of traffic along the two paths emanating from the separate eyes, up to the point of their convergence in the cortex. The changes in cortical function must therefore have been produced by the abnormal relationship between signals in the two paths. The nature of this faulty relationship can best be seen by considering what is known about binocular convergence at the cortical cell.

In the normal cat, the two receptive fields of a single cortical cell are similar in arrangement and occupy corresponding retinal positions in the two eyes. If the eyes fix normally on a flat object, the two retinal images, falling on corresponding parts of the retinas, will affect the cell in the same qualitative way by either eye, exciting it through both or inhibiting it through both. The amount of influence, excitatory or inhibitory, may differ for the two eyes, and when it does the direction and degree of the difference decides which ocular-dominance group the cell occupies in our rough and arbitrary scheme of classification. There is indirect evidence (3; and ref. 9, discussion) to suggest that impulses originating from the two eyes converge mainly upon simple cells in the cortex. If that is so, any changes in ocular dominance in a complex cell would merely reflect, in a passive way, interaction effects at the simple cell.

Now suppose that the retinas are exposed to an ordinary, real-life visual stimulus, and consider the response of a cell in group 2. In the normal animal the images fall on corresponding parts of the retinas (neglecting parallax) and the response will be determined mainly by impulses coming in from the dominant (here, the contralateral) eye, though there will be some help from the nondominant one. In the animal with strabismus this relationship is completely changed: the cell will tend to follow the commands of the dominant eye, and whether the other eye helps, hinders, or has no effect at all will be more or less a matter of chance, depending on the make-up of the stimulus and the amount of squint. It must be this lack of synergy between the two afferent paths that somehow, over a period of time, gives rise to the changes in over-all ocular-dominance distribution.

The new ocular-dominance distribution could result from a simple dropping out of binocularly driven cells. This seems unlikely experimentally, because of the wealth of responsive cells and absence of unresponsive cells, and because a dropping out of binocularly driven cells would leave short alternating sequences of group 1 and group 7 cells, rather than the very long sequences actually observed. A far more likely possibility is that the lack of synergy in the two paths causes the ocular dominance of cells to change, with an over-all increase in the number of group 1 and group 7 cells at the expense of the others. This would happen if there were a decrease in the effectiveness of the nondominant eye. There might also be an absolute increase in the effectiveness of the dominant eye, but that would be difficult to detect because of differences in the responsiveness from one cell to the next. In any case, given the initial normal tendency for grouping of cells by ocular dominance, a shift in ocular dominance, cells of groups 2 and 3 becoming group 1 and 5 and 6 becoming group 7, would explain very well the long sequences of cells of groups 1 or 7.

One may ask whether in these experiments it is the mere absence of synchronous visual input that produces the result, or whether it is the presence of asynchronous inputs. It seems reasonably clear that absence of synchrony by itself is not enough, since binocular occlusion in the early months of life did not give the marked loss of binocular driving found in strabismus. On the other hand, the alternating occlusion experiments gave substantially the same result as the squint experiments, showing that the result does not depend on simultaneous nonsynchronous activation of the two eyes. What does seem necessary to produce the result is absence of synchrony, and activation of at least one of the two afferent pathways at any one time.

Regardless of detailed mechanisms, the results of this paper are interpreted as suggesting that, in some systems at least, the maintenance of a synapse depends not only on the amount of incoming impulse activity but also on a normal interrelationship between activity in the different afferents. That two sets of synapses on the same cell can be interdependent is also suggested by a previous study comparing the effects of monocular and binocular eye closure (8, 9). In attempting to imagine how an organism can be influenced by experience—to account in synaptic terms for learning, imprinting, and other phenomena that demand neural plasticity—the possibilities would seem to be greatly increased by adding, to the ordinary use-disuse concept, that of the interdependence of different synapses on a single cell.

The plasticity demonstrated in the occlusion and strabismus experiments has two obvious limitations. First, it is probably confined to the early months of life. This was clearly shown for the occlusion experiments, inasmuch as three months of deprivation produced no changes in an adult cat (7, 8) and even several months, deprivation starting at 2–3 months was less severe in its effects than deprivation for a similar period from birth. Simi-

larly, the failure to obtain full recovery on opening the eyes after 3 months' deprivation from birth may be a matter of age rather than of irreversibility as such (10). The effects of cutting an eye muscle in older cats have not been studied, but one would probably find a similar age dependence, in view of the common clinical experience that strabismus acquired in the adult produces no permanent effects on mechanisms for fusion of images or for stereoscopic depth perception. A second limitation concerns the pathological nature of the changes. In all of the experiments of this series, both deprivation and strabismus, normal, fully formed connections were rendered abnormal by distorting the sensory input. The next step would be to look at more central parts of the visual path for changes in connections resulting from normal experience. The changes could involve the development of entirely new connections, or simply a modification—a relative strengthening or weakening—of innately determined ones, as in the present experiments. Here also the influence of age on plasticity would obviously be of interest.

In all of the experiments of this series there has been a certain correspondence between the sensory deprivation employed and the nature of the defect produced. Monocular form deprivation with only minor light deprivation led to an unresponsiveness of cortical cells to stimulation of the deprived eye, with very minor anatomical changes in the lateral geniculate body; whereas monocular deprivation of both form and light gave similar cortical unresponsiveness plus marked morphological changes in the lateral geniculate. This fits very well with the reactions of cells at the two levels to diffuse light—the virtual unresponsiveness of cortical cells and the brisk responses of most geniculate cells. With strabismus the result was similar: here the defect was precisely in the area of binocular interaction, with other cortical functions apparently intact. All of this makes one wonder whether more subtle types of deprivation—an animal brought up in isolation or a bird kept from hearing the call of another bird of the same species—may not likewise exert their ill effects through the deterioration of complex central pathways that either were not used or else were used inappropriately.

Finally, the results of these studies may have some bearing on the problem of strabismus in man.

It is recognized that a squint in a child must be corrected in the first few years of life if capability of using both eyes in binocular vision is to be retained. This correlates well with our finding that in cats a mechanical misalignment of the two eyes early in life produces a deterioration in cortical connections. We have made no attempt at testing the reversibility of the damage by straightening the eyes surgically, but our failure to produce any significant recovery in the occlusion experiments (10) would make us pessimistic. Furthermore, given even a normal mechanical apparatus for aligning the eyes, perfect binocular fixation presumably depends also upon a normal set of neural connections in the visual pathway, possibly the very connections concerned with binocular interaction that are lost in these experiments. In that case even a perfect mechanical repair would not guarantee the realignment necessary to promote recovery of binocular vision.

SUMMARY

In four kittens the right medial rectus was severed at about the time of normal eye opening, producing an obvious divergent squint. The animals were raised under normal conditions for periods of 3 months to 1 year. When the two eyes were then tested separately no behavioral visual defects were seen. Recordings from the striate cortex were normal, except for a marked decrease in the proportion of binocularly driven cells: instead of about 80%, only 20% could be influenced from the two eyes. The cortex appeared normal microscopically. In a given penetration there was a marked tendency for cells driven from a particular eye to occur in long uninterrupted sequences. These results suggest that the strabismus caused cells to shift in their ocular dominance, a given cell coming to favor more and more the eye that dominated it at birth, ultimately losing all connections with the nondominant eye. We conclude that a lack of synergy in the input from the two eyes is sufficient to cause a profound disruption in the connections that subserve binocular interaction.

In two kittens an opaque contact occluder was placed over one eye one day and the other eye the
next, alternating eyes each day from shortly after birth to an age of 10 weeks. This kept the eyes from working together without introducing the possibility of antagonistic interaction between them. Vision in either eye seemed normal. Penetrations in the striate cortex gave results similar to those obtained in squint animals; if anything, the shift in ocular dominance was more extreme, 91% of cells being driven by only one eye. Again cells were spatially aggregated according to ocular dominance.

Recordings from normal adult cats indicate that besides being grouped according to receptive-field orientation, cells in the striate cortex are grouped by ocular dominance into regions of ipsilateral, contralateral, and mixed dominance. The exaggeration of eye dominance of individual cells, in animals raised with squint or alternating monocular occlusion, produces an accentuation of these cortical subdivisions.

ACKNOWLEDGMENT

We express our thanks to Jane Chen, Janet Tobie, and John Tuckerman, for their technical assistance.

References

1. Hubel, D. H. Single unit activity in striate cortex of unrestrained cats. *J. Physiol.,* 1959, *147:* 226–238.
2. Hubel, D. H. and Wiesel, T. N. Receptive fields of single neurones in the cat's striate cortex. *J. Physiol.,* 1959, *148:* 574–591.
3. Hubel, D. H. and Wiesel, T. N. Receptive fields, binocular interaction and functional architecture in the cat's visual cortex. *J. Physiol.,* 1962, *160:* 106–154.
4. Hubel, D. H. and Wiesel, T. N. Shape and arrangement of columns in cat's striate cortex. *J. Physiol.,* 1963, *165:* 559–568.
5. Hubel, D. H. and Wiesel, T. N. Receptive fields of cells in striate cortex of very young, visually inexperienced kittens. *J. Neurophysiol.,* 1963, *26:* 994–1002.
6. Hubel, D. H. and Wiesel, T. N. Receptive fields and functional architecture in two nonstriate visual areas (18 and 19) of the cat. *J. Neurophysiol.,* 1965, *28:* 229–289.
7. Wiesel, T. N. and Hubel, D. H. Effects of visual deprivation on morphology and physiology of cells in the cat's lateral geniculate body. *J. Neurophysiol.,* 1963, *26:* 978–993.
8. Wiesel, T. N. and Hubel, D. H. Single-cell responses in striate cortex of kittens deprived of vision in one eye. *J. Neurophysiol.,* 1963, *26:* 1003–1017.
9. Wiesel, T. N. and Hubel, D. H. Comparison of the effects of unilateral and bilateral eye closure on cortical unit responses in kittens. *J. Neurophysiol.,* 1965, *28:* 1029–1040.
10. Wiesel, T. N. and Hubel, D. H. Extent of recovery from the effects of visual deprivation in kittens. *J. Neurophysiol.,* 1965, *28:* 1060–1072.

Extent of Recovery from the Effects of Visual Deprivation in Kittens[1]

TORSTEN N. WIESEL AND DAVID H. HUBEL • *Neurophysiology Laboratory, Department of Pharmacology, Harvard Medical School, Boston, Massachusetts*

INTRODUCTION

In kittens, deprivation of form and light over several months can lead to marked abnormalities in the visual pathway. These include behavioral blindness, morphological changes in the lateral geniculate body, and disruption of innately determined cortical connections (2, 6–8). This type of plasticity seems to be greatest in the early months of life and to decline rapidly with age; an adult cat deprived for similar periods showed no changes at all. We were naturally interested in whether the deprivation effects were permanent or whether they could be reversed by allowing normal stimuli to reach the retina again. Several kittens were therefore raised with the lids of one or both eyes sutured together for 3 months, as in previous experiments (6), and then the closed eye was reopened and the animals were allowed to live for another 3–14 months before making observations.

METHODS

Seven kittens were used, and the various procedures of deprivation and subsequent studies are summarized in Table 1. In six animals the lids of one eye were closed for the first 3 months of life. In the recovery period two of these kittens had the deprived eye opened. The other four had the deprived eye opened and the other (previously open) eye was closed. The seventh animal had both eyes closed for 3 months; the right eye was then opened. Recovery periods varied from 3 to 18 months. The animals were all kept together in a large, bright room, and were frequently played with by attendants and passersby.

Anatomical and physiological methods are described in other papers (1, 6, 8). Behavioral studies consisted mainly of observing the animal's use of vision to guide his activities. Tests of visual discrimination using operant-conditioning techniques are still being made on several animals; these will be reported elsewhere.

RESULTS

Behavior

The first kitten of this series had the right eye sutured shut from the tenth day up to 3 months of age. The lids were then separated under anesthesia. As with all the animals in this study the cornea was moist and clear; the fundus appeared normal, as were the direct and consensual pupillary light reflexes. At the outset the animal appeared to be blind in the deprived eye (7). The first signs of any recovery were noticed only after 2–3 weeks. With the good eye covered, the animal then seemed to be alerted by large objects moved in front of it, and at times would appear to follow them. These following movements showed some slight improvement with time, until after 3 months a large object was occasionally followed for several seconds. Even then, the animal did not always lock in on the object, but tended to lose it and go looking about wildly. Visual placing never returned. When put on the floor to roam freely, the animal would at times avoid large obstacles, but at other times would collide with them. It seldom avoided small objects such as chair legs. Placed on a chair, it would slide down, feeling its way with its forepaws. If the good eye was uncovered, the kitten would promptly jump to the floor.

This behavior was typical of all animals tested. Animal 2 (Table 1) was allowed to go for 18 months after the deprived eye was opened, but it showed little if any recovery after the first 3 or 4 months.

From *J. Neurophysiol.* 28:1060–1072

Received for publication December 23, 1964.

[1]This work was supported in part by Research Grants NB 02260-06, NB-05554-01, NB-02253-06 from the National Institutes of Health, and in part by Research Grant AF-49-638-1443 from the U. S. Air Force.

Table 1. Summary of Procedures Performed on the Seven Experimental Animals

Animal No.	DEPRIVATION			RECOVERY			PROCEDURE		
	Right eye	*Left eye*	*Time, months*	*Right eye*	*Left eye*	*Time, months*	*Anatomy*	*Physiology*	*Behavior*
1	Closed	Open	3	Open	Open	3	x		x
2	Closed	Open	3	Open	Open	18			x
3	Closed	Open	3	Open	Closed	3	x	x	x
4	Closed	Open	3	Open	Closed	8	x		x
5	Closed	Open	3	Open	Closed	14	x	x	x
6	Closed	Open	3	Open	Closed	18			x
7	Closed	Closed	3	Open	Closed	14	x	x	x

To test the possibility that, with both eyes open, the animals might in some way be "neglecting" the previously deprived eye, we sutured closed the normal eye at the time of opening the deprived one. This was done in four kittens (no. 3–6, Table 1). Following the eye reversal these animals did just as badly as the others, indicating that they could not be forced to use the deprived eye. The change in behavior was dramatic, especially for cat 6, which during the first 3 months had been the leader of about a dozen animals. This large, husky animal lost his prominent position in the group, became meek and cowardly, and even after 18 months is still subdued and anxious. Finally, the same kind of slow and inadequate recovery was seen in one animal (no. 7) that was initially deprived by bilateral suture, following which one eye was opened for over a year.

Single-Unit Recordings

Recovery After Monocular Deprivation. Cortical recordings were made from 3 of the 7 animals. In kitten 3 (Table 1) the right eye had been closed for the first 3 months, after which that eye was opened and the left eye closed for another 3 months. Two penetrations were made in striate cortex, one in each hemisphere, and 54 cells were recorded. The great majority of cells (45 of 54) were still driven exclusively from the left eye. Only 9 cells could be driven from the right eye; of these 8 were abnormal, and 7 were still strongly dominated by the left eye. Two cells were exclusively driven by the right eye. The ocular-dominance distribution, given in Fig. 1, was thus still highly abnormal; indeed it was probably not significantly

different from that of animals monocularly deprived for 3 months, as can be seen by comparing this figure with Fig. 2 in the paper on binocular deprivation (8). The 8 abnormal cells responded to a line stimulus regardless of its orientation; and showed a strong tendency to fatigue. That it was the connections between these cells and the right eye that were abnormal, rather than the cells themselves, is shown by the fact that the cells were driven in a perfectly normal manner by the left eye, having a precise receptive-field orientation and showing little tendency to fatigue. The 3 months' deprivation of the left eye immediately preceding the recording apparently had little or no effect on that eye's ability to drive cortical cells, despite the marked atrophy of the geniculate layers connected to the left eye (see below). In contrast to this, a simple closure of one eye following several months of normal vision produces a marked cortical defect (7). Taken together, these two results reinforce our conclusions from the binocular closures and strabismus experiments (8, 3) in suggesting a strong interdependence in the pathways originating from the two eyes.

Kitten 5 likewise had the right eye closed for the first 3 months, after which the right eye was opened and the left closed. It was then kept for over a year before recordings were made. The results of observing 72 cells in 2 penetrations are shown in Fig. 2. Again, the effects of the original deprivation to the right eye appear to have been irreversible or nearly so.

One result common to these two experiments is the absence of unresponsive cells. This contrasts with the usual monocular closure, in which some 10% of cells were not driven by either eye.

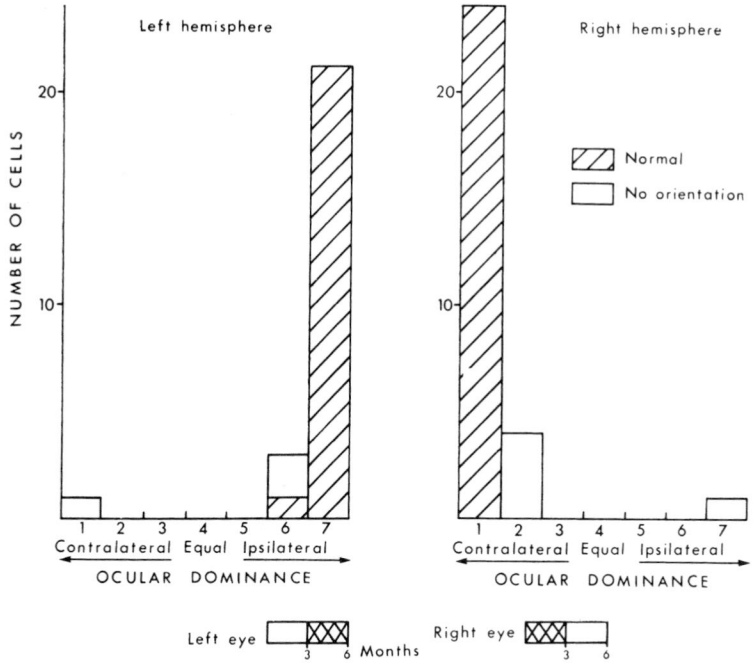

Fig. 1. *Ocular-dominance distribution of 54 cells recorded from a 6-month-old cat (no. 3) in which the right eye was closed for the first 3 months of life, following which the right eye was opened and the left eye closed for the next 3 months. (Definitions of the ocular-dominance groups are as follows: cells of group 1 are driven only by the contralateral eye; for cells of group 2 there is marked dominance of the contralateral eye; for group 3, slight dominance. For cells in group 4 there is no obvious difference between the two eyes. In group 5 the ipsilateral eye dominates slightly; in group 6, markedly, and in group 7 the cells are drive only by the ipsilateral eye.)*

RECOVERY AFTER BINOCULAR DEPRIVATION. It will be recalled that the cortical effects of depriving both eyes for the first 3 months of life are not at all what one would have predicted from the monocular deprivations (8): instead of only a very few responsive cells, 73% of the cells could be driven, and 41% responded normally. These results are summarized in the left-hand part of Table 2. In studying the cortical effects of reopening an eye one therefore begins with a totally different situation from that following monocular closure.

Cat 7 was brought up with both eyes closed for the first 3 months, at which time the right eye was opened. The animal then went for over a year with the left eye closed. Ninety-nine cells were studied in the two hemispheres, with the results shown in Fig. 3 and Table 2. The histograms show no striking predominance of the opened eye, indicating that, just as in the monocular closures, there was little tendency for recovery. On the other hand, an examination of Table 2 suggests that opening the eye did produce some changes. As in the other

recovery studies, unresponsive cells were diminished, amounting to 10% of the cells instead of 27%. At the same time, cells with abnormal responses (lack of receptive-field orientation) went from 32% to 60%. The abnormal responses came mainly from the right or opened eye, which accounted for twice as many abnormal fields as the left (52 as opposed to 25). Normal cells were, if anything, slightly reduced, and fewer of these were driven by the right eye (15%) than by the left (30%).

The asymmetry in the two eyes is further illustrated by the 31 cells that were driven from both eyes. Eight of these were driven normally from the left eye and abnormally from the right, having in that eye fields that lacked any clear orientation. The reverse was not true for any of the cells. Moreover, in our study of binocularly deprived animals without recovery there were none of these asymmetric cells, normal for one eye, but abnormal for the other. Here again it is as though the number of abnormal connections from the opened eye had greatly increased.

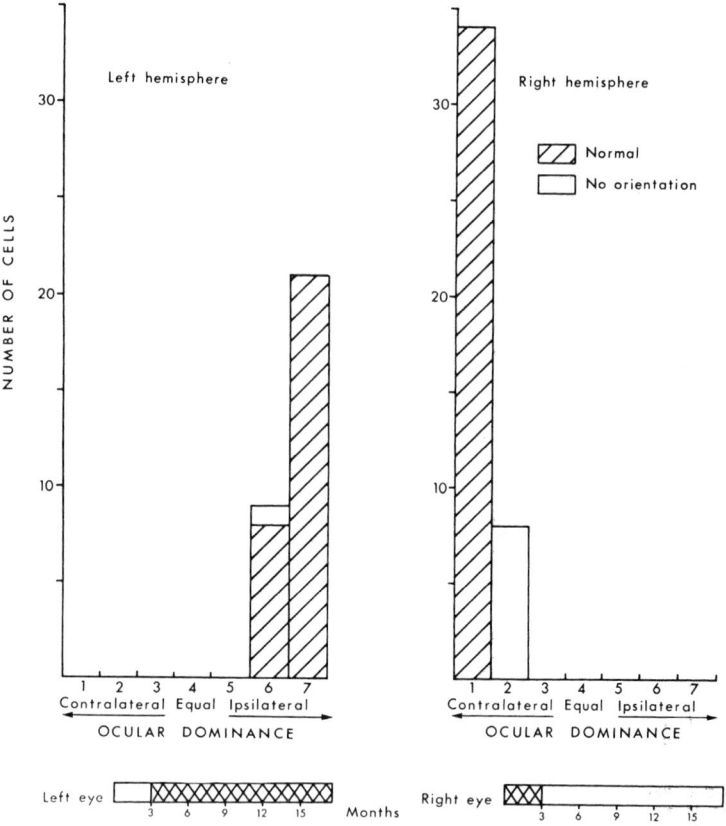

Fig. 2. Ocular dominance of 72 cells recorded from a cat (no. 5) in which the right eye was closed for the first 3 months of life, following which the right eye was opened and the left eye closed for the next 14 months.

In summary, it would seem that the recovery process had re-established connections between cortical cells and the opened eye, but that these connections were distorted ones. The fact that following recovery fewer cells were driven normally from the opened (right) eye than from the closed one is at first glance surprising. The "normal" category is, however, somewhat arbitrary and, in animals before the recovery period, it might include cells that had lost some connections and therefore responded less briskly than normal but with full specificity. If during the recovery process the lost

Table 2. Comparison of Single-Cell Responses Following 3-Month Binocular Deprivation, with and without Periods of Recovery

	3-MONTH BINOCULAR DEPRIVATION (8)		3-MONTH BINOCULAR DEPRIVATION FOLLOWED BY 14 MONTHS RECOVERY OF RIGHT EYE (CAT 7)	
	Cells	*Percent*	*Cells*	*Percent*
Normal cells	57	41	28	
Abnormally driven	45	32	61*	60
Unresponsive	37	27	10	10
Total cells	139	100	99	100

* Includes cells that were driven abnormally by one eye and normally by the other, as well as cells driven abnormally by both eyes.

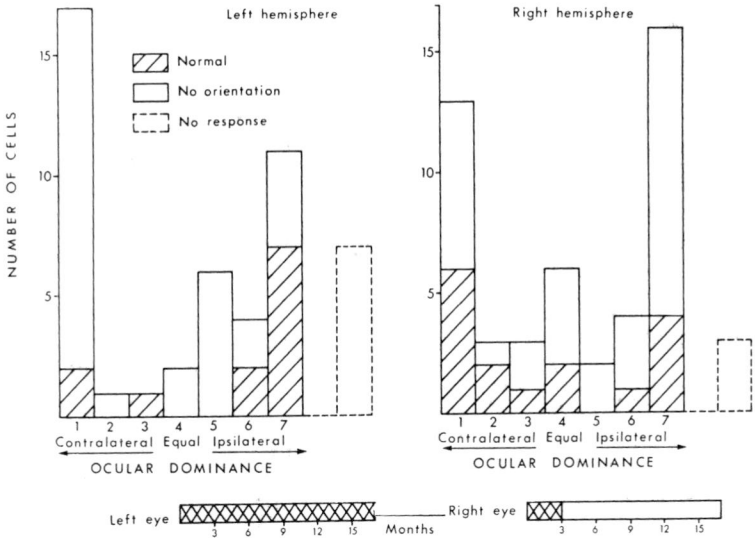

Fig. 3. Ocular-dominance distribution of 99 cells in a cat (no. 7) in which both eyes were closed for the first 3 months of life, following which the right eye was opened for the next 14 months.

connections were re-established, but in distorted form, one would have an increase of abnormal cells at the expense of the normal category. It does seem unlikely that opening an eye would cause abnormal connections to be established between that eye and otherwise normal cells.

Finally, this animal showed a marked increase in the proportion of cells driven only by one eye, cells of groups 1 and 7. The change resembles that seen in animals raised with squint or with alternating contact occluders (3), both conditions in which the synergic action of the two eyes is eliminated without the complication of complete disuse. Three months of binocular occlusion gave no comparable defect (8), suggesting that in the present experiment the relative increase in groups 1 and 7 must have taken place during the recovery period. Perhaps the process simply requires more time when the lack of synergy is produced by disuse, a point that could easily be settled by binocular deprivation for longer periods.

Morphology of the Lateral Geniculate Body

Of the 5 animals whose brains have been sectioned so far, 4 were studied by examining the Nissl-stained sections and by measuring cross-sectional areas of 50 cells in each geniculate layer. The results were unanimous in failing to show the least evi-

dence for any recovery. They are summarized in Table 3. For comparison, figures are included from an animal whose right eye was closed for the first 3 months. The average cell size of the dorsal pair of layers (A and A_1) in the normal cat at 3 months or older is about $300\mu^2$. (As discussed previously (6), cell sizes vary to some extent from one animal to the next, partly, no doubt, because of differences in fixation. We have found no evidence that cells increase significantly in size beyond 3 months of age. This seems to be confirmed by comparing in Table 3 the size of normal cells in the 3-month-old control cat with the normal cell size in the 6-month-old cat *1*.)

The simplest assessment of recovery can be made for cat *1*, in which the right eye was closed for the first 3 months and was open for the next 3, the left having been open at all times. Coronal sections of the two geniculates are shown in Fig. 4. The degeneration of layers A on the left and A_1 on the right is roughly the same as in animals with one eye closed for 3 months, and no recovery period (see ref. 6, Fig. 1). Cell sizes in corresponding layers on the two sides still differ by some 30%.

The other three animals confirm this finding, and show that if growth of cells is retarded by eye suture for the first 3 months, there is little or no subsequent recovery even if the eye is reopened for over 1 year. This is particularly impressive in cat 7 in

Table 3. Effects of the Various Experimental Procedures on Size of Cells in the Two Dorsal Layers of the Lateral Geniculate Body

Description of Cat	Layer	L. Side, μ^2	R. Side μ^2	Diff. Between Sides, %	DEV. FROM ASSUMED NORMAL OF 300μ^2, *%	
					Left	Right
Control: simple suture	A			37 (t = 4.8)	39	
R. eye closed 3 months						
L. eye open 3 months	A_1			38 (t = 5.6)		34
Cat 1: simple eye opening	A			28 (t = 6.3)	39	
R. eye closed 3 months, open 3 months						
L. eye open throughout	A_1			30 (t = 5.7)		34
Cat 3: eye reversal	A			11 (t = 0.6)	43	36
R. eye closed 3 months, open 3 months						
L. eye open 3 months, closed 3 months	A_1			25 (t = 1.2)	30	47
Cat 5: eye reversal	A			16 (t = 2.8)	47	36
R. eye closed 3 months, open 14 months						
L. eye open 3 months, closed 14 months	A_1	203 ± 11	172 ± 10	15 (t = 2.1)	33	43
Cat 7: binocular	A				43	38
R. eye closed 3 months, open 14 months						
L. eye closed throughout	A_1	201 ± 7	202 ± 9		33	33

* Assumed normal based on average of 10 cats ranging in age from 3 months to 1½ years. According to our measurements any growth in cells after 3 months is negligible.

which both eyes were closed for 3 months and the right eye was then opened for 14 months. Here there was no significant difference in corresponding geniculate layers on the two sides. A coronal section through the right lateral geniculate is shown in Fig. 5, and actual cell sizes are given in Table 3.

Finally, the eye-reversal results (cats 3 and 5) confirm our previous impression that late eye closure can produce an actual atrophy of cells (as opposed to the failure to grow produced by closure). The shrinkage is not as pronounced as that produced by initial closure, as can be seen directly in coronal sections of the geniculates of cat 5 (Fig. 6), and also from the actual measurements of cell size given in Table 3. A comparison of the atrophy in cats 3 and 5 indicates that the main atrophic changes occur within the first 3 months of the late closure. Comparing cats 5 and 7 suggests that it makes little difference to the abnormality produced, whether an eye is closed for the first 3 months or the first 17.

DISCUSSION

The absence of any great degree of recovery in this study was surprising, since previous reports on behavioral recovery following deprivation in man (5) and in animals (4) had led us to expect some return of function, slow and perhaps incomplete, to judge from human experience, and prompt and virtually complete, to judge from the animal experiments. It is difficult to reconcile these results. The human material is particularly hard to assess, since one frequently does not know certain crucial facts such as the age of onset of cataracts, the degree of reduction of retinal illumination, and the final extent of return of vision after cataract removal. In behavioral studies in animals a direct comparison of results is not possible, since schedules of visual deprivation and testing procedures have differed from those used in the present experiments. The evaluation of visual abnormalities in animals is in any case difficult, there being no generally accepted

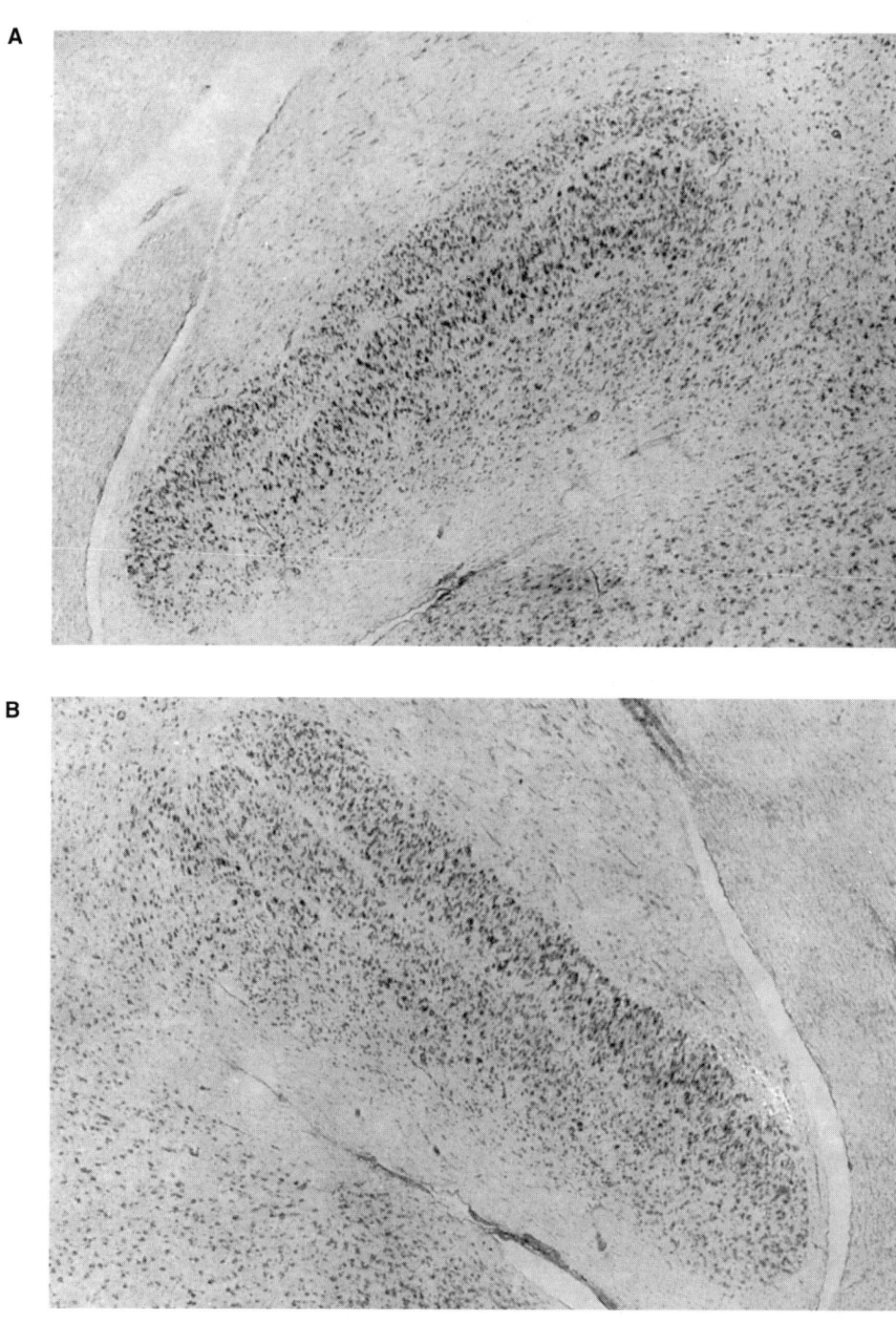

1 mm

Fig. 4. Coronal sections of left (A) *and right* (B) *lateral geniculate bodies of a 6-month-old kitten (no. 1) in which the right eye was closed for the first 3 months of life and open for the next 3, the left being open at all times. Celloidin, cresyl violet.*

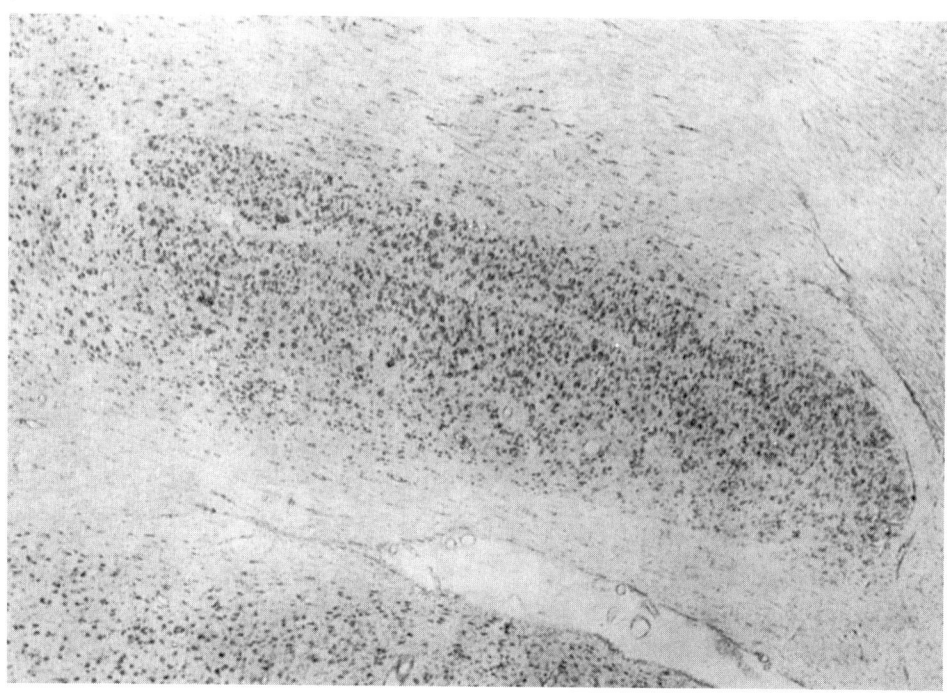

1 mm

Fig. 5. Coronal sections through right lateral geniculate body of a cat (no. 7) in which both eyes were closed for the first 3 months of life, and then the right eye was opened for the next 14 months. Note that cells in the middle layer (A₁), corresponding to the right eye, appear no different from those of the dorsal layer (A). Celloidin, cresyl violet.

or well-evaluated procedures for testing vision in normal animals.

All three phases of the present study—the behavioral, the physiological, and the morphological—agree in indicating only very minimal recovery from the effects of eye closure during the first 3 months of life. In the cortex such connections as did reform apparently did so in a distorted manner. There would seem to be two possible interpretations. Either connections, once lost, are incapable of properly re-establishing themselves, or the failure of recovery may simply be a matter of age— another manifestation of the decline in flexibility that occurs in the system some time between the third month and the first year. Experimentally it is difficult to know how to decide between these interpretations, since it probably requires a month or two to produce the abnormalities, by which time the period of flexibility may well be almost over.

SUMMARY

In kittens, monocular or binocular deprivation by lid suture for the first 3 months of life leads to virtual blindness, marked morphological changes in the lateral geniculate body, and a severe deterioration of innate cortical connections. In seven kittens whose eyes had been sutured at birth for 3 months, six unilaterally and one bilaterally, an attempt was made to assess the extent of recovery by reopening an eye and allowing the animals to live for another 3–15 months. In two of the monocular closures the deprived eye was opened and the normal eye closed.

In all kittens there was some slight behavioral recovery during the first 3 months, but the animals remained severely handicapped and never learned to move freely using visual cues. There was no morphological improvement in the lateral geniculate body. Our previous impression that atrophy can

A

B

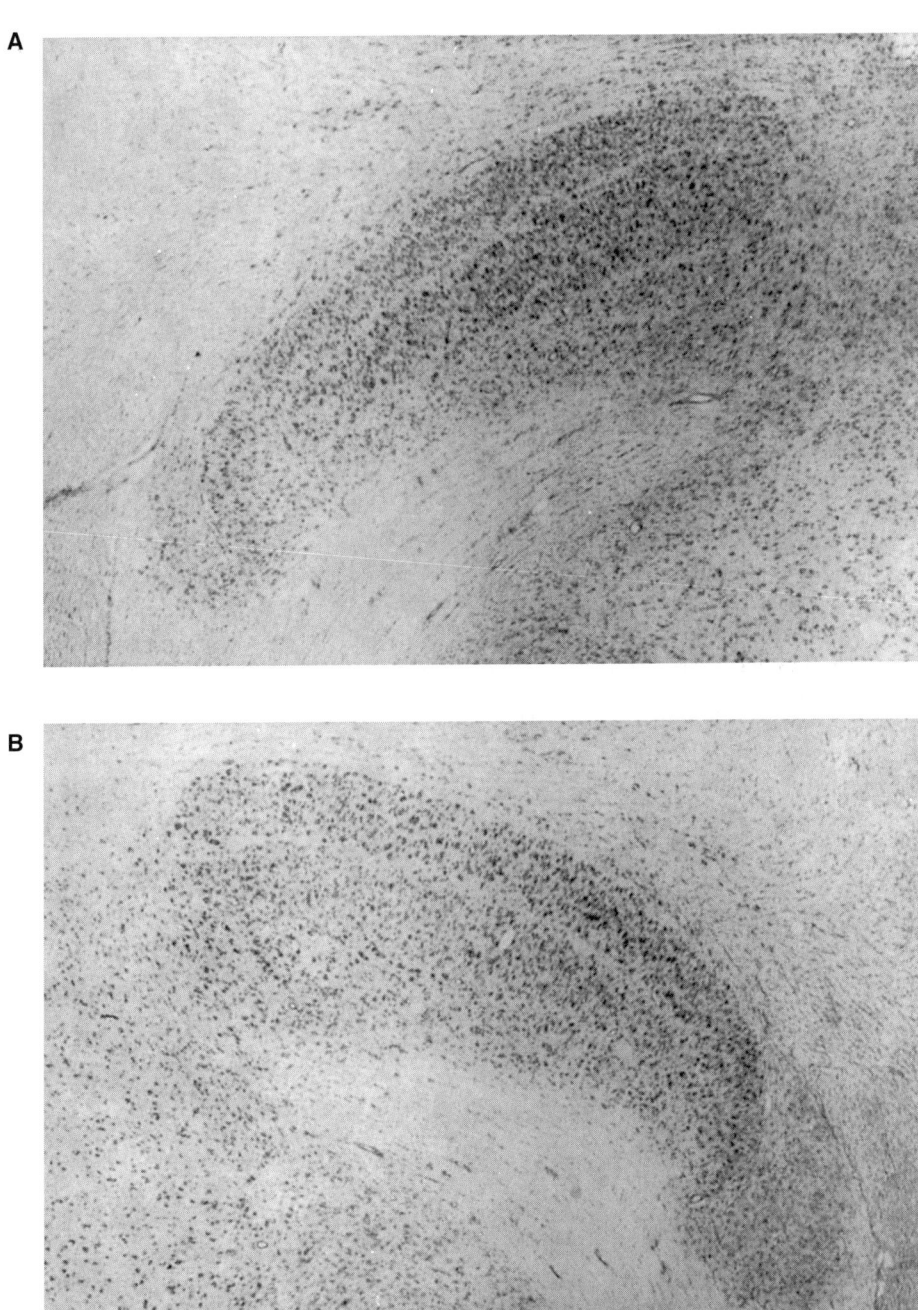

1 mm

Fig. 6. Coronal sections through left (A) and right (B) lateral geniculate bodies of a cat (no. 5) in which the right eye was closed for the first 3 months of life, following which the right eye was opened and the left eye closed for the next 14 months. Note the small size of cells in the dorsal layer of the left geniculate and the middle layer of the right, corresponding to the originally closed right eye. Celloidin, cresyl violet.

develop with deprivation beginning at 3 months was confirmed. In monocularly deprived animals a few cells in the striate cortex may have recovered responses to stimulation to the originally deprived eye, but in many of these cells the responses were abnormal. In the binocularly deprived kitten there was a marked increase in the proportion of cells responding abnormally to the eye that was re-opened, without any obvious increase in the total number of cells responding to that eye.

We conclude that the animals' capacity to recover from the effects of early monocular or binocular visual deprivation, whether measured behaviorally, morphologically, or in terms of single-cell cortical physiology, is severely limited, even for recovery periods of over a year.

ACKNOWLEDGMENT

We express our thanks to Jane Chen, Janet Tobie, and John Tuckerman for their technical assistance.

References

1. Hubel, D. H. and Wiesel, T. N. Receptive fields, binocular interaction and functional architecture in the cat's visual cortex. *J. Physiol.,* 1962, *160:* 106–154.
2. Hubel, D. H. and Wiesel, T. N. Receptive fields of cells in striate cortex of very young, visually inexperienced kittens. *J. Neurophysiol.,* 1963, *26:* 994–1002.
3. Hubel, D. H. and Wiesel, T. N. Binocular interaction in striate cortex of kittens reared with artificial squint. *J. Neurophysiol.,* 1965, *28:* 1041–1059.
4. Riesen, A. H. Stimulation as requirement for growth and function in behavioral development. In: *Functions of Varied Experience,* edited by D. W. Fiske and S. R. Maddi. Homewood, Ill., Dorsey Press, 1961, pp. 57–105.
5. Von Senden, M. *Raum-und Gestaltauffassung bei operierten Blindgeborenen vor und nach der Operation,* edited by J. Barth. Leipzig, 1932, English translation under the title: *Space and Sight.* Glencoe, Ill., Free Press, 1960.
6. Wiesel, T. N. and Hubel, D. H. Effects of visual deprivation on morphology and physiology of cells in the cat's lateral geniculate body. *J. Neurophysiol.,* 1963, *26:* 978–993.
7. Wiesel, T. N. and Hubel, D. H. Single-cell responses in striate cortex of kittens deprived of vision in one eye. *J. Neurophysiol.,* 1963, *26:* 1003–1017.
8. Wiesel, T. N. and Hubel, D. H. Comparison of the effects of unilateral and bilateral eye closure on cortical unit responses in kittens. *J. Neurophysiol.,* 1965, *28:* 1029–1040.

The Period of Susceptibility to the Physiological Effects of Unilateral Eye Closure in Kittens

D. H. HUBEL AND T. N. WIESEL • *Department of Neurobiology, Harvard Medical School, Boston, Massachusetts 02115, U.S.A.*

SUMMARY

1. Kittens were visually deprived by suturing the lids of the right eye for various periods of time at different ages. Recordings were subsequently made from the striate cortex, and responses from the two eyes compared. As previously reported, monocular eye closure during the first few months of life causes a sharp decline in the number of cells that can be influenced by the previously closed eye.

2. Susceptibility to the effects of eye closure begins suddenly near the start of the fourth week, remains high until some time between the sixth and eighth weeks, and then declines, disappearing finally around the end of the third month. Monocular closure for over a year in an adult cat produces no detectable effects.

3. During the period of high susceptibility in the fourth and fifth weeks eye closure for as little as 3–4 days leads to a sharp decline in the number of cells that can be driven from both eyes, as well as an over-all decline in the relative influence of the previously closed eye. A 6-day closure is enough to give a reduction in the number of cells that can be driven by the closed eye to a

From *J. Physiol.* (1970), **206,** *pp.* 419–436

Received 11 August 1969.

fraction of the normal. The physiological picture is similar to that following a 3-month monocular deprivation from birth, in which the proportion of cells the eye can influence drops from 85 to about 7%.

4. Cells of the lateral geniculate receiving input from a deprived eye are noticeably smaller and paler to Nissl stain following 3 or 6 days' deprivation during the fourth week.

5. Following 3 months of monocular deprivation, opening the eye for up to 5 yr produces only a very limited recovery in the cortical physiology, and no obvious recovery of the geniculate atrophy, even though behaviourally there is some return of vision in the deprived eye. Closing the normal eye, though necessary for behavioural recovery, has no detectable effect on the cortical physiology. The amount of possible recovery in the striate cortex is probably no greater if the period of eye closure is limited to 7 weeks, but after a 5-week closure there is a definite enhancement of the recovery, even though it is far from complete.

INTRODUCTION

Neurophysiological studies of single cells indicate that the highly specialized neurones in the cat visual cortex establish their proper connexions through innate mechanisms (Hubel & Wiesel, 1963). During the first months after birth these connexions are vulnerable, and can be disrupted through various procedures of visual deprivation such as closing the lids of one or both eyes, or surgically producing a strabismus (Wiesel & Hubel, 1963*b*; Hubel & Wiesel, 1965). For example, after an eye has been closed for the first 10–12 weeks of life only a small fraction of recorded cortical cells can be driven from that eye, while nearly all cells can be driven from the normal eye. In the adult cat, in contrast, there is no such sensitivity to deprivation; the cortical cells retain their inborn ability to respond to stimulation of an eye that has been closed for 3 months.

The disruption of cortical connexions following early eye closure is not accompanied by any anatomical changes that can be seen with stains for Nissl substance or myelin. In contrast, cells in the lateral geniculate body are virtually normal in their responses but show marked morphological changes

(Wiesel & Hubel, 1963*a*). Again, such abnormalities are not seen following a comparable period of closure in the adult.

These experimental results show that there must be a critical vulnerable period in the first 10–12 weeks, after which the animal is immune to deprivation procedures. In the present paper we set out to examine the timing more precisely. We wished to learn when the susceptibility was greatest, how long it lasted, the duration of deprivation necessary to produce a severe deficit, and the relation between timing of deprivation and ability to recover.

METHODS

Experiments were done on twenty-one monocularly deprived kittens and on two normal 4-week-old kittens. The deprived animals all had their right eyes closed by lid suture at various ages and for varying lengths of time. In some animals the right eyes were subsequently reopened to test recovery, and in some of these the left eye was closed at the time the right eye was opened ('eye reversal').

At the time of recording the kittens were anaesthetized with thiopentone and paralysed with intravenous succinylcholine to prevent eye movements. Recordings were made from single cells with extracellular tungsten micro-electrodes. Receptive fields were mapped by projecting white-light stimuli upon a wide flat white screen which the animal faced from a distance of 1.5 m. A white background light was kept at mesopic levels (–1 to +1 $\log_{10}$cd/m^2) and the intensity of the stimulating light was 1–1.5 log units brighter than the background. As in previous studies (Wiesel & Hubel, 1963*b*) recordings were usually made in the hemisphere contralateral to the previously closed eye. In the normal cat about twice as many cells are dominated by the contralateral eye as by the ipsilateral, so that a shift in favour of the ipsilateral eye is all the more significant.

At the end of the experiments the animals were perfused with normal saline followed by 10% formalin, the brains were embedded in celloidin, sectioned at 25 μ and stained with cresyl violet. The histological material was used for reconstruction of electrode tracks and for studies of morphologic changes in the lateral geniculate bodies.

RESULTS

In the normal adult cats about four fifths of the cells in the striate cortex can be influenced from both eyes (Hubel & Wiesel, 1962). The relative influence of the two eyes on cortical cells varies from one cell to the next. Some cells receive roughly equal inputs from the two eyes, while in others one eye is strongly dominant or completely so. Cells dominated by one eye show a tendency to be grouped in columns (Hubel & Wiesel, 1965), so that in any micro-electrode penetration perpendicular to the surface of the cortex most or all of the observed cells prefer one eye, though over half show some response to the other.

These findings apply also to kittens with no patterned visual experience, for example animals examined close to the time of birth (Hubel & Wiesel, 1963). We conclude from this that the connexions underlying the observed responses are innate. In the present study many of the deprived kittens were recorded from at an age of 4–6 weeks. We therefore began by recording from normal kittens at this age, to rule out the unlikely possibility that the ocular-dominance distribution might differ from that of either newborn kittens or adult

cats. Figure 1A shows the ocular-dominance distribution obtained in three micro-electrode penetrations in two normal kittens 3–4 weeks old. The composite histogram for all three penetrations is shown in Fig. 1B. As expected, the results are similar to those previously obtained in new-born kittens and in adult cats (Hubel & Wiesel, 1962, 1963).

Monocular Closure from Birth, for Periods of Varying Length

In ten kittens from five litters the lids of the right eye were sutured together at about 10 days and recordings were made at various times during the next 2–3 months. For any given period of deprivation during the sensitive period there was some variation in results from one kitten to the next, which was minimized by first comparing individuals within the same litter, and then comparing litters. The earliest recordings, made at about one month of age, were already abnormal. Figure 2A shows the results obtained from a kitten whose

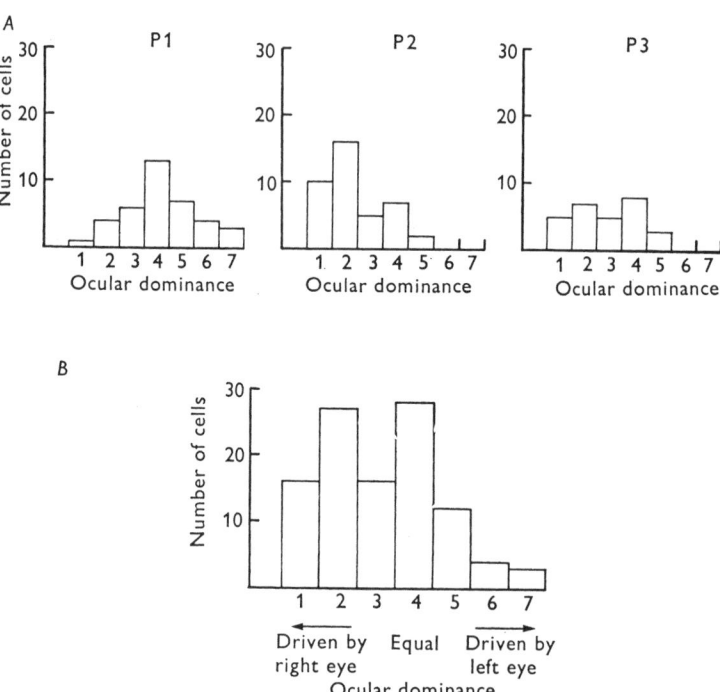

Fig. 1. Upper three histograms: ocular-dominance distributions of cells from three penetrations in striate cortex of two normal kittens, 3–4 weeks old. Lower histogram: sum of above three histograms. (Definition of ocular-dominance groups: cells of group 1 were driven only by the contralateral eye; for cells of group 2 there was marked dominance of the contralateral eye; for group 3, slight dominance. For cells in group 4 there was no obvious difference between the two eyes. In group 5 the ipsilateral eye dominated slightly; in group 6, markedly, and in group 7 the cells were driven only by the ipsilateral eye.)

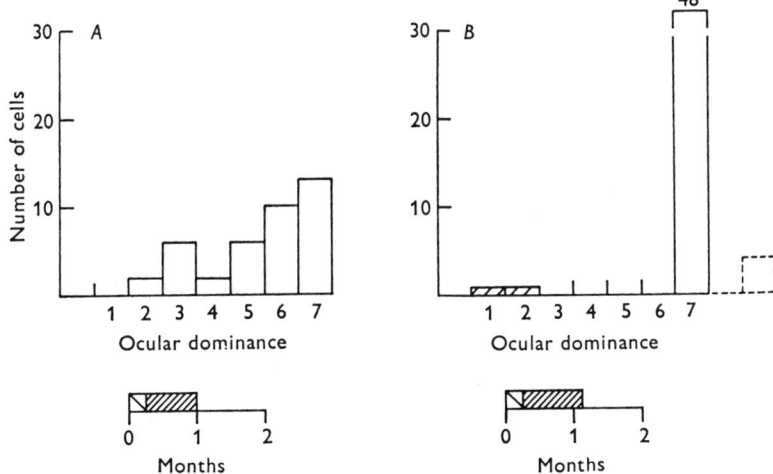

Fig. 2. *Ocular-dominance distribution of cells recorded in the left visual cortex of two kittens, litter-mates, in which the right eye was closed* (A) *from the 10th to 31st day;* (B) *from the 10th to 37th day.* □ *normal response;* [ ] *no orientation;* ▨ *no response. Coiling as in Fig. 1.*

right eye was closed from day 10 to day 31. The thirty-eight cells recorded in two penetrations gave a lopsided histogram showing clear dominance of the normal eye. Moreover, the responses from the right eye were generally more sluggish and fatigued more easily than those from the left, which seemed entirely normal.

Six days later, at 37 days, a litter-mate of this kitten gave the results shown in Fig. 2*B*. Now the

shift in favour of the left eye was virtually complete, with only two cells out of fifty-four driven by the closed eye. Four cells were uninfluenced by either eye, an abnormality commonly found in monocularly deprived kittens (Wiesel & Hubel, 1963*b*).

Results from a second litter, also with right eye closure from birth, are shown in Fig. 3. The first kitten in this litter (Fig. 3*A*) was studied at 37 days

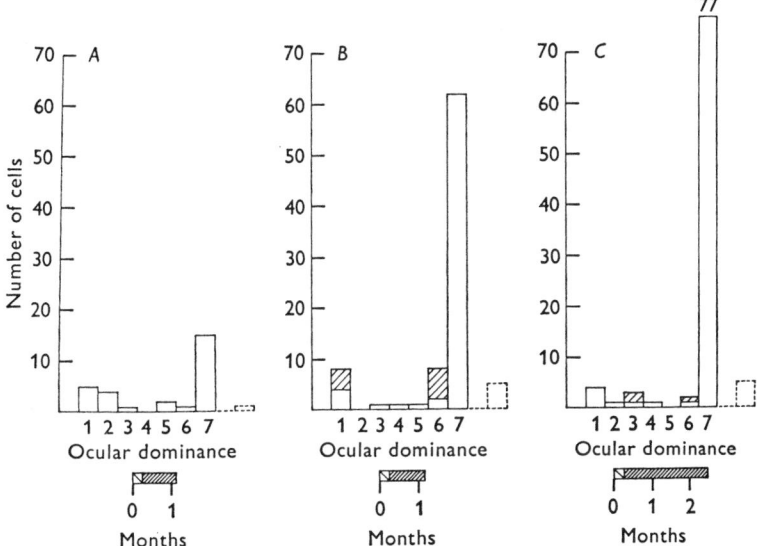

Fig. 3. *Ocular-dominance histograms for cells in the left visual cortex in three kittens, litter-mates, deprived by right-eye closure during days* (A) *10 to 37;* (B) *10 to 41;* (C) *10 to 75. Coding of responses as in Fig. 1.*

of age. Here the shift was not as marked as that of Fig. 2B, even though the duration of closure was the same. The histogram was nevertheless abnormal, with a shift in favour of the open eye and a dropping out of most binocularly driven cells. Four days later (41 days) a second member of the litter showed decidedly more advanced changes (Fig. 3B), though again some cells were still driven from the right eye. Many of these cells, however, responded sluggishly to the right eye and failed to show the usual selectivity to oriented line stimuli, whereas the responses seen from the left eye were normal. In a third animal, taken from the same litter at 75 days, the changes were still more pronounced (Fig. 3C). Now even fewer cells could be driven from the right eye, and with one exception all cells responded weakly from that eye, with none of the usual preference for a specific stimulus orientation. In this litter, then, the most dramatic changes seem to have occurred during the sixth week of life, between the recordings of Fig. 3A and B.

The results shown in Figs. 2B, 3B and 3C agree with our previous studies in 2–3 month deprived kittens. They are at variance with the findings of Ganz, Fitch & Satterberg (1968), who, using comparable durations of deprivation, found a roughly equal number of cells activated from the deprived and normal eyes. The reason for this difference in results is not clear, but in any case there is agreement that responses from the deprived eye are grossly abnormal.

Figures 2 and 3 illustrate the variations that can occur from one litter to the next. The earliest abnormalities were found in two litter-mates deprived from days 10–30 and 10–32 (not illustrated). In both of these kittens almost all the cells observed were driven by only the eye that had been open, giving a histogram similar to that of Fig. 2B.

The results from all five litters suggest that the changes begin by about the fifth week of life, and can become very marked in a matter of a few days.

Monocular Closure During the Sensitive Period

Our next step was to close an eye for only a few days in normal animals 3–5 weeks old, comparing various ages and durations of closure. The histogram of Fig. 4A shows the results of a 3-day closure in the 4th week (days 23–26). Even with such a brief period of deprivation the results were abnormal, comparable to those from an animal deprived from birth to 37 days (Fig. 3A). In this animal and in several others with eye closure from birth (e.g. the animals of Fig. 3A and B), there was not only some shift in favour of the normal eye, but also a marked decline in the number of binocularly driven cells, especially those in which the two eyes make almost equal contributions (groups 3 to 5). At this stage, before the normal eye has taken over completely, the ocular-dominance distribution thus tends to resemble that of animals with strabismus (Hubel & Wiesel, 1965). It is as though connexions from the open eye were in some way competing with connexions from the closed eye, hastening their disruption. By this line of reasoning, one

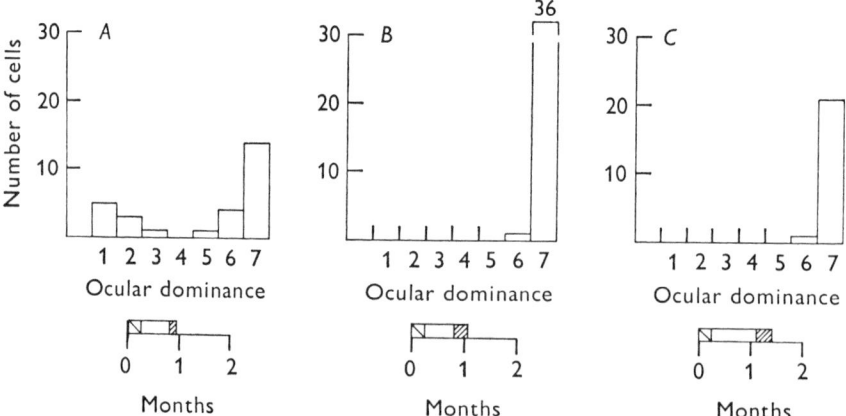

Fig. 4. Ocular-dominance histograms for cells in the left visual cortex in three kittens deprived by right-eye closure during days (A) 23 to 26; (B) 23 to 29; (C) 30 to 39. Kittens B and C were litter-mates. Coding as in Fig. 1.

might expect that cells with little or no input from the open eye (groups 1 and 2) would be less vulnerable to the effects of eye closure (Wiesel & Hubel, 1965*a*).

In a second animal, from a different litter, monocular deprivation from day 23 to 29 gave the result shown in Fig. 4*B*. Here the shift in ocular dominance was almost complete. A similar result was seen in a litter-mate deprived during days 30–39 (Fig. 4*C*). These experiments show that the sensitive period has a duration of at least several weeks, during which a few days of closure causes marked cortical changes.

Upper Limit of Sensitive Period

Our earlier work indicated that the period of sensitivity to monocular eye closure was limited (Wiesel & Hubel, 1963*b*). In an adult cat a 3-month closure produced no physiological or anatomical abnormalities. At two months of age, closure for 1 month gave the abnormal ocular-dominance distribution shown in Fig. 5*A*, but the changes were far from the extreme ones produced in the present study by much briefer periods of deprivation during the second month. Closure at 2 months for 4 months produced little additional damage (Fig. 5*B*), suggesting that the sensitive period may decline at about 3 months of age.

In the present series (Fig. 6) we closed an eye of a 4-month-old kitten for a period of 3 months.

This was followed by 16 months in which both eyes were open and during which extensive behavioural tests showed normal vision in the two eyes (Dews & Wiesel, 1970). When the animal was finally studied physiologically at almost 2 years of age the ocular-dominance histogram, shown in Fig. 6*A*, was also normal. The studies on recovery described previously (Wiesel & Hubel, 1965*b*) and in the next section make it most unlikely that any significant physiological recovery occurred after the deprived eye was opened.

A second kitten had one eye closed at 6 months of age for a period of 4 months. None of the receptive fields in the closed eye were abnormal, and the histogram, shown in Fig. 6*B*, is probably within normal limits. Finally, a 16-month closure in an adult cat likewise produced no abnormalities (Fig. 6*C*). A 6-month-old kitten and an adult cat were deprived for periods comparable to those of Fig. 6*B* and *C*, and then were tested behaviourally immediately after the deprived eye was opened. These animals had normal vision in the deprived eye.

We conclude that the susceptibility to the effects of deprivation, which appears rather suddenly near the beginning of the fourth week and is very great during that week, begins to fall some time between the sixth and eighth week, continues to decline during the third month, and has disappeared by the end of that month. An adult cat

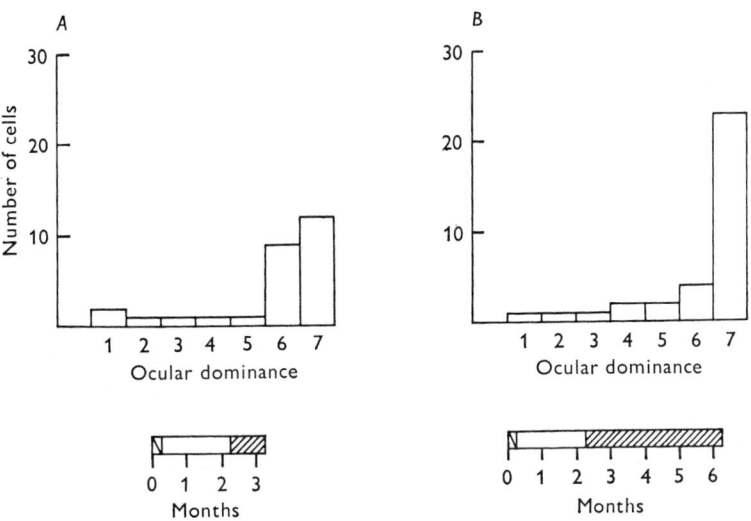

Fig. 5. Ocular-dominance histograms for cells in the left visual cortex of two kittens, not litter-mates, deprived by right-eye closure (A) from age 2 months to 3 months; (B) from age 2 months to 6 months. Coding as in Fig. 1. (From Wiesel & Hubel, 1963b.)

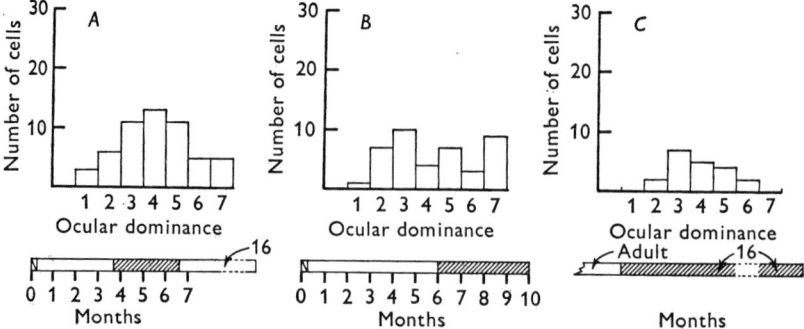

Fig. 6. Ocular-dominance histograms for cells in the left visual cortex of cats deprived by (A) right-eye lid suture at 4 months, eye opened at 7 months and recordings made at 2 years of age; (B) right-eye lid suture at 6 months, recording at 10 months; (C) right-eye lid suture in adult, recording 16 months later. Coding as in Fig. 1.

seems completely resistant to monocular deprivation.

Recovery from Monocular Deprivation of Various Durations

The effects of monocular deprivation for the first 3 months of life tend to be permanent, with very limited morphological, physiological, or behavioural recovery (Wiesel & Hubel, 1965*b*). It seemed important to ask whether the recovery would be greater in animals deprived only for the minimum time necessary to give severe physiological changes. For this purpose we used two litter-mates of the

kitten whose 10–37 day deprivation effects are shown in Fig. 2B. These kittens had their right eyelids sutured at 10 days and reopened at 37 days; one was studied physiologically after a 12-month recovery period, the other after 14 months. Recordings were almost identical in the two animals (Fig. 7A and B), and indicate a recovery that was clearly greater than that seen after 3 months deprivation, although it was still very limited. The degree of recovery is perhaps greater than indicated by the histograms alone, since a high proportion of the cells driven by the right eye were normal in their responses and stimulus requirements, and also

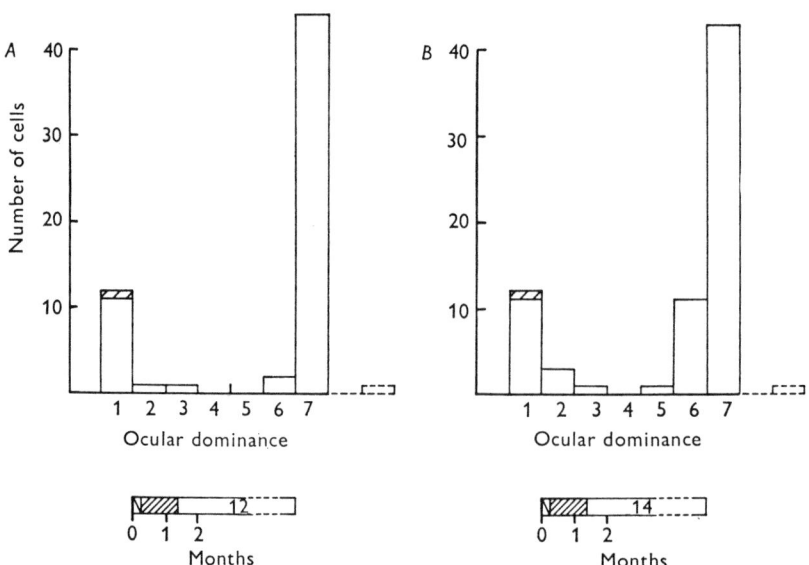

Fig. 7. Ocular-dominance histograms for cells in the left visual cortex of two litter-mates of kitten of Fig. 2B. Right-eye suture at 10 days, opened at 37 days. Recordings made at (A) 12 months (cat no. 13, Dews & Wiesel, 1970); and (B) 14 months after eyes were opened (cat no. 12, Dews & Wiesel, 1970). Coding as in Fig. 1.

since the number of cells that could not be driven by either eye was low compared with what is usually seen immediately after monocular deprivation. This decrease in unresponsive cells after a recovery period has been a consistent finding (Wiesel & Hubel, 1965*b*).

In both animals the scarcity of binocular cells is striking; only about one fifth of the cells, instead of the normal four fifths, received inputs from both eyes. Thus it appears that the normal binocular connexions are not only among the first to go (Figs. 3*A* and 4*A*), but are the least likely to recover. In these penetrations the cells that were driven exclusively by the closed eye tended to occur in groups, as though they were clustered together in the cortex. Normally cells tend to be grouped according to eye dominance (Hubel & Wiesel, 1965), so that presumably the cells that re-establish functional connexions with the deprived eye are those that were strongly dominated by that eye in the first place.

The effect of an additional 2 weeks of deprivation upon subsequent recovery is seen in Fig. 8. Here a pair of litter-mates were monocularly deprived between days 10 and 51, and then one was recorded from and the other allowed to recover after opening the lids for 11 months. As expected, the deprivation in the first kitten resulted in virtu-

ally complete domination by the left eye (Fig. 8*A*). After 11 months there was some minor recovery in the litter-mate, but considerably less than that seen in the animals of Fig. 7. Many of the cells driven by right eye showed abnormal responses. Thus in the critical period even a slight increase in duration of deprivation, to an age of 7 weeks as opposed to 5, may be important in further limiting the recovery. This is supported by the behavioural studies of some of these same animals (Dews & Wiesel, 1970).

Finally, in two kittens (not litter-mates) the right eyes were closed for the first 3–4 months of life and then opened. In one animal both eyes then remained open for the next 30 months. In the other, the left eye was closed for a year and then opened, and from then on both eyes were open for the next 58 months. When these animals were ultimately studied physiologically neither showed any spectacular recovery (Fig. 9), but just the usual slight increase in cells driven by the originally closed eye and a decline in the number of unresponsive cells. Eye reversal, comparable to patching an amblyopic human eye, thus had no detectable effects in the physiological studies. In contrast there was a clear difference in the behavioural recovery of the two animals, for the first (not reversed) cat remained completely and permanently form-blind in the

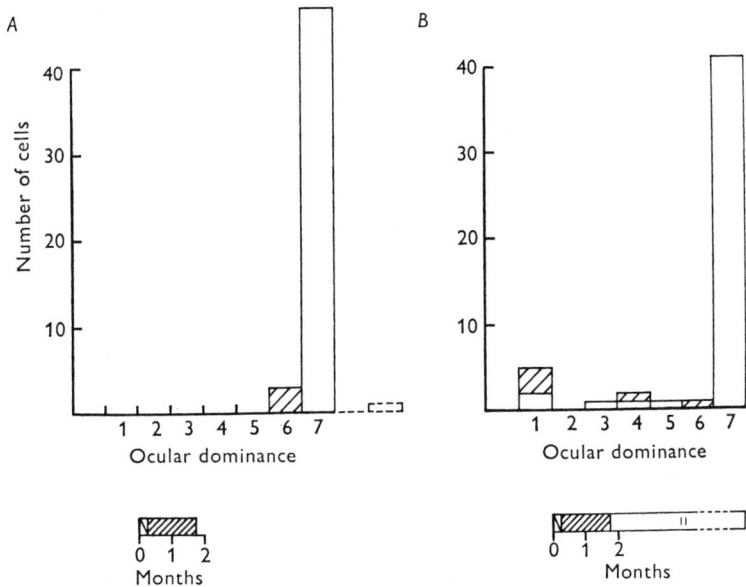

Fig. 8. Ocular-dominance histograms for cells in the left visual cortex of two litter-mates. (A) Right eyelids sutured from day 10 to day 51. (B) Right eyelids sutured from days 10 to 51, right eye than opened for 11 months.

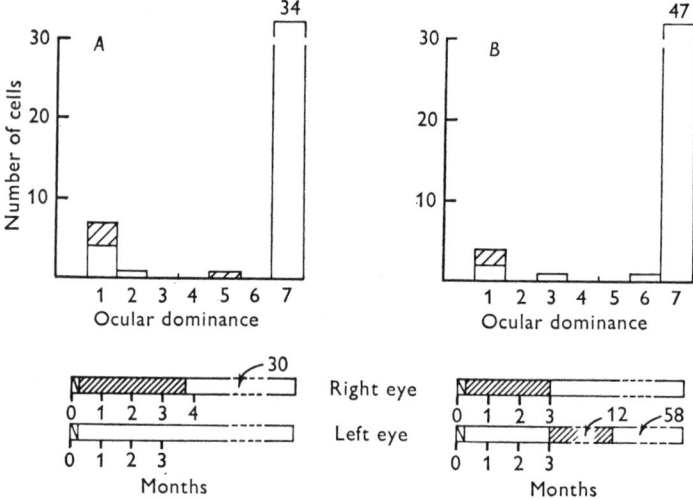

Fig. 9. Ocular-dominance histograms for cells in the left visual cortex of two kittens whose right eyes were closed for the first 3–4 months and then opened. (A) Both eyes were then kept open for 30 months (cat no. 10, Dews & Wiesel, 1970). (B) Left eye was then closed for 1 year, and then opened. From then on both eyes remained open for the next 4 years and 10 months. The cat was finally recorded from at age 6 years and 1 month (cat no. 1, Dews & Wiesel, 1970). Coding as in Fig. 1.

deprived eye whereas the reversal in the second cat led to some return of vision in the originally deprived eye (Dews & Wiesel, 1970). It is worth emphasizing this disparity between the physiological and behavioural recovery in the eye-reversed cat. Such an animal either learns to do very well with the few cortical cells that recover their connexions or else learns to use some other less damaged part of its visual system.

Morphologic Changes in Lateral Geniculate Body Following Monocular Deprivation

Our previous studies (Wiesel & Hubel, 1963a) showed that after three months of monocular closure from birth the geniculate layers receiving input from the deprived eye are thinner, and the cell bodies within these layers are smaller and stain less deeply with basic dyes. The atrophy was less marked the later the closure, with no changes in an adult cat deprived for 3 months. Most (though not all) of the cells in the affected layers responded well to visual stimulation and had the usual centre-surround receptive fields. There is considerable additional evidence that the physiological changes seen in cortical cells depend on cortical rather than on geniculate abnormalities; for example, form deprivation with a translucent occluder led to only

slight shrinkage in geniculate cells but gave a cortex just as abnormal physiologically as that following eye closure. Again, binocular occlusion gave surprisingly less cortical abnormality than would have been predicted from monocular closures, but resulted in just as severe shrinkage in all geniculate layers (Wiesel & Hubel, 1965a). The absence of geniculate abnormalities in animals raised with strabismus affords still another example of the lack of parallel between geniculate morphological and cortical physiological abnormalities.

The effects of deprivation on geniculate cells seem to involve both a retardation in normal growth and also atrophy in the usual sense (Wiesel & Hubel, 1963a; Kupfer & Palmer, 1964). At birth the cells are about one fourth adult size, in terms of cross-sectional area; they grow rapidly to about half size in 2–3 weeks and to full size in about 8–10 weeks. During the first 3 weeks eye closure seems to have little effect on this normal growth, not surprisingly perhaps, since even after the tenth day, when the eyes normally open, the animal sleeps or suckles most of the time, often in a dimly lit hiding place. After the third week sensory deprivation gives an irreversible arrest in growth, so that by the second month there is a 30–40% reduction in size relative to the normal. A kitten deprived at 2 months of age for one month shows a reduction in

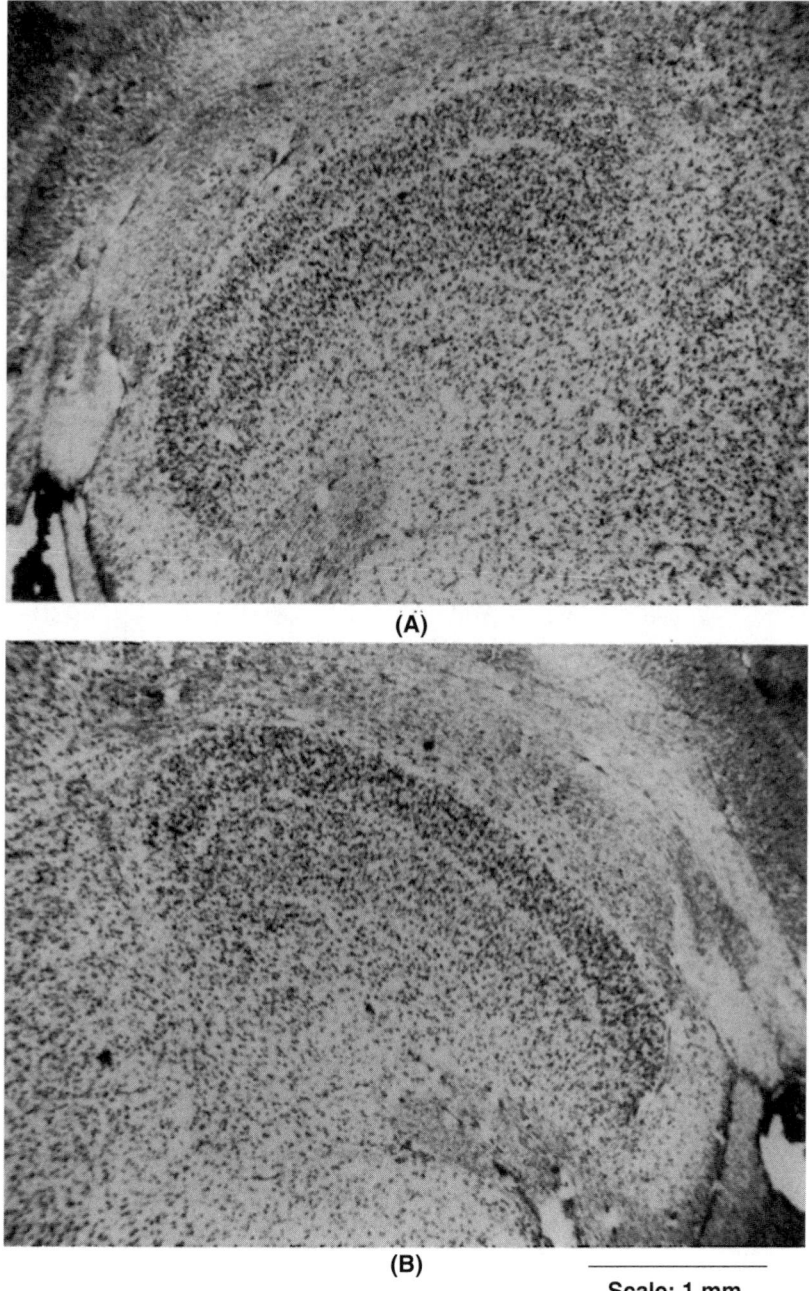

(A)

(B)

Scale: 1 mm.

Fig. 10. Coronal section through (A) *left and* (B) *right lateral geniculate bodies of a kitten whose right eye was closed from days 23–26; same cat as in Fig. 4A; cresyl violet.*

cell size (Wiesel & Hubel, 1963a) and this must be termed atrophy in the strict sense, since normal growth is practically complete at about 2 months.

During the most critical period for physiological changes in the cortex even a few days of deprivation gave a distinct difference between geniculate layers. Figure 10 gives the results of 3 days' deprivation (days 23–26) in the animal of Fig. 4A. While not approaching the shrinkage seen following a 3-month deprivation the effects are still obvious at a glance, particularly in the right geniculate, which was for some reason more seriously affected than the left. In Fig. 11 the deprivation lasted 6 days (days 23–29, same cat as in Fig. 4C); here the shrinkage was bilateral and more marked, though the change was still not so severe as that seen after a 3-month deprivation. It seems unlikely that differences as large as these could result simply from a cessation of growth during these brief periods, and we assume that there was in addition some atrophy.

Lateral geniculate bodies were examined histologically in both the animals of Fig. 9, in which the recovery period was protracted. Both showed the usual marked reduction in cell size and inability to take up Nissl stain in layers receiving input from the eye that was deprived in the first few months. This agrees with our previous findings (Wiesel & Hubel, 1965b). Even in the animal (Fig. 9B) whose right eye was closed only for the first 3 months and then the left eye closed for a year, the layers corresponding to the right eye were collapsed and the cells shrunken, compared to the other layers. It seems evident that the abnormalities produced by the original closure are virtually irreversible. Furthermore, the normal appearance of the layers receiving input from the left eye indicate that after 3 months of age, eye closure causes no appreciable changes. This fits well with the absence of any changes in the geniculate of a cat with an eye sutured at 4 months of age for 3 months (Fig. 6A), or in an adult cat with one eye shut for 16 months (Fig. 6C). Here the evidence is especially compelling since one can compare adjacent deprived and non-deprived layers. Burke & Hayhow (1968) have kept adult cats in darkness for over 2 years without finding any morphological changes in the lateral geniculate.

DISCUSSION

The most surprising result of this paper is the high degree of sensitivity a kitten shows to a few days of monocular deprivation during a very restricted period in life. The susceptibility begins suddenly near the start of the fourth week, at about the time a kitten begins to use its eyes, and persists until some time between the sixth and eighth weeks; it then begins to decline, disappearing ultimately around the end of the third month. After 4 months cats seem to be insensitive even to very long periods of monocular deprivation as tested by behavioural, physiological or morphological criteria.

An ability to recover from the physiologic effects of monocular deprivation seems to be closely related to this vulnerable period. Deprivation for the first 2–3 months produced virtually irreversible defects even when the normal eye was closed during the period of attempted recovery. When the deprivation period was shorter (Fig. 7) the recovery was greater, though it was still relatively slight. Perhaps this difference in ability to recover is simply an expression of a lesser degree of permanent damage from the shorter deprivation period. On the other hand, it may be that between the fourth and eighth weeks an animal's nervous system is better able to recover, just as it is more susceptible to damage. The immunity to deprivation effects after the third month and the failure to recover after that period may both be manifestations of a similar rigidity.

The observation of a critical period of susceptibility to deprivation or abnormal experience is by no means new. Examples have been found in many animals, including birds, dogs, monkeys, and man. The period of susceptibility to deprivation varies from animal to animal and no doubt from system to system within a given species. One extreme is seen in 'following responses' of certain birds, where the critical period peaks sharply within the first day of hatching (Lorenz, 1935). The other extreme is found in man, in whom language capabilities, for example, can be laid down in the non-dominant hemisphere following injury in the dominant one during early childhood, but not after the age of about 8–10. The present studies indicate an age of maximum susceptibility to visual deprivation between the fourth and eighth weeks. It is common experience that kittens handled extensively by humans during this period are subsequently tamer and more tractable than ones isolated from humans, and behavioural studies such as those of Scott & Fuller (1965) indicate a similar critical period for social development in dogs. It may be that the critical period coincides with the time when a particular system is being formed and developed and that use during this time is essential for its full maturation and sustenance.

One may reasonably ask whether mechanisms in which neural connexions become impaired through abnormal experience can possibly serve any use, or possess any survival value. Here one can only speculate, but it is worth emphasizing that in

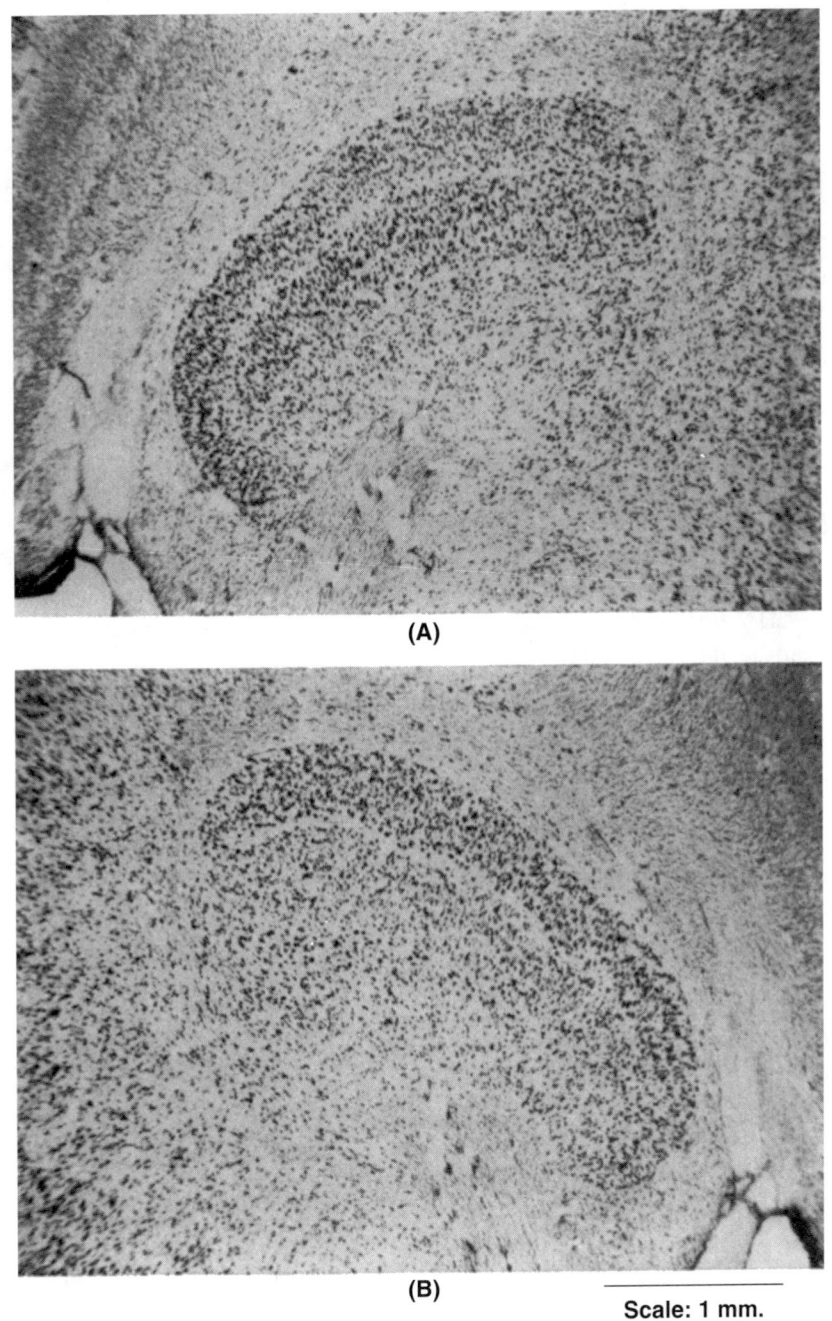

Scale: 1 mm.

Fig. 11. *Coronal section through* (A) *left and* (B) *right lateral geniculate bodies of a kitten whose right eye was closed from days 23–29; same cat as in Fig. 4C; cresyl violet.*

monocular deprivation the failure of cortical connexions from the closed eye may well be accompanied by an enhancement of connexions from the normal eye. It seems from the results of binocular closure that the failure of connexions from the closed eye is largely dependent on the other eye's being open (Wiesel & Hubel, 1965a). The abnormalities we see may thus be part of a larger process of adjustment to the loss or impairment of one eye. Similarly in animals reared with strabismus from birth, the falling out of connexions responsible for mixing of inputs from the two eyes may have the advantageous effect of overcoming double vision. But while it is easy to think of advantages to the animal in possessing some flexibility, it is difficult to understand why the sensitive period should decline so completely after a few months. A second possibility is that the flexibility is important for certain fine adjustments in the neural connexions from the eyes relative to each other. Such adjustments might be important early in life, and once made, might be sufficient to last a lifetime.

As yet we know nothing about the chemical changes and have only begun to learn about the morphologic changes that occur in the cortex as a result of visual deprivation. Light microscopic observations in dark-raised mice indicate that the visual cortex is thinner than in the normal animal (Gyllensten, Malmfors & Norrlin, 1965). It has been reported by Valverde (1967) that in such mice the number of spines on apical dendrites of layer V pyramidal cells are reduced in the parts passing through layer IV. Globus & Scheibel (1967), studying dark-raised rabbits, found that in the portions of the apical dendrite receiving geniculate input the spines were abnormal in size and shape but not reduced in numbers; otherwise cortical cells were normal in size and dendritic branching.

In considering the possible implications of studies like the present one for human development it is important to stress that in the cat, within the critical period between the fourth and eighth weeks, a deprivation as brief as a few days can have marked effects. This implies that for normal development normal environmental conditions must prevail throughout the critical period and not just during some small part of it. What an analogous critical period might be in man is of course not known though experience with squint would suggest that it is longer, possibly several years. We are now attempting to define this period in the macaque monkey; from the few animals already studied it is clear that 2 weeks of monocular deprivation during the first 5 weeks of life produces at least temporary blindness in the eye that has been closed and an absence of responses of cortical cells to stimulation of that eye. This suggests that the sensitive periods of cats and monkeys may not be too dissimilar.

We wish to thank Janet Wiitanen for her excellent technical assistance. This work was supported in part by N.I.H. Research Grants, No. 5 RO 1 NB 02260 and in part by No. 5 RO 1 NB 05554 Bell Telephone Laboratories Inc.

References

Burke, W. & Hayhow, W. R. (1968). Disuse in the lateral geniculate nucleus of the cat. *J. Physiol.* **194**, 495–519.

Dews, P. B. & Wiesel, T. N. (1970). Consequences of monocular deprivation on visual behaviour in kittens. *J. Physiol.* **206**, 437–455.

Ganz, L., Fitch, M. & Satterberg, J. A. (1968). Selective effect of visual deprivation on receptive field shape determined neurophysiologically. *Expl Neurol.* **22**, 614–637.

Globus, A. & Scheibel, A. B. (1967). Effect of visual deprivation on cortical neurons: a Golgi study. *Expl Neurol.* **19**, 331–345.

Gyllensten, L., Malmfors, T. & Norrlin, M.-L. (1965). Effect of visual deprivation on the optic centers of growing and adult mice. *J. comp. Neurol.* **124**, 149–160.

Hubel, D. H. & Wiesel, T. N. (1962). Receptive fields, binocular interaction and functional architecture in the cat's visual cortex. *J. Physiol.* **160**, 106–154.

Hubel, D. H. & Wiesel, T. N. (1963). Receptive fields of cells in striate cortex of very young, visually inexperienced kittens. *J. Neurophysiol.* **26**, 994–1002.

Hubel, D. H. & Wiesel, T. N. (1965). Binocular interaction in striate cortex of kittens reared with artificial squint. *J. Neurophysiol.* **28**, 1041–1059.

Kupfer, C. & Palmer, P. (1964). Lateral geniculate nucleus: histological and cytochemical changes following afferent denervation and visual deprivation. *Expl Neurol.* **9**, 400–409.

Lorenz, K. (1935). Der Kumpan in der Umwelt des Vogels. *J. Orn., Lpz.* **83**, 137–213.

Scott, J. P. & Fuller, J. L. (1965). *Genetics and the Social Behaviour of the Dog.* Chicago: University of Chicago Press.

Valverde, F. (1967). Apical dendritic spines of the visual cortex and light deprivation in the mouse. *Expl Brain Res.* **3**, 337–352.

Wiesel, T. N. & Hubel, D. H. (1963a). Effects of visual deprivation on morphology and physiology of cells in the cat's lateral geniculate body. *J. Neurophysiol.* **26**, 978–993.

Wiesel, T. N. & Hubel, D. H. (1963b). Single-cell responses in striate cortex of kittens deprived of vision in one eye. *J. Neurophysiol.* **26**, 1003–1017.

Wiesel, T. N. & Hubel, D. H. (1965a). Comparison of the effects of unilateral and bilateral eye closure on cortical unit responses in kittens. *J. Neurophysiol.* **28**, 1029–1040.

Wiesel, T. N. & Hubel, D. H. (1965b). Extent of recovery from the effects of visual deprivation in kittens. *J. Neurophysiol.* **28**, 1060–1072.

AFTERWORD

Before this work was done, we had considered that the deprivation effects we had found were ascribable to disuse, analogous to the muscular atrophy that results when an arm is put in a cast. The first three of these papers, and to some extent also the fourth, made it clear that the effects we were seeing must have involved more than simple disuse; that competition between the two eyes must be playing a major part.

It was hard for us to imagine that everything could be accounted for in terms of competition, however. The geniculate cell pallor and shrinkage especially were difficult to explain, given the fact that all the cells in any given layer were strictly monocular. The first hint that our reasoning was faulty came in 1970, when Guillery and Stelzner noticed, in examining our illustrations, that the shrinkage and pallor of the deprived layers was confined to the main body of the geniculates, and that the most lateral parts—the parts receiving input from the temporal crescents of the contralateral eyes only—were normal (*J Comp Neurol* 139:413–422). Needless to say, we felt slightly embarrassed not to have noticed this ourselves. Evidently we were so busy measuring cell sizes, in an effort to be quantitative, for once, that we had ignored the temporal crescents completely. The sparing of the temporal crescent representations strongly suggested that somehow or other, in the geniculates, the two eyes must be competing.

A further ingenious demonstration reinforced the evidence supplied by the normal temporal crescent representation. In 1972, Guillery (*J Comp Neurol* 144:117–130) made a destructive lesion in a small region of one temporal retina of a kitten, and then sewed closed the eyelids of the other eye. When he finally examined the lateral geniculate, he found the expected small patch of profound atrophy in the middle (A1) geniculate layer on the same side as the eye with the lesion, and the expected atrophy in the dorsal (A) geniculate layer on the side opposite the closed eye—except for a region immediately opposite the atrophic patch in the middle layer, where there was less atrophy than expected. So, clearly, making the retinal lesion had removed the competition from that small part of the retina. Later, Sherman, Guillery, Kaas, and Sanderson (*J Comp Neurol* 1974, 158:1–18) went even further, in showing that the focal retinal lesion prevented behavioral blindness and preserved single-cell responses in the corresponding region of visual field of the eye that had been closed.

All this seemed to uphold the idea of competetion at the geniculate level, but a fuller understanding of how that could happen only came when we finally established, in our 1977 papers with Simon LeVay, that at and around the time of birth the cortical ocular dominance columns are not yet completely segregated in layer 4C (pp. 493–539). This was clear from physiological recordings and from the autoradiography following eye injection. Evidently, at the time the deprivations took place, there was still mingling of the axons from the left- and right-eye geniculate layers, and hence the possibility of competition.

The squint result soon led us to examine the Siamese cat, which acquires squint honestly—at least without surgical intervention—with surprising and unexpected results, to be discussed in the next paper.

Our next step was obviously to repeat these experiments in monkeys, and we would have forged ahead sooner, except that writing up the cat work took time, and it was obviously economical to learn as much as possible from cats before graduating to monkeys, just as we had done in our work on normal physiology. Our postponing the monkey deprivation studies almost ended in disaster, however, because one of us (Torsten), carried away by our progress in cats, described the results of these first six papers to a colleague in a different department during a squash game. A short time later we learned that the colleague, and a colleague of his, were beginning to do monocular closures in monkeys. Such leap-frogging is not immoral, ("all is fair in love and ...") but it does have the effect of dampening one's tendency to talk openly and enthusiastically about current work. It lessens the fun. In the end this scare (if that is the right word) came to naught, perhaps because our interlocutors had not had the practice in closing eyes that we had had in cats.

As stated so frequently in this book, we cannot really complain about competition, having had the field of single-cell visual cortex neurophysiology largely ourselves for almost a full decade. Still, ideas are scarce, and often easy to carry out, and a few lessons like this one taught us to keep our cards closer to our chests.

All these deprivation experiments took many cats, and later many monkeys. Many of our kittens were born to pregnant cats in the lab, and cost us nothing. Today the increased cost of the kittens (close to $500 each), together with the endless number of forms to be filled out, protocols to be prepared and revised, cost of daily upkeep, and inspections would certainly put a severe damper on such a project. This seems ironic, given the importance of the work in clinical ophthalmology.

Some years later, an ingenious and thoughtful paper by Gunther Stent entitled "A physiological mechanism for Hebb's postulate of learning" (*Proc Natl Acad Sci USA* 1973, (4):997–100) drew attention to the support our deprivation experiments provided for Donald Hebb's ideas on synapse strengthening or weakening through experience. The arguments are spelled out in Stent's paper and in my later book (*Eye, Brain and Vision*). I had met Hebb in the early 1950s, when he was head of the Department of Psychology at McGill—we happened to sit together on a Westmount-NDG bus after a seminar at the Montreal Neurological Institute, and we met several times in subsequent years when I was invited to Montreal to give seminars. I may have been mistaken, but had the impression, in the 1950s, that there was little communication between the Montreal Neurological Institute and other departments at McGill. At that time, few would have dreamed that some day Hebb would be regarded as one of the most distinguished of Canadian scientists.

Chapter 23 • The Siamese Cat •

FOREWORD

We decided to study Siamese cats for several reasons. It is common knowledge that Siamese cats are often cross-eyed, and we wondered whether their strabismus would be accompanied by the same central defects that occurred in our artificially strabismic cats; namely, a marked decline in cells that could be driven from the two eyes.

In 1969, Ray Guillery had discovered that the lateral geniculate bodies of Siamese cats are anatomically strikingly abnormal. Part of the middle layer, which normally receives its input from the ipsilateral eye, instead receives input from the contralateral eye, not, as expected, from the contralateral visual field but from parts of the ipsilateral. Apparently some optic fibers that remain uncrossed in the chiasm of normal cats mistakenly cross to the opposite hemisphere in Siamese cats. We were anxious to learn how these aberrant optic fibers are mapped in the geniculate, and what happens to fibers from the abnormally connected parts of the geniculate when they get to the cortex. So we set out to record single cells in Siamese cats, mapping receptive field positions, first in the lateral geniculate and then in the striate cortex.

To someone not steeped in the vagaries of mammalian retinal projections, the onslaught in this paper of terms such as *nasal, temporal ipsilateral,* and *contralateral* may seem intimidating. Indeed, we, who must have had a grasp of this material at one time, have found the going rough after the relaxed intervening thirty years. We found that the best strategy in re-attacking this subject is to begin with the discussion section of the paper: the summary is too compressed for a beginner, and the results section will seem too detailed. We hope the richness of the subject and the bizarre nature of the results will make the effort worthwhile.

Aberrant Visual Projections in the Siamese Cat

D. H. HUBEL AND T. N. WIESEL • *Department of Neurobiology, Harvard Medical School, Boston, Massachusetts*

SUMMARY

1. Guillery has recently shown that the Siamese cat has a grossly abnormal lateral geniculate body. His anatomical study suggested that certain fibres originating in the temporal retina of each eye cross in the chiasm instead of remaining uncrossed. They thus reach the wrong hemispheres, but in the geniculate they terminate in the regions that the missing fibres from the ipsilateral eye would normally have occupied. The result is that each hemisphere receives an input from parts of the ipsilateral field of vision, this input being entirely from the opposite eye. The purpose of the present work was to study the physiological consequences of this aberrant projection, in the lateral geniculate body and visual cortex.

2. Single-cell recordings from the lateral geniculate body confirmed the presence of projections from the ipsilateral visual field of the contralateral eye. The part of layer A_1 receiving these projections was arranged so that the receptive fields of the cells were situated at about the same horizontal level and at the same distance from the vertical meridian as the fields of cells in the layers above and below (layers A and B), but were in the ipsilateral visual field instead of the contralateral. They thus occupied a region directly across the mid line from their normal position.

3. In the cortex of all animals studied, we found a systematic representation of part of the ipsilateral visual field, inserted between the usual contralateral representations in areas 17 and 18. When the visual cortex was crossed from medial to lateral the corresponding region of visual field moved from the contralateral periphery to the mid line, and then into the ipsilateral field for 20°. The movement then reversed, with a return to the mid line and a steady progression out into the contralateral field. The entire double representation was, with some possible exceptions, a continuous one. The point of reversal occurred at or near the 17–18 boundary, as judged histologically, and this boundary was in about the same position as in ordinary cats.

4. Cells in the part of the cortex representing the ipsilateral fields had normal receptive fields, simple, complex, or hypercomplex. These fields tended to be larger than those in corresponding parts of the contralateral visual fields. Receptive-field size varied with distance from the area centralis, just as it does in the normal cat, so that cells with the smallest fields, in the area centralis projection, were situated some distance from the 17–18 border.

5. Projections originating from the first 20° from the midvertical in both visual half-fields had their origin entirely in the contralateral eye, as would be expected from the abnormal crossing at the chiasm. Beyond this visual-field region, and out as far as the temporal crescents, there were projections from both eyes, but we found no individual cells with input from the two eyes. The cells were aggregated, with some groups of cells driven by one eye and some by the other.

6. From previous work it is known that ordinary cats raised with squint show a decline in the proportion of cells that can be driven binocularly, whereas animals raised with both eyes closed show little or no decline. A Siamese cat raised with both eyes closed had binocular cells in the regions of 17 and 18 subserving the peripheral visual fields, suggesting that the absence of binocular cells seen in the other Siamese cats was indeed secondary to the squint.

7. In two Siamese cats there were suggestions of an entirely different projection pattern, superimposed upon that described above. In the parts of

From *J. Physiol.* (1971), **218,** *pp.* 33–62
Received 15 February 1971.

17 and 18 otherwise entirely devoted to the contralateral visual field, we observed groups of cells with receptive fields in the ipsilateral field of vision. The electrode would pass from a region where cells were driven from some part of the contralateral visual field, to regions in which they were driven from a part of the ipsilateral field directly opposite, across the vertical mid line. The borders of these groups were not necessarily sharp, for in places there was mixing of the two groups of cells, and a few cells had input from two discrete regions located opposite one another on either side of the vertical mid line. The two receptive-field components of such cells were identical, in terms of orientation, optimum direction of movement, and complexity. Stimulation of the two regions gave a better response than was produced from either one alone, and the relative effectiveness of the two varied from cell to cell. These cells thus behaved in a way strikingly reminiscent of binocular cells in common cats.

8. The apparent existence of two competing mechanisms for determining the projection of visual afferents to the cortex suggests that a number of factors may cooperate in guiding development. There seems, furthermore, not to be a detailed cell-to-cell specificity of geniculo-cortical connexions, but rather a tendency to topographic order and continuity, with one part of a given area such as 17 able to substitute for another. Whether or not these tentative interpretations are ultimately proved correct, it seems clear that this type of genetic anomaly has potential usefulness for understanding mechanisms of development of the nervous system.

INTRODUCTION

Among animal breeders it is common knowledge that Siamese cats are frequently cross-eyed. A few years ago we showed that ordinary cats raised with squint from an early age develop marked abnormalities in the connexions subserving binocular interaction in the cortex (Hubel & Wiesel, 1965*b*), and we wondered whether Siamese cats would develop similar abnormalities, or if they might possibly show them at birth.

Recently Guillery (1969) has observed that Siamese cats possess a strikingly abnormal lateral geniculate body. Patterns of fibre degeneration following removal of one eye revealed that in each geniculate body parts of the layers that in the normal cat connect to the ipsilateral eye, in the Siamese received their input from the contralateral eye. Guillery suggested that some fibres from the temporal retina, which are normally uncrossed, become misdirected and cross to the opposite hemisphere during development.

If optic fibres that normally are uncrossed at the chiasm instead become crossed, there should be cells in the geniculate with receptive fields in the ipsilateral half-field of vision. One may then ask how these cells project to the cortex, whether, for example, there is in each hemisphere an added systematic topographic representation of part of the ipsilateral field of vision, or whether the aberrant projections become scrambled with the normal ones. What happens when the cortex is presented with an abnormal input could obviously be of interest for an understanding of normal development. Because of this, and our interest in the squint, we decided to investigate the central pathway of Siamese cats and kittens, particularly the topographic projections of the retinas to areas 17 and 18 of the visual cortex, and the receptive-field properties and binocular interaction of cells in these areas.

METHODS

Seven purebred Siamese cats were used: a litter of five kittens whose parents both had overt strabismus, and one additional adult cat and a 4-month-old kitten. The adult cat had no obvious squint. In the two kittens that were observed from birth to age 5 months, one developed a clear squint by about 2 months, though it was not nearly as marked as in some adult Siamese cats. The other kitten had only a suggestion of a squint by 5 months (as described below, however, both had a readily demonstrable convergent strabismus when the eyes were paralysed).

Methods of stimulating and recording from kittens and adult cats have already been described in detail (Hubel & Wiesel, 1962, 1963). The 5-month-old kittens were anaesthetized with thiopentone, but in two 2-week-old kittens xylocaine was used both as a general anaesthetic and for local infiltration of the skin wounds. The anaesthetized animal was placed in a stereotaxic head holder and the corneas protected with contact lenses, which also focused the eyes on a projection screen 1.5 metres away. The eye muscles were paralysed with succinylcholine, making it necessary to use artificial respiration. Tungsten electrodes were positioned in a closed-chamber system. Receptive fields were mapped with spots, slits, dark bars and edges, produced by a hand-held slide projector. Our main concern was to compare the responses of cells driven from the two eyes and to localize the receptive fields in the visual fields for as many cells and over as wide a region of visual cortex as possible, examining area 18 as well as 17. In each electrode track one or more electrolytic lesions were made, and the tracks were later reconstructed in the usual manner from serial Nissl-stained sections.

RESULTS

Recordings from the Lateral Geniculate Body

In the lateral geniculate body of the normal cat (Text-fig. 1) the nasal half-retina of the contralateral eye projects to the most dorsal layer (A) and to the most ventral (B), while the temporal half-retina of the ipsilateral eye projects to the intermediate

layer, A_1. (Guillery, 1970, has shown in the normal cat that there is a sublamina of layer B which also receives ipsilateral projections.) The contralateral half-field of vision is mapped on to each layer systematically, with the three maps in precise register, so that in any vertical penetration one first records cells driven from the contralateral eye, then cells driven from the ipsilateral, and then the contralateral, all with their receptive fields in the same part of the contralateral field of vision (Hubel & Wiesel, 1961; Bishop, Kozak, Levick & Vakkur, 1962). The further medial the penetrations, the closer the receptive fields are to the vertical meridian of the visual fields.

If, in the Siamese cat, part of layer A_1 is supplied by the temporal retina of the contralateral eye, rather than the ipsilateral, the sequence of events during a vertical penetration should be very different from the normal. To study this we made four penetrations in the lateral geniculate bodies of two Siamese kittens, one 5 months old (No. 3), and the other 4 months old (No. 7). In three of the pen-

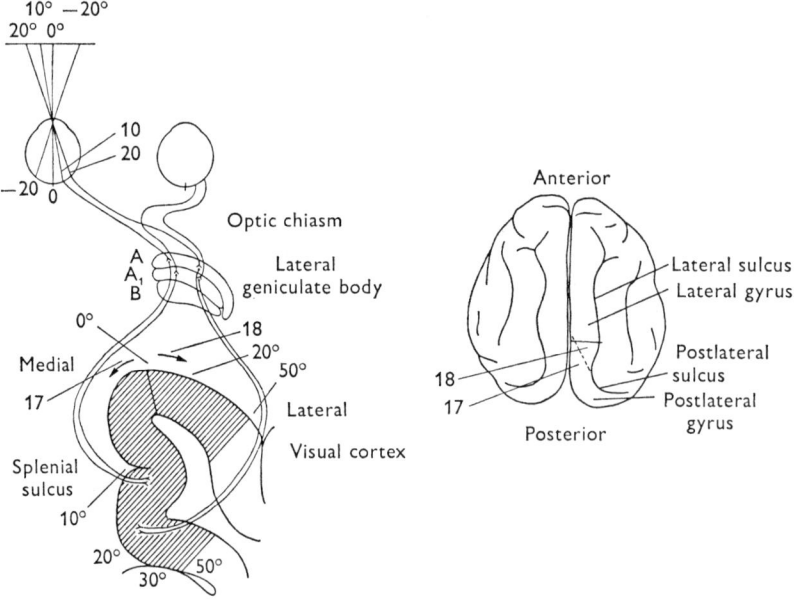

Text Fig. 1. Diagram to illustrate visual-field topography for areas 17 and 18 of normal cat cortex. The right-hand diagram shows a view of the cortex from above. The continuous line shows the level of the coronal section illustrated to the left. Geniculate and cortex are shown in coronal section, since for both structures a medio-lateral movement at a given coronal level corresponds roughly, in the visual field, to a movement to or away from the vertical mid line. (An anterior or posterior movement in geniculate or cortex corresponds to movement down or up in the visual fields.) For simplicity, connexions from geniculate to area 18, and from 17 to 18, are omitted.

etrations some of the cells had their receptive fields clearly in the ipsilateral field of vision, several degrees from the vertical meridian. Two of the three penetrations, however, were far forward in the geniculate, where the anatomy is not easily interpreted. The third, shown in Text-fig. 2, was near the middle of the left geniculate's antero-posterior extent.

The first group of cells in penetration 3, recorded from layer A, had fields some 5–6° from the mid line in the right (contralateral) field of the right eye. The next cells, from what we interpret to be A_1, instead of being in the right field of the left eye, were in the left field of the right eye, in a roughly mirror-symmetric position across the vertical mid line. The last cells, from layer B, were

driven from the right eye and right field, as would be expected in the dorsal part of this layer. The final electrode position was marked by a lesion (Text-fig. 2, Pl. 1). Except for their positions in the wrong visual field of the wrong eye, all of the cells recorded from layer A_1 behaved normally. These findings agree with Guillery's results concerning contralateral-eye input to A_1, and support his interpretation that the input originated from the temporal half of the contralateral retina.

Cortical Recordings

NORMAL CATS. The general topographic arrangement of the normal cat visual cortex is shown in Text-fig. 1 (Talbot & Marshall, 1941; Hubel &

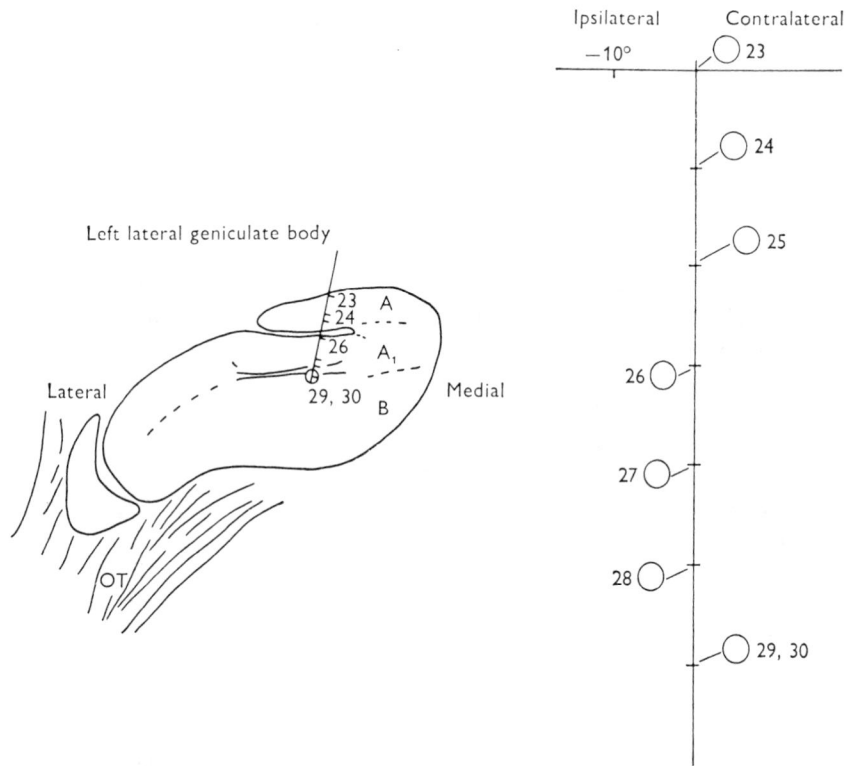

Text Fig. 2. Penetration through the left lateral geniculate body of a Siamese kitten (No. 7); Horsley-Clarke lateral 9.0, anterior 4.0. Each receptive field is shown relative to the area centralis, which is indicated, for each cell, by a short horizontal cross bar intersecting the long vertical line. The first cells, 23–25, were recorded from layer A, and had receptive fields in the right eye, 5–6° to the right of the mid-vertical and 1.5° above the horizontal meridian. Cells 26–28, recorded from layer A_1, and again driven from the right eye only, had fields 4–5° to the left of the mid line, 1° below the horizontal. Finally a cell recorded in the uppermost part of B had fields in the right eye in the same position as the fields of cells 23–25. The area centralis was not well defined, and no attempt was made to correct for eye rotation in the equatorial plane. OT = optic tract.

Wiesel, 1965*a*). The lateral geniculate body projects to the primary visual cortex in a systematic manner. There is also a direct projection from the main part of the lateral geniculate body to area 18 (Garey & Powell, 1967; Glickstein, King, Miller & Bailey, 1967). From Nauta-degeneration experiments in a series of normal cats, with small lesions confined to layers A or A_1 of the geniculate, we have shown that this projection to area 18 is a systematic one, consistent with the topographic representations as determined physiologically, and with the known anatomical projection from 17 to 18.

A given location in either 17 or 18 receives projections from a region in each of the three geniculate layers, one lying directly above or below the other, as would be expected from the fact that the three topographic maps are in register. As one explores the cortex from medial to lateral, at a given coronal level, there is a displacement in the corresponding positions in the visual fields, beginning in the contralateral visual field and moving inwards to the vertical mid line, and then out again to the contralateral periphery (Talbot & Marshall, 1941). The point of reversal at the vertical meridian is represented by the anatomical 17–18 border (Otsuka & Hassler, 1962; Hubel & Wiesel, 1965*a*). The ipsilateral field of vision, of course, projects to the other hemisphere. A forward movement along the cortex corresponds to a downward movement in the visual field. Within 50–60° of the vertical mid line, the projection to the cortex is from both eyes. The visual field beyond this (the temporal crescent) is represented by the contralateral eye only.

A vertical penetration entering the cortex near the medial border of the lateral gyrus (see Text-fig. 1) should thus record cells in 17 or 18 with fields close to the vertical meridian. If the penetration extends far down the medial bank of the gyrus the receptive fields should gradually move out further and further into the contralateral visual field. On the other hand a series of vertical penetrations beginning at successively more lateral positions along the lateral gyrus should record cells in area 18 with fields that again occupy progressively more peripheral positions in the contralateral field of vision.

SIAMESE CATS: TOPOGRAPHY AND BINOCULAR INTERACTION. In Seven Siamese cats, sixteen penetrations were made, and 303 cells were adequately studied. The first cat (No. 3) was examined at an age of 5 months. When awake and alert the animal was obviously strabismic. When it was anaesthetized and paralysed, the eyes took up a rest position with their axes converged by 12°, instead of the usual divergent separation of about 5° (Hubel & Wiesel, 1962; Bishop, Kozak & Vakkur, 1962). By this method of measurement there was thus about 17° of convergent squint.

Two cortical penetrations were made in this kitten, one in each hemisphere. Both penetrations were abnormal, in that all cells responded only to the contralateral eye and had abnormal receptive-field positions. Otherwise the cells responded normally, showing typical simple, complex, and hypercomplex properties. The first penetration (Text-fig. 3) entered the right post-lateral gyrus at a point that normally is well within area 17, and corresponds to a visual-field region 1–2° or less from the area centralis (Talbot & Marshall, 1941; Hubel & Wiesel, 1965*a*). In this cat, however, the fields began 15–20° in the ipsilateral field of vision, some 5–10° below the horizontal meridian. As the electrode descended along the medial bank there was a clear systematic trend first towards the vertical mid line, which was crossed at about cell 36, and then out into the contralateral field of vision, ending about 15° from the mid line. A second penetration down the medial aspect of the left hemisphere gave very similar results.

The ipsilateral-to-contralateral progression of receptive fields shown in Text-fig. 3 is what is normally seen with a lateral-to-medial movement of an electrode across area 17; what was most unprecedented was the inclusion of 15–20° of ipsilateral visual field in this progression. Clearly in this animal part of the cortex was devoted to a systematic representation of the medial part of the ipsilateral visual fields. The extent of the representation was not established, and the lateral parts of the lateral gyrus were not explored. In neither penetration was there any sign of responses from the ipsilateral eye in either field of vision; this was expected, given that the optic nerve fibres representing the central 30–40° of visual field were, in the Siamese cat, presumably virtually all crossed. From the morphological normality of the lateral parts of the lateral geniculate bodies in these animals one would predict a normal binocular input to parts of the cortex representing the contralateral

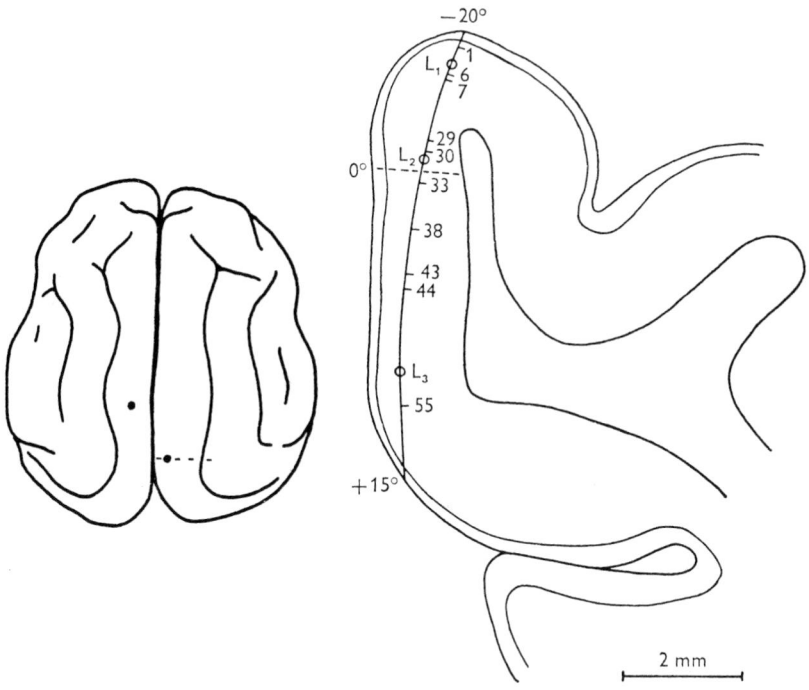

Text Fig. 3. First penetration in the right hemisphere of a 5-month-old Siamese cat (No. 3). The diagram at left shows a dorsal view of the brain surface, indicating the points of entry of two micro-electrode tracks. Right part of the Figure shows a reconstruction of the microelectrode track in the right hemisphere. The plane of section (Horsley-Clarke 0.0) is indicated on the brain surface map by a dotted line. Positions of units are indicated by numbered cross bars to the right of the electrode track. L_1, L_2 and L_3 refer to three electrolytic lesions made in the course of the penetration. Numbers just outside the cortical tracing refer to approximate azimuth positions of receptive fields, positive numbers standing for regions of visual field contralateral to the hemisphere recorded from; negative standing for ipsilateral.

In the diagram on p. 41 the position of each receptive field is shown relative to the area centralis, which is indicated for each cell or set of cells by a horizontal cross bar intersecting the long vertical line. Ipsilateral visual field is to the right, contralateral to the left, of each vertical line. All cells in this penetration were influenced only from the left (contralateral) eye. Orientations, for most receptive fields, are indicated by two short lines. Thus unit 1 had a 10 o'clock–4 o'clock orientation.

Note (1) the gradual drift of receptive-field positions from ipsilateral to contralateral as the electrode descended along the medial bank; (2) the decrease in field size with decreasing distance from the area centralis, for both ipsilateral and contralateral fields, and (3) the larger average size of ipsilateral fields, compared with contralateral ones. (continued)

visual fields beyond 20° or so. Obviously, what was needed next was an exploration of both 17 and 18, including parts representing the more peripheral contralateral visual fields.

Cat No. 4, a litter-mate of the previous cat, was also studied at 5 months of age. In this animal there was only a faint suggestion of a strabismus on simple inspection, but the convergent strabismus estimated from the rest position with muscles paralysed was 16°.

The entire lateral gyrus was explored at coronal level +5 by making five penetrations, as shown in Text-fig. 4. In the first, most medial penetration (P1) the first fields were 10–20° ipsilateral to the vertical meridian, and later ones, in the medial bank, showed a steady trend outwards beginning at the mid line and ending 30° in the contralateral visual field. Up to a point half way down the medial bank, near lesion 2 (unit 23), all cells responded only to the contralateral eye; here, how-

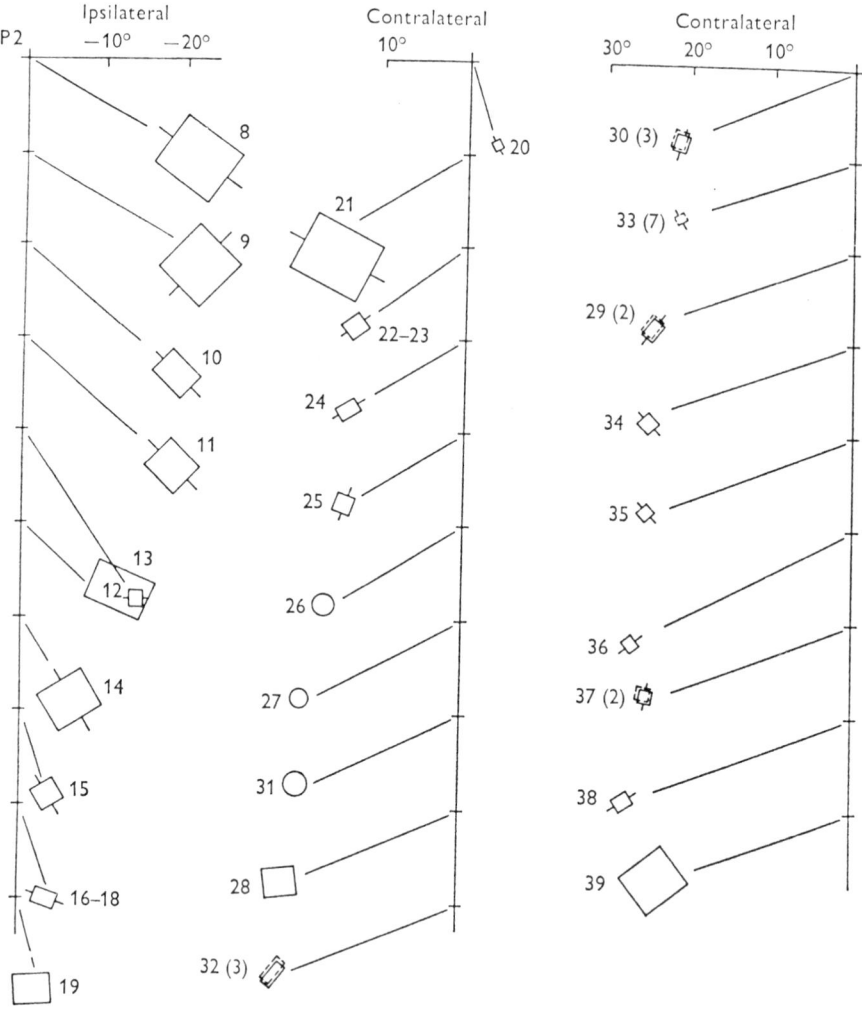

Text Fig. 3. (Continued)

ever, we came upon a group of cells driven only from the ipsilateral eye. Receptive fields were about 15° from the mid line, in about the same place as the fields of the contralateral-eye cells recorded just before. It can be seen in Text-fig. 4 that these cells occurred in groups (the fields are drawn in dashed lines): first units 23–26, later unit 32, and finally units 34–40. It seemed that we were going from regions where all cells were driven by one eye to regions where they were all driven by the other, an impression that was reinforced on noting that the background activity was influenced by one or the other eye, but not by both, except very briefly at the transition points.

In penetrations 2–5, as the recording site moved laterally, the fields shifted from the ipsilat-

eral visual field (penetration 2) into the contralateral (penetration 3), moving further and further out, as far as 30° in penetration 4, and 50° in penetration 5. All cells were driven from the contralateral eye except for two in penetration 4 which were influenced only from the ipsilateral eye and whose receptive fields were about 15–20° out from the mid line in the contralateral visual field.

We interpret these experiments as indicating that the extra 20° or so of ipsilateral visual field, in 17 and 18, had been, as it were, inserted into the cortex at the 17–18 boundary. It seemed that the extra piece was organized so that in a medio-lateral exploration of the cortex the visual-field representation proceeded not from the contralateral periphery to the vertical mid line and back out again, as it

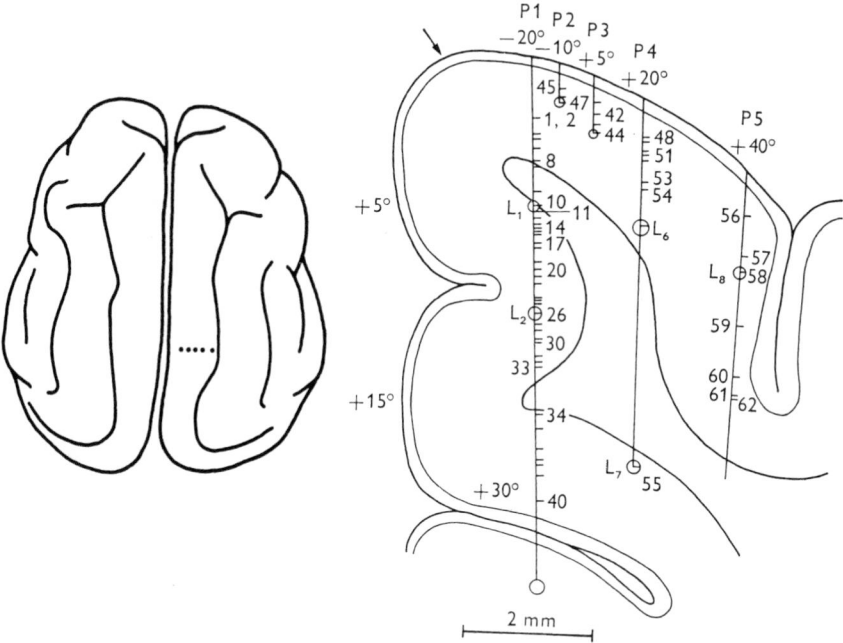

Text Fig. 4. Five penetrations in the right visual cortex of a 5-month-old Siamese cat (cat. No. 4, a litter-mate of Nos. 1, 2, 3, and 5). Horsley-Clarke anterior 5.0. Receptive fields drawn with continuous lines indicate that cells were driven from contralateral eye only; dashed lines, ipsilateral eye only. Penetration 1 (P1), from unit 10 on, shows a steady drift of receptive fields out into the contralateral field of vision; this is typical of area 17. Comparing field positions in the upper part of penetration 1 and penetrations 2–5, the movement from ipsilateral to contralateral in the visual field suggests that these recordings were all in area 18; this is supported by the large size of the fields and their wide scatter, in contrast to the smaller and better ordered fields in area 17. Up to cell 23 all responses were from the contralateral eye only. Beyond about 15°, in both 17 and 18, occasional cells were driven from the ipsilateral eye only. No cells were binocularly driven. Arrow shows the approximate position of the 17–18 border, as estimated from Nissl and myelin-stained sections. (Continued)

normally does (Text-fig. 9, left half), but instead progressed from the contralateral periphery to the mid line and beyond, into the ipsilateral field for some 20°. Then, in the region of cortex where the 17–18 border normally comes, there was a reversal in direction and, on traversing 18, a return to the mid line and a progression into the contralateral visual field (Text-fig. 9, right half). The prediction was confirmed that in the peripheral part of the visual fields, beyond about 20°, there should be input from both eyes. Even here, however, there was no evidence for binocular convergence upon single cells.

EFFECTS OF STRABISMUS ON SIAMESE CAT CORTEX. In ordinary cats reared with artificial strabismus, there is a striking decline in the number of cells driven by both eyes. One sees instead a mixture of cells, some driven by one eye, others driven

by the other (Hubel & Wiesel, 1965b). We naturally wondered if in Siamese cats the lack of binocular convergence in the periphery was secondary to the strabismus. The most direct way of settling this is to record from kittens at a very early age, before a critical period of susceptibility to deprivation begins. For eye closure the onset of this period is about 4 weeks of age (Hubel & Wiesel, 1970) and it seems reasonable to assume that for squint it is probably the same, though this has not been studied extensively. Two kittens (Nos. 1 and 2) were accordingly studied at 15 and 16 days of age, but neither survived long enough for examination of the outlying parts of the visual-field representations. We recorded from a total of fifty cells in the apex of the lateral gyrus, and, as expected from recordings in the older animals, all cells were driven exclusively from the contralateral eye. The responses seemed normal for animals at this age,

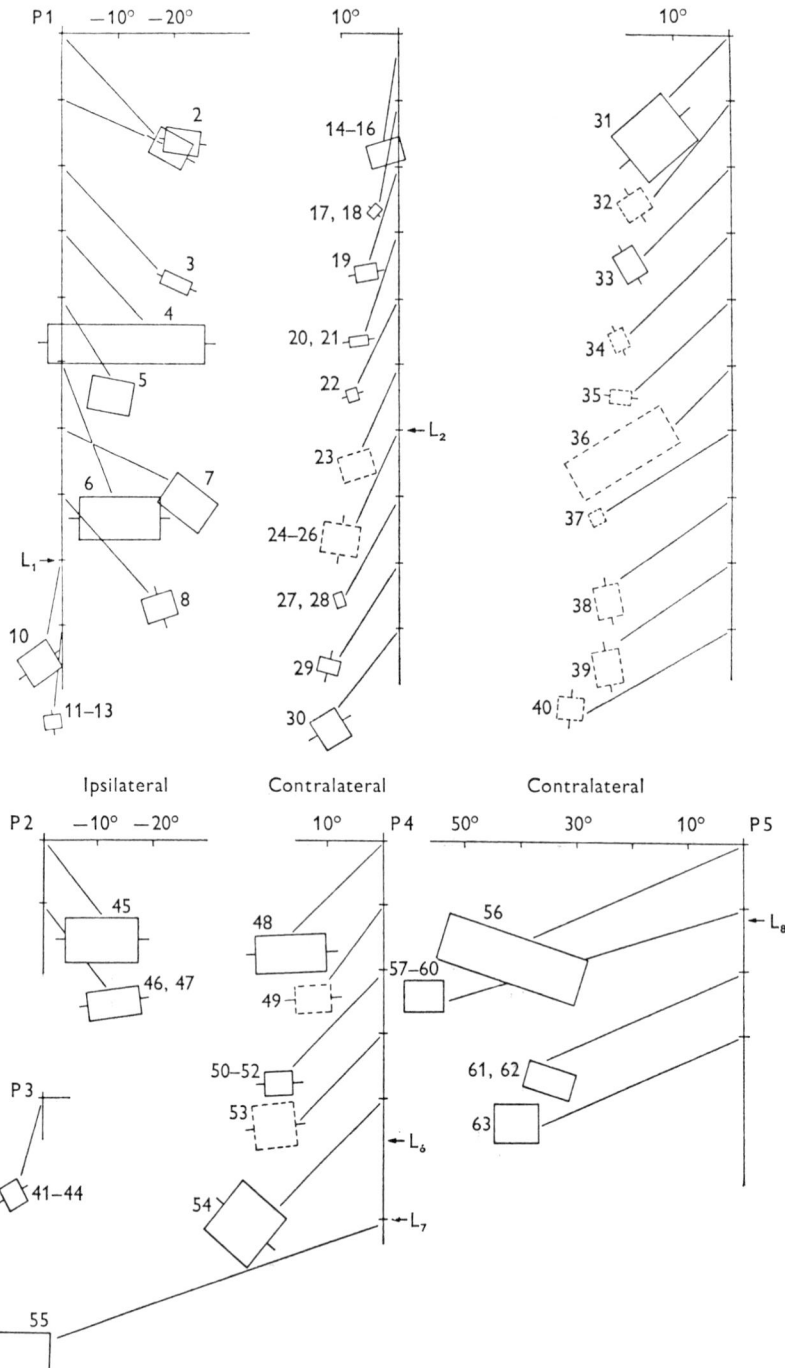

Text Fig. 4. (Continued)

but difficulties in seeing the retinal landmarks because of the cloudy ocular media prevented our localizing the receptive fields in relation to the area centralis and optic disk.

To circumvent the difficulties in working with very young animals, we brought up one of the kittens (No. 5) to an age of 5 months with both eyelids sutured. This procedure does not lead to any obvious change in binocular interaction in the cortex (Wiesel & Hubel, 1965), and with both eyes closed the proportion of binocularly driven cells should obviously not be influenced by the presence of a squint. When the eyelids were separated and the muscles paralysed there was a convergence of 2° and a vertical disparity of about 8°. Deviations as large as this are occasionally seen in normal cats

and in cats with binocular closures, after paralysis with succinylcholine. Clearly this cat differed from its littermates of the same age in having no marked convergent squint. Both this difference and the fact that the squint in the other animals developed only after several months of vision suggest that the squint is secondary to the neural abnormality.

A single penetration was made down the medial bank of the lateral gyrus at coronal level +3 (Text-fig. 5). Thirty-nine cells were recorded from, their fields localized, and responses to stimulation of the two eyes compared. As usual in binocularly deprived animals, about half the cells failed to respond, responded sluggishly, or showed other abnormalities such as a decline in orientation selectivity. Once more the initial fields were about 20°

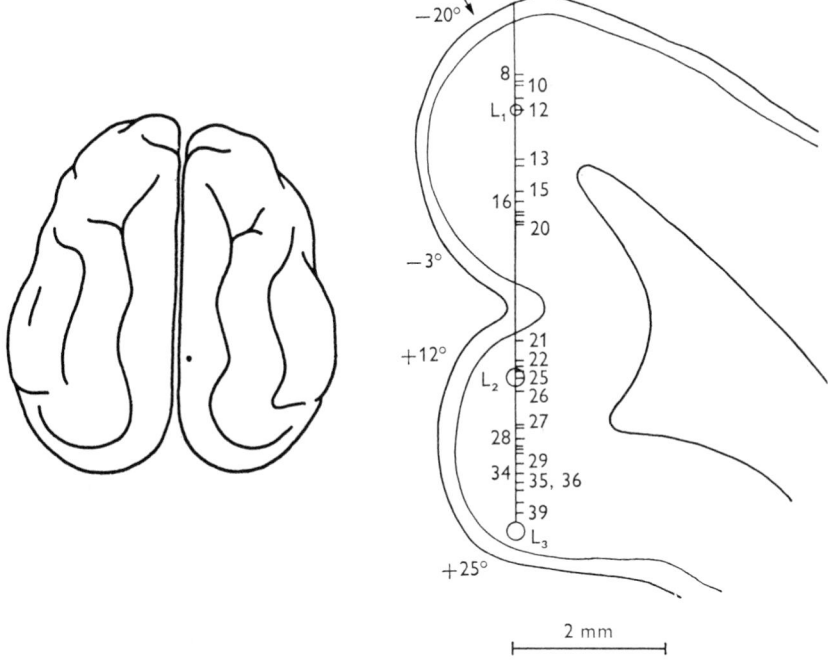

Text Fig. 5. *Five-month-old Siamese cat (No. 5) whose eyelids had both been sutured shut from birth. Thirty-nine cells were recorded from apex and medial aspect of lateral gyrus; all of these except possibly the very first were in area 17, to judge from the steady ipsilateral-to-contralateral progression in field position. Cells were influenced from the contralateral eye only, up to unit 32, whose field was 20° contralateral to the midvertical; from this point on there was a mixture of cells driven from both eyes (represented by dashed and continuous rectangles superimposed) and cells driven only from the contralateral eye. Numbers in parentheses following unit numbers refer to ocular-dominance groupings; e.g. '2' means that contralateral eye gave much stronger responses than ipsilateral, etc. (see Hubel & Wiesel, 1962). Note the relatively large size of ipsilateral receptive fields, and the very much smaller contralateral ones. Receptive fields represented by circles were not clearly oriented, a frequent finding in cats reared with both eyes closed from birth (cells 29–33 are out of sequence because electrode was withdrawn and then readvanced). (Continued)*

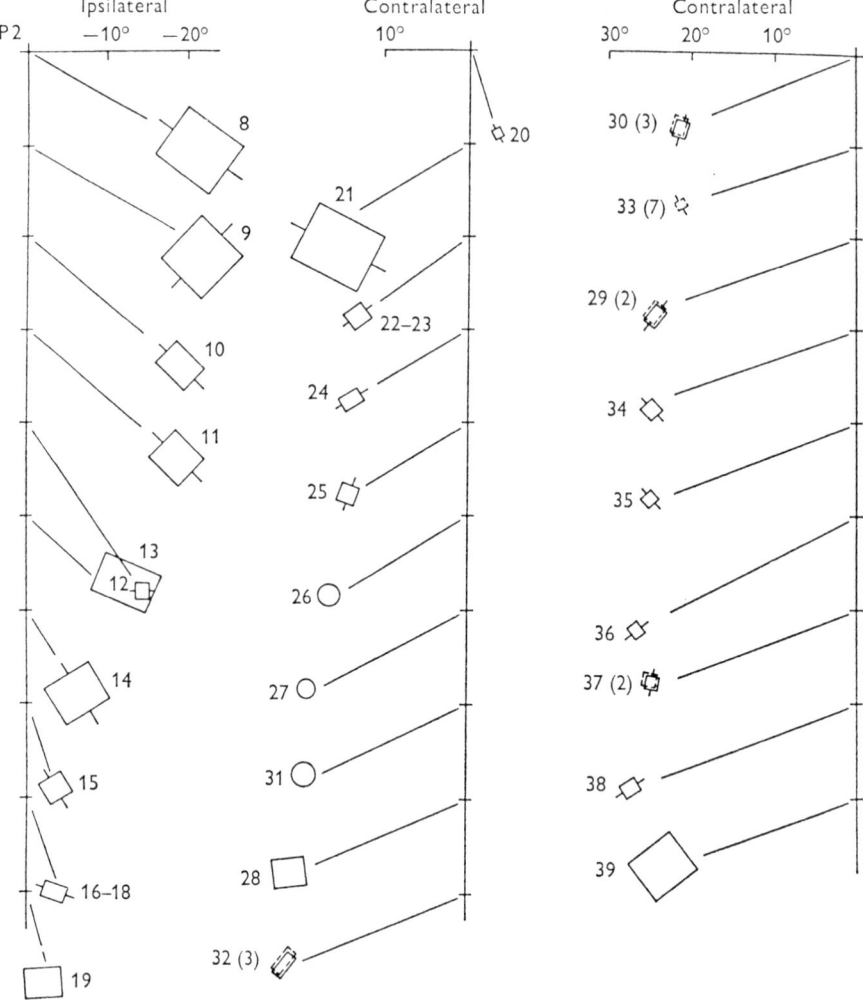

Text Fig. 5. (Continued)

out from the vertical in the ipsilateral field of vision and the cells were driven only by the contralateral eye; subsequent fields progressed steadily inwards to the vertical meridian. Following a gap between units 20 and 21, during which the electrode crossed layer I, the trend continued, with the first fields 15° contralateral and the final ones 30° contralateral. Ipsilateral fields in the first part of the penetration were several times larger than the contralateral fields recorded in the latter part, even though the two groups were about the same distance from the vertical meridian. This tendency was also seen, though not quite so compellingly, in the penetration of Text-fig. 3.

All cells were driven only by the contralateral (left) eye until unit 32, whose field was 20° contralateral; that cell was driven from both eyes, the left eye slightly dominating (group 3). We then observed a series of cells driven from both eyes, after which the cells, with one exception, again became monopolized by the contralateral eye. Thus this cat, unlike the previous two, showed clear convergence of input from both eyes on single cells. It is not possible to say whether the actual distribution of cells according to ocular dominance is normal, given such a small sampling of cells, but it seems clear that binocular convergence on to single cells is present at birth, and subsequently disappears because of strabismus, just as it does in ordinary cats or monkeys when a squint develops early in life.

ABERRANT INPUT. At this stage it appeared to us that the project of surveying the Siamese cat was reasonably complete, but since all the animals had been from the same litter we thought it wise to repeat the experiments in one or two unrelated Siamese cats. Accordingly the next experiment consisted of four penetrations made in an adult cat

(No. 6). The results, in terms of topographic representation and binocular interaction, were entirely consistent with the previous ones, with one interesting addition.

The first three penetrations were made at Horsley-Clarke coronal level 0.0 (Text-fig. 6). In the most medial penetration, P1, units 1–10 had fields in the vertical mid line area about 10° below the centre of gaze. This upper part of the penetration was slightly inclined so that there was a component of movement relative to the surface in a lat-

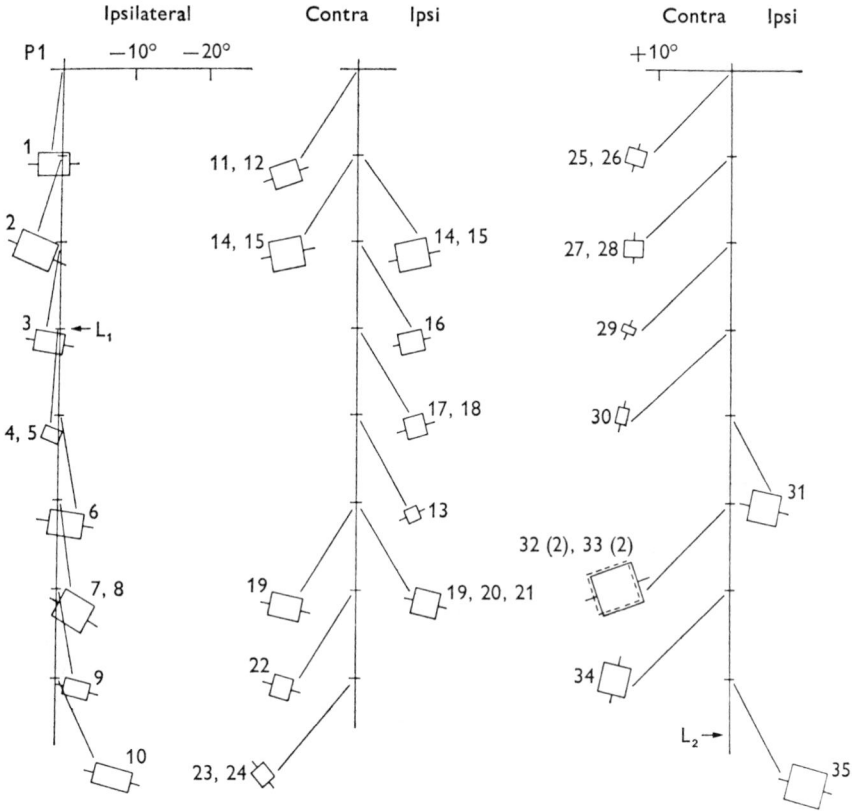

Text Fig. 6. First three penetrations in cat No. 6, an adult Siamese unrelated to cats 1–5. Horsley-Clarke 0.0. Upper part of penetration 1 and penetrations 2 and 3 were all in area 18, as judged by the histology and the ipsilateral-to-contralateral progression in receptive-field positions accompanying medio-lateral movement across the cortex. In the deeper half of penetration, and in penetration 3 there were occasions in which cells and background activity could be driven by stimuli in the ipsilateral visual field, roughly across the mid line from the part of the visual field from which the prevailing responses were obtained. In area 17, cells 14, 15, and 19 had dual fields, with components roughly symmetrically placed in each visual field. (Fig. 7 illustrates a recording from cell 14.) For these fields, the orientations of the two components, as well as the field sizes and directional preferences, were identical. (Fields 11–18 are numbered in the order in which they were recorded, but are illustrated in their anatomical order.) In area 18, background activity recorded simultaneously with unit 46 was again driven from the mirror-symmetric position in the ipsilateral field (46a). All cells were driven only from the contralateral eye, except for Nos. 32 and 33, which were driven also by the ipsilateral eye (group 2). (Continued)

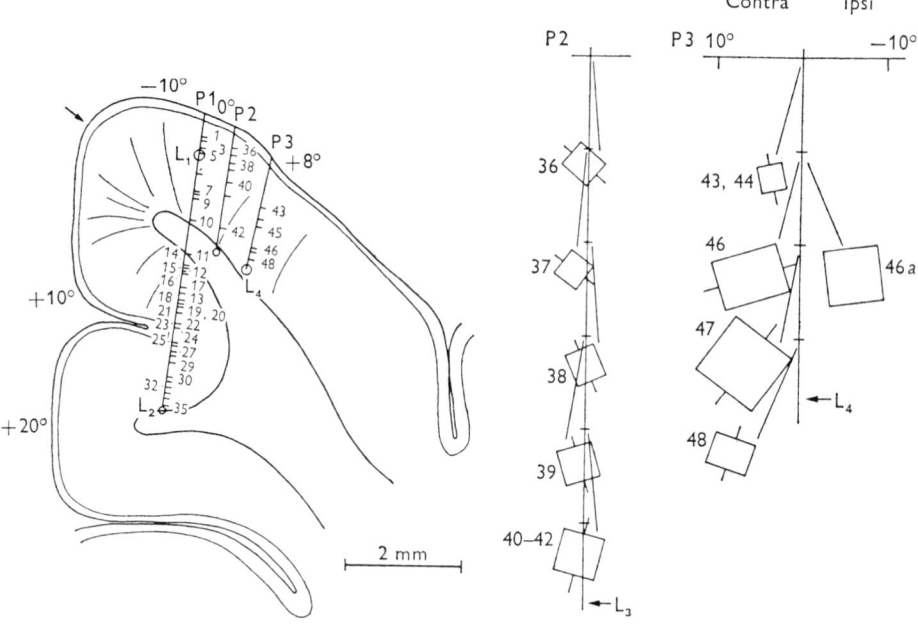

Text Fig. 6. (Continued)

eral-to-medial direction. The drift in receptive-field positions from contralateral to ipsilateral suggested that this region of cortex was area 18. After crossing white matter, the electrode, as expected, entered a region in which the first cells (Nos. 11 and 12) had fields in the contralateral visual field, in this case about 15° out; these cells were driven from the contralateral eye. Advancing the electrode rather rapidly, we suddenly entered a region in which the background activity was still driven by the contralateral eye, but now from the ipsilateral visual field, about the same distance out, and at about the same horizontal level. There was no trace of a response from the contralateral visual field. A well isolated cell, No. 13, had its field in this ipsilateral area. We withdrew the electrode slowly, to see if there was any overlap between these two mirror-symmetric cortical representations. A short distance back there was indeed a region in which activity was driven from both areas of visual field, with no response from the vertical mid line region between. Here we came upon a well isolated cell (No. 14) which was driven from both areas, a finding so unprecedented that we went to great pains to be sure that the recording was not from two differ-

ent cells. We finally convinced ourselves that it was a single cell by adjusting the electrode position back and forth, watching the spikes from the unit wax and wane, nevertheless remaining identical in size at any electrode position regardless of the region of visual field stimulated.

A recording from this cell is illustrated in Text-fig. 7. The two components of the field were exactly the same size, and both showed identical preferred stimulus orientations, with a moderate directional preference for downward movement. The situation was thus reminiscent of the usual cortical cell with a receptive field in each eye; all this time, however, the right eye was absolutely silent, and the fields, far from being in corresponding positions, were in virtual mirror-symmetry. What reinforced the analogy to the usual system of binocular interaction in cat cortex was the existence of clear summation when the two areas were stimulated together, and especially the fact that while the regions had similar properties in most respects, the responses were not equally brisk, the contralateral region giving slightly stronger bursts than the ipsilateral (the difference is not apparent in Text-fig. 7). In the normal cat it will be recalled

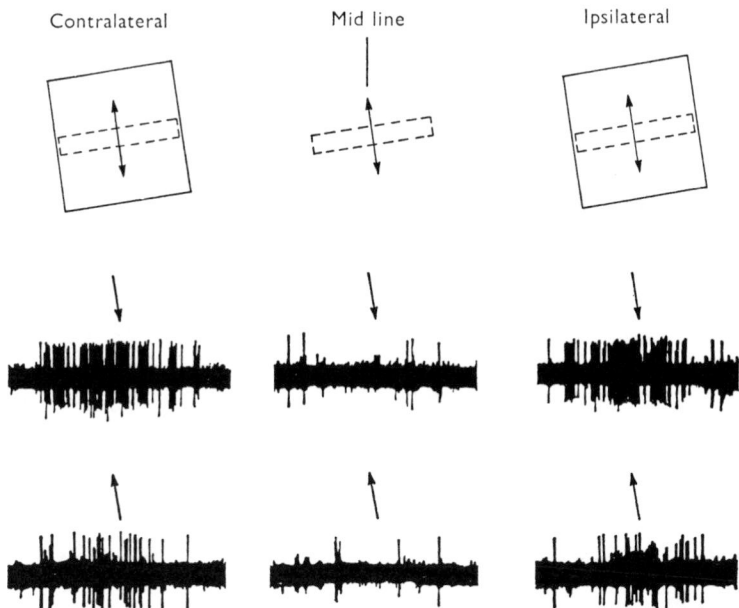

Text Fig. 7. *Responses of cell 14 of Text-fig. 6 (cat No. 6, penetration 1). The cell was driven from two regions, each 4° × 4° in size, one 9° to the left of the vertical mid line and 12½° below the horizontal (left records), the other 8° to the right of the vertical mid line and 13° below the horizontal (right records). Between these regions (middle set of records) no responses were evoked. Since this cat had a poorly defined area centralis, estimates of the vertical mid line could have been off by 2–3° in either direction. In each area the best responses were to a 2:30–8:30 slit moving downwards. Responses from the contralateral region were slightly brisker than those from the ipsilateral (though this does not show in the illustration). Duration of each trace, 4 sec.*

that cortical cells are not necessarily driven with equal vigour from the two eyes (Hubel & Wiesel, 1962).

Advancing the electrode, we recorded another unit with a double field (No. 15), whose components had the same positions and orientations as unit 14. Again the contralateral region dominated slightly. Cells 16–18 had fields only in the ipsilateral area, with no background activity evoked from the contralateral region. Cell 19 had a double field with the ipsilateral region now strongly dominant, while No. 20, recorded simultaneously, was driven only from the ipsilateral area. The next cell, No. 21, again responded only in the ipsilateral region. From that point on all activity disappeared from the ipsilateral area, and as cell after cell was mapped the receptive fields as usual moved gradually further into the contralateral visual field. Late in the penetration two more cells, Nos. 31 and 35, had receptive fields confined to the ipsilateral side. These fields were not as far out on

that side as were the fields of their neighbours on the contralateral side. All this time the ipsilateral (right) eye gave no hint of activity until cells 32 and 33, both of which were, however, strongly dominated by the contralateral eye (group 2), and were influenced only from the contralateral field of vision.

Cells recorded in penetration 2, lateral to 1 (Text-fig. 6), again had fields that were virtually in the mid line. In penetration 3 the fields of the initial cells were, as expected, further out in the contralateral field. A careful scrutiny of the ipsilateral visual field during the entire penetration again showed one small patch of cortex, containing cell 46, in which background activity was influenced both from the region of that cell's field and from the same eye in an area of ipsilateral field roughly opposite (No. 46a); cell 46 itself was driven only from the contralateral region. The two mirror regions were too close together for us to be absolutely certain that they did not merge across the mid line, but it was clear that in this part of area 18 there were patches in which there was input from the ipsilateral field.

In a final penetration made 6 mm further forward, a long traverse of the medial segment gave results very similar to those of Fig. 4, penetration 1. There were no patches of mirror representation.

Cat No. 7, a 4-month-old Siamese unrelated to the others (Text-fig. 8), was examined to confirm the existence of these ipsilateral patches of input. The animal already had a clear convergent squint. As in cat No. 6, the areae centrales were unusually poorly defined, and our estimate of their positions could have been off by several degrees in any direction. A penetration down the medial cortical bank revealed a topography virtually identical to that of previous experiments—an ipsilateral progression, a jump to the mid line after crossing white matter, and a subsequent progression into the contralateral field. Careful monitoring of the ipsilateral field during these recordings showed two portions of the penetration (cells 47–50; 54–56) in which responses were obtained from two separate regions of visual field, one on each side of the vertical meridian. On the first of these occasions two cells (47 and 48) were recorded together, one with a field about 12° in the contralateral visual field, the other with a field of slightly different orientation, about 7° in the ipsilateral visual field and slightly lower in position. There was abundant background activity influenced from both areas. Cells 49 and 50 were likewise simultaneously recorded. Two other cells, Nos. 54 and 56, had fields ipsilateral to the midvertical; in both recordings there was simultaneous activity driven from the contralateral field. At no point in the penetration were responses evoked from the ipsilateral eye.

This experiment, then, confirmed the presence of patches of input from the ipsilateral visual field superimposed on what was predominantly a representation of the contralateral field of vision. The lack of a strict mirror symmetry in the positioning of these receptive fields, and the relatively large scatter in their field positions, agrees with a similar finding in the previous experiment (Text-fig. 6, cells 31 and 35), but contrasts with the regularity suggested earlier in the same penetration (Text-fig. 6, cells 13–21). On the whole we had the impression that the ipsilateral-field input was less

well organized than the input from the contralateral field, which is as orderly as in the normal cat.

DISCUSSION

These experiments confirm Guillery's observation that the central visual pathway of the Siamese cat is highly abnormal, and they support his idea that the abnormality consists primarily of a mistake at the chiasm, with some optic fibres from the temporal retina crossing instead of remaining uncrossed. In this paper we have tried with the help of physiological tools to learn how the brain deals with the aberrant fibres, with the ultimate hope of gaining more insight into normal developmental processes.

At the geniculate level the problem of aberrant fibres is solved, it would seem, in the simplest and most obvious way. A medial segment of layer A_1 on one side should normally receive the innermost 15–20° of temporal fibres from the ipsilateral eye; these fail to reach the geniculate, which instead must deal with the innermost 15–20° of temporal fibres from the contralateral eye. Not surprisingly, the aberrant fibres project to just the gap in the geniculate that the absent optic fibres would have filled. Text-fig. 2 suggests that they do so in a systematic manner, since as the electrode crosses from layer A to A_1 the fields of cells jump from a region in the contralateral visual field to a region roughly in the corresponding part of the ipsilateral field, with mirror-like symmetry. Normally the site of termination of a retinal fibre relative to the medial border of the geniculate depends on the distance of its origin in the retina from the retinal vertical mid line, and the mirror-symmetry suggests that this is true even for aberrant fibres from the ipsilateral field. This ability of optic fibres to grow to precisely the right location in the geniculate, but on the wrong side with mirror symmetry, implying an absence of strict left-right specificity, is reminiscent of experiments in which Sperry (1945) obtained restoration of vision in frogs after crossing the optic nerves; his behavioural result seems to imply that the fibres had succeeded in growing back to the appropriate parts of the tectum, but on the wrong side.

The next question is how the cortex deals with such a complex input. In trying to predict the answer one may imagine several possibilities. The

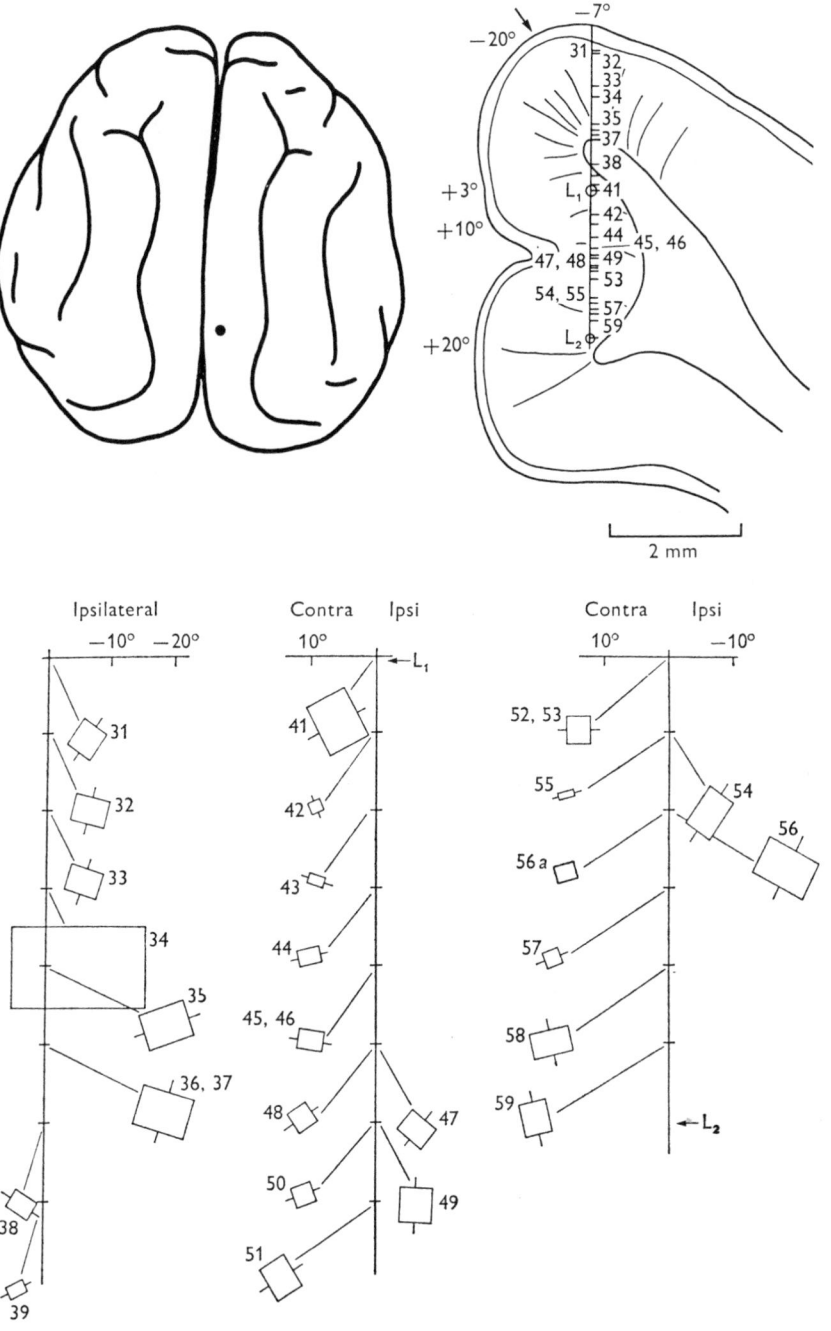

Text Fig. 8. Siamese kitten (No. 7) 4 months of age. A single penetration in the right visual cortex at coronal level 0.0. The first cells were recorded from area 18, as judged by the large size of receptive fields and progression out into the ipsilateral visual field. In the medial segment, presumably area 17, there was the usual regular contralateral drift of relatively small fields, broken only by two brief episodes of activity from the ipsilateral field of vision. No cells were seen with dual fields, but there were three examples in which the two simultaneously recorded cells were driven from regions to either side of the midvertical (47 and 48; 49 and 50; 54 and 55). All cells were driven from the contralateral eye only.

projections from layer A_1 of the geniculate might be organized very much as they are in the normal visual pathway, with groups of cells in A_1 connected to the same region of cortex as cells directly above, in layer A of the geniculate, and below, in the ventral set of layers (B). Or an entirely separate region of cortex might be set aside for the projections from the additional 15–20° of ipsilateral visual field, in which case neighbouring cells from A and A_1 would project to very different places. Finally, fibres from the abnormal part of A_1 could be mixed in with, and superimposed upon, the normal projection from the contralateral field in more or less random fashion.

The result, in fact, is a mixture of the first and second possibilities. Of these the second plan, in which part of the cortex of each hemisphere is devoted specifically to the 0–20° region of ipsilateral field, seems the dominant one, for it occurred in all of the Siamese cats in which topographic mappings were made. One of the most surprising findings in these experiments was the high degree of order shown by the new ipsilateral representations. Far from the scrambled topographic picture that one might have expected, the arrangement was almost as systematic as in the normal animal. In response to the problem of where in the cortex to represent an additional 20° of ipsilateral visual field, the answer has been to wedge it in neatly along the 17–18 boundary, which normally receives projections from the vertical meridian of the visual field. This is illustrated for the right hemisphere in Text-fig. 9: as the visual cortex is crossed from medial to lateral the visual-field representation begins as usual in the far left periphery and moves to the mid line. Instead of reversing here, it proceeds for another 20° into the right field. With further progression laterally across the cortex the movement reverses itself, going from 20° in the right field back to the mid line, and then advancing again across the left visual field. Presumably medial cortex, up to the reversal point, is area 17, and cortex lateral to this is area 18. Unfortunately, in none of the experiments was the point of reversal in the cortex precisely established, chiefly because the extreme curvature of cortex in this region makes it difficult to do so in a small number of electrode penetrations. Our estimates of it, however, coincided well with the anatomical 17–18 borders in Nissl and myelin sections, which are

marked by arrows in Text-figs. 4, 5, 6 and 8. These anatomical transition points were as usual not sharply defined, but they can be estimated with reasonable confidence to within a millimetre or so. The anatomical borders and reversal points were roughly the same in position as the 17–18 border in the common cat (Otsuka & Hassler, 1962; Hubel & Wiesel, 1965a).

The presence of an added 20° of course distorts the normal topography, so that in any coronal section a point in area 17 representing a given region of visual field is shifted medially by up to 4–5 mm, and similarly the representation in 18 is shifted laterally (see Text-fig. 9). There may also be some distortion in the anteroposterior direction, since all of our receptive-field positions seemed slightly low; a survey of much more of the striate cortex and area 18 would probably be necessary to learn whether such a distortion exists.

There are several hints that in the Siamese cat the topography is in places more complex and less regular than what we have described. Guillery's paper shows that, at least at some anteroposterior levels, there may be two segments of layer A_1 that receive aberrant contralateral-eye input, separated by a normal segment. In terms of topography a movement medially along A or A_1 corresponds to a visual-field displacement inward towards the vertical meridian. One would therefore expect that the part of temporal retina yielding crossed aberrant fibres would not necessarily extend uninterrupted to the mid line of the visual field, but might form several islands or strips in the ipsilateral field. In that case one would also expect in the cortex a corresponding discontinuity in the ipsilateral-field representation. This seemed not to be so in some of our cortical penetrations, such as that of Text-fig. 3, for in that experiment there was a continuous progression extending from 15° ipsilateral across the mid line to 15° contralateral. Text-fig. 5 likewise shows no gap. Moreover, there was no hint of any ipsilateral-eye input to the contralateral fields in their most medial parts, though Guillery's result might predict such an input. But the inner 10–20° of visual field, contralateral or ipsilateral, were in most experiments not thoroughly enough explored to rule out minor discontinuities, and it may be that the part of the temporal retina giving rise to crossed fibres extends uninterrupted to the mid line at some horizontal levels but not at others, or

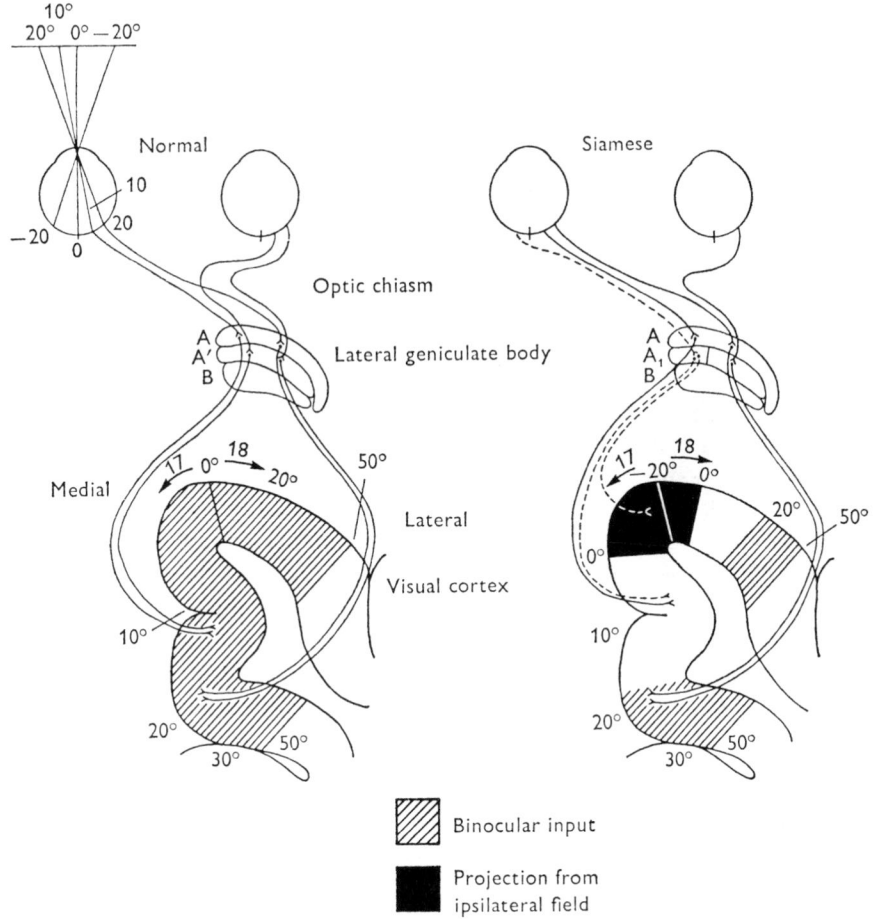

Text Fig. 9. Diagrams for normal and Siamese cats showing pathways from retina to cortex. Left diagram is the same as in Text-fig. 1. In the Siamese cat, abnormal projections are shown by dashed lines; note that the connexions from peripheral retina, beyond 15–20°, are normal. Shaded cortex represents areas receiving input from both eyes; unshaded regions receive input from contralateral eye only; black region in Siamese cat indicates the additional 20° of ipsilateral-field representation in 17 and 18 in the contralateral eye. The dashed pathway to the black region supplies this additional representation, whereas the dashed pathway to the unshaded area supplies the patches of ipsilateral field to the cortical region that otherwise mainly represents 0–20° in the contralateral field.

that all Siamese cats may not have the same number and distribution of aberrant fibres. It would be interesting to know the exact shape and extent of the retinal region or regions giving rise to the aberrant crossed fibres, and the variability in this from animal to animal.

The functional architecture of the Siamese cat's visual cortex may be of some value for understanding mechanisms of normal development. It is important, for example, to learn whether each geniculate cell is specifically connected to particular cortical cells. Our results seem to suggest that this is not so, but that the geniculate axons instead arrive at the cortex in a topographically ordered fashion and simply fill out the available space, connecting to certain classes of cells in highly specific groupings that produce simple-field and complex-field characteristics and so forth, but without absolute specificity for receptive-field position. In other words, a cortex that would normally receive fibres representing only the contralateral field of vision finds itself confronted with input from an additional 20° of ipsilateral field. The solution is to place the fibres with the furthest ipsilateral representation where the innermost ones would normally go, at the 17–18 border, and pack in the rest, as usual, in an ordered double representation. Even if the size of the visual field representation is larger for each hemisphere, the total number of incoming fibres is presumably not increased, since over the anomalous 20° there is input from the contralateral eye only.

This apparent lack of rigid specificity in geniculo-cortical connexions is reminiscent of the findings of Gaze, Jacobson & Székely (1963), in *Xenopus* embryos with compound eyes (double nasal or double temporal), that optic fibres which would normally have projected to only half of the contralateral tectum regenerate so as to fill the whole tectum. The analogy is of course a tenuous one since our results do not involve regeneration after surgical intervention, and furthermore the process is one of compression of a topographical representation after an addition of visual-field input rather than an expansion after a field deletion.

In the common cat, cortical receptive fields in or near the area centralis tend to be very much smaller than those in the periphery. The same is true in the Siamese cat, to judge from experiments like that of Text-fig. 3, even though the region of area 17 representing the area centralis is displaced. This suggests that the detailed interconnexions and transformations in the cortex are not very different from region to region of a given subdivision such as 17 or 18. In parts of cortex subserving the area centralis there is more cortex per degree of visual field than in peripheral parts (i.e. the magnification factor is larger), but there are also more entering geniculate fibres, whose receptive fields are smaller. If differences in precision of representation that occur in various parts of the visual field, in 17 and 18, are not reflected in differences in architecture, then any part of area 17 may substitute for any other, as the present results in the Siamese cat seem to imply. This idea is also supported by the relative histological uniformity of these regions.

If a new topographic order is the chief principle used to deal with the anomalous cortical input, there seems to be a second competing process in which cells of the anomalous segment of geniculate layer A_1 connect to the same regions as their immediate neighbours in layers A and B, above and below. In a normal animal, of course, these two tendencies need not compete, since the topographic maps of the visual fields in the three layers A, A_1 and B are in precise register. In the Siamese cat cortex, the second tendency results in alternating regions or patches (possibly columns) of two types: not left eye—right eye regions, as is found in common cats, but areas with contralateral-field input, mixed with occasional patches representing more or less mirror-symmetric ipsilateral-field regions. Here the two mirror-symmetric inputs are from the contralateral eye only. At boundaries between the two kinds of region, or where the two overlap, cells with receptive fields on one side of the vertical mid line may be inter-mixed with cells having fields on the opposite side, and an occasional cell may even be driven by one eye from two separate regions, one in the left and one in the right visual field. In the three cells of this type that were seen the orientations of the two regions were identical, showing that in some respects there was a high degree of specificity of connexions. Moreover, the responses from the two regions were not necessarily equal. This system thus strikingly resembles the system for binocular convergence in the cat, as would be expected if both systems depend on the same connexions.

The mirror-like patches of ipsilateral-field representation resemble even more closely the pattern of binocular convergence in ordinary cats brought up with strabismus, for here one sees especially sharp separation of left-eye and right-eye patches, with only a small proportion of cells receiving input from both eyes (Hubel & Wiesel, 1965*b*). In ordinary cats raised with strabismus the separation is the result of the long-term absence of correlated stimulation of corresponding regions in the two retinas. The same could well be true in the Siamese, for only by chance would identical stimuli ever fall upon points symmetrically disposed on either side of the vertical meridian of the visual field. In the present study we used an animal with eyes bilaterally occluded from birth to show that there is initially binocular convergence on cortical cells in the peripheral fields, from 20° to the temporal crescents, and that this convergence breaks down in the presence of squint early in life. A similar strategy might be used to test whether in

Siamese cats cells with double fields in one eye are more common in very young animals. Indeed, the question might have been asked in cat No. 5, but at that time we were not aware that such cells existed, and even if they had been more frequent in that cat, we may simply have missed them. In any case, the relative scarcity of ipsilateral patches seems to indicate that the main ipsilateral projections go to the topographically organized regions near the 17–18 border.

Patches of mirror-symmetric ipsilateral field representation were found in the predominantly contralateral-field region (in Text-fig. 9, the unshaded parts of the cortex), both in 17 and 18. We look upon this as a process reflecting a tendency for axons from adjacent parts of A, A_1 and B to travel to a common destination, namely the cortical region where contralateral fields are represented. There would be no reason to expect patches of contralateral-field input (from layers A and B) to be engrafted on the cortical ipsilateral-field representation (the black region in Text-fig. 9) and in fact no such mirror patches were found.

If all of the ipsilateral visual field input went to the new topographically ordered region (black, in Text-fig. 9), one might expect this projection to be just as detailed as its counterpart in the contralateral field. The ipsilateral input is divided, however, some going to the topographically ordered area, some to the patches in the otherwise purely contralateral region. The prediction from this would be that the ipsilateral projection should be cruder than the contralateral. The relatively larger size of receptive fields in the ipsilateral field representation in area 17 (see Text-fig. 3 and Text-fig. 6) may be one reflexion of a coarser representation.

All of these results indicate that the Siamese cat lacks any of the cortical mechanisms for binocular vision in the central 40° or so of its visual field. If these mechanisms play any part in binocular fixation it may not be surprising that a marked squint develops. The notion that the squint is secondary to the neural abnormality is supported by the absence of squint during the first few months in our animals, and the failure of a convergent squint to develop after 5 months when the eyes are kept closed. That the squint is convergent seems to make sense, since that would lead to a favouring of the nasal half retinas over the temporal halves. It is, of course, the temporal half retinas that give rise to

the aberrant projections, producing from the contralateral eye the crude ipsilateral-field representation in the cortex. With a marked convergent squint these projections may not receive much use. The fact that cat breeders have virtually eliminated squint in Siamese cats suggests that the extent of the neural abnormality may vary from one pedigree to the next.

Though as far as we know the visual capabilities of Siamese cats have never been tested behaviourally, the anatomical and physiological results suggest that this breed may be very defective. Surely even in the absence of squint there should be no stereoscopic depth perception for the first 20° of the visual fields in either direction out from the vertical mid line. Mirror-like patches of cortex, and cells such as the doublets of Text-figs. 6 and 8, are also hardly likely to enhance an animal's visual capacity.

In all of this discussion it has been assumed that the primary visual defect in the Siamese cat is an error occurring at the optic chiasm. At present, however, one has no idea what it is that causes such mistakes to occur in cat after cat. The real difficulty is that one does not know what guides the fibres in deciding whether or not to cross at the chiasm; if it is some kind of chemical attractant in the lateral geniculate, then the error in the Siamese cat may arise either from a misreading of the directions by a certain set of optic fibres, or a faulty specification of the geniculate cells. It would be of great interest to know why only certain fibres go astray. It hardly seems likely that one gene looks after a special set of temporal retinal fibres and another looks after a different set. Perhaps instead the error is one of programming, in which the timing of events is faulty. Thus the fibres that cross by mistake may do so because they arrive at the chiasm earlier or later than the others, before or after the normal signalling mechanism is in force.

It is of course surprising to find such anomalies in an animal that has been on the doorstep for so many centuries. Such a visual mutation in a species with a highly evolved visual system seems experimentally very useful, especially since the effects are mild enough not to destroy the visual system but severe enough to be interesting. Finally, one is encouraged to look for other mutants in higher mammals, and also to study the genetics of this one more thoroughly.

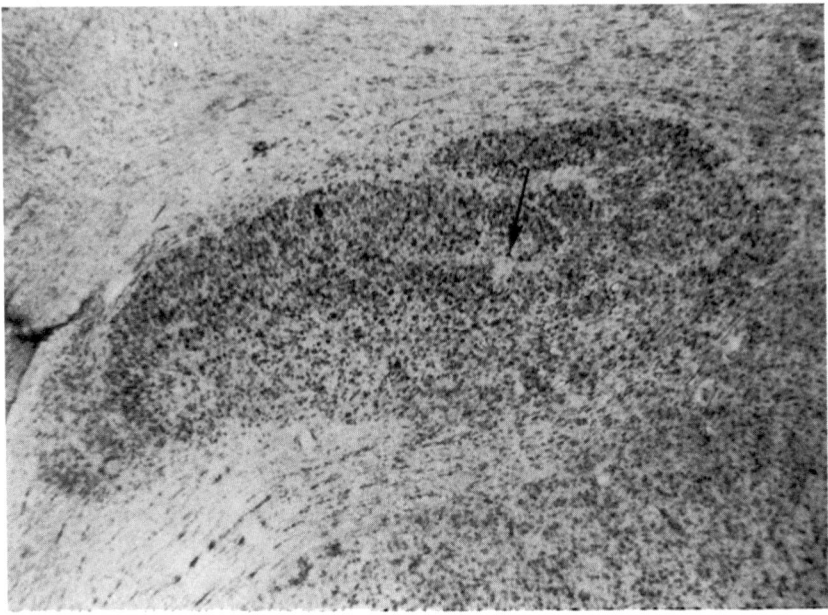

1 mm

Plate 1. Coronal section through left lateral geniculate body of a Siamese kitten (No. 7); compare Text-fig. 2. Electrolytic lesion made at the final position of the micro-electrode is indicated by the arrow, which shows the direction of the track. Nissl stain.

We wish to thank Janet Wiitanen and Mrs Stella Chow for their technical assistance, and Dr T. C. Jones for kindly supplying us with the Siamese cats. This work was supported by N.I.H. Research Grants, Nos. 5R01 EY00605-12 and 5R01 EY00606-07 and also by Grant No. 4916 from Bell Telephone.

References

Bishop, P. O., Kozak, W. & Vakkur, G. J. (1962). Some quantitative aspects of the cat's eye: axis and plane of reference, visual field co-ordinates and optics. *J. Physiol.* **163**, 466–502.

Bishop, P. O., Kozak, W., Levick, W. R. & Vakkur, G. J. (1962). The determination of the projection of the visual field on to the lateral geniculate nucleus in the cat. *J. Physiol.* **163**, 503–539.

Garey, L. J. & Powell, T. P. S. (1967). The projection of the lateral geniculate nucleus upon the cortex in the cat. *Proc. R. Soc.* B **169**, 107–126.

Gaze, R. M., Jacobson, M. & Székely, G. (1963). The retinotectal projection in *Xenopus* with compound eyes. *J. Physiol.* **165**, 484–499.

Glickstein, M., King, R. A., Miller, J. & Bailey, M. (1967). Cortical projections from the dorsal lateral geniculate nucleus of cats. *J. comp. Neurol.* **130**, 55–76.

Guillery, R. W. (1969). An abnormal retinogeniculate projection in Siamese cats. *Brain Res.* **14**, 739–741.

Guillery, R. W. (1970). The laminar distribution of retinal fibers in the dorsal lateral geniculate nucleus of the cat: a new interpretation. *J. comp. Neurol.* **138**, 339–368.

Hubel, D. H. & Wiesel, T. N. (1961). Integrative action in the cat's lateral geniculate body. *J. Physiol.* **155**, 385–398.

Hubel, D. H. & Wiesel, T. N. (1962). Receptive fields, binocular interaction and functional architecture in the cat's visual cortex. *J. Physiol.* **160**, 106–154.

Hubel, D. H. & Wiesel, T. N. (1963). Receptive fields of cells in striate cortex of very young, visually inexperienced kittens. *J. Neurophysiol.* **26**, 994–1002.

Hubel, D. H. & Wiesel, T. N. (1965*a*). Receptive fields and functional architecture in two non-striate visual areas (18 and 19) of the cat. *J. Neurophysiol.* **28**, 229–289.

Hubel, D. H. & Wiesel, T. N. (1965*b*). Binocular interaction in striate cortex of kittens reared with artificial squint. *J. Neurophysiol.* **28**, 1041–1059.

Hubel, D. H. & Wiesel, T. N. (1970). The period of susceptibility to the physiological effects of unilateral eye closure in kittens. *J. Physiol.* **206**, 419–436.

Otsuka, R. & Hassler, R. (1962). Uber Aufbau und Gliederung der corticalen Sehsphare bei der Katze. *Arch. Psychiat. NervKrankh.* **203**, 212–234.

Sperry, R. W. (1945). Restoration of vision after crossing of optic nerves and after contralateral transplantation of eye. *J. Neurophysiol.* **8**, 15–28.

Talbot, S. A. & Marshall, W. H. (1941). Physiological studies on neural mechanisms of visual localization and discrimination. *Am. J. Ophthal.* **24**, 1255–1263.

Wiesel, T. N. & Hubel, D. H. (1965). Comparison of the effects of unilateral and bilateral eye closure on cortical unit responses in kittens. *J. Neurophysiol.* **28**, 1029–1040.

AFTERWORD

The results were far more interesting and complicated than we expected. First, in each hemisphere, to accommodate the extra (nasal) part of the visual field, a region of cortex was co-opted in and around the normal vertical midline representation. Normally, in moving across the *left* visual cortex (area 17) from medial to lateral, one progresses in from the peripheral part of the *right* visual field until one reaches the vertical meridian; then as one proceeds further laterally into area 18 the progression stops and the ground is retraced, back into the right visual field. In our Siamese cats the progression instead continued well into the ispilateral (*left*) field of vision, before reversing and moving back out, as one continued into 18. Besides finding this additional very orderly (though extraordinary) representation of part of the ipsilateral piece of visual field, we found that the fields of cells subserving the part of the retina in and near the area centralis were just as tiny as they normally are, in spite of the cells' new locations centimeters away from the normal area centralis representation, where the receptive fields are normally much larger. (We did not examine magnification—this was a few years before our study of magnification and field size—but we can assume that it would also have dramatically changed.) So the cortex must have accepted the new geniculate inputs, whatever their field sizes and locations were, and simply handled them as if unaware that they were in any way different from normal. This is strikingly similar to the much more recent discovery by Sharma, Angelucci, and Sur (*Nature* 2000, 404:841–847), that a given part of the cortex, such as the auditory, can operate on an artificially introduced visual input so as to produce orientation selectivity. It is also reminiscent of our results obtained a few years later (and already described in this book) in which we found a parallel relationship between receptive field size and magnification in normal monkey cortex.

As if all that were not enough, we found in some cats a dramatically different solution coexisting with the one just described. It was as if some of the geniculate fibers from layer A1 had decided to blissfully proceed to the cortex, along with their neighbors from layer A, unaware that they were carrying the wrong and highly inappropriate messages. In the cortex one then ended up with a patches of cortical cells, some driven as usual from the contralateral visual field, via the contralateral eye, and others driven by the mirror-symmetric region in the ipsilateral field, via the ipsilateral eye. Most bizarre of all, we even found an occasional cell with two widely separated receptive subfields, in mirror positions to either side of the vertical midline.

There thus seem to be two competing tendencies in these animals: one, to make a continuous topographic representation of the visual fields in the cortex, and a second, in which cells lying opposite one another in neighboring geniculate layers insisted on sending their axons to the same parts of the cortex as they normally do, despite the outlandish consequences. In the second tendency, the clustering together, into patches, of cells with inputs from the same geniculate layer would seem to reflect the similar tendency in nor-

mal animals for cells of like ocular dominance to gather into ocular dominance columns. It is again as if the cortex were just doing its usual job with
the inputs coming in, unaware of their inappropriateness. Evidently the poor
Siamese cat is simply trying, one way or another, to make the best of the mess
bequeathed it by the abnormal crossing in the chiasm. We do not understand
the processes underlying these cats' problems—and still less can we imagine
what the outside world must look like to these creatures—but the abnormal
crossing of optic fibers is probably related to the abnormalities of pigment
epithelium that affect skin and fur coloring and also retinal pigment epithelium. Somehow the pigment epithelium must play a part in the crossing of
retinal ganglion cell axons at the chiasm.

To complicate the story even further, the two types of results we
describe in this paper are quite different from those obtained by Guillery and
Casagrande (*J Comp Neurol* 1977, 174:15–46) presumably in a different
breed of Siamese cats, which they call "Midwestern", in contradistinction to
our cats, which they call "Boston". Those authors have stressed that the differences are almost certainly in the breeds, not in the techniques used by the
two sets of workers.

In the Midwestern results, there is no systematically reorganized topography. Instead, the cortical inputs from the abnormal portions of the geniculate A1 layers, which receive their inputs from the ipsilateral visual fields and
temporal retinas, are suppressed in the cortex. These Siamese cats throw in
the sponge, at least figuratively: parts of the nasal visual fields in each eye are
blind. In their anatomy, Midwestern and Boston animals are clearly different: in the Midwestern animals the very most medial part of geniculate layer
A1 receives uncrossed optic fibers, just as it does in the normal animal. In
Boston cats this "medial normal segment" is lacking or very small. The disruption of the orderly progression in Midwestern cats, as one progresses
from medial to lateral along layer A1, is consequently more severe, with a
jump in representation on both sides of the aberrant segment. In our Boston
Siamese cats there is topographic continuity as one goes medially along the
most medial part of layer A, then down to the most medial part of A1, and
then laterally until the lateral part of the abnormal segment is reached. That
degree of continuity possibly makes it easier to establish order in the cortex.
Apparently the Midwestern animal abandons any attempt to produce an
ordered cortical topography for the ipsilateral eye.

The full story coming from the work of Guillery and his colleague is
long and fascinating, and includes raising their animals with lid closures,
and making cortical lesions to produce retrograde degeneration in the geniculates, to map the paths anatomically. It all makes for a rewarding weekend's
reading.

Carla Shatz, already mentioned in the context of normal callosal connections in the cat, also examined anatomically, with horseradish peroxidase
injections, the callosal connections in the Boston variety of Siamese cats. In
these animals the callosal projections from the 17–18 border regions of one
hemisphere were absent, or alomost so, from the border region of the other

side, but were instead located more medially, well within area 17, and also lateral to the border in 18.

Since we can think of little more to add to the already lengthy discussion in the paper, our readers may perhaps breathe a sigh of relief. Given that today even ordinary alley cats can cost around $800, it seems doubtful that much more work will soon be done on this even more expensive, special, and much-prized breed.

Chapter 24 • Cells Grouped in Orientation Columns in Newborn Monkeys •

FOREWORD

We were probably fortunate during the first decade of our working together in having our results virtually unchallenged by others in the field. This is no doubt because we were lucky enough to begin at a time when only a few groups had attempted to record from any part of the cortex, and those groups, especially the Mountcastle-Bard-Woolsey-Rose group at the Johns Hopkins physiology department, were close at hand and had already developed many of the important methods—the closed chamber, metallic electrodes, the use of curare-like agents to paralyze the eyes, and so on. We profited immensely from our interactions with them. Only by the end of the 1960s did the world begin to catch up and competition begin to develop. Within a few years almost no phase of our work had been unchallenged. There was considerable difference of opinion, especially in the area of the degree of specificity of cells in newborn kittens (Blakemore and Van Sluyters, *J Physiol* 1975, 248:663–716). Cats, to be sure, have poorly developed vision at birth (the eyelids are closed, the media are opaque), and in those animals we had to base our claims on a rather small number of cells that showed a grudging, if to us convincing, orientation selectivity. Later, in macaque monkeys, we were astonished at the degree to which a newborn or visually inexperienced monkey a few weeks old resembled an adult in the specificity of its responses. We had been convinced of the result in the 1963 kitten paper, but the challenges had continued unabated. Thus in the present study we felt that we needed to, so to speak, beat the matter into the ground. That was why we delivered a fetal monkey by caesarean section, to dispense with any arguments that an animal might have had a few moments of visual experience. It is also why we welcomed our evidence for regular sequences of orientation in newborn monkeys.

Nevertheless, one of the pleasures of science is the very existence of competition, especially when it is without rancor, and what made our dialogue with Colin Blakemore and others a pleasure was the total absence of ill-feeling, as far as we could judge. There was much admiration (we hope) on both sides, and we enjoyed the disagreements, just as one can enjoy a heated tennis game.

Ordered Arrangement of Orientation Columns in Monkeys Lacking Visual Experience

TORSTEN N. WIESEL AND DAVID H. HUBEL • *Department of Neurobiology, Harvard Medical School, 25 Shattuck Street, Boston, Massachusetts 02115*

ABSTRACT

The main object of this study was to see whether ordered sequences of orientation columns are present in very young visually naive monkeys. Recordings were made from area 17 in two macaque monkeys three and four weeks of age, whose eyes had been closed near the time of birth. The first monkey was born normally, but one day elapsed before eye closure could be done. The second was delivered by Cesarean section and the lids sutured shut immediately. The results in these two animals were very similar; in both, highly ordered sequences of orientation shifts were present, and were in no obvious way different from those seen in the adult. For example, average values for the size of orientation shifts, for the horizontal component of the distance between shifts, and for the slopes of orientation vs. track distance curves, were all similar to adult values. This indicates that the ordered column system is innately determined and not the result of early visual experience. In these two monkeys and a third one, sutured at two days and examined at 38 days, most of the cells seemed normal by adult standards, with simple, complex or hypercomplex receptive fields, showing about the same range in orientation specificity as is found in adults. About 10–15% of cells showed abnormalities similar to those seen in monkeys binocularly deprived of vision for longer periods. Furthermore, all three deprived monkeys showed a decided lack of cells that could be influenced from both eyes, whereas a normal three-week-old control animal seemed similar to the adult, with binocular cells comprising over half of the total population. A monkey deprived by binocular closure from the third to the seventh week also showed a diminution in number of binocularly influenced cells, suggesting that the deprivation from birth resulted in a deterioration of innate connections subserving binocular convergence. To be sure that the abnormalities in the deprived animals represented a deterioration of connections, we recorded from 23 cells in a normal two-day-old monkey: here the ocular dominance distribution of cells was about the same as in the adult, and the response characteristics of the cells were normal by adult standards.

In the past few decades evidence has steadily mounted for an astonishing degree of specificity of connections in the mature central nervous system. Not surprisingly, more and more attention has been given to the origin of this specificity and, in particular, to the relative importance of genetic as opposed to postnatal environmental factors. In the striate cortex of newborn and visually inexperienced kittens, we recorded several years ago from cells responding to specifically oriented stimuli,

From *Journal of Comparative Neurology*, Vol. 158, No. 3, December 1, 1974.

and found evidence suggesting that the orientation columns are already formed (Hubel and Wiesel, '63; Wiesel and Hubel, '65). Monkeys brought up for several months with both eyes sutured closed likewise have cells with orientation specificity in area 17 (Wiesel and Hubel, unpublished). In the first paper of the present series (Hubel and Wiesel, '74) we found in adult and juvenile monkeys a remarkable degree of orderliness in the arrangement of orientation columns: it was thus natural to push the question of innate specificity a step further by asking whether the entire system of columns is present at birth and hence probably genetically programmed. This is the purpose of the present study.

METHODS

Six monkeys were used. Of these, two were normal and four had both eyes sutured at various ages and for varying periods (Table 1). Techniques for stimulating and recording were generally the same as in previous papers (Hubel and Wiesel, '68, '74). For the experiment of Figure 4B, in the 2-day-old normal monkey, the moving-slit stimuli were generated on a television screen using a specially designed electronic stimulator, and the average responses for each orientation from 0° to 360° were plotted on-line using a PDP12 computer.

RESULTS

Because experiments designed to examine orientation-shift sequences tend to be protracted, we

decided against attempting them in newborn monkeys. In two monkeys we sutured both eyes closed and waited a few weeks before doing the acute experiments. One of these animals (Table 1, no. 1) had the eyes sutured two days after birth and was recorded from at 17 days. The second (Table 1, no. 2) was delivered by Cesarian section and the eyes sutured immediately; this monkey was born with the eyes closed, and the lids had to be pried open in order to trim the margins so that they could be sutured. Careful examination of the lids in the ensuing weeks showed the suturing to be completely successful (as was so for all animals in this series). Since no sign of the pupils or sclerae could be seen through the lids, it seemed unlikely that any images fell on the retinae. A third monkey was sutured at two days of age and studied at 38 days; in this animal our object was to examine receptive fields and ocular dominance.

Graphs of receptive-field orientation versus electrode-track position are shown for the first monkey in Figure 1 and for the second in Figure 2. These graphs are generally similar to those we obtained in normal adult (or juvenile) monkeys and indicate that the orientation-column system is present in the newborn monkey, with the same high degree of order.

Table 2 gives the results of measurements made from these graphs. This table is to be compared with a similar one for the normal adult (Hubel and Wiesel, '74, Table 1). As before, each straight-line sequence is listed separately. A com-

Table 1

Monkey	Type	Type of study	Figure
1	binoc closure 2–17 days	orientation shifts ocular dominance distribution	1, 3A
2	binoc closure (Cesarian) 0–30 days	orientation shifts ocular dominance distribution	2, 3B
3	binoc closure 2–38 days	receptive fields ocular dominance distribution	3C
4	21 day normal	ocular dominance distribution orientation specificity	3D
5	binoc closure 21–49 days	ocular dominance distribution orientation specificity	3F
6	2 day normal	ocular dominance distribution orientation specificity	4

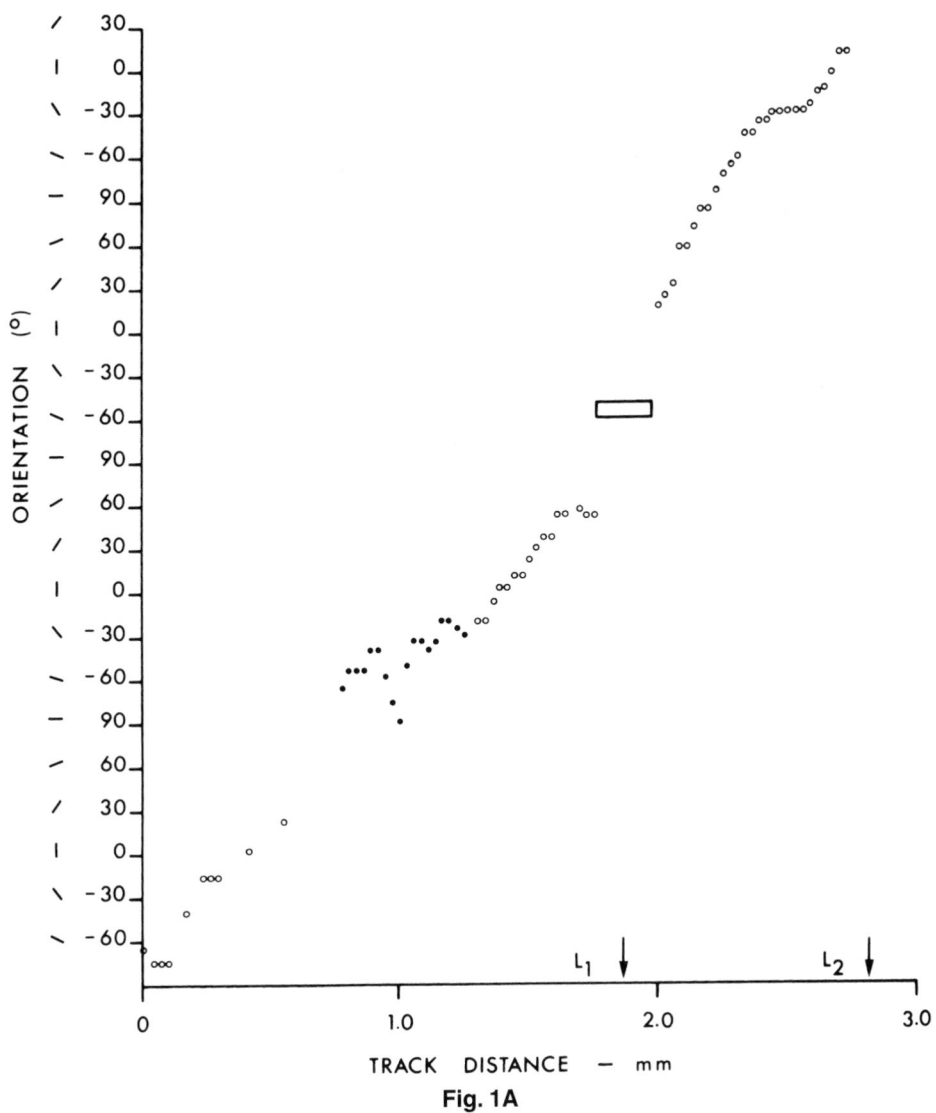

Fig. 1. Graphs of receptive-field orientation vs. electrode-track distance for two penetrations in the right striate cortex of a baby monkey whose eyes were sutured closed from the second to the seventeenth day (when the recordings were made). A Penetration no. 1. B. Penetration no. 2, about 0.6 mm from no. 1 and parallel to it. C. Reconstruction of the two electrode tracks. L_1–L_3 are lesions made to identify the tracks. Closed circles, ipsilateral eye; open circles, contralateral eye. Open bar, contralaterally dominated activity in layer IV C, unoriented. (continued)

parison of the four averages (uncorrected and corrected slopes, angle/shift, horizontal distance/shift) in adult and visually naive baby monkeys shows very little difference between the two, and in particular there is nothing to suggest that the system of orientation columns is any coarser in the visually naive monkeys. For example, the average shift in the baby monkey was 11.90°, compared with 11.91° for the adult. There is a suggestion that the hori-

zontal distance/shift may be smaller in the newborn monkey (33 μ compared with 43 μ for the adult), possibly indicating a thinner orientation-slab width in a brain that is smaller than adult size. In a previous study in monkeys (Hubel and Wiesel, '68), we observed that sharpness of tuning varies considerably, especially from one layer to the next. Similar variations were observed in these young visually naive monkeys. Our impression was that

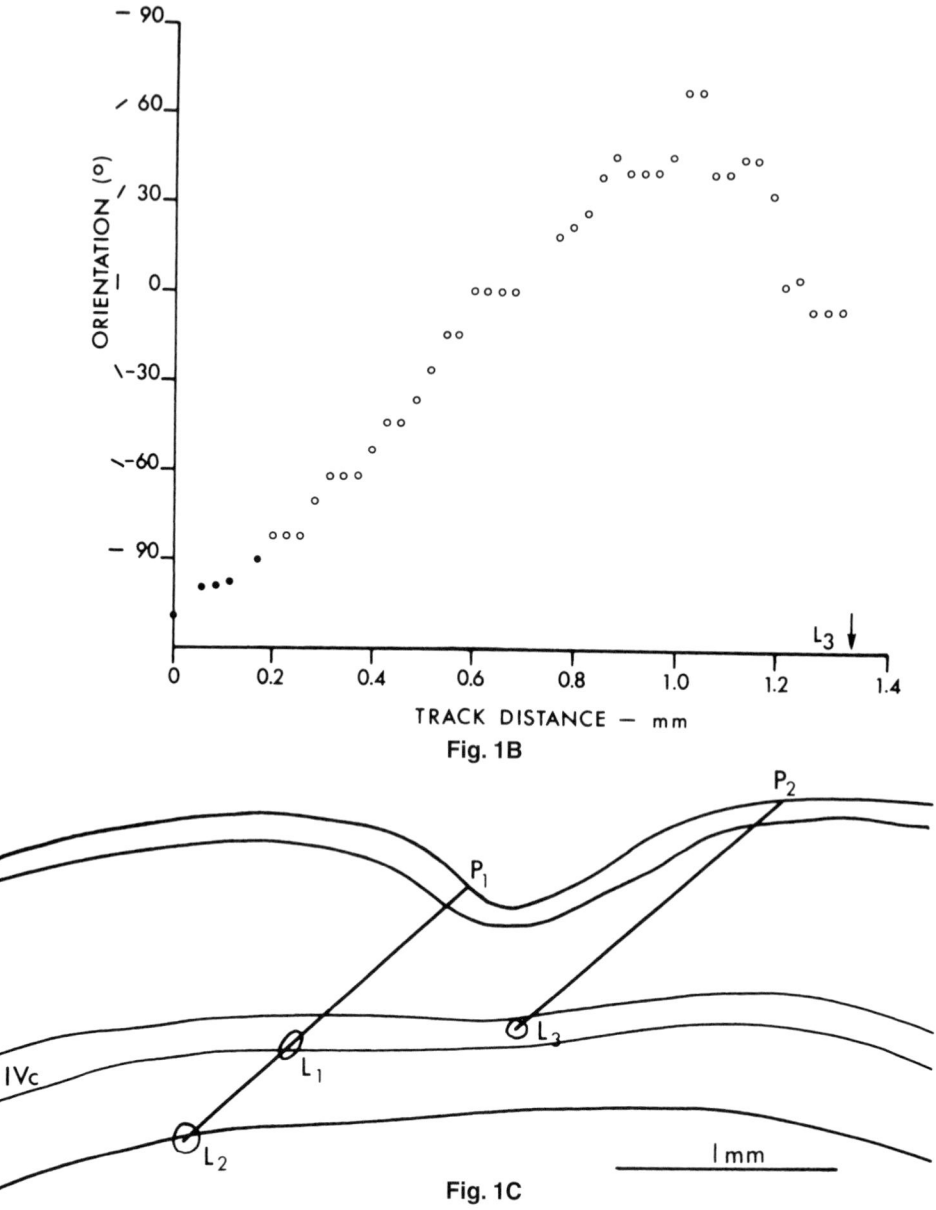

Fig. 1B

Fig. 1C

Fig. 1 (Continued)

the cells in these animals, except for 10–15% which appeared distinctly abnormal (see below), were on the whole no less sharply tuned than are cells in the adult. Otherwise sequences such as the initial ones in the two penetrations in monkey 1, or the second sequence of the first penetration in monkey 2, in which the average value of angle/shift was less than 10°, would have been difficult or impossible to plot.

Because of the claim that in kittens a few hours of visual experience can modify or affect the subsequent orientation preference of cortical cells (Blakemore and Mitchell, '73; Pettigrew et al., '73), it is perhaps worth mentioning that minutes after the eyes were reopened the very first cell recorded in the monkey born by Cesarian section (no. 2) showed a precise orientation preference from the outset. Moreover, if any orientation was used more than any other to stimulate this cell while testing it was the cell's own optimal orientation. Yet the next cell, recorded a few minutes after the first, showed

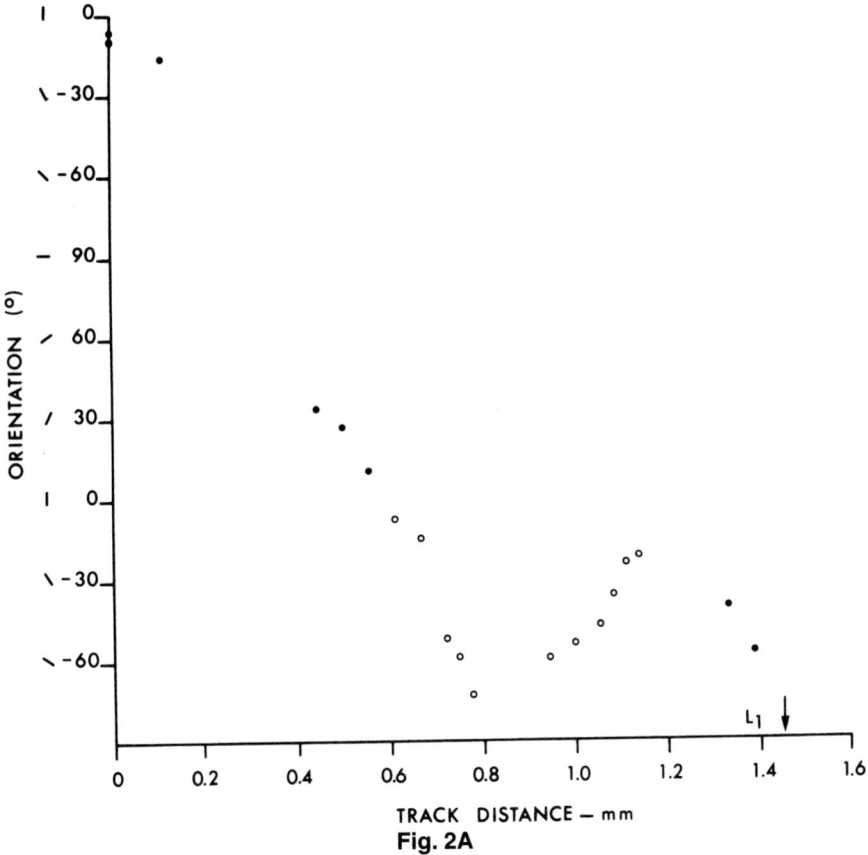

Fig. 2. Graphs of receptive-field orientation vs. electrode-track distance for two penetrations in the right striate cortex of a baby monkey whose eyes were sutured closed from birth (by Cesarian Section) to the thirtieth day (when the recordings were made). A. Penetration no. 1. B. Penetration no. 2, about 0.25 mm from no. 1 and parallel to it. C. Reconstruction of the two parallel electrode tracks, about 0.3 mm apart. (Continued)

a new optimum shifted in a counter-clockwise direction, the next showed a further shift, and so on. It would be difficult to imagine that the testing procedure was in any way responsible for producing the specificities that we observed.

In the course of recording from the first three monkeys there were several groups of cells, amounting to about 10–15% of the total, that could only be driven with difficulty, or whose orientation seemed less critical than usual. On one of these occasions, at the outset of penetration 1 in monkey no. 1, the level of CO_2 in the expired air was checked and found to be excessive. Within a few moments of correcting this the cells were responding with an orientation precision seen in normal adult cells. It is thus likely that at least some of the cells were abnormal because of the general state of the animal. On the other hand, monkeys, like cats,

when deprived by bilateral lid suture for several, rather than a few, weeks have substantial proportions of such abnormal cells (see Fig. 3, C and F); we therefore assume that some of the abnormal cells in the present series reflect the early stages of deprivation effects. That these abnormal cells are related to immaturity is unlikely, since no such cells were seen in the normal two-day-old monkey (see below).

In the present experiments our major aim was to establish whether or not the ordered orientation column system is present in visually naive animals, and we made no attempt to analyze receptive fields thoroughly or to make statistical comparisons between these monkeys and adults. In particular, we did not make careful measurements of receptive field size. Nevertheless, several general comments can be made concerning receptive fields. We

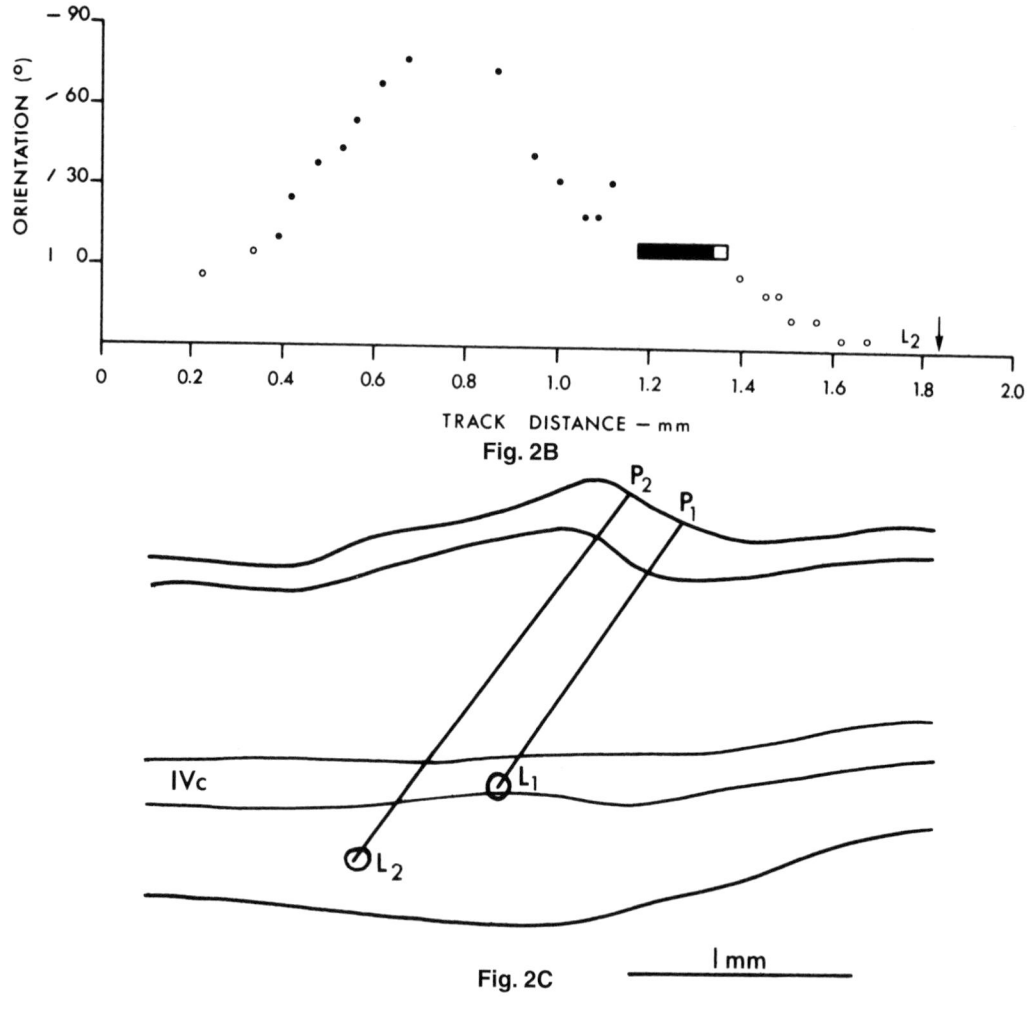

Fig. 2B

Fig. 2C

Fig. 2. (Continued)

found examples of all three receptive-field types, simple, complex, and hypercomplex. Complex cells, as in the adult, constituted the great majority of cells in the layers above and below layer IV. Simple cells were typical in firing brisk "on" or "off" responses to properly oriented stationary slits, dark bars, or edges. Orientation specificity to stationary stimuli, which we have also seen in visually inexperienced kittens, is of some interest in view of the assertion (Barlow and Pettigrew, '71; Pettigrew, '74) that it is direction specificity rather than orientation specificity that is present in visually naive kittens.

In Figures 1 and 2, the shifts in eye preference indicated by the periodic switching from contralateral eye (open circles) to ipsilateral eye (closed circles) and back indicate that the system of ocular-dominance columns develops by innate mechanisms and is present either at birth or within three to four weeks of birth. It would be worthwhile to test this further by anatomical methods (Hubel and Wiesel, '72).

What was very different in these two monkeys, compared with normal adults, was the overall degree of mixing of influence from the two eyes. Figure 3, A, B, and C shows ocular-dominance histograms for the three visually naive animals, as compared with the histogram for a normal three-week-old control (Fig. 3D) and for the adult (Fig. 3E). Compared with the normal monkey, the three deprived animals show a marked reduction in the number of cells that could be binocularly influenced. The few binocular cells that were found seemed quite normal, with fields in the two eyes in

Table 2

Experiment	Penetration no.	Sequence no.	Field distance from fovea	Span of sequence	Track length	Angle (θ)	Horizontal track length	Slope uncorrected	Slope corrected	Number of shifts	Angle/shift	Horizontal distance/shift	Figure no.
			deg	deg	mm	deg	mm	%/mm	%/mm		deg	μ	
1. binoc. closure	1	1	4	87	0.395	36	0.319	+219	+271	9	9.7	35	1
		2	4	174	0.776	36	0.628	+273	+337	16	10.8	39	
2–17 days	2	1	4	179	1.016	41	0.767	+183	+243	19	9.4	40	
		2	4	74	0.226	41	0.170	−284	−376	4	18.5	43	
2. Cesarian	1	1	8	107	0.339	48	0.225	−320	−478	7	15.0	32	2
bin. closure		2	8	51	0.225	48	0.150	+219	+327	6	8.5	25	
0–30 days	2	1	8	72	0.339	48	0.227	+219	+327	7	10.3	32	
		2	8	99	0.185	48	0.124	−134	−200	6	13.0	21	
Averages								231	320		11.90	33.38	
								±59	±86		±3.4	±7.5	
Averages, adult normals								222	281		11.91	43.26	
								±83	±93		±3.4	±11.5	

(Hubel and Wiesel, '74, Table 1)

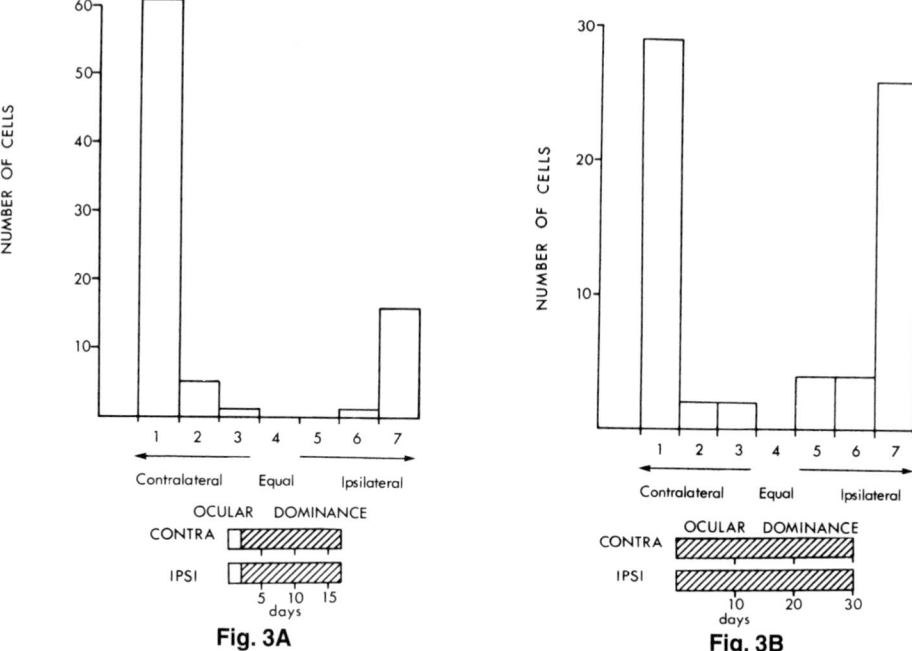

Fig. 3A   **Fig. 3B**

Fig. 3. Ocular-dominance histograms for the different monkeys. A. Monkey no. 1, binocular closure 2–17 days (Table 1). B. Monkey no. 2, binocular closure 0–30 days (Cesarian section). C. Monkey no. 3, binocular closure 2–38 days. D. Monkey no. 4, normal 21-day-old monkey. E. Ocular-dominance histogram for 1116 cells in area 17 in 28 normal adult (and juvenile) monkeys. F. Monkey no. 5, binocular closure 21–49 days. Definition of ocular-dominance groups: cells of group 1 were driven only by the contralateral eye; for cells of group 2 there was marked dominance of the contralateral eye; for group 3, slight dominance. For cells in group 4 there was no obvious difference between the two eyes. In group 5 the ipsilateral eye dominated slightly; in group 6, markedly, and in group 7 the cells were driven only by the ipsilateral eye. Shaded areas at the bottom of each histogram indicate period during which one or other eye was closed. Shaded areas in the histograms themselves represent cells that gave abnormal responses, for example, a lack of orientation specificity or unusual sluggishness. Dotted bins to the right of the histograms C and F represent cells that failed to respond to either eye.

corresponding positions and precisely tuned to the same orientation. We did not examine these cells using simultaneous stimulation of the two eyes. Taken at face value, the results suggest that binocular deprivation in the first three to four weeks has a markedly adverse effect on the convergence of influence of the two eyes on cortical cells. This is supported by Figure 3F, which shows a marked reduction in binocular cells in an animal in which both eyes were sutured from the third week to the seventh. Figures 3D and 3F together indicate that three weeks of closure in a baby monkey can lead to a marked decline in binocularly driven cells.

Despite this evidence, it seemed imperative to record from a newborn monkey to be sure that binocular cells were present, and to check, if possible, for the existence of orientation specificity. We

accordingly recorded from 23 cells in a two-day-old rhesus monkey. The histogram (Fig. 4A) shows the presence of binocular cells with about the same ocular dominance distribution as in the adult. In this monkey, cells were as precisely oriented as in the normal three-week-old monkey. A computer-generated graph of average number of impulses versus slit orientation from a complex cell is shown in Figure 4B; besides showing a very sharp tuning this cell responded to downward, but not at all to upward, movement. This graph indicates a high degree of specificity, but of course by itself it does not prove the presence of orientation specificity as distinct from directional specificity. Since the cell gave very little response to stationary stimuli, that criterion could not be used to differentiate the two types of specificity. Small moving spots, on the

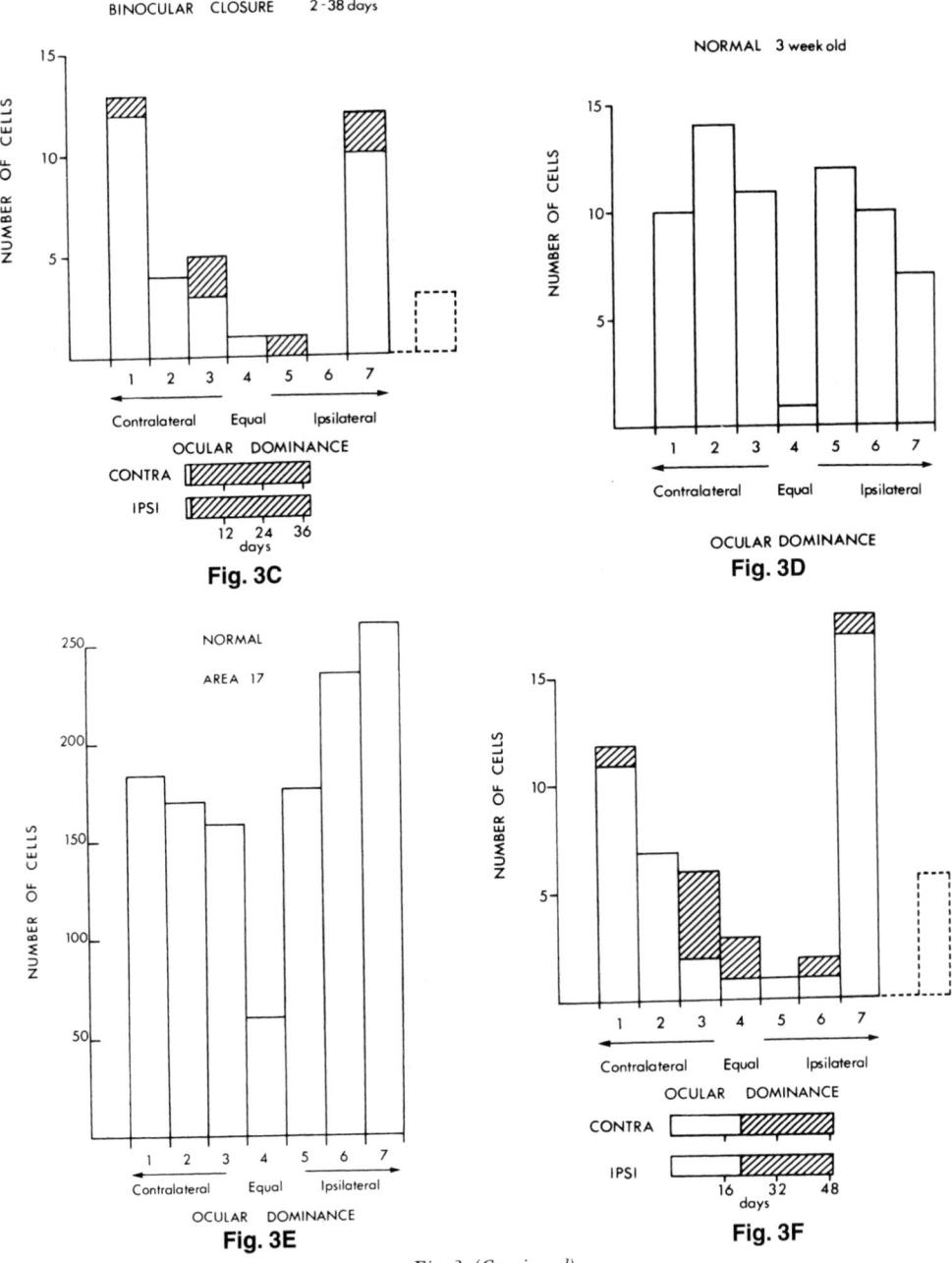

Fig. 3. (Continued)

other hand, evoked no responses; consistent responses were seen only to lines one-third to one-half the width of the field, and the responses improved steadily with increasing line length, suggesting that the cell was indeed selective for line orientation. In every way the behavior of this cell was typical of that seen in upper layer cells in adult monkeys.

During this penetration there were several sequences of regular shifts in orientation. For the binocular cells the positions of the fields in the two eyes seemed in exact correspondence, and to within

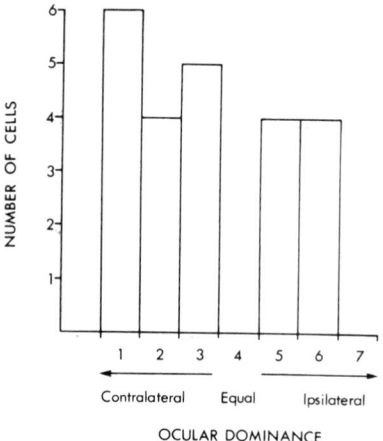

Fig. 4A. Ocular-dominance histogram for 23 cells in a normal two-day-old macaque monkey.

a few degrees the optimal stimulus orientations were identical. In these respects the cells were no less specific than cells in the adult monkey. Though it is not possible to make a detailed comparison between newborn cats and monkeys, given such a small sampling of cells, we were struck by the absence, in the two-day-old monkey, of unresponsive, very sluggish, or non-oriented cells in the upper and lower layers, in view of the presence of such cells in the ten-day-old kitten.

DISCUSSION

The present results show that the highly ordered system of orientation columns seen in adult monkeys is innately determined and not the result of visual experience early in life. Just as striking as the ordered sequences of orientation shifts was the precision with which the orientations of cells could be determined; evidently a newborn monkey is in this respect virtually mature. This is perhaps not surprising since already at birth a macaque monkey observes and follows objects. Anatomical studies on the birth days of cells in monkey visual cortex likewise indicate that, compared with other species, the macaque at birth is already well-developed (Rakic, '74).

The cat, in contrast, is visually very immature at birth. It does not open its eyes for about the first ten days of life, and at that time the optic media are quite cloudy, so that the fundus cannot be visualized. The cortex is likewise anatomically immature (Cragg, '72). Presumably this relative immaturity of the newborn kitten contributes to the difficulties one finds in observing orientation specificity. Nevertheless, the adult cat, like the monkey, has a well-ordered system of orientation columns (Hubel and Wiesel, '63a, '74, Fig. 13). The individual cells, except perhaps for those in layer 4C, are also remarkably similar in their basic properties in the two species. The similarity in the two visual systems

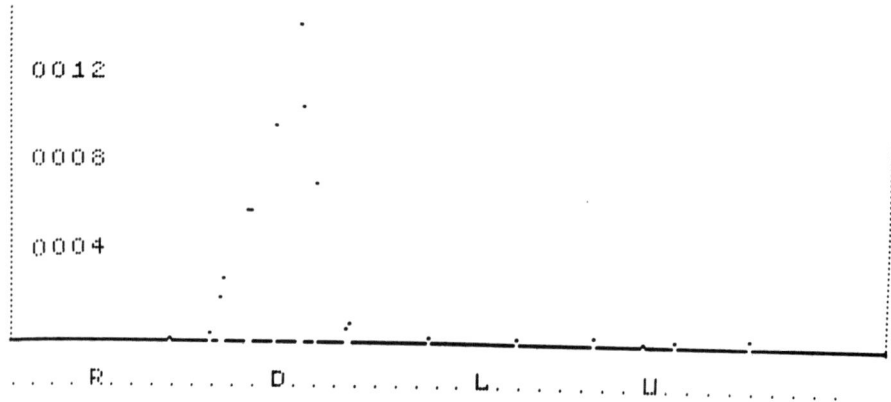

Fig. 4B. Computer graph, plotted on-line, of average response in impulses/stimulus (roughly 10 stimuli for each point) vs. orientation. Each stimulus consisted of a long narrow slit (6° × 1/4°) automatically swept in one direction across the receptive field in the orientation indicated. U = up. L = left. D = down. R = right. In addition to showing a high degree of orientation selectivity, this cell was completely unidirectional in its responses.

increases our confidence that the orientation specificity we saw in some cells in an eight-day-old kitten was genuine (Hubel and Wiesel, '63b), that its absence in other cells is a matter of maturation, and that the development of orientation specificity with all its orderliness is similarly determined in the two species, i.e., genetically.

At present this confidence is not shared by some others in the field (Barlow and Pettigrew, '71; Blakemore and Van Sluyters, '74; Pettigrew, '74). While is seems to be generally agreed that specificity of responses is present in some cells in newborn kittens, this has been said to take the form of a selectivity to direction of movement of virtually any shape of stimulus, whereas selectivity to line orientation is absent at birth and develops only with experience (Barlow and Pettigrew, '71). The present position of these authors is unclear, however, since both Pettigrew ('74) and Blakemore ('74) appear now to have found orientation specific cells in visually naive kittens. We have recently extended our experiments on visually naive kittens and have observed cells whose responses to a moving specifically oriented line improve as the line is lengthened and which also respond to the line if it is stationary, but only in the proper orientation (Hubel and Wiesel, unpublished). This is probably convincing enough evidence for orientation specificity as opposed to a directional specificity of the type seen in rabbit retina or cat tectum. In newborn monkeys the columnar arrangement seems to be identical to that found in the adult, and it is difficult to imagine that we are observing two distinct sets of cells, in newborn monkeys and in adults, arranged in the same architectural pattern, especially when their responses seem to be so similar.

An incidental and somewhat surprising finding in the present study was the marked decline in binocularly activated cells following a few weeks of binocular deprivation. The resulting ocular dominance histogram is very similar to that resulting from strabismus in cat (Hubel and Wiesel, '65) and in monkey (Hubel and Wiesel, unpublished; also Baker et al., '74). In binocularly deprived kittens there was some decline in the proportion of binocular cells in the middle groups, but certainly no change comparable to that seen in the present monkeys (Wiesel and Hubel, '65). This lack of any marked decline in binocular cells after binocular deprivation complicated the interpretation of the kitten squint histograms, as resulting simply from a chronic lack of synchronous input from the two eyes onto single cells (Hubel and Wiesel, '65); here it was necessary to add the stipulation that there be some on-going input from single eyes. In the monkey, this extra condition seems not to be necessary—apparently a simple lack of synchrony is enough.

ACKNOWLEDGMENTS

We are grateful for the use of the excellent facilities at the New England Regional Primate Center and to the staff for their assistance. In particular, we wish to thank Dr. F. Garcia for performing the Caesarian section. We thank Claire Wang and Sharon Mates for histological assistance and David Freeman for his help with electronics and computer programming. The work was supported by NIH Grants 5ROI EYO 0605 and 5ROI EYO 0606, and a grant from the Esther A. and Joseph Klingenstein Fund, Inc.

Literature Cited

Baker, F. H., P. Grigg and G. K. von Noorden 1974 Effects of visual deprivation and strabismus on the response of neurons in the visual cortex of the monkey, including studies on the striate and prestriate cortex in the normal animal. Brain Res., *66:* 185–208.

Barlow, H. B., and J. D. Pettigrew 1971 Lack of specificity of neurones in the visual cortex of young kittens. J. Physiol., *218:* 98–100P.

Blakemore, C. 1974 Development of the mammalian visual system. Br. Med. Bull., *30:* 152–157.

Blakemore, C., and D. E. Mitchell 1973 Environmental modification of the visual cortex and the neural basis of learning and memory. Nature, *241:* 467–468.

Blakemore, C., and R. C. Van Sluyters 1974 Reversal of the physiological effects of monocular deprivation in kittens: further evidence for a sensitive period. J. Physiol., *237:* 195–216.

Cragg, B. G. 1972 The development of synapses in cat visual cortex. Invest. Ophthal., *11:* 377–385.

Hubel, D. H., and T. N. Wiesel, 1963a Shape and arrangement of columns in cat's striate cortex. J. Physiol., *165:* 559–568.

——— 1963b Receptive fields of cells in striate cortex of very young, visually inexperienced kittens. J. Neurophysiol., *26:* 994–1002.

——— 1965 Binocular interaction in striate cortex of kittens reared with artificial squint. J. Neurophysiol., *28:* 1041–1059.

——— 1968 Receptive fields and functional architecture of monkey striate cortex. J. Physiol., *195:* 215–243.

——— 1972 Laminar and columnar distribution of geniculocortical fibers in the macaque monkey. J. Comp. Neur., *146:* 421–450.

——— 1974 Sequence regularity and geometry of orientation columns in the monkey striate cortex. J. Comp. Neur., *158:* 267–295.

Pettigrew, J. D. 1974 The effect of visual experience on the development of stimulus specificity by kitten cortical neurones. J. Physiol., *237:* 49–74.

Pettigrew, J., C. Olson and H. B. Barlow 1973 Kitten visual cortex: short-term, stimulus-induced changes in connectivity. Science, *180:* 1202–1203.

Rakic, P. 1974 Neurons in rhesus monkey visual cortex: systematic relation between time of origin and eventual disposition. Science, *183:* 425–427.

Wiesel, T. N., and D. N. Hubel 1965 Comparison of the effects of unilateral and bilateral eye closure on cortical unit responses in kittens. J. Neurophysiol., *28:* 1029–1040.

AFTERWORD

That the word 'genetic' occurs more than once in this paper is regrettable if understandable. What had not occurred to us was that a process resembling learning could possibly occur before birth. The fact that retinal ganglion cells are active before birth, and that their activity can be synchronized by waves of depolarization travelling across the retina, was undreamed of. We still have no idea whether the development of orientation selectivity depends on anything like that, but it is clear that 'innate' and 'genetic' are different by definition, and we should have been more careful. So for 'genetic' please read 'innate'!

We had had indications that orientation columns are present at birth but wanted to press the point. If orderly sequences could be demonstrated, orientation columns and orientation selectivity must exist *a fortiori*.

We were surprised to learn that a monkey brought up with both eyes closed for a few weeks would suffer a decline in binocularly driven cells. That, as we say in the paper, made us think a bit differently about the interpretation of our strabismus results, just as the alternating-occlusion experiments had.

And at last we had gotten started writing up monkey deprivation studies. Still on the near horizon were the new anatomical methods, especially autoradiography, waiting to be applied to the subject of visual deprivation in monkeys.

Chapter 25 • Plasticity and Development of Monkey Ocular Dominance Columns •

FOREWORD

These papers, two of our longest—and that is saying a lot—represent one of the first successful uses of modern methods of experimental anatomy in studying the cortex of the newborn monkey and the effects of visual deprivation. The previous work in kittens did not involve these newer anatomical methods, and only came a little later, with the collaboration of Carla Shatz, Sievert Lindstrom, and Torsten (*Brain Res,* 1977, 131:103–116). The first demonstration of ocular dominance columns using the Fink-Heimer-modified Nauta method, coupled with microlesions of identified geniculate layers, immediately suggested the extension of those methods to the deprivation work. That this took from 1969 to 1977 to accomplish is not too surprising: deprivation studies go slowly, especially if the experiments are done *seriatim* rather than all together. The photography alone required weeks in the darkroom and many hours of mounting the reconstructions.

These two lengthy papers represent an abandoning of our folie-à-deux in favor of making it a trio. We were very fortunate in being joined by Simon LeVay in this work: unlike ourselves he was a trained card-carrying anatomist, with a wonderful British sense of humor, a very gentle disposition, and a command of English as fluent as anyone we had ever met. (Not least of his accomplishments was the winning of many bicycle races, and the writing of his Ph.D. thesis in, of all languages, German.) We are lucky to have had the chance to work with him, and find it sad, for the field of neuroanatomy and the larger field of neuroscience, that a few years after leaving Boston for the Salk Institute in San Diego he left science to concentrate on social issues. The already underpopulated field of neuroanatomy could ill afford to lose someone with his talents.

Plasticity of Ocular Dominance Columns in Monkey Striate Cortex

D. H. HUBEL, T. N. WIESEL AND S. LEVAY • *Department of Neurobiology, Harvard Medical School,*

25 Shattuck Street, Boston, Massachusetts

Ocular dominance columns were examined by a variety of techniques in juvenile macaque monkeys in which one eye had been removed or sutured closed soon after birth. In two monkeys the removal was done at 2 weeks and the cortex studied at 1½ years. Physiological recordings showed continuous responses as an electrode advanced along layer IV C in a direction parallel to the surface. Examination of the cortex with the Fink-Heimer modification of the Nauta method after lesions confined to single lateral-geniculate layers showed a marked increase, in layer IV C, in the widths of columns belonging to the surviving eye, and a corresponding shrinkage of those belonging to the removed eye.

Monocular lid closures were made in one monkey at 2 weeks of age, for a period of 18 months, in another at 3 weeks for 7 months, and in a third at 2 days for 7 weeks. Recordings from the lateral geniculate body showed brisk activity from the deprived layers and the usual abrupt eye transitions at the boundaries between layers. Cell shrinkage in the deprived layers was moderate—far less severe than that following eye removal, more marked ipsilaterally than contralaterally, and more marked the earlier the onset of the deprivation. In autoradiographs following eye injection with a mixture of tritiated proline and tritiated fucose the labelling of terminals was confined to geniculate layers corresponding to the injected eye. Animals in which the open eye was injected showed no hint of invasion of terminals into the deprived layers. Similarly in the tectum there was no indication of any change in the distribution of terminals from the two eyes.

The autoradiographs of the lateral geniculates provide evidence for several previously undescribed zones of optic nerve terminals, in addition to the six classical subdivisions.

In the cortex four independent methods, physiological recording, transneuronal autoradiography, Nauta degeneration, and a reduced-silver stain for normal fibres, all agreed in showing a marked shrinkage of deprived-eye columns and expansion of those of the normal eye, with preservation of the normal repeat distance (left-eye column plus right-eye column). There was a suggestion that changes in the columns were more severe when closure was done at 2 weeks as opposed to 3, and

more severe on the side ipsilateral to the closure. The temporal crescent representation in layer IV C of the hemisphere opposite the closure showed no obvious adverse effects. Cell size and packing density in the shrunken IVth layer columns seemed normal.

In one normal monkey in which an eye was injected the day after birth, autoradiographs of the cortex at 1 week indicated only a very mild degree of segregation of input from the two eyes; this had the form of parallel bands. Tangential recordings in layer IV C at 8 days likewise showed considerable overlap of inputs, though some segregation was clearly present; at 30 days the segregation was much more advanced. These preliminary experiments thus suggest that the layer IV C columns are not fully developed until some weeks after birth.

Two alternate possibilities are considered to account for the changes in the ocular dominance columns in layer IV C following deprivation. If one ignores the above evidence in the newborn and assumes that the columns are fully formed at birth, then after eye closure the afferents from the normal eye must extend their territory, invading the deprived-eye columns perhaps by a process of sprouting of terminals. On the other hand, if at birth the fibres from each eye indeed occupy all of layer IV C, retracting to form the columns only during the first 6 weeks or so, perhaps by a process of competition, then closure of one eye may result in a competitive disadvantage of the terminals from that eye, so that they retract more than they would normally. This second possibility has the advantage that it explains the critical period for deprivation effects in the layer IV columns, this being the time after birth during which retraction is completed. It would also explain the greater severity of the changes in the earlier closures, and would provide an interpretation of both cortical and geniculate effects in terms of competition of terminals in layer IV C for territory on postsynaptic cells.

INTRODUCTION

Physiological experiments in cats and monkeys visually deprived from a young age indicate a certain amount of plasticity in central-nervous path-

From *Phil. Trans. R. Soc. Lond.* B. **278**, 377–409 (1977)

ways, especially at the cortical level. The nature of this plasticity is unclear. Connections present at birth can certainly be made nonfunctional as a result of deprivation, but whether there are actual morphological changes is not known. Neither is it known whether deprivation can lead to abnormal connections, either through sprouting or by the pathological persistence of connections that exist at birth and normally disappear postnatally.

In cats and monkeys deprived of vision in one eye by lid suture early in life, the cells in area 17 come to be strongly dominated by the eye that remained open (Wiesel & Hubel 1963, 1971; Baker, Grigg & von Noorden 1974). This is illustrated in Figure 1 (left), an ocular dominance histogram from a series of experiments in normal adult monkeys, and (right) in a histogram from a monkey deprived by monocular suture at 2 weeks of age for a period of 18 months. The takeover by the good eye at the expense of the bad seems to be due largely to competition between the two eyes, since closing both eyes produces effects that are far milder than would be predicted if the binocular closure were equal to the sum of two monocular

closures (Wiesel & Hubel 1965). The idea that competition is involved was borne out by the effects of monocular deprivation on geniculate responses, since here the physiological changes are rather mild, possibly because at this stage the inputs from the two eyes are largely kept separate, anatomically and physiologically, with little chance for competition. There is, to be sure, considerable cell shrinkage throughout the layers connected to the closed eye, except for the monocular crescent representation, but this may be secondary to a deterioration, through competition, of terminals in the cortex, and not a direct result of a lessening of input from the deprived eye (Guillery & Stelzner 1970; Guillery 1972*a*).

In the macaque monkey, binocular convergence in area 17 is delayed beyond what are probably the first and second synaptic stages (Hubel & Wiesel 1968). Cells representing both these stages, with concentric receptive fields and 'simple' fields, are located in layer IV and are perhaps confined to that layer. The bulk of the geniculate afferents terminate in the deep part of layer IV (layer IV C), where they segregate themselves into a series of

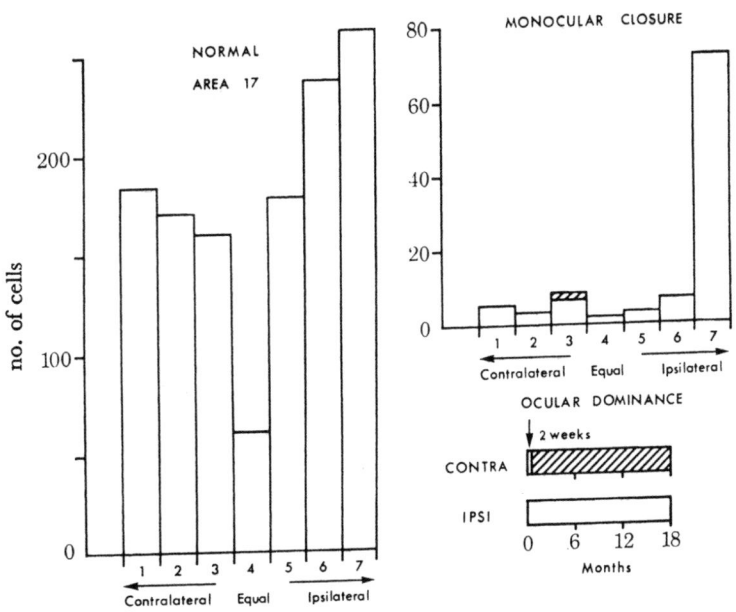

Fig. 1. Ocular dominance histograms in normal and monocularly deprived macaque monkeys. Histogram on the left is based on 1256 cells recorded from area 17 in normal adult and juvenile rhesus monkeys. Cells in layer IV C are excluded. Histogram on the right was obtained from monkey no. 3 of the present series; the right eye was closed from 2 weeks to 18 months, and recordings were then made from the left hemisphere. Shading in histogram indicates cells with abnormal responses. (Cells in group 1 are driven exclusively from the contralateral eye, those in group 7 exclusively from the ipsilateral, group 4 cells are equally influenced, and the remaining groups are intermediate.)

roughly parallel alternating stripes, one set connected to the left eye, the other to the right. Given the apparent lack of convergence of input from the two eyes onto single cells in layer IV, we were anxious to learn whether monocular deprivation would result in a redistribution of the afferent terminals to layer IV, or whether the boundaries would prove to be relatively immutable, as they seem to be in the lateral geniculate body. From the outset, in our studies of monocular deprivation in monkeys, we had been struck by the normality of the cortex in Nissl stains, and particularly by the absence of any hint of bands of cell atrophy in layer IV C to parallel the marked cell shrinkage in the deprived geniculate layers. This suggested that the geniculate and cortical layers were reacting in a very different way to deprivation.

We began by recording from layer IV C in monocularly deprived monkeys (lid sutured or enucleated). In addition to the technique of physiological recording there now exist three independent morphological methods for demonstrating ocular dominance columns (Hubel & Wiesel 1972; Wiesel, Hubel & Lam 1974; LeVay, Hubel & Wiesel 1975), and we were anxious to use these in examining the deprived cortex. It turned out that the physiological and the three anatomical methods all revealed very marked abnormalities, with clear evidence for an expansion of one set of columns at the expense of the other set. We also studied the distribution of geniculo-cortical terminals at birth, to learn whether the increase in the size of the columns corresponding to the open eye involved the formation of new connections or a regression of connections present at birth.

METHODS

Ten macaque monkeys were used, of which 9 were rhesus (*Macaca mulatta*) and one, no. 7, a pig-tailed macaque (*M. nemestrina*). The procedures used in these animals are summarized in table 1. Two monkeys had one eye removed at 2 weeks of age; three had the lids of one eye sutured at 2 days-3 weeks of age, and four served as controls. Results from one of the normal monkeys (no. 6) have already been published (Wiesel, Hubel & Lam 1974). In another control (no. 7), a 4½-year-old adult, the right eyelids had been sutured at 2½ years of age, and reopened 6 months later; behav-

ioural testing showed no visual defects in the eye that had been sutured, and this animal was therefore assumed, for our purposes, to be normal.

The lids of an infant monkey are surprisingly translucent; measurements showed that they attenuate light by about 0.5 log units. The lid tissue is nevertheless cloudy enough to prevent any dark-light contours from falling on the retinas.

Brains were examined by one or more of four procedures:

1. *Nauta method* (Hubel & Wiesel 1972). In some animals electrolytic lesions were placed with microelectrodes in single laminae of the lateral geniculate nucleus; the brains were perfused four days later, cut in frozen section at 30 µm and stained by the Nauta–Fink–Heimer–Wiitanen method (Wiitanen 1969).
2. *Autoradiography* (Wiesel *et al.* 1974). In six monkeys, one eye was injected with 2.0 mCi of a mixture of tritiated proline and tritiated fucose or with tritiated fucose alone. The brains were perfused 14 days later, and 25 µm thick frozen sections were prepared for autoradiography.
3. *Liesegang stain* (Le Vay *et al.* 1975). Other sections were examined by a reduced-silver stain, which has been shown to reveal ocular dominance columns in layer IV in normal juvenile or adult monkeys.

    In conjunction with these special morphological procedures, every fourth section was stained by a Nissl method (Cresyl Violet), and also some of the autoradiographs were counterstained for Nissl substance. Cell size was determined in the lateral geniculate and in layer IV of the cortex by measuring cross sectional areas of neuronal somata in which nucleoli were visible. Planimetry was done on the profiles traced in camera lucida, using an *X–Y* tablet.
4. *Neurophysiology*. Finally, most of these animals were recorded from. In the monkeys used for Nauta-degeneration studies, the geniculate lesions were placed by electrophysiological monitoring of the electrode position. On these occasions we also looked for possible abnormalities in the responses, and for any signs of spread of influence of the open eye beyond its normal territory. In the cortex, recordings were made at an acute angle to the surface, usually at 30–40°. Because of the gentle convex curvature of the

Table 1

no.	identifying nos. and dates	pages	figs.	procedure	age when procedure done	age studied	TECHNIQUES IN CORTEX			reduced silver
							physiology	Nauta	autoradiography	
eye removals:										
1	LM 50, 19 June 1972		2, 4b, 6, 7	eye removal (rt)	2 weeks	19 months	×	×	—	—
2	LM 57, 17 Jan. 1974		3	eye removal (rt)	2 weeks	18 months	×	×	—	—
lid closures										
3	LM 58, 23 Apr. 1974 157		1, 8a, 9, 11 14–18	lid closure (rt)	2 weeks	18 months	×	×	× (normal eye inj.)†	×
4	202, 23 Dec. 1974		8b, 10, 19–21, 27	lid closure (rt)	3 weeks	3 weeks 7 months	at 3 weeks at 7 months	—	— × (deprived eye inj.)†	—
5	201		22	lid closure (rt)	2 days reopened 7 weeks	7 months	—	—	× (deprived eye inj.)†	×
controls										
6	197, 28 Aug. 1973 (W. H. & L.)		—	normal	—	juvenile	—	—	× (left eye inj.)‡	—
7	186, 21 Aug. 1974		12, 13	late lid closure (rt)	2½ years reopened 3 years	4¼ years	—	—	× (rt eye inj.)†	×
8	209, 30 Jan. 1975		—	normal	—	juvenile (LGB cell size)	—	—	—	—
9	230		23–25	normal	left eye inj. at 1 day	1 week	—	—	× (left eye inj.)§	—
10	243, 30 Oct. 1975		26	normal	—	8 days	×	—	—	—

† 1 mCi L-proline [2,3-3H(N)], S.A. 30–50 Ci/mmol, and 1 mCi L-fucose [6-3H], S.A. 10–15 Ci/mmol, in 100 µl normal saline.

‡ 1.5 mCi proline and 1.5 mCi fucose.

§ 2 mCi fucose.

exposed part of area 17, the electrode tended to become more and more tangential as it advanced, so that if ideally positioned it took a course precisely tangential to layer IV or V (see Figure 3). This usually required several attempts, with the electrode either first missing layer IV completely or traversing it at too steep an angle to allow the recording of more than one eye-dominance shift. Each shift was marked by an electrolytic lesion (1 μA × 1 s; d.c., electrode negative). Recording procedures were otherwise the same as described previously (Hubel & Wiesel 1968).

RESULTS: PART I. EYE REMOVAL

In the first two monkeys of the present series one eye was enucleated rather than lid-sutured in order to maximize the likelihood of producing changes in the cortical columns. In retrospect such a drastic operation was not necessary, but it provided an opportunity to compare the effects of enucleation and eye closure. In these two animals the Nauta–Fink–Heimer was the only anatomical method used.

Lateral Geniculate Body

PHYSIOLOGY Recordings were made in the lateral geniculate bodies of the two eye-enucleated monkeys (nos. 1 and 2), primarily in order to position the electrode for making electrolytic lesions in the normal and deafferented layers, but also to learn whether the deafferented layers had been invaded by fibres from the normal eye. Without this knowledge it was obviously difficult to interpret any possible changes in the cortex.

In the geniculate contralateral to the normal eye, entrance of the electrode into the most dorsal layer was indicated by rich unit activity and brisk responses to visual stimulation. This persisted for about 0.5 mm; the electrode then suddenly entered a virtually silent region, with no hint of responses to stimulation of the normal eye and almost no spontaneous activity. As the electrode was further advanced a region of rich activity with brisk responses was again suddenly encountered, and was followed, again, by a silent region. This sequence of events of course reflected the passage of the electrode first through a normal layer, then through a deafferented one, and so on, as expected

from the well-known layering pattern of the geniculate. The position of the electrode in a given layer was later verified histologically. The results suggest that there was no significant reinnervation of cells in the deafferented layers by terminals from the normal eye.

HISTOLOGY As expected from previous studies (Minkowski 1920; Matthews, Cowan & Powell 1960) there was profound transneuronal atrophy of cells in the deafferented layers. This can be seen in Figure 2, Plate 1, for monkey 1, whose right eye was removed at 2 weeks and the brain examined at 18 months. The results of measurements of the cross sectional areas in the normal and deprived layers in the eye-removal and eye-sutured monkeys are given in table 2; the ratio of areas in the two sets of layers (average of the two sides) was 2.80 for monkey no. 1 and 1.86 for no. 2, the large values in both cases reflecting the severity of the atrophy. (We have no explanation for the difference in these values.) The atrophy was uniform through the entire thickness of each deprived layer, with an abrupt transition from atrophic to normal at the boundaries between layers supplied by opposite eyes. This by itself suggests an absence of any extensive reinnervation of the deprived layers by the remaining eye. Both physiological and anatomical results thus indicate that enucleation shortly after birth caused a permanent deafferentation of the corresponding geniculate layers, with no extensive sprouting between layers.

Striate Cortex

PHYSIOLOGY In the normal macaque monkey striate cortex the geniculate afferents associated with the two eyes are segregated as they terminate in the IVth layer in such a way that cells innervated by the left and right eyes form parallel alternating bands about 400 μm wide. This is the basis for the ocular dominance columns, regions in which one or other eye dominates, and which are most sharply defined in layer IV C but extend through all layers of the cortex. Thus in a typical tangential penetration the electrode moves from a region in which one eye gives the best responses to another in which the other eye dominates. In the IVth layer the cells are strictly monocular and their segregation according to eye input is very sharp; consequently transitions here are extremely abrupt. If

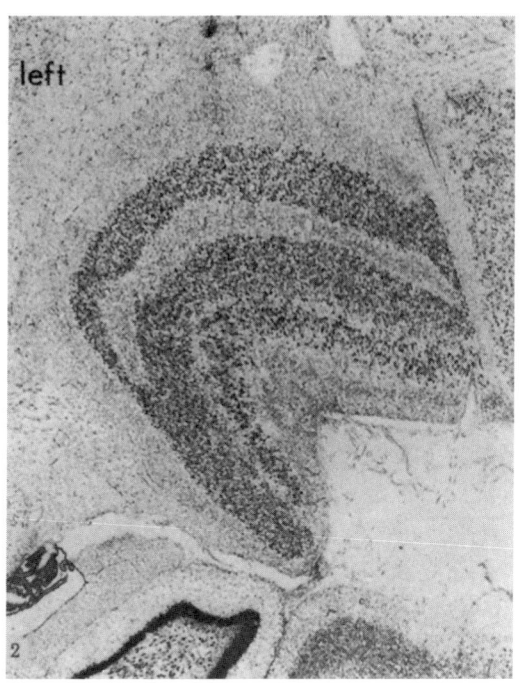
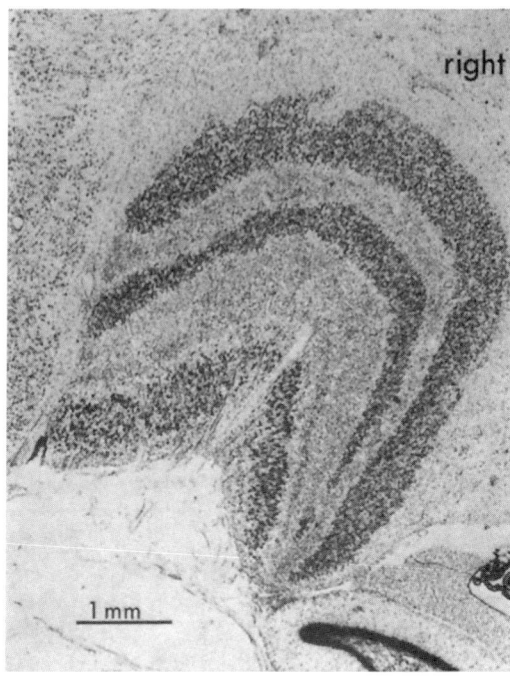

Fig. 2. Coronal sections through lateral geniculate bodies of monkey no. 1, whose right eye was removed at 2 weeks, and the brain examined at 19 months. Brain embedded in celloidin; cresyl violet stain.

there is any overlap at all, the regions must be 25 μm or less. In all our normal material we have seen no difference in widths of bands innervated by the contralateral as opposed to the ipsilateral eye: in the binocular part of area 17 (i.e. outside the representation of the temporal crescents) the two eyes seem to make almost exactly equal contributions. This equality is doubtless related to the symmetry suggested by the left histogram of figure 1, in which groups I–III are about as well represented as groups V–VII.

In the enucleated animals we were mainly interested in learning whether any changes had taken place in this arrangement of layer IV C ocular-dominance bands. If not, then in a tangential penetration one should expect an alternation between silent regions and regions of responsiveness to the remaining eye, as was found in the lateral geniculates of these animals. The results, in fact, were very different. Figure 3, Plate 1, shows the reconstruction of a long (13.3 mm) tangential penetration through the striate cortex of monkey no. 2. In the layers above IV all of the cells encountered responded normally to stimulation of the

remaining (left) eye. This was not entirely unexpected, since normally the majority of these cells are binocularly innervated. What was more surprising was to find that the cells in layer IV responded well to left-eye stimulation over the entire 3.7 mm during which the electrode was in that layer (3.0 mm entering the cortex, and 0.7 mm leaving). The recordings were typical for layer IV C, showing rich background activity, responsive cells with centre-surround receptive fields, and no clear tendency for the cells to prefer oriented line stimuli. There were no silent areas, only some waxing and waning of the evoked activity as the electrode advanced, perhaps more than is seen normally.

In the other eye-removal monkey (no. 1), the two penetrations in area 17 gave results that were consistent with this in showing continuous responses through the entire extent of layer IV C. The angle to the surface was too steep and the distance traversed in layer IV therefore too short to permit any conclusions to be drawn from this animal alone, but taken together, the results from monkeys nos. 1 and 2 suggested an expansion of the

Table 2. Comparisons of Geniculate Cell Sizes and of Cortical Column Areas

monkey no.	side	layer	mean area, μm^2	s.d., μm^2	ratio‖	significance†	cortex. ratio of column areas‡
			(LATERAL GENICULATE BODY 50 CELLS/LAYER)				
1. rt. eye removal	L	6	*51*§	12	2.65	<0.01	
		5	135	36			
	R	6	159	33	2.94	<0.01	
		5	*54*	14			
2. rt. eye removal	L	6	*91*	15	1.87	<0.01	
		5	170	33			
	R	6	171	28	1.84	<0.01	
		5	*93*	12			
3. rt. eye closure	L	6	*128*	31	1.44	<0.01	2.77
		5	184	45			
	R	6	150	29	1.48	<0.01	—
		5	*108*	28			
4. rt. eye closure	L	6	*156*	33	1.26	<0.01	1.60
		5	197	46			
	R	6	184	37	1.20	<0.01	1.97
		5	*154*	36			
7. 'control' (late closure right eye)	L	6	*196*	42	1.04	N.S.	
		5	188	39			
	R	6	229	53	1.18	<0.01	1.05
		5	*194*	48			
8. control	L	6	*268*	68	1.04	N.S.	
		5	258	68			
	R	6	248	70	1.12	<0.02	
		5	*280*	54			

† Welch test.

‡ Swollen/shrunken (see table 3).

§ Right eye layer italics.

‖ Larger/smaller.

territory occupied by the columns of the normal eye at the expense of the set corresponding to the enucleated eye. One might, of course, explain the continuous IVth layer activity by supposing that the electrode had approached this layer in a direction almost parallel to the borders separating the bands, and had stayed in a single left-eye band throughout the entire penetration. In many previous tangential penetrations in normal monkeys we have never, in fact, recorded so long a sequence of cells dominated by one eye. In any case, the anatomical results to be described below rule out such an explanation.

MORPHOLOGY An apparent disappearance of ocular-dominance stripes in layer IV C, in physiological recordings, could conceivably be due not to a takeover by the good eye, but rather to a simple dropping out (i.e. death) of the cells in these stripes, with either an absolute shrinkage of cortex to half its surface area or a spreading out of the remaining layer IV C cells together with an associated thinning of the layer. A routine examination of the morphology of the striate cortex using a Nissl stain failed to show any hint of such changes (Fig. 3); the total extent of the striate cortex was normal, there was no obvious reduction in thickness or cell den-

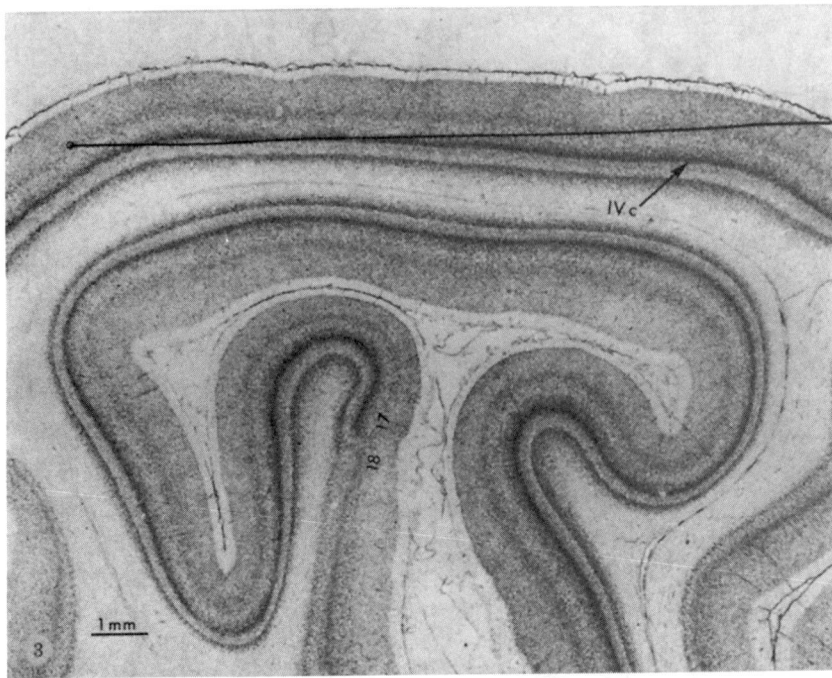

Fig. 3. Electrode track in a tangential penetration through the left striate cortex of monkey no. 2; right eye removed at 2 weeks and the recordings made at 18 months. The electrode passed antero-posteriorly through layer IV C for a total of 3.7 mm, during which responses were continuously obtained from the remaining (left) eye. Cresyl violet. Anterior is to the right; parasagittal section. Circle at end of track indicates electrolytic lesion.

sity in any of the layers, and layer IV C appeared uniform along its horizontal extent, with cells of normal size. In short, any reorganization had taken place in such a way as to leave no trace in routine histology.

In a previous study in normal monkeys the ocular dominance stripes in layer IV were visualized and reconstructed in serial sections by making lesions restricted to single laminae in the lateral geniculate body and later staining the cortex for degenerating terminals by a modified Nauta method (Hubel & Wiesel 1972). In any one section in these normal monkeys there were patches of terminal degeneration interrupted by equally wide patches with no degenerating terminals. Figure 4a, Plate 1, shows an example of the cortical degeneration pattern in a normal monkey after a small lesion restricted to the most dorsal geniculate layer. Regions of layer IV C containing terminals are sharply delineated from the terminal-free gaps, which are bridged by only an occasional degenerating afferent axon running between one zone of degenerating terminals and another. Figure 5

shows a serial reconstruction of the entire, necessarily relatively small, area of cortex containing degenerating terminals, to illustrate the characteristic striped pattern of normal ocular dominance columns, each with a width of about 400 μm (Hubel & Wiesel 1972, Figs. 8 and 10).

Similar single-layer lesions were made in both enucleated animals. Figure 4b shows the result of a geniculate lesion in layer 3 of monkey no. 1, on the left side, ipsilateral to (and innervated by) the normal eye. In contrast to what was found in the normal animals, the terminals in the cortex were distributed over virtually the entire region receiving input from the area of the lesion. Within this region there were variations in the density of degeneration, but gaps free of degenerating endings were only occasionally seen and were usually ill-defined and small, only a fraction of the size of the terminal-free gaps seen normally. A typical gap is shown in Figure 4b. Except for the waxing and waning and the small gaps in terminal degeneration, the picture was reminiscent of the continuous degeneration seen after a lesion in a normal mon-

Plate 1

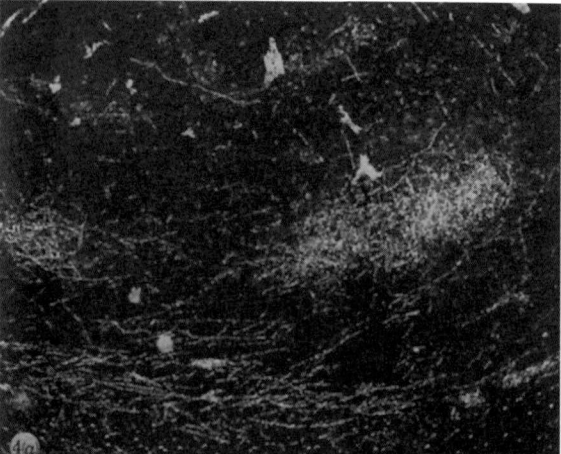

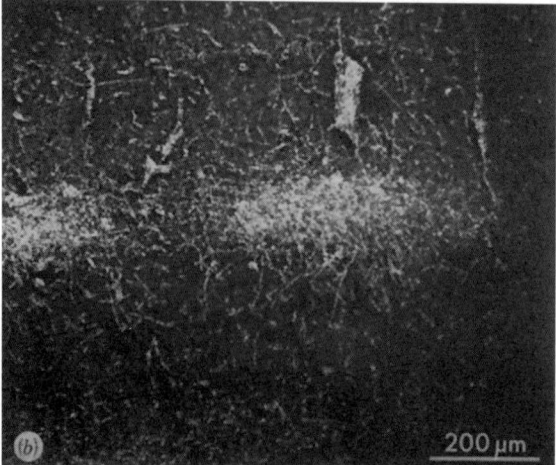

Fig. 4. Dark-field photographs of Nauta—Fink—Heimer stained striate cortex in monkeys following lesions confined to a single geniculate layer. (a) Normal monkey, following lesion in layer 6 of the left geniculate. (monkey no. 12 in Hubel & Wiesel 1972; cf. figure 5 of present paper and Figures 7–10 in Hubel & Wiesel 1972). (b) 19-month-old monkey in which right eye was removed at 2 weeks (monkey no. 1 of present paper.) Lesion was in layer 3 of left geniculate, this layer being innervated from the remaining (normal) eye; cf. figure 6. Each photograph includes white matter, near the bottom, but does not quite reach layer I above. In a the band of degeneration in IV C is about equal in width to the gap between. In b the gap between bands is ill defined and smaller than the band to the right.

key involving two adjacent dorsal layers (Hubel & Wiesel 1972).

A serial reconstruction of the entire region of terminal degeneration associated with this lesion, in monkey no. 1, is shown in Figure 6. No attempt has been made to illustrate the variation in terminal density; the regions free or almost free of degenerating fragments have simply been shown as gaps. A striped pattern is strongly suggested, with a drastic narrowing of one set of stripes and a probable widening of the other. The combined widths of the expanded and shrunken columns, assuming a 30% shrinkage in processing the tissue, is roughly 800 μm, a value close to the normal (see below).

Lesions in this monkey were also made in geniculate layer 6 on the side contralateral to the enucleated eye, i.e. a deafferented layer. The resulting degeneration in the cortex was very weak, and

was confined to small narrow patches separated by wide regions with no degeneration. The picture was thus the complement of that observed after a lesion in a layer corresponding to the surviving eye. A reconstruction of one of these projection areas is shown in Figure 7.

Very similar results were found in monkey no. 2 both for normal layer lesions and for deafferented layer lesions.

Thus in both the recordings and the Nauta degeneration studies it was as though the geniculate afferents serving the normal eye had invaded and virtually taken over the layer-IV territory of the enucleated eye. As Part II shows, similar results were found in animals with prolonged lid suture. Part III, however, will present evidence that casts doubt upon the notion of an invasion of one region by another, at least in any literal sense.

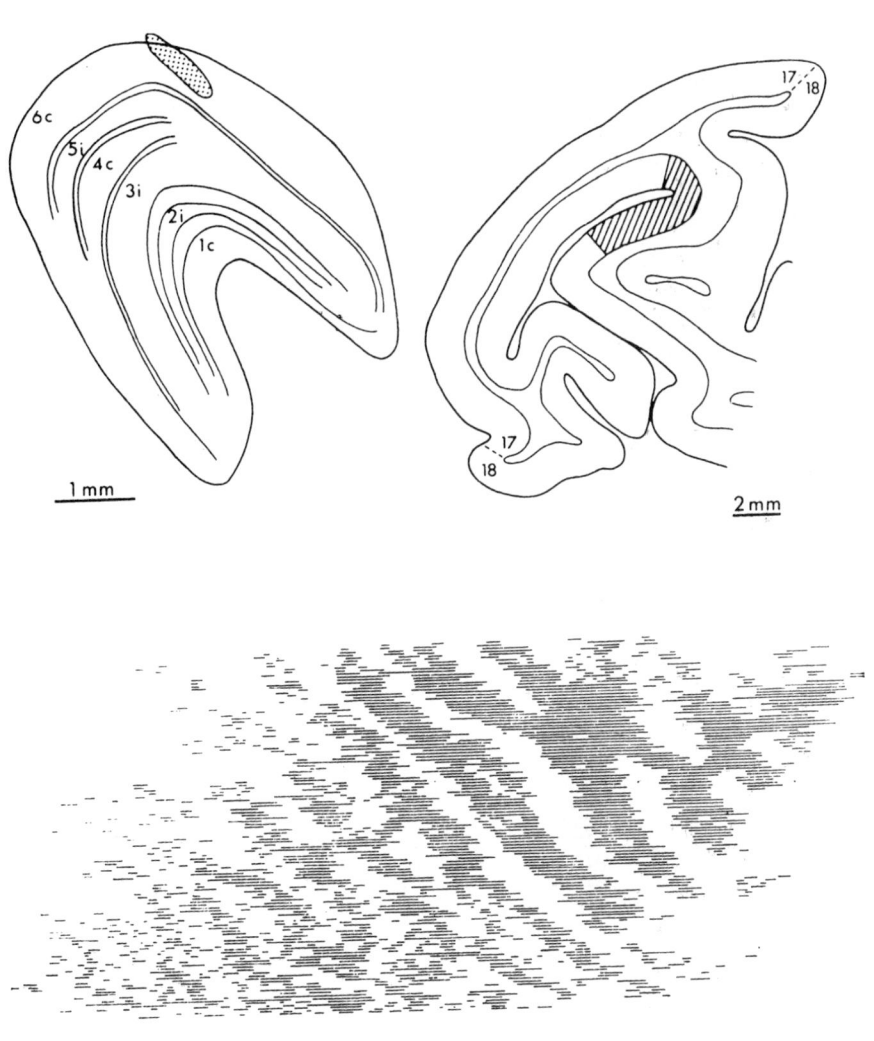

Fig. 5. Normal monkey. Reconstruction of cortical area of Nauta degeneration, made from 121 serial parasagittal sections. The projection site in area 17, shaded in the drawing on the upper right, corresponds to the layer 6 geniculate lesion on the upper left. Each interrupted horizontal line in the reconstruction is derived from a single cortical section, by graphically straightening the shaded part of the mushroom shaped calcarine cortex, and tracing the regions of degeneration (cf. Fig. 4a). When these lines are assembled the result is a surface view of layer IV C bands, which appear as roughly parallel stripes separated by equal-size gaps, with a repeat distance of about 0.8 mm (Hubel & Wiesel 1972, monkey no. 12, Figures 8–10).

Part II. Monocular Lid Suture

In three monkeys (Table 1, nos. 3–5) the lids of one eye were sutured closed in the first few weeks of life. Nos. 3 and 4 were expressly prepared to examine the results of long standing deprivation. No. 5 was part of a study on the time course of sensitivity to deprivation: an eye was closed from 2 days to 7 weeks and then reopened, and the animal was examined at 7 months. This monkey is mentioned in the present paper as a further illustration of monocular deprivation effects, because there is little likelihood that the reopening of the eye had any influence on the outcome.

Four control animals (nos. 6–10) are included: nos. 6 and 7 provide examples of normal cortical

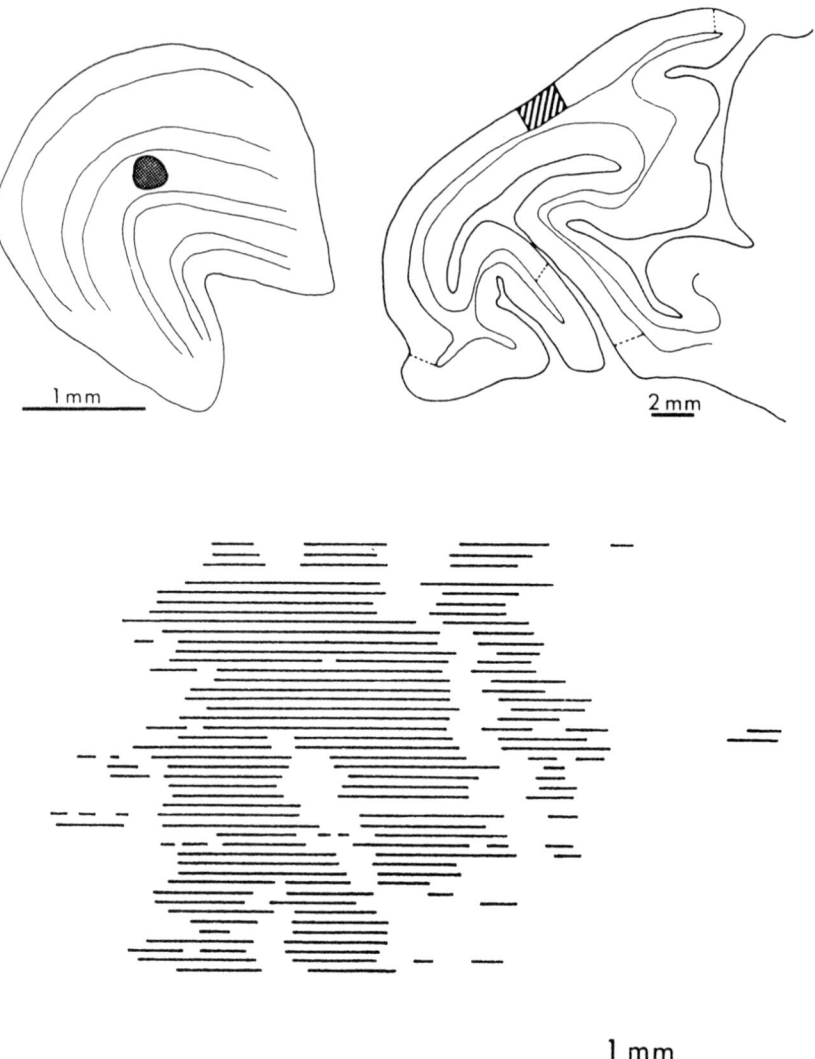

Fig. 6. Reconstruction of an area of terminal degeneration similar to that of Figure 5, but in a 19-month-old monkey (no. 1) in which the right eye was removed at 2 weeks. Lesion in layer 3 of the left lateral geniculate, supplied by the left (normal) eye. Compared with Figure 5, the regions of degeneration in the reconstruction are mostly much wider and the gaps narrower, the repeat distance being unchanged.

autoradiography; no. 7 (also part of the time-course study) had a six month period of monocular closure at 2½–3 years, but no abnormalities were found in a variety of behavioural tests; no. 8 was used for determination of normal geniculate cell size; nos. 9 and 10 represent a preliminary study of eye dominance columns in newborn and very young monkeys.

For the animals with eye closure two new methods were available for demonstrating ocular dominance columns, besides physiological record-

ing and Nauta degeneration. These were, first, transneuronal autoradiography (Wiesel, Hubel & Lam 1974), in which radioactive compounds are injected into one eye and the cortex later examined autoradiographically for label transported up to layer IV of the striate cortex. The second method depends on preparing of sections tangential to layer IVC with a reduced-silver stain (LeVay et al. 1975). The four methods—physiological recording, Nauta degeneration, autoradiogaphy, and reduced-

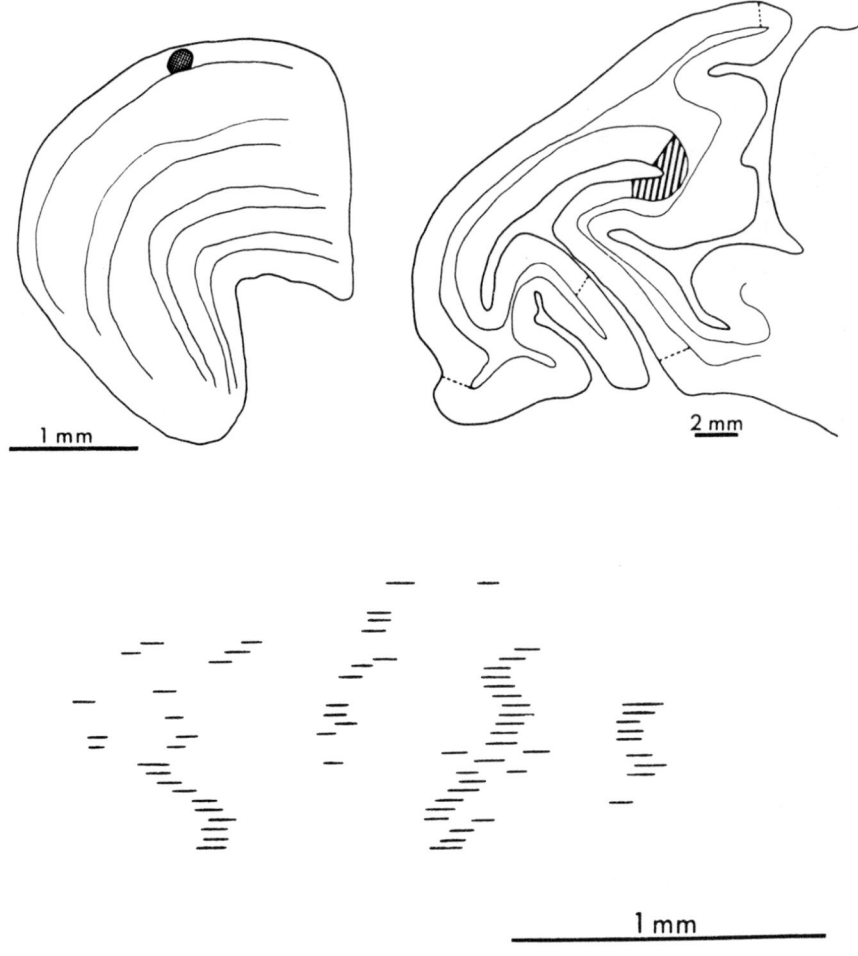

Fig. 7. Reconstruction similar to that of figure 6 and in the same monkey, following a lesion in a deafferented geniculate layer (no. 6 on the left side). Now the areas of degeneration are shrunken and the gaps widened.

silver stain—are entirely independent, relying as they do on a nerve fibre's ability to conduct impulses and on synaptic integrity, on degeneration following injury, on axonal transport, and on the ability of certain fibres to take up a particular stain.

Lateral Geniculate Body

PHYSIOLOGY In monkeys with monocular eye closure one could observe responses from the deprived geniculate layers to stimulation of the eye that had been closed—something that was obviously impossible in the eye removal animals. Lateral-geniculate recordings were made only in monkey no. 3, in the course of making lesions for the Nauta degeneration studies. About a dozen cells were recorded from the deprived layers: these seemed to have normal receptive field properties, giving vigorous responses to stimulation with small spots. Transitions from normal to deprived layers and back, as judged by responses, were abrupt, with no hint in the deprived layers of any driving from the normal eye. The sample of unit recordings was obviously too small and our examination too cursory to permit any conclusions except that there were no gross physiological abnormalities, and no signs of invasion of the deprived layers by the fibres from the normal eye.

HISTOLOGY: NISSL STUDIES Nissl stained sections through the lateral geniculate bodies of monkeys nos. 3 and 4 showed moderate pallor and shrinkage in the layers corresponding to the deprived eye. These results are thus similar to those seen by Headon & Powell (1973). Not surprisingly, the changes were far less marked than those following eye removal. The black and white photomicrographs of figure 8, plate 2, are perhaps deceptive, however, since they show the changes much less vividly than would be expected from simple inspection of the sections at low power, perhaps because the colours help bring out the differences in staining between normal and deprived layers. Measurements of cell size are given in table 2: the ratio of cross sectional areas in presumably normal *vs.* deprived layers was 1.46:1 for monkey no. 3 and 1.23:1 for no. 4. This is to be compared with an average of 2.33:1 for the two eye-removal monkeys.

That the deprivation effects were more severe in monkey no. 3 than in no. 4 can be seen both in figure 8 and in the cell measurements. In the cortex, as described below, the effects were likewise more severe in monkey no. 3. These differences could either be related to the week's difference in the time of eye closure or to the difference in duration of closure. Other results in the cortex of deprived and newborn monkeys suggest, however, that in eye closures lasting more than a few months the time of closure is more important than the duration.

In both of these eye sutured animals (nos. 3 and 4) the geniculate changes were most marked on the side ipsilateral to the suture—indeed, in the contralateral sections of monkey no. 4 (figure 8) it is not easy to see the changes at all. A similar asymmetry was seen by Headon & Powell (1973). Curiously, no difference between the sides showed up in the cell measurements, perhaps again because mild effects are expressed more in cell pallor than in shrinkage. A difference in susceptibility of the two sides, with more severe effects ipsilaterally, has been observed in many monkeys besides those of the present series. It also occurs in the cortical columns (see below), and there seems to be little doubt that it is genuine. (The interpretation of the apparently significant difference in a control monkey (Table 2, no. 7), in cell sizes of layers 5 and 6 on the right side, is not clear.)

In describing the differences in cell size in the various pairs of layers it has been tacitly assumed that it is shrinkage in the closed-eye layers that produces the disparity. Whether there is an enlargement of cells in the normal-eye layers is difficult to determine because of the large variations in average cell size from one brain to the next, related possibly to small differences in technique. Obviously this is a question of some interest, given the increase in width of the corresponding cortical columns, to be demonstrated below.

HISTOLOGY: AUTORADIOGRAPHY In monkeys nos. 3, 4 and 5 one eye was injected with radioactive label. The resulting autoradiographs in the lateral geniculate bodies are illustrated in darkfield, in Figure 9, Plate 3, for monkey no. 3 and Figure 10, Plate 4, for no. 4. There was heavy labelling of the appropriate layers, even in monkey no. 4, whose closed eye had been injected. In both animals the label in the layers corresponding to the non-injected eye was only slightly above background levels. This is well seen in Figure 11, Plate 4, a higher power light-field photomicrograph from the geniculate of monkey no. 3 (normal eye injected). Here the deprived layer, to the right, showed none of the grain clumps which indicate the positions of the optic nerve terminals belonging to the injected eye. Thus the autoradiography gave no indication of transgression of terminals beyond the normal boundaries. Obviously this was important in interpreting possible changes in the cortical columns.

A consistent finding in these autoradiographs of the lateral geniculate body was an accumulation of grains in several regions besides the classical 6 layers. In Figure 9 one can see a bilateral accumulation of grains in a narrow band between layers 2 and 3, best seen on the left in light field, and on the right in dark field. Also there is a band of grains of contralateral origin ventral to layer 1 on the right, best seen in light field, and a clump of ipsilateral origin near the hilum, interrupting and lying ventral to layer I (left, dark field). Higher power examination suggested that the grains were mostly in terminals rather than in fibres. These additional inputs to the geniculate were not seen at more caudal levels (Figure 9). They are discussed further in Part III, where similar aggregations are described in a normal newborn animal.

Plate 2

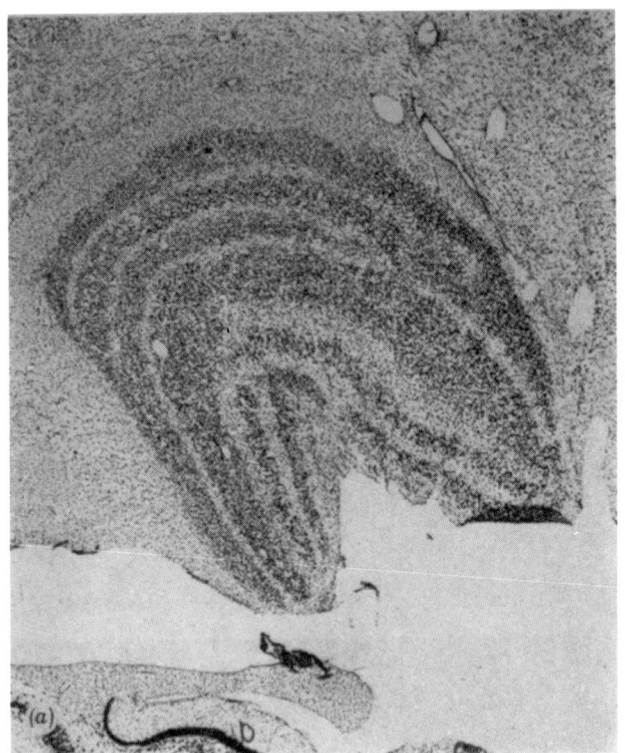

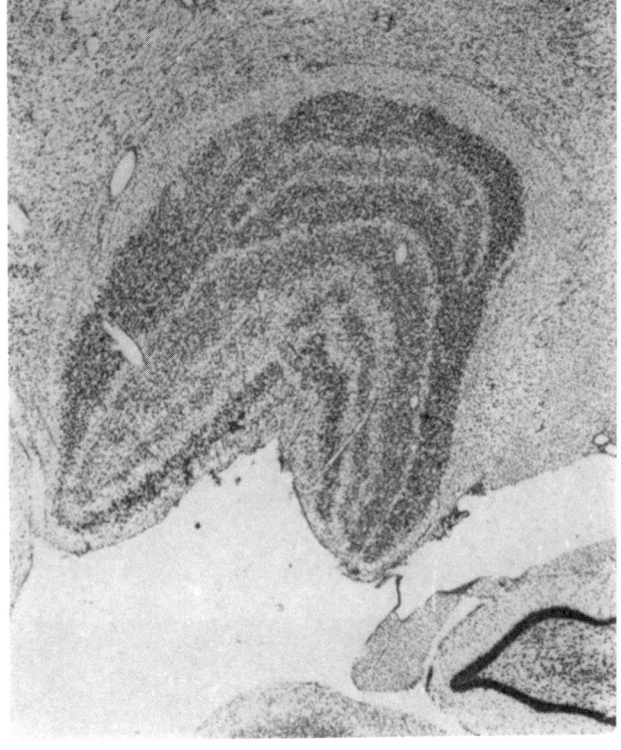

Fig. 8. Coronal Nissl-stained sections through lateral geniculates of (a) Monkey no. 3, right eye closed at 2 weeks for 18 months. (b) Monkey no. 4, right eye closed at 3 weeks for 7 months. Note that the atrophy of the layers receiving input from the closed eye is more marked on the ipsilateral (right) side and more marked in a than in b. Cresyl violet; frozen sections. (Continued)

Plate 2

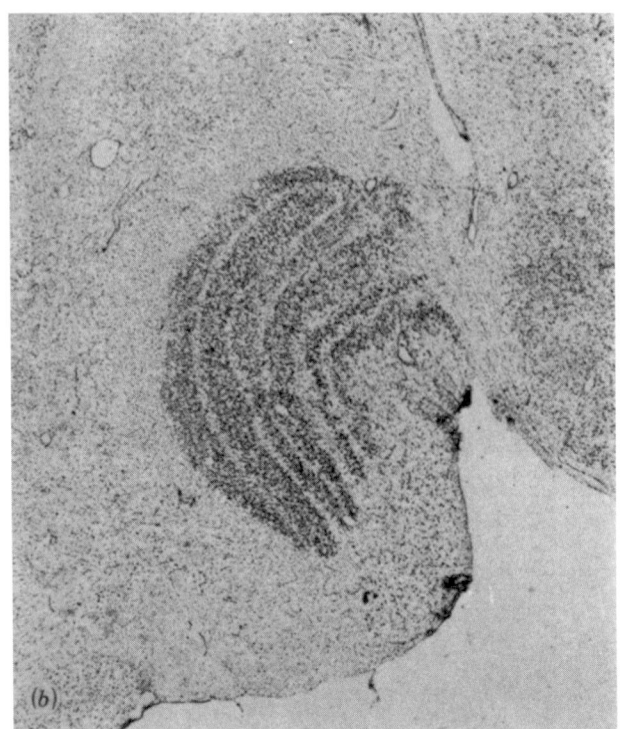

(b)

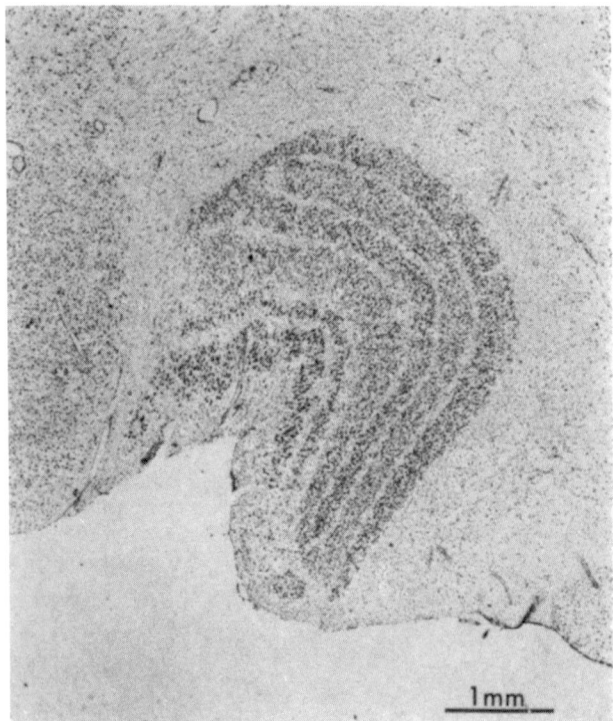

1mm

Fig. 8. (Continued)

Plate 3

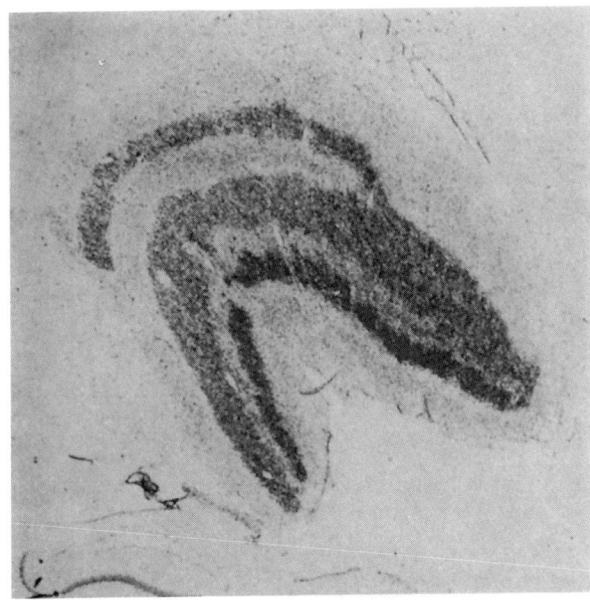

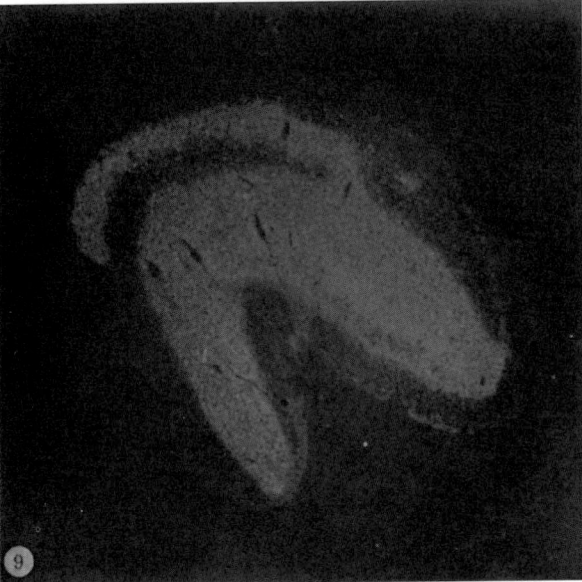

*Fig. 9. Autoradiographs of genicu-
lates from monkey no. 3 (right eye
closed at 2 weeks for 18 months) following injection of label into left
(normal) eye. Coronal sections.
Upper half, light-field, counterstained with cresyl violet. Lower
half, dark-field of same sections. Note
the band of label between classical
layers 3 and 2, in the dark-field picture on the right (compare figure 24,
layer* d). *(Continued)*

Superior Colliculus

The distribution of optic-nerve terminals from the two eyes in the superior colliculus takes a very special form (Hubel, LeVay & Wiesel 1975). In the superficial grey, where the bulk of the input ends, the contralateral terminals tend to make up a continuous band whose lower half frequently contains cavities, and whose lower border is irregular and scalloped. The ipsilateral terminals tend to form a row of clumps which are concentrated at a level matching these holes and scallops; thus they appear to be embedded in the deep part of the contralateral input. Towards the foveal representation the ipsilateral input also comes close to the surface, in patches that appear to alternate with the contralateral input. On the whole the contralateral input probably exceeds the ipsilateral, and while the extent to which the two overlap is not clear

Plate 3

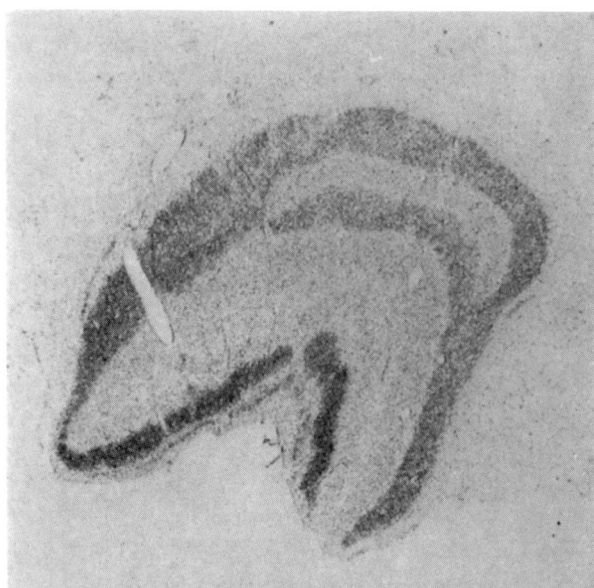

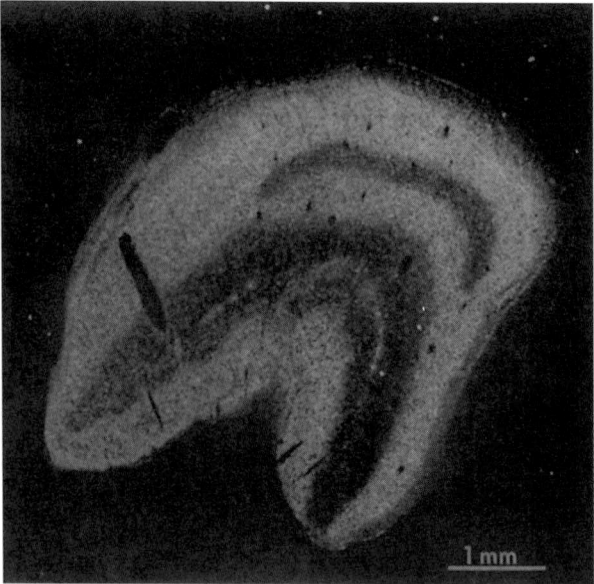

Fig. 9. (Continued)

anatomically, recordings indicate that the two eyes are not kept entirely separate.

We were curious to learn whether the eye closures had produced any changes in this patchy distribution of terminals, and especially whether there were signs of an expansion of the territory of one eye or contraction of that belonging to the other. Autoradiographs showed no hint of any changes: as in the geniculates, the distribution of terminals was normal in monkeys nos. 3 and 4. In sections counterstained with cresyl violet an examination of cells showed no hint of shrinkage or change in cell packing density in regions which from the autoradiography were known to receive input from the closed eye. Thus from the anatomical studies the superior colliculi seemed to be nor-

Plate 4

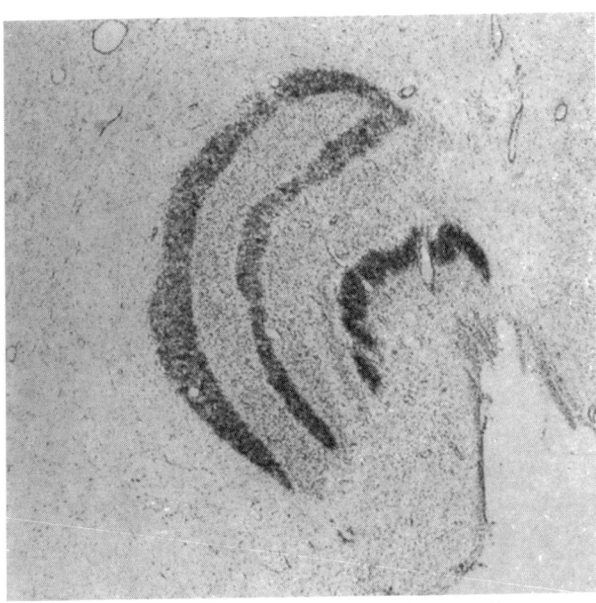

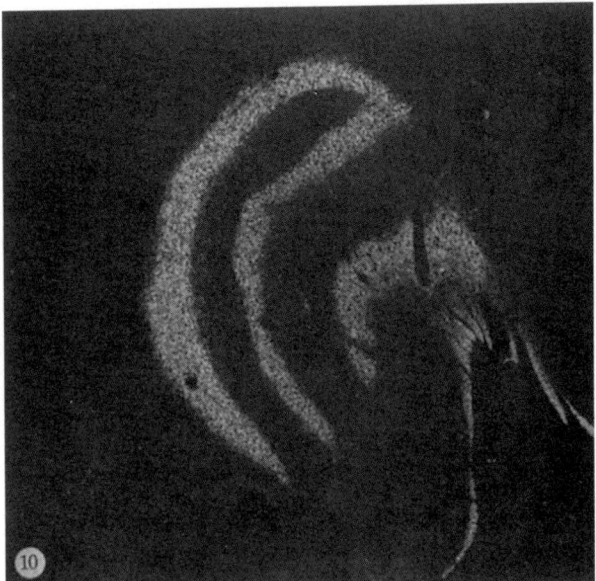

Fig. 10. Autoradiographs from geniculates of monkey no. 4 (right eye closed at 3 weeks, for 7 months) following injection of label into right (lid-sutured) eye. Upper half, light field; lower half, dark field, of same sections. Counterstained with cresyl violet. (Continued)

mal. We have not made recordings in the colliculi of deprived monkeys.

Striate Cortex

CONTROL MONKEYS (NOS. 6 AND 7): MORPHOLOGY The brains of monkeys nos. 3, 4 and 7 were cut in tangential sections in the region of the exposed striate cortex (the operculum). Brains of monkeys nos. 3, 4, 6 and 7 were also cut in sections that were either parasagittal or in a plane tipped back 45° from the coronal; in most places they were roughly perpendicular to cortex, and passed through the calcarine fissure. We begin by showing autoradiographs of presumably normal cortex (monkeys nos. 6 and 7) following injection of one eye.

The transverse section from monkey no. 7, shown in Figure 12a, Plate 5, is perpendicular to the occipital operculum (i.e. to the exposed surface

Plate 4

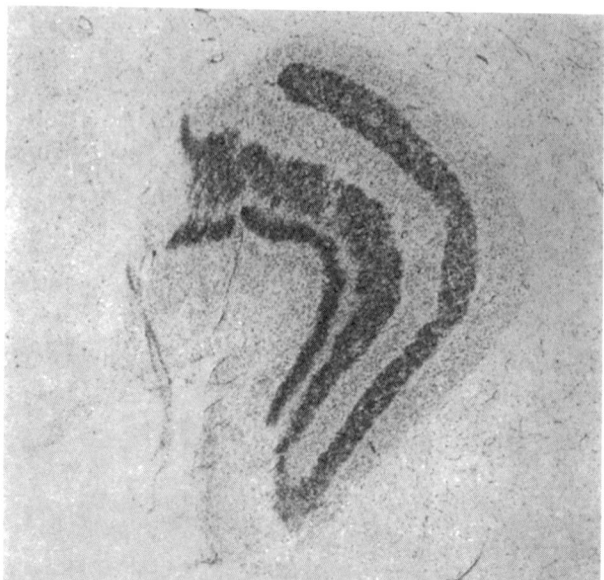

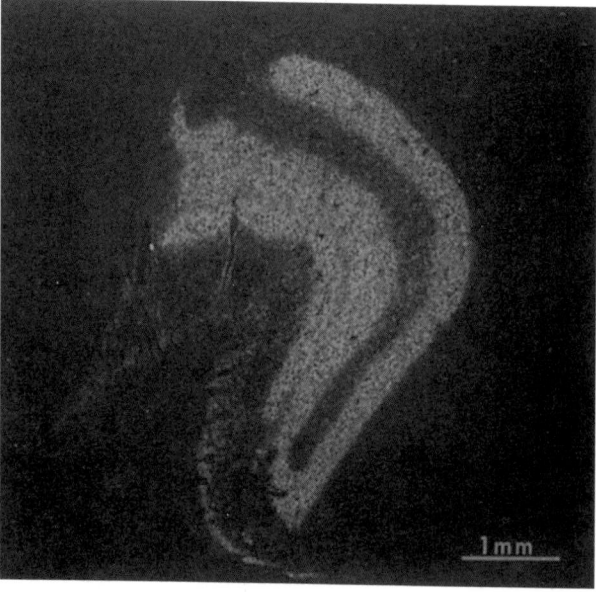

1 mm

Fig. 10. (Continued)

of the occipital lobe) and to part of the underlying calcarine fissure: almost all of the cortex in this section is striate, ipsilateral to the injected eye. Layer IV as expected shows a series of patches rich in label (brightly glowing in this darkfield photograph) interrupted by label free gaps. In this figure about 56 pairs of columns can be counted.

Figure 12*b* shows a parasagittal section through the calcarine fissure of monkey no. 6, con-

tralateral to the injected eye. Layer IV C is cut in most places transversely, forming a large irregular ring surrounding a smaller one, again with patches of label separated by gaps as in Figure 12*a*. To the lower right the two rings join, and here IV C is cut tangentially, forming parallel stripes arranged in an oval (as occurs in Figure 13). The upper right part of the outer ring of layer IV C in the figure is continuously labelled: this is the temporal crescent

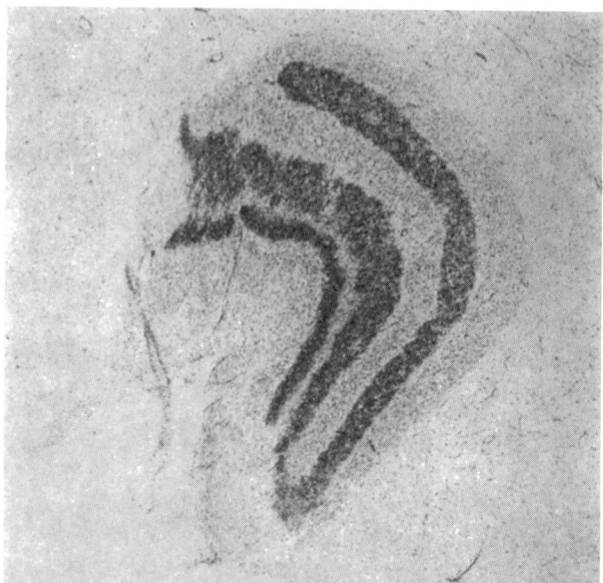

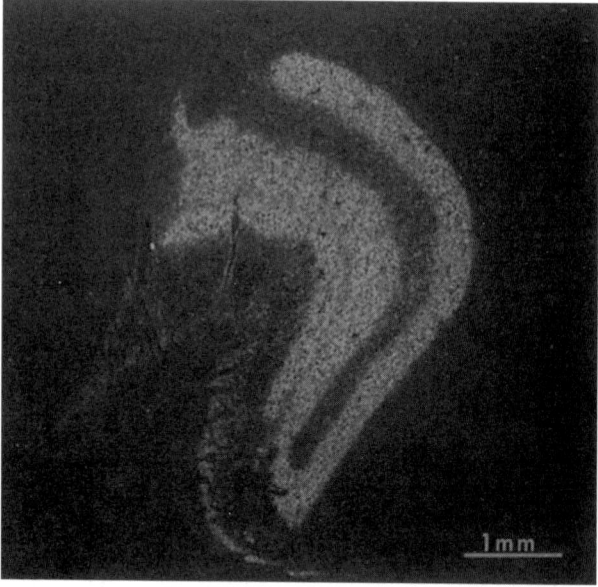

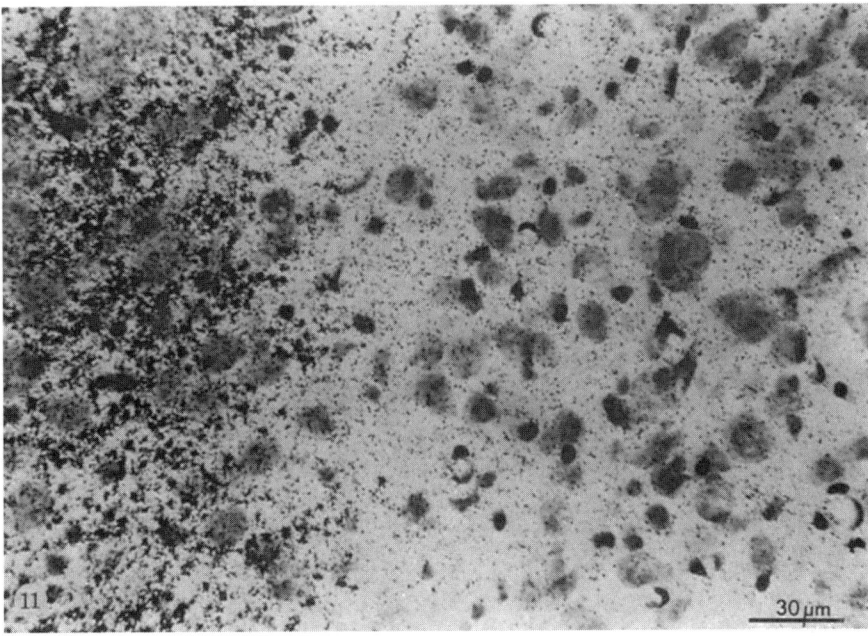

Fig. 11. Higher power light-field view of right lateral geniculate of monkey no. 3 (compare figure 9). Layer 6 (the most dorsal layer) is to the left, layer 5 to the right, with the relatively cell sparse interlaminar leaflet between. Note the abrupt fall-off in grains, particularly in the large clumps of grains presumably representing terminals, at the boundary between layer 6 and the leaflet, indicating a lack of any noticeable invasion of the deprived layer by terminals from the normal eye.

representation, with input entirely from the far peripheral temporal visual field of the contralateral eye.

Tangential sections through the operculum ipsilateral to the injected eye of monkey no. 7 are shown in Figure 13, Plate 6. The opercular cortex is dome shaped, and a plane of section that is tangential to a particular layer shows that layer as a circular patch or oval; deeper planes of section show the layer as an annulus. The section of Figure 13a just grazed layer IV C, which appears as an oval region of alternating dark and light stripes, surrounded by the more superficial layers. Figure 13b is taken at a slightly deeper level, and layer IV C appears as a ring made up of stripes, surrounding the deeper layers and surrounded by the more superficial ones.

Successively deeper sections through the operculum produced larger and larger IV C rings. By photographing every second or third section, cutting out layer IV C in each and superimposing

them, it was possible to reconstruct the columns over a considerable area. The result is shown in Figure 13c. The pattern is highly regular, with a tendency for the stripes to intersect the 17–18 border at a 90° angle. This border is near the top of Figure 13c, where the stripes end abruptly.

In this reconstruction, for comparisons with the deprived animals, calculations were made to determine the repeat distance for columns, i.e. the combined width of a left-eye column and an adjacent right-eye column. For this purpose we traced a number of regular roughly rectangular portions of the reconstruction, each containing an even number of stripes, between four and eight, avoiding areas where stripes forked or terminated. The two long edges of the block were chosen so that they fell along stripe borders. The areas of the blocks were determined by weighing. By dividing the area of each block by the total length of column pairs (number of pairs × length of block) one could estimate the repeat distance. Table 3 shows the

Plate 5

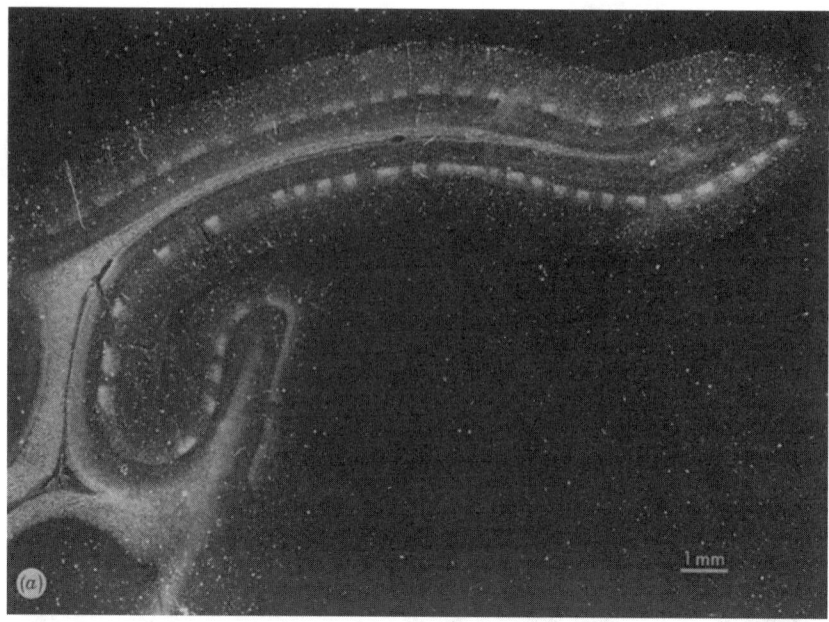

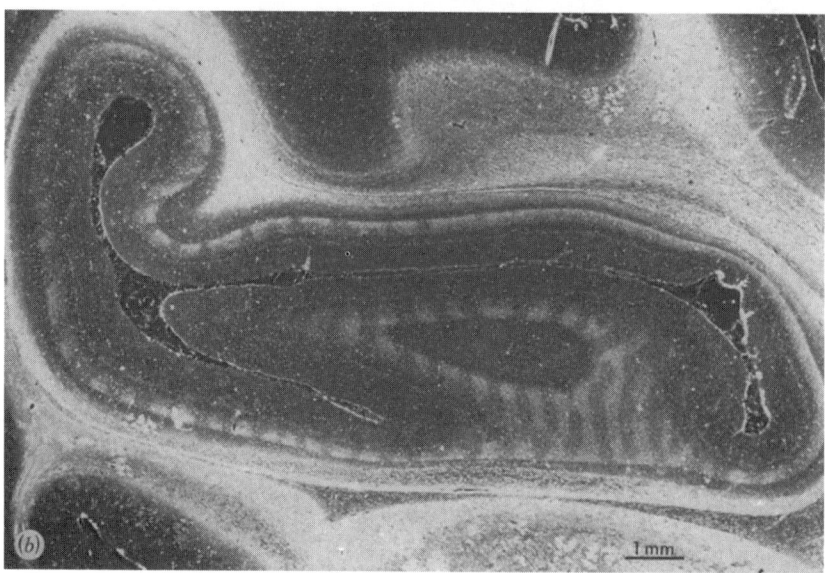

Fig. 12. Dark-field autoradiographs of striate cortex in normal adult monkeys following right-eye injection of radioactive fucose-proline mixture 2 weeks before. (a) Transverse section through right striate cortex, perpendicular to occipital operculum, in a plane normal to the sagittal, tipped back from coronal by about 45°. Labelled bands can be clearly made out in layer IV C. In the finger-like gyrus, the opercular cortex above and the superior bank of the calcarine fissure below are separated by a brightly labelled continuous band; this represents the optic radiations. (The lower bank of the calcarine fissure has fallen away.) Medial is to the right. (Monkey no. 7.) (b) Parasagittal section through the buried calcarine cortex contralateral to the injected eye; most of the cortex is cut in a plane perpendicular to the layers, but one fold is intersected tangentially, and here the layer IV C columns are seen as parallel bands. The upper tier in layer IV A can just be made out in most places. The stretch of continuous label in layer IV C in the upper right part of the ring represents the temporal crescent. Anterior is up and to the right; the operculum would be just to the left of the figure. (Monkey no. 6.)

Table 3. Estimation of Column Areas

monkey no.	hemisphere	eye injected	eye closed	combined width, μm	ratio†	shrinkage deprived columns (%)	ratio‡	shrinkage deprived columns (%)
3 (157)	left	left	right	892	2.24	38	2.77	47
4 (202)	left	right	right	817	1.45	18	1.60	23
	right	right	right	831	1.61	23	1.97	33
7 (186) ('control')	right	right	(right)§	848	1.05	—	1.05	—

† Determined from small regular patches within reconstruction.

‡ Determined from virtually the entire reconstructions (figures 13, 15, 20).

results for monkey no. 7 and also for eye-closed monkeys nos. 3 and 4 (see below). The repeat distance for monkey no. 7 was 848 μm.

The relative areas occupied by the two sets of columns were estimated from the reconstruction of figure 13c by tracing the borders, cutting apart the two sets, and weighing them. The difference in weight amounted to 5%, the contralateral set exceeding the ipsilateral (Table 3, ratio‡). This difference is probably not significant. Similar determinations were made from the selected regular blocks described above, with a difference again of 5% (Table 3, ratio†). This figure agrees well with a similar comparison made previously using the reduced silver method in another monkey (LeVay *et al.* 1975). Thus the anatomy and physiology both suggest that in the binocular representation of striate cortex the contributions of the two eyes are about equal.

MONKEY No. 3: PHYSIOLOGY In this monkey the right eye was closed from 2 weeks to age 18 months. The left eye was then injected. A week later 5 lesions were made in the right lateral geniculate body for Nauta studies. A week after that, finally, four penetrations were made in a direction almost parallel to the layers, in an effort to have long traverses through layer IV so that points of eye transition could be noted and marked with elec-

trolytic lesions. In two of the penetrations (nos. 2 and 3) the tilt was sufficient so that more than one eye transition occurred in layer IV.

As expected from the eye-removal results and from previous work in cats, the great majority of cells were strongly dominated by the normal eye. In the layers outside of IV only about one-fifth of cells were influenced from the deprived eye, many of these weakly but with the normal orientation specificity. The ocular dominance histogram from this monkey has already been shown in Figure 1. (A detailed account of the physiological properties of the cells in these animals will be presented elsewhere.)

In layer IV C, on the contrary, there were periods in which the activity was dominated strongly or completely by the deprived eye. The transitions from dominance by one eye to dominance by the other were as abrupt as in normal monkeys. In regions of domination by the deprived eye the responses seemed, surprisingly, to be quite normal, with the usual briskness and lack of any orientation specificity. These regions were nevertheless all distinctly shorter than those in which the normal eye dominated. Both the micromanipulator readings and the histological reconstruction showed that the spans in the left (normal) eye regions were 2–3 times as long as the spans in the right-eye regions. This is illustrated in Figure 14a,

Fig. 13. *(following page) Normal monkey (no. 7). Autoradiographs taken in dark field, of tangential sections through the dome shaped exposed surface of the right occipital lobe (operculum), ipsilateral to the injected (right) eye. The section shown in* (a) *passes tangential to layer IV C, which is seen as a series of light stripes, representing the labelled right-eye columns, separated by gaps of the same width representing the left eye.* (b) *is some 160 μm deeper than a, passing tangential to layer V and showing layer IV C as a ring of dark and light stripes into which the oval of a can be fitted.* (c) *is a reconstruction made by fitting together eight parallel sections including those of a and b. Anterior is up, medial to the left.*

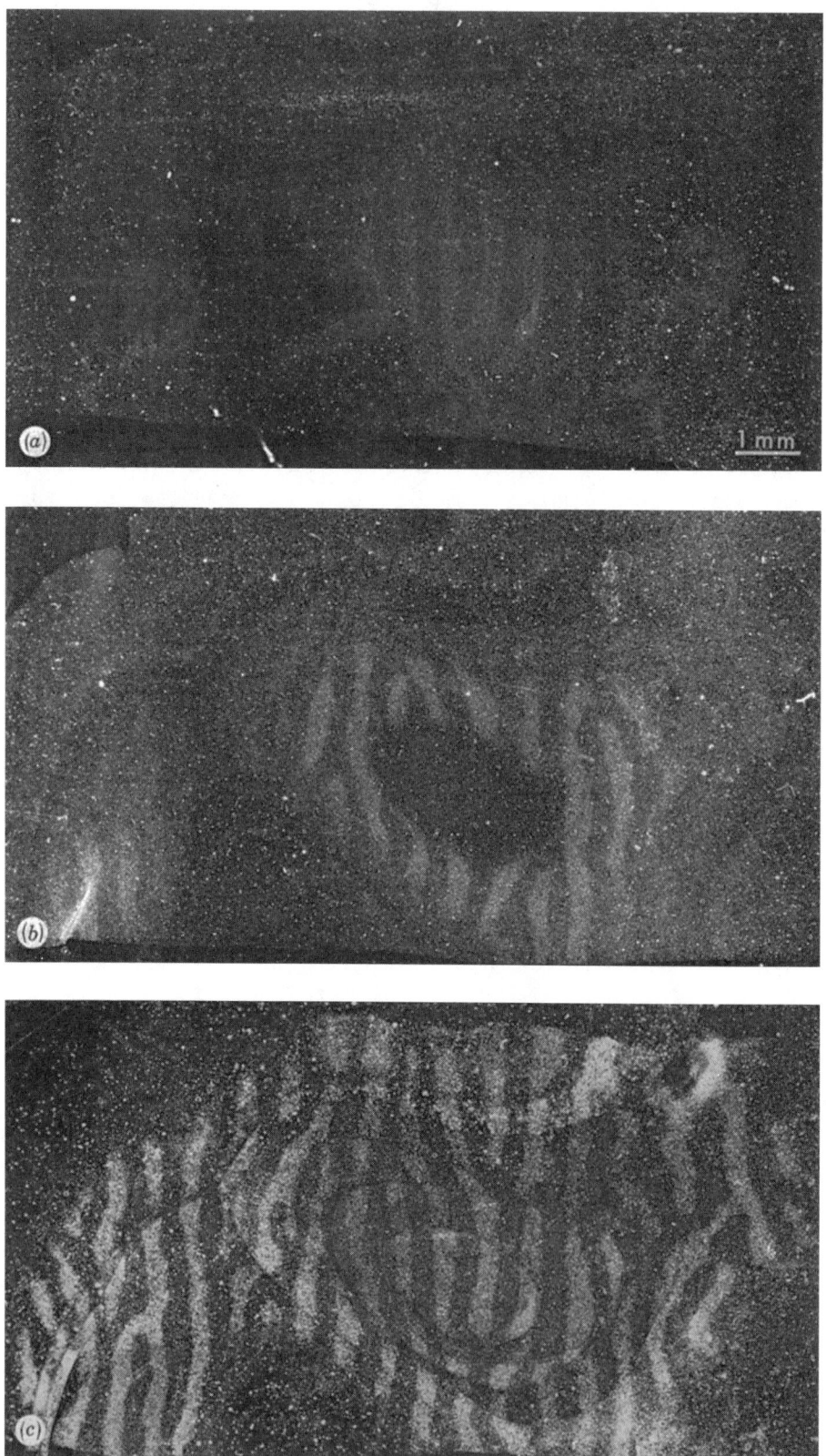

Plate 6

Fig. 13.

Plate 7

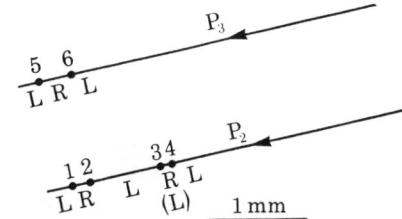

Fig. 14. Reconstruction of two penetrations, P_2 and P_3 through the left
striate cortex in monkey no. 3. Both
penetrations were almost tangential
to the surface, aimed in a roughly
mediolateral direction through the
operculum and placed 1 mm apart.
(Autoradiographs and reduced-silver
sections from the same region are
shown in Figures 15 and 17.) At the
top are shown the reconstructions
made from micrometer depth readings. Dots numbered 1–6 represent
lesions made in layer IV while withdrawing the electrode, at the points of
passing from one eye's territory to
that of the other eye. L and R indicate the dominant eye where only one
eye evoked responses: R(L) means
that the right eye dominated but the
left evoked a lesser response from the
multiunit activity. Middle portion
shows a cresyl-violet stained tangential section roughly in the plane of the
penetrations, passing through the
centre of lesion 6 and almost through
the centres of 1 and 5. No. 6 is clearly
in layer IV C, as were 1, 2 and 5,
when the appropriate sections were
examined. Lower section, a reduced-
silver fibre stain (LeVay et al. 1975),
passing through the centre of lesion 4
and just missing the centre of 3. Both
are at the border of layers IV B
(which contains most of the densely-
staining line of Gennari) and IV C.
This section is not ideally placed to
show the columnar banding: a more
superficial section at lower power
appears in figure 17.

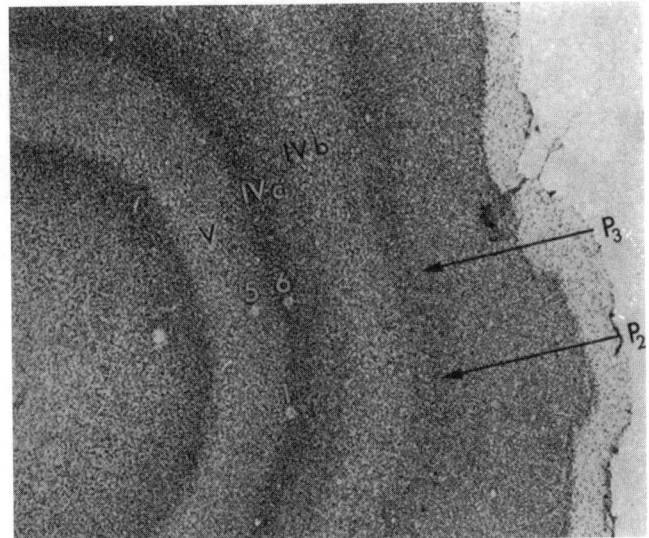

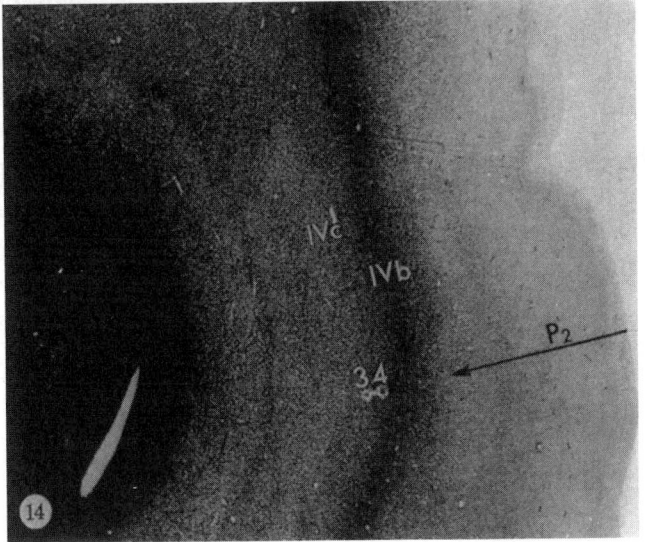

Plate 7, which shows the relation between penetrations 2 and 3, and the lesions made at the transition points. Both penetrations were made in the left hemisphere, from medial to lateral. The lesions were made on withdrawing the electrode so that the points of transition could be checked—hence the order of the lesion numbers. Figure 14*b* shows a Nissl-stained section almost in the plane of the penetrations and thus almost parallel to the surface, passing through the centre of lesion 6 and just missing the centres of 1 and 5. Appropriate sections through their exact centres demonstrated that lesions 1, 2, 5 and 6 were all well within layer IV C, and that lesions 3 and 4 were at the border between IV B and IV C, as seen in the fibre-stained section of Figure 14*c*.

Throughout all of the left-eye (nondeprived) columns no activity could be evoked from the right (deprived) eye. In the right-eye dominated columns weak but clearly audible responses could be heard in the span between lesions 3 and 4. This is not surprising, given that these lesions were made on the IV B–IV C border, since in normal animals the eye segregation in layer IV B is not as strict as in layer IV C. In the deeper right (deprived) eye segments (1–2 and 5–6) the left eye was silent.

In summary, there were small regions within layer IV in which cells were actively driven and strongly dominated by the deprived eye, in contrast to the virtual absence of influence of that eye in the upper layers. Within layer IV C there was a striking and consistent difference in the distances the electrode travelled in the two sets of columns.

MONKEY NO. 3: MORPHOLOGY Two neighbouring opercular sections are shown in Figure 15*a* and *b*, Plate 7, and a reconstruction from nine neighbouring sections including these two is shown in Figure 15*c*. Confirming the results of the recordings, the labelled columns (normal eye) are very much wider than normal, and the gaps (closed eye) are very much narrower. Comparing Figures 13 and 15 it is evident that the repeat distance—the combined widths of two neighbouring columns, one from each eye—is roughly the same in the two animals. Measurements made as described above for monkey no. 7 showed a combined width (repeat distance) of 892 μm, as opposed to 848 μm for the control (Table 3). (Unlike the millimetre scales on the illustrations, which refer to distances on the microscopic slides, these figures have been calculated from the histology by assuming a 30% shrinkage. This is only a rough estimate based on reconstructions of electrode tracks in other animals, but the comparison is valid, provided the brains have shrunk roughly equally.) The fact that the repeat distance was apparently unchanged in monkey no. 3 is consistent with the conclusion that the expansion of one set of columns is complemented by a contraction of the other. In addition to being reduced in width the deprived columns were pinched off at irregular intervals of a millimetre or so.

The relative areas occupied by the labelled columns and the gaps were estimated by the methods outlined above for the normal. Taking the entire reconstruction and cutting apart the left-eye and right-eye regions the result was a ratio of 2.77:1 for labelled columns to unlabelled ones, as compared with 1.05:1 for the normal (Table 3, ratio‡). The ratio from selected regular blocks, calculated as for monkey no. 7 (Table 3, ratio†, was lower, amounting to 2.24:1. The lower ratio presumably resulted partly from the omission of pinched off areas, in selecting these blocks.

We found that electrolytic lesions of the rather miniscule size necessary to mark the points of transition from one eye to the other, in the physiological recordings, were impossible to identify in dark-field autoradiographs. They were easily found, however, in the Nissl and reduced-silver sections that were interspersed between the autoradiographs (see Figure 14), so that comparison of adja-

Fig. 15. This figure is the counterpart of figure 13, in monkey no. 3, whose right eye was closed from age 2 week to 18 months. Left hemisphere operculum: (a) is tangential to layer IV C, (b) is 200 μm deeper, and (c) is the result of cutting and pasting 9 such sections, representing a total depth of 900 μm. Label in IV C, representing input from the normal eye, is in the form of swollen bands which in places coalesce, obliterating the narrow gaps which represent the columns connected to the closed eye. The thin, almost continuous belt of label in the upper tier (IV-A) is seen in all three parts. The six dots in (c) represent the positions of the six lesions of Figure 14, identified on neighbouring cresyl-violet or reduced-silver sections and superimposed on the autoradiographs. The lesions are clearly at or close to the column boundaries.

Plate 7

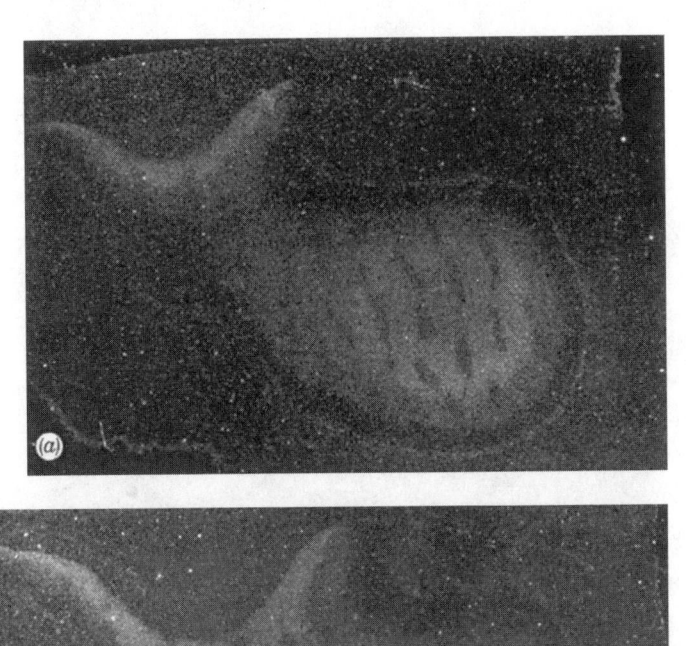

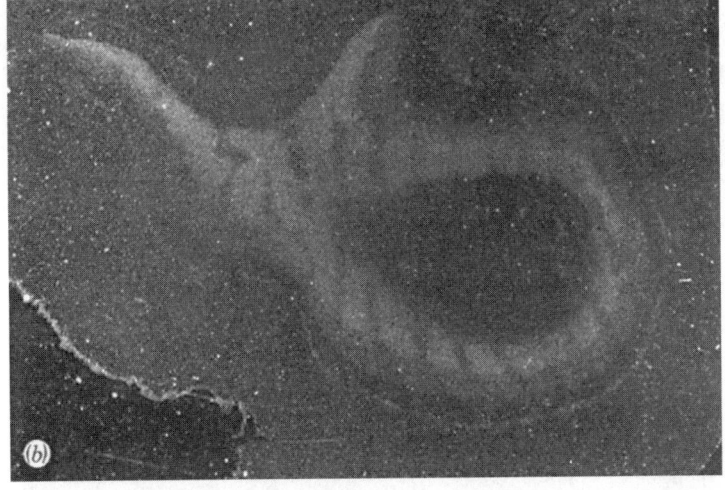

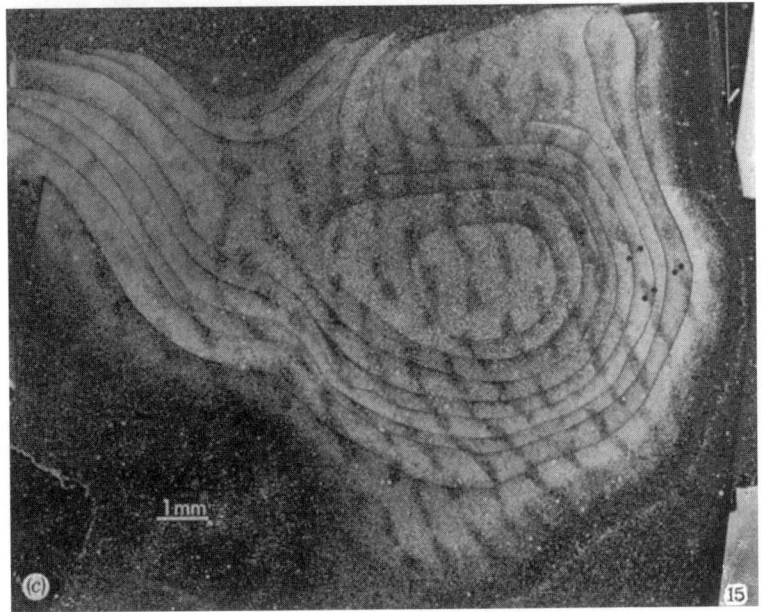

Fig. 15.

Plate 8

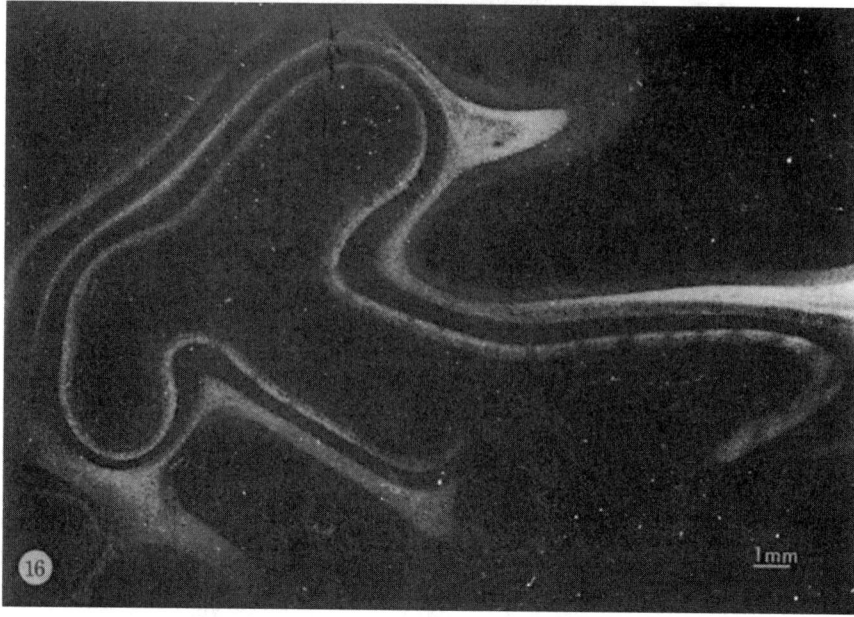

Fig. 16. Monkey no. 3; right eye closed from 2 weeks to 18 months. Left eye injected. Dark-field autoradiograph through right calcarine cortex. Over the mushroom, label representing input from the contralateral (normal) eye has almost obliterated the gaps, representing the deprived eye, and greatly narrowed them even where they are best preserved, in the dorsal stem. Anterior is up and to the right.

cent sections made it possible to determine their precise position on the autoradiographs, with respect to the column boundaries. These are marked in Figure 15c.

An autoradiograph through the calcarine fissure (Figure 16, Plate 8) likewise showed gaps, between labelled regions, that were markedly shrunk and in places almost obliterated. The section is taken from the side ipsilateral to the closed eye. Though it is difficult to compare the severity of shrinkage on the two sides, given the difference in planes of section, our impression from this and other examples is that deprivation effects were more marked on the side ipsilateral to the closed eye (compare Figures 21a and 21b).

The reduced-silver stains gave results that faithfully paralleled the autoradiographs and the physiology. The bands corresponding to columns in layer IV could be seen only in tangential or very oblique sections, and were seen best at very low power in the upper part of IV C, just beneath the line of Gennari. In Figure 17, plate 8, an alternation of wide (W) and narrow (N) dark bands can easily be seen. The narrow bands were clearly identified

as corresponding to the deprived columns, and the wide bands to the non-deprived, by noting their positions with respect to the lesions in penetrations 2 and 3, and to the columns as shown in the autoradiographs.

Another abnormality observed in the reduced-silver sections was the appearance of broad pale bands (P) in layer V, where normally no banding is visible. These bands, which stand out clearly in the central part of Figure 17, were in register with the set of shrunken ocular dominance columns just above, in layer IV C. Similar bands could be seen, though less clearly, in layer III. Close inspection of layer V showed that within the pale bands the tangential fibres were of abnormally fine calibre. The tangential fibre plexus of layer V consists largely of collaterals of the descending axons of layer III pyramidal cells (Spatz, Tigges & Tigges 1970; Lund & Boothe 1975). These observations thus suggest a deterioration of descending connections between layers III and V within the deprived-eye columns.

Finally, we were anxious to determine the degree of overlap (if any) between the widened and

Plate 8

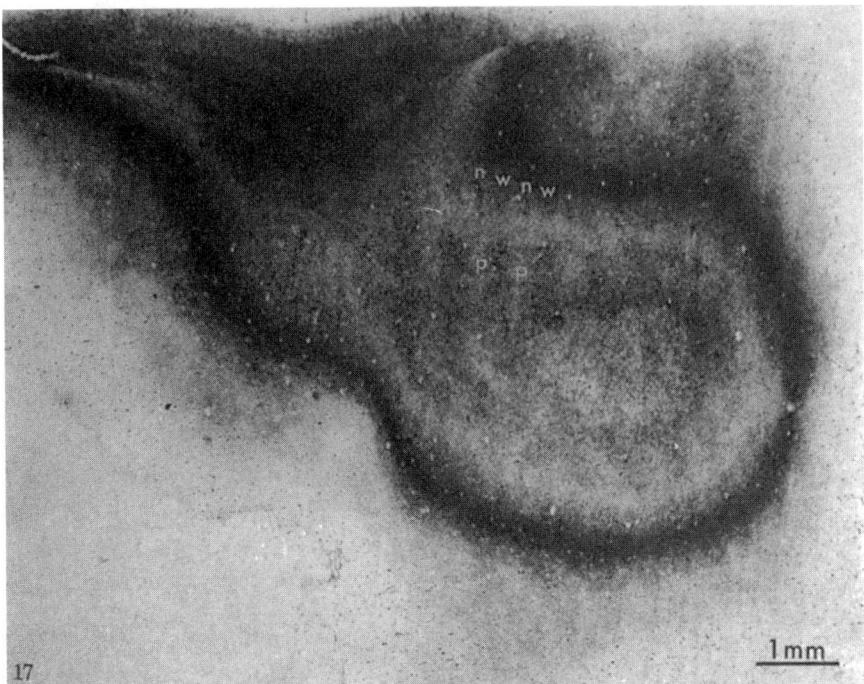

Fig. 17. Monkey no. 3. *Reduced-silver stained section parallel to those of Figure 15, and 40 μm deep to the section of Figure 15b. The Gennari Line, layer IV B, appears as the most densely stained black ring. Dark bands corresponding to the layer IV C columns are best seen in the most superficial part of IV C, i.e. just deep to IV B or the Gennari Line—in this section just inside the dark ring. These bands are alternatingly wide (W) and narrow (N). In autoradiographs neighbouring this section, such as the one shown in Figure 15b, the labelled (bright) columns were found to correspond precisely to the wide bands and the unlabelled (dark) gaps to the narrow bands. Still further inside the Gennari ring is a prominent light area, the cell-dense part of layer IV C; within this is layer V, with its pale bands (P) in register with the narrowed dark bands of IV C (N).*

the apparently narrowed columns of this animal. The recordings, as described above, indicated that the deprived-eye columns were reduced, and no activity was evoked from the deprived eye in the normal-eye columns in layer IVC, suggesting that there was little or no overlap. Autoradiographs from normal-eye injections by themselves could obviously prove nothing about the width of the stripes corresponding to the closed eye, and we wished to confirm morphologically the impression from the physiology-plus-lesions (Figure 14, 15c) that the gaps in the autoradiographic picture did actually represent the deprived-eye columns. Two studies in which deprived eyes were injected support this contention (see below), but for more direct evidence Nauta studies were made in monkey no. 3, and the results were correlated with the results of the autoradiography.

Five geniculate lesions were made in the hemisphere ipsilateral to the removed eye, 1 each in layers 1, 3, and 4, and two lesions in layer 6, and for three of these lesions the corresponding regions of degenerating terminals in the cortex were found. Figure 18a, Plate 8, shows a lesion in geniculate layer 3, which receives input from the closed eye, and Figure 18c (lower right) a Nauta-stained section from the corresponding region in the calcarine fissure. A single focus of degenerating terminals is conspicuous deep in layer IVC (arrow). This could be followed in neighbouring sections, and represented a wormlike structure 150 μm wide, extending some 400 μm in a direction normal to the plane of the section.

An autoradiograph made from the section immediately neighbouring that of Figure 18c is shown in Figure 18b. The gap between labelled

Plate 8

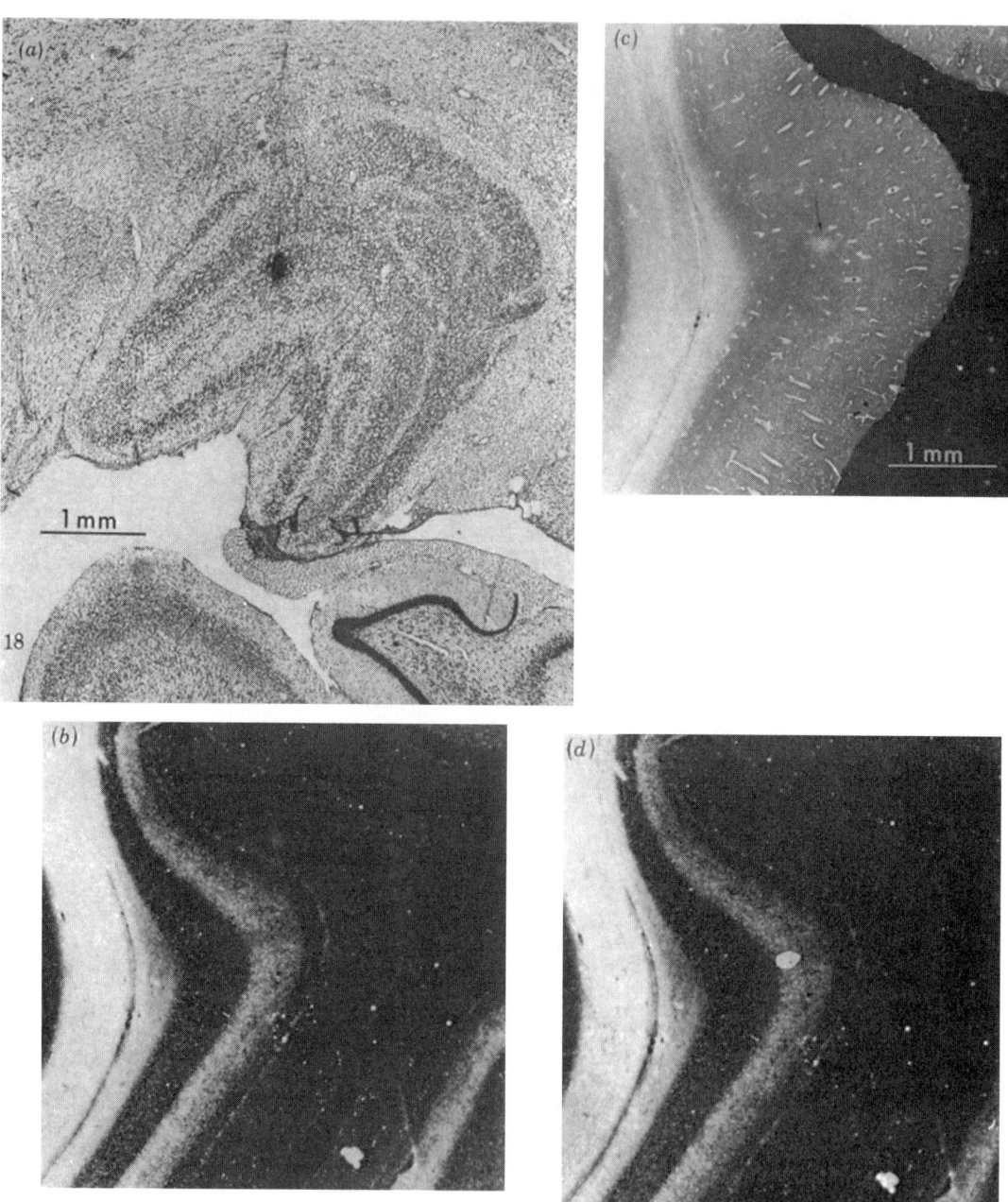

Fig. 18. Monkey no. 3. The results of making a lesion in the right lateral geniculate nucleus, confined to layer 3, a layer corresponding to the closed eye. The lesion and electrode track are shown in the cresyl-violet section in a. The resulting Nauta degeneration was deep in the calcarine fissure, no more than one or two small patches occurring in any one section. One such patch of terminals is shown in the dark field photograph in c. The next section to this was dipped for autoradiography, with the result shown in b: here layer IV C is almost continuously labelled except for a narrow gap at the knee where the calcarine stem joins the mushroom. Sections b and c were superimposed, and in d the region showing Nauta degeneration is indicated by white, in the autoradiograph. The two regions match precisely, except that the Nauta degeneration appears only in bottom half of IV C (IV C β), as expected following a parvocellular geniculate lesion.

columns corresponds precisely to the region of terminal degeneration (Figure 18*d*), providing a welcome mutual confirmation of the two methods. The fact that the space taken by degenerating fibres in the Nauta section and the size of the gap in the autoradiograph were roughly the same suggests, as had the recordings, that there was little if any overlap between the inputs from the normal and abnormal eyes.

Figure 18*d* shows that the terminal degeneration in layer IV following this dorsal-layer geniculate lesion was confined to the deeper half of layer IVC (IVCβ), in agreement with what was found in a previous study (Hubel & Wiesel 1972). The radioactive label following eye injection of course occupied the full thickness of IVC, since both dorsal and ventral geniculate layers were involved in the transport.

The remaining lesions were made in geniculate layers corresponding to the open eye. In all of these the corresponding degeneration in the cortex resembled that found in the eye-removal monkeys (Figure 6) and was present only in portions of layer IVC which, in the autoradiographs, were occupied by silver grains.

MONKEY NO. 4: PHYSIOLOGY The right striate cortex of this monkey was recorded from twice, at 22 days, at which time the right eye was sutured closed, and then at 7 months, after just over 6 months of deprivation. On the first occasion 66 cells were recorded in two penetrations. The ocular dominance histogram was entirely normal by adult standards, as may be seen by comparing the histogram from these two penetrations (Figure 19) with that of Figure 1 for the normal adult. The

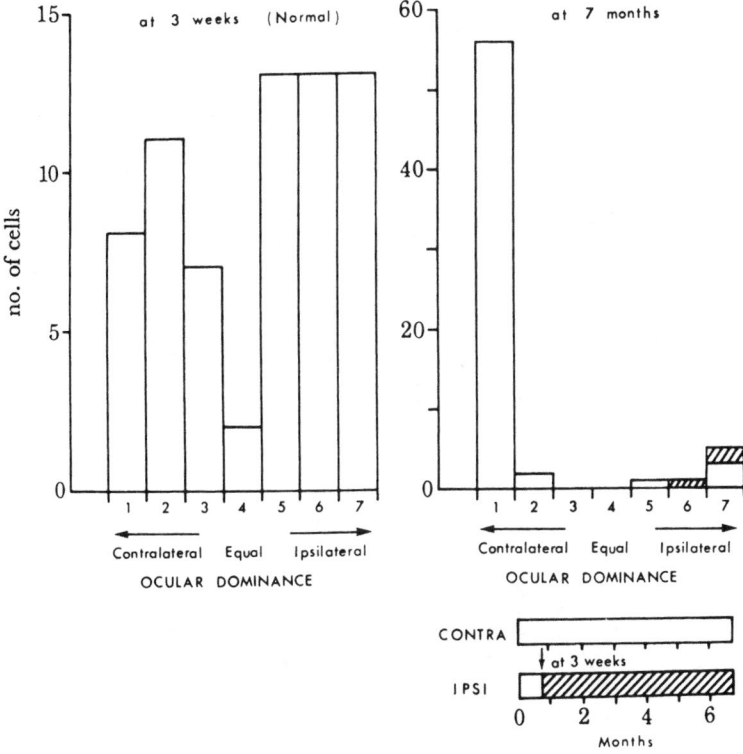

Fig. 19. Ocular dominance histograms from striate cortex of monkey no. 4, at 3 weeks, when the right eye was closed, and in a second recording session at age 7 months. The histogram at 3 weeks (right hemisphere) is similar to the adult histogram (Figure 1). After the deprivation the histogram is as expected strikingly abnormal, and almost identical to that of monkey no. 3 (see Figure 1). Here four penetrations were made, three on the right side and one on the left. 'Ipsilateral' refers to domination by the right (deprived) eye. Shading in histogram indicates cells with abnormal responses.

results of this recording session will be described in more detail in Part III.

The ocular-dominance histogram at 7 months is shown to the right in figure 19. Four penetrations were made, all tangential. Again, cells from layer IVC are not included. (We wished to study layer IV in detail, and therefore recorded as many cells as possible from it. The inclusion of these cells would have greatly increased the number of cells in groups 1 and 7.) The pronounced effects of the eye closure on the upper and lower layers is obvious, as can be seen by comparing the two parts of the figure.

In all four penetrations the activity recorded from layer IVC was strictly monocular, and in one of these penetrations the positions of six lesions made at the points of transition matched the column boundaries as revealed in subsequent autoradiography (compare Figure 15c).

MONKEY No. 4: MORPHOLOGY This monkey differed from monkey no. 3 in that the deprived (right) eye, rather than the normal one, was injected. Also the eye was closed at 3 weeks instead of 2, and the closure lasted 7 months rather than 18 (see Table 1). Sections of the operculum ipsilateral to the injected and deprived eye are shown in Figure 20, plate 9. Part a shows a single section which just grazed layer IVC, and b shows a slightly deeper section cutting layer V in two places, presumably reflecting some dimpling of the cortex; here IVC has the shape of an 8. These sections form the central part of the reconstruction shown in figure 20c. Cutouts of the two sets of columns on this side showed a ratio of areas, normal to deprived, of 1.97:1 (Table 3). On the contralateral side this ratio was 1.60:1, suggesting, as in monkey no. 3, that the side ipsilateral to the closed eye was the more severely affected.

The calcarine cortex of the two hemispheres is shown in Figure 21, Plate 10, contralaterally (A) and ipsilaterally (B); again there is a suggestion that in the ipsilateral hemisphere the labelled columns are narrower than in the contralateral. In addition one can see that the deep part of layer IVC (IVCβ) is labelled much more heavily than the superficial. This difference is seen in normal monkeys, but seems more pronounced here, while it might be taken to mean that the IVCα component is more

susceptible than IVCβ to deprivation effects, the results in monkey no. 3 (see Figure 16) suggest, if anything, the very reverse. In the geniculate, furthermore, there was no indication that the magnocellular layers, which correspond to IVCα, were more atrophic than the parvocellular. This is in agreement with the findings of Headon & Powell (1973).

In Figure 21a, Plate 10, a long continuous expanse of layer IV label can be seen over the anterior stem of the calcarine fissure in the region known to represent the part of the visual field temporal periphery that is visible only to one eye (temporal crescent). This label is at least as heavy as in any of the shrunken deprived-eye columns elsewhere on the same slide, and occupies as extensive an area of cortex as it does in the normal monkey. It thus seems that the temporal-crescent representation is little affected by the deprivation procedure. This again supports the suggestion that the effects of monocular deprivation depend on competition between the two eyes rather than simple disuse.

In this monkey the reduced-silver sections showed no banding, perhaps because the animal was too young. (The method has so far been successful only in animals a year or more old.) No geniculate lesions were made, and consequently no Nauta preparations were available.

MONKEY No. 5 (201): MORPHOLOGY This animal is included as a second example of monocular closure with deprived eye injected. The right eye was closed at 2 days and opened at 7 weeks, and the animal lived up to an age of 7 months. A more complete description of this monkey will be given as part of a separate paper on duration of the sensitive period and extent of recovery. The opercular autoradiographs were unsatisfactory, showing almost no label, probably because of uneven distribution of the injected material in the eye. A part of the calcarine cortex was labelled, however, and is shown in transverse section in Figure 22, Plate 10. We include this monkey here because it forms an almost exact complement to monkey no. 3 (Figure 16), with the deprived eye injected instead of the normal. Again, as in monkey no. 4, layer IVCα seems more severely affected than IVCβ, in apparent contradiction to what was seen in monkey no. 3.

Plate 9

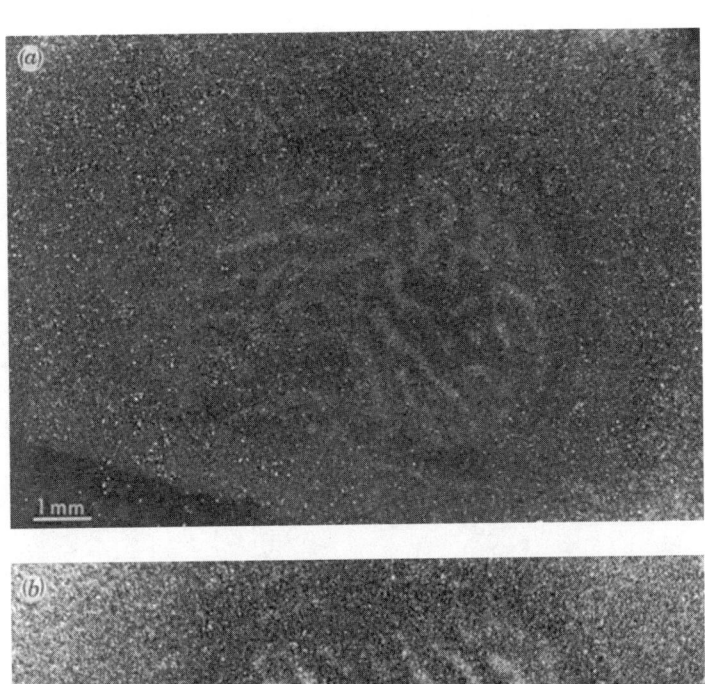

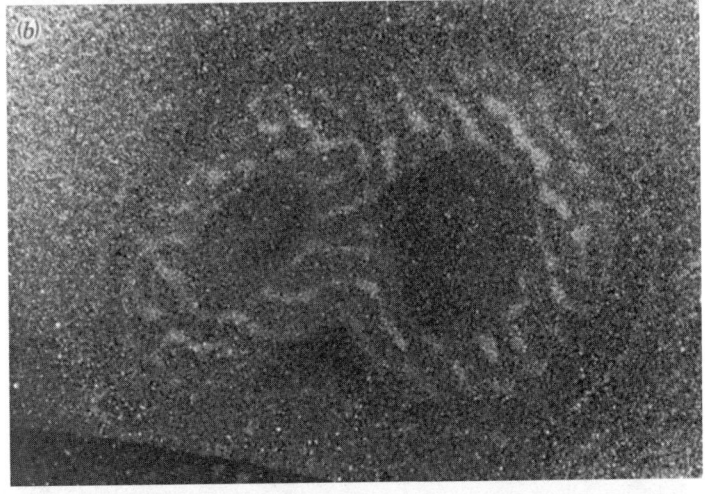

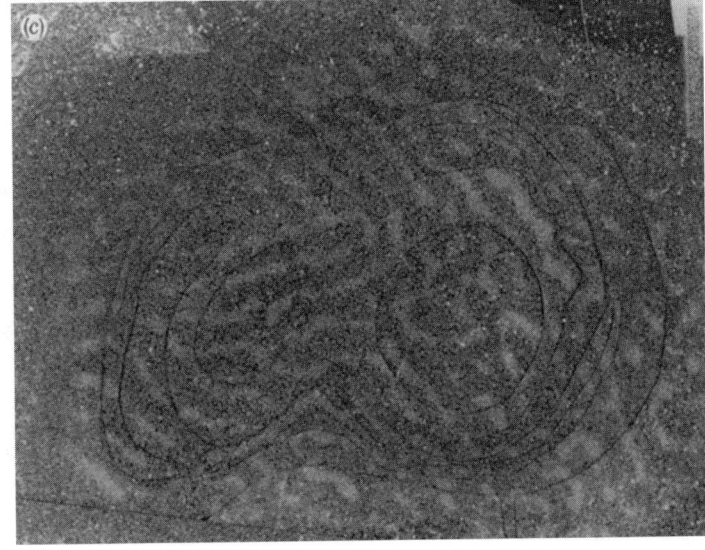

Fig. 20. This is the counterpart of Figures 13 and 15, for monkey no. 4; right eye closed at 3 weeks, until age 7 months; right eye injected. Dark-field autoradiographs of right occipital operculum. (a) tangential to layer IVC; (b) 120 μm deeper than a, tangential to layer V and intersecting it twice because of dimple in cortex. (c) reconstruction made up of 7 sections including a and b; total depth 640 μm. The labelled columns, corresponding to the closed eye, are markedly shrunken.

Plate 10

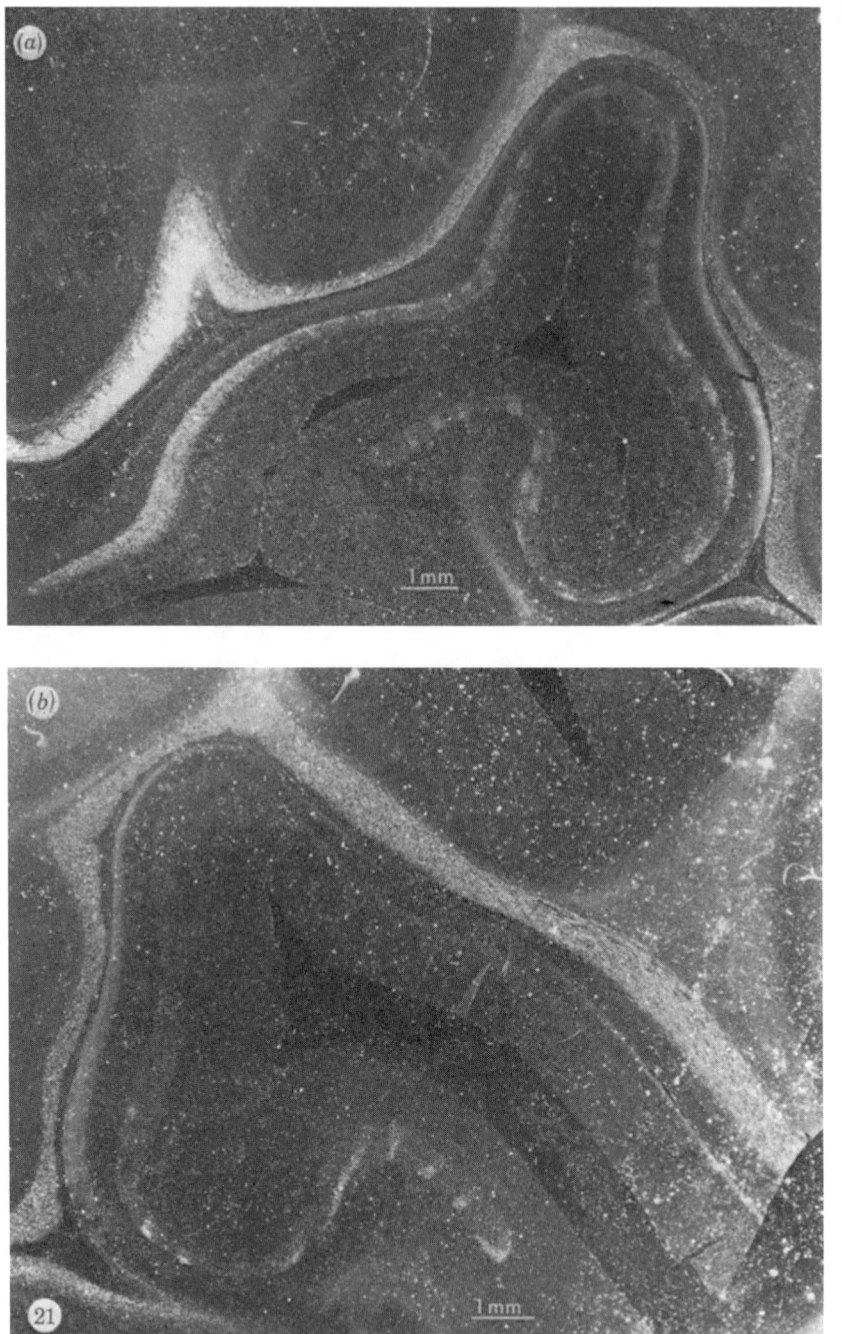

Fig. 21. Monkey no. 4, dark field autoradiographs through calcarine cortex, (a) contralateral to the closed, injected eye, (b) ipsilateral to the injected eye Note that the deprived columns are more severely shrunken on the ipsilateral side. The temporal-crescent representation is very conspicuous in a, and seems not to be affected at all.

Plate 10

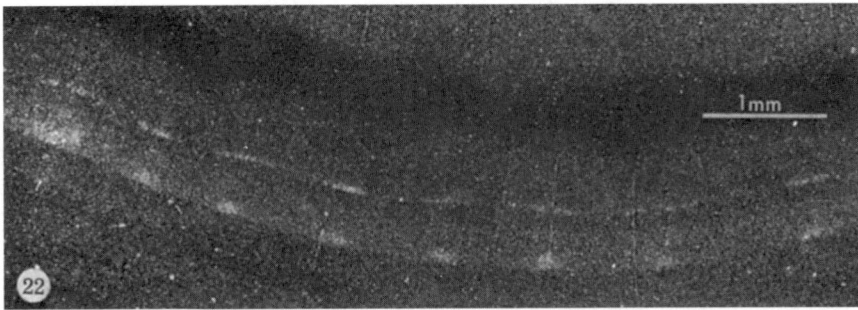

Fig. 22. Monkey no. 5; right eye closed at 2 days for a period of 7 weeks, then reopened up to the age of 7 months, when the right eye was injected and the brain examined 2 weeks later. Dark-field autoradiograph, transverse section through ipsilateral calcarine fissure. Labelled columns are markedly reduced in width in layer IVC, but comparatively intact in the upper tier, IV A.

GROSS ANATOMY AND NISSL STUDIES In monkeys nos. 1–4, there was no obvious change in the extent or overall shape of the striate cortex. No measurements were made of the total area of striate cortex, but the occipital lobes were not grossly shrunk as would be expected if half of the columns had been reduced to a fraction of their normal size; the extent of striate cortex in Nissl-stained sections, moreover, appeared quite normal. This strongly suggests that the shrinkage of one set of columns was compensated for by an expansion of the other set, supporting the conclusion already reached from measurements of the repeat distance. For the same reason it is unlikely that one set simply failed to grow following the eye closure. Indeed, if the differences in column width in monkey no. 3 had been due to a failure of one set to grow, the striate cortex of a 2 week old monkey would have been about one-third its adult size. Far from this, comparisons between newborn and adult show that the newborn brain is closer to 80% of the adult size.

In marked contrast to the lateral geniculates, the Nissl-stained cortex in all of the experimental monkeys appeared normal. In particular, layer IVC gave no hint of any fluctuations in thickness, cell size or cell density, to parallel the changes seen in the autoradiography or degeneration studies. Measurements of cell density and cell size were made in monkey no. 3 to learn whether any minor variations, too subtle to be seen by mere visual inspection under the microscope, might be present. In an autoradiographic section counterstained for Nissl substance, squares were selected in the mid-dle of four normal-eye columns, midway between the borders, and these were compared with squares similarly centred in the neighbouring deprived-eye columns. Each square measured 50 μm × 50 μm. The locations of column boundaries were determined directly from the autoradiography by examining the same slide under dark-field illumination. Table 4 shows the results of these measurements: no significant differences were seen in cell density or cell size.

Part III. Newborn Monkeys

An interpretation of the findings just described depends heavily on a knowledge of the state of the ocular dominance columns at the time an eye was closed or removed. Some preliminary studies were therefore made on three very young monkeys. The first of these (no. 9) was studied anatomically following eye injection; the second and third were recorded from, the second (no. 10) at 8 days and the third (no. 4) at 22 days.

MONKEY No. 9: AUTORADIOGRAPHY This monkey was injected in the right eye with 2.0 mCi of tritiated fucose the day after it was born. Though we normally allow 14 days for transport, the animal died of a respiratory infection at 6 days and was perfused probably less than an hour after death.

The geniculates seemed to be fully developed by adult standards. The layers corresponding to the injected eye were heavily labelled, as shown in Figure 23, Plate 11. On each side the three layers corre-

Table 4. *Cell Density and Size, Monkey No. 3, Layer IVCβ, R.H.†*

| Column Type | Density (Cells/2500 μm²) | MEAN AREA | | Significance (Welch test) |
		(μm²)	(s.d)	
normal	31	48	8.9	
deprived	30	48	11.1	N.S.
normal	33	50	11.8	
deprived	23	41	10.7	p < 0.05
normal	22	54	12.9	
deprived	37	54	14.6	N.S.
normal	29	50	9.6	
deprived	26	49	8.4	N.S.
total:	(cells/10000 μm²)			
normal	115	50		
deprived	116	49		N.S.

† 4 pairs of samples from normal and deprived columns. Each consists of all the neurones in a 2500 μm² square in the middle of the column and the middle of the layer.

sponding to the uninjected eye showed some label in excess of background, perhaps somewhat more than was seen in monkeys nos. 3 and 4. Comparisons are difficult, however, given the large amount of label injected relative to the size of the eye or the monkey's weight, the use of fucose alone instead of a fucose-proline mixture, the differences in the time allowed for transport, and a number of other variables that could not be completely controlled.

In addition to the six classical layers, Figure 23 shows four subsidiary groups of terminations. These are labelled in Figure 24, Plate 11. From ventral to dorsal they consist of: (1) a thin layer *a* ventral to layer 1, contralaterally supplied, and separated from most of 1 by a thin label-free gap. (2) A clump of label *b* near the hilum, supplied ipsilaterally and sandwiched between *a* and layer 1. This is seen as a small aggregation of label on the left, and its position is marked by a space on the right. (3) A thin leaflet *c* just dorsal to layer 1, contralaterally innervated, and, like, *a,* separated from layer 1 by a label free gap. (4) A thin leaflet *d* sandwiched between layers 2 and 3, contralaterally innervated so that it stands out clearly between these two, especially in dark-field illumination (Figure 23, lower right). This layer is probably also ipsilaterally innervated as shown in light field (see also Fig-

ure 9). *c* and *d* appear to be joined in some sections by bands of label that pass through layer 2. Layers *a, b* and *d* are also shown in Figure 9. *a* and *b* probably correspond to the single lamina 'S', described by Campos-Ortega & Hayhow (1970), and thought by them to receive only ipsilateral innervation.

The findings in the striate cortex came as a surprise. At first glance no columns were evident at all. Sections cut in the parasagittal plane through the calcarine fissure contralateral to the injected eye showed almost continuous moderately dense label in layer IVC. This is shown in Figure 25a, Plate 12. The minor fluctuations in density of layer IV label were hard to evaluate in these sections and we were tempted to dismiss them until we examined tangential sections through the dome of the mushroom of the calcarine fissure on the ipsilateral side (Figure 25b). Though the parallel bands in the central oval region through IVC are faint their regularity is very clear, with a repeat distance of about 700 μm, or 20% less than our value for the normal adult. Even in the regions of minimum label the density is considerably higher than outside IVC. It is difficult to compare the sides ipsilateral and contralateral to the injected eye because of differences in the planes of section, but our impression is that the fluctuations in density were more marked ipsilaterally.

Plate 11

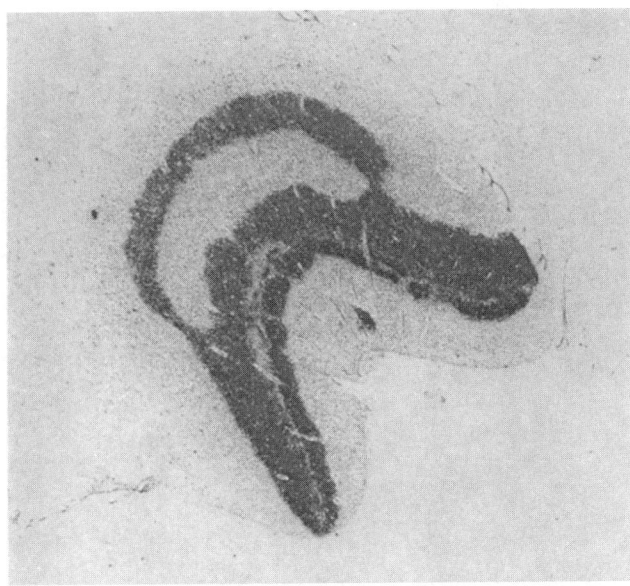

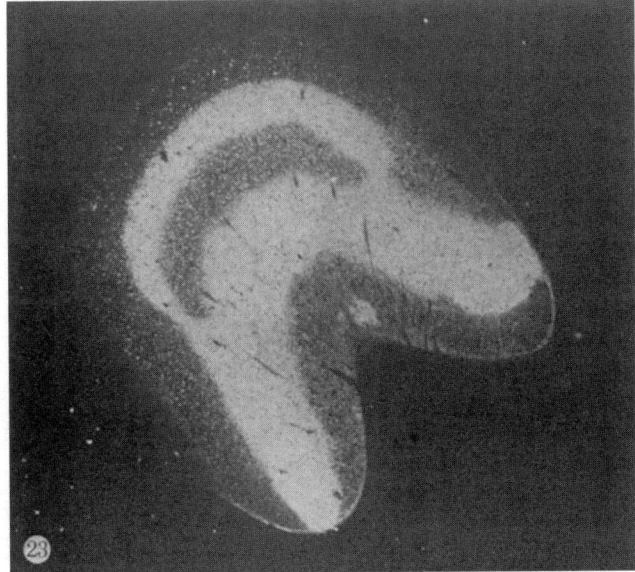

Fig. 23. Normal newborn monkey (no. 9). Autoradiographs of lateral geniculate bodies. The left eye was injected at 1 day of age and the brain examined at 1 week. Upper part, light field, lower, dark field. The label in the layers corresponding to the right, non-injected eye is denser than the background but is in fibres rather than terminals. Several layers other than the six classical ones can be identified; these are indicated in Figure 24. (Continued)

There are two possible explanations for this result. The first is that label may have leaked from the path originating in the injected eye to the non-injected path. The geniculates would be the most likely site of spillover. Some leakage of this sort may indeed occur in the normal adult, as is shown in Figures 12 and 13 by the above-background levels in the gaps between labelled columns. It may be that any such leakage is more serious in the new-

born. The second possibility is that the columns are indeed not fully formed at birth, the full extent of layer IV being occupied by terminals from the two eyes, with only minor but regular variations in density representing the precursors of the columns.

MONKEYS NOS. 10 AND 4: PHYSIOLOGY One obvious method for resolving this impasse was to record from a newborn monkey. No. 9, unfortunately,

Plate 11

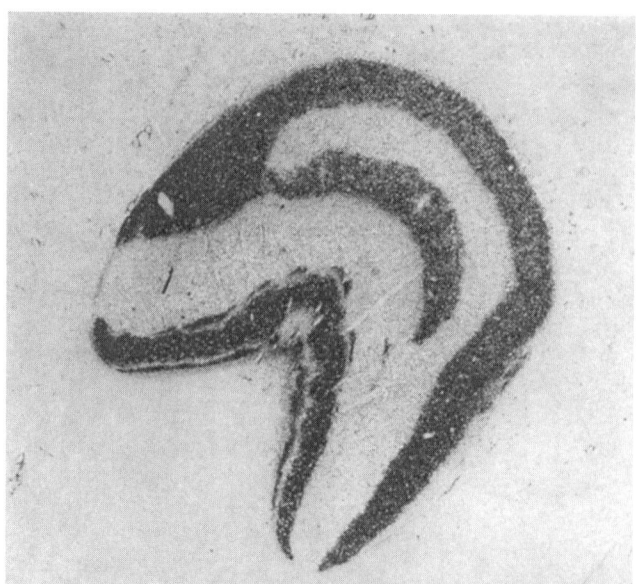

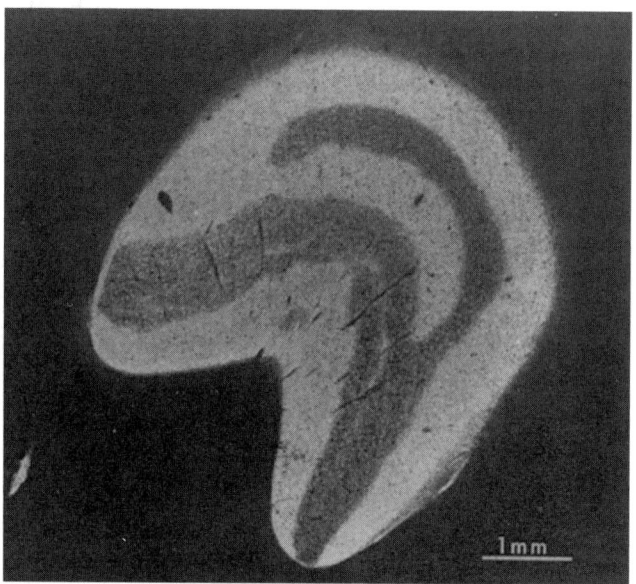

Fig. 23. (Continued)

died before recordings could be made. No. 10 was not injected, but was recorded from at 8 days of age, having been in a normally lit nursery up to that time.

Four penetrations were made in monkey no. 10, in area 17 of the left hemisphere. They were made very obliquely so as to explore as great a span of layer IVC as possible. The reconstruction of these penetrations is shown in Figure 26, Plate 12, with the ocular dominance of the cells indicated below. Points to the left of the gap in the diagram indicate units or unit clusters in layer IVC. The smaller dots, to the right of the gap, indicate cells in the upper layers. Our main concern was of course to learn whether single cells or local groups of cells in IVC were fed from one eye or from both.

The first penetration was normal by adult standards: in the layers above IVC most cells had sharp orientation specificity and most were driven from both eyes, one or other being preferred. The

Plate 11

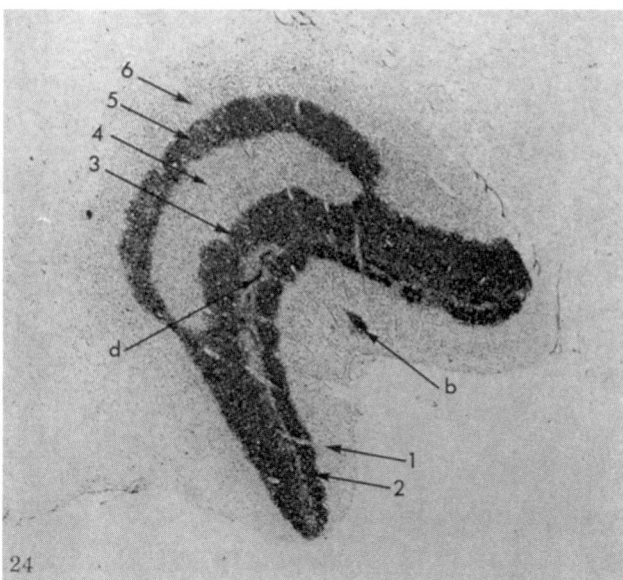

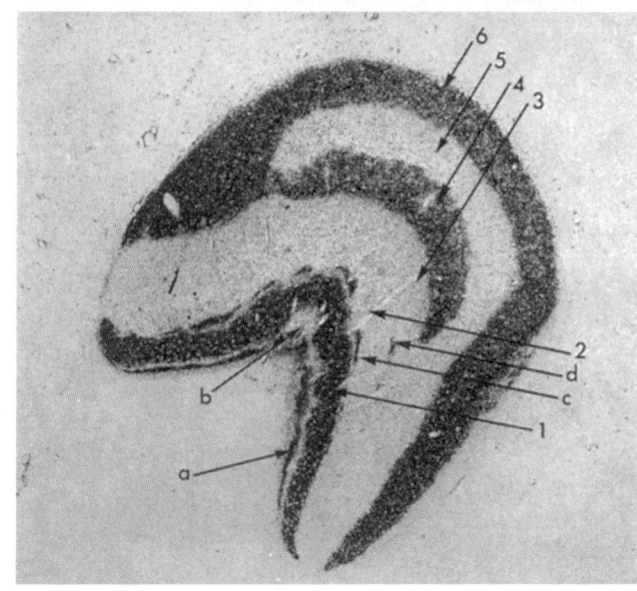

Fig. 24. Monkey no. 9; same as light-field part of Figure 23. Nine regions of input have been identified. In addition to the two classical magnocellular layers, 1 and 2, and the four parvocellular (dorsal) layers, 3, 4, 5, and 6, one can see two thin leaflets a and c, both contralaterally supplied, the one dorsal to 1 and the other ventral to it; a thin leaflet d, sandwiched between the dorsal four and the ventral two classical layers, and probably receiving input from both eyes; and finally a clump of label b (ipsilaterally supplied) between a and 1, which shows up as a labelled region on the left, and a label-free space on the right.

contralateral eye dominated at first, then came a span of about 1 mm in which the ipsilateral eye dominated, and finally, in IVC, all cells had unoriented fields and were activated from the contralateral eye only. In the other three penetrations, binocular cells similarly prevailed in the upper layers, but in IVC a variable amount of binocular input was also found. Thus in penetrations 2 and 3 the ipsilateral eye dominated but the contralateral contributed weakly or moderately throughout the traverse through IVC, while in penetration 4 the two eyes were almost equal. These observations refer mostly to the unresolved multiunit activity, since single units are hard to resolve in IVC. Nevertheless, there were in layer IVC several clear examples of binocularly driven cells with no preferred orientation. In this monkey, then, layer IVC showed the usual variation in eye emphasis, but much more binocular mixing than we have ever found in juvenile or adult monkeys.

Plate 12

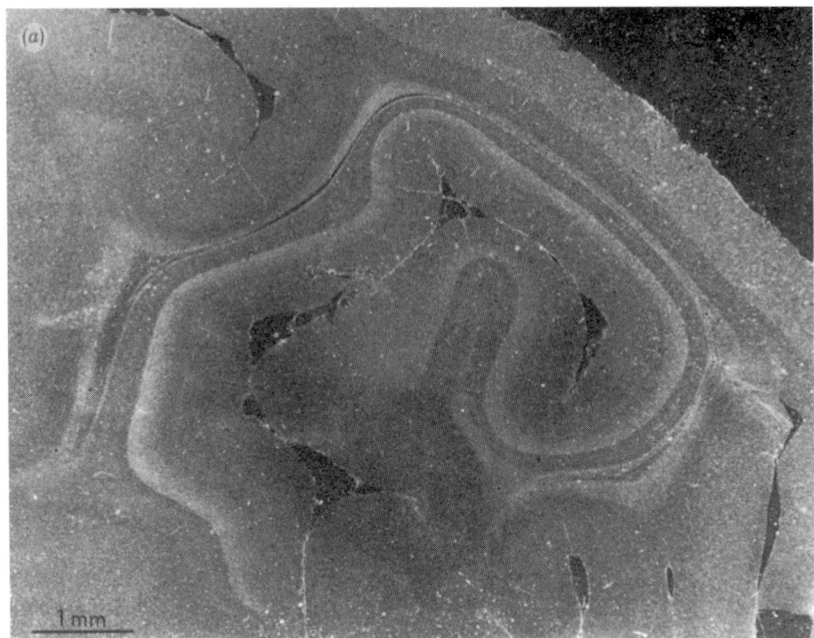

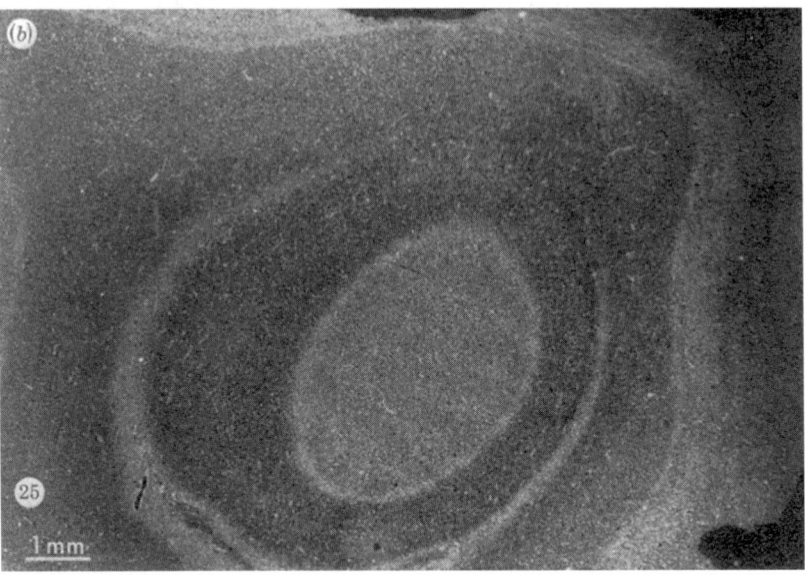

Fig. 25. Newborn monkey, no. 9, Autoradiographs in dark field. (a) Transverse section through calcarine fissure and operculum on the right side, contralateral to the injected eye. Label is virtually continuous, both in the fissure and over the convexity, though there is some suggestion of fluctuations in density over the dorsal calcarine stem. (The part of this stem furthest to the left is probably the temporal crescent representation, where one expects continuous label; compare Figure 21a.) Anterior is up and to the left. (b) Tangential section through operculum of left occipital lobe (ipsilateral to the injected eye). Section passes deep to the outer convexity, and cuts the buried mushroom-like calcarine convexity, grazing layer IV C which appears as an oval near the centre. Throughout this area levels of label are well above background, but there is nevertheless a definite regular banding with a periodicity of about 0.7 mm. 1–2 mm outside of the oval is a ring of label formed by the optic radiations. Still further out is a continuous double ring of label in layers IV C α and β of the outer exposed convexity.

Plate 12

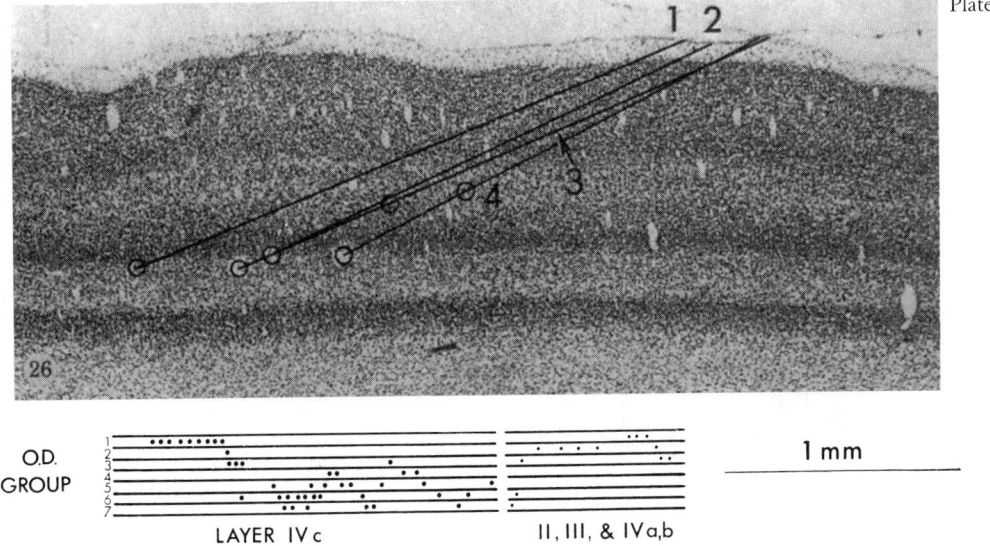

Fig. 26. *Reconstructions of four penetrations made in striate cortex of an 8-day-old monkey (left hemisphere). The object was to explore as long an extent of layer IV C as possible, determining how much binocular mixing was present. Circles indicate points at which electrolytic lesions were made. The lower diagram indicates, on the left, the ocular dominance of the multiunit activity in layer IV C. The right hand portion, with smaller dots, indicates ocular dominance of the cells in the upper layers, in the early parts of the penetrations. The points are pooled from all four penetrations, preserving the cortical position of each recording site. In the region explored, obviously the contralateral (right) eye dominated in the portions to the left and right and the ipsilateral eye dominated in the middle. For the left hand region the input was almost exclusively contralateral; in the middle region, however, there was considerable mixing of inputs from the two eyes. In adult monkeys virtually no mixing is found in layer IV C.*

A recording was also made in monkey no. 4 at 3 weeks of age, up to which time both eyes had been normally exposed. (After the recording the monkey was resurrected and the right eye was sutured closed.) In this animal the results were very similar to those previously obtained in the adult, and are illustrated in Figure 27. In both penetrations (each at about 45°) binocularly driven cells were present in abundance above and below layer IVC, with the normal swings in dominance from eye to eye. The short passage through layer IVC in penetration 1 (between arrows) showed monocular influence only, but a subsequent experiment in a 3-week-old monkey has indicated a lack of complete segregation in this layer; another at 6 weeks suggests that by then segregation is virtually complete. (These experiments are part of a separate study on the time course of columnar development.)

Thus early in life layer IVC probably contains a mixture of inputs from the two eyes, perhaps at most points along its length; by 3 weeks, on the other hand, segregation seems to be fairly well advanced but probably still not complete.

DISCUSSION

The chief finding of the present study concerns the effects of early eye removal or monocular lid closure on the ocular dominance stripes in layer IVC. Deprivation in the first few weeks of life resulted in a change in the relative sizes of the two sets of stripes, with a shrinkage of stripes receiving input from the deprived eye and a corresponding expansion of those with input from the normal eye.

In discussing the nature of these changes a number of possibilities can be quickly dispensed with. The first of these is the notion that in the shrunken columns the reduction is only apparent: that in the areas invaded by the normal-eye terminals, the terminals from the deprived eye remain

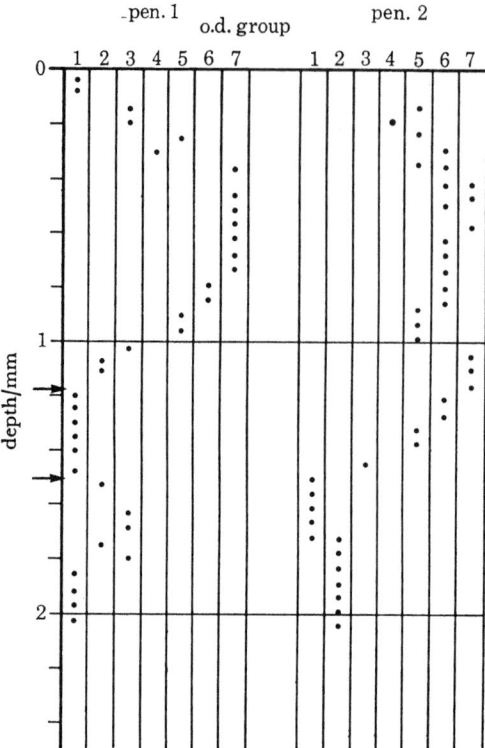

Fig. 27. Ocular dominance in two penetrations made at 45° through right striate cortex of a normal 3-week-old monkey (no. 4, first recording, compare figure 19). Penetration 1 passed through layer IV C in the region indicated by the arrows; this activity was strictly monocular. There are clear regular fluctuations in ocular dominance, just as is found in adult monkeys.

occupied by each entire band, cells and all. This could only happen if the cell packing density deviated markedly from normal, increasing in the shrunken columns and decreasing in the expanded ones, or if cells died in large numbers in one set and proliferated in the other. But a fluctuation in packing density of the magnitude necessary to fit the changes in width that we see can be ruled out by direct counts (Table 4), while cell proliferation ceases altogether in the cortex 2 months before term (Rakic 1974), and a cell death sufficient to equalize the cell counts would produce a radical drop in cell numbers which in fact does not occur.

Thirdly, there is a possibility that the brain of the newborn monkey is much smaller than that of the adult, and that the columns in area 17 are present at birth and also correspondingly smaller. The disparity in column size would then arise if the columns connected to the deprived eye simply failed to grow. It appears, however, that in overall size the striate cortex increases very roughly 20% after birth—it certainly does not double or triple in area as would be required to explain the discrepancies in column width. Consistent with this, the columns in the newborn show a periodicity not very different from that of the adult, to judge from direct anatomical (Figure 25b) and physiological (Figures 26 and 27) observations. Finally, there is the finding that in the deprived animals the columns associated with the open eye are larger than normal, and the combined width of a left eye-right eye pair is unchanged. None of this would be consistent with an explanation based on failure to grow.

With these possibilities out of the way, a discussion of the pathogenesis of the changes due to deprivation hinges strongly on a knowledge of the state of the columns at birth. If one assumes that in the newborn monkey (or within a few days of birth) the geniculocortical fibres have already taken up their final positions in the form of clearly defined parallel IVth-layer stripes, then it is hard to avoid the conclusion that in the final state one set of terminals has extended its territory, possibly by sprouting, while the other set has retracted. If sprouting were involved here it would be of some interest. Although a number of examples of sprouting have been reported, all of them were brought about by a destructive deafferentation of one source of input to a structure. In the present

but are non-functional. The concept of non-functional synapses in the nervous system is not unheard of, the best established example probably being botulinum poisoning at the nerve-muscle junction. In the present experiments, given the variety of techniques we have used to demonstrate the abnormalities, one would have to suppose in this model not only that the synapses were physiologically non-functional, but that the fibres did not degenerate after geniculate lesions in such a way as to show up with Nauta-Fink-Heimer methods, did not transport materials normally, and were not revealed with reduced silver stains. Such an interpretation thus seems most improbable.

Secondly, we must consider the idea that there is not only an abnormal distribution of terminals in layer IV, but also a change in the territory

series even eye enucleation amounts to a lesion one synapse away from the site of the changes, and the eye closures involve no direct destruction of any neural tissue. If the changes in layer IV are indeed produced by sprouting and retraction the result is in marked contrast to what is seen in the geniculate or colliculus, for there we have no hint of invasion of terminals from the normal eye into the deprived or deafferented territory. This may simply be a matter of timing with respect to normal developmental events, since it is known that in enucleated cats there is no invasion of afferents into a deprived geniculate layer unless the enucleation is done in the first week after birth (Kalil 1972; Guillery 1972b). Even then the invasion is modest and occurs only near the laminar borders; that it occurs at all is probably related to the immaturity of the cat visual system at birth, compared with that of the monkey.

Up to the time when we saw the results of autoradiography in the newborn, described in Part III, we regarded a sprouting of terminals as the strongest contender in explaining the cortical changes. Our previous physiological recordings in young monkeys (Hubel & Wiesel 1974) had actually tended to support the idea that ocular dominance columns were present at birth. By the second day, for example, there was a clear grouping of upper-layer, mostly binocular, cells according to ocular dominance, and in an animal with both eyes closed up to 3 weeks there was an almost complete segregation of eye inputs even in the upper and lower layers, reminiscent of the picture obtained with artificial strabismus. Tangential penetrations were not used in either of these animals, however, so that no clear idea was obtained of the state of affairs in layer IVC.

In the present paper both the physiological recordings and the anatomy in monkeys in the first week or so of life strongly suggest that the sets of terminals associated with the two eyes have arrived at layer IVC but have not yet separated themselves out completely into distinct bands. There is, to be sure, a clear banding visible in the autoradiographs in tangential sections (monkey no. 9, Figure 25b), but these are produced by mild fluctuations in levels of label, rather than a series of abrupt rises and falls from maximum to minimum and back. The physiology in monkey no. 10 confirmed this mixing of inputs, though there was perhaps more seg-

regation than would have been expected from the autoradiographic picture.

The notion that the columns are not fully formed at birth in this species can at present be only rather tentative; what is still needed is a set of injections and recordings at various ages in the first 6 weeks. But our results so far receive support from the findings of Rakic (1976a, b), in foetal monkeys in which one eye was injected with radioactive label at different times during gestation. At 6 weeks before term label was present in IV C but appeared uniform, with no hint of columns. Three weeks before term there were fluctuations in label density that were only barely discernable on visual inspection of transverse sections, but were clearly confirmed by grain counts. As with our eye-injection results, one must keep in mind the possibility of leakage of label in the geniculate.

If the columns do, as it were, crystallize out only in the few weeks before and after term, the process presumably occurs by a retraction of the two sets of terminals. One may imagine that in any areas occupied by both sets of terminals there is a competitive mechanism in which the weaker set at any point tends to regress. Given such an unstable equilibrium, the normal end result of any initial inequalities would be a complete segregation of terminals. Such a model for the normal development, based on competition, is illustrated schematically in the left half of Figure 28. In this figure the terminals dominated by one eye in layer IV C are blackened, and the other set is represented by open areas. (Obviously the two sets should be superimposed, but are shown one under the other for clarity.) The thickness of these representations suggests the relative density of label at each point along IV C. If we suppose that at birth there exist some mild periodic out-of-phase fluctuations (which may be less than portrayed here) the density of the weaker inputs at any point will decline, with consequent production of a series of ever widening gaps until all overlap is eliminated.

On this model for the normal development, the deprivation results in layer IV can be predicted. One has only to assume that lack of use of a set of terminals puts them at a competitive disadvantage which transcends that related to mere numbers, so that at any point along IV C the terminals from the opposing normal-eye set take over, provided they have not already retracted. This is illustrated in the

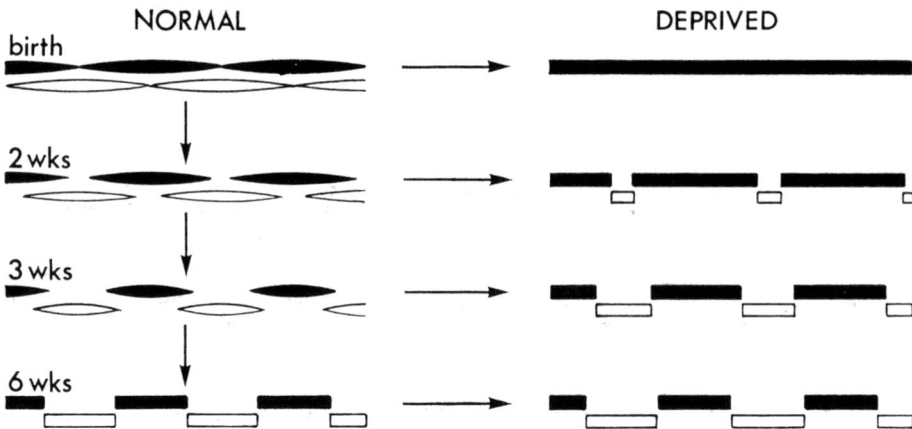

Fig. 28. Scheme that might explain the effects of eye closures on columns in layer IV C, on the assumption that the segregation of the eyes is not complete until some weeks after birth. The thick dark lines represent the terminations of geniculate afferents in layer IV C corresponding to one eye; the open lines, the terminations from the other eye. In each, the width is intended to represent the presumed density of the terminals. At birth there is some periodic and regular variation in density (Figure 25b): it is unlikely that the minimum is zero, as the drawing suggests, and in any case the fluctuations are probably different in different parts of the striate cortex. In this scheme we suppose that competition normally occurs between the eyes, with the weaker input at any given point declining and the stronger being fortified. The result is a progressive retraction as the sparse terminals die out entirely. For purposes of the drawing we assume that the retraction process has the time course illustrated and that it takes about 6 weeks; again, the exact time course is far from clear.

right half of Figure 28. Where no competition is possible, because the other set has already disappeared (or in the case of the temporal crescent representation, where only one set was present from the beginning—see Figure 21a) the deprived set survives and is apparently intact. The end result of the deprivation thus depends on the amount of overlap that still existed at the time of eye closure or removal.

It should be emphasized that the details of Figure 28, such as the ages assigned to the four illustrated stages of development or the amount of fluctuation of label density at birth, should not be taken literally. We do *not* know, for example, that closure of an eye from birth produces a complete takeover by the open eye. The illustration merely provides, at present, the best fit with the results from the few deprivation and control monkeys available (nos. 1–5, and 9 and 10). We are still uncertain of the variation to be expected from one animal to the next, even under experimental conditions that are as similar as possible.

One advantage of the scheme of Figure 28 is that it removes some of the mystery connected with the 'critical period'—the period of susceptibility to monocular deprivation. At least as far as layer IV is concerned the flexible state would, by this model, involve not some kind of ill-defined vulnerability to insult, or capacity for nerve-terminal proliferation, but merely the period of development from birth to the final consolidation of the columns.

If the idea of a post-natal retraction of inputs is correct, it would be interesting to know whether there are consistent differences in the timing of the process, in different parts of area 17 (for example, foveal *vs.* more peripheral representations) and, in a given hemisphere, between terminals belonging to the ipsilateral and contralateral eyes. As far as laterality is concerned, deprivation effects have consistently been more severe in the hemisphere ipsilateral to the eye that was closed; this has been true both for the shrinkage of cortical columns and the attendant geniculate atrophy (see also Headon & Powell 1973). On the model of Figure 28 this would be readily explained if it were found that the fibres from the contralateral eye were slower in retracting than their counterparts from the ipsilateral. We have fragmentary hints that this may indeed be so, since in the layer IV C recordings from monkey no. 10 (Figure 26) at 8 days the contralateral eye had already gained exclusive possession of some territory in IV C, whereas the ipsilateral eye had not. On the competition model a closure of the contralatera eye would find ipsilateral terminals available only in the designated ipsilateral territory; a closure of the ipsilateral eye would find terminals from the contralateral eye available to take over everywhere. The autoradiography (Figure 25) tended to support this idea, although comparisons were difficult since the planes of section in the two hemispheres were different.

The model of course says nothing about changes in connections beyond layer IV C. That such changes almost certainly occur is shown by the scarcity in deprived animals of cells in layers outside IV that can be influenced from the closed eye, a scarcity more severe than would be expected from the extent to which deprived stripes in IV C are spared, and the relative normality of responses within those stripes. (We were, in fact, surprised when we first recorded from layer IV C to find any significant number of cells responsive to the deprived eye.) Also it is clear that monocular deprivation can produce changes in the ocular dominance of cells outside layer IV when closures are done well beyond 6 weeks—effects are seen as late as 4 months and possibly even later, if an eye is closed for a long enough time. We have some indication, from reduced silver stains, that such late deprivation leaves the layer IV band widths unchanged. Thus eye-dominance changes in higher order cells may have to be explained in terms of competition between different groups of afferents for territory on a single postsynaptic cell, as has been proposed previously (Wiesel & Hubel 1965). Indeed, an important reason for doing the present experiments was a curiosity to learn what would happen in layer IV C, where competition between eyes on a single-cell level seemed impossible. This is in contrast to the situation in the cat, in which the physiology suggests that there is a direct convergence of geniculate afferents from the two

eyes on cortical cells. It now appears that the mechanisms for the layer-IV changes in the monkey could also involve competition, since before the columns are fully formed terminals from the two eyes may likewise converge on single cells in that layer. The presence of a few resolvable binocular cells in layer IV C of monkey no. 10 (at 8 days) tends to support this, although we admittedly have no guarantee that the particular cells we recorded received direct input from the geniculate. The question would have to be resolved by intracellular or morphological (EM) techniques. In any case, it is probably easier to imagine competition between afferents for territory on a single cell than a competition between entire columns or large groups of afferents.

Since the notion of competition between eyes is now a dominant one in visual deprivation, and a recurring theme in the present paper, it may be useful to review some of the evidence in its favour. It was originally suggested to account for the surprising finding that binocular deprivation in cats produced defects in cortical cell responses that were far milder than predicted from monocular closures (Wiesel & Hubel 1965). This seemed to rule out simple disuse as a mechanism for the unresponsiveness of cells when one eye was deprived. In 1970 Guillery & Stelzner observed that in the geniculate of monocularly deprived cats the part of layer A representing the temporal crescent did not show the same defect in cell growth as the rest of this layer: a possible explanation advanced to explain this was competition between the two eyes, with a sparing of the part of the geniculate in which there could be no competition. Since convergence of input from the two eyes occurs first (for all practical purposes) in the cortex, it was suggested that the cell shrinkage in the geniculate might reflect a failure of axon terminals to compete effectively for synaptic surface of cortical cells. Subsequent experiments have strengthened this idea: (1) In cats deprived of vision in one eye, focal retinal lesions in the open eye produced a protection from deprivation effects, of just those geniculate cells whose competition had been removed (Guillery 1972a). (2) Behavioural tests after monocular deprivation showed relatively normal responses to visual cues in the temporal crescent of the deprived eye (Sherman 1973). (3) Sherman, Guillery, Kaas & Sanderson (1974), finally, showed that focal retinal lesions in the eye that remained open protected the closed eye from defects in behavioural and cortical-cell responses in the corresponding part of the visual field.

To this accumulated evidence the present paper has added the anatomical observation that the temporal-crescent input to the monkey cortex is largely spared on the side opposite to the closed eye, compared to the severe effects on cortical columns in the binocular part of area 17. One would expect also to see a sparing of the corresponding geniculate cells, as is found in the cat, but for this problem parasagittal sections would probably be necessary. In a study of the geniculate in monocularly deprived monkeys, von Noorden, Middleditch & Crawford (1975) saw no sparing in the monocular segment representation.

It is worth noting, in this context, that in the foetal eye-injection experiments of Rakic (1976a, b) the optic afferents both to the geniculates and to the superior colliculi occupied their entire targets for an extended period between their first arrival and their eventual segregation into layers (geniculates) or clumps (colliculi). In both targets segregation occurred during the middle period of gestation and was apparently complete by birth. A similar process, then, may well take place in geniculate, colliculus and cortex, though in the cortex it seems to occur later, and to be still incomplete at birth. This would suggest that the apparent reluctance of optic terminals in geniculate and tectum to extend their territory in monocular deprivation is a reflection of the complete segregation of the terminals at birth: the deprivation simply comes too late to produce an effect.

Though direct proof is still lacking, there are strong indications that the formation of ocular dominance columns does not require visual experience, even though some of the formation takes place postnatally and can be rendered abnormal by binocular closure. At present there are two kinds of evidence for this: (1) the autoradiographs at and before birth, i.e. the bands seen on tangential sections (Figure 26b) or the fluctuations in grain counts 21 days before term (Rakic 1976b); and (2) physiological recordings at 4 weeks in monkeys with both eyes closed at birth (Wiesel & Hubel 1974), where layer IV was not examined carefully, but extreme eye segregation was present in the layers outside IV, and therefore, *a fortiori*, in IV. We

have examined one macaque dark raised to an age of 6 weeks, and found the responses in layer IV C to be strictly monocular. What is still needed is autoradiography after eye injection in a monkey dark reared, or with both eyes sutured, for the first six weeks or more.

The model involving mutual competition to explain the normal process of post-natal IVth layer segregation presupposes some initial inequality that starts the process. It would be most interesting to know what causes this, and what forces lead to a pattern of parallel lines roughly 0.4 mm apart. If the model is correct it must explain the obliteration of the deprived columns at irregular intervals along the bands, seen in cases of early eye closure (see Figure 15), and hinted at in the eye-removal reconstructions (Figure 6). Perhaps the process begins at multiple foci along the future bands and spreads in two directions forming line segments which then join similar segments, while simultaneously widening. (On a sprouting model one is tempted to conclude that the obliteration of columns here and there reflects an instability in the columns when they shrink beyond some limiting width.)

An intriguing problem arises from a consideration of the topographic representation of the visual field upon layer IV C (Hubel, Wiesel & LeVay 1974). This topography is detailed enough so that in crossing a single eye-dominance column one can observe a precisely corresponding displacement of receptive fields through the visual field. A displacement of equal magnitude, but in the visual field as seen by the other eye, takes place when the next column is crossed. The representations seem to be interlaced, so that on crossing a boundary between columns the receptive fields in the second eye jump back to about the midpoint of the territory just traversed in the first eye. All of this means that the magnification (mm/deg) across a column must be one-half that along its length. What happens, then, when two neighbouring columns are distorted, one compressed and the other expanded? How do the magnifications change during development? Answers to these questions may lead to a deeper understanding of the developmental mechanisms by which topographic representations arise.

Finally, one may ask again whether there is any benefit to the animal in having a critical period of postnatal flexibility. Does a virtual doubling of the IVth layer territory devoted to one of the eyes in any way improve the capabilities of that eye? Until behavioural tests can be made this question must be left open, but one would hardly expect to find an improvement in acuity, which is presumably limited by such things as the optics of the eye, the inter-receptor spacing, and the number of bipolar and ganglion cells. If an eye is lost early in life a number of cortical cells are clearly kept in use rather than being allowed to lie fallow, but how this helps the animal, if it does at all, is a complete mystery.

We wish to thank Claire Wang, Gail Grogan and Sharon Mates for histological assistance, and Carolyn Scott for help with photography.

Supported by National Institutes of Health Grants EY00605 and EY00606, The Esther A. and Joseph Klingenstein Foundation, Inc. and The Rowland Foundation, Inc.

References

Baker, F. H., Grigg, P. & von Noorden, G. K. 1974 Effects of visual deprivation and strabismus on the response of neurons in the visual cortex of the monkey, including studies on the striate and prestriate cortex in the normal animal. *Brain Res.* **66**, 185–208.

Campos-Ortega, J. A. & Hayhow, W. R. 1970 A new lamination pattern in the lateral geniculate nucleus of primates. *Brain Res.* **20**, 335–339.

Guillery, R. W. 1972*a* Binocular competition in the control of geniculate cell growth. *J. Comp. Neur.* **144**, 117–130.

Guillery, R. W. 1972*b* Experiments to determine whether retinogeniculate axons can form translaminar collateral sprouts in the dorsal lateral geniculate nucleus of the cat. *J. Comp. Neur.* **146**, 407–420.

Guillery, R. W. & Stelzner, D. J. 1970 The differential effects of unilateral lid closure upon the monocular and binocular segments of the dorsal lateral geniculate nucleus in the cat. *J. Comp. Neur.* **139**, 413–422.

Headon, M. P. & Powell, T. P. S. 1973 Cellular changes in the lateral geniculate nucleus of infant monkeys after suture of the eyelids. *J. Anat. (Lond.)* **116**, 135–145.

Hubel, D. H., LeVay, S. & Wiesel, T. N. 1975 Mode of termination of retinotectal fibers in macaque monkey: an autoradiographic study. *Brain Res.* **96**, 25–40.

Hubel, D. H. & Wiesel, T. N. 1968 Receptive fields and functional architecture of monkey striate cortex. *J. Physiol., Lond.* **195**, 215–243.

Hubel, D. H. & Wiesel, T. N. 1972 Laminar and columnar distribution of geniculo-cortical fibers in the macaque monkey. *J. Comp. Neur.* **146**, 421–450.

Hubel, D. H., Wiesel, T. N. & LeVay, S. 1974 Visual field representation in layer IVC of monkey striate cortex. *Soc. Neurosci., 4th Annual Meeting (Abstracts)* 264.

Kalil, R. E. 1972 Formation of new retino-geniculate connections in kittens after removal of one eye. *Anat. Rec.* **172**, 339–340.

LeVay, S., Hubel, D. H. & Wiesel, T. N. 1975 The pattern of ocular dominance columns in macaque visual cortex revealed by a reduced silver stain. *J. Comp. Neur.* **159**, 559–576.

Lund, J. S. & Boothe, R. G. 1975 Interlaminar connections and pyramidal neuron organisation in the visual cortex, area 17, of the macaque monkey. *J. Comp. Neur.* **159**, 305–334.

Matthews, M. R., Cowan, W. M. & Powell, T. P. S. 1960 Transneuronal cell degeneration in the lateral geniculate nucleus of the macaque monkey. *J. Anat.* **94**, 145–169.

Minkowski, M. 1920 Über den Verlauf, die Endigung und die zentrale Repräsentation von gekreuzten und ungekreuzten Sehnervenfasern bei einigen Säugetieren und bei Menschen. *Schweiz. Arch. Neur. u. Psychiat.* **6**, 201–257.

Rakic, P. 1974 Neurons in rhesus monkey visual cortex: systematic relation between time of origin and eventual disposition. *Science, N.Y.* **183**, 425–427.

Rakic, P. 1976*a* Prenatal genesis of connections subserving ocular dominance in the rhesus monkey. *Nature, Lond.* (in press).

Rakic, P. 1976*b* Prenatal development of the visual system in the rhesus monkey. *Phil. Trans. R. Soc. Lond.* B **278**, 245–260 (this volume).

Sherman, S. M. 1973 Visual field defects in monocularly and binocularly deprived cats. *Brain Res.* **49**, 25–45.

Sherman, S. M., Guillery, R. W., Kaas, J. H. & Sanderson, K. R. 1974 Behavioral, electrophysiological and morphological studies of binocular competition in the development of the geniculo-cortical pathways of cats. *J. Comp. Neur.* **158**, 1–18.

Spatz, W. B., Tigges, J. & Tigges, M. 1970 Subcortical projections, cortical associations and some intrinsic interlaminar connections of the striate cortex in the squirrel monkey (*Saimiri*). *J. Comp. Neur.* **140**, 155–174.

von Noorden, G. K., Middleditch, P. R. & Crawford, M. L. J. 1975 Disuse or abnormal binocular interaction in the etiology of amblyopia. *Proc. A.R.V.O.* p. 79.

Wiesel, T. N. & Hubel, D. H. 1963 Single-cell responses in striate cortex of kittens deprived of vision in one eye. *J. Neurophysiol.* **26**, 1003–1017.

Wiesel, T. N. & Hubel, D. H. 1965 Comparison of the effects of unilateral and bilateral eye closure on cortical unit responses in kittens. *J. Neurophysiol.* **28**, 1029–1040.

Wiesel, T. N. & Hubel, D. H. 1971 Long-term changes in the cortex after visual deprivation. *Proceedings of the International Union of Physiological Sciences.*

Wiesel, T. N. & Hubel, D. H. 1974 Ordered arrangement of orientation columns in monkeys lacking visual experience. *J. Comp. Neur.* **158**, 307–318.

Wiesel, T. N., Hubel, D. H. & Lam, D. N. K. 1974 Autoradiographic demonstration of ocular-dominance columns in the monkey striate cortex by means of transneuronal transport. *Brain Res.* **79**, 273–279.

Wiitanen, J. T. 1969 Selective silver impregnation of degenerating axons and axon terminals in the central nervous system of the monkey (*Macaca mulatta*). *Brain Res.* **14**, 546–548.

The Development of Ocular Dominance Columns in Normal and Visually Deprived Monkeys

SIMON LEVAY, TORSTEN N. WIESEL AND DAVID H. HUBEL • *Department of Neurobiology, Harvard Medical School, 25 Shattuck Street, Boston, Massachusetts 02115*

ABSTRACT

The main purpose of this study was to examine the normal postnatal development of ocular dominance columns in the striate cortex of the macaque monkey and to determine how this developmental process is influenced by monocular lid-suture. The physiological pattern of ocular dominance was studied in long, tangential electrode penetrations. For anatomical demonstration of the distribution of afferents we relied principally on the transneuronal transport of [³H]proline injected into one eye, and to a lesser extent on the Liesegang silver method. The effects of deprivation on cell size in the lateral geniculate nucleus (LGN) were also studied. Twenty-six monkeys, divided into 5 groups (A–E), were used.

A) The process of normal columnar development was examined in four monkeys aged from 1 to 6 weeks. At one week, there was both an anatomical and a physiological mixing of left- and right-eye inputs to layer IVC, but the basic columnar pattern was evident, and some small regions were already monocular. At three weeks the columnar pattern resembled that seen in the adult, except for a suggestion that the borders between columns were not so sharply demarcated. By six weeks an adult degree of columnar segregation was established.

B) A series of ten monkeys had monocular suture performed at successively later ages, ranging from 2 days to adult, and they were allowed to survive for a long period. It was found that deprivation begun at any age from birth to about 6 weeks had approximately the same effect: the afferents for the open eye formed greatly expanded columns in layer IVC, and the columns for the closed eye were shrunken and fragmented. In the layers above and below IVC the open eye dominated almost completely. At 10 weeks, closure had only a mild effect on columnar size in layer IVC. With closures at 7–14 months there was no change in the size of columns in layer IVC, but when stained with the Liesegang silver method the deprived-eye columns were paler than those for the open eye, suggesting a lower density of fibers. These late deprivations still caused a shift of ocular dominance in the upper cortical layers but not such an extreme change as with earlier closures. Lid suture in an adult had no detectable anatomical or physiological effects. Even monocular enucleation, in an adult, failed to induce sprouting of the geniculocortical afferents for the remaining eye.

C) In order to investigate the rate at which monocular deprivation produces its effects, six monkeys were examined after short periods of deprivation in infancy. Eye-closure from birth to 3 weeks was sufficient to produce the full anatomical and physiological effects. A nine-day closure at 3 weeks, followed by reopening of the eye, also produced the full effects. A two-week period of deprivation begun at five weeks of age, however, caused relatively mild columnar expansion in layer IVC, suggesting that late closures may require more time to produce anatomical changes than early closures.

D) The effects of reopening the deprived eye and closing the experienced eye (reverse suture) were studied in three monkeys. The initial lid sutures were performed in the first few days of life. With reverse suture at 3 weeks the relative sizes of the two sets of columns were reversed. This anatomical reversal was, however, limited to the afferents from the parvocellular laminae of the LGN; the magnocellular afferents remained in the pattern induced by the early deprivation. The layers outside of IVC were strongly dominated by the initially deprived eye. Reverse suture at 6 weeks allowed an anatomical recovery of the parvocellular afferents to a normal columnar size, but not a complete reversal. Again, the magnocellular afferents for the initially deprived eye were not induced to enlarge their territory. Reverse suture at 1 year of age did not lead to any recovery.

E) One monkey was reared in complete darkness from 3 days of age until 7 weeks of age. This animal, studied autoradiographically, showed a normal columnar pattern in layer IVC.

We draw four conclusions from these experiments. i) Ocular dominance columns are only partially formed at birth but develop rapidly in the first few weeks of postnatal life. The process of segregation of the left- and right-eye afferents in layer IV occurs in the presence or absence of visual experience. ii) This developmental process may be redirected by early monocular deprivation, causing the segregation of the two sets of afferents into columns of unequal width. iii) A rearrangement of the afferents can be induced for a short period after their segregation is complete. This is true of both normal and deprived animals. iv) The eye preference of neurons in the upper and lower layers may be changed even after plasticity in layer-IVC is no longer detectable.

Visual experience seems not to play a major role in the development of the mammalian visual system, at least up to the level of the striate cortex. This is most obvious for animals that are visually competent at birth: neurons in the visual cortex of newborn macaque monkeys (Wiesel and Hubel, '74) and lambs (Ramachandran et al., '77) have receptive field properties hardly distinguishable from those of mature animals. In cats, born with closed eyes and immature brains, cortical receptive field properties are not adult-like at birth, but continue to develop normally for several weeks postnatally, whether or not the eyes are permitted to open (Sherk and Stryker, '76).

In spite of this innate tendency towards a normal functional organization, certain forms of visual deprivation in early life lead to alterations or deficits in cortical structure and function. Binocular deprivation, if continued for several months, causes a secondary deterioration in the responsiveness and selectivity of cortical neurons. Monocular deprivation—the main subject of the present study—causes a loss of responsiveness to stimulation of the deprived eye and a corresponding increase in the influence of the experienced eye (Wiesel and Hubel, '63). An anatomical basis for this effect has been demonstrated (Hubel et al., '77) by the use of techniques that permit the visualization of ocular dominance columns, the cortical domains innervated by geniculo-cortical afferents serving the left and right eyes (Hubel and Wiesel, '72; Wiesel et al., '74; LeVay et al., '75; Shatz et al., '77). In normal monkeys the columns for the left and right eyes are, in surface view, bands of equal width (about 400 μm) that alternate with each other to form a rather constant overall pattern in area 17. In animals reared with one eye closed the overall pattern of columns is normal but the columns for the experienced eye are abnormally wide (about 550 μm), whereas those for the deprived eye are shrunken and interrupted (Hubel et al., '77; Shatz and Stryker, '78).

Such plasticity is certainly related to development since it is limited to a relatively short period in the animal's early life (Hubel and Wiesel, '70), yet the nature of the developmental processes that permit it, and later terminate it, is obscure. A clue to the problem, at least as it relates to the effects of monocular deprivation, is offered by recent observations on early stages in the growth of geniculocortical afferents. In 1-week-old monkeys (Hubel et al., '77) we found by use of the autoradiographic method that the afferents for the two eyes are partially intermixed in layer IVC, and recordings showed a mixing of left- and right-eye responses, although the basic columnar pattern was already evident. Rakic ('76) has extended the autoradiographic observations to fetal monkeys: initially the two sets of afferents are completely intermingled, but traces of a columnar organization are detectable by about 3 weeks before birth. A similar sequence of events has been observed in the cat (LeVay et al., '78). In this species complete overlap of left- and right-eye afferents persists until 2 weeks postnatally. Segregation into columns begins at about 3 weeks and is completed by about 7 weeks of age. Before segregation begins most fourth-layer neurons are about equally responsive to stimulation of either eye, suggesting that afferents establish functional connections in the early, overlapping pattern. In adult cats many fourth-layer neurons are monocular. Columnar development therefore seems likely to involve the breakage and re-formation of functional synapses.

In an attempt to link the plastic and developmental processes, it was suggested (Hubel et al., '77) that geniculocortical afferents connected to a seeing eye could hold on to an abnormally large amount of cortical territory, at the expense of the closed eye, but could not sprout back into regions that they had already vacated. This would mean that monocular deprivation can affect the course of columnar segregation but cannot alter an established pattern. According to this hypothesis the effects of monocular deprivation on the fourth layer of the cortex would depend on the anatomical distribution of the afferents at the time that lid suture is performed, and the event that terminates the plasticity of the afferents would be the completion of their segregation into ocular dominance columns. Of course, on the evidence then available, it was not possible to choose between this and a number of other possibilities.

In the present study we have further explored the relationship between developmental processes and plasticity. First, we have studied the time course of postnatal columnar development and compared this with the effects of monocular lid suture performed at successively later ages. Second, we have examined whether, once the afferents for a deprived eye have settled out into their narrow, fragmented columns, they can be induced to sprout back into the territory that they have relinquished. We attempted to do this by opening the deprived eye and closing the experienced eye (reverse suture). This procedure is known to permit a recovery of the physiological influence of the initially deprived eye, if done early enough (Blakemore and Van Sluyters, '74).

Of the several techniques now available for the study of ocular dominance columns, we have relied primarily on two. We have used the transneuronal autoradiographic method (Specht and Grafstein, '73; Wiesel et al., '74) to demonstrate the anatomical distribution of the afferents serving one eye, and microelectrode recording, usually in long tangential penetrations, to determine the eye preference of the target neurons in the fourth layer, as well as that of higher-order neurons in the upper and lower cortical layers. We have also made use, in the more mature animals, of the Liesegang reduced-silver method (LeVay et al., '75). In addition to the study of cortical columns, we have examined the effects of visual deprivation on cell size in the lateral geniculate nucleus.

METHODS

The experimental animals were 26 macaque monkeys, bred at the New England Regional Primate Center. All were rhesus monkeys (Macaca mulatta) except for one pigtailed macaque (M. nemestrina). They fall into five groups, as detailed in Table 1. Group a consisted of four normal animals, ranging in age from 6 days to 6 weeks. The main purpose of studying these animals was to determine the time course of the development of ocular dominance columns. Group B consisted of 12 monkeys that were monocularly deprived, starting at successively later ages, ranging from 2 days to adult. In ten of these, deprivation was produced by lid suture, and in two (both adults), by monocular enucleation. The period of deprivation ranged from 7 weeks to 4 years and was followed in a few cases by the reopening of the deprived eye and a further survival period of 4 to 12 months. The intention with this group was to follow the decline in susceptibility to the effects of lid suture with increasing age, and to compare the time course of the decline with that of normal columnar development. The third group (C—five monkeys) underwent short periods of monocular deprivation in the first few weeks of life. The object here was to determine how fast the anatomical effects of monocular deprivation developed. The animals in group D (three monkeys) were also monocularly deprived from the first week of life, but at varying times thereafter the deprived eye was reopened and the experienced eye sutured shut. The animals were then allowed to survive until 9 months to 3.5 years of age. It was intended, by comparing results in this group with those from the third group, to determine whether reverse suture could cause a reexpansion of shrunken columns. Finally, one monkey (E) was raised in complete darkness from 3 days to 7 weeks of age.

Most of the animals were studied both autoradiographically and physiologically. In a typical case, the monkey received an injection of ^{3}H-proline (2 mCi of 2,3-[^{3}H]L-proline, specific activity 20–40 Ci/mmole, in 50 μl of normal saline) into the vitreous of one eye, 1–2 weeks before a terminal physiological experiment. The eye injection was done under combined ketamine/pentobarbital anesthesia, and the labeled compound was delivered over 5–10 minutes through a 27-gauge needle, which was inserted through the sclera just behind the ora serrata at the lateral margin of the eye. In some experiments, a mixture of tritiated proline and fucose was injected. When lid-sutured eyes were injected, the lids were not reopened: The injection was made through a skin inci-

Table 1. Summary of Experimental Protocols and Key to Figures

No.	Age at closure	Age at reopening	Age at reversal	Age at death	Eye injected	Side of recording	Figures
A 230	—	—	—	6 days	L	—	1
243	—	—	—	8 days	—	R	2
256	—	—	—	3 weeks	R	R	3, 4
257	—	—	—	6 weeks	R	L	5–7
B 201	2 days	7 weeks	—	7 months	R	—	8
206	11 days	—	—	6 months	R	L	9, 10
157	2 weeks	—	—	18 months	L	L	11–13
202	3 weeks	—	—	6 months	R	L,R	14, 15
282	5.5 weeks	16 months	—	20 months	L	R	16–18
365	10 weeks	—	—	6 months	L	R	19–21
198	7 months	4 years	—	5 years	R	—	22
185	1 year	—	—	2 years	—	L	25
286	14 months	28 months	—	33 months	L	—	23, 24
280	6 years	—	—	7.5 years	L	R	26, 27
150	adult (enucl.)	—	—	6 months post-op.	—	L	—
269	adult (enucl.)	—	—	4 months post-op.	L	—	28
C 164	8 days	—	—	20 days	L	R	30
308	2 days	—	—	24 days	R	L	31, 32
316	2 days	—	—	23 days	L	—	—
307	4 days	—	—	47 days	R	R	33, 34
195	21 days	30 days	—	4 years	—	L	35, 36
213	5 weeks	7 weeks	—	10 weeks	L	—	37
D 240	2 days	—	3 weeks	9 months	R	R	38–40
194	3 days	—	6 weeks	6 months	R	L	41–43
203	7 days	—	1 year	3.5 years	R	R	44, 45
E 266	3 days (darkness)	—	—	7 weeks	R	—	46

sion lateral to the lateral canthus. Methods for physiological recording were as described previously (Hubel and Wiesel, '68). Usually an attempt was made to aim the electrode penetrations so that they ran for some distance tangentially in the fourth layer of the exposed, opercular region of area 17 (LeVay et al., '75; Hubel et al., '77). Points of transition in ocular dominance were marked with small electrolytic lesions (1 µA for 1 second).

The animals were perfused with 10% formol-saline. Blocks taken from area 17 and from the lateral geniculate nucleus were left in the same fixative for a week, sunk in 30% sucrose in formol-saline, and frozen-sectioned at 20 µm. The cortical blocks were usually taken in such a way as to permit sectioning in a plane tangential to the exposed opercular region of area 17. The sections were processed for autoradiography, using Kodak NTB2 emulsion and Kodak D19 developer. Exposure times were from 1 to 6 months. Development conditions were adjusted so as to maximize labeling density while keeping background at acceptable levels. A 3-minute development at 23°C was often found best. Interspersed with the autoradiographs, sections were stained with thionin and sometimes with the Liesegang reduced-silver method (LeVay et al., '75).

Low-power, dark-field micrographs were obtained from the tangential autoradiographs with a high intensity light source (Sage Instruments model 281) and a camera equipped with a macro lens and bellows extension. Prints were made of every fourth section (i.e., every 80 µm). Reconstructions of the columnar labeling pattern were made by carefully tearing the region out of each print that included layer IVC and gluing the series together to make a montage, which was rephotographed without retouching.

For the measurement of columnar area, the labeling pattern was traced from the original montages onto heavy acetate film of uniform thickness, cut into left- and right-eye columns, and weighed. The area measured was generally the same as that shown in the figures—about 50 mm^2 in most cases.

For the reconstruction of electrode tracks a separate series of micrographs was taken at higher magnification, from both the autoradiographs and the interspersed Nissl sections. It was generally necessary to photograph every section that included a portion of the track. In these micrographs, large, transversely sectioned blood vessels were visible, and these were used as fiducial marks for the subsequent tracing of the track, the electrolytic lesions, and the autoradiographic labeling pattern. Finally, the position of all recording sites was calculated from the readings on the electrode advancer and from the positions of the lesions, and the ocular dominance of the activity recorded at each site (while the electrode was traveling tangentially in layer IVC) was added to the reconstruction.

The eye preference of neurons recorded in layers above and below layer IVC was tabulated in the form of ocular dominance histograms. From each histogram was derived a figure (ocular dominance index) representing the overall balance between the two eyes in that animal. The ocular dominance index is simply the mean ocular dominance value for all neurons recorded outside of layer IVC. The index is somewhat artificial, based as it is on a nonquantitative estimate of ocular dominance for each cell, but it is a useful means of comparison between different animals.

For the measurement of cell size in the LGN, coronal sections from the middle of the anteroposterior extent of the nucleus were stained with cresylviolet. The outlines of 100 cells in the middle of lamina 6 were drawn at a magnification of 2,000 ×, using a microscope with a camera lucida attachment, and the same number were drawn in the adjacent region of lamina 5. Thus for most animals a total of 400 cells were measured. In a few animals the measurements were extended to the other laminae, making a total of 1,200 cells per animal. The mean cross-sectional area for cells in each lamina was then determined with the help of a PDP-11 computer equipped with a graphic tablet. It should be stressed that preparative techniques varied considerably (for example, celloidin rather than frozen sections were occasionally used), and absolute differences in cell size between animals probably reflect these variations.

RESULTS

A. Normal Development

In order to establish the time course of normal development of ocular dominance columns, five monkeys, extending in age from 6 days to 6 weeks, were examined.

SIX DAYS (No. 230). Results for the two youngest monkeys, examined at 6 and 8 days of age, have been described in detail previously (Hubel et al., '77) and will only be summarized here. The 6-day-old monkey (No. 230) had received an eye injection of [^{3}H]fucose on the day after birth, and it died 5 days later. Autoradiography of tangential sections of area 17, ipsilateral to the injected eye, showed a banding pattern suggestive of ocular dominance columns (Fig. 1), but it was an extremely blurred pattern compared with that seen in the adult. The density of grains in layer IVC waxed and waned gently without ever dropping towards background levels. On the contralateral side only parasagittal sections were taken. In these sections layer IVC appeared uniformly labeled throughout its extent, with no hint of any columnar pattern of labeling (not illustrated; see Fig. 25A of Hubel et al., '77).

EIGHT DAYS (No. 243). This monkey was studied physiologically at 8 days of age, but no eye injection was made. A reconstruction of the four electrode penetrations, along with the ocular dominance of units or unresolved background activity recorded, is shown in Figure 2. Just as one might have imagined from the autoradiographic results in the previous animal, there was much more mixing of right- and left-eye activity in the fourth layer than there is in the adult, and at some of the recording sites binocularly activated single cells were recorded. These cells, like those recorded in layer IVC in the adult monkey, lacked orientation specificity. Nevertheless, there was on the whole a clear grouping of cells according to eye preference, and for one stretch of about 300 μm the contralateral eye dominated completely. It should be emphasized that, with the electrodes used in the present study, single units were not often isolated in layer IVC. The ocular dominance values given in the figures refer mostly to the overall eye preference of the multi-unit activity recorded at each site.

THREE WEEKS (No. 256). The right eye of this monkey was injected with [^{3}H]proline when it was 13 days old, and recordings were made 8 days later when it was 3 weeks old. In this and subsequent

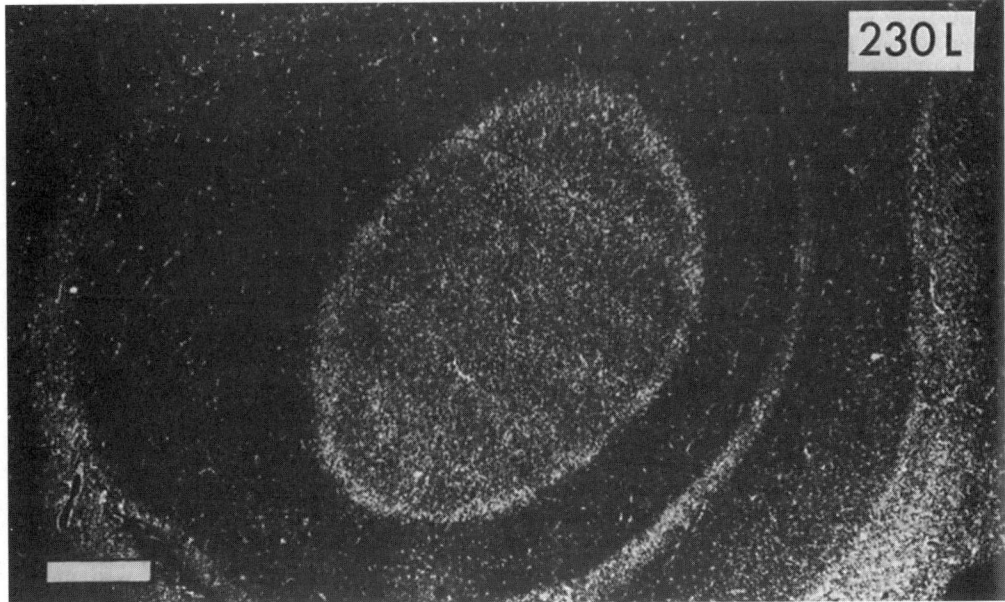

Fig. 1. Dark-field micrograph of autoradiographic labeling pattern in the striate cortex of a normal 6-day-old monkey, ipsilateral to the eye that had been injected with [³H]fucose 5 days earlier. This is a single section that grazes layer IVC tangentially in the central oval region. Silver grains are distributed continuously over layer IVC, but there are bands of alternating higher and lower grain density, indicating that afferents for the two eyes are already in the process of columnar segregation. In this and subsequent figures, the number and letter give the animal's identification number and the side of the brain illustrated. The unlabeled bar is 1 mm in all figures. From Hubel et al. ('77).

monkeys the autoradiographic results will be presented first, because the findings from the tangential electrode penetrations can be best understood in terms of the distribution of left- and right-eye afferents existing in that animal.

Ocular dominance columns were clearly visible in layer IVC on both sides of the brain (Fig. 3). On the right side (ipsilateral to the injection) the columnar pattern was almost as clear as it is in adults, while on the left (contralateral) side the pattern was still rather blurred.

Two tangential electrode penetrations were made into the right hemisphere. During the passages through layer IVC eye preference swung between complete contralateral (O.D. group 1) and complete ipsilateral (group 7) eye dominance. This is illustrated for penetration No. 2 in Figure 4, which shows a Nissl preparation with two marking lesions, autoradiographs of two neighboring sections, and a reconstruction of the same region of the electrode track, with the ocular dominance of the neuronal activity recorded at each site. The

transitions in eye preference were slightly less abrupt than is seen in adult monkeys. At one recording site a binocular single unit was recorded (O.D. group 5), but most of the recordings were of the massed background activity ('hash') that is characteristic of layer IVC.

THREE WEEKS (No. 202). Another monkey (No. 202) was studied physiologically at the same age. It did not receive an eye injection and after the recording session it was resuscitated to be used as part of the deprivation series (see section B). A single short pass-through layer IVC yielded strictly monocular responses (see Fig. 27 of Hubel et al., '77), and in other layers an adult-like pattern of ocular dominance was also evident. The results from this animal were useful, not only in confirming that the development of ocular dominance columns is complete, or nearly so, by 3 weeks of age, but also in demonstrating that the eye injections do not themselves cause any obvious alteration in the rate of columnar development.

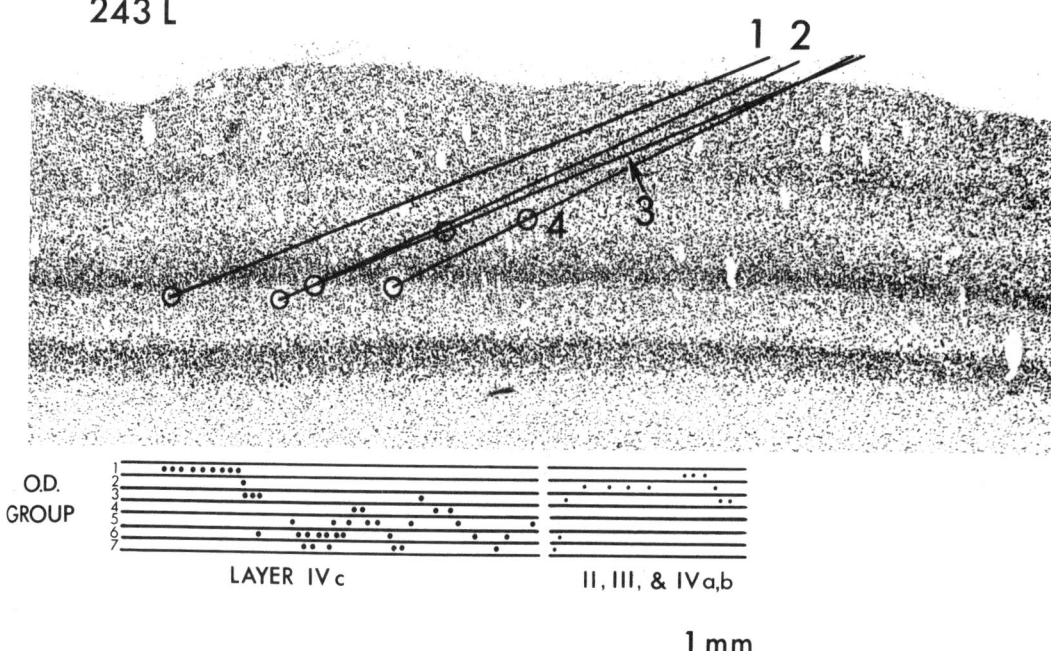

Fig. 2. Reconstruction of four electrode penetrations into the striate cortex of a normal 8-day-old monkey. The four penetrations were made in the same parasagittal plane. The circles indicate the positions of marking lesions. The ocular dominance of all activity recorded in layer IVC has been plotted as a function of cortical position, below left. Unlike the situation in adults, binocular multi-unit activity could be recorded at many sites, although a columnar organization was already evident, and the region at the extreme left was already influenced only by one eye (the contralateral eye). The smaller right-hand portion of the graph shows the ocular dominance of units recorded in the upper cortical layers during the same penetrations. A columnar organization is suggested here too. From Hubel et al. ('77).

SIX WEEKS (No. 257). The final monkey of this group, No. 257, received an injection of [³H]proline into the right eye at 30 days of age, and recordings were made 12 days later when it was 6 weeks old. The autoradiographic labeling pattern in the visual cortex (Figs. 5 and 6) was very similar to that seen in the adult. The pattern was slightly less sharp in the left hemisphere than in the right hemisphere: this was due to the presence of more label in the gaps between the labeled columns.

One penetration was made into the left hemisphere (Fig. 7). The electrode traveled 2.26 mm tangentially in layer IVC, recording only non-oriented responses. For the first 1.50 mm of this pass, activity was completely dominated by the left eye (group 7). Then (lesion No. 1) there was a rapid shift to the right eye, which dominated completely for 600 μm, after which there was another reversal, shortly before the electrode entered the fifth layer. The marking lesions, accompanying autoradiographs and track reconstruction are shown in Figure 7. It may be noted that the changeover between the two eyes occurred over a distance of not more than 100 μm. Such very narrow zones of

Fig. 3. Autoradiographic labeling pattern in the right and left hemisphere of a normal 3-week-old monkey. The upper half of the figure is a montage of tangential sections from the right hemisphere (ipsilateral to the injected eye); the lower half is a single section from the left hemisphere. The autoradiographs show a columnar pattern that is much advanced over that seen at 1 week (Fig. 1). The only difference from the normal adult pattern is a slight blurring of the margins of the labeled bands, suggesting a modest intermixing of left- and right-eye afferents at the borders of ocular dominance columns. The boxed area indicates the region of an electrode penetration, reconstructed in Figure 4.

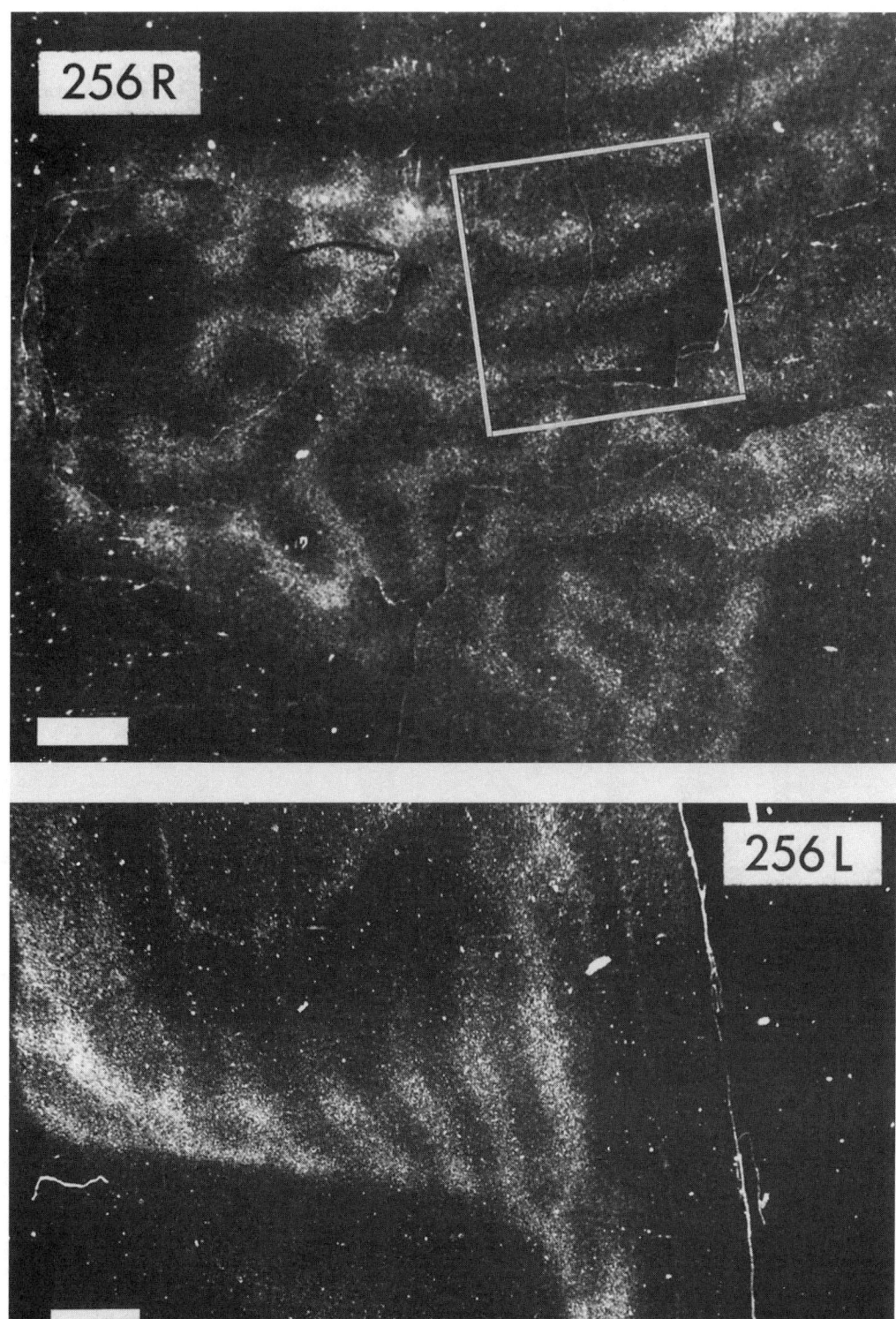

Fig. 3.

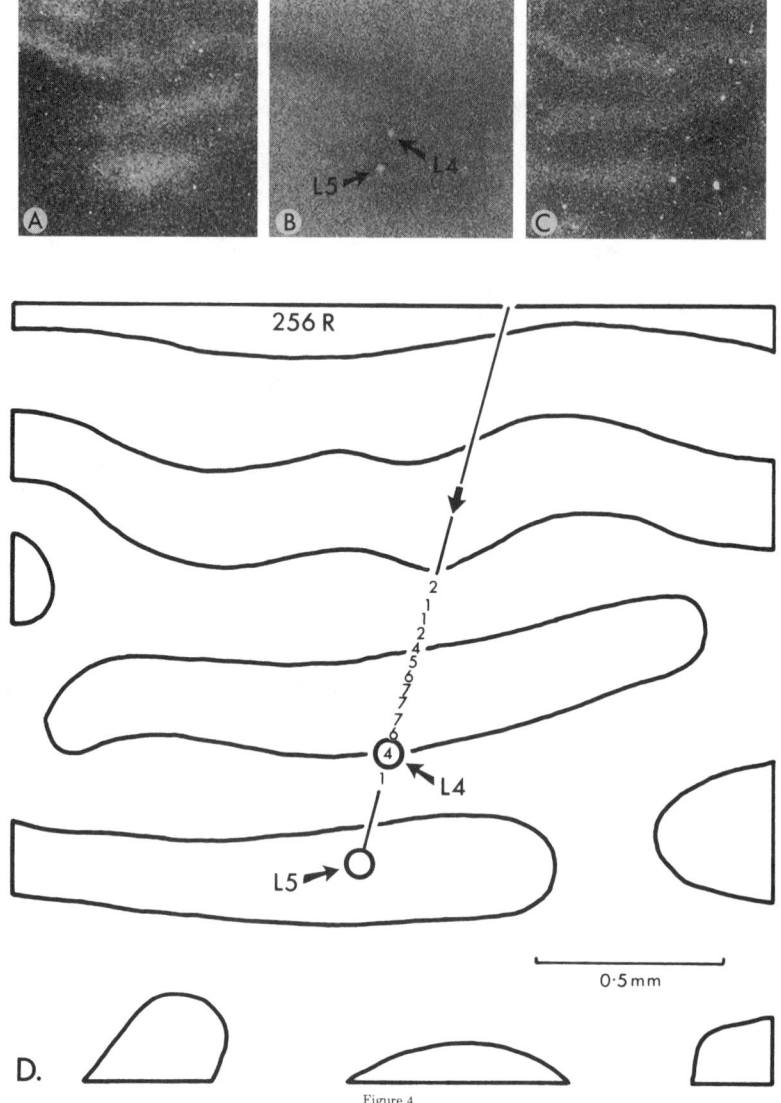

Figure 4

Fig. 4. Reconstruction of a tangential electrode penetration in a normal 3-week-old monkey (see boxed area in Fig. 3). In this and all subsequent track reconstructions the following conventions are adopted. The track is shown as a straight line except for the region where it traverses layer IVC, where it is shown as a string of numbers. Each of these numbers indicates the ocular dominance of a unit or (more commonly) the multi-unit activity recorded at that position on the track. The circles indicate the positions of electrolytic lesions. Often (as with lesion 4 in this figure) the lesions were placed to mark the transition in ocular dominance from one eye to the other. Lesions were also often placed at the ends of penetrations (as with lesion 5 in this figure). The pattern of autoradiographic labeling in the region of the track is also reconstructed. The labeled regions are closed off at the edges of the figure; the unlabeled regions are left open. The micrographs (A–C) are part of the series on which the reconstruction is based. B is a cresylviolet-stained section showing the positions of lesions 4 and 5. A and C are autoradiographs of neighboring sections. Registration between sections was achieved by lining up large, vertically oriented blood vessels.

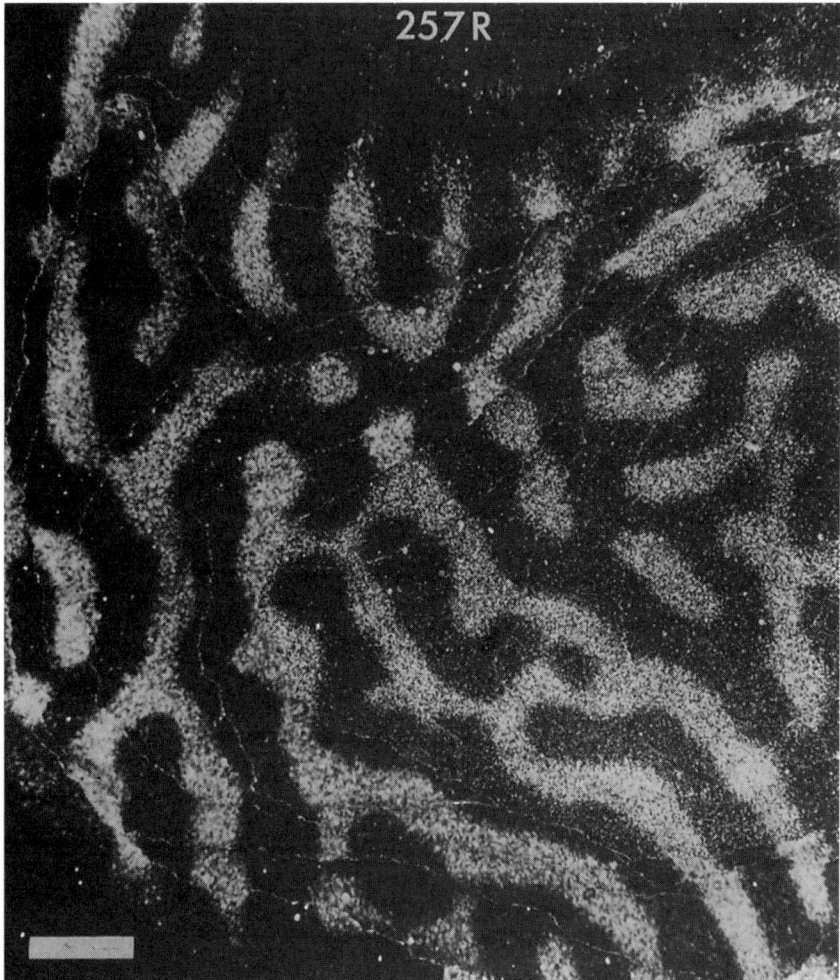

Fig. 5. Autoradiographic montage from a 6-week-old normal monkey, ipsilateral to the injected eye. The labeled bands are as sharply defined as in adults.

overlap are seen in normal adults and may represent an actual mixing of left- and right-eye activity at the border or, more likely, may mainly reflect the size of the uninsulated electrode tip.

Comment

These findings indicate that geniculocortical afferents for the left and right eyes show substantial overlap at birth, are nearly completely segregated at 3 weeks of age, and have reached the mature columnar organization at 6 weeks of age. There are some reasons to think that the process of segregation occurs rather more rapidly than is suggested by the autoradiographs. First, there is evidence

from work on the cat that the leakage of label between laminae of the lateral geniculate nucleus degrades the cortical labeling pattern in young animals, especially on the side contralateral to the injected eye (LeVay et al., '78). Second, the physiological results, while generally in good agreement with the anatomy, gave no hint of a residual presence of contralateral eye afferents in ipsilateral eye columns at 6 weeks of age (see Fig. 7). These issues will be taken up more fully in the Discussion.

B. Effects of Monocular Deprivation begun at Successively Later Ages

This section describes the results of experiments on monkeys that had one eye closed at ages ranging

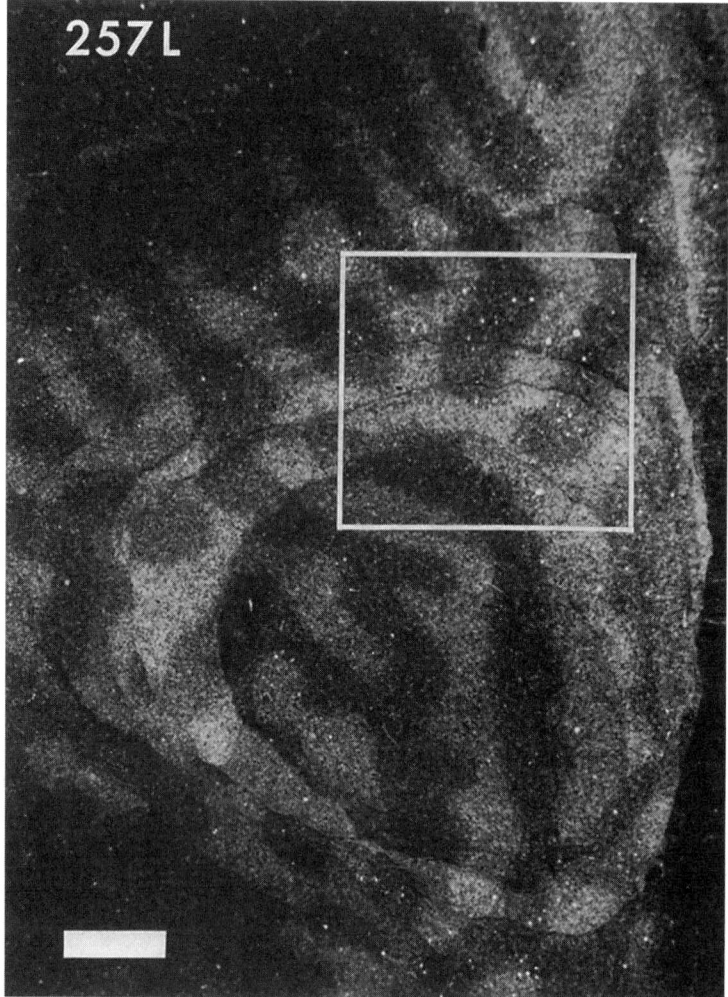

Fig. 6. Autoradiographic montage for the same 6-week-old monkey, contralateral to the injected eye. The labeled bands are slightly less well defined than ipsilaterally, owing to the presence of a certain amount of label in the gaps between them. This may be attributable to spillover of radioactivity between laminae of the LGN (see text). An electrode penetration was made in the boxed area (see Fig. 7).

from 2 days to adult, and that were allowed to survive for a substantial period thereafter. The right eye was closed in every case. The intent was to determine whether there was a clear relationship between the effects of eye closure and the state of columnar segregation existing at the time of operation, as predicted by our hypothesis (see introduction). Although the exact length of the survival period varied from animal to animal, and was even in some cases followed by a surgical reopening of the deprived eye, for the purpose of behavioral test-

ing (see Table 1 for details) we believe that the age at which the initial operation was performed was the most important variable and was responsible for most if not all of the differences observed in the different experiments (see Discussion). The major quantitative results from these monkeys—the ocular dominance index derived from recordings (excluding layer IVC), the ratio of column areas derived from the autoradiographic montages, and the mean size of cells in laminae 5 and 6 of the LGN—are summarized in Table 2.

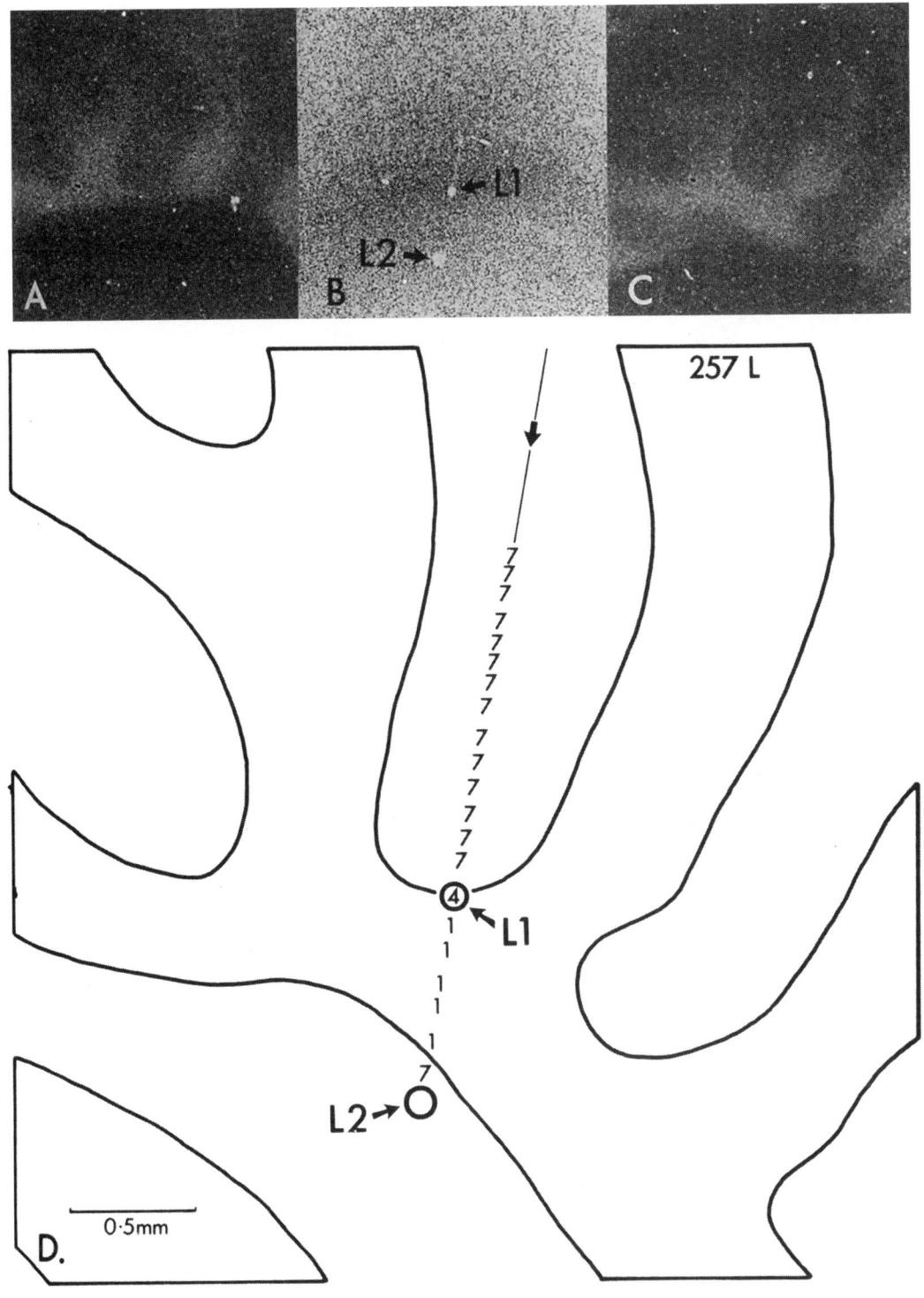

Fig. 7.

Table 2. Quantitative Physiological and Anatomical Results for the Animals in Section B

| No. | OCULAR DOMINANCE INDEX | | RATIO OF COLUMN AREAS | | LGN CELL SIZE (μM²) | | | |
	L	R	L	R	L6 (dep.)	L5	R6	R5 (dep.)
201	—	—	—	—	(unavailable)			
206	1.42	—	3.8:1	3.3:1	140	204	198	140
157	2.05	—	3.2:1	—	128	184	150	108
202	1.80	2.03	1.6:1	2.2:1	156	197	184	154
282	—	1.10	3.2:1	3.8:1	171	250	213	151
365	—	1.80	1.0:1	1.6:1	172	191	210	177
198	—	—	—	—	144	182	175	137*
185	2.75	—	—	—	165	172	172	173
286	—	—	1.0:1	1.0:1	198	202	183	168
280	—	3.95	0.9:1	1.1:1	192	194	199	204
150	—	—	—	—	(unavailable)			
269	—	—	1.0:1	1.0:1	128	186	177	103

The headings L and R refer to the side of the brain studied, not the left and right eyes. The ocular dominance index is a measure of average ocular dominance of all cells recorded in each hemisphere *with the exception of those in layer IVC*. Figures from recordings in the left hemisphere have been reversed, so that in all cases an index of 1.0 would represent complete dominance of the left (experienced) eye and an index of 7.0 would represent complete dominance of the right (deprived eye). The ratio of column areas is the ratio of left-eye to right-eye areas in the autoradiographic reconstruction (usually the same reconstructions that are reproduced in the illustrations). The ratio was obtained by tracing the original photomontage onto acetate film, and cutting and weighing the labeled and unlabeled areas. The LGN cell sizes were obtained tracing 100 cells from the middle of each lamina onto a graphic tablet connected to a PDP-11 computer. The laminae innervated by the deprived eye are indicated (dep.)

* The apparent deprivation effect on cell size in monkey No. 198 is probably an artifact reflecting damage to the retina of the right eye during the injection of isotope (see text).

TWO DAYS (No. 201). The first monkey in this series underwent lid suture of the right eye at 2 days of age, that is, at an age when there exists a pronounced overlap of the left- and right-eye afferents in layer IVC. The eye was reopened at 7 weeks of age, and at 7 months of age the same eye was injected with tritiated proline and fucose. The monkey was perfused 15 days later, without recordings being made. (From our previous experience we would expect the left eye to be strongly dominant in the cortex of this animal; the later reopening of the right eye was not likely to have affected the physiological balance between the eyes.)

The eye injection was only partially successful: a small part of the ipsilateral LGN, and a corresponding region of cortex in the ipsilateral calcarine fissure, were labeled. Nevertheless the labeling in this region of cortex was excellent (Fig. 8). The labeled patches were about 200 μm across and separated by gaps about 600 μm in width (uncorrected for shrinkage). In addition, the labeled patches seemed mostly to be confined to the lower part of layer IVC, called IVCβ, which

Fig. 7. Electrode penetration in the cortex of a normal 6-week-old monkey (enlargement of boxed area in Fig. 6). B is a cresylviolet-stained section showing two lesions. A and C are neighboring sections processed for autoradiography. D is a reconstruction of the track (conventions the same as for Fig. 4). For the first part of the traverse through layer IVC the electrode was moving lengthwise along the middle of an unlabeled band (column for the ipsilateral eye), and responses were completely dominated by that eye (O.D. group 7). At the point marked by lesion 1 equal activity from both eyes was recorded (O.D. group 4). The lesion lay exactly on the border of a labeled band. Group 1 activity was recorded as the electrode crossed that band, followed by another reversal to group 7 (not marked by a lesion) as it moved into a second unlabeled band. Shortly thereafter (lesion 2) the electrode entered layer V.

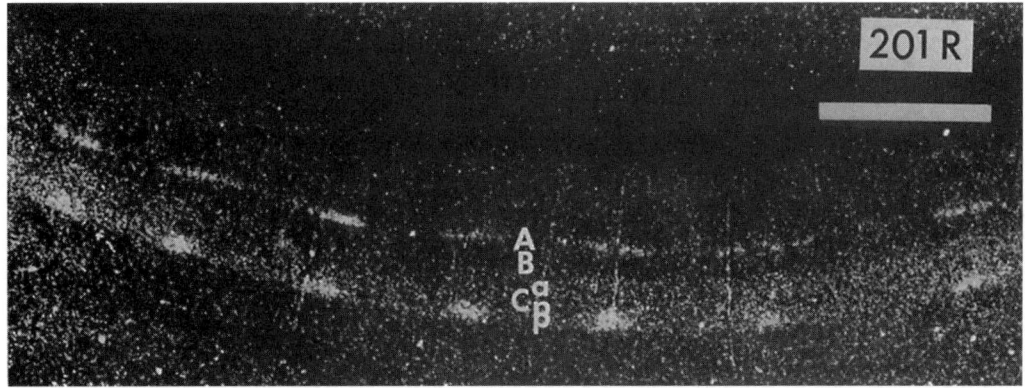

Fig. 8. Autoradiograph from the right cortex of a monkey (No. 201) whose right eye was closed from 2 days of age to 7 weeks of age. The eye was then reopened, and at 7 months it was injected with [³H]proline. This is a single section, cut perpendicular to the layers in the cortex of the calcarine fissure, i.e., in the representation of the far periphery of the visual field. The columns for the deprived eye are markedly reduced in width in layer IVC but appear comparatively intact in the upper tier, layer IVA. From Hubel et al. ('77).

receives afferents from the parvocellular laminae (3–6) of the LGN (Hubel and Wiesel, '72). Many of the patches did not extend up into IVCα, which receives input from the magnocellular laminae (1 and 2) of the LGN. This picture suggested that the deprived magnocellular afferents had been even more severely affected than the parvocellular afferents. It should however be borne in mind that in normal animals layer IVCα is more lightly labeled than is IVCβ, so that the residual input from the deprived magnocellular lamina may have been somewhat more extensive than is suggested by Figure 8. The input to layer IVA (whose innervation is from the parvocellular laminae of the LGN) seemed relatively less affected by the closure. We have, however, observed changes in column width in this layer in other monocularly deprived monkeys.

ELEVEN DAYS (No. 206). This monkey's right eye was closed at 11 days of age. At 6 months an injection of tritiated proline and fucose was made into the same eye, and recordings were made 14 days later.

The autoradiography showed marked shrinkage of the right-eye columns on both sides of the brain (Fig. 9, Table 2). The shrinkage was perhaps not quite so severe as in the previous monkey: In particular, the labeled columns were clearly visible in both sublaminae of layer IVC.

Two penetrations were made into the left hemisphere. In both penetrations the experienced (left) eye dominated almost completely in the layers outside of layer IVC, as shown in histogram form in Figure 10. The few cells responsive to the right eye were encountered in the upper part of layer IV. In layer IVC a combined traverse of 5 mm yielded only four short regions (50–150 μm long) in which response to stimulation of the right eye could be obtained, and even within these regions the influence of the left eye never entirely disappeared. It is not clear whether this overlap of activity was caused by a true extension of the left-eye afferents through the right-eye regions, or whether it was due to limited electrophysiological resolution within the diminutive right eye columns.

TWO WEEKS (No. 157). Monkey No. 157 has been described in detail previously (Hubel et al., '77—monkey No. 3). The right eye was closed from 2 weeks to 18 months of age. The left eye was injected with tritiated proline and fucose, and lesions were made in single laminae of the LGN (for the purpose of demonstrating cortical columns for both eyes with the Nauta method). Recordings were made from the right hemisphere.

The autoradiographic labeling pattern is shown for the left hemisphere in Figure 11. The labeled bands—corresponding to ocular dominance columns for the open eye—were about 2.5

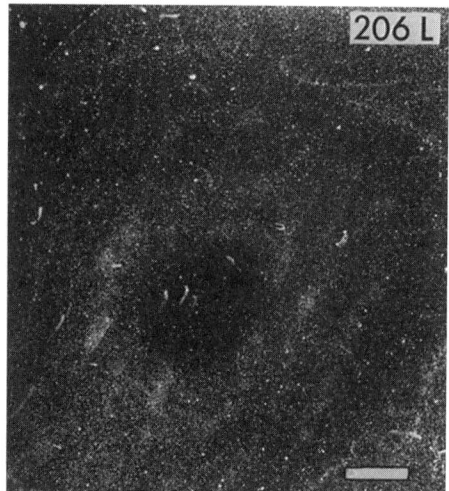
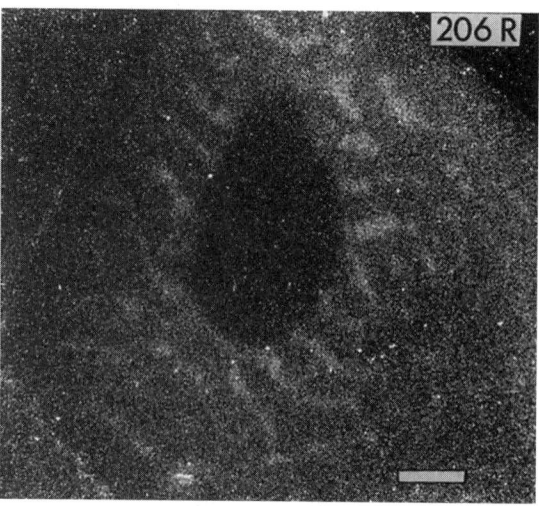

Fig. 9. Autoradiographs of single tangential sections from the left and right opercular cortex of a monkey (No. 206) whose right eye was closed at 11 days of age. The same eye was injected with [³H]proline at 6 months of age. There is clear shrinkage of the right-eye columns. The shrinkage appears somewhat less than in monkey No. 201 (Fig. 8), but this may be due to the difference in the region of cortex studied and the plane of section, rather than to the difference in the age at suture.

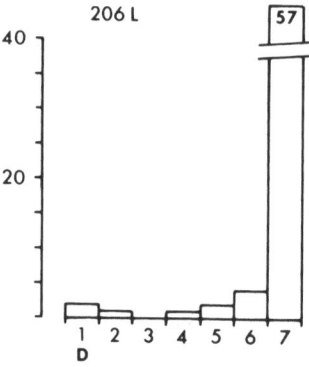

Fig. 10. Ocular dominance histogram for cells recorded in monkey No. 206. In the compilation of this and subsequent O.D. histograms, cells recorded in layer IVC have been excluded. The letter D indicates the side of the histogram corresponding to dominance by the deprived eye. Of the 67 neurons recorded only 10 were influenced by the deprived eye, and these were situated in the upper part of layer IV.

hemisphere only parasagittal sections were taken. These showed a deprivation effect that was if anything even more marked, but in the absence of tangential sections the ratio of the areas could not be measured. On this side it was possible to trace afferents for the deprived eye also, by making use of the single-lamina lesions in the LGN. These projected exactly to the narrow gaps in the band of autoradiographic label (not illustrated—see Fig. 18 of Hubel et al., '77).

The physiological results for this animal have also been described previously. To summarize: most cells in the upper layers were driven exclusively from the left eye (Fig. 12). In layer IVC there were alternations between complete right-eye and complete left-eye dominance. The stretches in which the right eye dominated were very short, and lesions showed them to correspond exactly to the gaps in the autoradiographic labeling pattern (Fig. 13).

THREE WEEKS (No. 202). The next monkey was also described in our previous paper (Hubel et al., '77—monkey No. 4). Its right eye was closed at 3 weeks of age, i.e., at a time when the columnar system has very nearly reached its mature state of

times wider than the unlabeled bands, and the latter were not only shrunken but also markedly fragmented. The overall ratio of labeled to unlabeled areas (open-eye to deprived-eye columns) in the reconstruction was 3.23, compared with a figure of 1.05 obtained from a normal adult. In the right

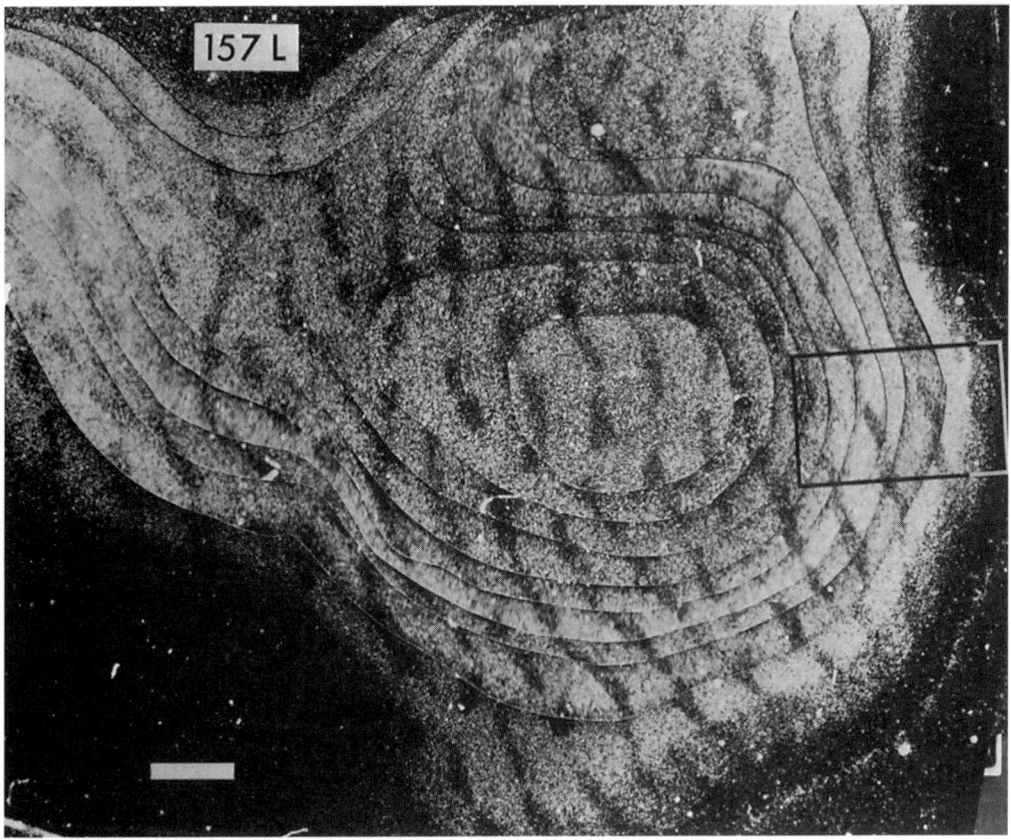

Fig. 11. Autoradiographic montage from a monkey (No. 157) whose right eye was closed at 2 weeks of age. The left eye was injected 18 months later. The reconstruction shows expansion of the labeled columns for the open eye and shrinkage of the unlabeled columns for the deprived eye, with preservation of the normal columnar periodicity (about 750 μm for a left-right pair). The overall pattern is also normal: the columns are oriented orthogonal to the 17–18 border, which runs along the top of the figure. The boxed area indicates the region of an electrode penetration that is reconstructed in Figure 13.

development (compare normal monkey No. 256, Figs. 3 and 4). This is the animal, mentioned in section A, from which we recorded twice: once at 3 weeks, immediately before the lid suture, and once in a terminal experiment when it was 6 months old.

Before the final experiment the right (deprived) eye was injected with tritiated proline and fucose. The labeling pattern in the right cortex is shown in Figure 14. There was again a marked deprivation effect, although it was less pronounced than in the previous animals, particularly on the left side. The ratio of unlabeled to labeled areas (columns for experienced and deprived eyes) was 2.16:1 on the right side and 1.6:1 on the left side.

Long tangential penetration was made in both hemispheres. As with the previous monkey, the experienced (left) eye dominated very strongly in the upper layers (Fig. 15), and in layer IVC there were alternations in eye preference that could be matched to the autoradiography (not illustrated).

FIVE AND ONE-HALF WEEKS (No. 282). Since monkey No. 202 showed a marked effect of deprivation, even though columnar segregation was probably all but complete at the time of lid suture, we went on to study animals deprived at even later ages. Monkey No. 282 had its right eye closed at 5.5 weeks of age, i.e., at a time when we are confident

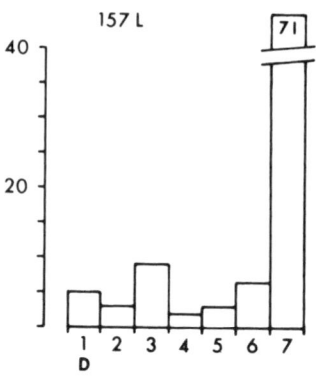

Fig. 12. Ocular dominance histogram for 100 cells recorded on four penetrations in monkey No. 157 (cells in layer IVC excluded).

that columnar segregation is complete (compare normal monkey No. 257, section A). This eye was reopened at 16 months of age and recordings were made 4 months later. The left eye was injected with [³H]proline 18 days before the experiment.

The autoradiography showed a very marked expansion of the left-eye columns on both sides of the brain (Fig. 16, Table 2). The unlabeled areas were not only narrow but also very fragmented, especially on the right side of the brain where the columnar pattern was all but obliterated. The ratio of labeled to unlabeled areas (experienced- to deprived-eye columns) was 3.2:1 on the left side and 3.8:1 on the right side.

This markedly abnormal picture was fully supported by the physiology. Two penetrations were made into the right hemisphere. In both, activity in the upper layers was driven almost exclusively by the left eye (Fig. 17), and in layer IVC there were regular alternations between left-eye and right-eye dominance, with the left-eye stretches about 3 times longer than those for the right eye. Figure 18 illustrates one of these penetrations. All in all, the results from this monkey were almost identical to those obtained from monkeys deprived at earlier ages.

TEN WEEKS (No. 365). This animal's right eye was closed at 10 weeks of age. Its left eye was injected with [³H]proline at 6 months of age, and recordings were made 10 days later.

Figure 19 shows the labeling pattern in the cortex. On the left side the labeling pattern was normal (ratio of labeled to unlabeled areas: 1.04:1). On the right side there was a slight but definite expansion of the labeled (open-eye) columns. The ratio of labeled to unlabeled areas in the reconstruction shown in Figure 19 was 1.55:1. This figure was confirmed for a second reconstruction of another region of cortex, also on the right side.

In the recording session 4 penetrations were made into the right hemisphere. In the layers outside of layer IVC there was a strong dominance of the open eye, with 99 out of the 118 recorded cells belonging to O.D. groups 1 or 2 (Fig. 20). The four traverses through layer IVC were all rather short; one of them, which passed through a left-eye column, is reconstructed in Figure 21.

The mild anatomical effects in layer IVC are supported by the measurement of cell size in the LGN (Table 2). On the right side (ipsilateral to the closure) cells in the deprived lamina 5 were 16% smaller than cells in lamina 6. On the left side cells in lamina 6 were 10% smaller than those in lamina 5. In addition, cells in the deprived laminae were noticeably paler than those in laminae innervated by the open eye.

SEVEN MONTHS (No. 198). This monkey's right eye was closed at 7 months of age. It was reopened at 4 years, and 1 year later the same eye was injected with [³H]proline and [³H]fucose. The monkey was perfused 15 days later; no recordings were made.

The eye injection successfully labeled only a small part of the cortex, in the calcarine fissure on the left side. In this region the labeling pattern appeared completely normal (Fig. 22).

ONE YEAR (Nos. 185 AND 286). Two monkeys had lid sutures at about 1 year of age (Table 1). One of these (No. 286) was studied autoradiographically after an injection of [³H]proline into the left (non-deprived) eye. Reconstruction from these autoradiographs (Fig. 23) showed a completely normal cortical labeling pattern. This was confirmed by area measurements: the ratio of labeled to unlabeled areas was 1.00:1 on the left side and 1.05:1 on the right (Table 2).

In spite of the normal autoradiographic pattern in monkey No. 286, the application of the

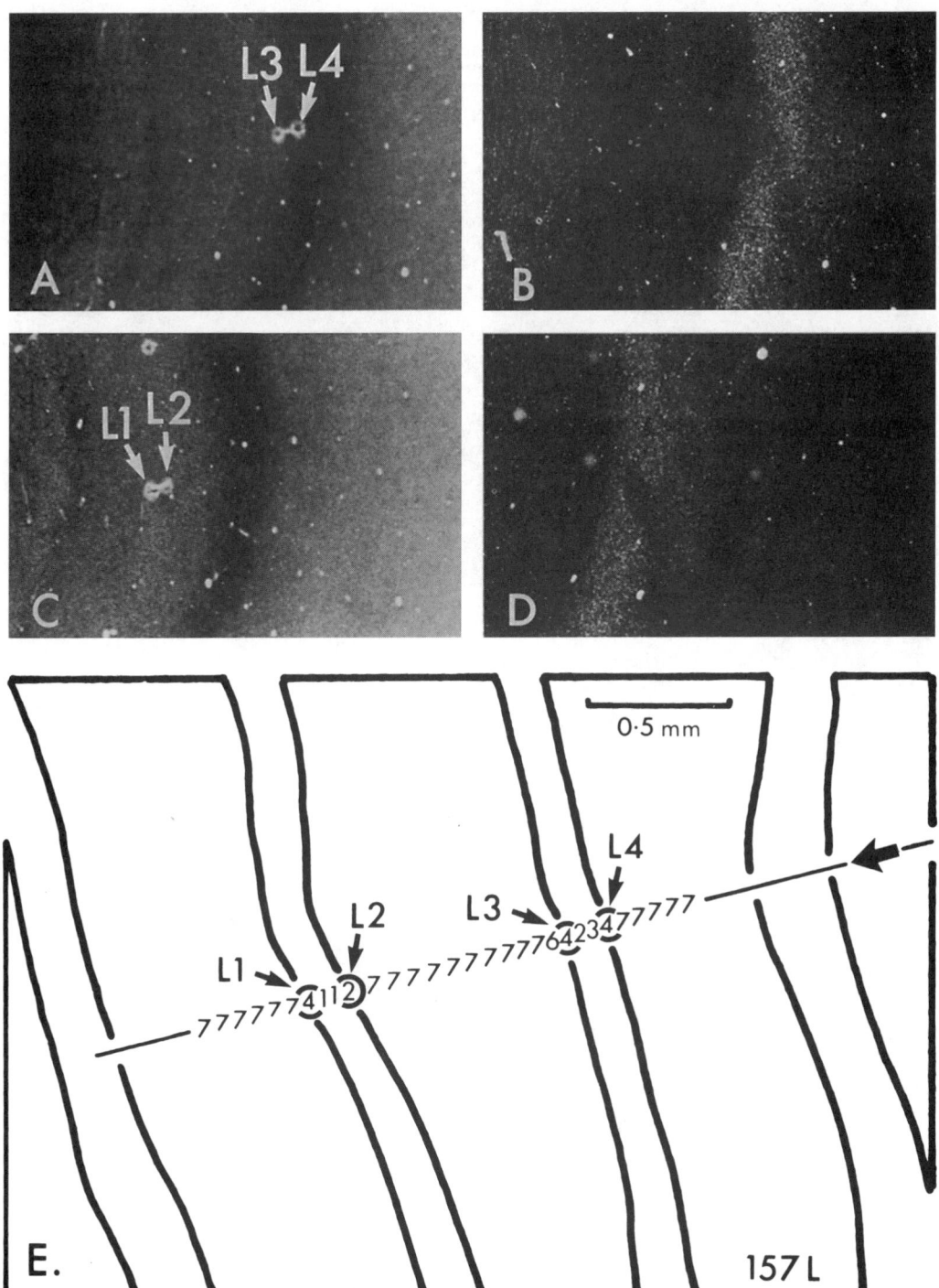

Fig. 13. Reconstruction of a tangential electrode penetration in monkey No. 157. The region illustrated corresponds to the boxed area in Figure 11. A to D are selected sections stained with the Liesegang silver method to show lesions (A and C) or processed for autoradiography (B and D). The Liesegang sections do not show the columnar pattern because the section plane is insufficiently tangential to the layers in this region. E is a reconstruction of the track and the columnar pattern in the area. The electrode advanced from right to left; the four lesions are numbered in reverse order because they were made during withdrawal of the electrode (a procedure sometimes used to permit the physiological observations to be repeated before the lesions were placed).

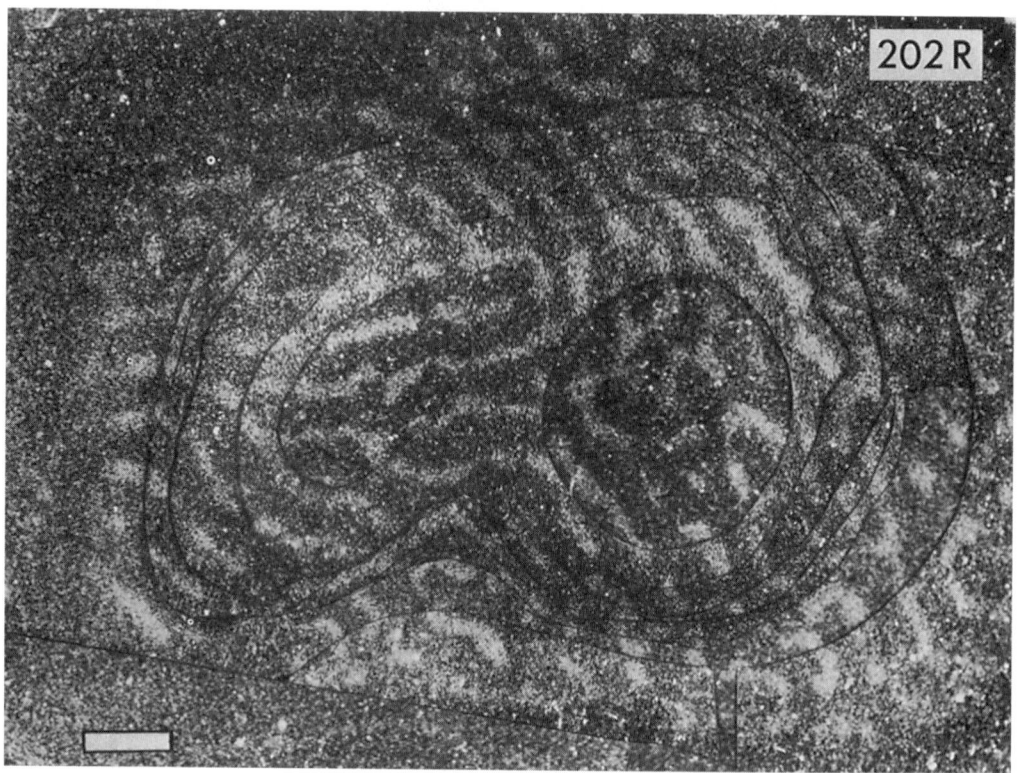

Fig. 14. Autoradiographic montage from the right hemisphere of monkey No. 202, whose right eye was closed at 3 weeks of age. The same eye was injected with [³H]proline at 6 months of age. The montage shows marked shrinkage of columns for the deprived eye. The picture is roughly complementary to that seen in monkey No. 157 (Fig. 11). The overall pattern of columns is different from Figure 11 because the specimen was taken from a different region of opercular cortex (well removed from the 17–18 border), where the bands are more confluent and irregular (LeVay et al., '75). From Hubel et al. ('77).

Liesegang silver method (LeVay et al., '75) revealed a clear abnormality in the fourth layer, both in monkeys No. 286 and 185. The bands for the deprived eye, as revealed with the fiber method, were distinctly lighter in color than the bands for the normal eye. This effect is illustrated in Figure 24 for monkey No. 286. In normal animals the border zones between left- and right-eye columns show up in Liesegang preparations as thin, pale bands about 50–100 μm wide, and the columns themselves appear as darker bands about 300 μm wide. In these late-deprived monkeys the paleness of the deprived columns caused them to merge visually with the thin 'borderline' bands adjacent to them, making them appear wider than normal. Thus the main impression sustained on inspection of these sections at low power (Fig. 24B) is of the remaining dark bands, corresponding (as

shown by autoradiography and recording) to the columns for the non-deprived eye. Whatever the basis for this effect (see Discussion), it does not seem to be reflected in any abnormality in geniculate cell size (Table 2).

Recordings made from monkey No. 185 also indicated a physiological effect of late deprivation, but it was restricted to the layers outside of layer IVC. In these layers the left (open) eye dominated strongly, as may be seen in the histogram (Fig. 25). In layer IVC there was alternation in eye preference at what seemed to be normal intervals, and these corresponded to the columnar boundaries as determined anatomically.

Six Years (No. 280). Monkey No. 280 had its right eye closed when it was 6 years old, i.e., fully adult. After a survival period of 17 months the left eye

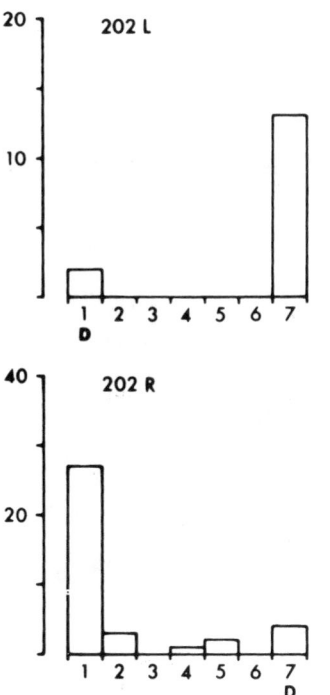

Fig. 15. *Ocular dominance histograms for penetration in the left and right hemispheres of monkey No. 202. There is a strong dominance of the open eye in both hemispheres, although the samples are rather small. As before, the letter D indicates the side of the histogram corresponding to dominance of the deprived eye.*

was injected, and recordings were made 21 days later.

As expected, the autoradiographic labeling pattern was entirely normal on both sides of the brain; Figure 26 shows a reconstruction from the left hemisphere. In Liesegang silver preparations, the columnar pattern was also normal.

Recordings were made from the right hemisphere. They showed a normal balance of the eyes in the layers outside of layer IVC (Fig. 27), and in layer IVC there were recorded the usual monocular responses with sharp transitions from one eye to the other.

ADULT ENUCLEATION (NOS. 150 AND 269). Although lid suture is clearly ineffective in causing columnar reorganization in the adult, we thought that the more drastic operation of monocular eye enucleation might produce an effect. This was

because, unlike lid suture, eye nucleation leads to rapid transneuronal atrophy in the LGN, even in adult monkeys (Minkowski, '20; Matthews et al., '60; LeVay, '71). We therefore removed the right eye from two adults (Nos. 150 and 269) and allowed them to survive for 4 months (No. 269) and 6 months (No. 150).

Monkey No. 150 did not receive an eye injection, but we made recordings from the left hemisphere (contralateral to the enucleation) 6 months after the operation. In the upper layers there were continuous responses to stimulation of the remaining eye, with some waxing and waning in the level of responsiveness. There were orderly shifts in orientation preference as found in normal monkeys.

There were four traverses through layer IVC, the longest being about 5 mm in length. The level of responsiveness to visual stimulation waxed and waned periodically, as the electrode advanced, but there were only two short stretches, about 50 μm long, where absolutely no visual responses could be elicited. This pattern suggested that the enucleation had permitted a definite expansion, even in layer IVC, of the physiological columns for the remaining eye.

The other enucleated monkey (No. 269) was studied autoradiographically 4 months after the operation. The remaining eye was injected with [³H]proline 12 days prior to perfusion. No recordings were made.

Somewhat to our surprise the labeling pattern in this animal was entirely normal in both hemispheres. A reconstruction of the labeling pattern in the left hemisphere is shown in Figure 28. This reconstruction is made from an area of cortex in the roof of the calcarine fissure, and it includes part of the representation of the optic disc in the contralateral (enucleated) eye. In this area (just as in normal animals) the afferents for the ipsilateral eye form a uniform, roughly circular patch without any gaps. This figure points up the difference between the labeling pattern produced when optic nerve fibers for one eye are missing during fetal development (complete filling-in by the other eye) and the pattern produced when one set is removed in the adult, after all development is complete (lack of reinvasion by fibers for the other eye).

We do not understand the reason for the apparent discrepancy between the results from these two monkeys. Clearly one needs to do the

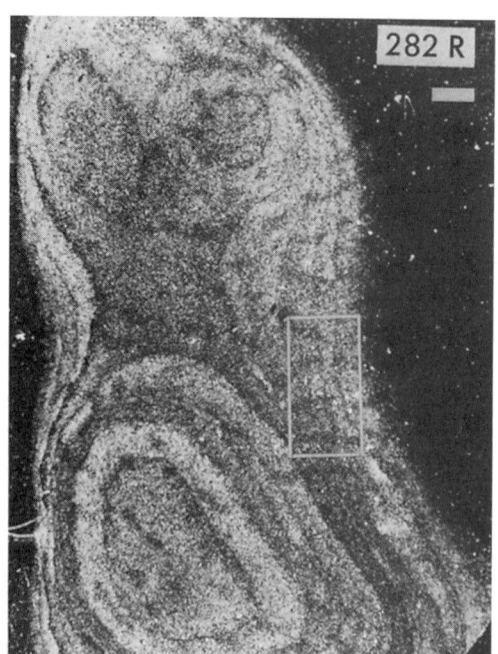
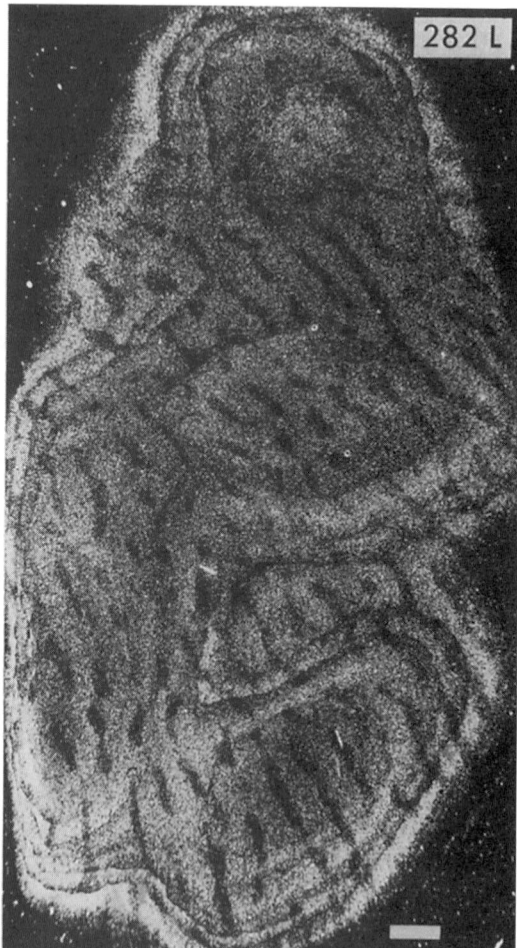

Fig. 16. Autoradiographic montages from the right and left hemispheres of monkey No. 282, whose right eye was closed at 5.5 weeks of age. The left eye was injected. The autoradiographs show an expansion of the left-eye columns on both sides of the brain; the effect is rather more marked on the right than on the left side. An electrode penetration in the right hemisphere (boxed area) is reconstructed in Figure 18.

physiological and autoradiographic experiments in the same animal. In addition, we need to examine the distribution of geniculo-cortical afferents for the enucleated eye. In the deafferented laminae of the LGN there was marked cell shrinkage (Table 2) as well as an intense gliosis. This atrophy may well be reflected in a shrinkage of cortical columns for the missing eye, or at least a thinning-out of the synapses in those columns, but further experiments—for example, an injection of [³H]proline into a single denervated lamina of the LGN, or the use of the Nauta method, as was applied to the

neonatally enucleated monkeys (Hubel et al., '77)—will be needed to resolve this point.

Comment

It has long been known from experiments on cats that the end of the critical period is not an abrupt cessation but rather a gradual decline in susceptibility (Hubel and Wiesel, '70). The present results demonstrate this to be true for the monkey, and also show that different aspects of the deprivation effect have different time courses. Three such effects have been quantified and plotted as a func-

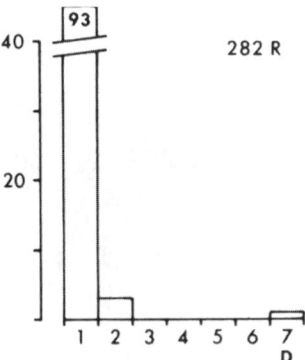

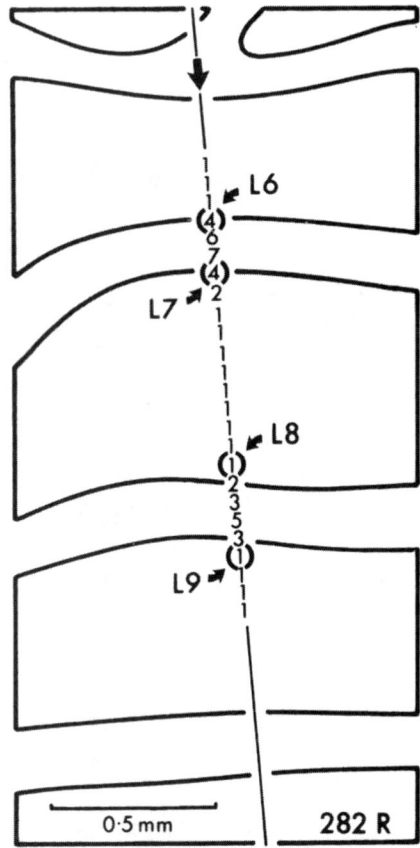

Fig. 17. *Ocular dominance histogram for 97 neurons recorded on two tangential penetrations into the right striate cortex of monkey No. 282. The three cells that were slightly influenced by the deprived eye (group 2) were grouped together in a small region at the bottom of layer III. The one group 7 cell was found in layer VI, close to the white matter. Layer IVC cells are excluded.*

tion of age in Figure 29. These are 1) changes in cell size in the LGN, expressed as the ratio of the mean cell area for the non-deprived lamina 6 to the sum of the means for laminae 6 and 5, on the side ipsilateral to the lid suture; 2) changes in the size of ocular dominance columns in layer IV of area 17, expressed as the fraction of the total cortical area occupied by afferents for the non-deprived eye; and 3) the changes in eye preference in the layers above and below layer IVC, expressed as the mean ocular dominance group for all recording sites (excluding IVC) for each animal.

As far as the anatomical effects of deprivation in layer IVC are concerned, susceptibility to monocular deprivation begins to decline between 6 and 10 weeks of age. Ocular dominance in the upper layers, however, is still subject to alteration by deprivation begun at 1 year of age, and in fact we have not pinned down the termination of this kind of susceptibility other than to show that it is not present in fully mature animals.

Comparison of the results from this series with those from the normal animals described in part A suggests that anatomical changes in the fourth layer can be produced by lid suture at an age when the segregation of the left- and right-eye afferents is already complete. Nevertheless, plasticity of these afferents probably outlasts the period of overlap by a relatively short time. This conclusion

Fig. 18. *Reconstruction of an electrode penetration in monkey No. 282 (corresponds to boxed area in Fig. 16). The picture is very similar to that obtained in monkey No. 157 (compare Fig. 13), even though the right eye was closed at 5.5 weeks rather than at 2 weeks of age. In the first deprived-eye column traversed by the electrode (between lesions 6 and 7), the deprived eye dominated completely at one recording site (O.D. group 7). During the traverse of the second deprived-eye column (between lesions 8 and 9), the influence of the open eye was never completely lost. Note that lesions 8 and 9 were placed at the last group 1 recording sites before and after the deprived-eye column. They are therefore farther apart from each other than are lesions 6 and 7, which were placed at recording sites where the two eyes were balanced (O.D. group 4).*

is subject to a number of qualifications which will be considered in the Discussion.

C. Short-Term Deprivation

So far we have described experiments in which one eye was closed for a long period of time, in order that the maximum effect of lid suture performed at

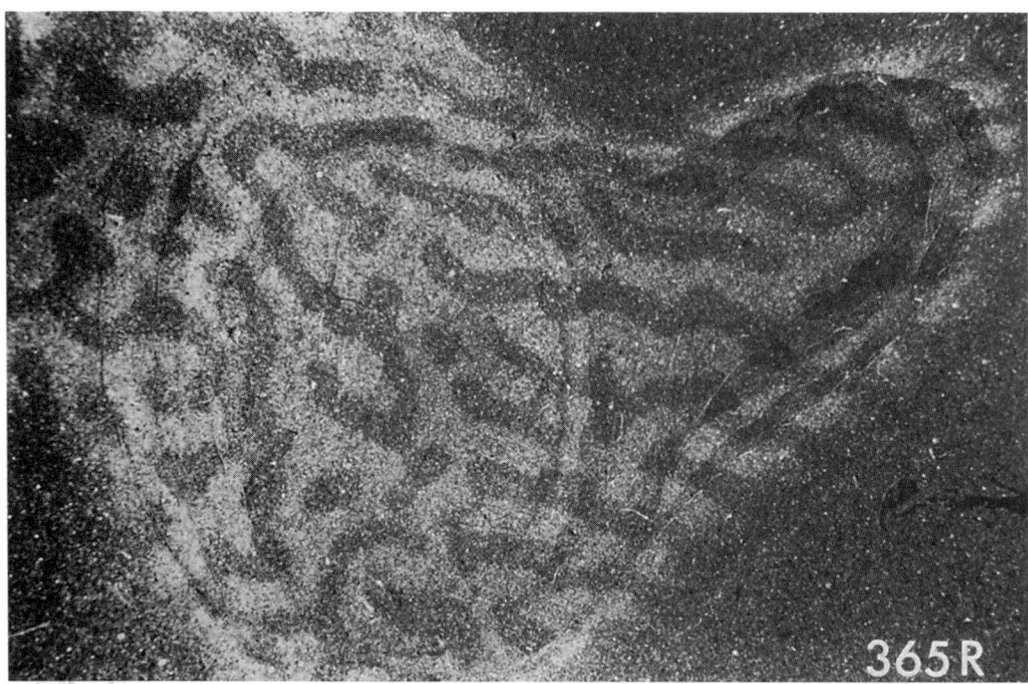

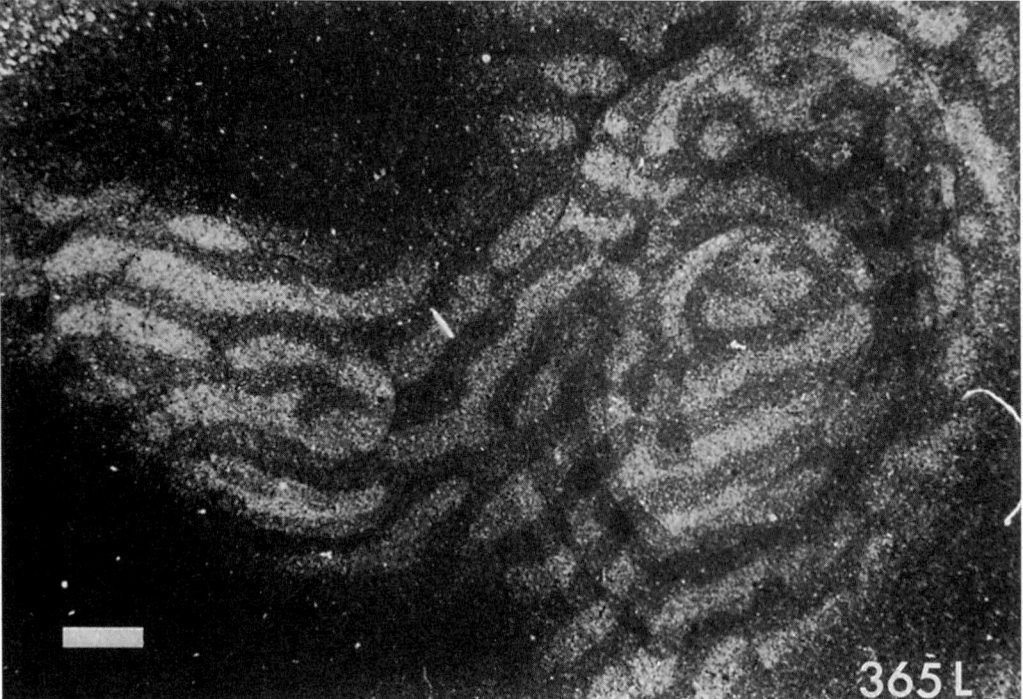

Fig. 19. Autoradiographic montages from the right and left opercular cortex of a monkey (No. 365) whose right eye was closed at 10 weeks of age. The left eye was injected at 6 months. On the right side the labeled columns show a modest expansion. On the left side the labeled and unlabeled columns are of the same size. The anatomical effects of deprivation in this animal are thus restricted to the hemisphere ipsilateral to the sutured eye.

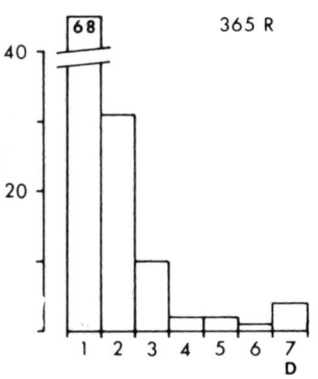

Fig. 20. *Ocular dominance histogram for 118 cells recorded on four penetrations into the right striate cortex of monkey No. 365.*

dominance, with the regions responding to the left (experienced) eye being twice as long as those for the right eye. The physiology in this animal, which was deprived for only twelve days, already resembled that seen after long-term deprivation.

Two to 24 Days (No. 308). Wishing to obtain the anatomical picture for a case of short-term deprivation, we closed the right eye of another animal (No. 308) at 2 days of age, injected the same eye with [³H]proline at 16 days, and recorded from the cortex at 24 days of age.

The autoradiographic labeling pattern for the left hemisphere is shown in Figure 31. The labeled areas were very shrunken and fragmented, with few elongated, band-like structures remaining. There was considerable label above background between the patches of grains, which gave the reconstruction a rather blurred appearance. This may well be due to spillover of label in the LGN (see Discussion). Shrunken columns were also visible in the right cortex, but the labeling was too faint to illustrate satisfactorily. The abnormality of the autoradiographic picture was matched by cell-size changes in the LGN; cells in the deprived laminae were already obviously shrunken and pale-staining (Table 3).

The physiological results were very similar to those obtained in the previous animal. A single penetration was made in the left hemisphere (contralateral to the deprived eye). In the layers outside of IVC, the left eye dominated strongly (Fig. 32), although not quite so completely as was seen in some long-term deprived animals such as No. 157 (compare Fig. 32 and Fig. 12). In one 1-mm traverse through layer IVC, responses to both eyes were obtained for the first 200 μm, and for the remaining 800 μm responses were obtained only to stimulation of the left (experienced) eye. Because of the rather poor quality of the autoradiographs (Fig. 31) it proved impossible to match the physiological responses to the autoradiographic labeling pattern, but it appeared that the electrode had been traveling obliquely to the columns.

a given age might be revealed. We also wished to know how fast the observed effects develop, when lid suture is performed in early life. In particular we were interested by the question of whether the process of normal segregation is itself modified, or whether, even in deprived animals, the columns first develop normally and are later reorganized. A second reason for studying the effects of short-term deprivation has to do with the reverse-sutured animals to be described in part D. In order to understand those results it will be necessary to know the state of the ocular dominance columns at the time when the reverse suture was performed.

There were six monkeys in this series. Four of them (Nos. 164, 308, 316, and 307) had lid suture performed within the first 8 days of life and were allowed to survive until 20–47 days of age. Two had short periods of deprivation a little later in life (Nos. 195 and 213, Table 1).

Eight to 20 Days (No. 164). Monkey No. 164 had its right eye closed at 8 days, and it was studied physiologically at 20 days. An eye injection of [³H]lysine was made but it did not label the cortex satisfactorily. The physiological results were, however, very clear. In all three penetrations made into the right hemisphere the left eye dominated very strongly. The ocular dominance histogram for cells recorded above and below layer IVC is shown in Figure 30. In layer IVC responses alternated between complete left-eye and complete right-eye

Two to 23 Days (No. 316). The deprivation schedule in the next animal (No. 316) was very similar to that for No. 308. The right eye was closed from 2 to 23 days. The difference was that the left, rather than the right, eye was injected. No recordings

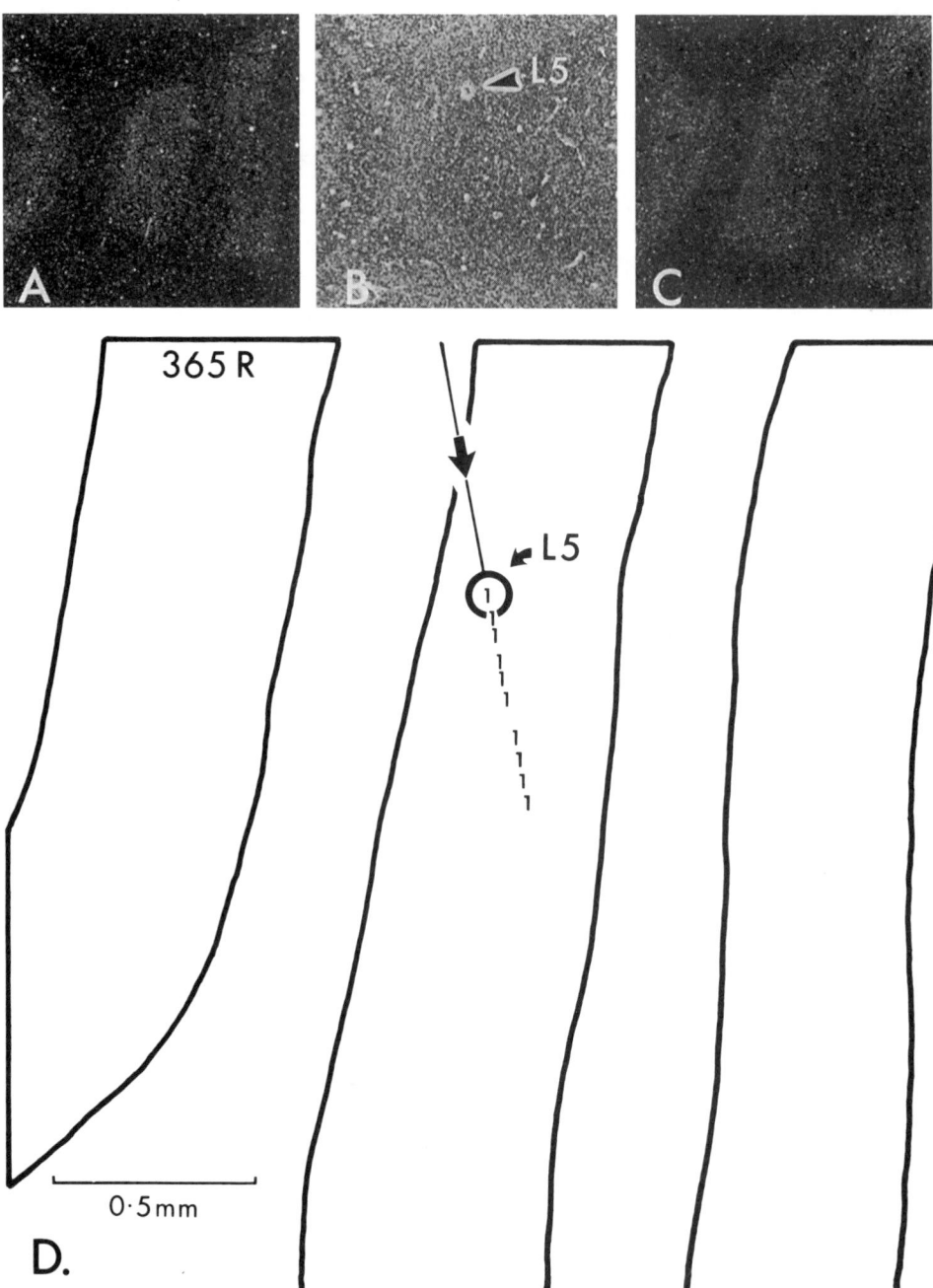

Fig. 21. Reconstruction of part of an electrode penetration in monkey No. 365. The reconstructed area is in the roof of the calcarine fissure and is not included in the montage of Figure 19. The electrode remained within a single labeled band (column for the nondeprived eye) during its traverse of layer IVC, and responses were exclusively to stimulation of that eye. The labeled columns are wider than the gaps in this area of calcarine cortex, just as they are in the opercular cortex. The unlabeled gap to the left of the central labeled column in A appears larger than it really is, because the section passes out of layer IVC in this region. Compare with the Nissl-stained adjacent section (B) and the next autoradiograph (C) which shows the gap at its correct size.

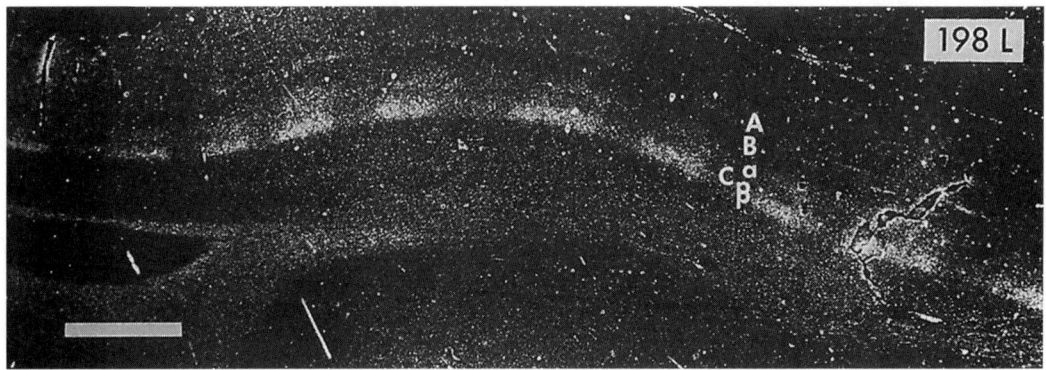

Fig. 22. Autoradiograph of a single section from the calcarine fissure of a monkey (No. 198) whose right eye was closed at 7 months of age. The same eye was injected at 5 years of age. The labeled patches and gaps are of about the same width, indicating that the late eye closure did not affect column size in layer IVC.

were made. The labeling pattern in the right hemisphere was the converse of that seen in monkey No. 308, with wide labeled columns separated by shrunken, rather indistinct gaps (not illustrated). Again, we suspect that the clarity of the columnar pattern was degraded to some extent by spillover of label in the LGN. The labeling in the left hemisphere was too faint for the columnar pattern to be discerned. (This was probably due to damage to the temporal retina of the left eye during injection of isotope, since there was poor labeling of the left LGN as well as a shrinkage of cells in the left-eye laminae on that side.)

FOUR TO 47 DAYS (No. 307). This monkey had its right eye closed at 4 days of age. The same eye was injected with [³H]proline at 33 days of age and recordings were made from the right hemisphere at 47 days of age. This is an age at which, in normal animals, the process of columnar segregation is complete (compare animal No. 257, section A).

In the autoradiography (Fig. 33) both hemispheres showed marked shrinkage of the labeled columns. The ratio of unlabeled to labeled areas (open-eye to deprived-eye columns) was 3.18:1 on the right side and 2.3:1 on the left. There were many fewer silver grains between labeled columns in this animal than in the animals deprived until 3 weeks (308 and 316). This clearing of the labeling pattern parallels what is seen in normal animals between 3 and 6 weeks of age, and, as in normal animals, we are inclined to attribute it to a progressive reduction in spillover in the LGN (see Discussion).

In the recording session, a complete dominance of the left eye was found in the layers outside of IVC (Fig. 34). On both of the first two penetrations, 500-μm-long traverses through layer IVC yielded exclusively left-eye activity. The third penetration was aimed too superficially to enter layer IVC, but a 2.2-mm traverse through IVB again only gave left-eye responses. Finally on the fourth attempt we encountered a right-eye column in IVC: the 680-μm-long traverse began in the left eye, then right-eye responses were obtained over about 120 μm (but without ever entirely losing the left eye), and finally there was another stretch of pure left-eye activity before the electrode passed out of the layer.

The LGN also showed marked cell-size changes (Table 3). Thus in all respects the results in this animal resembled those obtained in monkeys deprived for much longer periods of time.

TWENTY-ONE TO 30 DAYS (No. 195). We went on to study two monkeys that had a few days of monocular deprivation after some period of normal vision. The first of these, No. 195, was allowed normal vision up to 21 days of age. At this time the right eye was closed, and it was reopened 9 days later. The animal was then permitted to survive with both eyes open for 4 years. The intent here was to determine whether the short period of deprivation had long-lasting effects or whether the reopening would permit a functional or morphological recovery. A strabismus developed as a result of the monocular deprivation. As part of a separate study, visual acuity was measured repeatedly dur-

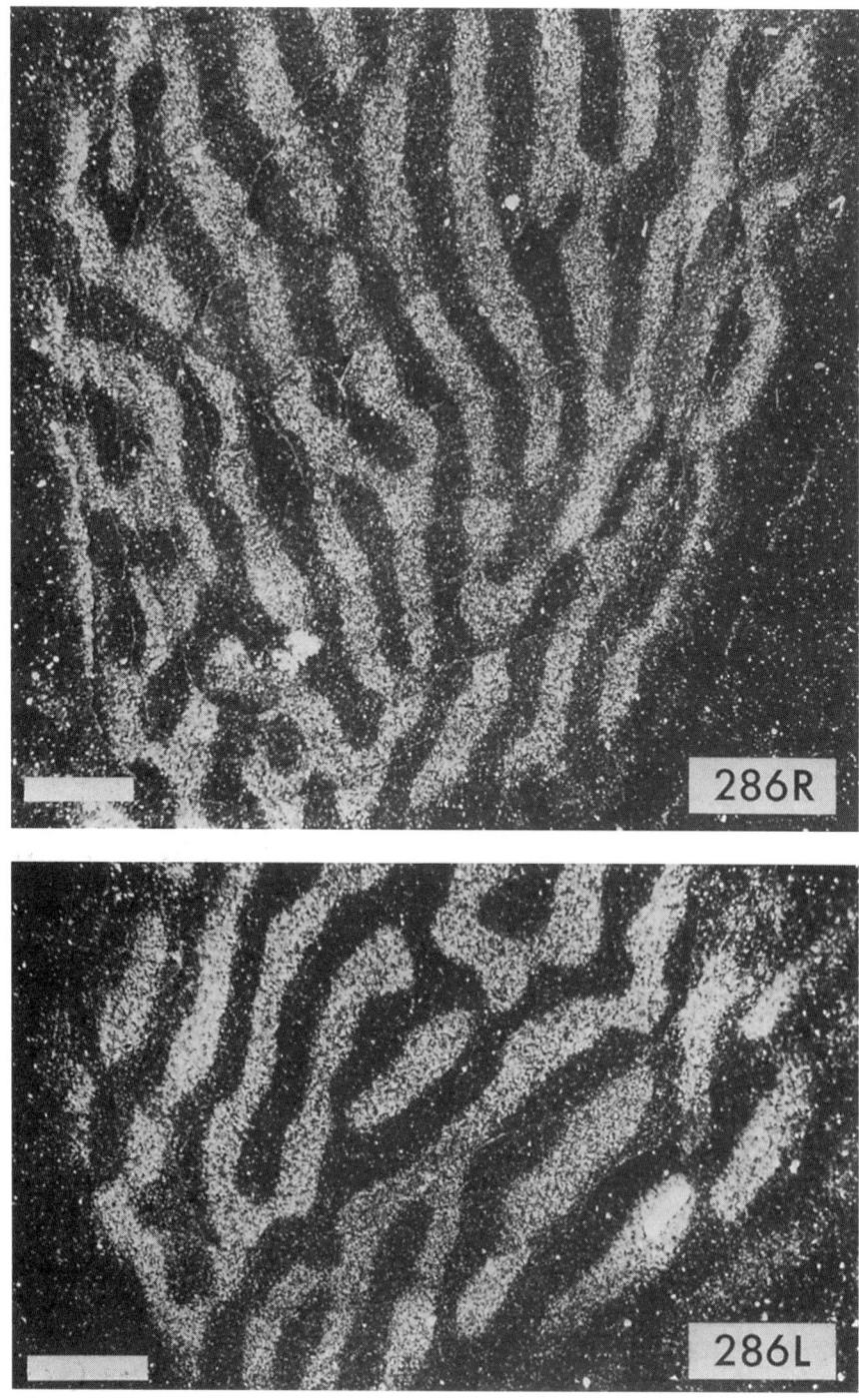

Fig. 23. Autoradiographic montages from the right and left hemispheres of monkey No. 286, whose right eye was closed at 14 months of age. The left eye was injected 19 months later. The labeling pattern is normal in both hemispheres.

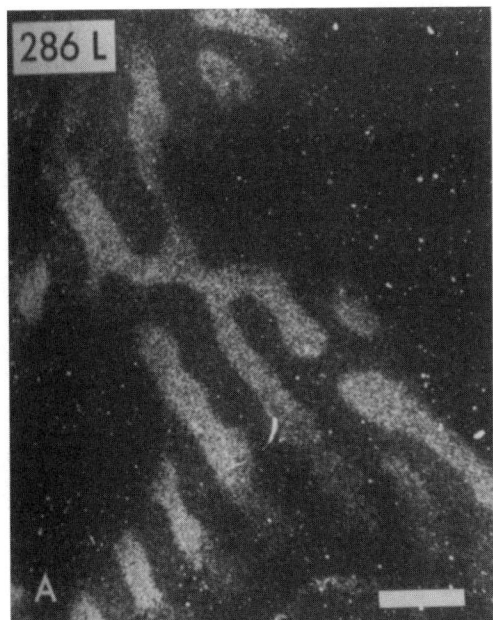
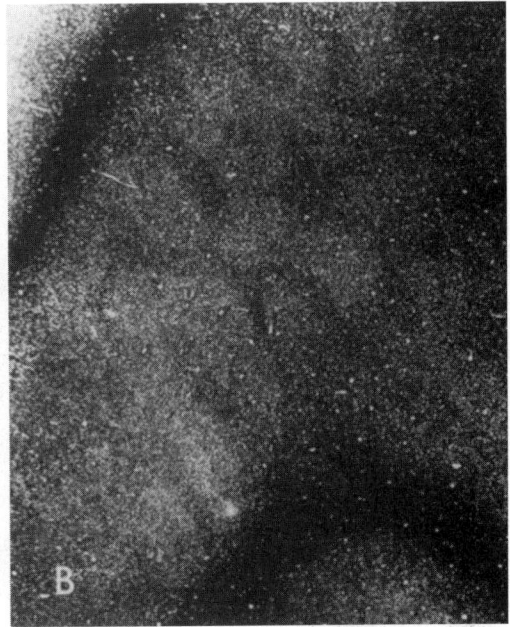

Fig. 24. *Two adjacent sections from the left striate cortex of monkey No. 286, to illustrate an anatomical abnormality revealed only by the Liesegang silver method. A is an autoradiograph, and B is a Liesegang preparation. The labeled areas in A (columns for the nondeprived eye) are in register with dark bands in B, while the unlabeled areas in A (columns for the deprived eye) are in register with lighter bands in B. The correspondence is seen most clearly for the chromosome-shaped labeled area in the center of the micrograph. The banding in B is quite subtle: it is best appreciated when the page is held at some distance from the observer. The prominent dark zones at the top left and bottom right of B are portions of the stria of Gennari (corresponding roughly to layer IVB). See text for further interpretation.*

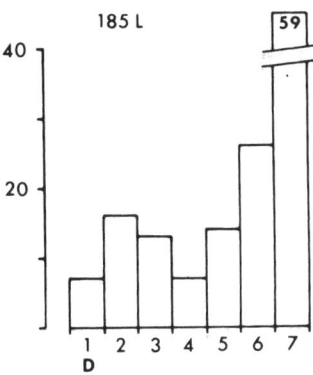

Fig. 25. *Ocular dominance histogram for 142 cells recorded on two tangential penetrations in monkey No. 185. The closure of the right eye at 1 year has caused quite a pronounced skewing of the histogram towards the open eye. Most of the recording sites were in layers II-IVB; there was some suggestion of a relatively greater preservation of deprived-eye activity in layers V and VI.*

ing the recovery period. Acuity in the deprived eye was poor when measured soon after reopening, but gradually improved to a near-normal level.

Recordings were made from the left hemisphere. In spite of the brevity of the deprivation and the long period allowed for possible recovery, the left eye dominated the upper layers; there were just a few patches in which right-eye activity was recorded (Fig. 35). In layer IVC we encountered one stretch, about 500 μm long, in which cells were driven from the deprived eye.

An eye injection was not done, so the columnar pattern could not be studied autoradiographically. It was, however, well shown with the Liesegang silver method (Fig. 36). These preparations showed a clear shrinkage of one set of columns, identified by the lesions made during the recording session as belonging to the right (deprived) eye. The electrode had passed very

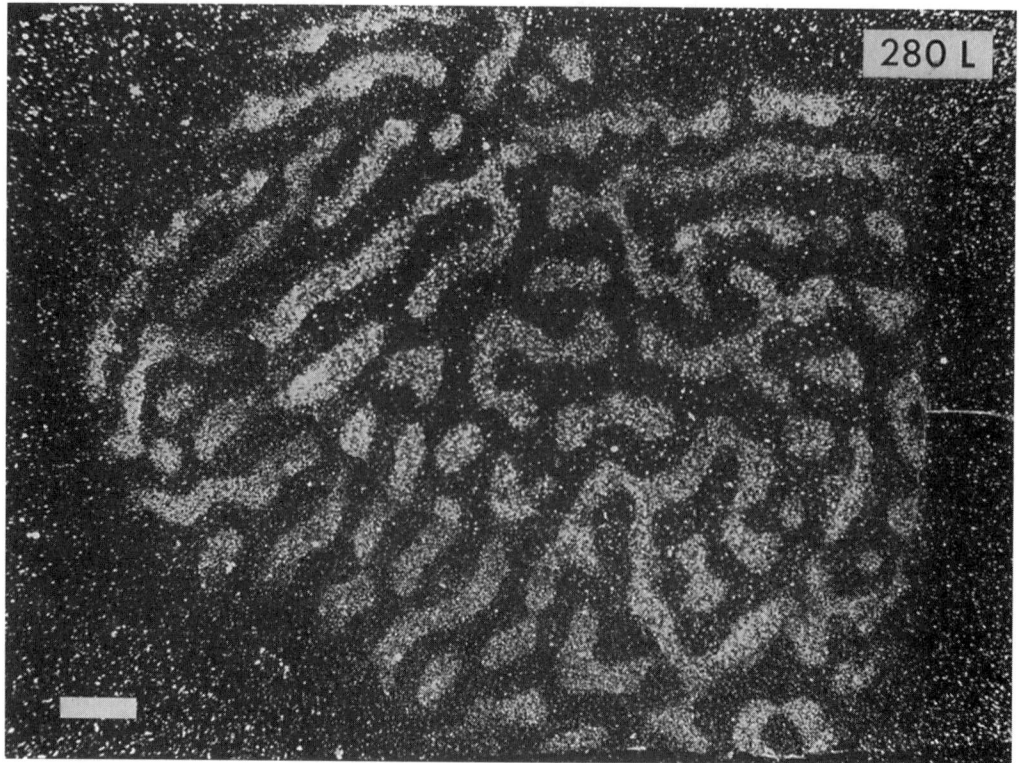

Fig. 26. Autoradiographic montage from a monkey (No. 280) whose right eye was closed when it was adult. The left eye was injected 17 months later. The labeled bands and gaps are of normal size. The rather irregular layout of the columns is also normal: the region reconstructed is well away from the 17–18 border, where the bands are most orderly.

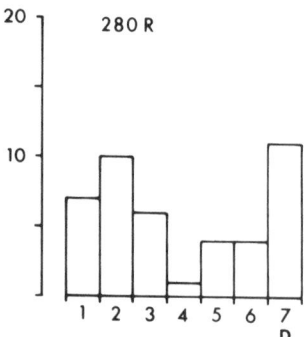

Fig. 27. Ocular dominance histogram for monkey No. 280. Among the 43 cells recorded (admittedly rather a small sample) the influence of the two eyes was about equal.

obliquely to the direction of the columns, thus explaining why such a long traverse through a right-eye column was obtained. The actual widths of the two sets of columns, as measured in the silver preparations, were 500 μm (left eye) and 200 μm (right eye). An unusual feature of the silver preparations, compared with what was seen in long-term deprived monkeys, was that the columns for the deprived eye were darker, not paler, than those for the open eye (Fig. 36). It is not clear whether this effect was related to the strabismus that developed subsequent to the deprivation or to the apparent functional recovery suggested by the gradual improvement of visual acuity in the right eye.

THIRTY-FIVE TO 47 DAYS (No. 213). The last animal in this group had its right eye closed at 5 weeks of

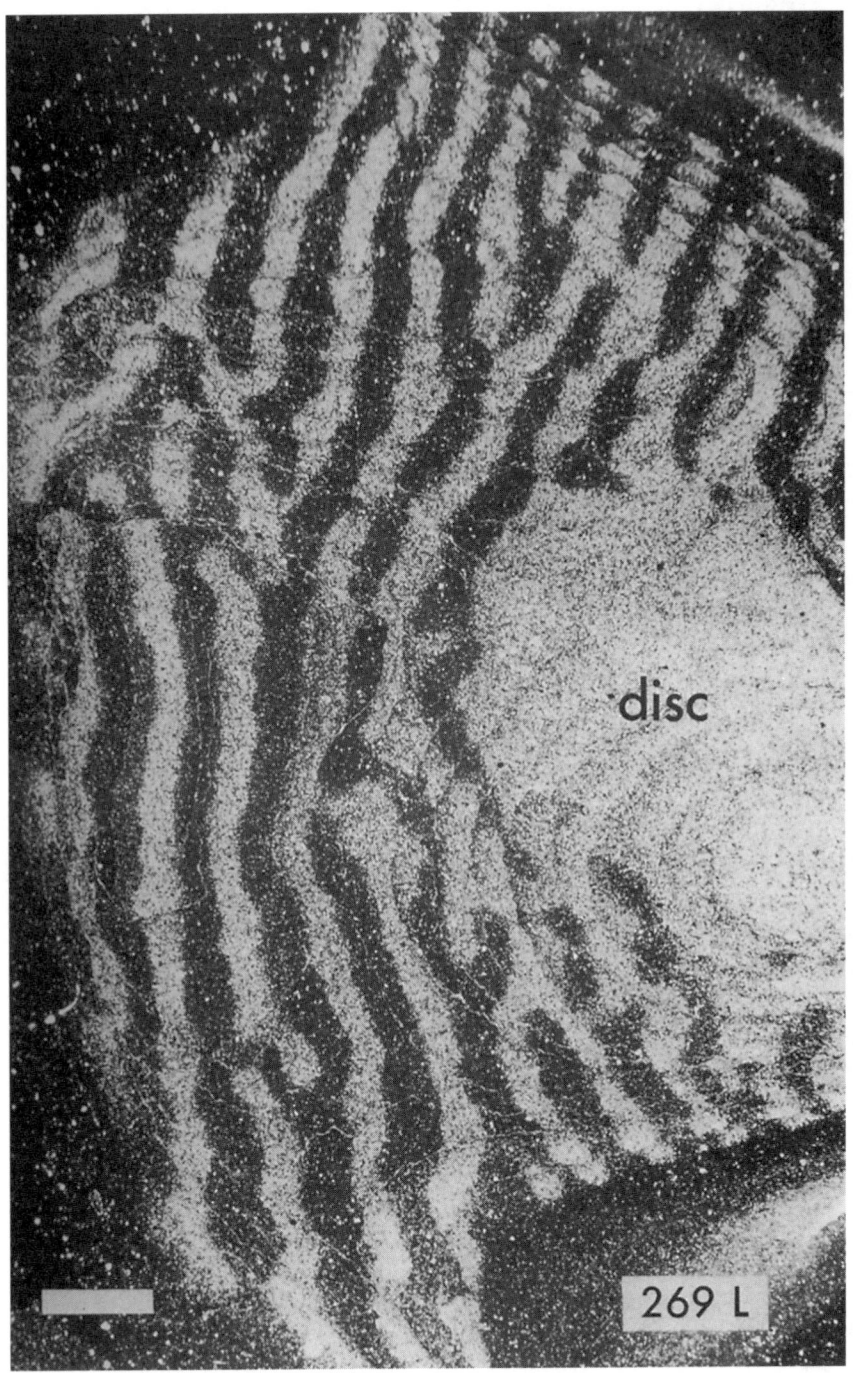

Fig. 28. Autoradiographic montage for a monkey (No. 269) whose right eye was removed when it was adult. The left eye was injected 4 months later. The reconstructed area comprises the lateral part of the roof of the calcarine fissure (medial is to the left, anterior is above). The montage shows a normal pattern, with bands and gaps of equal width. The uniformly labeled zone (right center) is the representation of the optic disc of the enucleated contralateral eye. As in normal animals the zone is completely filled in by afferents serving the ipsilateral eye. (The faint striations in parts of the disc region result from uneven illumination of successive layers of the montage.) The labeling pattern in the opercular cortex was also normal.]

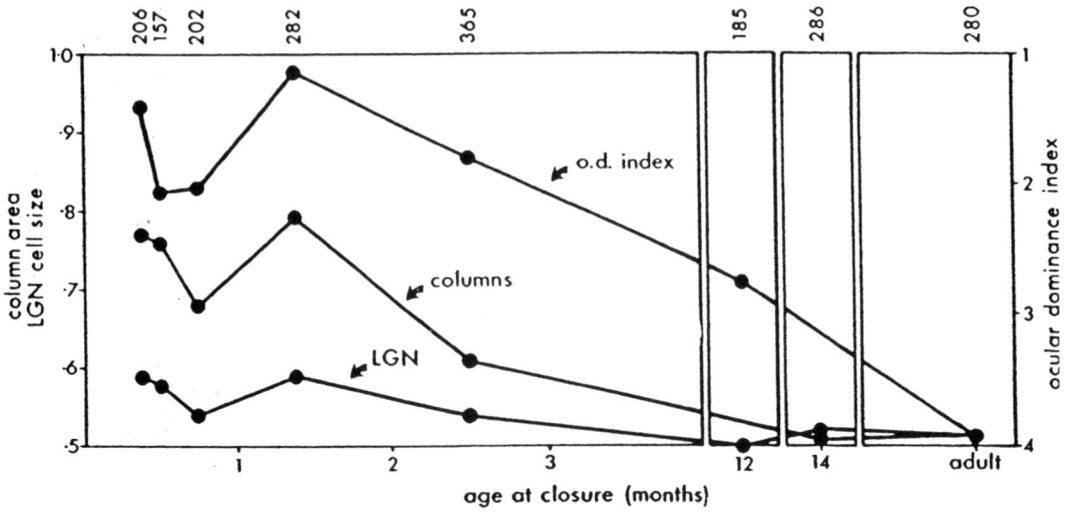

Fig. 29. Effects of monocular deprivation on three parameters related to ocular dominance as a function of age at suture. Note the interruptions in the abscissa.

Upper curve: the ocular dominance index. This index is simply the average of the ocular dominance groups of all the cells recorded outside of layer IVC in a given animal. In the case of recordings from the left hemisphere the ocular dominance values have been reversed. Thus an index value of 1 would indicate that every cell responded exclusively to stimulation of the nondeprived eye, and a value of 4 (bottom of graph) indicates that the overall influence of the two eyes was equal. Each point is derived from a single animal, whose identification number is given at the corresponding position at the top of the graph. The individual histograms from which these points are derived have all been illustrated in previous figures.

Middle curve: This shows the effect of deprivation on the relative areas of the two sets of columns in layer IVC, as measured on the autoradiographs. Each point gives, for a single animal, the area occupied by the open-eye afferents as a fraction of the total area of the reconstruction. Thus a value of 1.0 would indicate that the open-eye afferents had taken over the entire cortex, and a value of 0.5 (bottom of graph) represents the normal situation where both eyes' afferents occupy equal areas. Measurements from the cortex ipsilateral to the deprived eye (right hemisphere) were used.

Lower curve: This shows the effect of deprivation on cell size in the LGN. Each point gives the mean cross-sectional area of cells in the nondeprived parvocellular lamina 6 as a fraction of the sum of the mean areas of cells in laminae 6 and 5. Thus a value of 1.0 would correspond to total elimination of neurons in the deprived lamina 5, and a value of 0.5 corresponds to equal sizes of cells in the two laminae, the normal situation.

age. The eye was reopened at 7 weeks and the animal was perfused at 10 weeks of age. The left eye was injected with [³H]proline 16 days before death.

The autoradiographic picture in this animal is shown in Figure 37. There was a definite expansion of the labeled columns: the ratio of labeled to unlabeled areas was 1.76:1 on the left side and 1.19:1 on the right. As usual in young animals, the picture on the side contralateral to the injected eye was partially blurred by label in the inappropriate columns, and again we are inclined to attribute this to spillover of label in the LGN.

Comment

The results from this group of animals show that very early lid suture causes a redirection of the normal process of columnar development. The afferents segregate from each other at something close to their normal rate (being segregated, or very nearly so, by 3 weeks, and definitely mature by 6 weeks), but they segregate into an abnormal pattern. A short period of deprivation at 3–4 weeks can also produce marked effects, however, and a short period of deprivation at 5–7 weeks can still produce a mild effect. Comparing the results

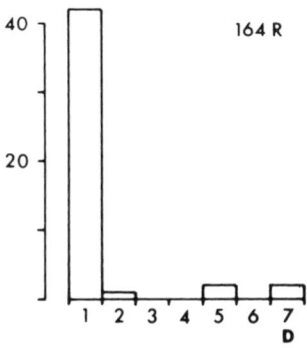

Fig. 30. Ocular dominance histogram for 47 neurons recorded in a 20-day-old monkey (No. 164) whose right eye had been closed since 8 days of age. The physiological picture is similar to that seen after months of deprivation (compare for example the histogram from monkey No. 206, Fig. 10).

obtained in monkeys No. 307, 282, and 213, it appears that monocular suture performed after five weeks of age requires a longer time to produce its anatomical effects in layer IVC than does closure soon after birth.

D. Effects of reverse suture

Having obtained some idea of the time course of the deprivation effects, we went on to study the effects of reopening the deprived eye and closing the experienced one. Besides a natural interest in the reversibility of the deprivation effects, we particularly wished to seek further evidence for or against the hypothesis stated in the introduction. If that hypothesis is correct, reverse suture performed at 3 weeks of age should produce little if any effect on the size of ocular dominance columns in layer IVC, since the afferents for the deprived eye have already retracted into their narrow, fragmented

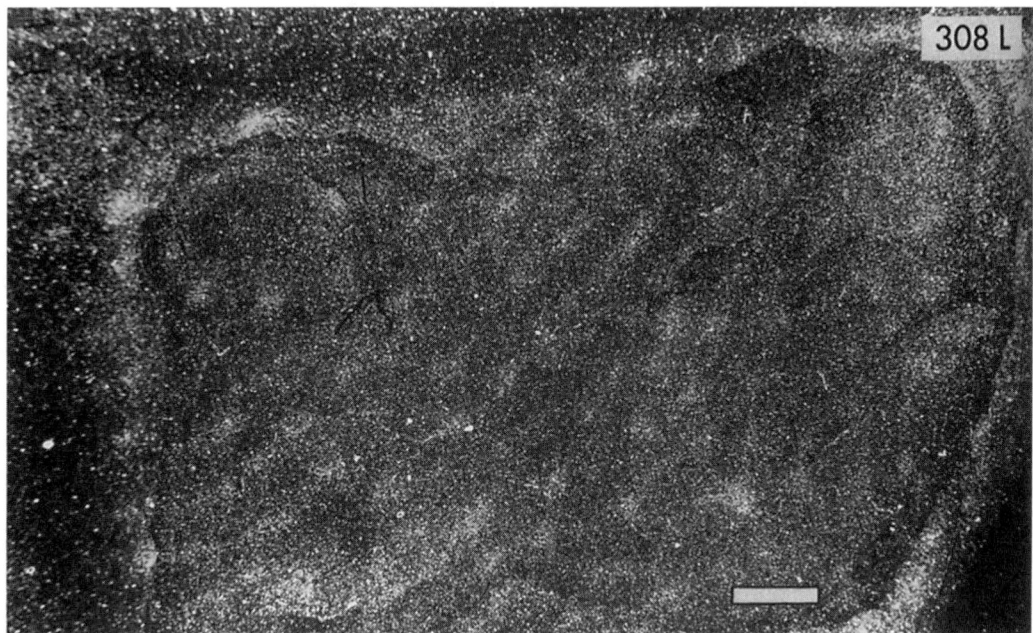

Fig. 31. Autoradiographic montage from monkey No. 308, studied at 24 days of age. The deprived right eye was injected, and the reconstruction shows shrinkage and fragmentation of the right-eye bands. As with normal monkeys at this age (cf. monkey No. 256, Fig. 3) the bands are less sharply defined than in adults, suggesting a certain amount of overlap of the two sets of afferents at columnar borders. There is also label above background in the gaps between the deprived-eye columns. This may be due to leakage of label between laminae of the LGN during transneuronal transport (see Discussion).

Table 3. Quantitative Physiological and Anatomical Results for the Animals in Section C

No.	OCULAR DOMINANCE INDEX		RATIO OF COLUMN AREAS		LGN CELL SIZE (μM^2)			
	L	R	L	R	L6	L5	R6	R5
164	—	1.40	—	—	234	217*	265	217
308	1.90	—	3.8:1	—	318	366	356	252
316	—	—	—	—	285	256*	291	254
307	—	1.00	2.3:1	3.2:1	204	250	254	166
195	1.73	—	—	—	141	183	189	166
213	—	—	1.8:1	1.2:1	300	345	345	341

For explanation of the indices, see Table 1.

* Cell sizes in the left LGN of monkeys No. 164 and 316 probably reflect damage to the temporal retina of the left eye during injection of isotope, rather than a deprivation effect (see text).

columns (section C, animals No. 164 and 308). Reverse suture at 6 weeks or later should definitely not lead to any recovery in layer IVC, whatever might occur in the layers above or below it. There were three monkeys in this series, and the quantitative results are presented in Table 4.

REVERSAL AT 3 WEEKS (No. 240). The first animal had its right eye closed at 2 days, and reverse suture was performed at 3 weeks of age. At 9 months [^{3}H]proline was injected into the right eye, and recordings were made 9 days later.

The autoradiographic labeling pattern observed in this animal (Figs. 38 and 39) was most unusual in that it showed completely opposite effects in the two sublaminae of layer IVC. In the

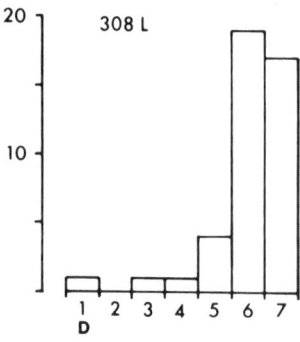

Fig. 32. Ocular dominance histogram for monkey No. 308. The skewing of the histogram towards the experienced eye, though quite clear, is for some reason less extreme than in monkey No. 164 (Fig. 30) or No. 307 (Fig. 34).

lower part, IVCβ, which receives the afferents from the parvocellular LGN (laminae 3–6— Hubel and Wiesel, '72), the labeled columns were greatly expanded, producing a picture similar to a long-term mon-ocular deprivation with injection of the open eye (compare section B, monkey No. 157). In the upper part, layer IVCα, which is innervated by the magnocellular laminae (1 and 2) of the LGN, very shrunken labeled bands were seen, with wide gaps between them. In this layer the picture resembled a long-term monocular deprivation with an injection of the deprived eye (e.g., section B, monkey No. 202). The shrunken labeled columns in IVCα lay in exact register with the centers of the expanded labeled columns in IVCβ. This could be seen in single sections simply by following a labeled band as it passed from one sublamina to the other (Fig. 38A and B). It was also obvious when sections at different levels were compared. In the right hemisphere, a reconstruction was made of the labeling pattern in layer IVCβ (this is the sublamina that we have generally used for preparing reconstructions, because it is thicker and more heavily labeled than IVCα). In this reconstruction (Fig. 38C) the ratio of labeled to unlabeled areas was 2.54:1. On the left side separate reconstructions were made of the labeling pattern in layer IVCβ (Fig. 39A) and in IVCα (Fig. 39B), working from the same set of micrographs. These reconstructions clearly illustrated the opposite results produced by the reverse-suture experiment in the two sublaminae. In layer IVCβ the ratio of labeled to unlabeled (right- to left-eye) areas was

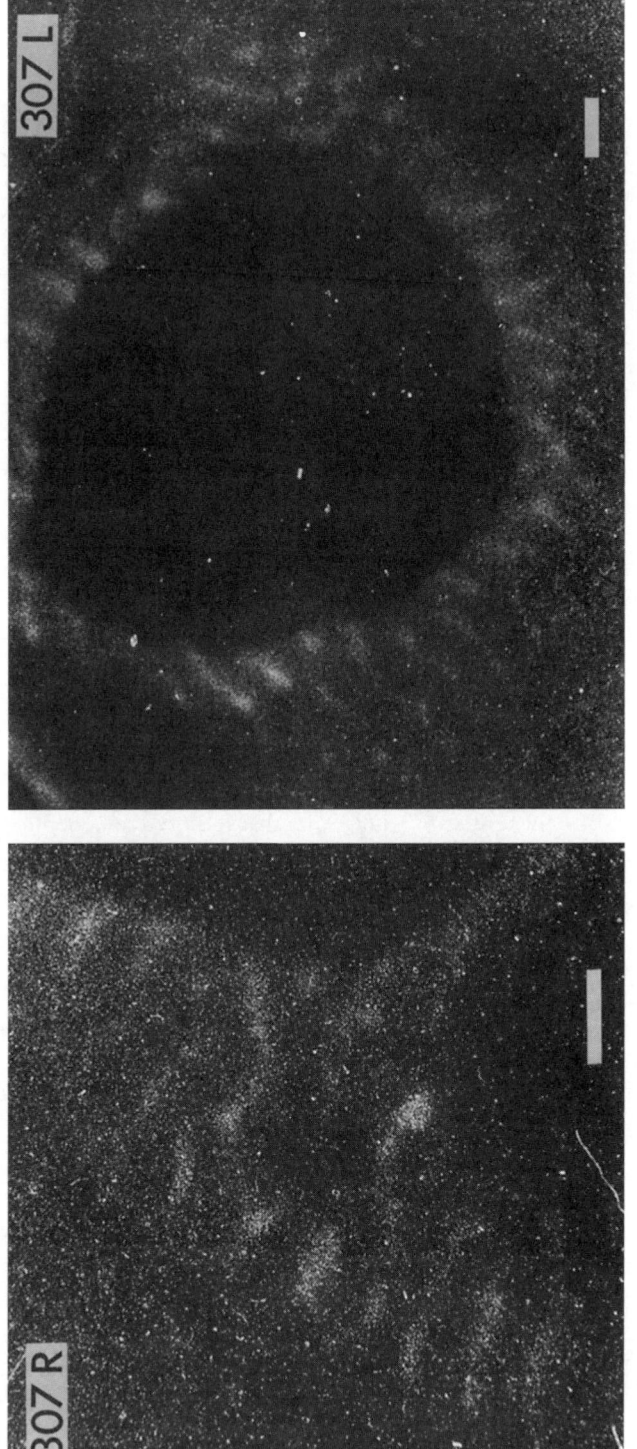

Fig. 33. Autoradiographs of single sections from the right and left hemispheres of a monkey (No. 307) that was studied at 47 days of age. The deprived right eye was injected, and the labeling pattern is similar to that seen in long-term deprivation (compare monkey No. 202, Fig. 14). Note the difference in magnification between the two micrographs.

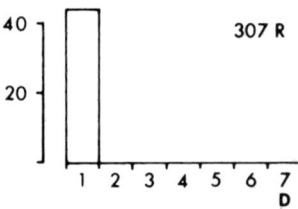

Fig. 34. Ocular dominance histogram for cells recorded in monkey No. 307. None of the 43 cells recorded outside of layer IVC responded to stimulation of the deprived right eye.

3.09:1, while in IVCα the ratio of unlabeled to labeled (left- to right-eye) areas was 2.96:1. Thus in layer IVCβ reverse-suture appeared to have permitted not merely a recovery of the deprived-eye columns but an actual reinvasion of the territory belonging to the initially open eye. In layer IVCα, however, it seems that reverse suture came too late to effect any change in the distribution of afferents.

Because of this strange labeling pattern in area 17 we made a more than usually (for us) thorough study of cell sizes in the LGN. The results are presented in Table 5 with the corresponding measurements from monkey No. 308. (Numbers from monkey No. 308 are included to give an indication of the situation existing in the LGN of the reverse-sutured monkey at the time reversal was performed.)

The results were only partially in accordance with what one might have predicted on the suppo-

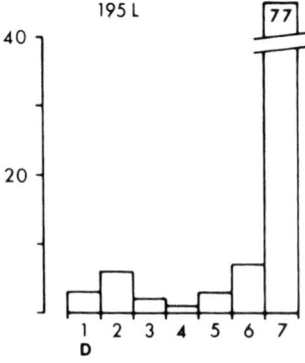

Fig. 35. Ocular dominance histogram of 99 cells recorded in a monkey (No. 195) whose right eye was closed from 21 to 30 days of age. In spite of a subsequent 4 years of binocular vision, most cortical neurons were unresponsive to stimulation of the right eye.

sition of a strict relationship between column area and LGN cell size. The parvocellular laminae in the right hemisphere (R3-R6) did show a reversal: cells in the laminae innervated by the initially deprived right eye were about 25% larger than those in layers innervated by the left eye. Cells in the two magnocellular laminae in the right hemisphere were about the same size, however, suggesting a partial recovery that was not reflected in the cortical autoradiographs. In the left hemisphere cells in all four parvocellular laminae were about the same size, as were those in the two magnocellular laminae. Thus the LGN showed a greater reversal effect in the right hemisphere, whereas the cortical autoradiographs showed a very similar picture on the two sides. This appears to be an instance in which the degree of spread of terminal arbors in the cortex was not completely reflected in the size of cell bodies in the LGN (see Discussion).

Recordings were made in the right hemisphere of monkey No. 240. In all three penetrations, the right eye dominated almost completely in the upper layers (Fig. 40). When one considers that at the time of reverse suture, the left eye must have dominated almost completely—see histogram for monkey No. 164 (Fig. 30) and No. 308 (Fig. 32)—it appears that most of the upper-layer cells were induced by the reverse suture to change their eye preference from one extreme (group 1) to the other (group 7). Of course, a large part of these changes may have been a passive reflection of events occurring in the fourth layer. If so, it is of some interest that the physiology was apparently so strongly dominated by layer IVCβ as opposed to IVCα.

REVERSAL AT 6 WEEKS (No. 194). In monkey No. 194 the right eye was closed from 3 days to 6 weeks of age. Reverse suture was performed at this age and when the animal was 6 months old the right eye was injected with [³H]proline and [³H]fucose. Recordings were made 13 days later. The results from monkey No. 307 (Fig. 33) assure us that at the time of the reverse suture the right-eye afferents had already settled out into shrunken columns.

In the autoradiographs (Fig. 41) the labeling pattern was at first glance normal, suggesting that a full recovery had occurred. Closer examination, however, showed that the labeled bands had their normal width only in layer IVCβ, the parvocellular receiving lamina. In IVCα they were definitely

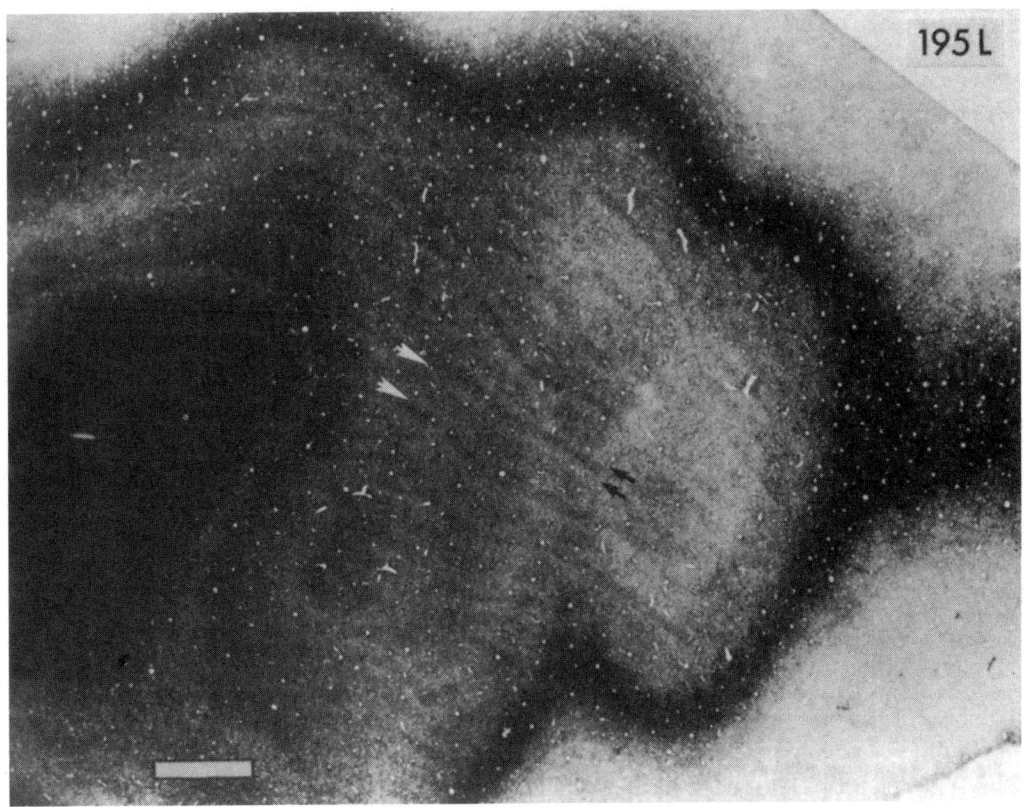

Fig. 36. Anatomical abnormality of ocular dominance columns in monkey No. 195, revealed by the Liesegang silver method. This is a single tangential section of opercular cortex, contralateral to the deprived eye. Layer IVC is the central area traversed by bands that lies within the dark-staining stria of Gennari. To the left of the figure the section grazes the white matter, which is stained black.

    The banding pattern in layer IVC is grossly abnormal. The thin pale bands, which correspond to the borders between adjacent ocular dominance columns (LeVay et al., '75), are not evenly spaced but grouped into pairs. Each pair encloses a 200-μm-wide, dark-staining band. These dark bands were shown by recording to correspond to shrunken ocular dominance columns for the right eye. Alternating with these are 500-μm-wide bands, somewhat lighter in color, that are the columns for the left eye. The black arrows indicate two thin pale bands enclosing a right-eye column; the white arrow, two bands enclosing a left-eye column. The picture in this animal thus differs from that seen in most deprived animals, in which the columns for the deprived eye stain less strongly with the silver method than the columns for the open eye. (Compare with Fig. 17 of Hubel et al. ('77) and Fig. 24 of this paper.)

shrunken, although the relative weakness of labeling and other technical problems made this less obvious than in monkey No. 240.

    Two penetrations were made into the left hemisphere. In the upper layers, the right (initially deprived) eye dominated (Fig. 42). As with the previous animal, then, there must have occurred an almost complete reversal of eye preference in these layers. The two passages through layer IVC gave alternations between exclusively left-eye and exclusively right-eye responses, at what seemed to

be normal intervals. One of these passages is reconstructed in Figure 43.

    Although the autoradiography showed only a recovery of the right-eye afferents to a normal columnar size (in layer IVCβ) and not an expansion beyond this, the sections stained with the Liesegang silver method (Fig. 43B) were not normal. They showed a relative paleness of the columns belonging to the left eye, reminiscent of the pattern seen in late monocular deprivation (e.g., monkey No. 286, section B, Fig. 24). It may

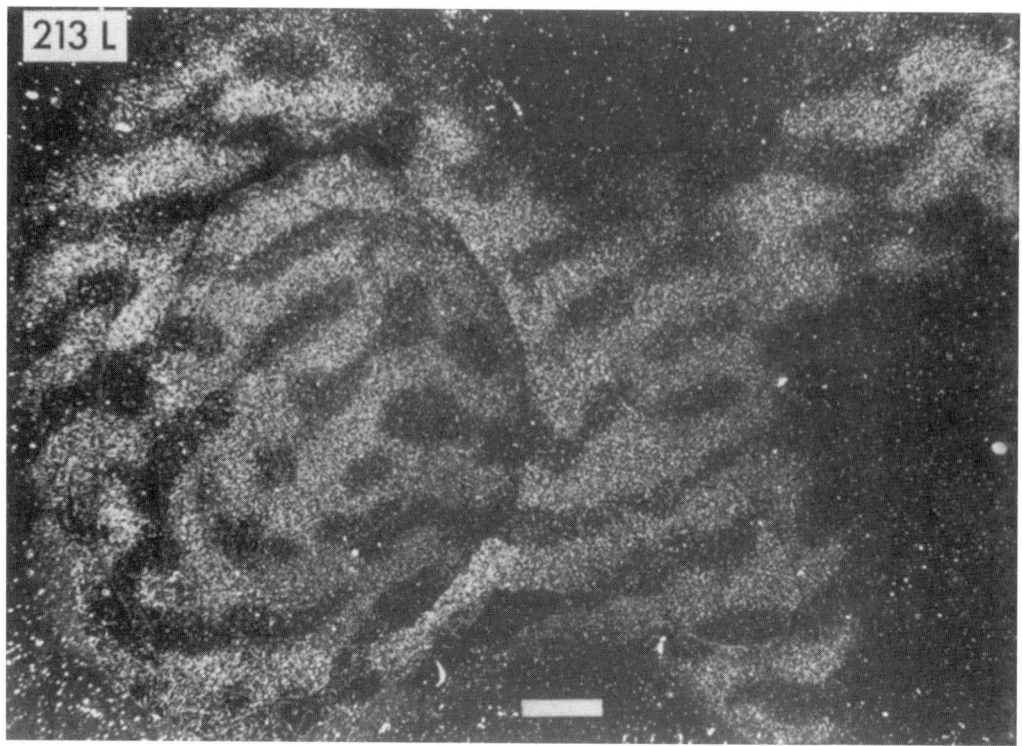

Fig. 37. Autoradiographic montage from the left cortex of monkey No. 213, whose right eye was closed from 5 to 7 weeks of age. The left eye was injected, and the labeled left-eye columns have expanded. The expansion is not, however, as great as in monkey No. 282 (Fig. 16), whose right eye was closed from 5.5 weeks to 16 months. It appears therefore that later closures require more time to produce changes in column size than do closures soon after birth.

therefore be that the afferents for the later-deprived left eye had suffered in some way beyond what was suggested by the autoradiographs.

REVERSAL AT 1 YEAR (No. 203). The last animal in this series had its right eye closed at 7 days of age

and reverse suture was not performed until 1 year of age. After a further year the left eye was opened and a further 18 months of binocular vision were allowed. The right eye was injected with [³H]proline and [³H]fucose, and recordings were made 12 days later.

Table 4. Quantitative Physiological and Anatomical Results for the Animals in Section D

No.	OCULAR DOMINANCE INDEX		RATIO OF COLUMN AREAS		LGN CELL SIZE (μM2)			
	L	R	L	R	L6	L5	R6	R5
240	—	6.82	0.32:1(IVCβ) 3.0:1(IVCα)	0.39:1(IVCβ)	253	241	185	229
194	6.09	—	1.1:1	—	(unavailable)			
203	—	1.34	1.4:1	2.2:1	140	181	180	158

For explanation of the indices, see Table 1. Note that a high O.D. index means a dominance of the initially deprived right eye, and a low index a dominance of the later deprived left eye. The column area ratios are expressed as left eye:right eye. The headings L and R refer to the side of the brain studied, not the left and right eyes.

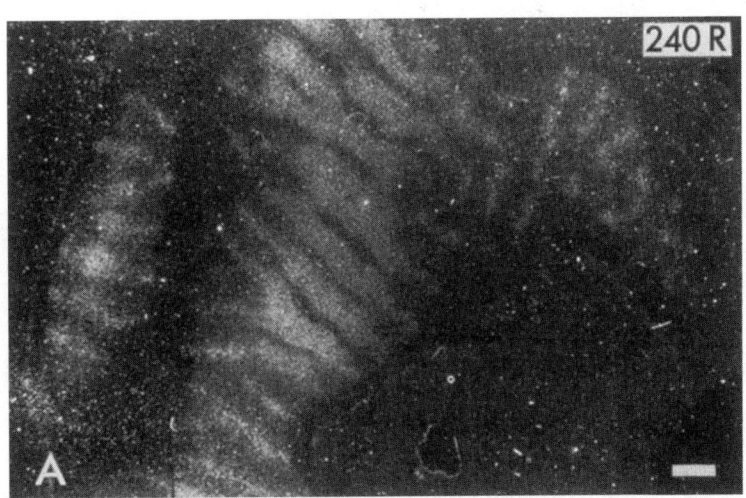

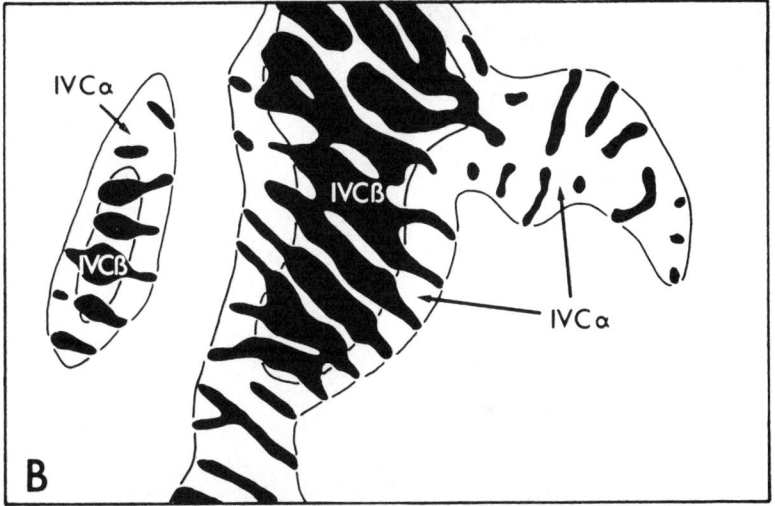

Fig. 38. Effect of reverse suture at 3 weeks of age on the labeling pattern in the right cortex of monkey No. 240. The right (initially deprived) eye was injected with [³H]proline.

A: A single tangential section. In the central region the labeled bands are expanded. In a surrounding belt they are contracted. These two regions correspond to the β and α sublaminae of layer IVC.

B: Key to A, showing the distribution of label (in black) and the boundaries of the sublaminae IVCβ and IVCα, traced from an adjacent section stained with cresylviolet. The reverse-suture protocol has led to opposite anatomical effects in the two sublaminae. Note that the thin labeled bands in IVCα run into the centers of the enlarged bands in IVCβ, meaning that the two sets of bands, though of very different widths, are still in register with each other just as they are in normal animals.

C: Autoradiographic montage of the same area. Only the regions of each micrograph that include layer IVCβ have been used in the reconstruction. Thus the montage shows expanded labeled columns throughout

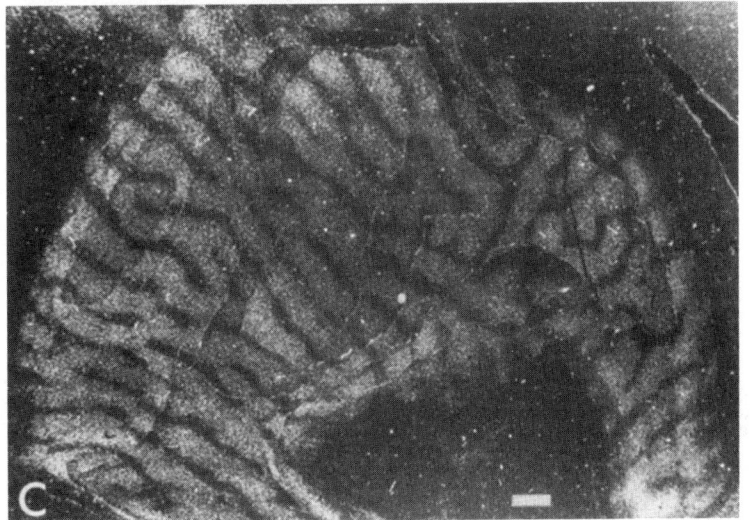

577

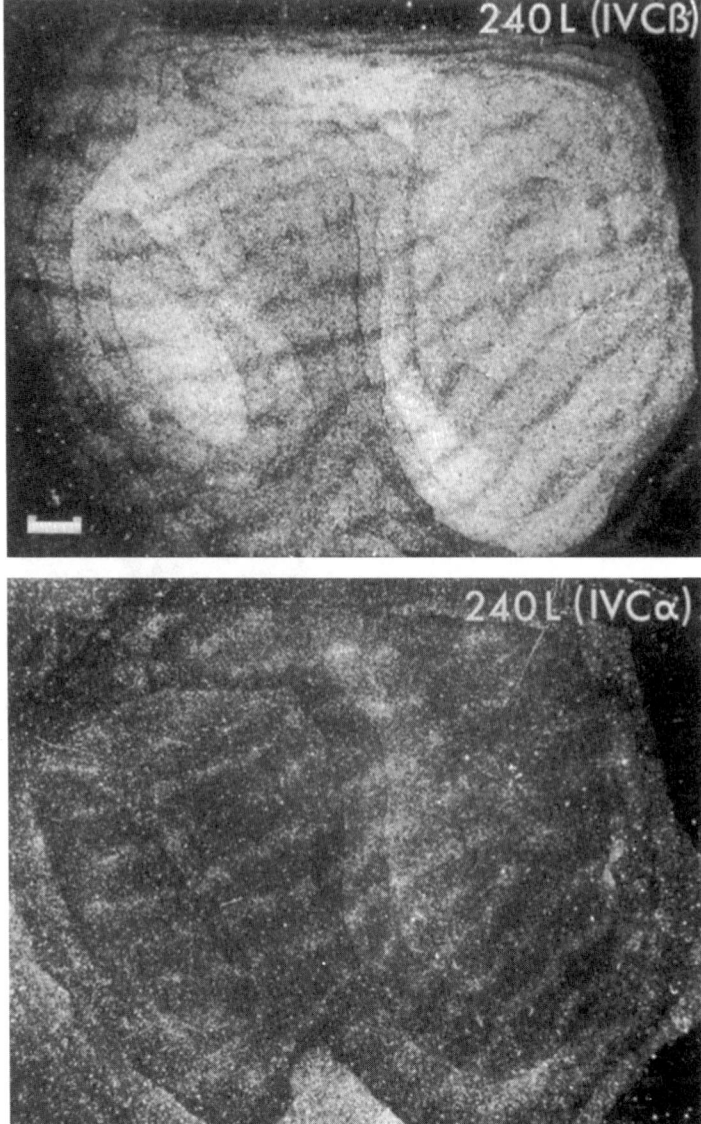

Fig. 39. Autoradiographic montages from the left cortex of monkey No. 240. The upper and lower montages were prepared from the same set of micrographs, the difference being that in one case (above) the labeling pattern in layer IVCβ was reconstructed, and in the other (below) the pattern in IVCα. Just as in the right hemisphere (Fig. 38) the shrunken labeled bands in IVCα lie in register with the enlarged bands in IVCβ.

The autoradiographs (Fig. 44) showed a strong deprivation effect, with the labeled columns (for the initially deprived eye) being about as shrunken as would be produced by a simple long-term monocular deprivation. The ratio of left- to right-eye column areas was 2.2:1 in the right hemisphere and 1.4:1 in the left hemisphere. These figures are not quite as high as in some of the cases of simple monocular deprivation (see Tables 2 and 3). We therefore cannot exclude the possibility that some recovery had occurred, although if so it was very modest in extent.

Recordings were made in the right hemisphere. The left eye dominated strongly in the

Table 5. Cell Sizes in all Laminae of the LGN for the Reverse-Sutured Monkey, No. 240, and for a Short-Term Deprived Monkey, No. 308 (See Section C)

MONKEY NO. 240				MONKEY NO. 308			
L6	253	R6	185	L6	318	R6	356
L5	241	R5	229	L5	366	R5	252
L4	243	R4	190	L4	274	R4	348
L3	254	R3	238	L3	351	R3	238
L2	407	R2	366	L2	531	R2	385
L1	386	R1	355	L1	384	R1	517

Monkey No. 308 was examined at 3 weeks, the same age at which the reverse suture was performed in No. 240. The laminae innervated by the right eye are shown in italics.

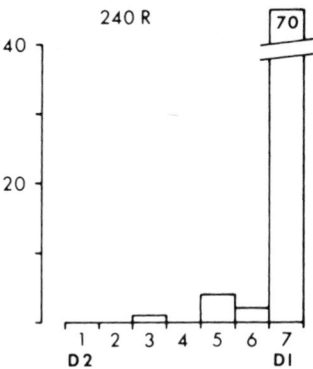

Fig. 40. Ocular dominance histogram for 77 neurons recorded in the right cortex of monkey No. 240. As with all other O.D. histograms in this paper, neurons recorded in layer IVC have been excluded. D1 and D2 mark the sides of the histogram corresponding to dominance by the initially closed eye, and the eye closed later, respectively. Nearly all neurons responded only to the initially deprived right eye.

upper layers (Fig. 45), and in layer IVC there were alternations between the two eyes, with the left eye regions about three times longer than those for the right eye. Lesions made in regions of left-eye dominance were found to coincide with the narrow bands of label in the autoradiographs. Thus the physiology supported the anatomical findings in layer IVC and indicated further that the reverse suture at 1 year had not caused any significant reversal in eye preference in the upper layers.

Comment

The results for these animals indicate that opening the deprived eye and suturing closed the other eye can cause a reversal of the anatomical and physiological effects of monocular deprivation. When performed at 3 weeks the reversal is virtually complete for the parvocellular afferents in layer IVCβ, but the magnocellular afferents in layer IVCα seem no longer capable of recovery. Performed at 6 weeks, reverse suture allowed a recovery of the normal pattern in IVCβ (i.e., equal widths for the two sets of columns) but not a complete reversal. Performed at 1 year, the reverse suture had no obvious effect.

We have already shown in section C that monocular deprivation produces its full effect by 3 weeks of age. The present results therefore indicate that reverse suture can induce changes in an established columnar pattern, and not merely a redirection of their development. Just as with simple monocular deprivation (section B) the period of susceptibility to reverse suture probably outlasts the developmental period by only a relatively short time.

E. Binocular Deprivation

It has been shown previously by physiological techniques (Wiesel and Hubel, '74) that ocular dominance columns will develop in monkeys deprived by binocular lid suture from birth. Indeed the breakdown of binocularity, which occurs as a normal process in layer IVC, extends in these animals to the upper and lower cortical layers, leading to a cortex almost devoid of binocular convergence, and possessing sharp columnar boundaries in all layers. Nevertheless, we wished to confirm with the autoradiographic technique that the segregation of afferents in layer IVC can occur independently of visual experience. We therefore reared one monkey (No. 266) in complete darkness from 3 days until 5 weeks of age, and then injected one eye

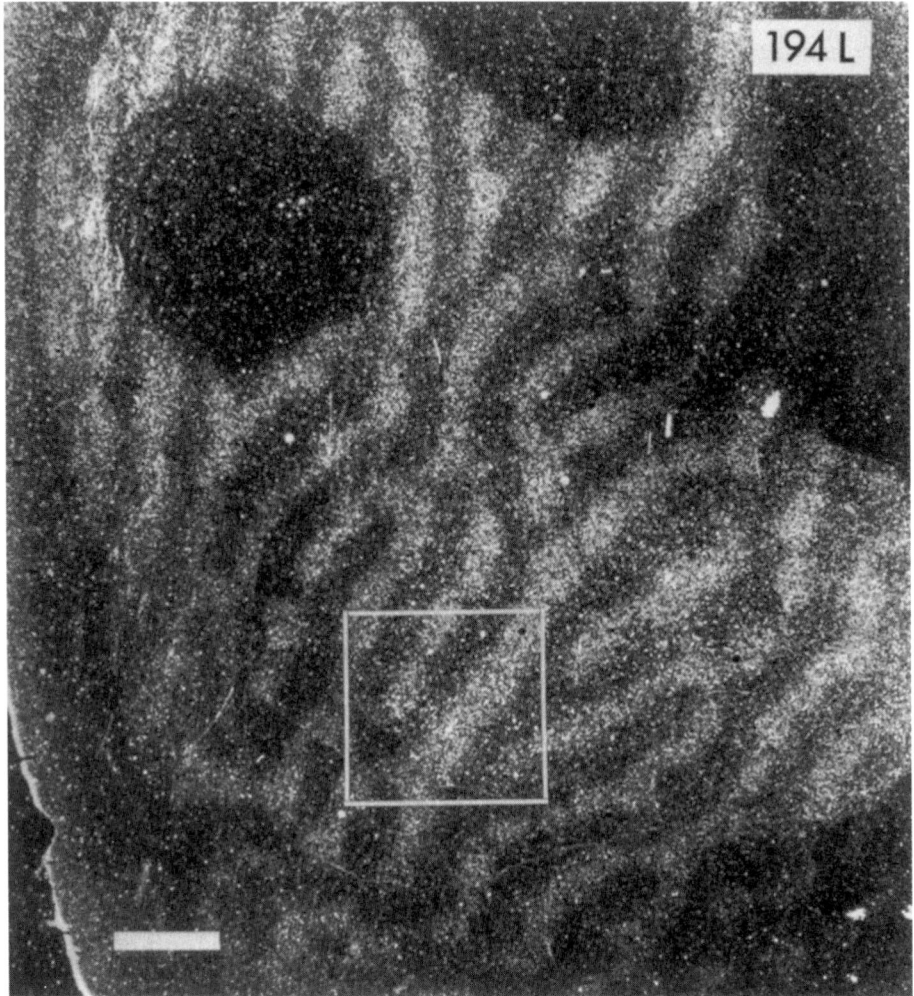

Fig. 41. Autoradiographic montage of the labeling pattern in a monkey that underwent reverse suture at 6 weeks of age (No. 194). Again, the initially deprived right eye was injected. The labeled bands are of about normal width, indicating a recovery from the effects of the early deprivation but not a complete reversal. Most of the montage shows layer IVCβ, but a small region of IVCα is visible, lower left. In this area the labeled columns have remained shrunken. An electrode penetration was made in the boxed area (Fig. 43).

with [³H]proline. The animal was allowed to survive a further 2 weeks in darkness, and perfused, without recording, at 7 weeks of age.

The injection successfully labeled only a part of the LGN on each side, so that the geniculocortical afferents were labeled only in the corresponding regions, which were in the calcarine fissure. Nevertheless in these regions a completely normal pattern of labeled patches and gaps was evident (Fig. 46). We conclude that complete darkness does not prevent columnar development. Since we have only one binocularly deprived animal, we cannot say whether the rate of segregation is accelerated, retarded, or normal.

DISCUSSION

This study extends previous work (Hubel et al., '77) on the development and plasticity of ocular dominance columns in the macaque monkey. Four main conclusions may be drawn from it. The first is that ocular dominance columns, although only partially formed at birth, develop rapidly in the first few postnatal weeks by segregation of the left-

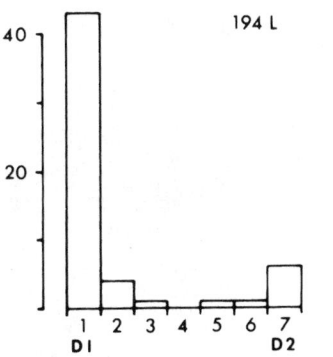

Fig. 42. Ocular dominance histogram of 56 neurons recorded on two tangential penetrations in monkey No. 194. As with monkey No. 240, most neurons have come to be driven exclusively by the initially deprived eye.

and right-eye afferents in cortical layer IV. This process seems to occur in the presence or absence of visual experience. Second, the process may be redirected by early monocular deprivation, causing the segregation of the two sets of afferents into columns of unequal width. Third, a rearrangement of the afferents can be induced for a short period after their segregation is complete. This kind of plasticity can be demonstrated both in normal animals, by later eye closure, and in monocularly deprived animals, by reverse suture. Fourth, the eye preference of neurons in the upper layers of the cortex may be changed even after plasticity in layer IV is no longer detectable.

Normal Development

Our observations suggest that, at 1 week of age, the left- and right-eye afferents overlap extensively with each other in the fourth layer, but have already begun the process of segregation into alternating bands. Physiologically, this is reflected in a mixing of left- and right-eye responses, even if some monocular regions are already present. By 3 weeks segregation is nearly complete, but there is still a slight overlap at the borders of columns. By 6 weeks the afferents are fully segregated, and physiologically the ocular dominance columns have their mature organization.

Before accepting this description of columnar development, however, it is necessary to consider the validity of the two methods on which we have principally relied: the autoradiography of transneuronally transported [³H]proline, and electro-

physiological recordings made during long tangential penetrations.

There are several reasons for doubting that the autoradiography gives a totally faithful image of the distribution of geniculocortical terminals for the injected eye. The most important reason is the possibility of 'spillover' in the LGN: the spread of labeled material to neurons in the inappropriate laminae of the LGN and its transport to their terminals in the wrong set of ocular dominance columns in area 17. In the cat this leakage has been measured and its effect on the cortical labeling pattern has been calculated (LeVay et al., '78). From that study it appeared that spillover seriously degraded the cortical labeling pattern in young animals, especially on the side contralateral to the eye injection. It was concluded that in the cat the two sets of afferents *were* intermixed initially— since spillover would not have been sufficient to mask a columnar pattern, had it been present—but that the process of segregation occurred more rapidly than was suggested by direct inspection of the autoradiographs. In the present study the preparative technique (frozen-sectioning) precluded measurement of spillover. Our impression on simple inspection of the geniculate autoradiographs was that, as in the cat, labeling of neurons in the inappropriate laminae of the LGN was much heavier in infant than in adult animals.

A second point is that some unknown fraction of the autoradiographic label must be present in preterminal fibers rather than synaptic boutons. In adult monkeys, preterminal fibers are known to be less rigorously confined to their appropriate columns than are the boutons (Hubel and Wiesel, '72). It is possible that at early stages of development the boutons are relatively few and that their columnar distribution is therefore masked to some extent by the labeled fibers. A third, perhaps more fanciful, source of error is that eye injections done 1–2 weeks before the animal's death might give a distribution of cortical label corresponding to the columnar pattern existing, not at the time of death, but at a slightly earlier time. These three possible sources of error would tend to have a common effect: they would make the pace of columnar development seem slower than it is.

In spite of these problems, we do not doubt the basic conclusion derived from the autoradiography in infant (Hubel et al., '77) and fetal (Rakic,

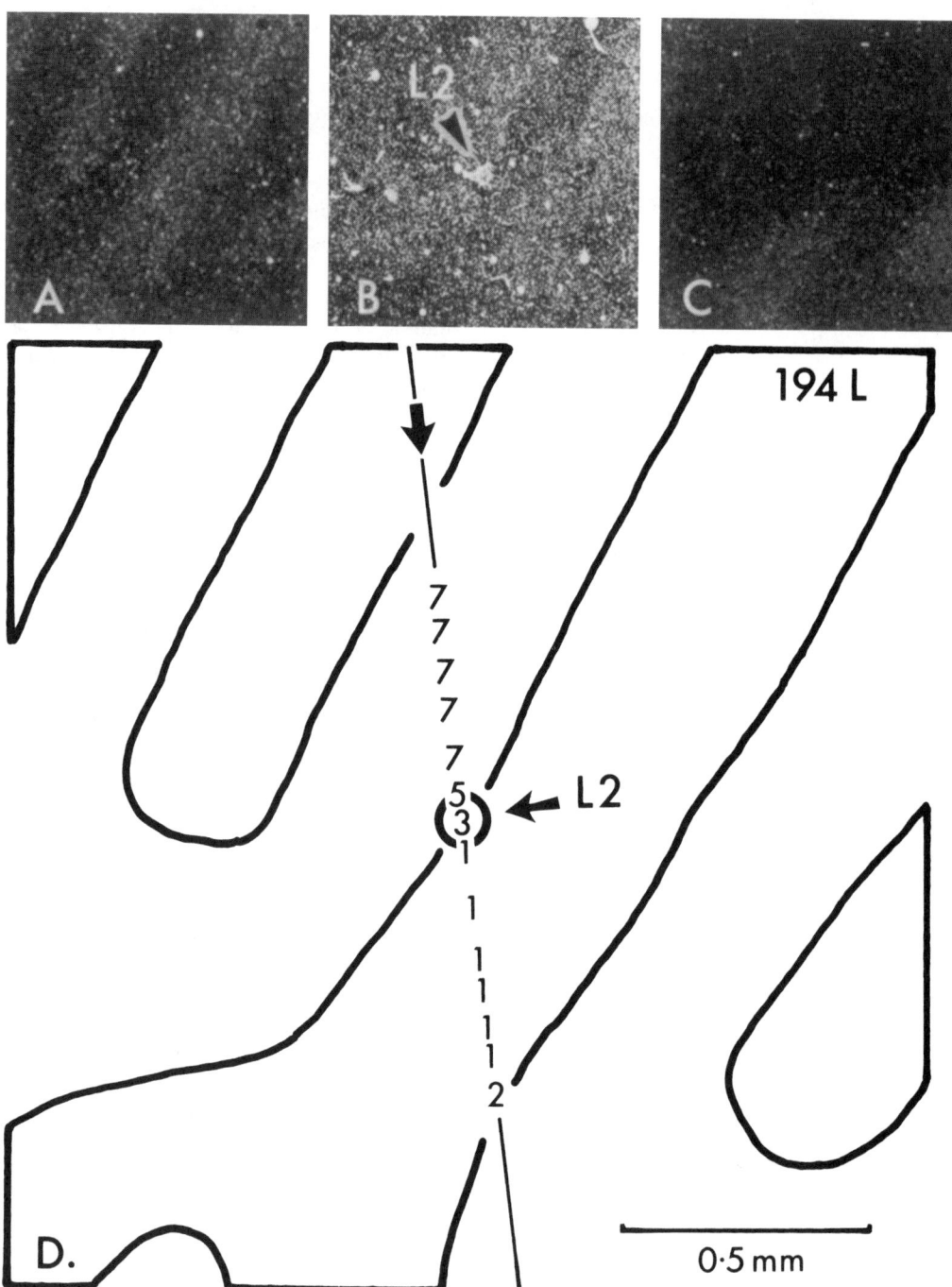

Fig. 43. Reconstruction of an electrode pass-through layer IVC in monkey No. 194 (see Fig. 41). A and C are autoradiographs, and B is an intervening section stained with the Liesegang silver method. Besides showing the position of a lesion, this section illustrates that the columns for the initially deprived right eye stain more darkly with the silver method than do the columns for the left eye (the oblique dark bands in B are in register with the labeled bands in A). D is the track reconstruction, showing a sequence of left-eye responses, an abrupt transition at the column border (lesion 2), and another sequence of right-eye responses. This is the normal physiological picture in layer IVC. Only the first two or three recording sites were in IVCα, the rest in IVCβ.

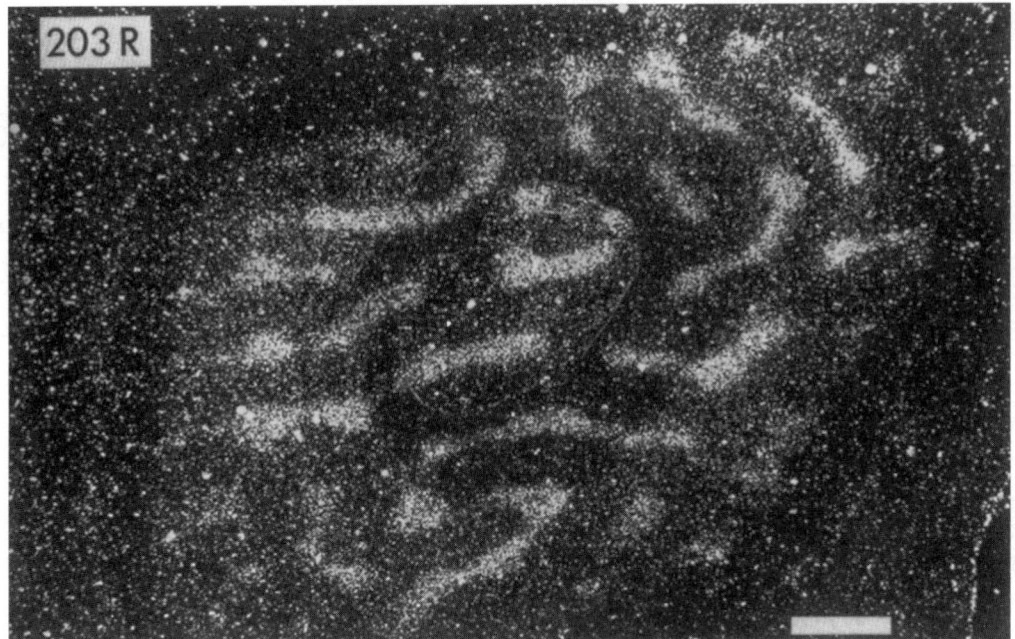

Fig. 44. Autoradiographic montage from monkey No. 203, which was reverse-sutured at 1 year of age. The labeled columns (for the initially deprived right eye) show a marked deprivation effect, indicating that the late reversal did not permit any anatomical recovery.

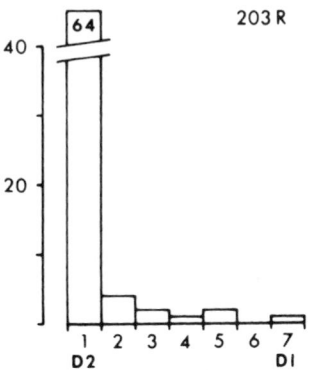

Fig. 45. Ocular dominance histogram of 74 neurons recorded on two tangential penetrations in monkey No. 203. Most cells responded only to stimulation of the eye that had initially been open.

'76) monkeys, namely that ocular dominance columns do develop by a process of segregation of the afferents out of an initially intermixed state. This conclusion is supported by a second and independent line of anatomical evidence. In cats, it has proved possible to reconstruct the entire terminal arborizations of single geniculocortical afferents, both in young kittens, by the use of the Golgi method (LeVay and Stryker, '79), and in adults, by bulk-filling with horseradish peroxidase (Ferster and LeVay, '78). In two-week-old kittens, at an age when transneuronal autoradiography still shows completely uniform and continuous labeling (LeVay et al., '78), single afferents have arborizations that span a large cortical territory—regions as large as 2 mm in diameter in surface view. Within this area, which would be large enough to house several ocular dominance columns in an adult cat, the arborization is uniform and shows no local clumping or gaps (LeVay and Stryker, '79). In adult cats, by contrast, these large arborizations are broken up into clumps of terminal-bearing branches, about 0.5 mm across, separated by terminal-free gaps of about the same size (Ferster and LeVay, '78). These clumps correspond in all probability to a number of ocular dominance columns for the same eye, and the gaps to the intervening columns for the other eye. Thus the uniform distribution of the axonal arborizations in young kittens agrees well with the autoradiography and suggests that left- and right-eye afferents overlap extensively with each other at this age.

The physiological recording technique is immune to the problems just mentioned, but it has

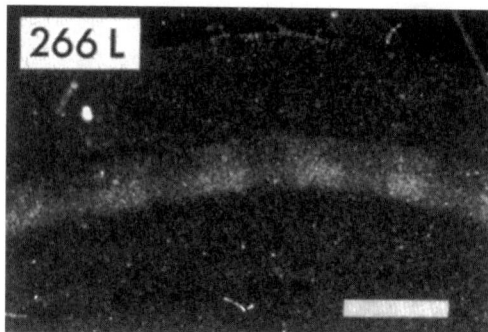
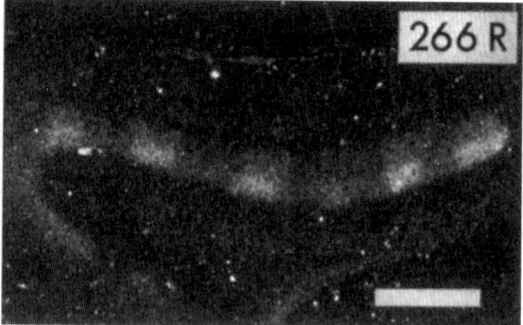

Fig. 46. Autoradiographs of single transverse sections from the left and right cortex of monkey No. 266, which was reared in complete darkness from 3 to 49 days of age. In spite of the monkey's lack of vision, the columns have a normal autoradiographic appearance. For physiological evidence for normal development of ocular dominance columns in dark-reared monkeys, see Wiesel and Hubel ('74).

others of its own. First, we are not entirely sure whether the activity recorded in layer IVC arises predominantly from cortical neurons or geniculate afferents, although we believe the former to be the more likely source. Certainly the recording of even occasional binocular single units in this layer in young animals supports this assumption. Another problem concerns the spatial resolution of the technique. When an electrode crosses a column border in layer IVC of an adult monkey's cortex, the eye-preference of the multi-unit activity shifts from group 1 to group 7 (or vice versa) over a distance of about 50 μm, depending partially on the angle between the electrode track and the column traversed. At least some of this apparent mixing of left- and right-eye cells at the borders between columns must be due to technical factors, in particular to the recording of neuronal activity at some distance from the electrode tip and to the actual uninsulated tip length of the electrode. It is conceivable that the recording situation in infant monkeys differs from that in adults in such a way as to increase the artifactual mixing of left- or right-eye activity—perhaps because of the lack of myelin. Since we cannot eliminate this possibility we must lay particular emphasis on the finding, in the 8-day-old monkey, of binocular single units in layer IVC. Such units, with a center-surround receptive field organization and no orientation preference, are never binocularly activated in the adult (Hubel and Wiesel, '68). Although other explanations for their binocularity are possible, the simplest is that it arises from an overlap of the left- and right-eye afferents as suggested by the autoradiography.

Further insight into the physiology of ocular dominance columns in infant monkeys has been provided by the use of the [^{14}C]deoxyglucose method. Sokoloff and his collaborators (Des Rosiers et al., '78; Sokoloff, personal communication) have studied the uptake of [^{14}C]deoxyglucose in 1-day-old monkeys during monocular vision. In these animals, just as in adults, autoradiography showed alternating columns of high and low uptake, but the columns were somewhat less sharply defined than in adults, particularly in layer IV. Within the binocular region of area 17, there was no difference between the labeling patterns in the hemispheres ipsilateral and contralateral to the stimulated eye. This result is in agreement with our physiological observations; but contrasts with the transneuronal autoradiography in our youngest monkey, which showed forming columns on the side ipsilateral to the injected eye but none on the contralateral side. Thus it strengthens our belief that the failure to see any columns by transneuronal transport of [^{3}H]proline, in the hemisphere contralateral to the injected eye, was caused by leakage of label between laminae of the LGN.

By 3 weeks of age segregation is very nearly complete, as judged both from the autoradiographic and the physiological results. There is a discrepancy, however, between the results obtained by the two methods. While both methods indicate a slight blurring of the borders of columns, the autoradiography also showed some label above background in the gaps between labeled columns, particularly on the side contralateral to the injected eye, as if the afferents for the contralateral eye had not yet completely cleared from the ipsilateral eye's columns. Indeed, even at 6 weeks of age there was a noticeably higher grain density in the gaps between labeled bands on the contralateral side than on the ipsilateral side or in either hemisphere of adults. The physiology, however, gave no hint of such an asymmetry: in the two animals recorded from at 3 weeks (Nos. 256 and 202) as well as in the 6-week-old animal (No. 257) neuronal activity in layer IVC swung between complete ipsilateral-eye and complete contralateral-eye dominance. In one of the 3-week-old monkeys (No. 256) there was a suggestion in the physiology that the column borders were less sharply defined than in the adult (Fig. 4), and this observation was strengthened by the finding, in layer IVC, of one binocular single unit at a column border. In the 6-week-old monkey the physiological picture in layer IVC suggested complete segregation as in the adult. In view of the evidence, discussed above, that the autoradiography can give a false impression of the rate of columnar development, we believe that the actual timetable of segregation is that suggested by the physiology: that both sets of afferents segregate out at the same pace, are largely separate from each other at 3 weeks, and are completely so by 6 weeks.

The alternative possibility is that changes in the eye preference of cortical neurons (from binocular to monocular responses) precede the anatomical segregation of the afferents. In a very limited and local sense this may well be so: a particular axon terminal that is destined for withdrawal may lose its physiological effectiveness while it is still in contact with the postsynaptic cell, and certainly will do so once it is separated by a few microns. But the overall process of columnar development occupies several weeks, and there is more than enough time for normal growth processes to bring about a redistribution of terminals as the physiological columns mature. We think, it unnecessary to postulate any detectable mismatch between the distribution of the afferents and the ocular dominance of the cortical cells at any given time.

Columnar Development in Binocular Deprivation

The process of columnar development, in the monkey at least, does not seem to require visual experience. Segregation of left- and right-eye afferents

begins in utero (Rakic, '76). As mentioned above, the presence of functional columns, although less well defined than in adults, was demonstrated in 1-day-old monkeys by the [^{14}C]deoxyglucose method (Des Rosiers et al., '78) and in a 1-week-old monkey by microelectrode recording (see above). That postnatal columnar maturation also occurs independently of visual experience is indicated by the result from the dark-reared monkey, No. 266 (Results, section E). This monkey was put in the dark at 3 days of age and at 7 weeks showed an autoradiographic labeling pattern similar to that of a normal adult. Physiologically, binocularly deprived monkeys show an even more pronounced segregation according to eye preference than is seen in normal animals (Wiesel and Hubel, '74). Most cells are monocularly activated, both within and outside of layer IVC, and columnar borders are very sharp (see especially Figs. 2B and 3B of Wiesel and Hubel, '74). The picture thus resembles that obtained by raising animals with artificial strabismus (Hubel and Wiesel, '65; Baker et al., '74). Normal binocular experience, far from promoting columnar segregation, therefore seems necessary for the maintenance of connections (outside of layer IVC) that mediate binocular convergence.

Misrouting of Development by Early Monocular Deprivation

According to the working hypothesis stated earlier, the critical period for the production of anatomical changes in the fourth layer would be the period of overlap of the left- and right-eye afferents. This idea was partially borne out, to the extent that anatomical changes could be produced during this period. The results of short-term deprivation (part C) show that if one eye is closed soon after birth segregation of the afferents continues, with the difference that most of the retraction is done by the afferents for the closed eye. Patterned visual input to one eye, with the other eye closed, does therefore seem to allow that eye's geniculocortical afferents to hold on to synaptic targets that they would normally abandon, and conversely, the afferents for the deprived eye relinquish more territory than they normally would.

Just as with the young normal animals, the short-term deprived monkeys showed a slight discrepancy between the autoradiography and the physiology. In the monkey deprived until 3 weeks of age (No. 308) injection of the deprived eye led to labeling of shrunken, fragmented bands in layer IVC, but the large gaps between these bands also contained some label above background levels. In the recording, however (monkeys No. 308 and 164), responses to stimulation of the deprived eye were recorded only for short segments in layer IVC: the greater part of the passages through the layer was taken up by neurons that responded exclusively to the experienced eye. We believe that the physiology gives a more truthful picture of the state of columnar development, and that the presence of label above background throughout layer IVC results from spillover in the LGN. As with the normal animals at the same age, however, we have not fully excluded the alternative possibility, that the deprived eye's afferents maintain some (nonfunctional) terminals in the open eye's columns. This possibility could be investigated with the Nauta method after single-lamina lesions in the LGN (Hubel and Wiesel, '72). Whether the label in the gaps between columns is artifactual or not, it had largely disappeared by 27 days of age (monkey No. 307): the picture in this animal was very similar to that seen in long-term deprivation.

Rearrangement of Columns after Segregation

A more decisive test of our ideas about the relationship between plasticity and development was offered by the series of experiments in which monkeys had one eye closed at successively later ages (part B). Given the information now available about normal development, we would have predicted that lid suture at 3 weeks would produce at most quite a modest effect on the relative size of left- and right-eye columns in layer IVC, and at 6 weeks it would produce no effect in this layer. In fact, lid suture at 5.5 weeks of age produced a marked effect—just as great as at 2 weeks of age. Even when begun at 10 weeks, monocular deprivation still produced a measurable effect in layer IVC, although it was a mild one and was restricted to the side ipsilateral to the lid suture. The period of anatomical plasticity therefore seems to outlast the period of overlap, even if only by a few weeks.

Although the evidence is fragmentary, we suspect that changes in column width induced after completion of segregation take longer to develop than do the effects of early closure. Thus a 2-week closure begun at 5 weeks had a milder effect than a similar period of deprivation begun at 1 week (compare monkeys No. 213 and 164, section C), while a 15-month closure begun at 5.5 weeks had an effect as great as a 3-week closure begun at 1 week (monkeys No. 282, section B, and No. 308, section C). The greater time required for reexpansion may reflect a reduced opportunity for competition between left- and right-eye afferents for synaptic targets, once they have segregated into columns. Clearly, though, segregation is not a complete barrier to effective competition.

The Liesegang reduced-silver method (LeVay et al., '75) revealed an additional effect of monocular deprivation even when begun as late as 1 year of age. This was the relative paleness (reduced argyrophilia) of the fourth-layer bands representing the deprived eye in the absence of any abnormality of column width (see Fig. 24). We do not know the basis for this curious effect; it could be due to a lowered density of deprived-eye afferents, a reduction in their caliber, or some weakening of intracortical connections within the deprived-eye columns. It should be mentioned that the silver method was used primarily on tissue from older animals, since it did not satisfactorily stain sections from animals under about 7 months of age.

We have concentrated our attention on the fourth layer of the cortex—in fact on one sublamina, IVC, which receives most of the geniculocortical afferents. Our motivation for this was, of course, the availability of the anatomical methods for studying the columnar pattern in this layer. It is very clear, however, that susceptibility to monocular deprivation is also exhibited in the upper and lower cortical layers, and that in these regions it persists for a longer time, perhaps for well over a year after birth. Thus the projections from layer IVC to the upper layers are probably also capable of modification by visual deprivation, even though we have not as yet examined the question anatomically.

Reverse Suture

The conclusion that a reorganization of the columnar pattern can be induced after segregation is complete is strengthened by the results of the experiments involving reverse suture (part D). Reverse suture done at 3 weeks—an age at which the initial deprivation had already caused the segregation of the afferents into bands of unequal width—caused reversal of the autoradiographic and physiological picture in layer IVC, although the effect was limited to the zone of termination of the parvocellular geniculate afferents (layer IVCβ). Reverse suture at 6 weeks, while not permitting a reversal of the autoradiographic picture, did allow a re-expansion of the deprived eye's afferents (in IVCβ) to their normal width. Here too was demonstrated an ability of geniculocortical afferents to regain cortical territory that they had previously relinquished. Only the third animal in this group, which was reverse-sutured at one year of age, failed to show any recovery.

Why the magnocellular afferents (to lamina IVCα) were not induced to re-expand by reverse suture is something of a puzzle. The differential effect may be related to the observation that very early closure seems to cause a more dramatic loss of territory by the deprived eye in layer IVCα than in IVCβ (monkey No. 201, section B). Alternatively, whatever process terminates anatomical plasticity in layer IV may simply exert its effects earlier on the magnocellular than on the parvocellular afferents. If this explanation is correct, one would expect to be able to find an age at which simple monocular closure also would affect selectively the parvocellular afferents. We do not have a clear example of such a result among the series of animals in section B, having on the whole paid less attention to lamina IVCα than IVCβ (the reconstructions illustrated in this paper—except for Figure 39B—are all from IVCβ, principally because of its greater labeling density).

Our physiological observations on the effects of reverse suture are in general agreement with those of Blakemore et al. ('78) in showing a reversibility of eye preference after the effects of the initial deprivation have taken place. The autoradiography suggests that this process involves a contraction and later re-expansion of the afferents for the deprived eye in layer IVC. The alternative model, by which deprived-eye synapses are 'suppressed' and later 'de-repressed' (Blakemore et al., '78) seems less likely (one would have to invoke a failure of axonal transport in the suppressed afferents), but more precise anatomical methods will be required to resolve the issue.

We believe, then, that the geniculocortical afferents *can* re-expand into territory they have previously relinquished. A definitive experiment to verify this conclusion would involve examining the columnar pattern in the same animal twice: before and after a period of monocular deprivation, or before and after a reverse suture. This was actually done physiologically in monkey No. 202, and the results from this animal certainly support the idea that established columns can be rearranged. Nevertheless, it would be most convincing to have autoradiographic evidence of the columnar structure at the two ages. Although we have not done such an experiment, it would probably be feasible to biopsy the cortex of a young monkey before closing one of its eyes and then to examine it again after a long period of deprivation. In the absence of this kind of evidence our present conclusion remains strong but perhaps falls short of certainty.

In considering how such a re-expansion of afferents could occur, it may be significant that the preterminal portions of the axonal arborizations, even in adults, are not entirely restricted to columns for the appropriate eye. This was shown initially by degeneration methods (Hubel and Wiesel, '72). Since then, as mentioned above, it has been possible to bulk-fill entire arborizations (in the cat) with horseradish peroxidase by extracellular (Ferster and LeVay, '78) or intracellular (Gilbert and Wiesel, '79) injections. Some of these arborizations spanned several ocular dominance columns. Their terminal-bearing portions were arranged in clumps, and these clumps were joined by myelinated preterminal segments that ran tangentially in the fourth layer, apparently traversing columns for the other eye. For axons of this type, re-expansion might involve nothing more than local sprouting of boutons from preterminal segments. The application of the HRP bulk-filling method to normal and deprived monkeys might well throw more light on the exact nature of the rearrangement that is induced by eye-closure.

Cell Size in the LGN

Our previously published results (Hubel et al., '77) suggested that the relative size of cells in left- and right-eye laminae of the lateral geniculate nucleus was related to the relative size of left- and right-eye ocular dominance columns in area 17. The larger number of animals in the present study allows us to examine the relationship quantitatively (Fig. 47).

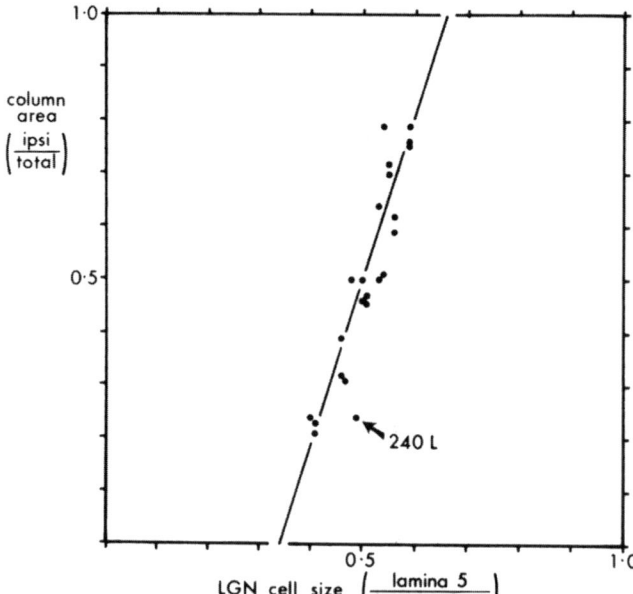

Fig. 47. Relationship between LGN cell size and cortical column size. The ordinate is the fraction of total cortical area occupied by afferents for the ipsilateral eye (derived from measurement of the autoradiographic montages). The abscissa is the ratio of the mean cell size in LGN lamina 5—a lamina supplying ipsilateral eye columns in area 17—to the sum of the means for laminae 5 and 6. Each point is derived from one hemisphere in one animal. The solid line is the calculated regression line. The point lying farthest from the regression line (left hemisphere of monkey No. 240—see text) has been labeled.

There is indeed a good correlation between the two variables (r = 0.91). This result supports Guillery's ('72) hypothesis that the size of neurons in the LGN is a reflection of the size of the axonal arborizations they must sustain in the visual cortex. It is important, though, to point out the existence of exceptions. The most glaring of these was the left hemisphere of monkey No. 240, the animal reverse-sutured at 3 weeks of age (see Results, section D). In the left visual cortex the parvocellular afferents for the initially deprived right eye had re-expanded to occupy most of the area of their target lamina, but the neurons in all the parvocellular laminae of the left LGN were about the same size. An exception of the opposite kind was provided by the monkey subjected to monocular enucleation as an adult (No. 269, not plotted in Fig. 47). This animal showed dramatic cell shrinkage in the de-afferented laminae of the LGN, but the columnar pattern in the cortex appeared normal. There may well be relatively simple explanations for these exceptions (perhaps the density of synapses, as well as the overall column area, needs to be taken into account) but they are a reminder that one should be cautious about predicting conditions in the cortex from geniculate cell size alone.

Columnar Development and the Critical Period

It seems from our results that the completion of columnar segregation is not responsible for the end of susceptibility to monocular deprivation in layer IVC. A similar conclusion has been reached for the cat's cortex (LeVay et al., '78), but for a different reason. In that species segregation stops short of completion: the edges of columns in the adult cat are more blurred than in the monkey, and plenty of binocular cells are found in the regions of overlap. If our hypothesis were to be the complete explanation for the critical period and its termination, there should be a substantial anatomical effect of lid suture even in the adult cat. This there is not; even monocular enucleation fails to induce re-expansion of columns for the other eye in adult cats (LeVay, unpublished observations). There are other species in which ocular dominance columns are even less clearly defined, such as the squirrel monkey (LeVay et al., '76; Hubel and Wiesel, '78), or not present at all, such as the mouse (Dräger, '74, '75). The effects of lid suture in adults of these species have not been described, but we doubt that they would show any more plasticity than do adult cats or monkeys. We therefore suspect that some other developmental process acts to terminate the critical period. There are a number of possible candidates for this. One might cite, as an example, the myelination of the terminal arborizations of the geniculocortical afferents. Myelination occurs after columnar segregation is completed, and it is quite a gradual process. In their fully mature state, the arborizations are clad with myelin throughout their extent, and only the boutons and the very short and fine preterminal segments are free of it (Ferster and LeVay, '78). The relocation of an axon, thus ensheathed, might well be more difficult than if it were bare. Still, the image of a myelin sheath as a straitjacket is probably simplistic: there are reports of sprouting from nodes of Ranvier (Speidel, '42, Barker and Ip, '66), and demyelination might also occur.

It should also be kept in mind that the postsynaptic cortical neurons, as well as the afferents, undergo morphological changes during postnatal development. Boothe et al. ('79) have examined, in the monkey, the development of dendritic spines on the spiny stellate cells of layer IVC. They reported an increase in spine density during the first two postnatal months, followed by a more gradual decline. These spines are the main synaptic target for the geniculocortical afferents (Garey and Powell, '71). The continued generation of new synaptic sites during the first two months might therefore be the process which permits re-expansion of afferent arborizations in response to lid suture, and the cessation of synaptogenesis might terminate the period of plasticity. It should be pointed out, though, that the synapses formed by geniculate afferents constitute only a minority of the total axospinous synapses, even within layer IV (Garey and Powell, '71; LeVay and Gilbert, '76). More information is needed on the numbers and distribution of the synapses formed by geniculate afferents during postnatal development. Further study of the morphological development of the layers above and below layer IVC might also be helpful for an understanding of why sensitivity to deprivation, in these layers, extends so much longer into postnatal life.

ACKNOWLEDGMENTS

We are grateful to the staff of the New England Regional Primate Center for care of the animals. We also thank Neil Segil, Birthe Storai, Karen Larson, and Edward Coughlin for the histology, autoradiography, and cell measurements; Marc Peloquin for assistance with photography; David Freeman for computer programming; and Olivia Brum for assistance with the manuscript.

This study was supported by NIH grants EY00605, EY00606, and EY01960, and NIH Core grant EY01995. S.L. is the recipient of an NIH Research Career Development Award.

Literature Cited

Baker, F.H., P. Grigg, and G.K. von Noorden (1974) Effects of visual deprivation and strabismus on the response of neurons in the visual cortex of the monkey, including studies on the striate and prestriate cortex in the normal animal. Brain Res., *66:*185–208.

Barker, D., and M.C. Ip (1966) Sprouting and regeneration of mammalian motor axons in normal and deafferented skeletal muscle. Proc. R. Soc. Lond. B, *163:*538–554.

Blakemore, C., L.J. Garey, and F. Vital-Durand (1978) The physiological effects of monocular deprivation and their reversal in the monkey's cortex. J. Physiol., *261:*423–444.

Blakemore, C., and R.C. Van Sluyters (1974) Reversal of the physiological effects of monocular deprivation in kittens: Further evidence for a sensitive period. J. Physiol. *237:*195–216.

Boothe, R.G., W.T. Greenough, J.S. Lund, and K. Wrege (1979) A quantitative investigation of spine and dendrite development of neurons in visual cortex (area 17) of *Macaca nemestrina* monkeys. J. Comp. Neurol., *186:*473–489.

Des Rosiers, M.H., O. Sakurada, J. Jehle, M. Shinohara, C. Kennedy, and L. Sokoloff (1978) Functional plasticity in the immature striate cortex of the monkey shown by the [^{14}C]deoxyglucose method. Science, *200:*447–449.

Dräger, U.C. (1974) Autoradiography of tritiated proline and fucose transported transneuronally from the eye to the visual cortex in pigmented and albino mice. Brain Res., *82:*284–292.

Dräger, U.C. (1975) Receptive fields of single cells and topography in mouse visual cortex. J. Comp. Neurol., *160:*269–290.

Ferster, D., and S. LeVay (1978) The axonal arborizations of lateral geniculate neurons in the striate cortex of the cat. J. Comp. Neurol., *182:*925–944.

Garey, L.J., and T.P.S. Powell (1971) An experimental study of the termination of the lateral geniculo-cortical pathway in the cat and monkey. Proc. R. Soc. Lond. B, *179:*1–63.

Gilbert, C.D., and T.N. Wiesel (1979) Morphology and intracortical projections of functionally characterised neurones in the cat visual cortex. Nature, *280:*120–125.

Guillery, R.W. (1972) Binocular competition in the control of geniculate cell growth. J. Comp. Neurol., *144:*117–130.

Hubel, D.H., and T.N. Wiesel (1965) Binocular interaction in striate cortex of kittens reared with artificial squint. J. Neurophysiol., *28:*1041–1059.

Hubel, D.H., and T.N. Wiesel (1968) Receptive fields and functional architecture of monkey striate cortex. J. Physiol., *195:*215–243.

Hubel, D.H., and T.N. Wiesel (1970) The period of susceptibility to the physiological effects of unilateral eye closure in kittens. J. Physiol., *206:*419–436.

Hubel, D.H., and T.N. Wiesel (1972) Laminar and columnar distribution of geniculo-cortical fibers in the macaque monkey. J. Comp. Neurol., *146:*421–450.

Hubel, D.H., and T.N. Wiesel (1978) Distribution of inputs from the two eyes in striate cortex of squirrel monkeys. Soc. Neurosci. Abstr., *4*:632.

Hubel, D.H., T.N. Wiesel, and S. LeVay (1975) Functional architecture of area 17 in normal and monocularly deprived macaque monkeys. Cold Spring Harbor Symposia, *40*:581–589.

Hubel, D.H., T.N. Wiesel, and S. LeVay (1977) Plasticity of ocular dominance columns in monkey striate cortex. Phil. Trans. R. Soc. Lond. B., *278*:377–409.

LeVay, S. (1971) On the neurons and synapses of the lateral geniculate nucleus of the monkey, and the effects of eye enucleation. Z. Zellforsch., *113*:396–419.

LeVay, S., and C.D. Gilbert (1976) Laminar patterns of geniculocortical projection in the cat. Brain Res., *113*:1–19.

LeVay, S., D.H. Hubel, and T.N. Wiesel (1975) The pattern of ocular dominance columns in macaque visual cortex revealed by a reduced silver stain. J. Comp. Neurol., *159*:559–576.

LeVay, S., and M.P. Stryker (1979) The development of ocular dominance columns in the cat. Soc. Neurosci. Symp., *4*:83–98.

LeVay, S., M.P. Stryker, and C.J. Shatz (1978) Ocular dominance columns and their development in layer IV of the cat's visual cortex: A quantitative study. J. Comp. Neurol., *179*:223–244.

Matthews, M.R., W.M. Cowan, and T.P.S. Powell (1960) Transneuronal cell degeneration in the lateral geniculate nucleus of the macaque monkey. J. Anat., *94*:145–169.

Minkowski, M. (1920) Über den Verlauf, die Endigung und die zentrale Repräsentation von gekreuzten und ungekreuzten Sehnervenfasern bei einigen Säugetieren und bei Menschen. Schweiz. Arch. Neurol. Neurochir. Psychiatr., *6*:201–257.

Rakic, P. (1976) Prenatal genesis of connections subserving ocular dominance in the rhesus monkey. Nature (London), *261*:467–471.

Ramachandran, V.S., P.G.H. Clarke, and D. Whitteridge (1977) Cells selective to binocular disparity in the cortex of newborn lambs. Nature (London), *268*:333–335.

Shatz, C.J., S.H. Lindström, and T.N. Wiesel (1977) The distribution of afferents representing the right and left eyes in the cat's visual cortex. Brain Res., *131*:103–116.

Shatz, C.J., and M.P. Stryker (1978) Ocular dominance in layer IV of the cat's visual cortex and the effects of monocular deprivation. J. Physiol., *281*:267–283.

Sherk, H., and M.P. Stryker (1976) Quantitative study of cortical orientation selectivity in visually inexperienced kitten. J. Neurophysiol., *39*:63–70.

Specht, S.C., and B. Grafstein (1973) Accumulation of radioactive protein in mouse cerebral cortex after injection of ^{3}H-fucose into the eye. Exp. Neurol., *41*:705–722.

Speidel, C.C. (1942) Studies of living nerves. VII. Growth adjustments of cutaneous terminal arborizations. J. Comp. Neurol., *76*:57–69.

Wiesel, T.N., and D.H. Hubel (1963) Single-cell responses in striate cortex of kittens deprived of vision in one eye. J. Neurophysiol., *26*:1003–1017.

Wiesel, T.N., and D.H. Hubel (1974) Ordered arrangement of orientation columns in monkeys lacking visual experience. J. Comp. Neurol., *158*:307–318.

Wiesel, T.H., D.H. Hubel, and D.M.K. Lam (1974) Autoradiographic demonstration of ocular-dominance columns in the monkey striate cortex by means of transneuronal transport. Brain Res., *79*:273–279.

AFTERWORD

There seems to be little to add to these papers. A missing aspect of this work is knowledge of the time course of the strabismus animals, cats or monkeys, and in monkeys the possibilities of recovery—but that would have required many more monkeys, and one cannot do everything. To repair an artificial strabismus would probably exceed the limitations of our ophthalmologic surgery, unfortunately, considering how useful that type of knowledge would be to clinical ophthalmology.

Our showing that at birth the monkey ocular dominance columns have begun to form but are still not fully formed was entirely compatible with the results of Pasco Rakic (*Phil Trans R Soc Lond B,* 1977, 278:245–260), who had seen no hint of columns six weeks before the expected date of birth, but mild fluctuations in grain counts three weeks before. Subsequent work by Carla Shatz (*J Neurosci* 1983, 3:482–499) has shown that during development in cats, optic nerve fibers from the two eyes invade the entire geniculate, showing no respect for the alternating layers, which comes about only late in the prenatal period with the shedding of connections from the inappropriate eye and the further development of connections from the appropriate one.

Our delay in writing up our strabismus results in monkeys seems strange. We must simply have forgotten, and it was not until it came time to prepare the Nobel papers that we became aware of the oversight and repaired it in Torsten's final Nobel report. Since the results were so similar in cats and monkeys, it must have seemed to us a bore to have to set pen to paper yet again. There was one major item to add to the monkey study; namely, that we at last succeeded in producing an animal with amblyopia, which was the original object of the strabismus work.

PART V
THREE REVIEWS

Chapter 26 • Ferrier Lecture, 1977 •

FOREWORD

This paper must hold a record for the greatest lapse of time between the delivery of a lecture (London, March 2, 1972), and the submission of the manuscript (November 1976). Much work went into its preparation, to be sure, but perhaps not three and a half years of uninterrupted labor! Of all the reprints in the present collection, except for the Nobel lectures, this is the only one that is a summing up of other papers, and the result is doubtless some duplication of figures and text. But we felt it might be useful as a summary of much of the work, and as a chance to express the thoughts of some of the main papers in a different, more relaxed way.

Ferrier Lecture
Functional Architecture of Macaque Monkey Visual Cortex

D. H. HUBEL AND T. N. WIESEL • *Harvard Medical School, Boston, Massachusetts*

CONTENTS

From *Proc. R. Soc. Lond.* B. **198**, 1–59 (1977)

Lecture delivered 2 March 1972—*typescript received* 10 November 1976.

Of the many possible functions of the macaque monkey primary visual cortex (striate cortex, area 17) two are now fairly well understood. First, the incoming information from the lateral geniculate bodies is rearranged so that most cells in the striate cortex respond to specifically oriented line segments, and, second, information originating from the two eyes converges upon single cells. The rearrangement and convergence do not take place immediately, however: in layer IVc, where the bulk of the afferents terminate, virtually all cells have fields with circular symmetry and are strictly monocular, driven from the left eye or from the right, but not both; at subsequent stages, in layers above and below IVc, most cells show orientation specificity, and about half are binocular. In a binocular cell the receptive fields in the two eyes are on corresponding regions in the two retinas and are identical in structure, but one eye is usually more effective than the other in influencing the cell; all shades of ocular dominance are seen.

These two functions are strongly reflected in the architecture of the cortex, in that cells with common physiological properties are grouped together in vertically organized systems of columns. In an ocular dominance column all cells respond preferentially to the same eye. By four independent anatomical methods it has been shown that these columns have the form of vertically disposed alternating left-eye and right-eye slabs, which in horizontal section form alternating stripes about 400 μm thick, with occasional bifurcations and blind endings. Cells of like orientation specificity are known from physiological recordings to be similarly grouped in much narrower vertical sheeet-like aggregations, stacked in orderly sequences so that on traversing the cortex tangentially one normally encounters a succession of small shifts in orientation, clockwise or counterclockwise; a 1 mm traverse is usually accompanied by one or several full rotations through 180°, broken at times by reversals in direction of rotation and occasionally by large abrupt shifts. A full complement of columns, of either type, left-plus-right eye or a complete 180° sequence, is termed a hypercolumn. Columns (and hence hypercolumns) have roughly the same width throughout the binocular part of the cortex.

The two independent systems of hypercolumns are engrafted upon the well known topographic representation of the visual field. The receptive fields mapped in a vertical penetration through cortex show a scatter in position roughly equal to the average size of the fields themselves, and the area thus covered, the aggregate receptive field, increases with distance from the fovea. A parallel increase is seen in reciprocal magnification (the number of degrees of visual field corresponding to 1 mm of cortex). Over most or all of the striate cortex a movement of 1–2 mm, traversing several hypercolumns, is accompanied by a movement through the visual field about equal in size to the local aggregate receptive field. Thus any 1–2 mm block of cortex contains roughly the machinery needed to subserve an aggregate receptive field. In the cortex the fall-off in detail with which the visual field is analysed, as one moves out from the foveal area, is accompanied not by a reduction in thickness of layers, as is found in the retina, but by a reduction in the area of cortex (and hence the number of columnar units) devoted to a given amount of visual field: unlike the retina, the striate cortex is virtually uniform morphologically but varies in magnification.

In most respects the above description fits the newborn monkey just as well as the adult, suggesting that area 17 is largely genetically programmed. The ocular dominance columns, however, are not fully developed at birth, since the geniculate terminals belonging to one eye occupy layer IVc throughout its length, segregating out into separate columns only after about the first 6 weeks, whether or not the animal has visual experience. If one eye is sutured closed during this early period the columns belonging to that eye become shrunken and their companions correspondingly expanded. This would seem to be at least in part the result of interference with normal maturation, though sprouting and retraction of axon terminals are not excluded.

INTRODUCTION

Anyone who glances at a human brain can hardly fail to be impressed by the degree to which it is dominated by the cerebral cortex. This structure almost completely envelopes the rest of the brain, tending to obscure the other parts. Though only 2 mm thick it has a surface area, when spread out, of about 2000 cm^2. Even more impressive is the number of elements it contains. Under every square millimetre there are some 10^5 nerve cells, making a total of around 10^{10} cells. The number of synaptic connections in the cortex is certainly several orders of magnitude greater than this. For sheer complexity the cortex probably exceeds any other known structure.

To reveal this complexity special methods are necessary. Certain stains such as the Nissl make it possible to count and classify the cells, but help little in unravelling the wiring diagram, to say nothing of revealing what the cells are doing in the daily life of the animal. For these problems one needs a combination of approaches such as the Golgi method, autoradiography and the electron microscope, in anatomy, and single-cell recordings in physiology. Since many of these methods have been developed only recently, it is not surprising that beginnings have been made in understanding only a few areas of cortex.

Much of the work on cortex in the past 20 years has concentrated on sensory areas, which are more accessible to the neurophysiologist since they are close to the input end of the nervous system. For these few cortical regions some understanding of function in terms of structure seems to be evolving. An interesting and certainly a surprising result of this work is the discovery of structural patterns that were not apparent at all with the standard morphological techniques. One particular type of order, which we term 'functional architecture', seems only to be revealed by a combination of physiological and morphological approaches. What we mean by functional architecture will, we hope, become evident in the course of this paper, which presents a description of the known functional architecture of the primary visual cortex of the macaque monkey.

The Geniculo-Cortical Pathway

Cells in the visual cortex tend to be grouped together according to their physiological properties. On the crudest level, all of the cells in this part of the cortex are obviously concerned primarily with vision. But within the visual cortex finer functional groupings of several kinds also occur, and the functional architecture is a description of these groupings. To understand the architecture one must therefore have some knowledge of the physiological properties of the individual cells. We

accordingly begin with a summary of the single-cell physiology of the striate cortex, as it is presently understood. We propose to give only a rough sketch of the subject: those who wish to read further may consult the original papers (Kuffler 1953; Hubel & Wiesel 1959, 1962, 1968).

The position occupied by the striate cortex in the visual pathway is illustrated in Figure 1, a diagram taken from Polyak (1957). The brain in this figure is seen from below. It is from a human rather than a macaque, but the pathways are very similar in the two species. The main components of the visual pathway are the retinas, the lateral geniculate bodies, and the striate cortex. About a million optic nerve fibres (axons of retinal ganglion cells) issue from each eye and pass uninterrupted through the optic chiasm to the lateral geniculate bodies. (Some of the fibres end in the brain stem, especially in the superior colliculus.) At the chiasm a little over half of the optic fibres cross, and the other half (or slightly less) remain uncrossed. The redistribution takes place in such a way that the left lateral geniculate body receives axons from retinal ganglion cells in the two left half retinas, and hence is concerned with the right visual field; the right geniculate is similarly concerned with the left visual field. The lateral geniculate is in some respects quite complex; anatomically there are several cell types, and a variety of synaptic categories are seen (Guillery & Colonnier 1970). But compared with many other structures in the brain, and in particular with the cortex, the lateral geniculate body is simple: most geniculate cells receive synaptic input directly from optic nerve fibres, and most of these cells in turn send their axons directly to the cortex. Thus it is not unfair to say that it is basically a one-synapse station.

The axons that form the output of the geniculates pass back in the white matter of the cerebral hemispheres to the striate cortex. The striate cortex is clearly more complicated, with at least 3 or 4 synapses interposed between the input and the output. The organization of this structure will be the subject of most of this paper. Finally, the axons that leave the cortex make their way to a number of different destinations: to other nearby cortical regions such as area 18, to the optic tectum, and, in a recurrent path, to the lateral geniculate bodies. The striate cortex should thus not be regarded in any sense as the end of the visual path—in fact it is probably

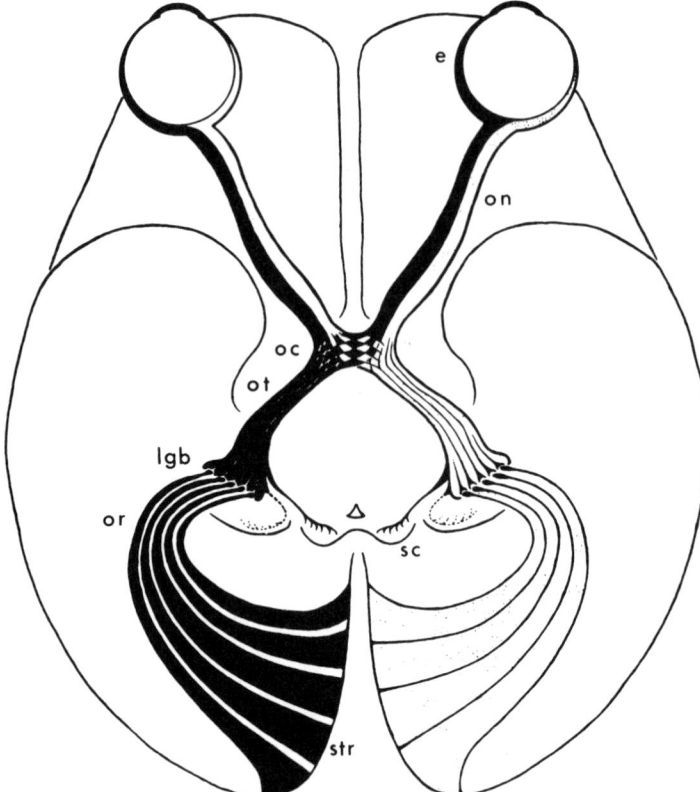

Fig. 1. Diagram of the retino-geniculo-cortical pathway in a higher mammal. The brain is viewed from below; by skilful dissection the eyes and optic nerves have been removed from the orbits, and kept in their normal relationship to the brain. Up, in the diagram, is anterior. The right halves of each retina, shown in black, project to the right hemisphere (to the left, in the figure, since it is viewed from below): thus the right hemisphere receives input from both eyes and is concerned with the left half-field of vision. e, eye; on, optic nerve; oc, optic chiasm; ot, optic tract; lgb, lateral geniculate body; sc, superior colliculus; or, optic radiations; str, striate cortex. (Figure from Polyak, 1957.)

very close to the beginning, and, as we will see, the behaviour of the cells, though it tells us the outcome of the first five or six steps in the processing of visual information, does not take us very far toward solving the ultimate problem of visual perception.

In studying the physiology of the visual pathway we have made use of methods developed by Hartline (1940), Kuffler (1953), Talbot & Marshall (1941), and others. Our general strategy has been to stimulate the retina in a natural way (i.e. with patterns of light) and to record the responses of single cells at one stage after the next, starting with retina, going on to the geniculate, and finally to the cortex. In this type of work we record with extracellular microelectrodes because our main interest is in the all-or-none impulses of the cells, and because firing patterns tend to be seriously distorted if a cell is penetrated by an electrode; to make such extracellular records from single cells for periods of many hours is today relatively easy. At any given stage one studies cell after cell, observing how each reacts to spots and patterns of light, gradually forming an overall idea of the behaviour of the cells in that

structure. The procedure is then repeated at the next stage, and by comparing the two sets of results one may learn what kinds of analysis the second stage has made upon the input that it received from the first.

The primary visual cortex (also called 'striate cortex' and 'area 17'—the three terms are synonymous) can be said to have two main functions—there are certainly others, some known and perhaps many still to be discovered, but the two to be described here are very important. First, the visual input from the lateral geniculate body is rearranged in such a way as to make the cortical cells responsive to specifically oriented short line segments. Second, the cortex is the first point in the retino-geniculo-cortical path at which fibres carrying information from the two eyes converge upon single cells. Let us discuss each of these functions in turn.

Receptive Field Orientation

A retinal ganglion cell or a geniculate cell responds best to a roughly circular spot of light, the optimal size of spot varying from cell to cell, and for any one cell the spot must be presented in a particular part of the visual field (i.e. of the retina). The response may consist of a speeding up of the resting train of impulses, or a slowing down. Because of the concentric, mutually antagonistic centre-surround receptive field arrangement (Kuffler 1953), a spot occupying exactly the centre of the receptive field is always more effective than one of larger size, and consequently more effective than diffuse light. The responses to various shapes of stationary stimuli are to a large extent predictable from the receptive-field maps; for example a slit whose width is the same as the diameter of the receptive field centre will excite an on-centre cell (Figure 2) even though some of the surround is illuminated. Apparently the centre and surround interact in such a way that a stimulus covering all the centre but only a fraction of the surround produces a strong centre-type response.

These cells have fields with circular symmetry, and consequently respond roughly equally to all orientations of a line stimulus.

In the cortex we first find cells with orientation specificity. By this we mean that a cell responds to a specifically oriented stationary or moving straight line segment presented within a restricted receptive field. An example of the behaviour of such a cell is shown in Figure 3. This cell, recorded, say, from the right hemisphere, responds only to stimuli within a roughly rectangular area in the left half field of vision. To evoke consistent strong responses it is not enough to use a circular spot of light, however: the region must be crossed by a slit of light in 01h30–07h30 orientation. The slit may be kept stationary and presented anywhere within the rectangle, or it may be swept across the receptive field in the direction of the arrow. Changing

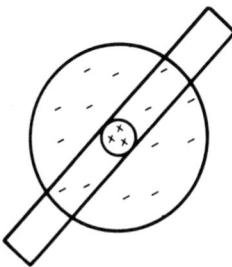

Fig. 2. Centre-surround receptive field of a typical on-centre retinal ganglion cell. The diagram represents a small portion of the retina, or, what is equivalent, a small portion of the visual field. In the case of the retina, the retinal ganglion cell body is situated close to the centre of the region, and the region itself is the territory of retina containing receptors that make functionally effective connections (via other interposed retinal cells) with the ganglion cell. In a monkey the entire receptive field occupies a region a degree or so in diameter (about 0.3 mm, on the retina). The field centre varies from a few minutes of arc, for cells near the fovea, up to a degree or so, for peripheral cells. Shining light anywhere within the centre region (×) causes the cell to increase its firing rate, whereas shining light in the annular surround (—) produces a slowing in firing rate, with a transient discharge when the light is turned off (the off-response). Because of this antagonism between the two regions, a light shining over the entire field gives a much weaker response than light confined to the centre; the centre usually dominates, so that the response is 'on' in type. The slit-shaped stimulus illustrated gives a strong on-response, since it covers all of the centre region and only a fraction of the opposing surround. Cells in the lateral geniculate body have similar receptive fields. Many cells in retina and geniculate have just the reverse configuration, with inhibition from the centre of the receptive field and excitation from the surround.

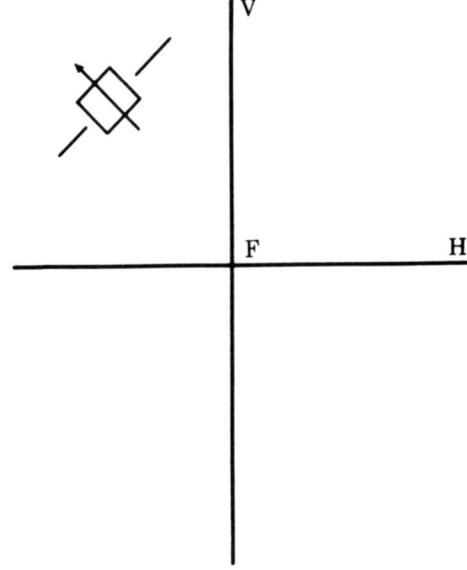

Fig. 3. Receptive field of a complex cell in the striate cortex. Axes represent the vertical (V) and horizontal (H) meridian of the visual field, crossing at the centre of gaze F (the projection of the fovea). The cell is recorded from the right hemisphere, so that the receptive field, represented by the rectangle, is in the left field of vision. No responses are observed when this region is illuminated diffusely, and small circular spots produce at most only weak or inconstant responses. An appropriate line, however, gives strong reproducible responses. The cell in this example gives optimal responses to a long narrow slit oriented in a 01 h30–07 h30 manner; responses are especially strong if the line is swept over the area in the direction indicated by the arrow.

the orientation so that the slit is misoriented by more than 10°–20° usually results in a marked decline in the response. The sensitivity to variations in orientation differs to some extent from cell to cell, but almost all cells fail to respond long before the misorientation reaches 90°. A moving stimulus is generally very powerful in evoking a discharge (i.e. in raising the impulse frequency of the cell above the resting level). In many cells movement of a slit, or even a small spot, in one direction (here, up-and-left) evokes a much more vigorous response than movement in the reverse direction (down-and-right), and often movement in one of the two directions will evoke no response at all. The mechanism for this directional selectivity for movement is still unknown, but must depend on connections within the cortex, since in cat and monkey such selectivity has not been described at the geniculate level (see, for example, Wiesel & Hubel 1966). In lower vertebrates such as frog (Lettvin, Maturana, McCulloch & Pitts 1959), and even in some mammals such as the rabbit (Barlow, Hill & Levick 1964) and cat (Cleland & Levick 1974; Stone & Fukuda 1974), some retinal ganglion cells show directional selectivity, but these cells probably project mainly to the superior colliculus. The ideas proposed by Barlow *et al.* to explain directional selectivity in the rabbit retina may also apply to the cat and monkey cortex, but there are important differences which make it unlikely that exactly the same mechanisms are used. While retinal cells in frog and rabbit may be directionally selective, they show no selective responses to specifically oriented line segments. In cat and monkey cortex, directional selectivity is intimately bound up with orientation specificity, since the optimum orientation of a slit is always 90° to the optimum direction of movement.

The optimal orientation of the line varies from cell to cell, some cells preferring vertical, others horizontal, and still others oblique. All possible orientations are represented roughly equally— there being no obvious preponderance of cells tuned, for example, to vertical or horizontal stimuli. The line stimulus may be produced in any one of three ways: most cells respond best to a light line on a dark background; many others, however, respond selectively to dark lines on a light background, and some prefer borders between light and dark.

Cells in the primary visual cortex are not all specifically sensitive to particular orientations. Roughly four classes of cells can be distinguished, in a series of ascending complexity (Hubel & Wiesel 1959, 1962, 1965, 1968). These are termed 'circularly symmetric', 'simple', 'complex' and 'hypercomplex'. We assume that cells at each stage receive their major input from cells at the previous stage, with the circularly symmetric cells receiving their inputs predominantly from geniculate cells. Circularly symmetric cells, as their name implies, show no preference to any particular orientation of lines, and, indeed, seem similar in their properties to geniculate cells. Simple cells are the first in the hierarchy to show orientation specificity, so that the rearrangements responsible for orientation specificity are presumed to take place between the circularly symmetric and the simple cells. A simple cell responds to an optimally oriented line in some narrowly defined position: even a slight displacement of the line to a new position, without change in orientation, renders the line ineffective. A complex cell, on the contrary, is probably just as specific in its orientation requirements as the simple cell, but is far less particular about the exact positioning of the line. Such a cell will respond wherever a line is projected within a rectangle such as that of Figure 3; if the cell responds to a dark or light line (rather than to an edge), increasing the line's thickness beyond some value that is far less than the width of the receptive field renders it ineffective. Thus a patch of light as large as the entire receptive field evokes no response at all. This is equivalent to saying that diffuse light is ineffective. As mentioned above, sweeping the line over the receptive field usually evokes a sustained discharge from the cell. Hypercomplex cells, finally, resemble complex cells in all respects but one: extending a line beyond the region from which responses are evoked produces a marked reduction or complete abolition of the response. A few years ago Bishop & Henry (1972) described in cat cortex a type of cell whose properties resembled those of simple cells, except that extending the line led to a drop in the response. Schiller, Finlay & Volman (1976) and we have seen such cells in monkey cortex, and Gilbert (1977) has confirmed their presence in the cat striate cortex. It is thus clear that there are two categories of hypercomplex cells. Different cells show different degrees of suppression when a line is made very long, suggesting that the distinction between hypercomplex cells on the one hand and simple and complex on the other may not be very sharp; rather there seems to be a continuum, from cells that respond very well to cells that do not respond at all, to long lines.

In this paper no attempt will be made to describe these different cell types in detail. It is enough to point out that a complex cell can most easily be understood by supposing that it receives inputs from many simple cells, all with the same orientation preference. Similarly a hypercomplex cell's properties can be explained by assuming that it receives inputs from complex cells (or, for the less common type, from simple cells) all with the same preferred orientation. One would therefore predict that cells whose fields are in a particular part of the visual field and which prefer the same stimulus orientation would be highly interconnected, whereas cells of different orientation preference would not be expected to be interconnected except possibly by inhibitory synapses. These predictions will be referred to again in interpreting the significance of the orientation columns described below.

One may add, parenthetically, that the organization suggested here, while hierarchical in a rough sense, is certainly not rigidly so. For example, complex cells probably do not all project to hypercomplex cells; many of those situated in layer V, for example, project to tectal cells (Palmer & Rosenquist 1974; Toyama, Matsunami, Ohno & Takashiki 1974), while many VIth layer cells project back to the lateral geniculate body (Gilbert & Kelly 1975; Lund *et al.* 1975). Despite a certain degree of dissension over the idea of an underlying hierarchy, there is considerable evidence to support it (Kelly & Van Essen 1974; Gilbert (1977).

Binocular Convergence

To understand the second main function of the striate cortex, the combining of influences from the two eyes, we must return for a moment to the lateral geniculate body, for this, as already mentioned, is the first structure in the path to receive input from both eyes. The geniculate nevertheless seems to go well out of its way to avoid any significant mixing of the inputs from the two eyes. Figure 4*a,* Plate 1, shows a coronal section through the right lateral geniculate of a macaque monkey, in which cell bodies are stained by the Nissl method. The

geniculate consists of six layers stacked one above the other rather like a club sandwich, each plate being many cells thick. The terminals coming in from the two eyes distribute themselves to these six layers in such a way as to produce six topographic maps of the contralateral half field of vision; all six maps are in register so that in a radial pathway traversing the six layers, as indicated by the arrow, all the receptive fields of the cells encountered will have virtually identical positions in the visual fields (Brouwer & Zeeman 1926; Bishop, Kozak, Levick & Vakkur 1962; Hubel & Wiesel 1961).

In the geniculate of many primates including man the distribution of the terminals from the two eyes takes a very special form. Each of the six layers receives input from one eye only. For the right lateral geniculate the most dorsal layer has input from the left eye, and beginning with this layer the sequence proceeds left-right, left-right, right-left. Why a reversal should occur between the dorsal four and the ventral two layers is a mystery, but, for that matter, why there is any sequence at all is still an unsolved riddle. The important point for our present purposes is that each layer, and consequently each individual cell in each layer, receives input from only one eye. The geniculate in the monkey, then, consists almost entirely of monocular cells. Layer VI of the visual cortex sends a strong projection to the geniculate (Lund *et al.* 1975), and many cells in that layer are binocular. There is therefore some reason to expect an indirect influence of some kind on a geniculate cell from both eyes, by way of the cortex. Such an influence has been demonstrated in the cat geniculate, where there are also opportunities for direct interchange of information across the layers (Sanderson, Darian-Smith & Bishop 1969; Guillery 1966), but not, so far, in the monkey. The original evidence that the different layers correspond to single eyes was based on the degeneration of cells that occurs on eye removal, as shown by Minkowski in 1920. An example of a result similar to Minkowski's is shown in Figure 4*b*. There is now very much additional evidence to support Minkowski's finding, both physiological and anatomical (see Figure 21).

The fibres carrying information to the cortex are thus for all practical purposes strictly monocular. The process of convergence of information from the two eyes occurs first in the primary visual cortex. It is, however, delayed to a point beyond the

Plate 1

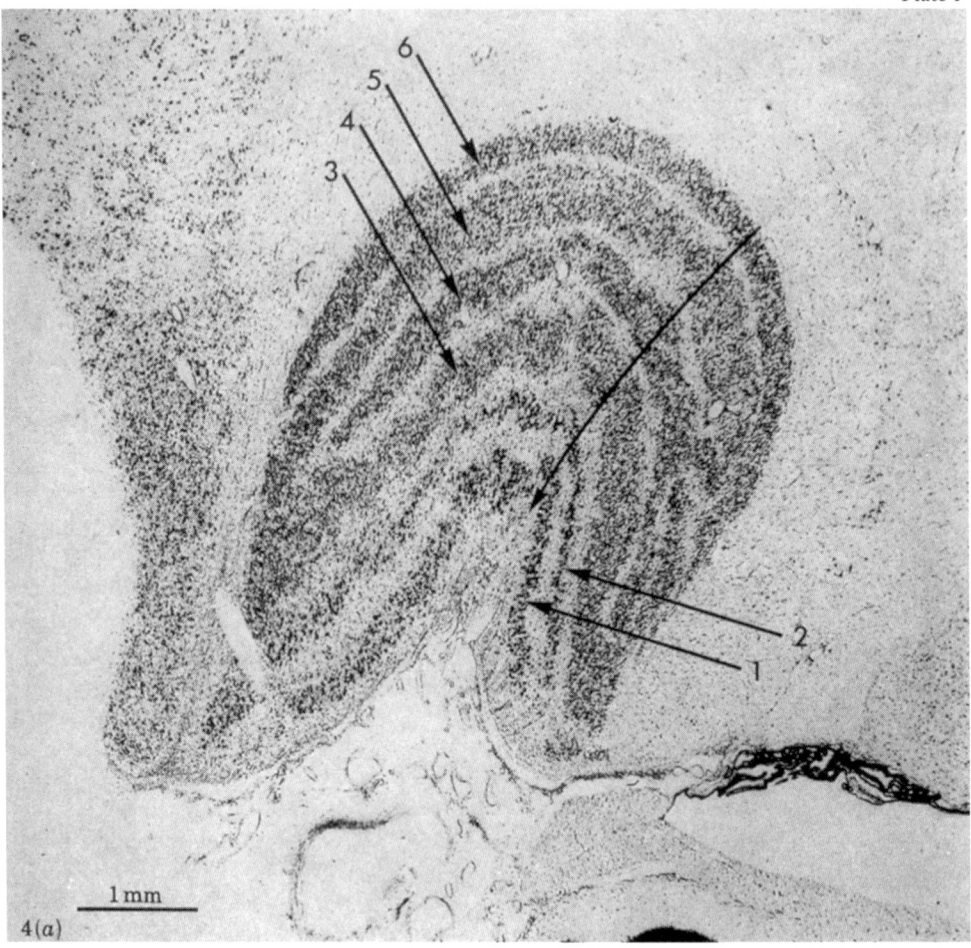

1 mm

4(a)

Fig. 4. (a) *Coronal section through the right lateral geniculate body of a normal adult inacaque monkey, cresyl violet stain. Cells are divided into six layers: Nos. 1, 4, and 6 receive input from contralateral (left) eye; 2, 3, and 5 from the ipsilateral. Each layer contains a detailed and orderly representation of the contralateral field of vision; moving along one layer thus implies a movement through the visual field dictated by this representational map. The six maps of the visual field are in precise register, so that corresponding to movement along a radial line, such as the arrow, there is no movement in the visual field.* (b) *One form of evidence that certain geniculate layers receive input from the contralateral eye, and others from the ipsilateral. The right eye of this rhesus monkey was removed at the age of 2 weeks, and the brain examined at 19 months. Coronal sections, Nissl stain (cresyl violet). On each side cells in layers with input from the right eye are markedly atrophic and appear pale. Compare Figure 4a. (From Hubel, Wiesel & LeVay 1977.)*

first two cortical stages, for the circularly symmetric cells and the simple cells are almost all monocular, whereas among the complex and hypercomplex cells binocular input is very common. Nevertheless even at these stages binocular cells make up only a little more than half of the population.

Now we can ask a very specific question designed to reveal more about the way in which the inputs from the two eyes combine. If we record from a binocular cortical cell, a complex cell for example, we may map its receptive field in one eye, meanwhile keeping the animal's other eye closed. Suppose the result is a map like that of Figure 3. We then transfer the mask to the other eye and repeat the procedure. If the cell is a binocular cell, how similar will the receptive fields be in the two

Plate 2

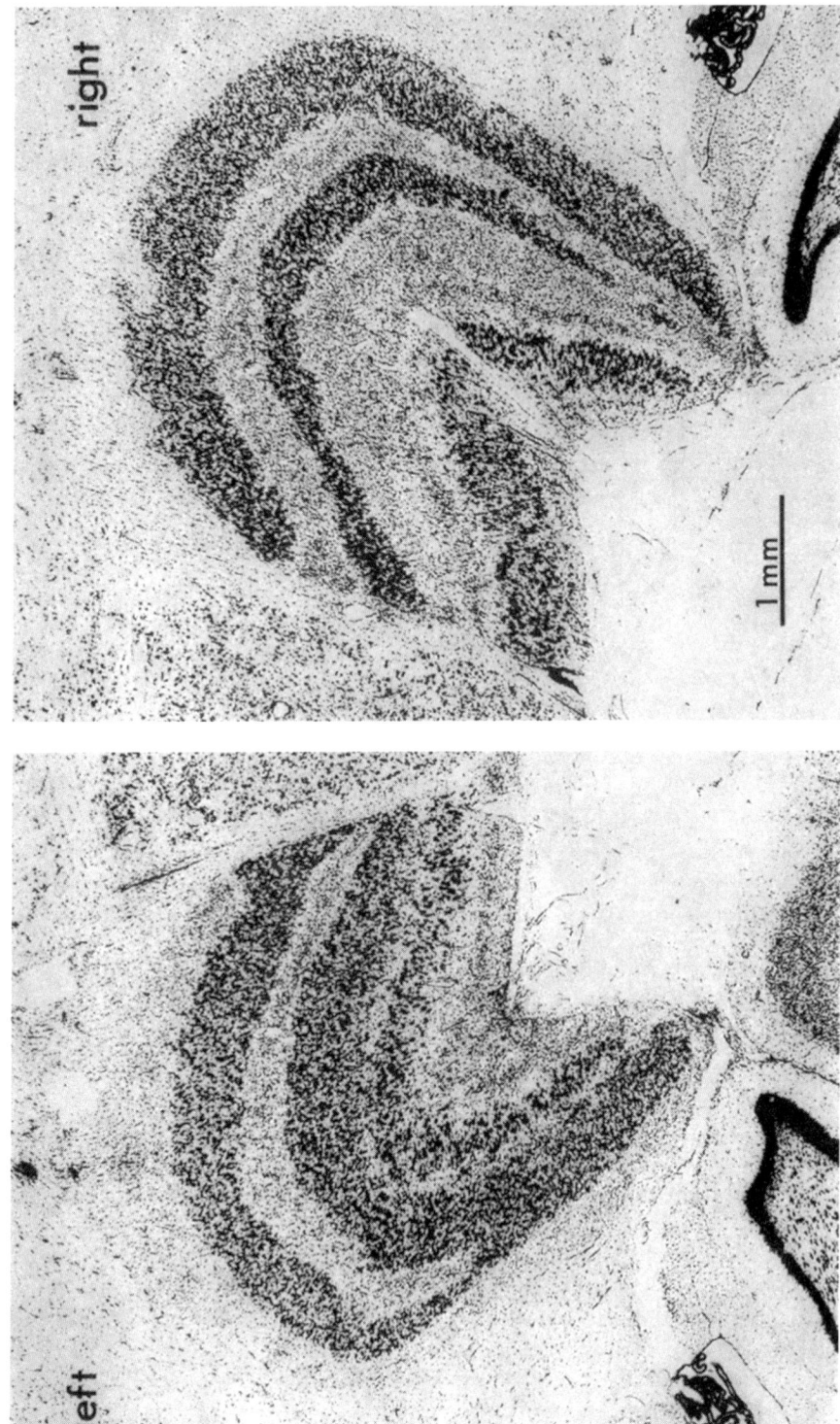

left

right

1 mm

Fig. 4 (Continued)

left eye   right eye

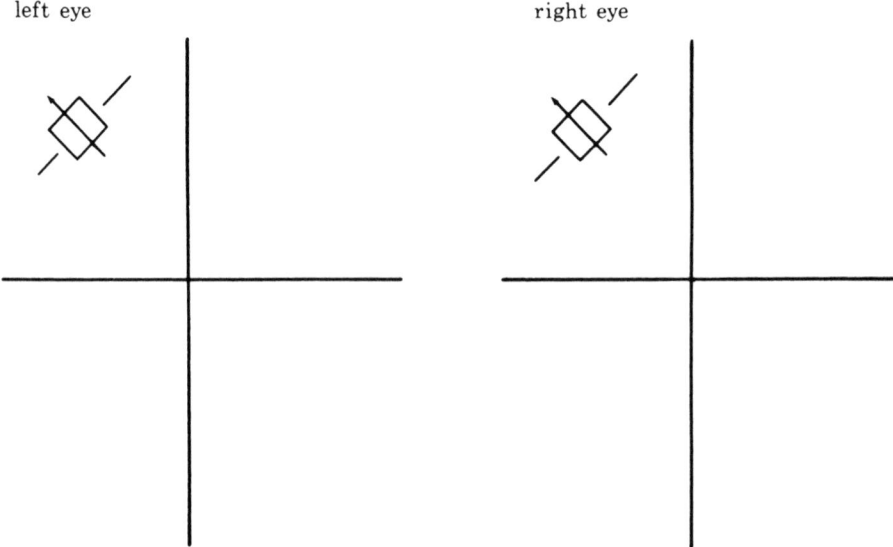

*Fig. 5. Receptive fields of a binocular cell in area 17. Each diagram shows the visual field as seen by one eye; nor-
mally the two would be superimposed, but they are drawn separately here for clarity. The fields in the two eyes
are, as closely as one can measure, similar in size, shape, position and orientation, and respond to the same form
of stimulus, in this case a moving slit.*

eyes? The answer is that they are practically identical (Hubel & Wiesel 1959; 1968). This is illustrated in Figure 5. The positions of the receptive
fields in the two retinas match as perfectly as one
can measure: the fields are the same distance from
the fovea and in the same direction, and thus in the
visual fields the two receptive fields are superimposed. The receptive-field complexity is the same,
the orientations are identical, the direction preferences, if any, are the same. In short, everything one
learns about the cell through one eye matches precisely what one learns through the other. It is therefore no surprise to find that when both eyes are
used together and properly lined up, a stimulus
usually evokes a much more vigorous response
than when either eye is used alone.

We can say, then, that the cell receives inputs
from the two eyes and that these inputs are qualitatively virtually identical—which means that the
wiring in the two paths, up to their point of convergence, must be very similar. Only in one respect
are there differences: the responses that are
obtained on comparing identical stimuli in the two
eyes may not be equal. For many cells the responses
from one of the two eyes are consistently greater
than those from the other; some cells, the monocular ones, receive input only from one of the eyes;

some receive equal inputs. There are, in fact, all
shades of relative ocular dominance in the population, from complete dominance by one eye,
through equality, to complete dominance by the
other. We can sum this up by saying that cortical
cells receive qualitatively similar inputs from the
two eyes but that for any given cell the densities of
the two inputs are not necessarily the same.

Everything we have said up to now applies
not only to the normal adult macaque monkey, but,
with one minor exception to be discussed below,
also to the newborn monkey, lacking any visual
experience (Wiesel & Hubel 1974). It is hard to
escape the conclusion that the connections responsible for the findings so far outlined, and indeed
also for the architecture to be described, are genetically determined. At least their formation is not
dependent on visual experience. This will be discussed in more detail later in the paper.

To sum up this abbreviated account of the
physiology, we may think of a cell in area 17 of the
monkey as responding optimally when a number
of stimulus variables are correctly specified. The
cell may be described, then, by its degree of complexity, the *x–y* coordinates of the position of the
receptive field, the receptive field orientation, the
ocular dominance, and the degree to which there is

directional preference to movement. Such a list of specifications is analogous to the tag showing the price, sleeve length, percentage of wool, and so on, attached to a suit in a department store.

The drawing up of such a list allows us to pose a key question that leads to new information on the architecture of the cortex. Are cells with similar qualities—similar orientations or similar field positions—aggregated together in the cortex, (as suits often are in a store), or are they scattered at random through the cortex with respect to these variables? The answer to this question provides some strong hints as to how the cortex carries out its functions.

FUNCTIONAL ARCHITECTURE

1. Anatomy

Before addressing directly the subject of functional architecture we must look briefly at the anatomy of the striate cortex. The entire cortex is a plate of cells about 2 mm thick and in the macaque monkey about 13 cm² in surface area. Figure 6*a*, Plate 3, shows a view of the macaque brain from behind. The visual cortex is partly buried, and partly exposed on the outer surface of the occipital lobe and visible in the picture. The exposed part extends forward to the dotted line (the 17-18 border),

Plate 3

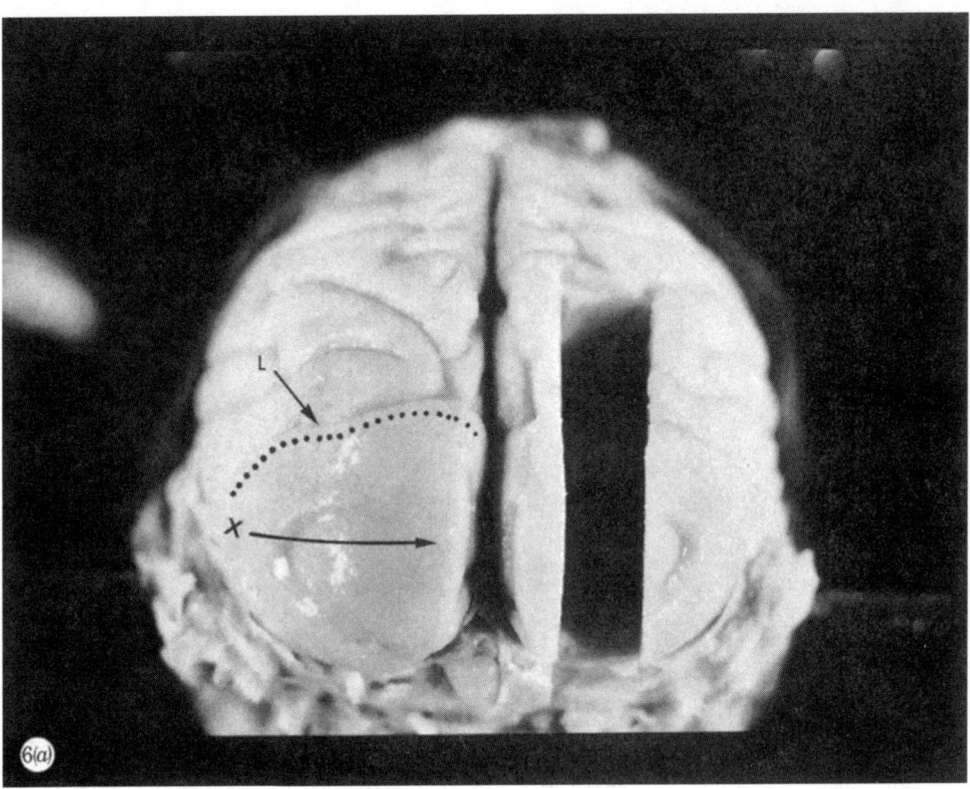

Fig. 6. (a) *Brain of a macaque monkey, perfused with formalin, viewed from above and behind. The occipital lobe is demarcated in front by the lunate sulcus (L) and consists mainly of the striate cortex, which occupies most of the smooth surface, extending forward to the dotted line (the 17–18 border). If followed medially area 17 curves around the medial surface of the brain and continues in a complex buried fold, a part of which lies underneath the convexity and parallel to it. X marks the projection of the fovea; movement in the direction of the arrow corresponds to movement out along the horizon; movement along the dotted line, to movement down along the vertical midline of the visual field. The groove in the right hemisphere was made in removing a parasagittal block of tissue to produce the cross section of Figure 6b.* (b) *Low power Nissl-stained section from a parasagittal block such as that of Figure 6a. It is what would be seen if one could stand in the groove of 6a and look to the left. A marks the outer convexity; B the buried fold, and arrows indicate the 17-18 borders, the upper right one of which is indicated by the dotted line in Figure 6a.*

Plate 4

6(b)

2 mm

A

B

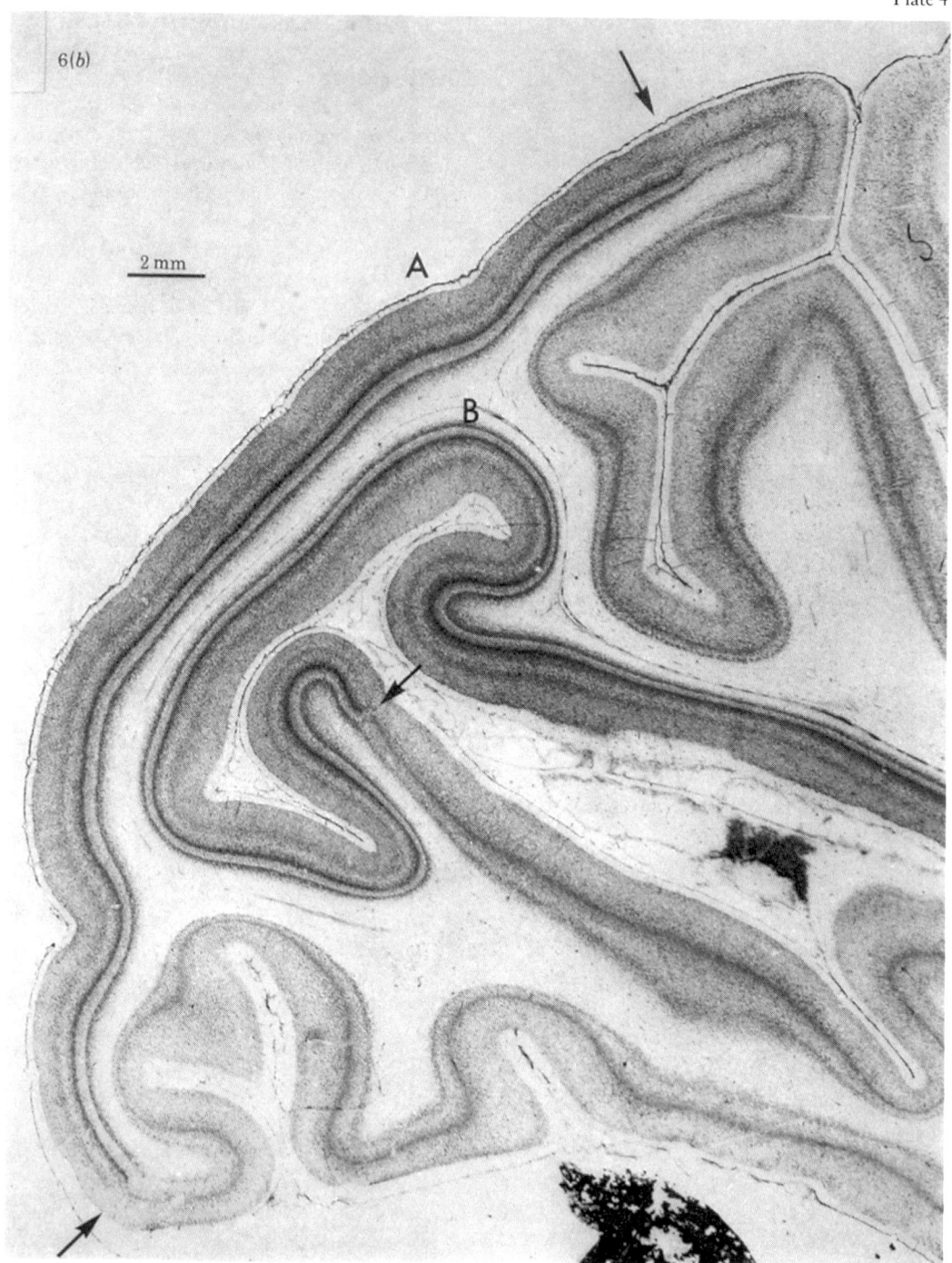

Fig. 6b.

which lies a millimetre or so behind the lunate sulcus (L). As one proceeds medially to the midline the striate area bends around and continues as a complicated buried fold, some of which is roughly parallel to the exposed surface but one level deeper. The contralateral half visual field is mapped systematically onto the striate cortex, just as it was in the case of the lateral geniculate. The foveal projection is far lateral, roughly at x in Figure 6*a*, and as one moves from x in the direction of the arrow the corresponding points in the visual field move out from the foveal projection along the horizon. As one moves medially from x along the dotted 17-18 border the corresponding points in the visual field move downwards from the fovea along the vertical midline.

The deep groove in the right hemisphere represents a knife cut made in blocking the cortex for histology. If one were to stand in this groove and look to the left one would see in cross section the smooth outer part of area 17 as well as the buried fold: this is shown, in a Nissl stained section, in Figure 6*b*, Plate 4. The arrows mark the 17-18 boundaries. The outer convexity (A) and the buried fold (B) are of course all part of the same folded continuous surface.

The topography of the macaque visual cortex is in itself not of major interest, but the landmarks just pointed out will be needed in the descriptions that follow.

2. Position in the Visual Field

Besides the richness of the layering pattern formed by alternating zones of concentration and rarefaction of cells, the most striking feature of this part of the cortex is its remarkable uniformity as one proceeds in a direction parallel to the surface. There are no great differences in layering pattern or thickness that cannot be accounted for by the folding or by the oblique angle at which the cortex is inevitably cut in some regions. This uniformity is at first glance surprising. Physiologically it is clear that at every level up to and including area 17 the visual fields are analysed in much more detail in regions near the fovea than in the periphery. The most obvious manifestation of this non-uniformity of analysis is the variation of receptive field size with distance from fovea (with 'eccentricity'). In retinal ganglion cells and in cells of the geniculate, for example, the receptive fields, and especially the

receptive-field centres, are very small in the most central region and become progressively larger with increasing eccentricity (Wiesel 1960; Hubel & Wiesel 1960, 1961; Wiesel & Hubel 1966; Hoffman, Stone & Sherman 1972). This of course has a psychophysical parallel in the greatly heightened visual acuity in the foveal region compared with the periphery. From all of this it is only to be expected that the neural machinery necessary to take care of one square degree of fovea should be much more massive than that subserving the same area of visual field periphery. In the retina the difference is obvious histologically. Figure 7, Plate 5, shows that near the primate fovea the ganglion cell layer is many cells thick, whereas peripherally there are not enough cells to make up a single continuous layer (Van Buren 1963). In the cortex one might similarly expect a relative thickening in parts subserving regions of visual field in or near the fovea, but if there is any at all it is so subtle that careful control of plane of sectioning would be required to be certain of it: certainly there is no variation in thickness remotely approaching what is seen in the layer of retinal ganglion cells.

The cortex, in fact, finds an entirely different way of devoting proportionately more machinery to central visual field areas than to peripheral. The amount of retinal surface devoted to a degree of visual field is of course constant; it must be for obvious optical reasons. In the cortex the corresponding amount of surface is far from constant, being large in the foveal region and falling off progressively as eccentricity increases. This variation in magnification (mm cortex/degree visual field) was first systematically analysed by Daniel & Whitteridge (1961). Magnification in fact seems to vary with eccentricity in such a way as to guarantee a uniform thickness of cortex (Hubel & Wiesel 1974*b*). Instead of being heaped up in the region representing central vision, the cortex is spread out, to just the amount required to preserve uniformity.

The orderliness of this arrangement can be seen by examining the positions of receptive fields as an electrode moves through the cortex sampling cell after cell. In a vertical penetration (here and elsewhere we mean vertical not in a literal sense, but simply in the sense of perpendicular to the surface) the fields are all clustered in some particular part of the visual field—not surprisingly, given the precise map of the field of vision on the cortex. The

Plate 5

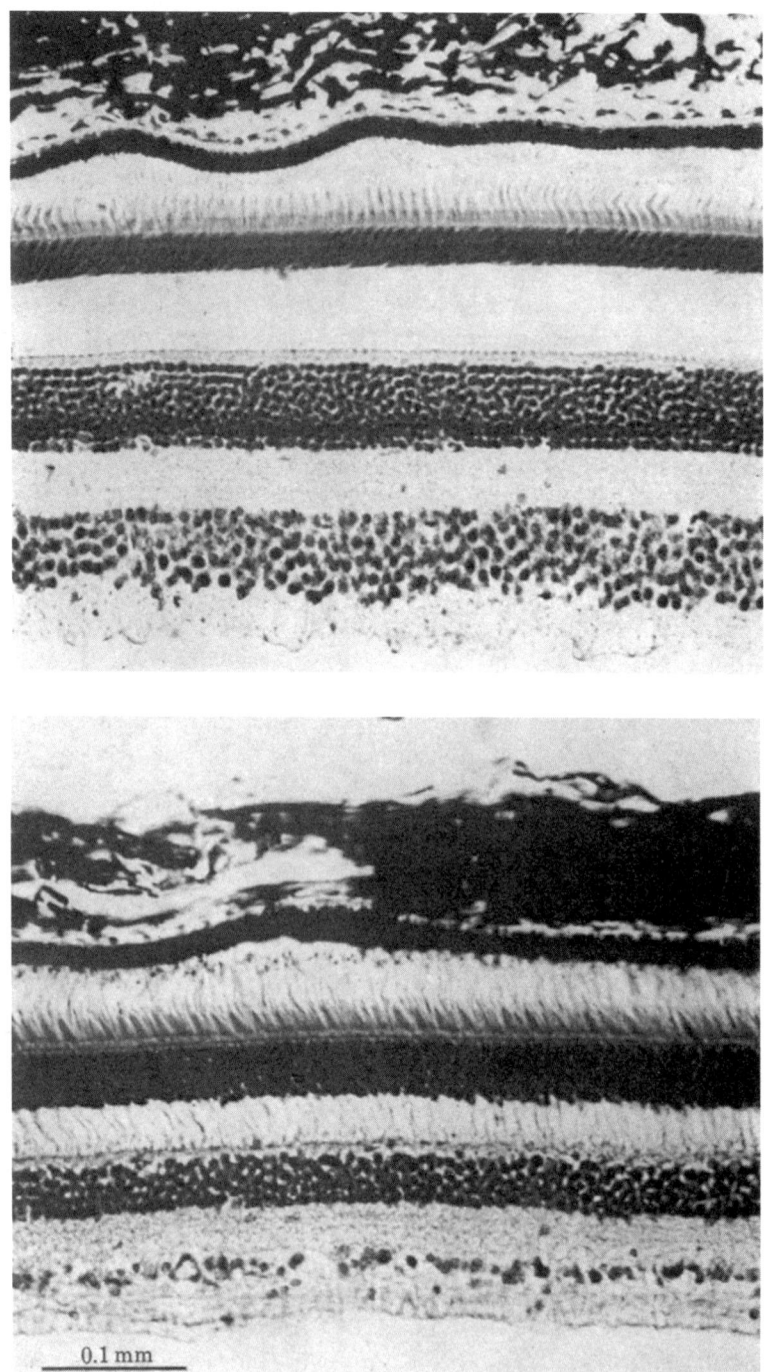

Fig. 7. Comparison of ganglion cell layer of monkey retina near fovea and in the periphery. Cross sections of a macaque monkey retina, stained with hematoxylin-eosin, from the parafoveal region and the far periphery. on, outer nuclear layer; in, inner nuclear layer; g, ganglion cell layer. Note how retinal ganglion cells form a layer about five cells deep in the parafoveal region, but constitute only a thinly populated layer in the periphery.

receptive fields recorded in a vertical penetration in fact show considerable overlap. They are not precisely superimposed, however: there is not only some variation in size, but also a certain amount of apparently random scatter in position. In any one penetration the fields collectively cover an area several times the size of an average receptive field, as illustrated in Figure 8*a*. For convenience we can refer to this areas as the *aggregate field* of any point on the cortical surface.

Both field size and the amount of scatter vary from layer to layer, being smallest in layer IVc, largest in layer V and intermediate in the others. Thus for any point on the cortex we can obviously speak of the aggregate field for an individual layer. (The aggregate field for the full cortical thickness will then be about the same as the aggregate field for layer V.)

Now consider what happens as an electrode is moved not vertically, but horizontally through the cortex, sampling cell after cell in a given layer. Over a short distance one will again find a random scattering of receptive fields, again over a territory several times the size of any one field; the exact size, as just mentioned, will vary with the layer one is traversing. Let us suppose, to be specific, that the electrode is recording from layer III, where the field sizes and scatter are not huge, as in layer V, nor tiny as in IVc, but somewhere in between. As the penetration progresses one begins to detect an overall drift in field position, superimposed on the random scatter, in a direction dictated by the topographic map of the visual field upon the cortex. It requires a traverse of about 1–2 mm through the cortex to produce a drift equal to the size of the aggregate field, that is, a drift sufficient to produce a displacement of the receptive fields into territory completely distinct from the original one (Figure 8*b*). The interesting thing is that 1–2 mm is what is required for such a displacement regardless of where in area 17 the penetration is made (Figure 9). For a more peripheral part of the visual field, receptive-field sizes and scatter are both larger and consequently the aggregate field is larger; a 1–2 mm traverse along the cortex gives a drift in fields that is likewise larger, in exact proportion. At an eccentricity of 45° the aggregate field is about 3° and a 1–2 mm displacement shifts this territory by about 3°. At 22° the figure is 1½°, at 7° it is about 0.5°, and in the fovea about 0.1°. The overall law is

that for this layer a 1–2 mm displacement along the cortex is about enough, on the average, to displace the aggregate field into an entirely new terrain. The figure of 1–2 mm will be somewhat greater if one studies the deep part of layer III or layer V, and much less for layer IVc or layer II. This suggests that over the entire visual field a region whose size is that of the aggregate field is subserved by the machinery contained in a block of cortex with a surface area of about 2 mm × 2 mm. The block everywhere subserves the same function—the field sizes and scatter for the incoming geniculate fibres vary, but the number of fibres is probably constant (Clark 1941), and what is done with the input by the cortical machine is probably the same everywhere. Thus diagrams such as those of Figure 8 will be similar wherever the penetration is made in the striate cortex, except that the scale will differ.

The dimension of 1–2 mm is an interesting one, for studies of the cortex by silver degeneration methods (Fisken, Garey & Powell 1973) show that the longest intracortical connections extend only for a few millimetres, and most are under 1–2 mm. (The longest connections probably involve cells of layer V and deep III, and the shortest, cells in IV c.) This means that there is little or no opportunity for signals entering the cortex in one place to make themselves felt at points more than 1–2 mm away. As a corollary to this it may be added that the striate cortex must be analysing the visual world in piecemeal fashion: information about some region in the visual field is brought to the cortex, digested, and the result transmitted on with no regard to what is going on elsewhere. Visual perception, then, can in no sense be said to be enshrined in area 17—the apparatus is simply not made to analyse a percept that occupies more than a small region of visual field. All of the single cell physiology in fact suggests that area 17 is concerned simply with what may be thought of as building blocks for perception.

To sum up, a 1–2 mm square of cortex subserves an area of visual field roughly equal to the aggregate field in that part of the cortex. In this way magnification is adjusted to receptive field size so that the cortex can be everywhere uniform. In the paragraphs that follow it will be shown that each 1–2 mm block of cortex contains just enough machinery to analyse its region of visual field, for all line orientations and for both eyes.

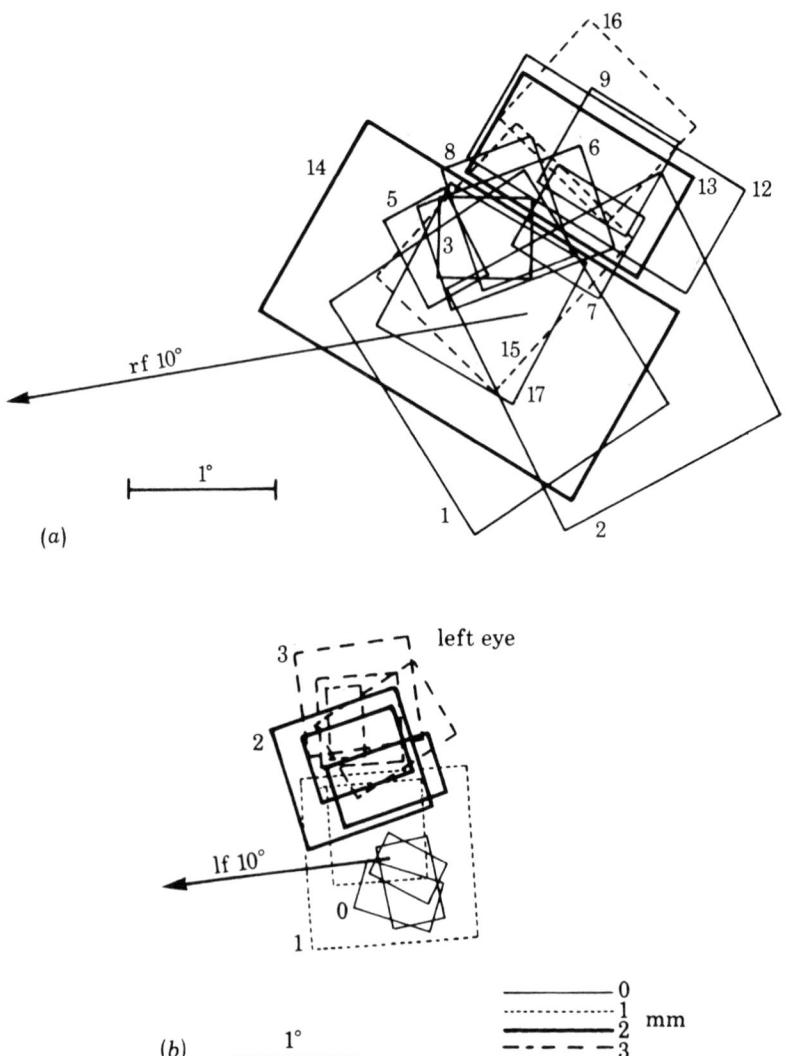

Fig. 8. (a) *Receptive-field scatter: Receptive-field boundaries of 17 cells recorded in a penetration through monkey striate cortex, in a direction perpendicular to the surface. Note the variation in size, and the more or less random scatter in the precise positions of the fields. The penetration was made in a part of the cortex corresponding to a visual field location 10° from the centre of gaze, just above the horizontal meridian. Fields are shown for one eye only. Numbers indicate the order in which the cells were recorded. (From Hubel & Wiesel 1974b.) (b) Receptive-field drift: Receptive fields mapped during an oblique, almost tangential penetration through striate cortex, in roughly the same region as in a. A few fields were mapped along each of four 100 μm segments, spaced at 1 mm intervals. These four groups of fields were labelled 0, 1, 2 and 3. Each new set of fields was slightly above the other, as predicted from the direction of movement of the electrode. Roughly a 2 mm movement through cortex was required to displace the fields from one region to an entirely new region. (From Hubel & Wiesel 1974b.)*

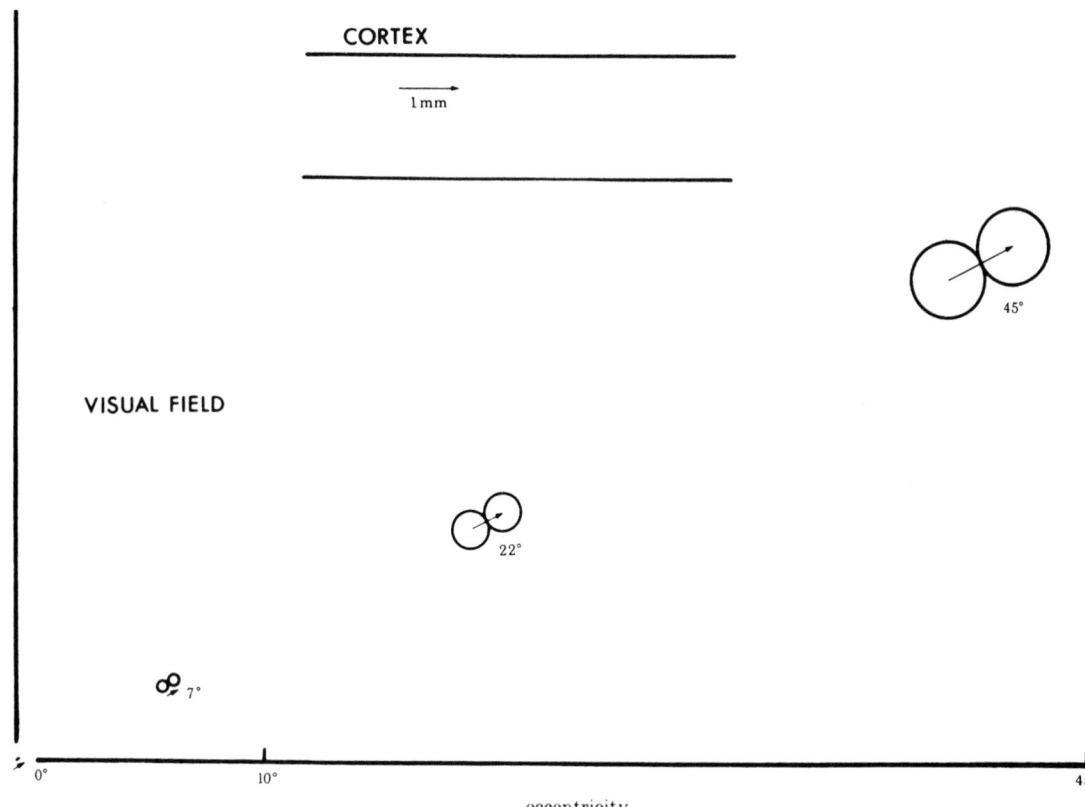

Fig. 9. *Variation of receptive-field drift with eccentricity: The diagram represents one quadrant of the field of vision, and the circles represent aggregate receptive fields, the territory collectively occupied by receptive fields of cells encountered in a micro-electrode penetration perpendicular to the cortical surface. Each pair of circles illustrates the movement in aggregate receptive field accompanying a movement along the cortex of 1–2 mm. Both the displacement and the aggregate field size vary with distance from the fovea (eccentricity), but they do so in parallel fashion. Close to the fovea the fields are tiny, but so is the displacement accompanying a 1–2 mm movement along the cortex. The greater the distance from the fovea, the greater the two become, but they continue to remain roughly equal. (From Hubel & Wiesel 1974b.)*

3. Complexity and Binocularity According to Laminae

We turn now to the layering of area 17, which is shown at higher power in Figure 10, Plate 6. The afferents coming from the lateral geniculate terminate at several levels—layers IVa, IVc and VI, and perhaps also layer I (Hubel & Wiesel 1972). The great majority of terminations are, however, in IVc. The subsequent wiring is not fully known, but several synapses are required before the information reaches cells whose axons project out of the cortex (Lund 1973). If we examine the properties of cells layer by layer, two salient findings emerge. First, there is a correlation between complexity and layering, at least to the extent that the least complicated cells, the circularly symmetric geniculate-like cells, are located mainly in layer IVc. Simple cells seem to be located mainly in IVb; they are perhaps also present in VI—at least they have been found there in the cat (Hubel & Wiesel 1962; Gilbert 1977). Complex and hypercomplex cells are found, in our experience, only in II, III, V, and VI. It is a relief, at any rate, to find the simplest cells at the input end of the cortex.

The second fact about lamination involves binocular convergence. Cells in layer IVc are almost exclusively monocular. This of course is consistent with our previous statement that the

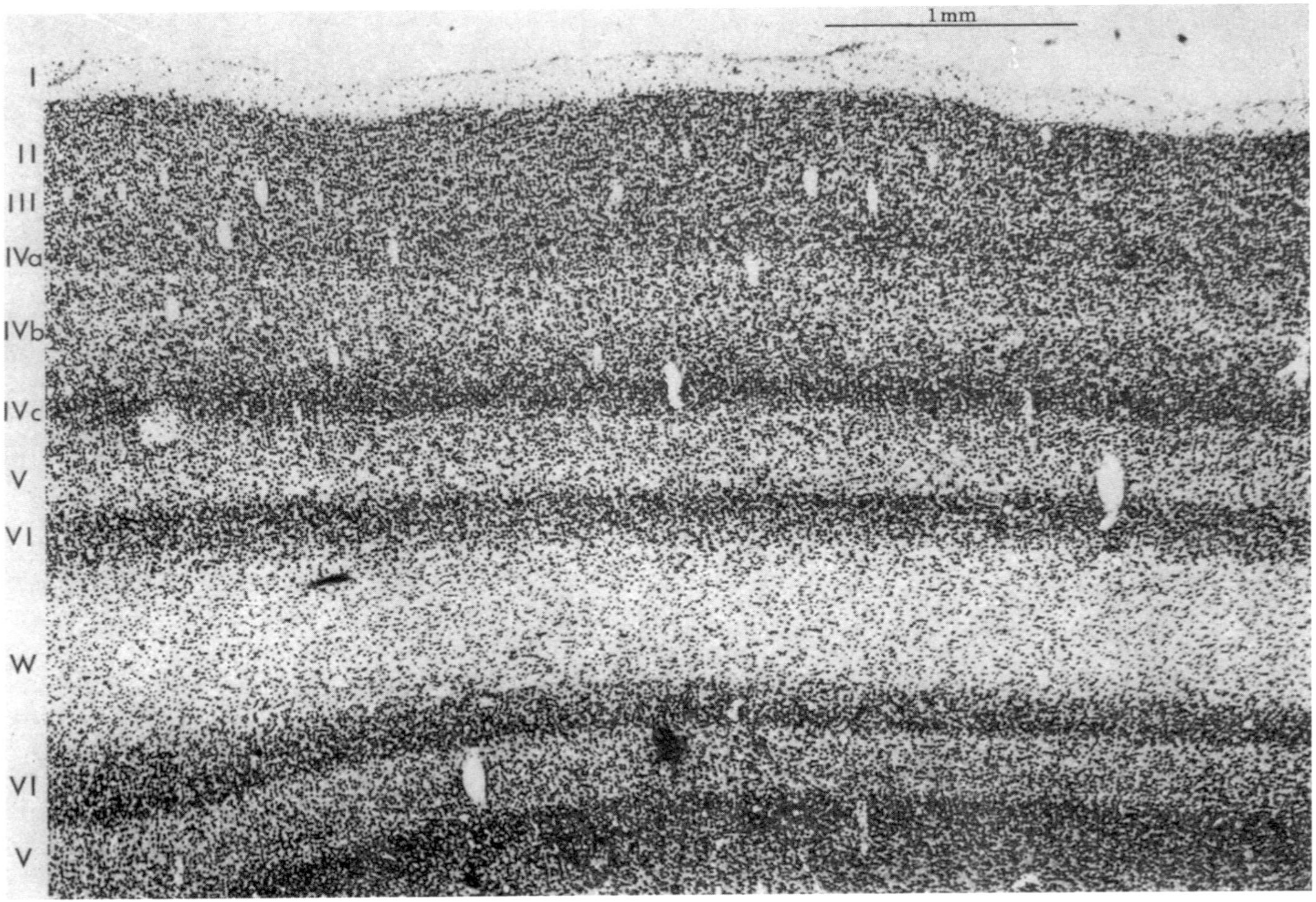

Plate 6

Fig. 10. Cross section through monkey striate cortex showing conventional layering designations. W, white matter. Deeper layers (VI, V) of the buried fold of cortex are shown in the lower part of the figure (compare Figure 6b). Cresyl violet.

concentric cells are almost all monocular. Cells in IVb, including the simple cells found there, are predominantly monocular, whereas over half of those in II, III, V, and VI are binocular.

4. Ocular Dominance Columns

We next consider the distribution of cells in the cortex according to ocular dominance. We begin by asking whether two cells sitting side by side in the cortex are likely to have the same ocular dominance. The answer is that they almost always do. Either both prefer the left eye or both prefer the right. Furthermore, if an electrode penetration is made perpendicular to the cortical surface all of the cells encountered, from the surface to the white matter, will with high probability respond preferentially to the same eye (Figure 11). If we pull out the electrode and reinsert it at a point a millimetre or so away, the same eye may again be dominant all the way down, or the other eye may now dominate. In a horizontal or oblique penetration there is an alternation of eye dominance: first one eye prevails, then the other. By making a large number of penetrations in various directions one reaches the conclusion that the striate cortex is subdivided into regions whose cross-sectional width is in the order

of 0.4 mm and whose walls are perpendicular to the cortical surface and to the layers. We term these subdivisions *ocular dominance columns*. The word 'column' as applied to vertically organized cortical subdivisions was coined by Mountcastle (1957) for a system of aggregations in the somatosensory cortex, corresponding to cutaneous versus deep sensory sub-modalities. The cross-sectional appearance of the ocular dominance columns does indeed suggest a pillar-like three-dimensional shape, but as we will see the actual shape in area 17 is not at all pillar-like. In retrospect, for the visual system, the term 'column' may be somewhat misleading, but to change the term seems undesirable, since whatever the exact geometric shape there is no doubt that the subdivisions in the visual and somatosensory systems are to a large extent analogous. In both systems, one may add, the discovery of the subdivisions came as a complete surprise, since the classical neurophysiological procedures, Golgi, Nissl and fibre stains, had given no hint of their presence.

Given these ocular dominance columns, we may imagine that a binocular cell results from wiring of the sort shown, very schematically, in Figure 12. Suppose a cell X in layer II or III lies above the centre of a right-eye ocular-dominance

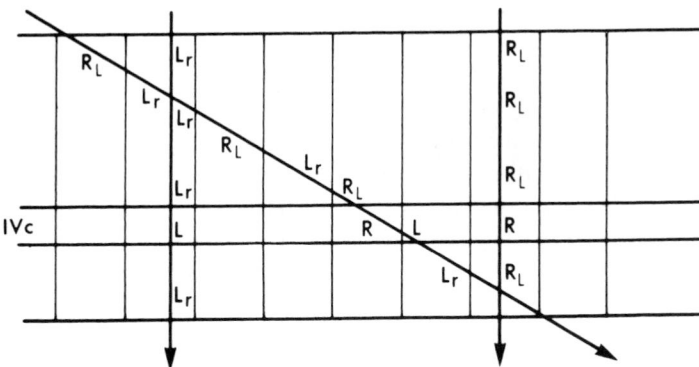

Fig. 11. Illustration of ocular dominance columns in macaque monkey. The diagram represents a cross section through striate cortex, with surface at top and border between layer VI and white matter below. Two vertical penetrations and one oblique are illustrated. Letters refer to expected eye dominance at various stages in each penetration. R_L stands for a region in which there is a mixture of binocular cells preferring the right eye, and monocular cells responding to the right eye. R stands for a region containing only cells driven exclusively from the right eye. Layer IVc contains only monocular cells, grouped separately in patches according to eye affiliation. Layers above and below IVc contain binocular cells, grouped in columns according to eye preference. When a vertical penetration reaches IVc the eye that has been preferred all along comes to monopolize. In an oblique or horizontal penetration there is a regular alternation of eye preference as the electrode goes from column to column.

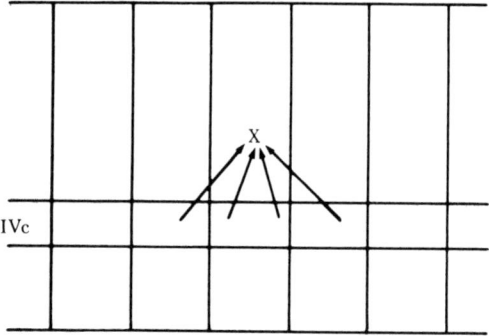

Fig. 12. Scheme to illustrate the wiring of a binocular cell in a layer above (or below) layer IVc. The bulk of the afferents to the striate cortex from the lateral geniculate body, themselves monocular, are strictly segregated by eye affiliation in layer IVc, and thus the cells in this layer are strictly monocular. A cell outside of IVc, labelled X in the diagram, receives its input connections, directly or indirectly, by one or more synapses from cells in IVc (to some extent also, perhaps, from layers IVa and VI). Cells in IVc will be more likely to feed into X the closer they are to it; consequently X is likely to be binocular, dominated by the eye corresponding to the nearest patch in IVc. The degree of dominance by that eye is greater, the closer X is to being centered in its ocular dominance column, and cells near a boundary may be roughly equally influenced by the two eyes (see also Figure 13).

patch. We know from the Golgi anatomy that this cell receives its input, either directly or over a few synapses, from a region of layer IV having a horizontal extent of 1 or a few millimetres. The cell will be most richly connected to cells in IVc lying directly below it. It can therefore be predicted that cell X will have stronger links with the eye that feeds the IVc patch directly beneath it, than with the other eye. The nearer X is to being centered over (or under) a particular patch the stronger will be its domination by the corresponding eye; the closer to a columnar border, the more nearly equal will be the influence of the two eyes. This expectation is borne out experimentally, for in a horizontal penetration through the upper or lower layers (i.e. the layers above or below layer IV) there is a strong tendency to systematic fluctuation in dominance back and forth, from one extreme through equality to the other extreme. This is illustrated in the left part of Figure 13, which shows the variations in ocular dominance with electrode distance for a penetration passing horizontally along layer III. It should be stressed that the ocular-dominance col-

umn, as we define it, refers to the full thickness of cortex and is defined by eye *preference*. The part of the column in layer IVc contains monocular cells only; at the borders of the columns in IVc there is little intermixing of the two cell populations, and the borders themselves are consequently very sharp, more so than in the other layers. This is illustrated in the right half of Figure 13. Even outside of IVc, however, the boundaries are far from nebulous, and can generally be specified to within 50–100 μm.

Just why the two eyes should be brought together in this elaborate but incomplete way is not yet clear. What the ocular dominance columns appear to achieve is a partial mixing of influences from the two eyes, with all shades of ocular dominance throughout the entire binocular field of vision. The columns may represent a way of making sure that this special kind of mixing occurs in the same way everywhere. That monocular complex cells are kept aside in all parts of the visual fields is perhaps related to stereoscopy. It seems that cells whose fields in the two eyes show positional disparity in a horizontal direction are absent or rare in area 17 but rather common in 18 (Hubel & Wiesel 1970; 1973). Area 17 projects in a topographically faithful way to 18. To build up such depth cells in 18, with all the degrees of disparity required for stereopsis, probably requires keeping aside monocular cells in area 17 which can later be combined in various ways, producing a complete range of field disparities: to commit all cells in area 17 by combining them with zero disparity would preclude this procedure later. Presumably the machinery required to produce all degrees of disparity is too ponderous for it to be included in area 17, which perhaps has enough to worry about as it is. While stereopsis provides a plausible explanation for the existence of monocular cells at the output end of area 17, the question of why binocular cells should exist in all shades of eye preference remains an open one.

5. Orientation Columns

Let us now turn to the final variable on our list, receptive-field orientation. Here again we first ask whether neighbouring cells tend to favour the same stimulus orientation. Again, the answer is that they almost invariably do. And as with ocular dominance, a penetration exactly perpendicular to

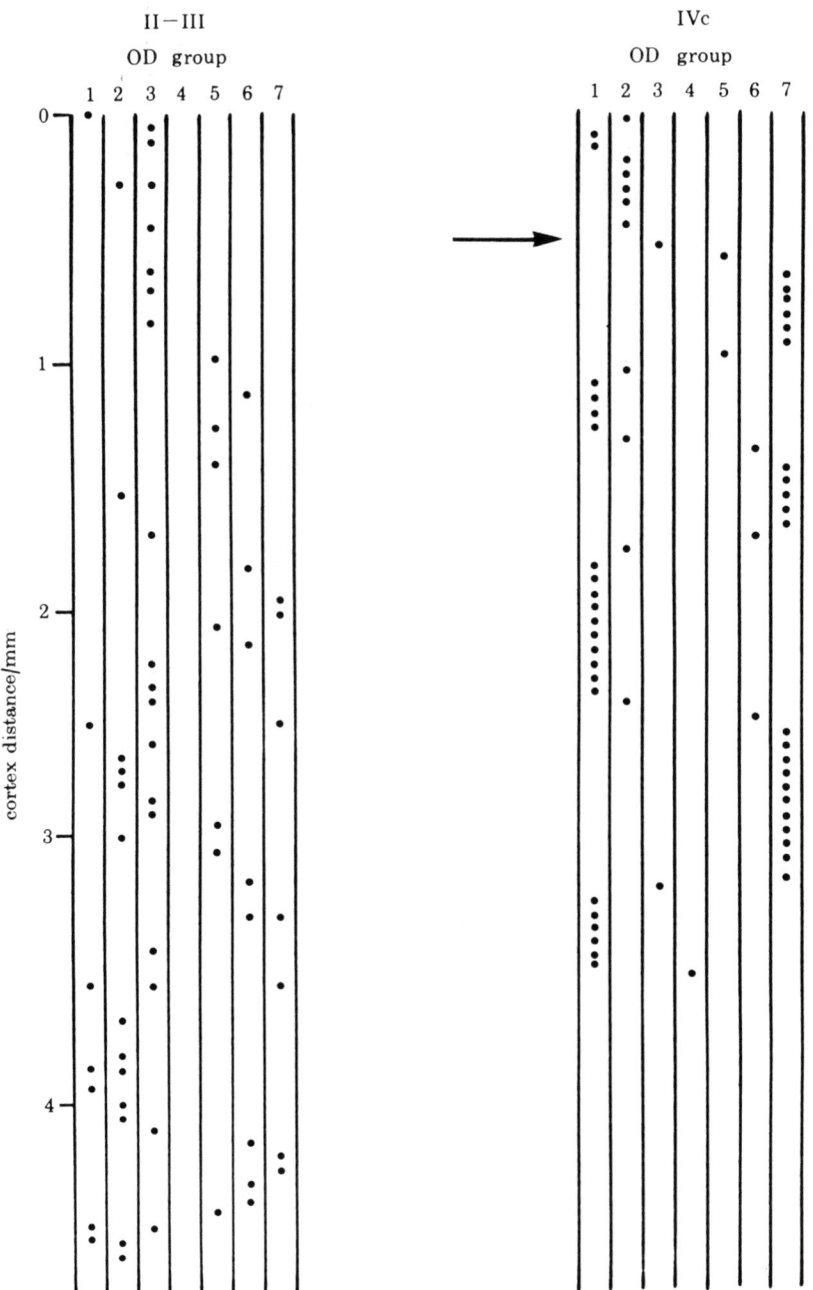

Fig. 13. Variation of ocular dominance with distance in two penetrations made at a very oblique angle to area 17, in the parasagittal plane in macaque monkey striate cortex. The part of the penetration illustrated on the left side is entirely in layers II and III. The portion of the penetration illustrated on the right begins in IVb, but enters IVc at the arrow and remains in IVc to the end. The two penetrations were about 1 mm apart. In layers II and III (and also in V and VI) most cells are binocular but show some eye preference. As the electrode passes through 8 or 9 dominance columns, the cells first show marked preference for one eye, then are more nearly equally driven by the two eyes, and finally the other eye gains the ascendancy; the dominance thus swings back and forth in a smooth fashion. In IVc, on the other hand, the transitions are more abrupt and complete, from regions dominated exclusively by one eye to regions monopolized by the other.

the cortical surface and to the layers reveals cells all of which favour the same orientation, except of course those in layer IVc, which have no orientation preference at all (Figure 14). In a horizontal or oblique penetration one sees a succession of preferred orientations. The shifts occur so frequently that even the smallest advance one can make, and be sure that the electrode has indeed moved (that is about 20 μm), is accompanied by a detectable change in optimal orientation (Hubel & Wiesel 1974*a*). The shifts are generally small and occur usually, though not always, in an amazingly orderly sequence, with many clockwise or counterclockwise steps that add up finally to total rotations of up to 180° or more. From time to time, unpredictably, the direction of rotation may reverse.

A typical sequence is shown in Figure 15*a*. Here the anaesthetized and paralysed monkey was facing a tangent screen 1½ m distant. The directions of gaze for the two eyes in these circumstances are seldom parallel, and here they even crossed so that the left foveal projection (lf) lay to the right of the right projection (rf) (as determined with an ophthalmoscope). The recording was almost tangential to the surface of the striate cortex of the right side, so that the aggregate receptive

fields in the two eyes were in the left visual fields, as indicated by the interrupted circles. The first unit recorded (which happened to be the 96th in this entire experiment) was binocular but with the right eye dominant, and for this cell the fields were mapped in both eyes. The preferred orientations were almost identical, roughly 1 o'clock–7 o'clock. Advancing the electrode produced a slight counterclockwise shift (no. 97), and from this point on each advance was accompanied by a similar shift, always counterclockwise. To save time, from cell 97 on we mapped fields only in the dominant eye. At no. 111 the eye dominance suddenly shifted to the left eye, indicating that the electrode had crossed over into a new eye-dominance column: the orientation sequence nevertheless went its own way, quite unaffected by the dominance shift. By the end of the sequence the orientation had rotated through some 160°.

This result is shown as a graph in Figure 15*b*, where orientation is plotted against distance traversed by the electrode. The relation is virtually linear, with only a small offset where the dominance changed from right eye (filled circles) to left eye (open circles), caused by a slight relative eye rotation in the equatorial plane. Figure 16 shows a

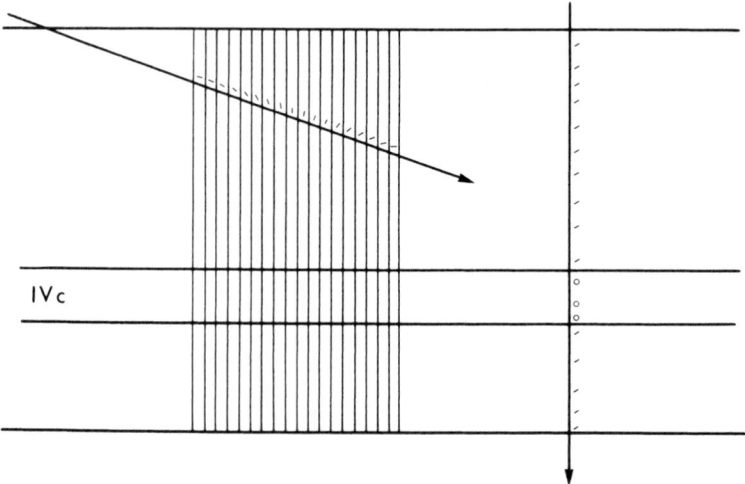

Fig. 14. Diagram to illustrate orientation columns in monkey striate cortex. Two penetrations are illustrated, one vertical, the other oblique. In the vertical penetration orientation is clearly defined and constant, from cell to cell, in layers above and below IVc. In layer IVc the cells have fields with circular symmetry, and there is no orientation preference. In an oblique penetration there is a systematic variation in orientation, clockwise or counterclockwise, in steps of about 10° or less, that occur roughly every 50 μm. (That the variation is in some sense continuous is not ruled out—see text.)

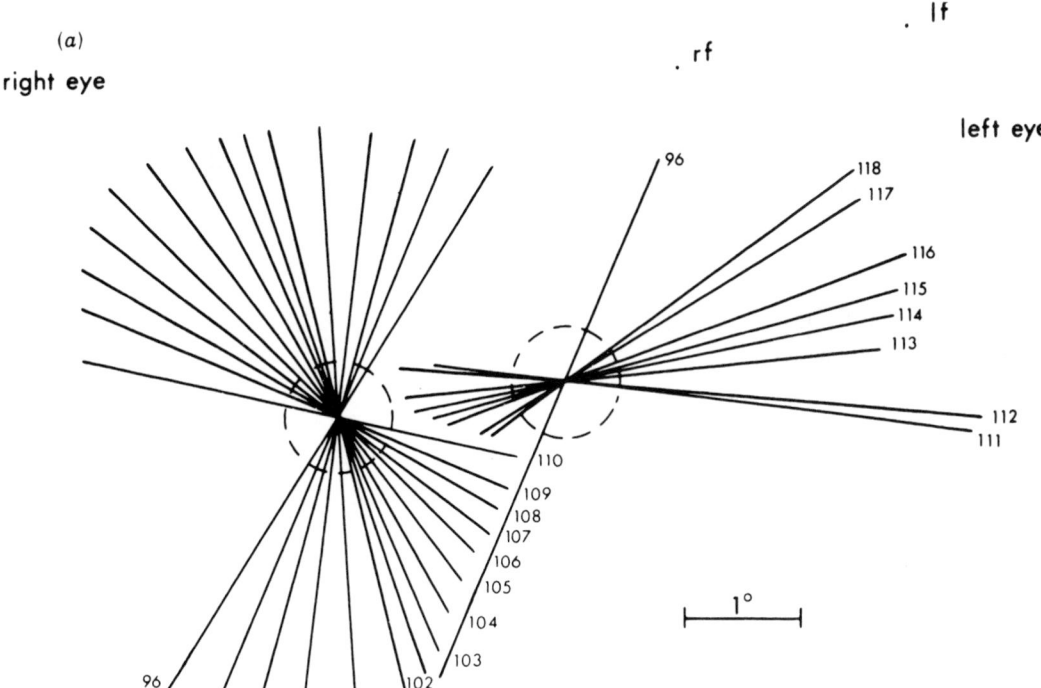

Fig. 15. (a) Illustration of results obtained in a typical experiment during part of an almost tangential penetration through area 17 in the right hemisphere. The figure represents the tangent screen on which fields were mapped. rf and lf represent projections of the two foveas—the paralysed eyes had their axes crossed at a point in front of the screen. Receptive fields, collectively occupying the regions outlined in dashed circles, were about 4° below and to the left of the centre of gaze. At the beginning of the sequence shown here (cell no. 96) the orientation was about 1 o'clock–7 o'clock, and responses were evoked from both eyes, the right better than the left. As the electrode was advanced the orientation shifted in a counterclockwise direction in small steps at a rate of about 280°/mm. The right eye continued to dominate, and fields were therefore mapped only in that eye, up to cell no. 111. Here eye dominance abruptly changed to favour the left eye, and fields were mapped in that eye up to no. 118, when the penetration was terminated. Note that when eye dominance changed there was no interruption of the orientation sequence.

second graph from a different experiment. The penetration was long and very oblique, almost tangential, as shown in the reconstruction at the upper right. Several reversals were seen, with the largest uninterrupted sequence totalling 267°.

The conclusion from these results is that the cortex is subdivided by a second set of vertical partitions into columns which are very slender. For technical reasons (see Hubel & Wiesel 1974a) one cannot be sure that orientation does not vary in some sense continuously with horizontal position

(see also Albus 1975). If the steps are discrete they occur every 20–50 μm and correspond to orientation shifts of about 10°. Whether or not they are discrete, one can say that roughly 180° rotation corresponds to a 1 mm displacement along the cortex. To judge from a number of penetrations made in different parts of area 17, this law probably holds true throughout the cortex. Thus the columns probably have the same thickness everywhere.

It is hard to imagine that such an elaborate and highly patterned organization as this would

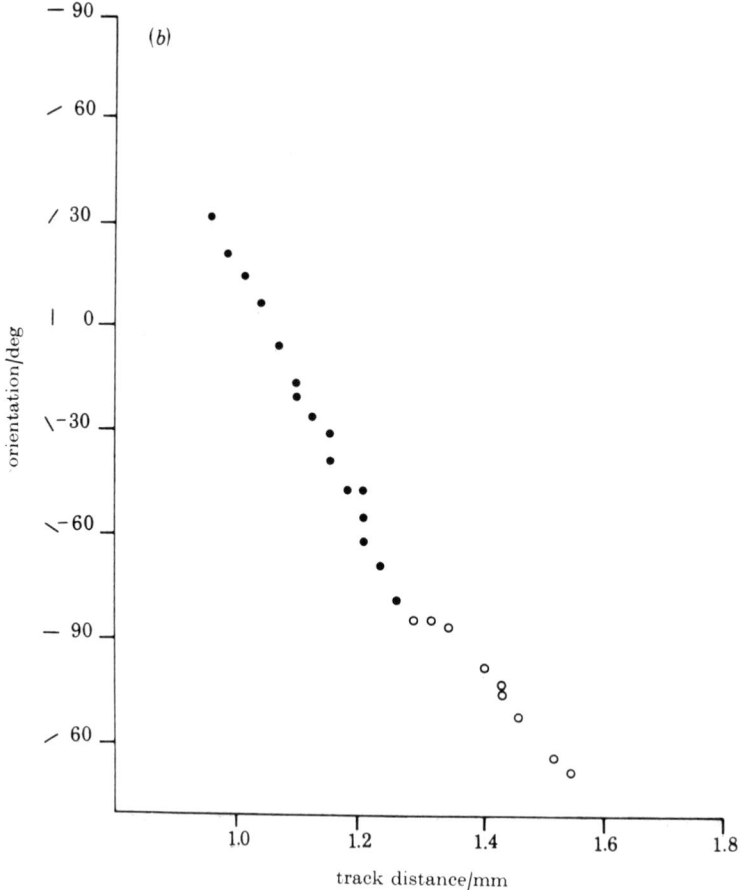

Fig. 15(b). Graph of orientation in degrees plotted against electrode track distance in millimetres, for the sequence illustrated in 15a. ●, cells dominated by right eye; ○, left eye.

have evolved if orientation were not important. The significance of the organization is suggested by the physiology. Within each column are housed cells with concentric fields together with simple, complex, and hypercomplex cells, having the same orientation preference and all having more or less the same receptive-field position. These are the very cells which the physiology tells us are probably interconnected—certainly there is no suggestion that cells with very different receptive field positions or very different orientations have major excitatory interconnections. One may thus look upon a column as a functional unit of cortex, a means of bringing into one place the cells that are to be interconnected, and of separating them from cells with which they have few or no connections. The alternative, of having cells mixed at random

without regard to preferred orientation, would surely be less efficient in terms of length of connections and specificity, for any cell could then not simply reach out to its nearest neighbour or to cells directly above or below, but would instead have to search out the axons or dendrites of other cells having just the correct orientation, while ignoring all the others. It is indeed hard to contemplate the nightmare of interconnections that would have to exist if the cells were distributed at random with respect to orientation.

Probably there is functional importance not only in the orientation columns themselves, but also in the regularity of their arrangement. Having such a regularity presumably guarantees that all orientations are represented everywhere in the field of vision, with no omissions or redundancies.

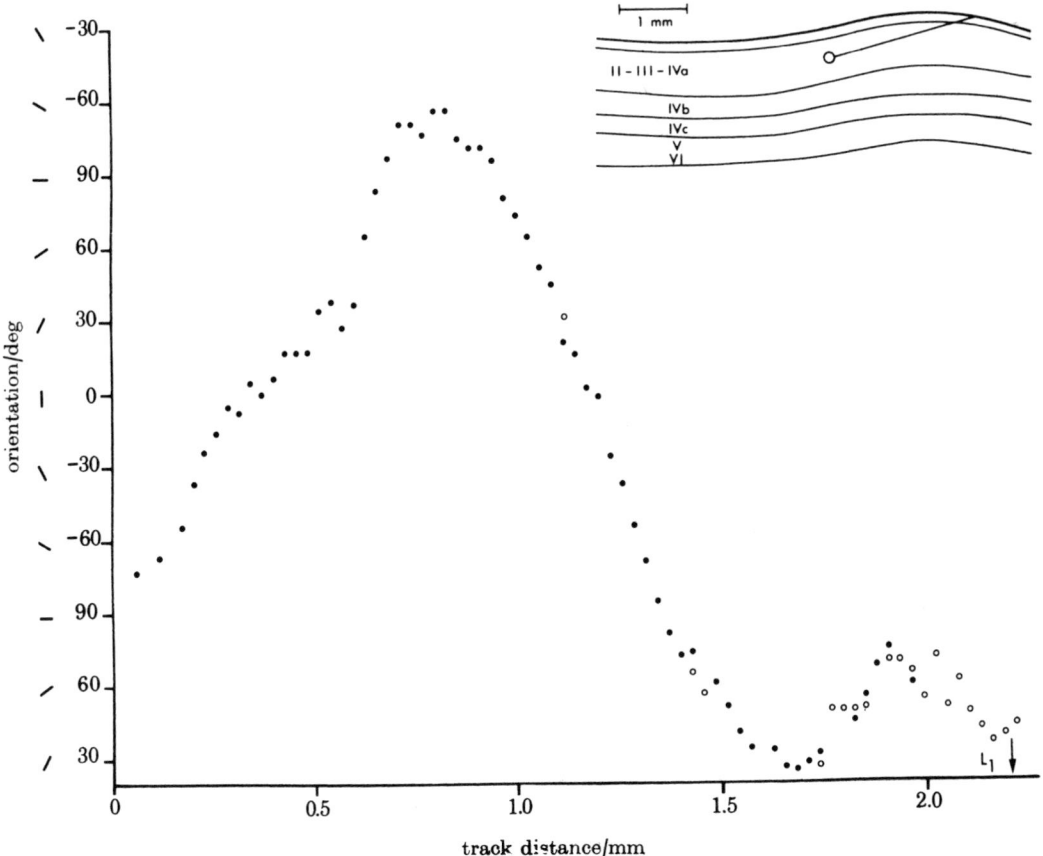

Fig. 16. Graph similar to that of Figure 15b, but from a different experiment. Again, the penetration was almost horizontal and was restricted to layers II and III (see inset). Several reversals in the direction of rotation occur, with two very long, almost linear, sequences followed by two short ones. The right eye was dominant until almost the end of the sequence.

There is probably also an improved economy in the connections that are required to manufacture simple cells from circularly symmetric ones (Hubel & Wiesel 1974a). Finally, orientation specificity may be enhanced by mutual inhibition between cells whose orientations differ by a small angle (Blakemore & Tobin 1972); having such cells close together in neighbouring columns would shorten the connections responsible for this inhibition.

In a cross section such as that represented in Figure 14 the orientation columns appear as pillar-like structures, just as the ocular dominance columns do, but several lines of evidence indicate that they are not columns at all, in the usual sense of that word. Direct observation by means of mul-

tiple parallel electrode tracks, which can be reconstructed in three dimensions (Hubel & Wiesel 1974a), indicate that the shape is actually that of narrow parallel slabs lined up vertically (perpendicular to the surface) like slices of bread. Cross sections of such arrays would then give the appearance of Figure 14 unless the plane of section happened to be parallel to the slabs. Only rarely, in fact, does orientation remain constant in a horizontal penetration (resulting in a zero slope in graphs of the type shown in Figures 15b and 16), and such constancy would indeed be expected only rarely, given the unlikelihood of an electrode's threading its way along such narrow slabs. Moreover, the slabs may be swirls rather than parallel planes, and a swirling pattern would easily explain the reversals in direction of rotation seen in Figure 16.

An entirely different argument that the columns are actually slabs comes from considerations of continuity. If we suppose that throughout a particular region of cortex there is order everywhere—that for all directions of penetrations the orientation changes in small steps, or does not change at all—then the regions of constant orientation must be slabs. The argument runs as follows: When we say there is order everywhere, geometrically we mean that if orientation in degrees is plotted on the z-axis against the two-dimensional $x - y$ cortical surface position, the graph forms some kind of surface. The surface is smooth if orientation is a continuous function of position along the cortex, as discussed above, and finely terraced if orientation changes in small steps. Such a surface in a three-dimensional graph yields the curves of Figures 15b and 16, when cut by any plane perpendicular to the cortex. On the other hand if the surface in the three-dimensional graph is cut by a plane parallel to the cortical surface, corresponding to a particular z-value of orientation, the intersection between surface and plane yields a contour line of constant orientation. Sets of such contour lines correspond to the tops of the slabs, as seen when one looks down on the cortex from above. The shape of the surface would of course be fascinating to know. The reversals seen in Figure 16 could be produced by mountains and valleys, corresponding to the swirling columns mentioned above, or by a surface with ridges like a washboard or a camera bellows or a series of mountain ranges.

These two lines of evidence, from parallel penetrations and from the argument based on the orderliness of the shifts, are obviously less direct than an actual anatomical visualization of the slabs, but so far no such anatomical method has been found. This is in part because the orientation columns (or slabs, as we may now term them) are produced not by any special distribution of the afferent terminals, but by interconnections within the cortex. What the precise connections are that lead to orientation specificity is not known, and as mentioned already none of the common methods for examining nervous tissue, such as Nissl or Golgi or fibre stains, or the use of the electron microscope, has yet shown anything that could be convincingly construed as representing the orientation columns. The ocular dominance columns, on the other hand, actually result from the specific patchy terminal distribution of afferents from the geniculate to layer IV. In this respect they differ profoundly from the orientation columns, and are more akin to the superficial vs. joint columns described for the somatosensory cortex by Mountcastle. This dependence on afferent distribution has made it possible to visualize the dominance columns anatomically, as we shall describe in the next section.

6. Geometry of Ocular Dominance Columns

Here again our problem was to determine the three-dimensional shape of columns when the physiological recordings told us only that the walls separating the columns were perpendicular to the surface. A cross-sectional appearance of the sort indicated in Figure 11 might result from several very different geometries. The columns seen from above could, for example, consist of alternating squares of right and left eye affiliation, forming a sort of checker board (Figure 17a). They could consist of islands of right-eye dominance in a sea of left-eye dominance, or the reverse, or of some combination of these two (Figure 17b). Or, finally, they could consist of a set of alternating left-eye and right-eye stripes (Figure 17c). Cut in cross section any of these topologies would result in the alternating sequence of Figure 11. To distinguish among the three possibilities (or any others that one might conjure up) with a microelectrode is possible in principle, for example with reconstructions of multiple parallel penetrations, but to attack such a three-dimensional problem with a one-dimensional weapon is a dismaying exercise in tedium, like trying to cut the back lawn with a pair of nail scissors. And so it turned out—after one or two attempts we decided that it would be more rewarding to turn to farming (with modern implements) as a career.

Fortunately (for American agriculture) over the last few years four entirely independent anatomical methods have become available, and it has been possible to approach the problem of dominance-column geometry directly and answer it unequivocally. The first of these was the Nauta silver-degeneration method, which relies on the possibility of staining selectively axons that degen-

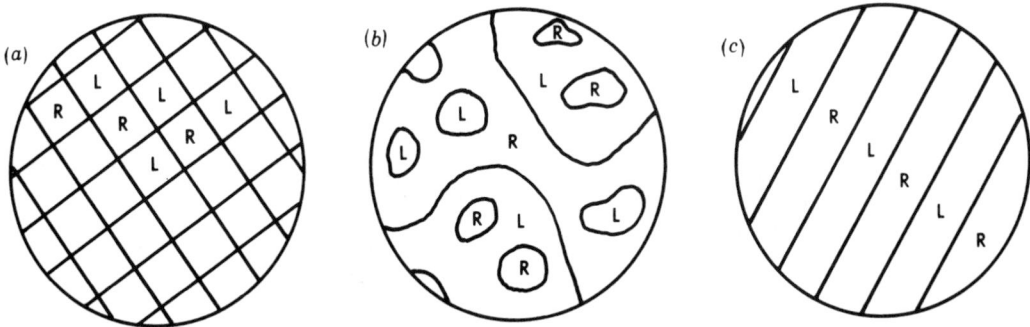

Fig. 17. *Three possible ways in which a plane surface might be partitioned into two types of region; here, left eye (L) and right eye (R).*

erate when they are cut proximally or when the parent cell bodies are injured. A subsequent modification of this method, by Fink & Heimer (1967) and later by Wiitanen (1969), made possible the selective staining of degenerating axon terminals. With this method a large lesion in the lateral geniculate body would be expected to produce a forest of stained terminals, appearing as dense 5–10 μm brown dots, precisely in layer IV. In 1965 (Hubel & Wiesel) we had begun to adapt the Nauta method to microelectrodes, making minute lesions in single cortical layers or single subdivisions of deep nuclei, recording from the electrode to help guide its precise placement prior to making the lesion. It occurred to us that if we were to place a small lesion in a single geniculate layer (corresponding to a single eye) the degeneration of terminals in IVc of the cortex should be in discrete regular patches with gaps between, unless our deductions from the physiology were completely faulty.

The results of one of our first attempts at this are shown in Figure 18, Plate 7 (Hubel & Wiesel 1972). The geniculate penetration was luckily almost tangential to the most dorsal of the geniculate layers, which allowed us to make a long cigar-shaped lesion entirely within this layer. This produced a rather wide region (4 × 8 mm) of cortical degeneration in the mushroom-like buried fold of cortex, shown diagrammatically in the upper right of Figure 18a. A photomicrograph of a typical section is shown in Figure 18b in dark field; here regions rich in degenerating terminals glow brightly. The existence of regular alternations of patches of terminals and terminal-free gaps was

thus confirmed. Now to get at the three-dimensional shape of these patches it was only necessary to prepare a few hundred serial sections and stack them next to each other at the correct spacing. This was done graphically as shown below in Figure 18c. Each horizontal broken line in the diagram represents the patches and gaps from a single section, artificially (graphically) straightened out into a line. The entire reconstruction thus represents a face-on view of the cortex, or, to be more specific, of the degenerating terminals in layer IVc.

From this reconstruction and a number of others it was clear that to a first approximation the IVth layer terminals have the distribution of parallel stripes. The stripes have a width of about 0.4 mm and are in most regions remarkably regular. There is, to be sure, a certain degree of irregularity, especially a tendency for two stripes corresponding to one eye to join, leaving the intervening stripe from the other eye to end blindly. Near the fovea the anastomoses are very frequent and form a lattice-like series of cross linkings (Figure 19). Perhaps the most striking feature of the stripes is the regularity of their spacing; it is difficult to find a point in layer IVc that is more than about 0.2 mm from the nearest stripe border.

As a by-product of these experiments it was shown that geniculate terminals do not occur in layer IVb (Line of Gennari), confirming an old observation of Clark & Sunderland (1939), and that the parvocellular layers (the four dorsal layers) project to layer IVa and to the deeper half of IVc, whereas the magnocellular (ventral two) layers project to the superficial half of IVc. This was the

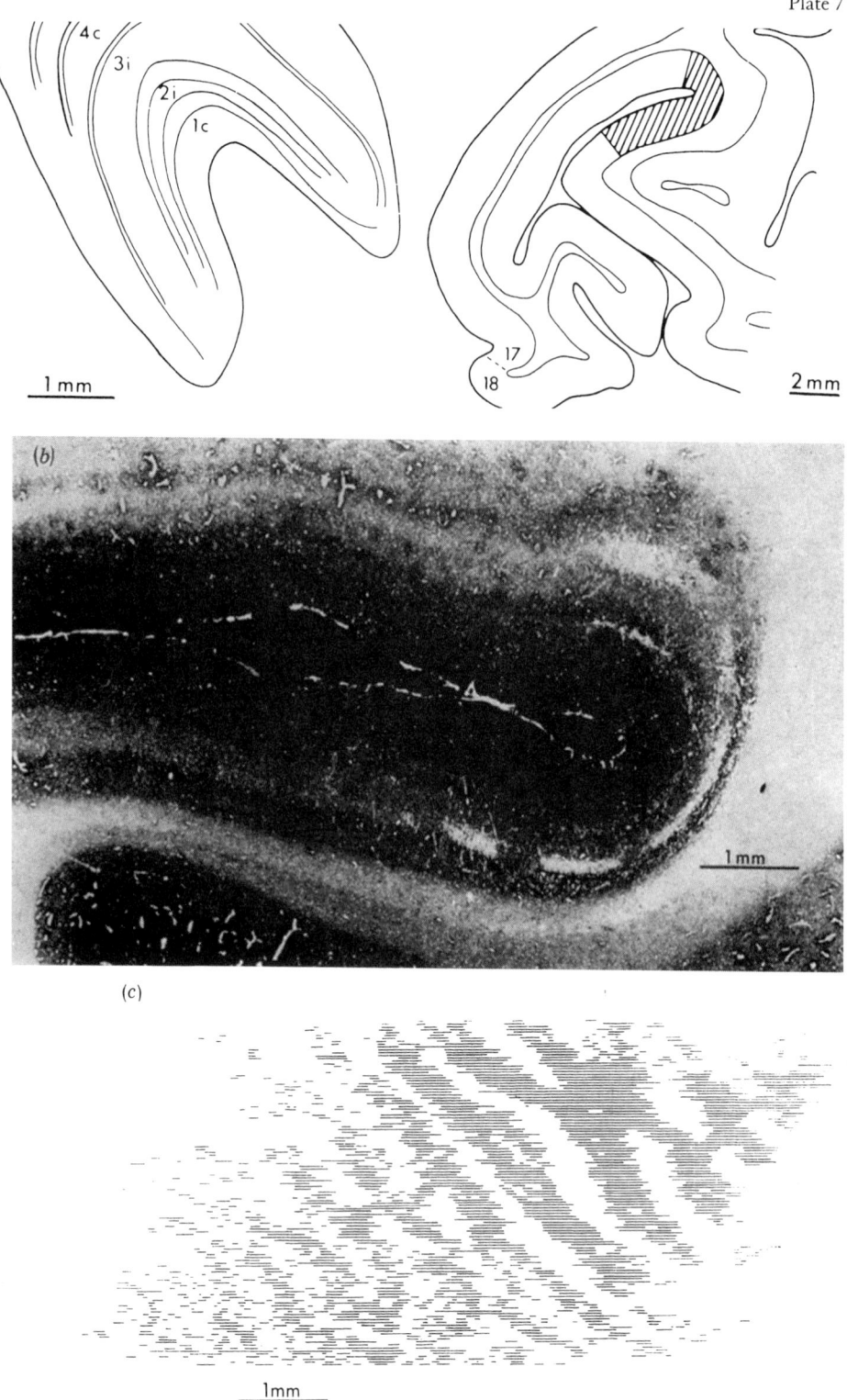

Plate 7

4 c

3 i

2 i

1 c

17

18

1 mm

2 mm

(b)

1 mm

(c)

1mm

Fig. 18.

622

Fig. 18. (a) *Distribution of degenerating terminals in macaque monkey striate cortex following a focal lesion confined to the most dorsal layer (no. 6) of the left lateral geniculate body. At the upper left the position of the lesion is shown (stippled) on a tracing of a coronal section through the geniculate. At the top right the shaded region indicates the part of area 17 in which degenerating terminals were found, in layers IVa and c; this drawing is traced from a parasagittal section through the occipital lobe (compare Figure 6). Within the shaded region the degenerating terminals occurred in patches about 0.5 mm wide, separated by terminal free gaps of about the same size; each section contained about 5–6 patches and gaps. (b) Dark field photomicrograph through region of cortex to which degenerating fibres projected. Bands of densely packed degenerating endings can be seen as light patches in the highly curved portion of the buried part of area 17. (c) Reconstruction drawn from 118 sections parallel to the one in b, and including it. Each horizontal interrupted line is obtained from a photograph like that shown in b, by graphically flattening the part of layer IVc containing degenerated terminals and tracing the patches of degeneration. The resulting pattern represents the view one would get looking at layer IVc face on. The columns are thus for the most part parallel stripes. The vertical lines indicate the position of the crease in the cortex.* (Hubel & Wiesel 1972, Figures 8–10.

first evidence that the ventral and dorsal layers have different projections. The significance of this pattern of projection is still quite obscure.

The Nauta method as applied to this problem had one severe limitation. For a lesion to be confined strictly to a single geniculate layer it had to be small, so that the consequent overall size of the cor-

responding region of striate cortical degeneration was only a few mm in diameter. To visualize a wider area, to say nothing of the entire striate cortex, a new method was needed. One day Simon LeVay, who had recently joined our laboratory, was examining tangentially sectioned striate cortex of macaque using a reduced silver stain, in the hope

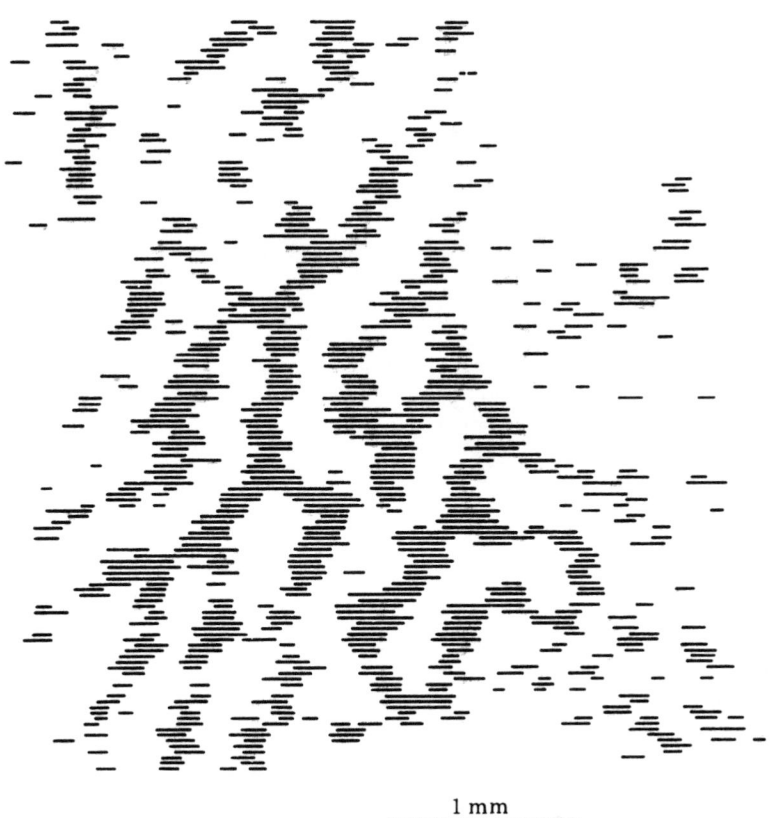

1 mm

Fig. 19. *Reconstruction similar to that of Figure 18c, but here the geniculate lesion was made a few degrees from the foveal representation in the most ventral geniculate layer (no. 1). The lattice-like appearance, with a large number of blind endings and cross linkings, seems to be a characteristic of the foveal and parafoveal region.* (Hubel & Wiesel, 1972, Fig. 17.)

of seeing something that might correlate with orientation columns. He noticed high in layer IVc a series of dark parallel stripes about 400 μm wide, separated by narrow paler interbands about 50 μm wide (Figure 20, Plate 8). Clearly these dark bands could not be orientation columns—they were much too wide. Could they represent the eye dominance columns? Close examination showed that occasionally two dark stripes joined, but never two adjacent ones; there was always a dark stripe between the two, which ended blindly. LeVay recognized that this was just what was to be expected in a twofold system, since by definition if two columns joined they must correspond to the same eye. To establish that the stripes were, in fact, the dominance columns we made very oblique penetrations down to layer IVc, cutting it tangentially or nearly so, and then made lesions each time the electrode tip crossed from a region dominated by one eye to a region dominated by the other. When the brain was later sectioned tangentially and stained by the reduced silver method the lesions matched precisely the narrow pale regions separating the dark bands. This established beyond any doubt that the dark bands do indeed represent the eye dominance columns. The bands are produced by large and medium sized horizontally running fibres in upper IVc; they are somewhat more concentrated in the dark bands than in the narrow lighter interbands. Exactly what these fibres are is not known; some of them are probably geniculate afferents, since some of the afferents run in this region and are more numerous within columns than between them (LeVay, Hubel & Wiesel 1975).

At the same time as LeVay's method was developed a third method for demonstrating the columns became available, this one based on autoradiography and axonal transport. The method of mapping pathways by injecting radioactive amino acids or other compounds in the vicinity of nerve cell bodies, and identifying the axon terminals autoradiographically, was already well known (Goldberg & Kotani 1967; Lasek, Joseph & Whitlock 1968; Cowan et al. 1972). In applying it to the monkey visual system one simply injected the label into the vitreous humour of the eye, whereupon the retinal cells took it up and in the case of retinal ganglion cells transported it (probably in the form of proteins) down their axons. An accumulation

of radioactive compounds in the axon terminals led to the dense accumulation of silver grains on autoradiographs in the layers receiving input from the injected eye. A typical result for macaque monkey is shown in Figure 21, Plate 9, confirming once again the original deduction of Minkowski. (The power of the autoradiographic method is shown by its ability to reveal four aggregations of optic nerve terminals besides the six classical layers. These are described in Figure 21 (Hubel *et al.* 1976). The targets to which these aggregations project are unknown, and their significance is quite obscure.)

A few years before our studies, Grafstein & Laureno (1973) had observed that in a mouse whose eye had been injected with a mixture of radioactive proline and fucose, some of the label was transported all the way to the striate cortex of the opposite hemisphere. Since in the mouse the visual pathway is predominantly crossed, they concluded that some of the radioactive compounds had passed out of the optic nerve terminals in the geniculate, had been taken up by the cell bodies there and transported by the geniculate-cell axons to the striate cortex. We reasoned that if the same thing could be made to happen by using autoradiography in the monkey we should be able to see the distribution, in layer IV, of the geniculate-cell terminals corresponding to the injected eye. These should then appear in cross section as patches of silver grains, about 0.4 mm wide, separated by gaps corresponding to the eye that had not been injected.

The result of such an experiment is shown in Figure 22, Plate 10 (Hubel *et al.* 1976). Dark-field techniques had to be used since the grains were too sparse to be obvious on cursory inspection by light field illumination. The layer IVc columns stand out clearly everywhere, and this section by itself shows some 56 pairs of columns.

Though requiring an eye injection and the use of large amounts of radioactive substances, which are expensive and not free of danger, this method has several advantages over LeVay's reduced silver technique, for the latter only reveals stripes in sections that are tangential or almost tangential to layer IV, and does not seem to work at all in monkeys under about 6 months old.

To reconstruct the pattern of columns over a wide area and to visualize them *en face,* one can

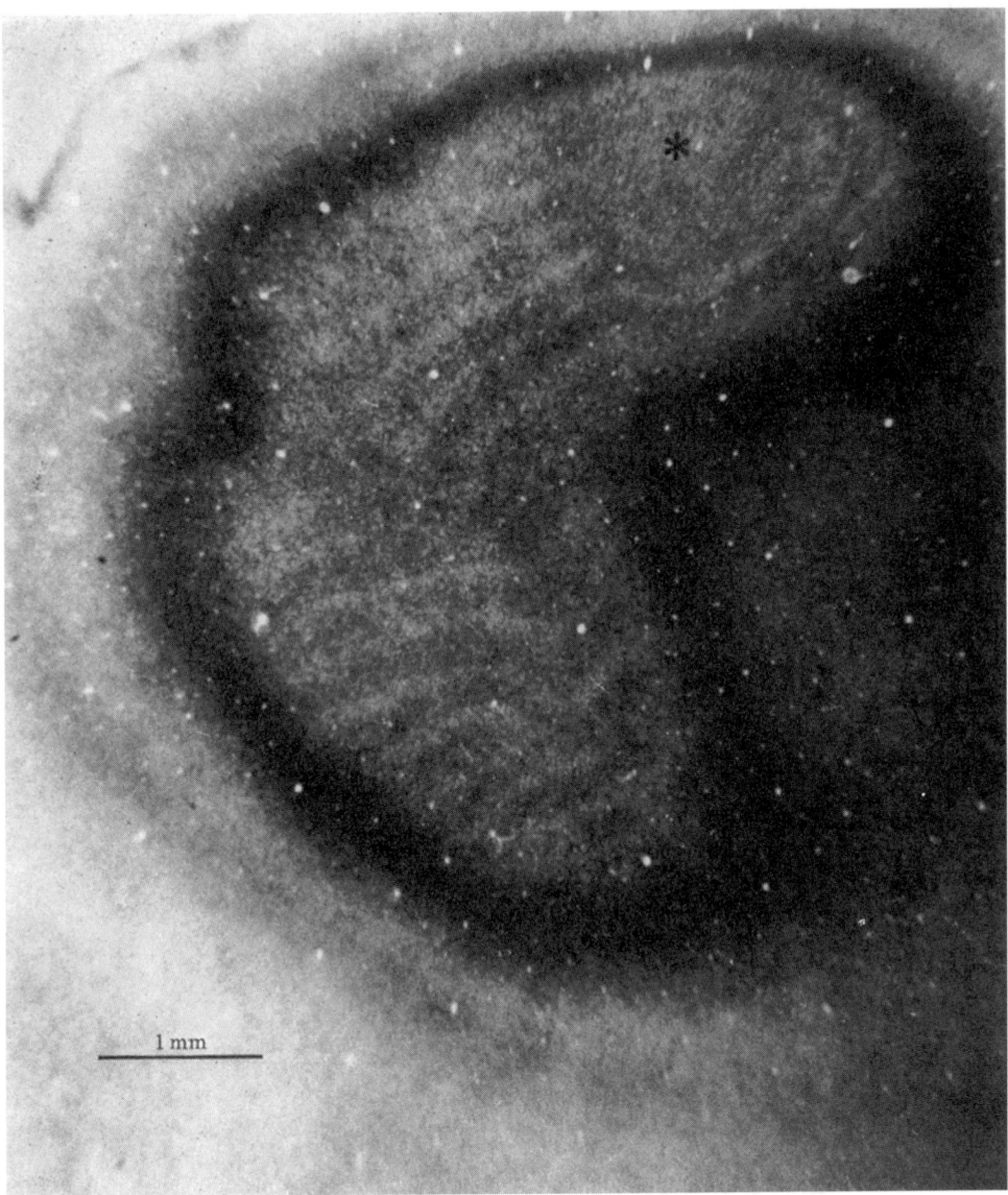

Plate 8

Fig. 20. *Pattern of ocular dominance columns seen in a tangential section through layer IVc of normal macaque striate cortex, stained by the reduced-silver method of Liesegang. The cortical surface is seen on the upper left of the figure. The very dark ring is layer IVb, the line of Gennari. Within this is layer IVc with the alternating dark and light bands, except for a small area marked by the asterisk, which grazes layer V. The dark bands represent the columns. These contain relatively fewer horizontally running fibres near their borders, resulting in the light bands. The actual column boundaries are thus the centre lines of these light bands (LeVay et al. 1975, Fig. 2).*

Plate 9

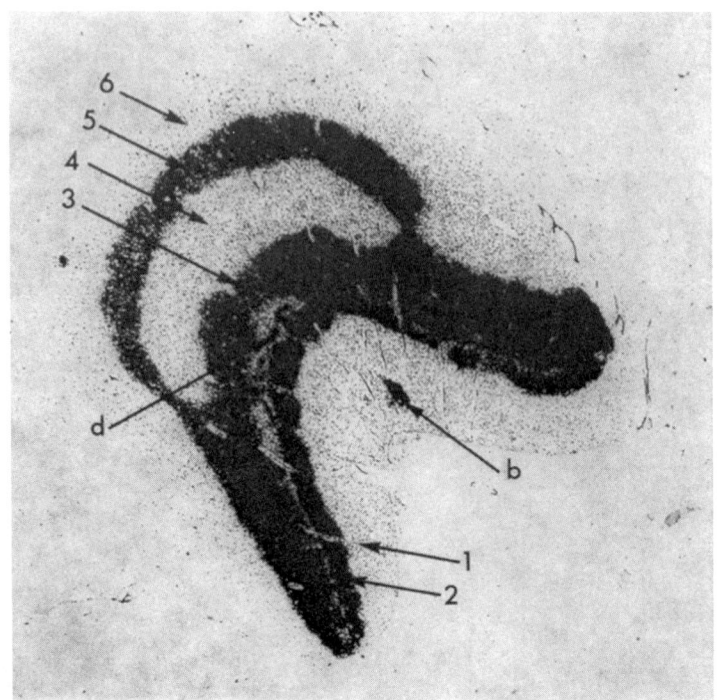

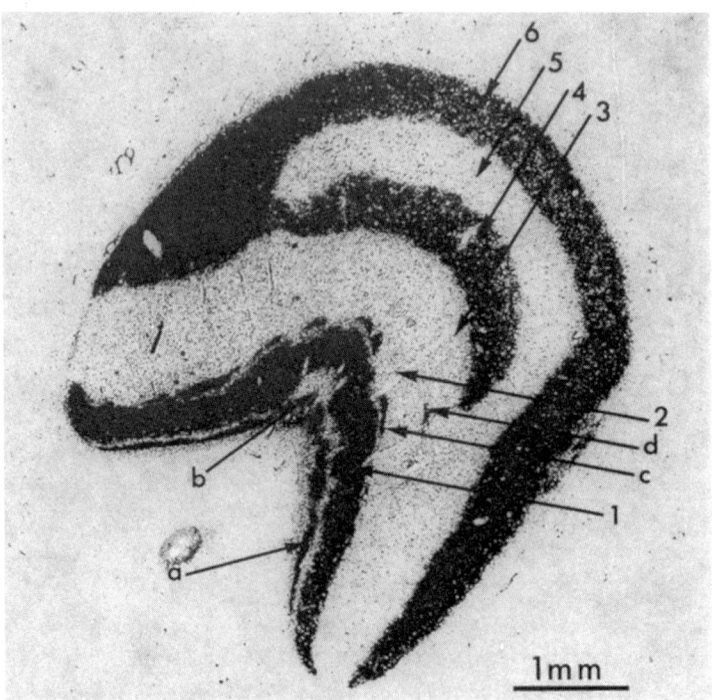

Fig. 21. Autoradiographs of left and right lateral geniculate bodies of a 1-week-old monkey whose left eye was injected at birth with tritiated fucose. Light field: labelled regions are black. 1–6 are the classical six layers, numbered from ventral dorsally. a–d represent four additional regions of input: a and c are supplied from the contralateral eye, b from ipsilateral, and d is apparently supplied by both eyes, possibly as alternating band-like monocular regions.

Plate 10

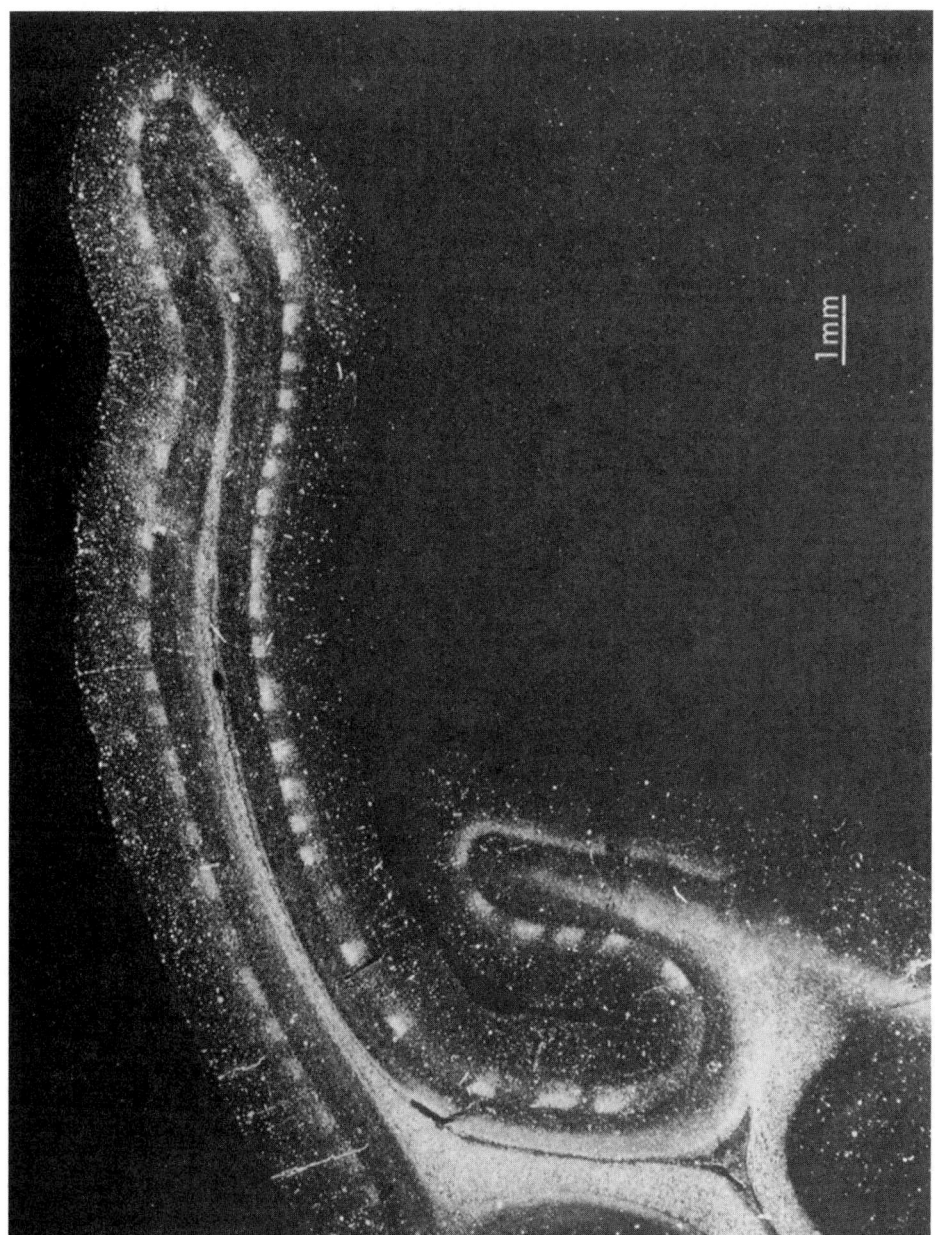

1mm

Fig. 22. Dark-field autoradiograph of striate cortex in an adult macaque in which the ipsilateral eye had been injected with tritiated proline-fucose 2 weeks before. Labelled areas show as white. Section passes for the most part in a plane perpendicular to the surface. Photo-graph shows part of the exposed surface of the striate cortex and the buried part immediately beneath; some of the buried part has fallen away during sectioning. In all, some 56 columns can be counted in layer IVc.

stack many serial sections such as that of Figure 22 one above the other just as was done in preparing Figures 18c and 19. A more direct alternative is to section the cortex tangentially—something that was impractical in the Nauta studies because one never knew exactly where in the cortex the small patch of degenerating terminals would be found. If the microtome knife cuts the dome-shaped exposed part of area 17 so as to graze layer IVc, this layer appears as an oval. A slightly deeper section cuts layer V in an oval, and layer IVc then appears as an annulus. Such a section, showing layer IVc as an annulus, is shown in Figure 23a, Plate 11, from the same monkey as that of Figure 20, but the opposite hemisphere. By taking deeper and deeper sections a series of larger and larger annuli results. These can then be cut and superimposed, giving the reconstruction shown in Figure 23b. Again the general arrangement of the layer IVc patches as parallel stripes is very clear, as are the occasional bifurcations and blind endings.

By using LeVay's reduced-silver technique (the autoradiographic technique could have been used equally well) it has been possible to reconstruct the columns over the entire exposed part of the occipital lobe (the operculum), and, with small gaps where curvature is extreme, their continuation in the calcarine fissure. The reconstruction of the operculum is shown in Figure 24a (LeVay et al. 1975). This diagram represents the same part of area 17 as is shown in the right side of Figure 6a, with the foveal representation to the extreme right and the left boundary representing roughly a semi-circle 9° distant from the fovea. To visualize more easily the actual size of the stripes in Figure 24, a fingerprint of one of us (D.H.) is reproduced in Figure 24b, to the same scale.

Several conclusions can be drawn from this reconstruction and from results using the other two anatomical methods. First, the stripes are roughly of equal width in all parts of 17, except for a few stripes at the extreme peripheral binocular region and, of course, the monocular region. Thus it seems that for both systems of columns the widths are constant throughout most of the cortex. For the monocular part of the cortex, i.e. the representation of the outlying temporal parts of the visual field, which can be seen by one eye but not the other (the temporal crescents), there is in the autoradiographs the expected continuous band of

label in the hemisphere opposite the injected eye, and nothing on the ipsilateral side. We have not sectioned this part of the cortex tangentially and stained with the reduced silver method because tangential sections here are difficult to obtain. We will refer again to the temporal crescent representation in discussing effects of deprivation.

Secondly, from hemisphere to hemisphere, even on the two sides in the same monkey, the patterns of stripes differ in their details. Identical patterns would indeed not be expected, any more than one would expect the stripes of all zebras to be identical. Nevertheless, as with zebras' stripes (Portmann 1948) certain general rules seem to be obeyed in all the monkeys we have so far looked at. For example, the stripes seem always to interest the 17-18 border at approximately 90°. At least in the mid-periphery and periphery of the visual fields the stripes when projected into the visual fields turn out to be approximately semi-circles (Figure 25); see also Hubel & Freeman (1977). This figure also shows strikingly the distortion in size that occurs as a consequence of the variation in magnification with eccentricity. The number of dominance columns in each hemisphere is about 150.

A final demonstration of ocular dominance columns comes from the 2-deoxyglucose method developed in recent years by Sokoloff's group (Sokoloff 1975, 1977) The method is based on the increase in uptake of glucose or deoxyglucose by active cells, and the inability of the metabolic end product of deoxyglucose to pass out of a cell. In animals injected intravenously with radioactive glucose, previously active cells thus show on autoradiography a surfeit of silver grains. Macaque monkeys in which one eye has been removed or closed show in area 17 a beautiful pattern of ocular dominance columns (Sokoloff 1975; Kennedy et al. 1975). In contrast to the eye injection technique, this method reveals the entire column from layer I down to layer VI, rather than just the part in layers IVa and c.

7. Representation of Visual Fields in Layer IVc

In one important respect Figure 25 may be misleading, since taken literally it could give the impression that only half of the visual field is represented in each eye. If black stripes represent right eye, for example, one could infer that the right eye

Plate 11

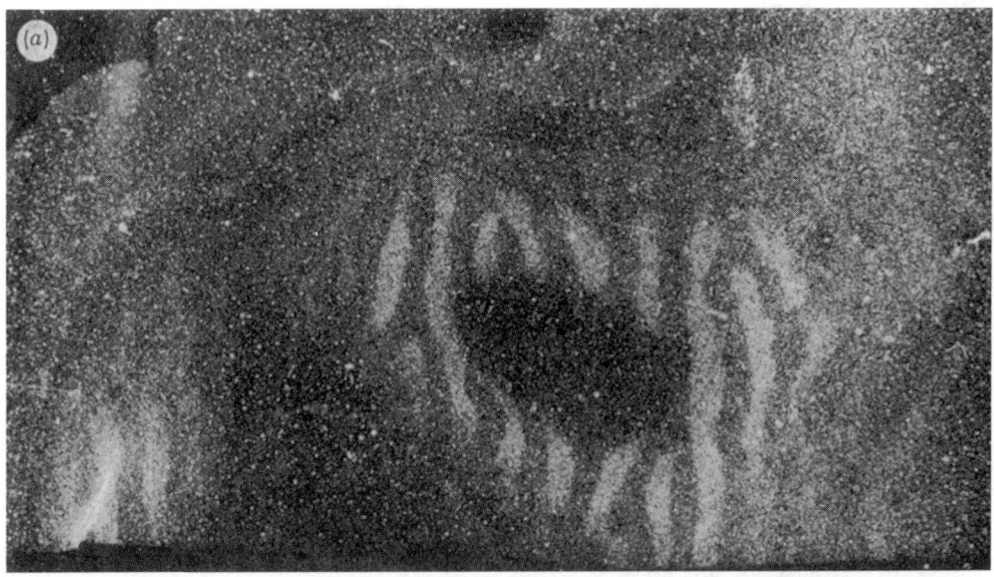

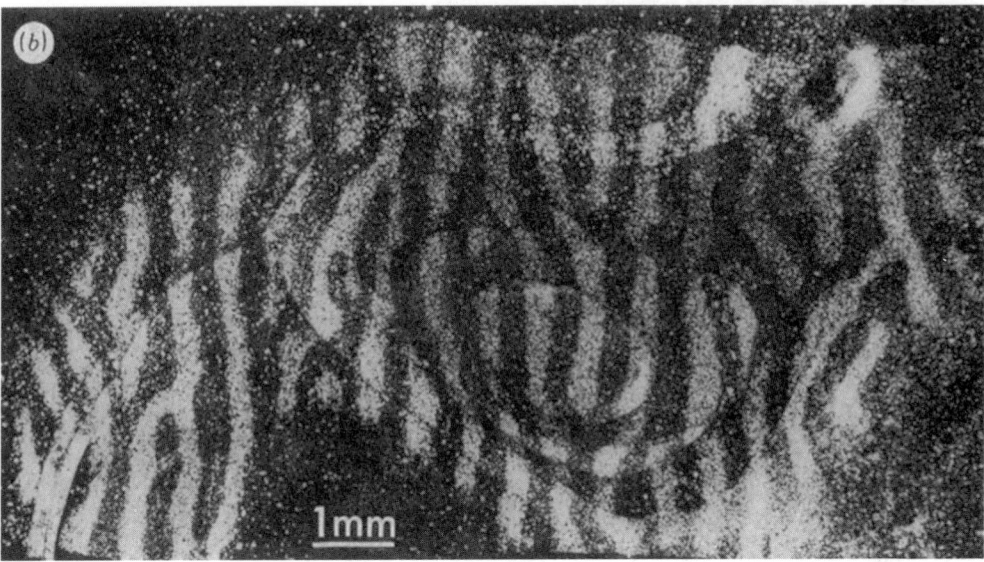

Fig. 23. Autoradiograph from the same (normal) animal as Figure 22, but hemisphere contralateral to the injected eye (dark field). (a) shows a section tangential to the exposed dome-like surface of the occipital lobe, just grazing layer V, which appears as an oval, surrounded by layer IVc, which appears as a ring containing the labelled parallel bands; these appear as light against the dark background. (b) a composite made by cutting out layer IVc from a number of parallel sections such as the one shown in (a), and pasting them together to show the bands over an area some millimetres in extent.

629

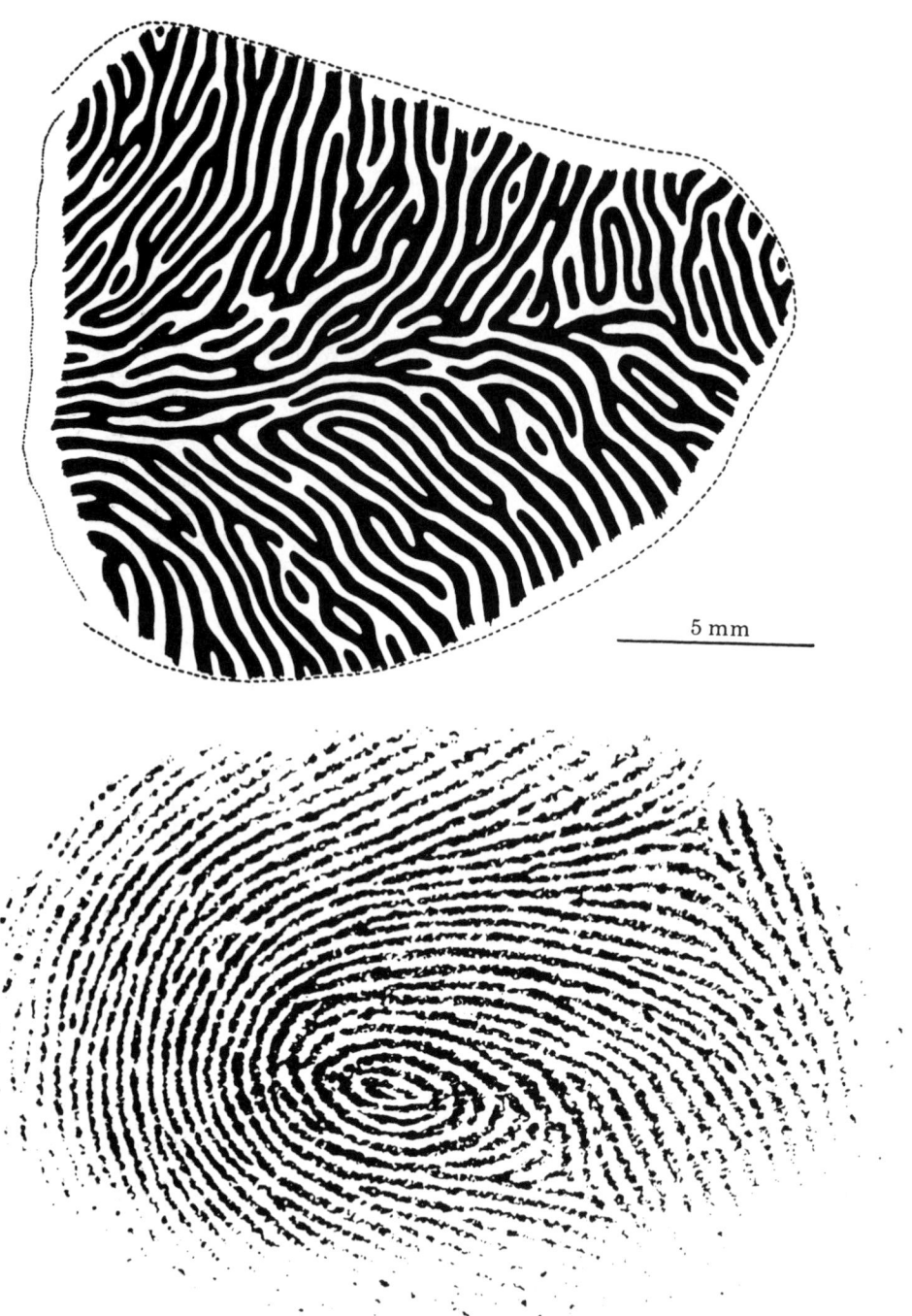

Fig. 24. (a) Reconstruction of layer IVc ocular dominance columns over the entire exposed part of area 17 in the right occipital lobe, made from a series of reduced-silver sections (LeVay et al. 1975). Dotted line on the left represents the midsagittal plane where the cortex bends around. Dashed c-shaped curve is the 17–18 border, whose apex, to the extreme right, represents the fovea. Every other column has been blackened in, so as to exhibit the twofold nature of the set of subdivisions. Note the relative constancy of column widths. (b) Fingerprint of human index finger, to scale, for comparison.

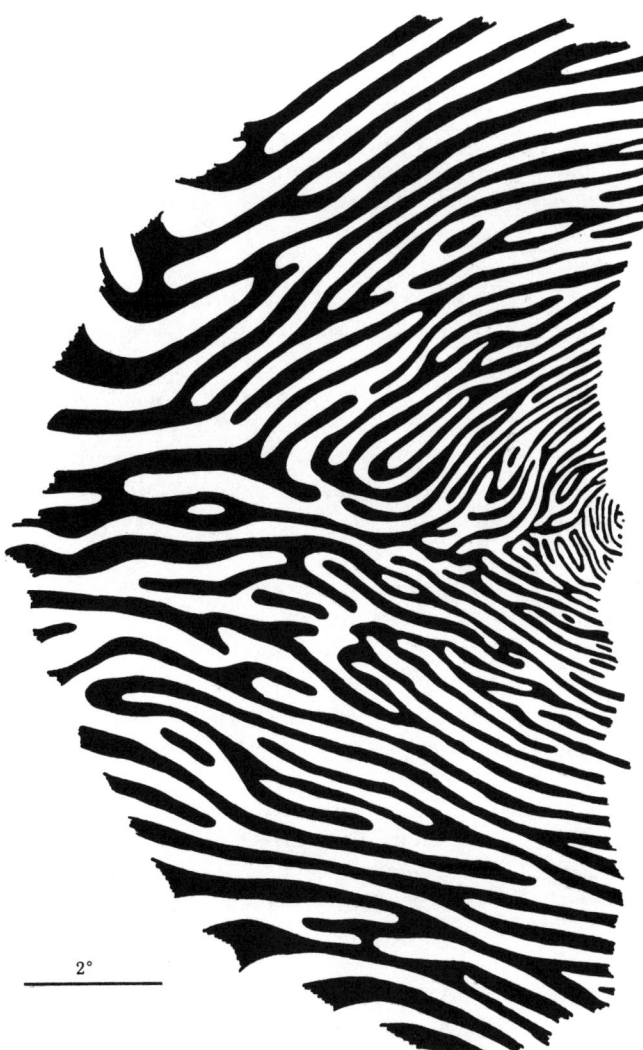

2°

Fig. 25. Translation of the reconstruction of Figure 24a into the visual field. Since this is the right hemisphere, the translation is into the left visual field. With the aid of a computer each point along the diagram in Figure 24a has been projected into the visual field. Note that projected stripes are narrowest around the point of fixation and become progressively broader with increasing eccentricity. The projection is shown out to 9°. (Hubel & Freeman 1977.)

sees the black regions but is blind to the white, which are seen only by the left eye. Intuitively, this would seem most unlikely. To resolve the problem the most direct procedure is to ask what happens to the positions of receptive fields as an electrode moves horizontally through the cortex from one eye dominance column to the next.

In the layers above and below IVc, in crossing through the 0.4 mm occupied by a single column, it is very difficult to make out any appreciable drift in receptive field position against the random scatter; one records a number of binocular cells all dominated by one eye, intermixed with some monocular cells especially near the column borders, all of these

cells varying slightly and rather unpredictably in receptive-field position. As described above, a displacement in the cortex several times this size is required to detect any clear overall movement in the visual field. In the upper and lower layers, at least, there is no doubt that any given part of the visual field is represented in both eyes.

In layer IV, however, the receptive field centres are very much smaller than the fields in the upper and lower layers. The positions of the individual fields can therefore be specified far more accurately. The scatter in field positions is also very much less—the cells seem to obey the rule that we have found to apply wherever we have recorded in the visual system, namely that receptive-field scatter is of the same order of magnitude as the size of the fields that are scattered, so that the aggregate field for any one layer is several times the size of an average field. It occurred to us that in crossing from one side of an ocular dominance slab to the other, within layer IVc, the precision of representation might be sufficient to permit the detection of a corresponding movement through the visual field. Experimentally this is, in fact, possible (Hubel, Wiesel & LeVay 1974) and there turns out to be a very special and highly ordered topography within layer IVc. As an electrode crosses from one side to the other of a single column there is a clear progression through the visual field in a direction predicted by the topographic map of the visual fields. All of this movement of course takes place in one eye only; as long as the electrode tip is within a layer IVc column no responses are detected from the other eye. When the border of the column is reached the eyes switch, and one now looks to see the positions of the receptive fields of the first cells recorded in the newly dominant eye. If the receptive fields were to continue their march through the visual field uninterrupted by the change of eyes, and if this were to occur at every column border crossing, then the visual field would obviously end up being shared by the two eyes in the manner suggested by Figure 25. This is not at all what happens. As the border is crossed there is an abrupt discontinuity in the visual-field representation. The position of the receptive fields suddenly jumps back in the visual field through a distance equal to about half of that crossed in the preceding column, when the other eye was used. As the electrode is advanced the fields resume their march forward, recovering the lost territory and then going on for an equal distance into new ground. This is illustrated in Figure 26. The visual field is traversed completely in each eye, but in an intermittent 'two steps forward and one step back' fashion, in which each eye must take its turn. The corollary of this is that within a single column the magnification—the number of degrees traversed for each millimetre of cortex—must be double the overall local cortical magnification: in crossing column after column each eye is heard from only half the time, and if the fields are to keep up with the movement of the receptive fields in the other layers the movement must occur at twice the overall rate. Across a

given column magnification (mm cortex/degree visual field) must be half that along the length.

The main point, however, is that the field of vision in layer IV is represented completely in each eye. The peculiar interlaced way in which this is accomplished is necessitated by the very special side-by-side manner in which the cortex is shared by the two eyes.

8. The Cortical Machinery

If we now step back and survey the different components of area-17 architecture just reviewed, we find that they fit together rather like the pieces of a Chinese puzzle. The orientation columns, if discrete, are some 50 μm in width, and each represents a shift in angle of about 10°. To cover the full 180° therefore requires a movement across the cortex of the order of 1 mm. Similarly each ocular dominance column is about 0.4 mm in width, and to take care of both eyes requires two such columns—again roughly 1 mm. In each case we designate one complete set of columns, subserving all orientations on the one hand or both eyes on the other, as a *hypercolumn* (Hubel & Wiesel 1974b). We now ask what happens to the position of receptive fields in the visual field as an electrode moving horizontally through the cortex traverses one hypercolumn, of either type. Obviously, it would make no sense at all if movement through one orientation hypercolumn were associated with a movement through the visual field that was large compared to aggregate field size, for that would mean that some regions of visual field must be specialized to handle certain orientations and others other orientations. There is certainly no hint, from psychophysics, of any such specialization in our own visual fields. Similarly crossing a single eye-dominance column outside of layer IVc produces a displacement of aggregate field considerably less than the local aggregate field size. In fact, as we have seen, it takes a 1–2 mm traverse through the cortex to produce a movement in the visual field that is comparable to the aggregate field size. What this means is that contained in a 2 mm × 2 mm block there is more than enough machinery to digest such a region of visual field (the aggregate size), examining it for light-dark contours in all orientations and with both eyes.

A block of cortex containing a hypercolumn of each type is illustrated schematically in Figure

cortex

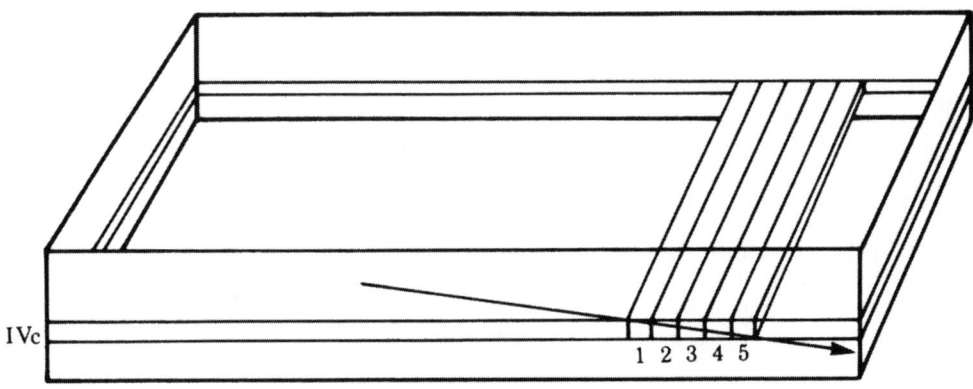

IVc

1 2 3 4 5

visual field

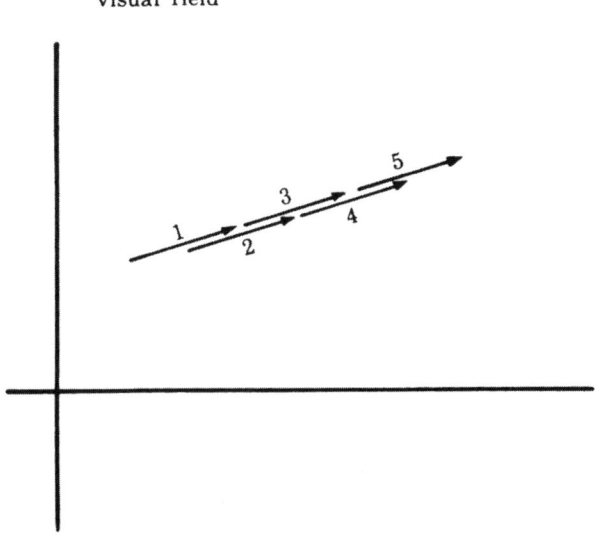

Fig. 26. Diagram to illustrate topographic representation in layer IVc. An electrode passes through cortex obliquely, almost parallel to the layers; it enters layer IVc, crosses five ocular dominance stripes, and then leaves that layer. During this traverse there is a progressive movement of receptive-field centres through the visual field: the fields in this layer are small enough, and the topography precise enough, to make this movement obvious. Suppose arrow 1, in the lower part of the figure, represents the movement as measured in the eye that feeds into column 1—say the left eye. On crossing over to column 2, the right eye becomes the one that evokes responses. The receptive-field position jumps back in the visual field by half the distance just traversed, moves forward so as to retrace the lost ground and then an equal distance further (arrow 2). The left eye then takes over again, with a jump back to its previous position and a similar progression (arrow 3)—and so on. The overall rate of movement is the same as that measured in the upper and lower layers (Figure 8b). Thus layer IVc has a complete representation of the visual fields.

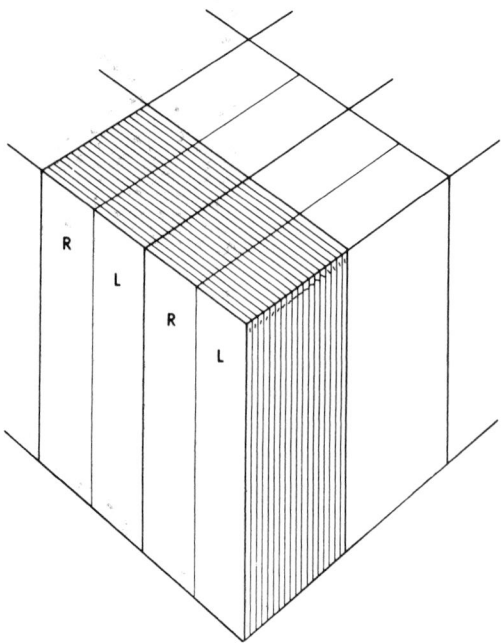

Fig. 27. Model of the striate cortex, to show roughly the dimensions of the ocular dominance slabs (L, R) in relation to the orientation slabs and the cortical thickness. Thinner lines separate individual columns; thicker lines demarcate hypercolumns, two pairs of ocular dominance columns and two sets of orientation columns. The placing of these hypercolumn boundaries is of course arbitrary; one could as well begin at horizontal or any of the obliques. The decision to show the two sets of columns as intersecting at right angles is also arbitrary, since there is at present no evidence as to the relationship between the two sets. Finally, for convenience the slabs are shown as plane surfaces, but whereas the dominance columns are indeed more or less flat, the orientation columns are not known to be so, and may when viewed from above have the form of swirls.

27. For purposes of illustration we have drawn the two sets of columns orthogonal to each other, but it should be stressed that there is at the moment no direct evidence to suggest how the two sets are related, if indeed there is any consistent relation. There would seem to be advantages, however, for them to intersect at some angle, and preferably at 90°. There is good reason to expect cells that are interconnected to have the same orientation preference, at least if the connections are excitatory, and our notion of the significance of the orientation column is that it houses together groups of cells with like orientation preference in the interests of efficiency of connections. At the same time we

imagine that a binocular cell in the cortex, complex or hypercomplex, receives its input directly or otherwise from two sets of simple monocular cells, one set for each eye (Figure 12). The connections subserving this binocular convergence must by definition extend beyond the borders of a single ocular dominance column. If the two column systems were parallel these connections would at the same time have to link up at least two orientation columns with the same orientation affiliation, separated by all the intervening orientation columns. This cumbersome wiring could largely be obviated if the two sets of columns were to intersect, since then the fibres could cross ocular dominance columns while remaining within the same orientation column.

The probable pattern of activity of cells in area 17 in response to a contour in the visual field is illustrated in Figure 28. We suppose that the contour is a short horizontal line segment, and is viewed by the left eye only: this is shown to the right in Figure 28. For the sake of specificity we place the line in the upper left visual quadrant. The general region of cortex affected is predictable from the topographic map of the visual field; let us suppose the line projects to the elongated region in the right striate cortex shown by the broken lines in the left part of the figure. Within this area the dispositons of the boundaries of the two types of columns will, given the limitations of our present knowledge, be unpredictable; let us assume that the boundaries are more or less orthogonal and have the shape shown—for the present discussion the precise shape and relationship to the cortical topography are immaterial. The regions of cortex maximally affected will be those areas within the broken-line boundary that represent horizontal lines and also represent the left eye. The pattern produced by the active cells should therefore be something like that shown in heavy lines. Of course, a truer representation would show fuzziness both at the edges, since orientation specificity is for most cells relaxed enough so that neighbouring columns will be weakly stimulated, and at the ends, since many cells in the right-eye columns will be influenced from the left eye, though again rather weakly. (In layer IVc, of course, the ocular dominance column boundaries are rigidly respected, but the orientation columns are irrelevant, so here all of the left-eye territory within the bro-

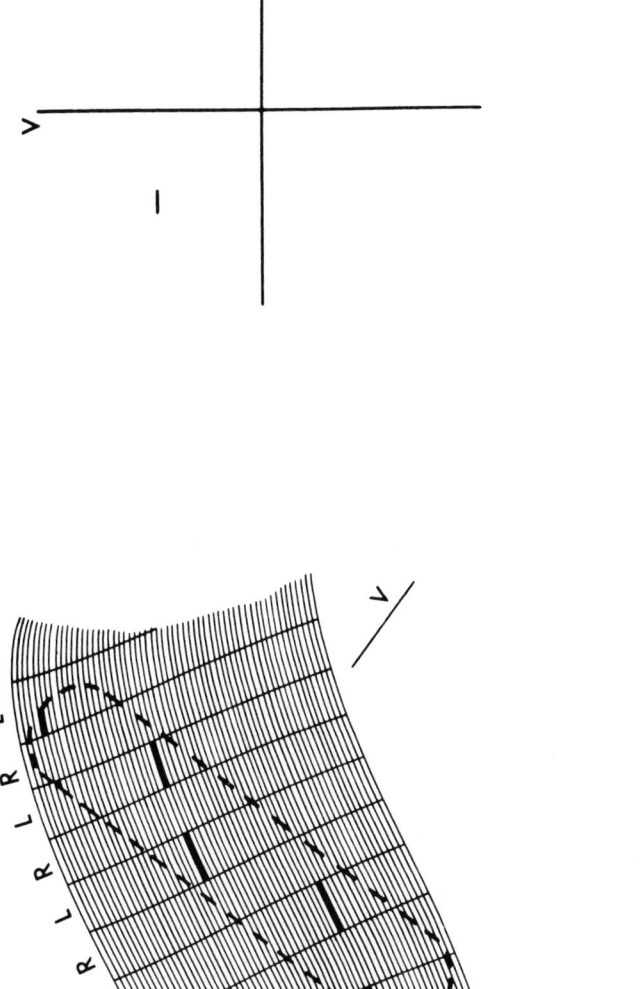

Fig. 28. Diagram illustrating the pattern of cortical activity that might follow from stimulation of the left eye with a short line in the visual field, say a horizontal line in the left visual field, as shown in the diagram on the right. To the left is drawn an area of cortex including the activated region as it might appear if one stood above and looked down at it. Let V and H represent the vertical and horizontal directions—their position will of course be determined by the topographic map of the visual fields on the cortex. Let the region outlined by dashes be the area receiving input from the illuminated part of the visual field (i.e. the sum of aggregate fields of all the points along the line stimulus). Suppose, finally, that the eye-dominance and orientation columns are as shown; for the argument, any other directions would do just as well; as in Figure 27, the decision to make the boundaries of the two sets of columns orthogonal is arbitrary. Then the regions of activation will be those marked by heavy lines—the areas corresponding to horizontal stimuli and left eye. See text for additional comments.

ken lines will be active, instead of only the territory belonging to one specific orientation, and no right-eye territory will be affected.) Such a diagram can, in principle, be prepared for any line or curve in the visual scene: one first draws the swath of activated territory on the cortex, as determined from the topographic map, and then fills in the squares according to the local orientation and the eye that is being used. The interesting conclusion is that a continuous line in the visual field produces a very discontinuous activity pattern in area 17.

Parenthetically we may emphasize here how absurd it is to think of a simple or complex cell as a 'straight-line detector'. What is detected is the orientation of a short line-segment. A straight line long enough to be seen as straight (or for that matter a curved line) would have to be 'detected' by some cell receiving input from populations of area-17 cells, presumably scattered in regions such as those shown in Figure 28. Whether such cells exist is not known.

It is perhaps worth stressing once more that the cortical machinery is highly uniform, as far as is known, at least throughout the binocular part of the cortex. Both sets of columns have roughly constant width. In the temporal crescent representation, where only the contralateral eye has input, there are obviously no ocular dominance columns. It is also likely that certain kinds of analysis, for example those involving colour, are selectively emphasized in the fovea, while others, like movement, are best developed in the periphery. Thus the uniformity may not be absolute. Aside from these probable differences, what seem to be the main preoccupations of area 17, orientation selectivity and binocular convergence, probably depend on the same apparatus throughout. This is supported, as mentioned earlier, by the similarity of the histology everywhere, and the tailoring of aggregate field size to magnification.

The cortex, then, seems to solve the problem of analysing the visual field in great detail centrally and in much less detail peripherally, in a very special way. The same basic units of cortical function (Figure 27) seem to be used throughout, but more of them are used per degree of visual field the greater the detail of analysis. The alternative to this would be to vary the machinery, for example by having a thicker cortex in the region subserving the fovea, with more cells and more connections in a

unit area. Intuitively one suspects that that would be a far more difficult and cumbersome solution. The disparity in magnification between fovea and periphery is very large, so that if magnification were uniform the corresponding regions of cortex would presumably have to be very different in thickness.

The development of the cortex, finally, must pose a much easier problem if the structure is uniform, since the instructions need only be specified once, for a block roughly 2 mm × 2 mm; and then repeated again and again—perhaps about 300–400 times, since the surface area of the macaque striate cortex is probably in the neighbourhood of 1300–1400 mm^2 (Clark 1941; Daniel & Whitteridge 1961).

STUDIES IN NEWBORN MONKEYS

In addressing the problem of the development of area 17, it seemed to us that the first question to ask was whether the system as we know it in the adult, with its hierarchy of cells, its topographic map and its intricate architecture, is all present at birth and thus presumably determined genetically, or whether some or all of the specificity depends on the details of postnatal experience. Our previous work in cats (Hubel & Wiesel 1963) had led us to conclude that in that species genetics was the main, if not the sole determinant in the formation of area 17, but the problem was complicated by the immaturity of the cat's visual system at birth and a difficulty in knowing whether binocular deprivation effects were a result of holding back postnatal maturation or of withholding specific experience. By now almost everyone seems to agree that one can find cells with strict orientation specificity in visually naïve cats (Blakemore & Van Sluyters 1975), but it is still difficult to interpret the large number of non-oriented cells in these animals. Any slight deterioration in an animal's condition during recording can lead to a disappearance of orientation specificity, and very young animals are especially hard to keep in good condition during acute experiments.

The newborn macaque monkey is visually much more advanced than the cat. The eyes are open, and by the day after birth the baby monkey fixes visually and follows objects with its eyes. One would expect, then, that for interpretations of dep-

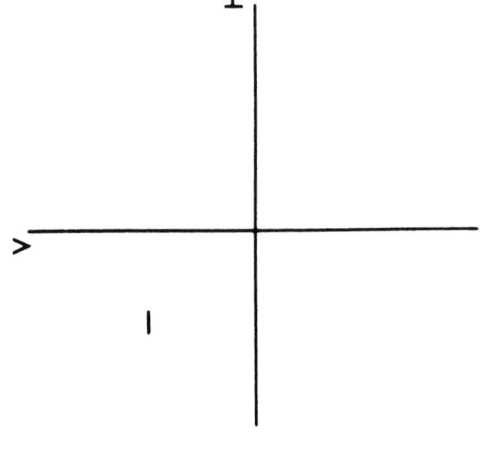

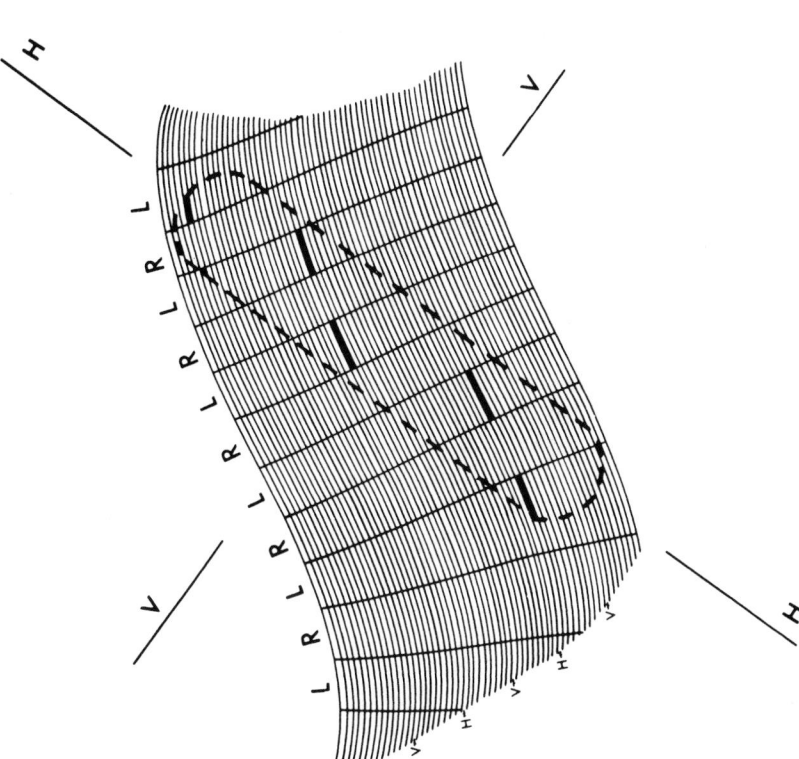

Fig. 28. Diagram illustrating the pattern of cortical activity that might follow from stimulation of the left eye with a short line in the visual field, say a horizontal line in the left visual field, as shown in the diagram on the right. To the left is drawn an area of cortex including the activated region as it might appear if one stood above and looked down at it. Let V and H represent the vertical and horizontal directions—their position will of course be determined by the topographic map of the visual fields on the cortex. Let the region outlined by dashes be the area receiving input from the illuminated part of the visual field (i.e. the sum of aggregate fields of all the points along the line stimulus). Suppose, finally, that the eye-dominance and orientation columns are as shown; for the argument, any other directions would do just as well; as in Figure 27, the decision to make the boundaries of the two sets of columns orthogonal is arbitrary. Then the regions of activation will be those marked by heavy lines—the areas corresponding to horizontal stimuli and left eye. See text for additional comments.

ken lines will be active, instead of only the territory belonging to one specific orientation, and no right-eye territory will be affected.) Such a diagram can, in principle, be prepared for any line or curve in the visual scene: one first draws the swath of activated territory on the cortex, as determined from the topographic map, and then fills in the squares according to the local orientation and the eye that is being used. The interesting conclusion is that a continuous line in the visual field produces a very discontinuous activity pattern in area 17.

Parenthetically we may emphasize here how absurd it is to think of a simple or complex cell as a 'straight-line detector'. What is detected is the orientation of a short line-segment. A straight line long enough to be seen as straight (or for that matter a curved line) would have to be 'detected' by some cell receiving input from populations of area-17 cells, presumably scattered in regions such as those shown in Figure 28. Whether such cells exist is not known.

It is perhaps worth stressing once more that the cortical machinery is highly uniform, as far as is known, at least throughout the binocular part of the cortex. Both sets of columns have roughly constant width. In the temporal crescent representation, where only the contralateral eye has input, there are obviously no ocular dominance columns. It is also likely that certain kinds of analysis, for example those involving colour, are selectively emphasized in the fovea, while others, like movement, are best developed in the periphery. Thus the uniformity may not be absolute. Aside from these probable differences, what seem to be the main preoccupations of area 17, orientation selectivity and binocular convergence, probably depend on the same apparatus throughout. This is supported, as mentioned earlier, by the similarity of the histology everywhere, and the tailoring of aggregate field size to magnification.

The cortex, then, seems to solve the problem of analysing the visual field in great detail centrally and in much less detail peripherally, in a very special way. The same basic units of cortical function (Figure 27) seem to be used throughout, but more of them are used per degree of visual field the greater the detail of analysis. The alternative to this would be to vary the machinery, for example by having a thicker cortex in the region subserving the fovea, with more cells and more connections in a

unit area. Intuitively one suspects that that would be a far more difficult and cumbersome solution. The disparity in magnification between fovea and periphery is very large, so that if magnification were uniform the corresponding regions of cortex would presumably have to be very different in thickness.

The development of the cortex, finally, must pose a much easier problem if the structure is uniform, since the instructions need only be specified once, for a block roughly 2 mm × 2 mm; and then repeated again and again—perhaps about 300–400 times, since the surface area of the macaque striate cortex is probably in the neighbourhood of 1300–1400 mm^2 (Clark 1941; Daniel & Whitteridge 1961).

STUDIES IN NEWBORN MONKEYS

In addressing the problem of the development of area 17, it seemed to us that the first question to ask was whether the system as we know it in the adult, with its hierarchy of cells, its topographic map and its intricate architecture, is all present at birth and thus presumably determined genetically, or whether some or all of the specificity depends on the details of postnatal experience. Our previous work in cats (Hubel & Wiesel 1963) had led us to conclude that in that species genetics was the main, if not the sole determinant in the formation of area 17, but the problem was complicated by the immaturity of the cat's visual system at birth and a difficulty in knowing whether binocular deprivation effects were a result of holding back postnatal maturation or of withholding specific experience. By now almost everyone seems to agree that one can find cells with strict orientation specificity in visually naïve cats (Blakemore & Van Sluyters 1975), but it is still difficult to interpret the large number of non-oriented cells in these animals. Any slight deterioration in an animal's condition during recording can lead to a disappearance of orientation specificity, and very young animals are especially hard to keep in good condition during acute experiments.

The newborn macaque monkey is visually much more advanced than the cat. The eyes are open, and by the day after birth the baby monkey fixes visually and follows objects with its eyes. One would expect, then, that for interpretations of deprivation effects the problems of postnatal maturation might be less troublesome in the monkey than in the cat.

Recordings from newborn monkey cortex are in fact very similar to those obtained in the adult (Wiesel & Hubel 1974). Cells in layers outside IVc occur in simple, complex and hypercomplex types, with orientation and directional specificity that appear to be about as well developed as in the adult. To be certain that there are *no* differences between newborn and adult would require a statistical survey, with automated stimuli and averaged responses. This has not yet been done. Histologically the cortex of the newborn macaque is indeed not fully mature (though it is far advanced by comparison with the cortex of the newborn cat), so that some differences between it and adult cortex might well be expected. Receptive field size, for example, may be larger. But what strikes one most forcibly in these records is the similarity to the adult, not the differences. One exception to this, in the case of ocular dominance columns, is taken up below.

To record in area 17 from a monkey on the day of its birth is technically difficult and risky. In most cases we have therefore sutured the eyes closed at birth, to avoid visual experience, and recorded after about 2–4 weeks. The eye closures allow some diffuse light to reach the retinas but almost certainly exclude any light-dark contours. Records from area 17 in these animals were virtually indistinguishable from those of adults. One problem posed by this procedure was the delay between the birth of the monkey and our notification of the birth, during which time the animal usually received a few hours of visual exposure. It seemed hardly likely that a few hours' experience in dim light would by itself produce an adult-like cortex, but it seemed important to avoid all possibilities of this. We accordingly did a Caesarean section in a mother monkey near term, immediately sutured the eyes of the baby, and waited 2 weeks before recording. This animal's primary visual cortex showed just as high a degree of specificity as was seen in the cortex of other less stringently controlled monkeys. A graph of optima orientation against track distance in this monkey is shown in Figure 29. The graph points up another aspect of the recordings: in addition to the regular small orientation shifts indicated by the graph, there were periodic alternations in ocular dominance. This indicates that both the orientation and ocular dominance columns are present, though, as we will see, the development of the dominance columns is not quite complete at birth. That area 17 is in so many respects wired up and ready to go when the animal is born is perhaps not so surprising if one remembers that the machinery of area 17 represents building blocks of vision, used in a piecemeal analysis of the visual fields and required whatever the detailed environment of the animal is to be. One would not expect experience to be important in the development of area 17 any more than it is in the development of retinal connections: the striate cortex extends the kinds of analysis already begun in the retina, and what takes place there is not much more sophisticated, relative to the tasks that still remain to be solved in perception. Nevertheless, our original finding that specificity of various types, particularly orientation specificity, was already present in the newborn was greeted with surprise and some considerable scepticism. The reason for this is a partly justified conviction that the cerebral cortex of all parts of the brain is the structure most important for perception, memory, and in fact for mentation in general. A structure that is involved in learning must change in some way with experience. Hence to find some part of the cortex for all intents and purposes formed at birth seems to fly in the face of all one's preconceptions about that structure. Too little is known about other cortical areas to permit guesses as to the importance of experience in forming and organizing them, but, to take an extreme case, one would certainly expect regions such as the speech areas of man to be modified by the details of postnatal experience. The striate cortex seems to represent an extreme in the other direction, and the lesson, if any, is that very different rules may apply in the development of different regions of the cerebral cortex.

DEPRIVATION STUDIES

A detailed account of the studies we and others have made on the effects of early deprivation on the visual system is beyond the scope of this article. Some recent results, nevertheless, bear strongly on the problem of the origin of the ocular dominance columns, and illustrate the possibility of deforming the columns. To describe these results it will be

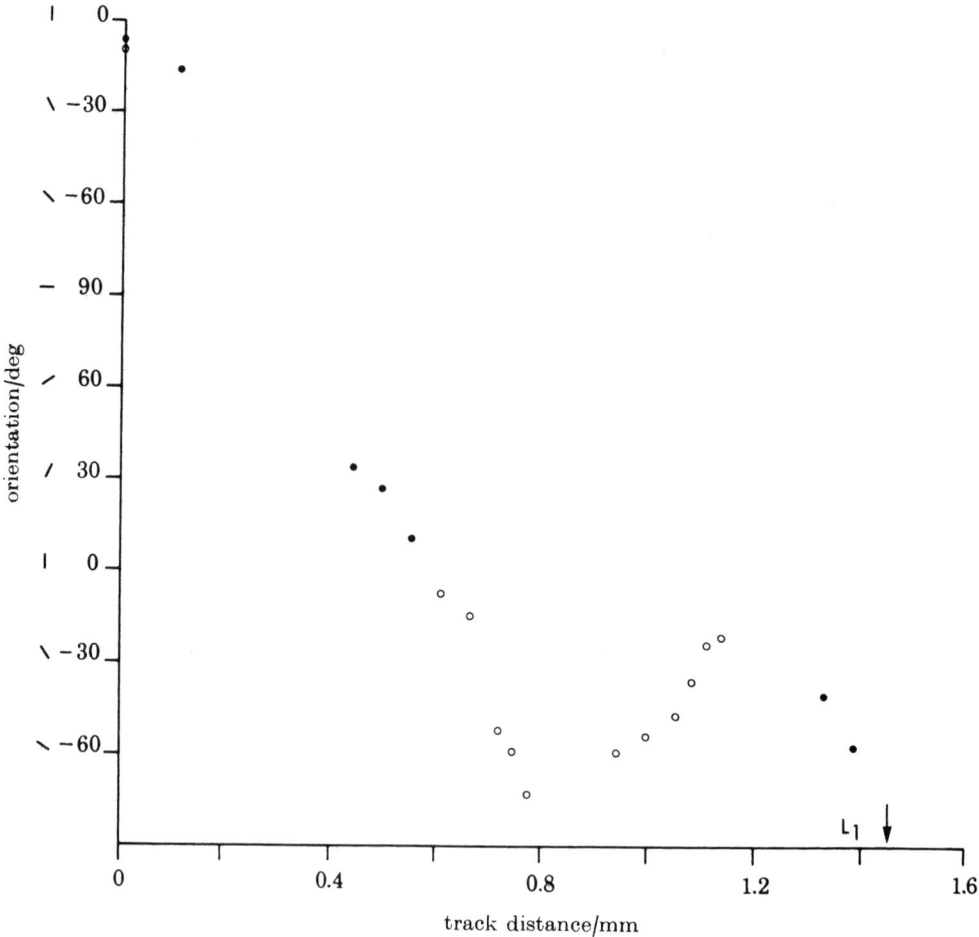

Fig. 29. Graph of orientation plotted against electrode position similar to those of Figures 15b and 16, but for a 30-day-old monkey that was delivered at term by Caesarean section and both eyes immediately sewn shut. The animal thus had no patterned visual experience. Orientation specificity in this animal showed no obvious lack of precision, compared with what is seen in the adult.

necessary to review at least some of the deprivation work. Some years ago we observed that if one eye of a kitten was sewn closed for the first few months of life a marked change occurred in the cortical physiology (Wiesel & Hubel 1963). Instead of most cells' responding to both eyes, the great majority of cells lost all ability to respond to the eye that had been closed, while remaining normally responsive to the eye that had been open. Recordings from retina and geniculate were relatively normal, so that the major defect was clearly in the cortex. We

found that to obtain the changes the eye had to be closed some time during the first few months, and the most marked changes were produced by closures between about the fourth and eighth week of life. Closures in adults produced no obvious defects. Our first guess was that the defects resulted simply from disuse of the closed eye. This guess was incorrect, as we found on examining cats in which both eyes had been sewn shut from birth, for here there were far less severe defects than would have been predicted on any naïve expectation that the separate lid-closure effects add in a simple way (Wiesel & Hubel 1965). Evidently monocular closures produced such striking results because of some kind of binocular competition; if the right eye was closed the pathway belonging to the left eye could presumably take over the right eye's territory at some point along the pathway. The idea of a competitive interaction between the two paths was subsequently reinforced by anatomical findings at the geniculate level by others (Guillery & Stelzner 1970; Guillery 1972; Sherman 1973; Sherman, Guillery, Kaas & Sanderson 1974).

Similar experiments in monkeys have given almost the same results. The critical period for monocular-closure effects is probably the first 6 weeks or so, though eye closure produces defects for a period of up to a year or more if the closure is sufficiently prolonged.

The macaque monkey provides an opportunity to test the idea of binocular competition, since in area 17, as described in the first part of this paper, convergence of inputs from the two eyes does not occur until after the first two stages of integration. There is thus little or no convergence in layer IV, and one might not expect to see a profound disturbance of responses in this layer following monocular deprivation. For the layers above and below IVc our early studies in monkeys had shown a takeover by the normal eye that was just as impressive as that which occurs in the cat, but until a few years ago we had not looked specifically at layer IV itself. Obviously the time was ripe to study layer IV in deprived monkeys, using the same tools we had employed in the normal physiological recordings, i.e. tangential penetrations, the Nauta method, the reduced silver method and transneuronal autoradiography (Hubel, Wiesel & LeVay 1977).

We began with the rather radical procedure of removing one eye in each of two 2-week-old monkeys and waiting 1½ years before experimenting. We felt that if this did not produce a change in layer IV nothing would! We were not disappointed, for when we made long tangential penetrations through the cortex we found that there was in layer IVc almost continuous activity evoked from the normal eye as the electrode moved forward, instead of responses for about 0.4 mm alternating with silence for 0.4 mm, as would be expected if no change had occurred. This sug-

gested that there had been a rearrangement in layer IVc, with the retinogeniculate fibres belonging to the normal eye occupying space normally allotted to the deprived eye.

This was confirmed anatomically. In one of the animals, for example, we made several geniculate lesions 5 days before the recording; some were made in layers fed by the normal eye, some in the deafferented layers, which were electrically silent. On examining the cortex with Nauta stain we were able to find the projections from two of the normal-layer lesions and from one of the deprived-layer lesions. The reconstruction of two of these projections is shown in Figures 30 and 31; they are analogous to the reconstructions from a normal monkey shown in Figure 18. What the diagrams show is that the terminals from the geniculate layers fed by the normal eye have occupied virtually the entire extent of layer IVc, instead of exactly half of it, while the bands representing the removed eye are less than one-third normal size. This anatomical result was obtained in both monkeys, and confirms the physiological findings.

We have done similar experiments over the past few years in monkeys with monocular eye suture from an early age. The results have been generally similar to those obtained after eye removal. For example, one monkey had its right eye sutured closed at 2 weeks of age and was allowed to live for 18 months. Two weeks before the records were made, the left (normal) eye was injected with radioactive amino acids, and a week before recording, geniculate lesions were made for Nauta studies. The results of making several tangential penetrations were similar to what we had found after eye removal, but not so extreme; rather to our surprise there were regions in layer IVc in which brisk responses were obtained only from the right (closed) eye. The spans over which these responses were recorded were clearly short compared with the normal 0.4 mm. In striking contrast, the regions dominated by the normal eye were much wider than normal. At each point where a shift of eyes occurred a small electrolytic lesion was made in order to correlate the points of transition, in the recordings, with the autoradiographic results.

Transneuronal autoradiography fully confirmed this impression of an extreme departure

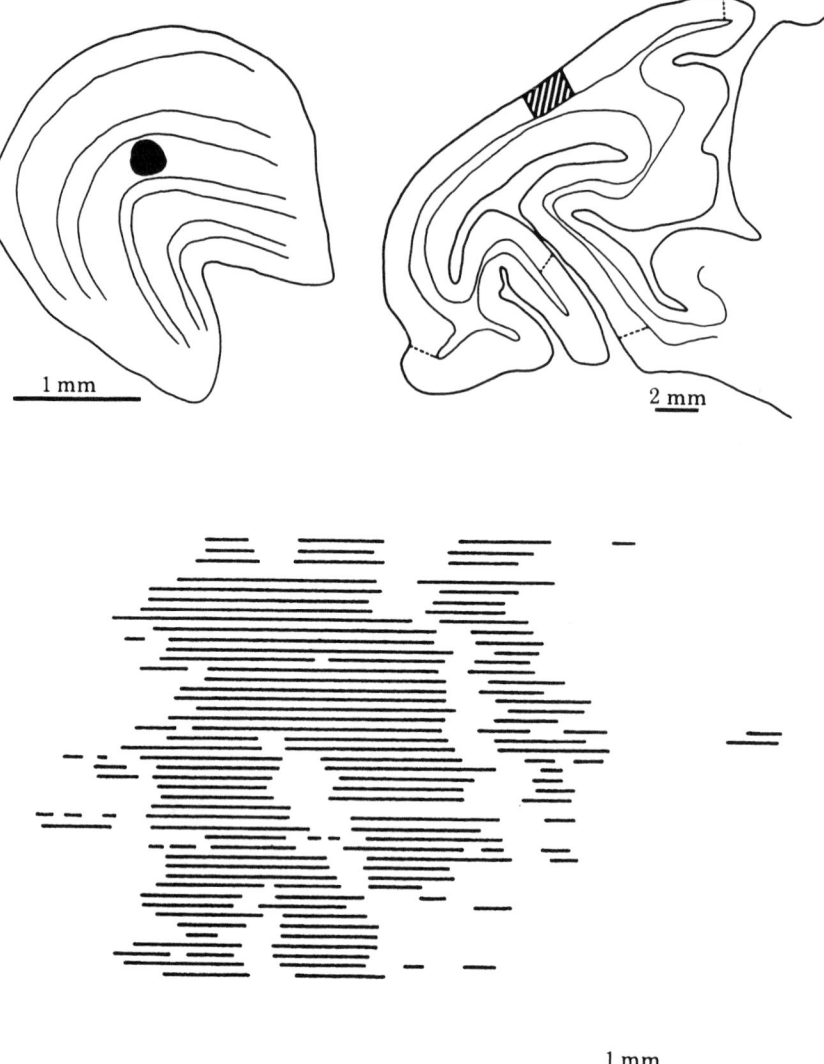

Fig. 30. *Distribution of degenerating terminals in layer IVc of a macaque monkey whose right eye was removed at 2 weeks of age and the experiment carried out at an age of 18 months. At that age lesions were made in two layers of the left lateral geniculate body, and the brain sectioned 5 days later and stained by the Fink–Heimer method (compare Figure 18). Here the lesion was made in layer 3, whose input was from the surviving eye. Bands of terminal degeneration are wider than normal, whereas gaps between the bands, corresponding to the eye that was removed, are markedly shrunken.*

from the normal balance in the distribution of geniculate terminals. Figure 32a, Plate 12, shows a photograph of a section made tangential to layer IVc, analogous to the normal section of Figure 23a. The picture is again taken under dark-field illumination, so that the bright regions produced by silver grains represent terminals of afferent genicu-late fibres belonging to the injected, normal eye. A montage from a number of sections parallel to this one is shown in Figure 32b. The deprived columns not only show marked shrinkage, but seem in places to be pinched off entirely. Actual measurements of area in this montage indicate a shrinkage of about 50%. To the right in (b) the lesions made

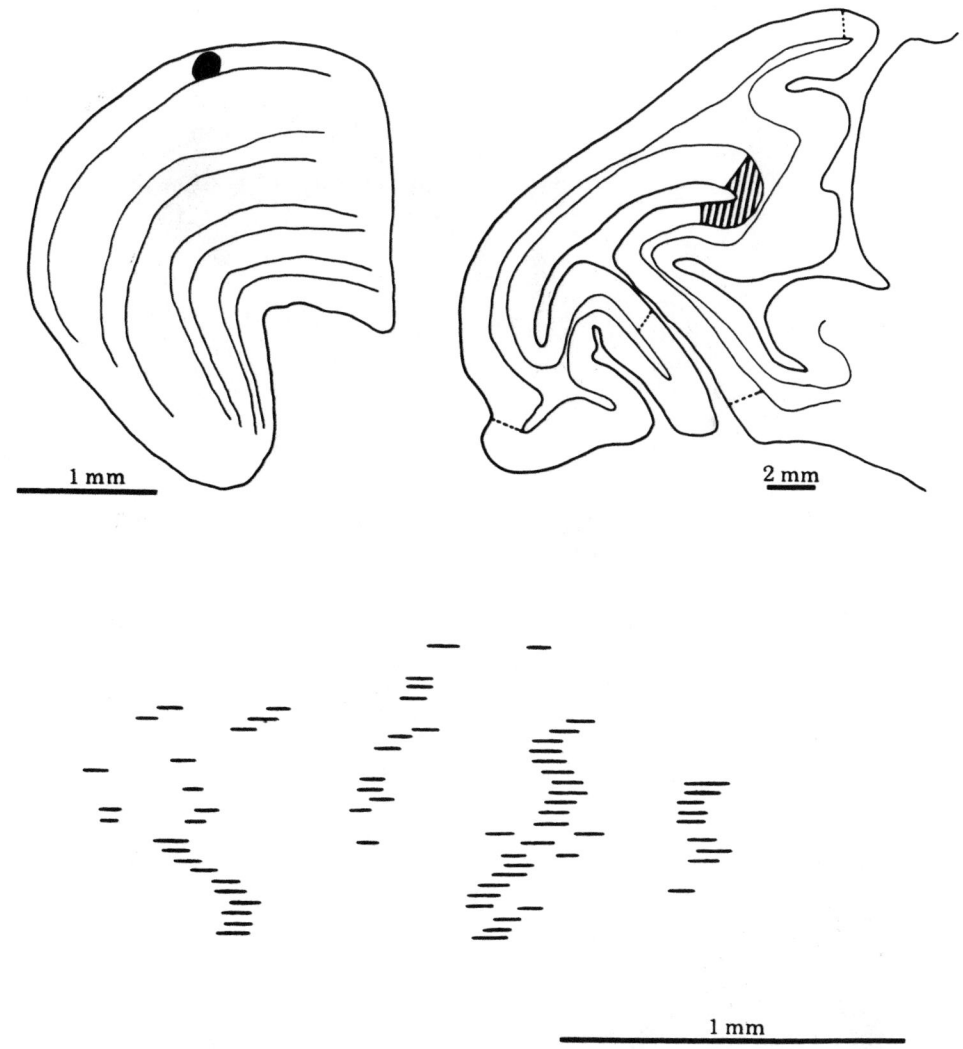

Fig. 31. *Same monkey as in Figure 30. Lesion in layer 6, the most dorsal layer, deafferented. Bands of degeneration in IVc are markedly shrunken, and the gaps between widened. This is thus the complement of Figure 30. (Figures 30 and 31 are from Hubel et al. (1977).)*

during the recording are indicated, traced from neighbouring fibre-stained sections. Each lesion is just where the recordings had predicted it should be, on the border separating two bands. The agreement between the physiologic and anatomic results tends to strengthen one's confidence in both approaches.

Finally, another monkey had its right eye sutured at 2 days of age, for a period of only 7 weeks; the eye was then reopened and the animal kept to an age of 7 months, at which time the right (deprived) eye was injected with a tritiated proline-and-fucose mixture and the brain examined two weeks later. A transverse section through the left striate cortex is shown in Figure 33, Plate 13. Here the labelled portions of layer IVc, corresponding to the deprived eye, are markedly shrunken. This experiment thus forms the complement of the previous one. In addition, in agreement with other anatomical and physiological studies, it shows that even a very brief clo-

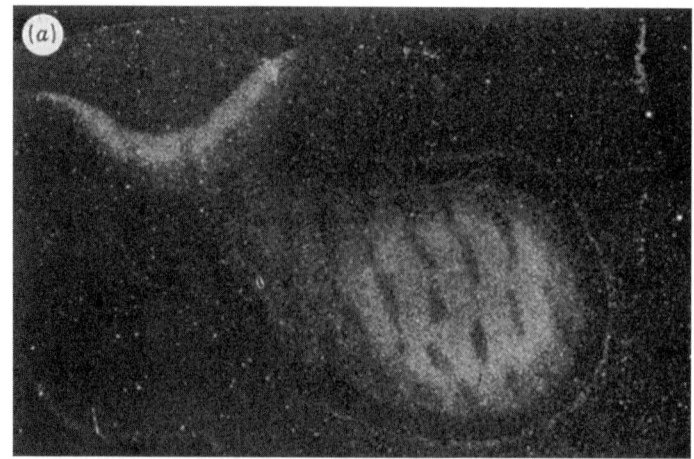

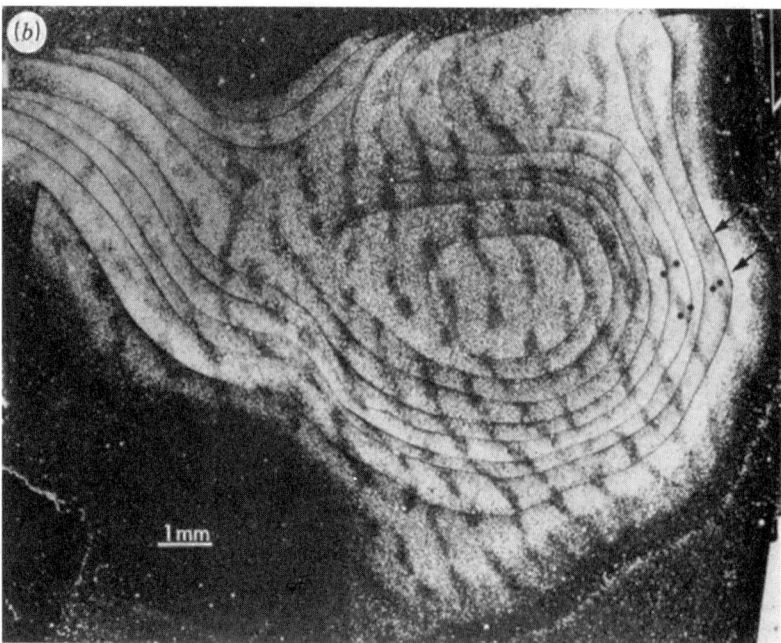

Fig. 32. Transneuronal autoradiography of left occipital lobe of macaque monkey whose right eye was sutured closed at 2 weeks, and studied at 18 months. Left (normal) eye injected with tritiated proline-fucose mixture 2 weeks before brain was sectioned. (a) Section tangential to layer IVc, dark field, as in Figure 23. Note expansion of labelled columns and shrinkage of the gaps. The serial reconstruction, (b), was made from a number of sections parallel to a and including a. The positions of six lesions, determined from neighbouring sections, are shown near the right border. These lesions were made during the electrical recordings, in two penetrations (arrows), at points of eye transition. Note how each lesion falls on a column border. (From Hubel et al. 1977.)

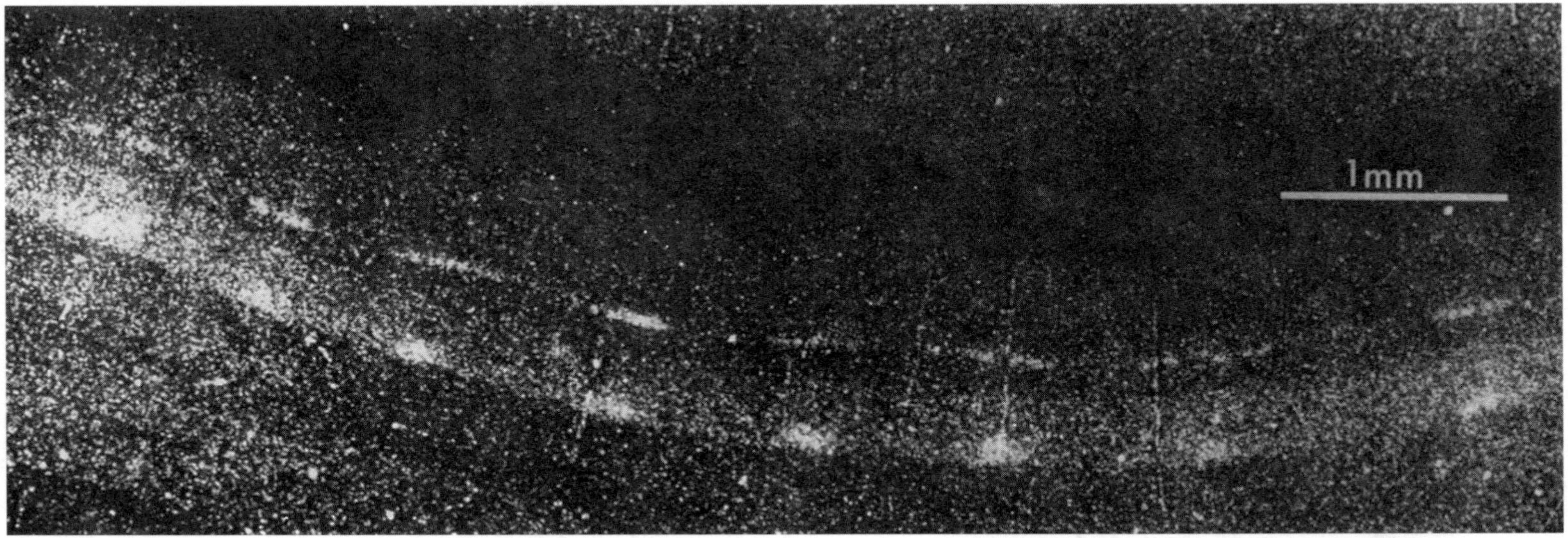

Plate 13

Fig. 33. Autoradiograph of transverse sections through striate cortex of a 7-month-old macaque monkey whose right eye was closed at 2 days of age, for a period of 7 weeks; the eye was then reopened and kept open till an age of 7 months, when the right (deprived) eye was injected with radioactive proline–fucose mixture and the brain examined 2 weeks later. The labelled columns in layer IVc are shrunken, and the gaps between enlarged. (Label is seen at two distinct horizontal levels, thin in layer IVa above and thicker in IVc below.) This figure forms the complement of Figure 32, in which the normal eye was injected. (From Hubel et al. 1977.)

sure is enough to disturb the columns, and further that the recovery resulting from simply reopening the eye is very disappointing.

DOMINANCE COLUMNS IN NEWBORN MONKEYS

On first seeing the results described in the preceding section our natural tendency was to assume that monocular closures had led to an invasion of the deprived columns by geniculate terminals belonging to the eye that had been open. A process of proliferation of terminals and spread beyond their normal territory when a competing set of terminals is put at a disadvantage has been observed in many situations, and is usually termed 'sprouting', though that term has normally been used in cases where the competition has been destroyed by a lesion, surgical or electrolytic. The notion that sprouting can occur by an insult as mild as merely covering one eye would in itself be of considerable interest. If this were indeed a matter of sprouting one would have to modify the idea of competition, for here one can obviously only talk about competition between columns, i.e. sets of terminals in layer IVc, and not about competition between two inputs for territory on a single cell. How one set of terminals would know that it should extend its domain, whether by a chemical signal or some other action at a distance, is a matter for speculation.

A recent set of findings (Hubel *et al.* 1977) has made us reconsider the whole question of sprouting. In accounting for the IVth layer changes following deprivation we had assumed that the ocular dominance columns were present at birth, or at least at 2 weeks, when the closures were made. There was some reason for this assumption, since recordings from layers outside IVc in newborn animals had shown regular fluctuations in ocular dominance. What we needed, however, was autoradiographic proof that in the newborn monkey the geniculate terminals were sharply segregated in layer IVc. Accordingly, we injected the eye of a monkey the day after birth and examined the visual pathway autoradiographically at one week. The lateral geniculate bodies were well labelled, and showed a layering as distinct as in the adult. This result has already been illustrated in Figure 21. The cortical picture was, on the contrary, not at all what

we had expected. Layer IVc, as seen in transverse section, was virtually continuously labelled, with only the vaguest of fluctuations in density here and there (Figure 34*a*, Plate 14). Tangential sections did, however, show periodic stripe-like variations in density, but with levels of label that were well above background throughout (Figure 34*b*), suggesting that at that age terminals belonging to one eye were not restricted in any clear-cut way to one set of stripes. This would mean that a particular geniculocortical fibre, which in the adult would enter the cortex, subdivide, and have its branches run selectively to several stripes of its own set, over an area of perhaps 1–2 mm, would in the newborn distribute its branches over the entire area, perhaps favouring its own set of stripes but not confining itself to them.

In a series of eye injections of foetal monkeys Rakic (1977) has extended these observations by showing that when the geniculate afferents from one eye grow into the cortex they occupy layer IVc continuously, whereas a week or so before term there are periodic fluctuations in density too subtle to see by naked eye, but obvious from grain counts.

Interpretation of these eye-injection experiments is complicated by the likelihood that a smearing of input to the cortex from one eye results from leakage of label at the geniculate level by diffusion from one set of layers to the other. We have therefore felt it necessary to crosscheck the results in the newborn in as many ways as possible. For example, physiological recordings in the first days after birth support the anatomical results in showing a binocular input to layer IVc at most points along its extent. By 6 weeks, however, this binocularity has disappeared, and the distribution of input from the two eyes seems to be identical to that found in the adult. (This postnatal change, incidentally, takes place even if both eyes are sutured closed, and hence is not dependent on visual experience.) The physiological findings thus appear to support the autoradiography.

In the normal development of ocular dominance columns, then, what seems to happen first is a complete occupation of layer IVc all along its length by fibres from both eyes and, with time, a gradual retraction and segregation until the process is complete, at about 6 weeks. What produces the orderly retraction is not known, but one might imagine a competition between terminals

Plate 14

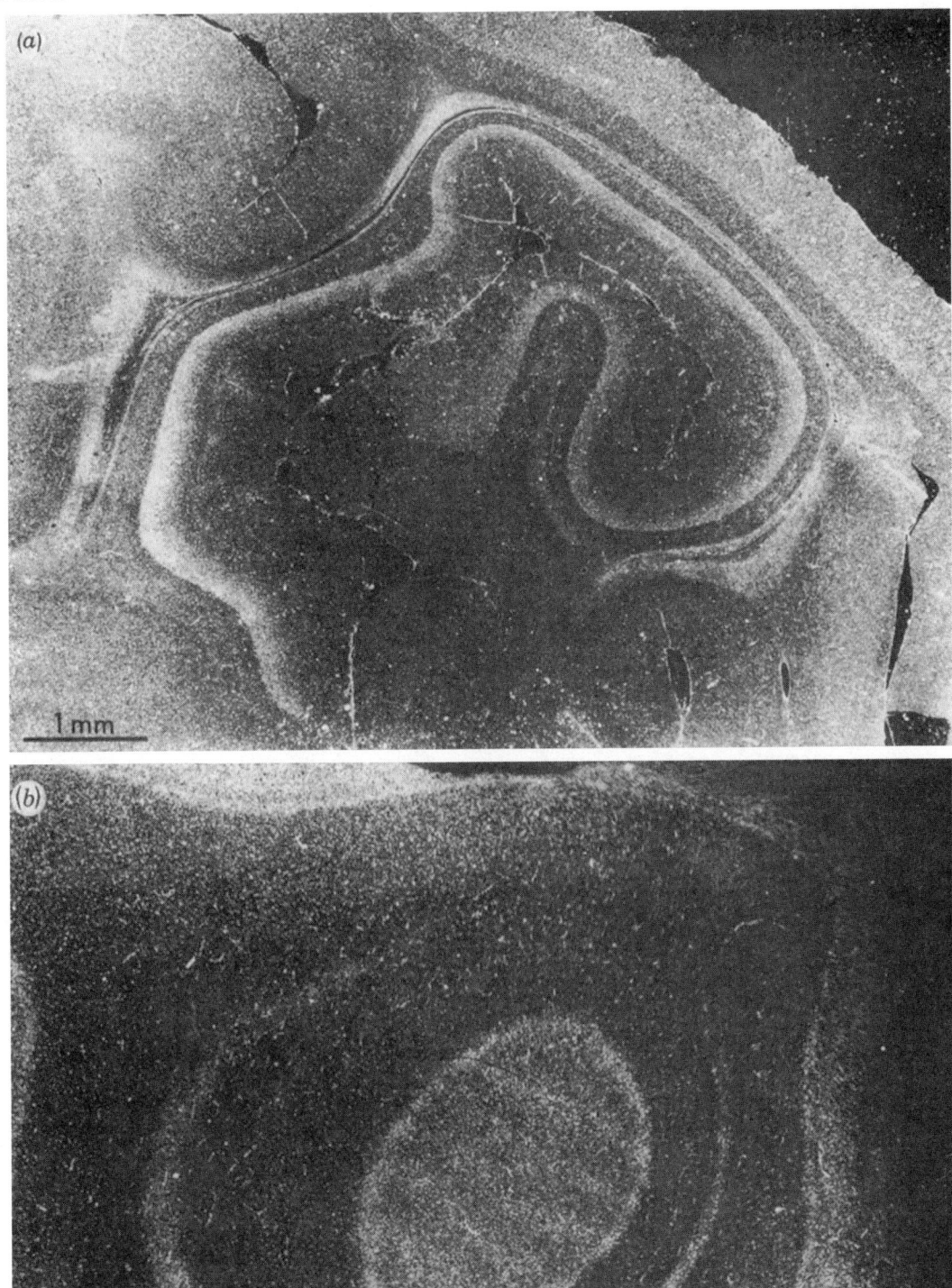

(a)

1 mm

(b)

1mm

Fig. 34.

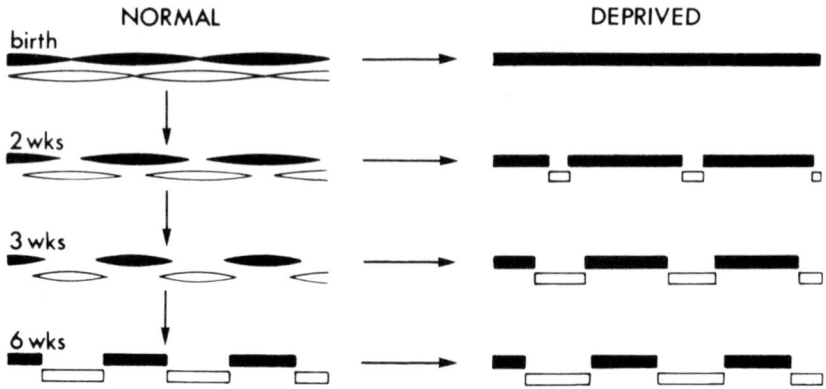

Fig. 35. *Scheme that might explain the effects of eye closures on columns in layer IVc, on the assumption that the segregation of the eyes is not complete until some weeks after birth. The solid lines represent the terminations of geniculate afferents in layer IVc corresponding to one eye; the open lines, the terminations from the other eye. In each, the width is intended to represent the presumed density of the terminals. The left half of the diagram illustrates the course of normal development suggested by our results. At birth there is some periodic variation in density (see Figure 34): it is unlikely that the minimum is zero, as suggested here, and the fluctuations may be different in different parts of the striate cortex. In this scheme we suppose that competition normally occurs between the eyes, with the weaker input declining progressively and the stronger becoming fortified. The result is a progressive retraction as the sparse terminals die out entirely. For purposes of the drawing we assume that the retraction process takes about 6 weeks, but the exact times are not known. On the right, the illustration shows what happens if at any stage in this process one eye (here, the eye corresponding to open lines) is sutured closed. We suppose that this inflicts a competitive disadvantage on the terminals from the closed eye so that they die out at those places where terminals from the normal eye are still present. Where normal-eye terminals have already retracted, their adversaries meet no competition and survive. The final outcome thus depends on when the deprivation was inflicted. (From Hubel et al. 1977.)*

from the two eyes, in which the rules are that the denser of the two sets proliferates and the less dense regresses. In such an unstable equilibrium the final result would be complete segregation. This is schematized in the left half of Figure 35.

To explain the deprivation effects, then, one need only suppose that closing one eye puts the corresponding IVc terminals at a competitive disadvantage, so that they retract completely from any point provided their adversaries have not themselves already retracted. The later the closure in the first 6 weeks the less would be the final apparent

shrinkage. This process is shown in Figure 35 on the right.

Thus there seems to be a good possibility that the monocular deprivation results involve not so much a pathological proliferation of terminals as a persistence and perhaps strengthening of inputs that are present at birth and normally regress in the first 6 weeks. If this proved to be true it would neatly explain two otherwise puzzling problems. First, the 'sensitive period' would become simply the time of normal consolidation of columns, the period between birth and the final maturation of

Fig. 34. *Autoradiographs through striate cortex of a baby monkey whose right eye was injected with radioactive fucose the day after birth, and the brain examined at 1 week of age. (From Hubel et al. 1977.) (a) Transverse section through hemisphere contralateral to injected eye, shows virtually no hint of fluctuation in label density along layer IVc. (The extreme lower left tail of label, deep in the calcarine fissure, is temporal crescent representation; here no fluctuations are expected.) (b) Tangential section through top of mushroom-like part of calcarine fissure, intersecting layer IVc in an oval. A strong suggestion of stripes is seen, but the entire region is labelled, rather than having virtually label-free gaps between dense stripes, as was seen in the normal adult (Figure 23)*

this part of the visual system. Second, if at and shortly after birth layer IVc were supplied all along its length by fibres from both eyes, it would be possible to explain the effects of monocular deprivation on a model that presupposes competition for space on the postsynaptic cell. Such a model would assume that a large number of afferent fibres make transitory synaptic contacts in IVc. One should emphasize, however, that the existence of temporary synapses in IVc is not established. Competition is in any case easier to imagine among fibres that are interwoven than between groups that are separated by a sizeable fraction of a millimetre.

Meanwhile, we do not exclude sprouting as a contributing mechanism in the process of columnar shrinkage and expansion. Eye closures after the sixth week seem not to affect the columns in layer IVc, but whether sprouting can be produced by removals or reversing the suturing—opening the closed eye and closing the open one—remains to be tested.

COMPARATIVE STUDIES OF ARCHITECTURE

Obviously an important motive for investigating the brains of mammals is the possibility of understanding the brain of man. It is partly for this reason that one seeks to learn as much as possible about the brains of higher mammals, especially of primates. To avoid making false generalizations it is important to survey as broad a range of mammals as possible. We were therefore interested in looking at physiology and architecture in striate cortex of a number of other species.

Our experiments in cats preceded the work in monkeys, but since about 1962 the two sets of studies have gone in parallel. In striate cortex of adult cats orientation specificity is just as common as in monkeys, and indeed it is likely that some cells in layer IVc have simple receptive fields (with orientation specificity) rather than circularly symmetric ones. Orientation columns are well developed. Ocular dominance columns, on the other hand, while present, are more subtle, and it was only after seeing accentuated versions of them in cats brought up from an early age with artificial squint that we were fully convinced of their presence. Eye injection studies (Shatz, Lindström & Wiesel 1977) have since revealed their presence clearly (Figure 36,

Plate 15). They are well defined on the ipsilateral side, but less well on the contralateral, where the input is stronger but also more diffuse. In tangential section they are less stripe-like, more chaotic, than those of the macaque. The cat is unique among known mammals in having a strong projection to area 18 from the geniculate. Eye dominance columns are seen also in 18 where they are well defined and probably coarser than in 17.

In the mouse (Dräger 1975) cells with orientation specificity are common but in contrast to the cat and monkey form only about 50% of the population. There may be some kind of grouping of cells with like orientation preference, but no clear columns have been observed. Compared with cat and monkey, the mouse has a much higher proportion of fibres crossing in the optic chiasm. Eye injection studies (Dräger 1974) show the expected disparity on the two sides, with the contralateral hemisphere far more strongly labelled (Figure 37, Plate 16). There is no hint, from physiology or autoradiography, of dominance columns. Results in the rat (Dräger, unpublished) are similar to those in mouse except that the ipsilateral input seems even weaker (Figure 38, Plate 17).

The tree shrew shows no hint of ocular-dominance columns (Hubel 1975; Casagrande & Harting 1975). The main difference in labelling on the two sides is an absence of label in the narrow cell-sparse cleft which subdivides layer IVc into three sublaminae (Figure 39, Plate 18).

In the prosimian, Galago, orientation specificity is as common as in macaque, and orientation columns are well developed and orderly (Hubel & Ginzler, unpublished). Both studies with Nauta degeneration (Glendenning & Kofron 1974) and eye injection (Hubel, unpublished) reveal clear eye dominance columns, again better defined ipsilaterally (Figure 40, Plate 19). Finally in the squirrel monkey, a New World species, one animal whose eye was injected showed no hint at all of eye-dominance columns, both hemispheres showing uniform label in layer IVc (Hubel *et al.* 1976). If this result is confirmed physiologically it will form an amazing departure from what otherwise seemed like a tendency for columns to be better defined the higher one looked in phylogeny. One is reluctant to accept this result without physiological confirmation, however, since the lamination of the lateral geniculate in this animal is not so well defined as in

Plate 15

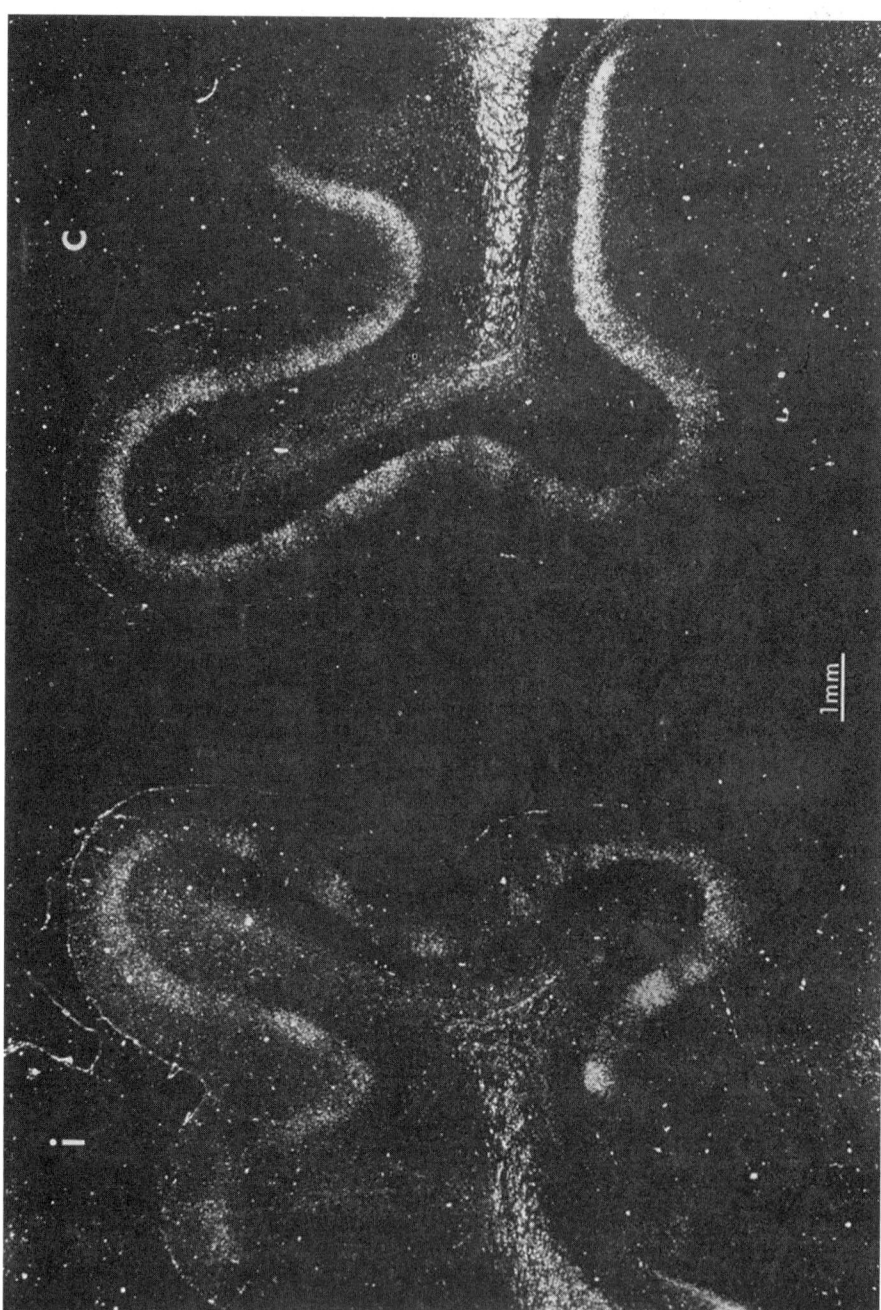

Fig. 36. Distribution of label in layer IV of cat cortex following injection of left eye with a tritiated proline-fucose mixture. Autoradiograph, coronal section through postlateral gyri; darkfield. The label in most of the dorsal part of the postlateral gyrus and sulcus is in area 18; the medial surfaces (which face each other) are area 17. Columns are more obvious ipsilater- ally (i). On the contralateral side (c) the label is in places almost continu- ous. The intensely and continuously labelled inferior portion on the con- tralateral side is the temporal crescent representation; it is of course absent ipsilaterally.

Plate 16

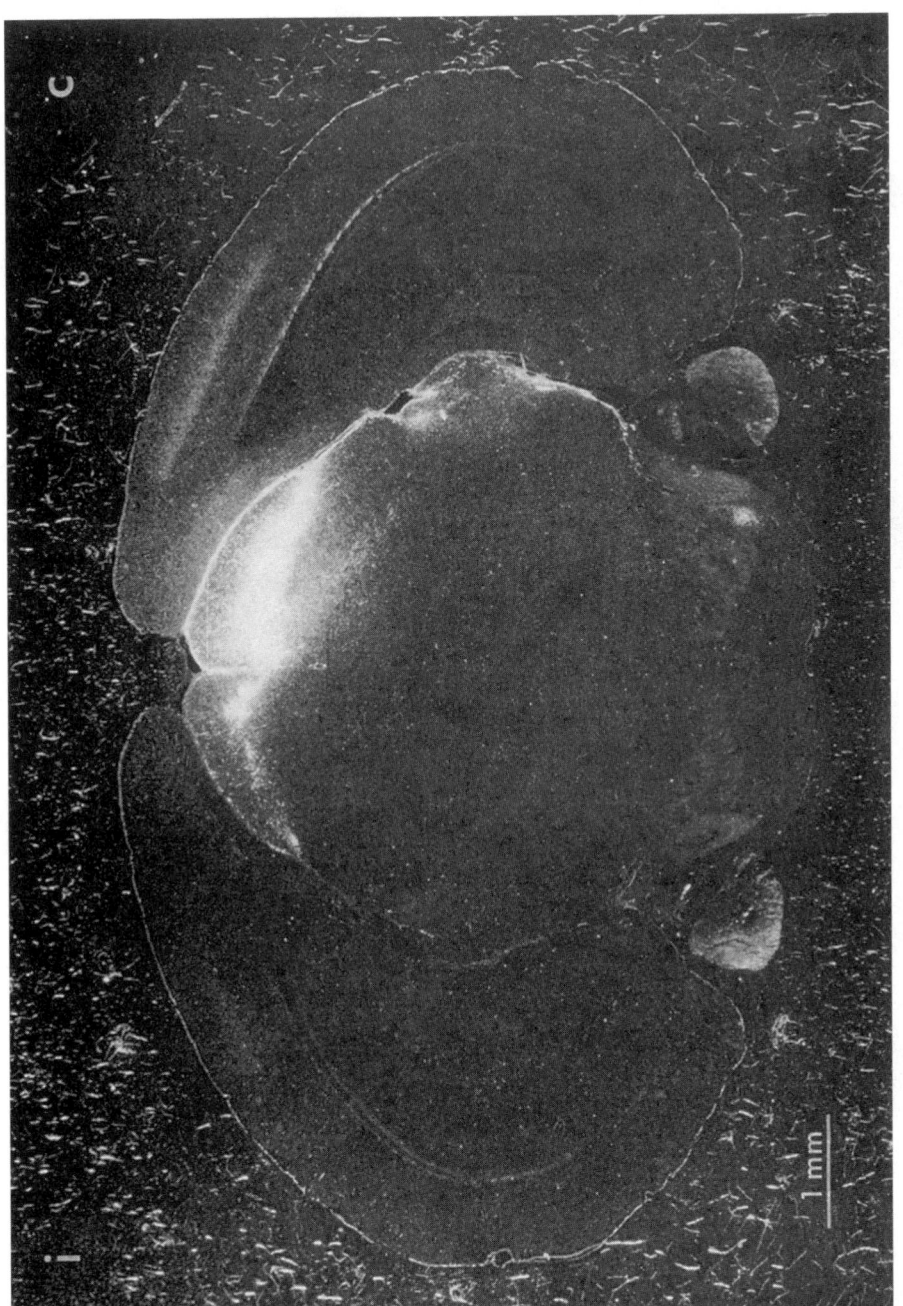

Fig. 37. Coronal section through mouse brain; autoradiograph, dark field, showing visual cortex following injection of a tritiated proline-fucose mixture into the left eye. Label in layer IV of contralateral cortex (c) is very obvious, in contrast to the ipsilateral cortex (i) in which the label is only barely visible. There is no suggestion of ocular dominance columns.

There is probably some label in area 18 (which in the mouse is termed 18a), just lateral to the densely labelled area 17 on the side contralateral to the injection. The optic tectum as expected is intensely labelled. (From Dräger 1974.)

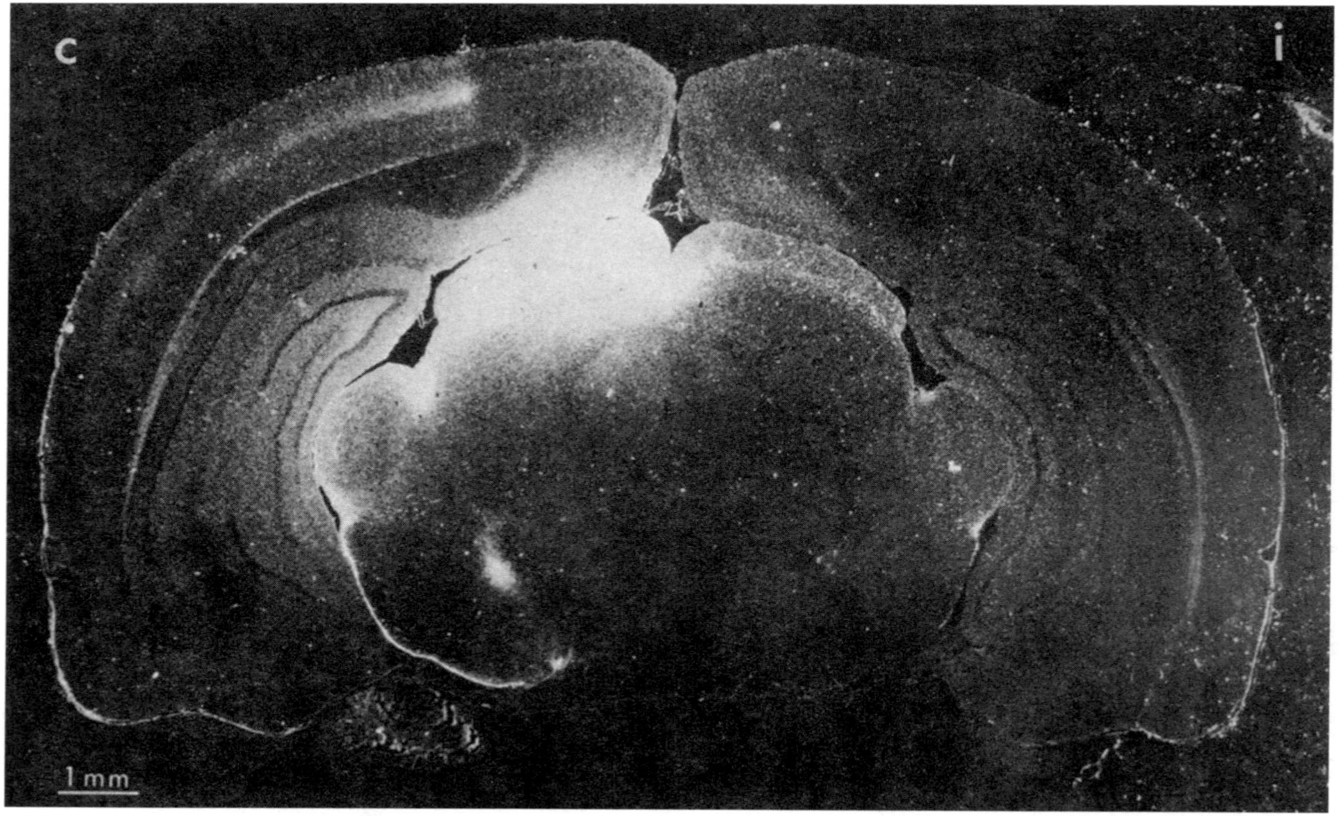

Plate 17

Fig. 38. Autoradiograph of rat brain; right eye was injected with a tritiated proline-fucose mixture; coronal section, dark field. As in the mouse the cortical label is much heavier in the contralateral cortex (c), and no columns are present. (Indeed, in this section there is virtually no label in the ipsilateral cortex (i).) Label in contralateral area 17 is concentrated mainly in layer IV, but some faint label may be seen in layers I and VI (Ribak & Peters 1975). Lateral to area 17 two fainter areas of label can be made out. Again, the contralateral optic tectum is intensely labelled. (Dräger, unpublished.)

Plate 18

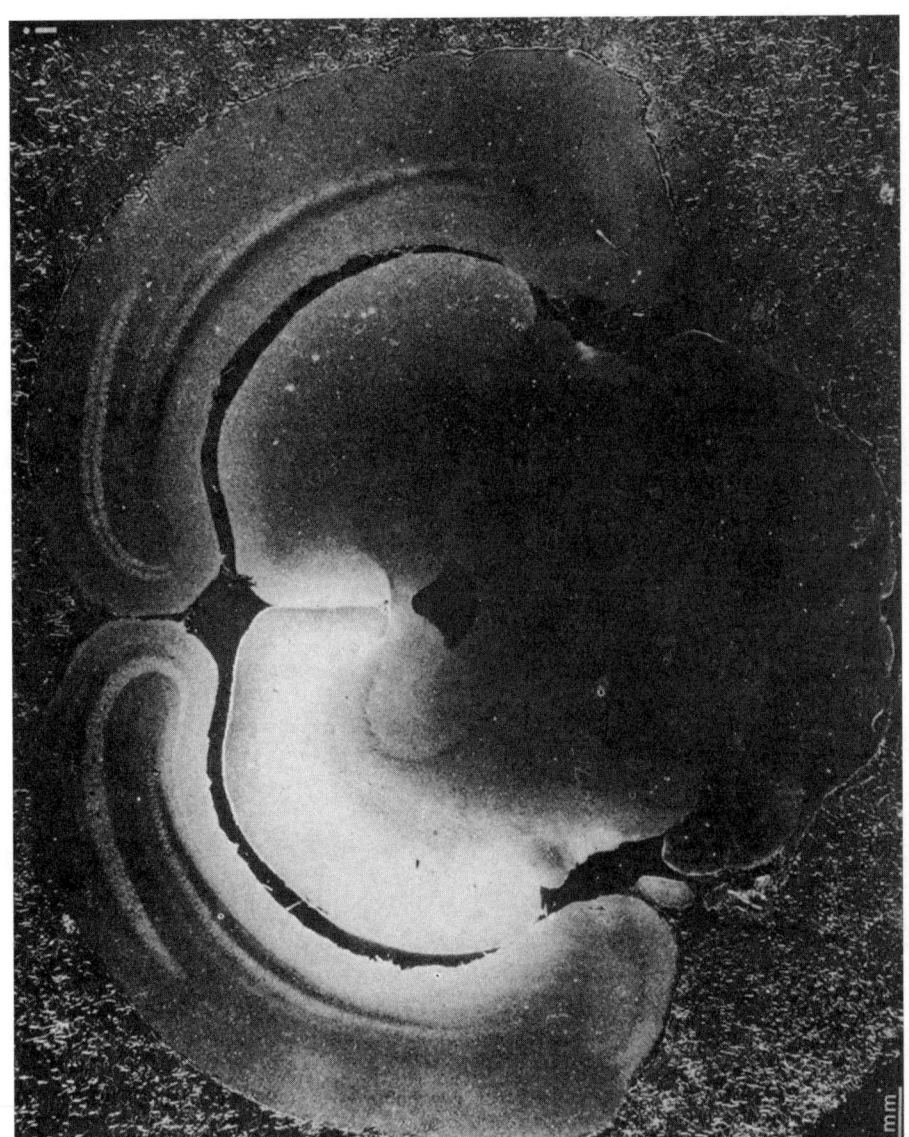

Fig. 39. Autoradiograph of the brain of a tree shrew whose right eye was injected with a tritiated proline-fucose mixture; dark field, coronal section (c) (Hubel 1975). On the contralateral side layer IVc is labelled throughout its entire thickness; an upper tier of label can be seen in layer IVa (to use a terminology analogous to that employed in the macaque). Ipsilaterally (i) there is a narrow label free cleft dividing layer IVc, and IVa is not labelled. In the optic tectum label is almost confined to the contralateral side; only a few tiny clusters of label are seen ipsilaterally

Plate 19

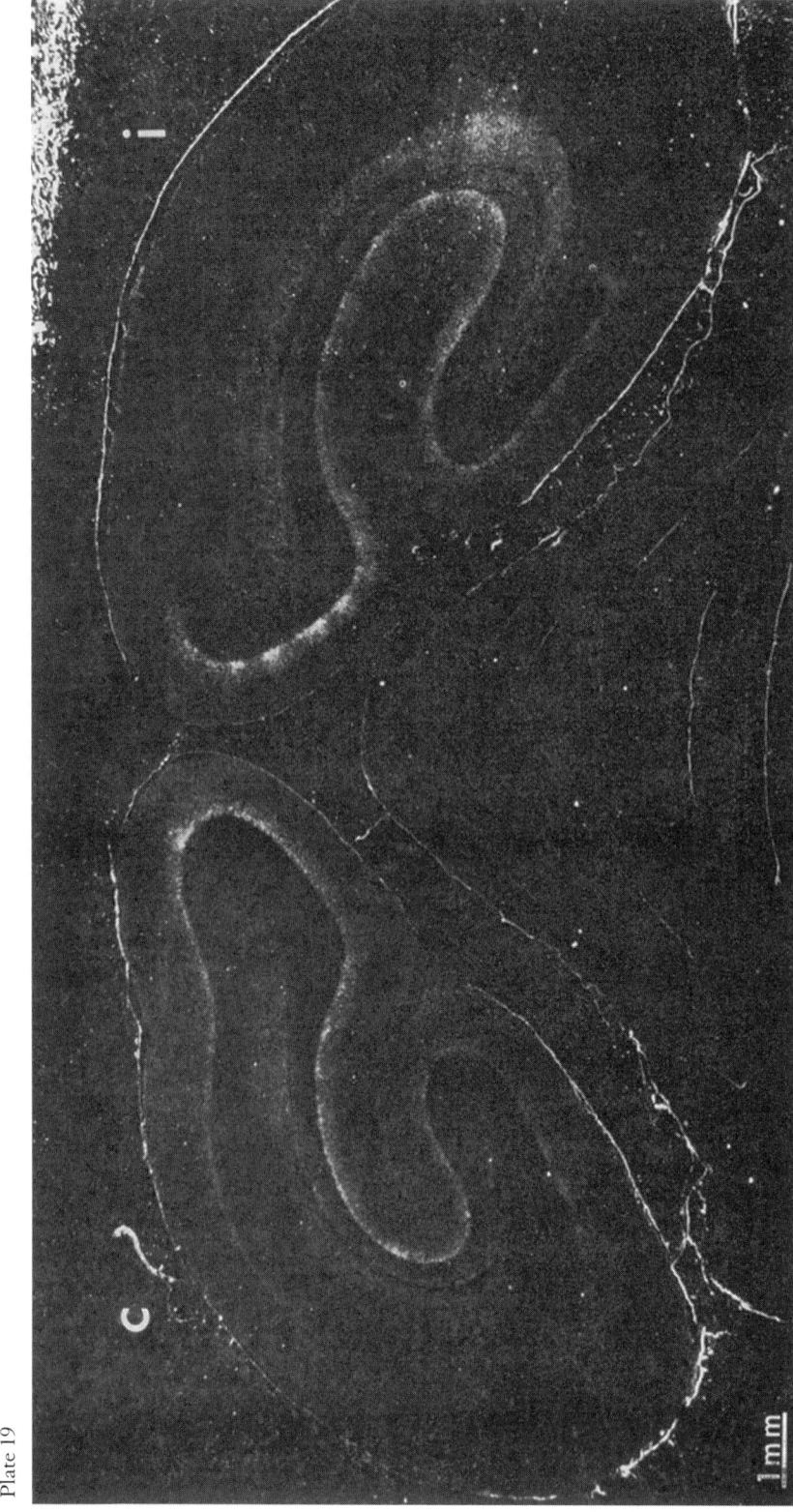

Fig. 40. Autoradiograph of the brain of an old world prosimian, Galago crassicaudatus, whose right eye was injected with a tritiated proline-fucose mixture. Ocular dominance columns are obvious in both hemispheres, but, as in the cat, are better defined ipsilaterally (i)

the old world monkey, and opportunity for label to leak from one set of layers to the other is greater.

In man the methods of physiology and autoradiography are of course unavailable and will remain so. We had hoped that LeVay's reduced silver technique might be used to demonstrate bands, but so far the method has failed to show any. The apparent difference between squirrel monkey and macaque should, however, make one cautious in assuming that all higher primates have ocular dominance columns.

CONCLUSION

We end up, then, with a view of the cortex as containing a thousand small machines of more or less identical structure. Each machine contains two types of hypercolumns, whose functions are dovetailed with each other and with the topographical map. This dicing up into subdivisions is the way the cortex handles or represents two variables (orientation and ocular dominance) besides the two obvious visual-field positional variables. Undoubtedly the picture is incomplete and, given the indirectness of much of the evidence, perhaps in places also incorrect. Colour information is not taken into account at all, for example, nor is black vs. white. Both of these may be associated with columns. What makes the architecture encouraging and attractive to us, however, has nothing to do with the relative completeness of the picture but the reinforcement it gives to much of the physiological findings. Orientation specificity, for example, might be just a curious property of cortical cells, shown, to be sure, by the majority of cells, but merely one among twenty or thirty competing properties. The existence of such an intricate edifice of orderly columns subserving this variable suggests, on the contrary, that it is of very great importance in area 17.

Another interesting aspect is the very orderliness of the architecture. It would be surprising if other regions of cortex did not use some similar orderly principles. If area 18 is largely devoted to mechanisms related to stereopsis (Hubel & Wiesel 1970), one might expect to see the eyes brought together in a whole range of different horizontal disparities in all parts of the visual field, and it would seem reasonable to find this done again in

repetitive units. At the moment there is no conclusive evidence for such an arrangement but it would surely be reasonable to look for one. What orderly arrangements one should expect in a structure like auditory cortex, where time sequences might conceivably be expected to form some vague counterpart to orientation, is difficult to imagine; on the other hand, our ideas about frontal lobes or speech areas are so vague as to make the auditory cortex seem like home territory. At least it can be said that with some years of work a few regions of cortex are capable of being understood, even if incompletely.

We wish to thank all those who have been so helpful over the past few years: Jane Chen, Janet Wiitanen, David Freeman, Claire Wang, Carolyn Scott, and many others. Supported by National Institutes of Health Grants EY 00605 and EY 00606, The Esther A. and Joseph Klingenstein Foundation, Inc. and The Rowland Foundation, Inc.

References

Albus, K. 1975 A quantitative study of the projection area of the central and paracentral visual field in area 17 of the cat. II. The spatial organization of the orientation domain. *Exp. Brain Res.* **24**, 181–202.

Barlow, H. B., Hill, R. M. & Levick, W. R. 1964 Retinal ganglion cells responding selectively to direction and speed of image motion in the rabbit. *J. Physiol., Lond.* **173**, 377–407.

Bishop, P. O., Kozak, W., Levick, W. R. & Vakkur, G. J. 1962 The determination of the projection of the visual field on to the lateral geniculate nucleus in the cat. *J. Physiol. Lond.* **163**, 503–539.

Bishop, P. O. & Henry, G. H. 1972 Striate neurons: receptive field concepts. *Investigative Ophthalmol.* **11**, 346–354.

Blakemore, C. & Tobin, E. A. 1972 Lateral inhibition between orientation detectors in the cat's visual cortex. *Exp. Brain Res.* **15**, 439–440.

Blakemore, C. & Van Sluyters, R. C. 1975 Innate and environmental factors in the development of the kitten's visual cortex. *J. Physiol., Lond.* **248**, 663–716.

Brouwer, B. & Zeeman, W. P. C. 1926 The projection of the retina in the primary optic neuron in monkeys. *Brain* **49**, 1–35.

Casagrande, V. A. & Harting, J. K. 1975 Transneuronal transport of tritiated fucose and proline in the visual pathways of tree shrew *Tupaia glis. Brain Res.* **96**, 367–372.

Clark, W. E. LeGros 1941 The laminar organization and cell content of the lateral geniculate body in the monkey. *J. Anat.* (*Lond*) **75**, 419–433.

Clark, W. E. LeGros & Sunderland, S. 1939 Structural changes in the isolated visual cortex. *J. Anat.* (*Lond.*) **73**, 563–574.

Cleland, B. G. & Levick, W. R. 1974 Properties of rarely encountered types of ganglion cells in the cat's retina and an overall classification. *J. Physiol., Lond.* **240**, 457–492.

Cowan, W. M., Gottlieb, D. I., Hendrickson, A. E., Price, J. L. & Woolsey, T. A. 1972 The autoradiographic demonstration of axonal connections in the central nervous system. *Brain Res.* **37**, 21–51.

Daniel, P. M. & Whitteridge, D. 1961 The representation of the visual field on the cerebral cortex in monkeys. *J. Physiol., Lond.* **159**, 203–221.

Dräger, U. C. 1974 Autoradiography of tritiated proline and fucose transported transneuronally from the eye to the visual cortex in pigmented and albino mice. *Brain Res.* **82**, 284–292.

Dräger, U. C. 1975 Receptive fields of single cells and topography in mouse visual cortex. *J. Comp. Neurol.* **160**, 269–290.

Fink, R. P. & Heimer, L. 1967 Two methods for selective silver impregnation of degenerating axons and their synaptic endings in the central nervous system. *Brain Res.* **4**, 369–374.

Fiskin, R. A., Garey, L. J. & Powell, T. P. S. 1973 Patterns of degeneration after intrinsic lesions of the visual cortex (area 17) of the monkey. *Brain Res.* **53**, 208–213.

Gilbert, C. D. & Kelly, J. P. 1975 The projections of cells in different layers of the cat's visual cortex. *J. Comp. Neurol.* **163**, 81–106.

Gilbert, C. D. 1977 Laminar differences in receptive field properties of cells in cat primary visual cortex. *J. Physiol., Lond.* (In the press.)

Glendenning, K. K. & Kofron, E. A. 1974 Projections of individual laminae of the lateral geniculate nucleus in the prosimian. *4th ann. meet. Soc. Neurosci. (St Louis) Abstr.* p. 229.

Goldberg, S. & Kotani, M. 1967 The projection of optic nerve fibers in the frog, *Rana catesbeiana*, as studied by autoradiography. *Anat. Rec.* **158**, 325–332.

Grafstein, B. & Laureno, R. 1973 Transport of radioactivity from eye to visual cortex in the mouse. *Exp. Neurol.* **39**, 44–57.

Guillery, R. W. 1966 A study of Golgi preparations from the dorsal lateral geniculate nucleus of the adult cat. *J. Comp. Neurol.* **128**, 21–50.

Guillery, R. W. 1972 Binocular competition in the control of geniculate cell growth. *J. Comp. Neurol.* **144**, 117–130.

Guillery, R. W. & Colonnier, M. 1970 Synaptic patterns in the dorsal lateral geniculate nucleus of the monkey. *Z. Zellforsch.* **103**, 90–108.

Guillery, R. W. & Stelzner, D. J. 1970 The differential effects of unilateral lid closure upon the monocular and binocular segments of the dorsal lateral geniculate nucleus in the cat. *J. Comp. Neurol.* **139**, 413–422.

Hartline, H. K. 1940 The receptive fields of optic nerve fibers. *Amer. J. Physiol.* **130**, 690–699.

Hoffman, K.-P., Stone, J. & Sherman, S. M. 1972 Relay of receptive-field properties in dorsal lateral geniculate nucleus of the cat. *J. Neurophysiol.* **35**, 518–531.

Hubel, D. H. 1975 An autoradiographic study of the retinocortical projections in the tree shrew (*Tupaia glis*). *Brain Res.* **96**, 41–50.

Hubel, D. H. & Freeman, D. C. 1977 Projection into the visual field of ocular dominance columns in macaque monkey. *Brain Res.* **122**, 336–343.

Hubel, D. H. & Wiesel, T. N. 1959 Receptive fields of single neurones in the cat's striate cortex. *J. Physiol., Lond.* **148**, 574–591.

Hubel, D. H. & Wiesel, T. N. 1960 Receptive fields of optic nerve fibres in the spider monkey. *J. Physiol., Lond.* **154**, 572–580.

Hubel, D. H. & Wiesel, T. N. 1961 Integrative action in the cat's lateral geniculate body. *J. Physiol., Lond.* **155**, 385–398.

Hubel, D. H. & Wiesel, T. N. 1962 Receptive fields, binocular interaction and functional architecture in the cat's visual cortex. *J. Physiol., Lond.* **160**, 106–154.

Hubel, D. H. & Wiesel, T. N. 1963 Receptive fields of cells in striate cortex of very young, visually inexperienced kittens. *J. Neurophysiol.* **26**, 994–1002.

Hubel, D. H. & Wiesel, T. N. 1965 Receptive fields and functional architecture in two nonstriate visual areas (18 and 19) of the cat. *J. Neurophysiol.* **28**, 229–289.

Hubel, D. H. & Wiesel, T. N. 1968 Receptive fields and functional architecture of monkey striate cortex. *J. Physiol., Lond.* **195**, 215–243.

Hubel, D. H. & Wiesel, T. N. 1970 Cells sensitive to binocular depth in area 18 of the macaque monkey cortex. *Nature, Lond.* **225**, 41–42.

Hubel, D. H. & Wiesel, T. N. 1972 Laminar and columnar distribution of geniculo-cortical fibers in the macaque monkey. *J. Comp. Neurol.* **146**, 421–450.

Hubel, D. H. & Wiesel, T. N. 1973 A re-examination of stereoscopic mechanisms in area 17 of the cat. *J. Physiol., Lond.* **232**, 29–30 P.

Hubel, D. H. & Wiesel, T. N. 1974a Sequence regularity and geometry of orientation columns in the monkey striate cortex. *J. Comp. Neurol.* **158**, 267–294.

Hubel, D. H. & Wiesel, T. N. 1974b Uniformity of monkey striate cortex: a parallel relationship between field size, scatter, and magnification factor. *J. Comp. Neurol.* **158**, 295–306.

Hubel, D. H., Wiesel, T. N. & LeVay, S. 1974 Visual-field representation in layer IV C of monkey striate cortex. *4th ann. meet. Soc. Neurosci. (St. Louis) Abstr.* p. 264.

Hubel, D. H., Wiesel, T. N. & LeVay, S. 1976 Functional architecture of area 17 in normal and monocularly deprived macaque monkeys. *Cold Spr. Harbor Symp. Quant. Biol.* **40**, 581–589.

Hubel, D. H., Wiesel, T. N. & LeVay, S. 1977 Plasticity of ocular dominance columns in monkey striate cortex. *Phil. Trans. R. Soc. Lond.* B **278**, 131–163.

Kelly, J. P. & Van Essen, D. C. 1974 Cell structure and function in the visual cortex of the cat. *J. Physiol., Lond.* **238**, 515–547.

Kennedy, C., Des Rosiers, M., Sokoloff, L., Reivich, M. & Jehle, J. 1975 The ocular dominance columns of the striate cortex as studied by the deoxyglucose method for measurement of local cerebral glucose utilization. *Trans. Am. Neurol. Ass.* **100**, 74–77.

Kuffler, S. W. 1953 Discharge patterns and functional organization of mammalian retina. *J. Neurophysiol.* **16**, 37–68.

Lasek, R., Joseph, B. S. & Whitlock, D. G. 1968 Evaluation of a radioautographic neuro-anatomic tracing method. *Brain Res.* **8**, 319–336.

LeVay, S., Hubel, D. H. & Wiesel, T. N. 1975 The pattern of ocular dominance columns in macaque visual cortex revealed by a reduced silver stain. *J. Comp. Neurol.* **159**, 559–576.

Lettvin, J. Y., Maturana, H. R., McCulloch, W. S. & Pitts, W. H. 1959 What the frog's eye tells the frog's brain. *Proc. Inst. Radio Engrs. N.Y.* **47**, 1940–1951.

Lund, J. S. 1973 Organization of neurons in the visual cortex, area 17, of the monkey (*Macaca mulatta*). *J. Comp. Neurol.* **147**, 455–496.

Lund, J. S., Lund, R. D., Hendrickson, A. E., Bunt, A. H. & Fuchs, A. F. 1975 The origin of efferent pathways from primary visual cortex, area 17, of the macaque monkey as shown by retrograde transport of horseradish peroxidase. *J. Comp. Neurol.* **164**, 287–304.

Minkowski, M. 1920 2. Über den Verlauf, die Endigung und die zentrale Repräsentation von gekreuzten und ungekreuzten Sehnervenfasern bei einigen Säugetieren und beim Menschen. *Schweiz Arch. Neurol. Psychiat.* **6**, 201–252.

Mountcastle, V. B. 1957 Modality and topographic properties of single neurons of cat's somatic sensory cortex. *J. Neurophysiol.* **20**, 408–434.

Palmer, L. A. & Rosenquist, A. C. 1974 Visual receptive fields of single striate cortical units projecting to the superior colliculus in the cat. *Brain Res.* **67**, 27–42.

Polyak, S. 1957 *The vertebrate visual system* (ed. H. Klüver), Chicago, Ill.: University of Chicago Press.

Portmann, A. 1948 *Tiergestalt—Studien über die Bedeutung der tierischen Erscheinung*. Basel: Reinhardt.

Rakic, P. 1977 Prenatal development of the visual system in the rhesus monkey. *Phil. Trans. R. Soc. Lond. B.* **278**, 245–260.

Ribak, C. E. & Peters, A. 1975 An autoradiographic study of the projections from the lateral geniculate body of the rat. *Brain Res.* **92**, 341–368.

Sanderson, K. J., Darian-Smith, I. & Bishop, P. O. 1969 Binocular corresponding receptive fields of single units in the cat dorsal lateral geniculate nucleus. *Vision Res.* **9**, 1297–1303.

Schiller, P. H., Finlay, B. L. & Volman, S. F. 1976 Quantitative studies of single cell properties in monkey striate cortex. I. Spatiotemporal organization of receptive fields. *J. Neurophysiol.* **39**, 1288–1319.

Shatz, C. J., Lindström, S. H. & Wiesel, T. N. 1977 The distribution of afferents representing the right and left eyes in the cat's visual cortex. *Brain Res.* (In the press.)

Sherman, S. M. 1973 Visual field defects in monocularly and binocularly deprived cats *Brain Res.* **49**, 25–45.

Sherman, S. M., Guillery, R. W., Kaas, J. H. & Sanderson, K. J. 1974 Behavioral, electro-physiological and morphological studies of binocular competition in the development of the geniculo-cortical pathways of cats. *J. Comp. Neurol.* **158**, 1–18.

Sokoloff, L. 1975 Influence of functional activity on local cerebral glucose utilization. In *Brain work. The coupling of function, metabolism and blood flow in the brain* (ed. D. H. Ingvar and N. A. Lassen), pp. 385–388. New York: Academic Press.

Sokoloff, L. 1977 Measurement of local glucose utilization and its use in mapping local functional activity in the central nervous system. *Proc. 4th World Congress of Psychiatric Surgery,* Madrid, Sept. 7–10, 1975, pp. 111–121.

Stone, J. & Fukuda, Y. 1974 Properties of cat retinal ganglion cells: a comparison of W-cells with X- and Y-cells. *J. Neurophysiol.* **37**, 722–748.

Talbot, S. A. & Marshall, W. H. 1941 Physiological studies on neural mechanisms of visual localization and discrimination. *Am. J. Ophthal.* **24**, 1255–1263.

Toyama, K., Matsunami, K., Ohno, T. & Takashiki, S. 1974 An intracellular study of neuronal organization in the visual cortex. *Exp. Brain Res.* **21**, 45–66.

Van Buren, J. M. 1963 *The retinal ganglion cell layer.* Springfield, Ill.: Charles C. Thomas.

Wiesel, T. N. 1960 Receptive fields of ganglion cells in the cat's retina. *J. Physiol., Lond.* **153**, 583–594.

Wiesel, T. N. & Hubel, D. H. 1963 Single-cell responses in striate cortex of kittens deprived of vision in one eye. *J. Neurophysiol.* **26**, 1003–1017.

Wiesel, T. N. & Hubel, D. H. 1965 Comparison of the effects of unilateral and bilateral eye closure on cortical unit responses in kittens. *J. Neurophysiol.* **28**, 1029–1040.

Wiesel, T. N. & Hubel, D. H. 1966 Spatial and chromatic interactions in the lateral geniculate body of the Rhesus monkey. *J. Neurophysiol.* **29**, 1115–1156.

Wiesel, T. N. & Hubel, D. H. 1974 Ordered arrangement of orientation columns in monkeys lacking visual experience. *J. Comp. Neurol.* **158**, 307–318.

Wiitanen, J. T. 1969 Selective silver impregnation of degenerating axons and axon terminals in the central nervous system of the monkey (*Macaca mulatta*). *Brain Res.* **14**, 546–548.

AFTERWORD

We seize this opportunity to make a few minor amendments and corrections. As discussed in our comments on papers on deprivation and development, we may have used the word *genetic* too freely in dealing with the innate quality of the specificity of cortical responses. Today we would simply say "innate" and leave it at that. One amusing error occurs in Fig. 24 of the Ferrier lecture, in which the ocular dominance columns and the fingerprint are presented supposedly at the same scale, whereas they obviously cannot be, unless the human had an exceptionally large index finger, or the monkey an exceptionally small brain.

This account comes many years before one knew of the existence of blobs, and when double-opponent cells had only been briefly mentioned in our 1968 monkey cortex paper. The machinery contained in a few square millimeters of cortex would have to include the blobs and a description of double-opponent cells, and our ice-cube model in Fig. 27 would have to show the blobs (as was done in Fig. 34 of Livingstone and Hubel (*J Neurosci* 1984, 4, 309–356). Luckily, perhaps, we did not yet know of the complex swirling of the orientation columns that the optical mapping later revealed—as perfectly parallel stripes they were hard enough to portray even with a ruler and drafting machine. Close scrutiny of the ice-cube model will show a difference, in the orientations of successive lines, of one degree, without which the cube seemed severely distorted. We did realize at the time that orientation columns could hardly be perfectly parallel stripes, given the reversals and fractures, but we had to draw them some way, and chose the simplest possible.

Chapter 27 • Nobel Lecture, David H. Hubel
Nobel Lecture, Torsten N. Wiesel •

FOREWORD

When the word came at 6:30 in the morning, in the form of a hearty and loud American voice on the telephone saying "Congratulations!", I was shivering and annoyed, having been rousted out the shower by the incessant ringing. I had to sit on the edge of the bed to digest the news. A Nobel prize could not have been further from my mind (or, I'm sure, Torsten's). We had heard a few rumors over the years that our names had been proposed, but we looked on our chances of ever winning it as about the same as winning a state lottery. Given the incredible progress in the field of molecular biology at that time, the chances for a neurobiologist seemed remote. Not that we were all that modest. We looked on our work as being the first to show what some area of cerebral cortex was doing with the information coming into it, and we supposed that someone must appreciate its importance. But, that fall of 1981, a Nobel prize was far from our minds. We had no champagne on ice!

People ask if the prize changed our lives. Of course it must have, but to find out exactly how we would have to go back and do a control. It certainly led to more invitations, more travel, more pressure to take on administrative tasks. But for me, the money meant some freedom from taking on loans to put our children through college. That November, at the Neuroscience Meeting in Los Angeles, a big celebration was held for us in a huge church, which thousands of our fellow members attended. At one point Torsten was asked to say a few words and with typical modesty remarked that he felt the prize was really to honor everyone in the field and that he would love to share it with everyone present. I couldn't quite agree, and broke in to say that given the size of the crowd, sharing the prize would net each person present about $10.00. Generosity had to have its limits.

We hesitated to include the published Nobel lectures, again because of their obvious overlap with the other reprints, but as in the case of the Ferrier lecture we felt that a summing up might be helpful. As with all such published lectures, the correspondence between what one said and what was published was minimal. We had always felt that a lecture and a paper were

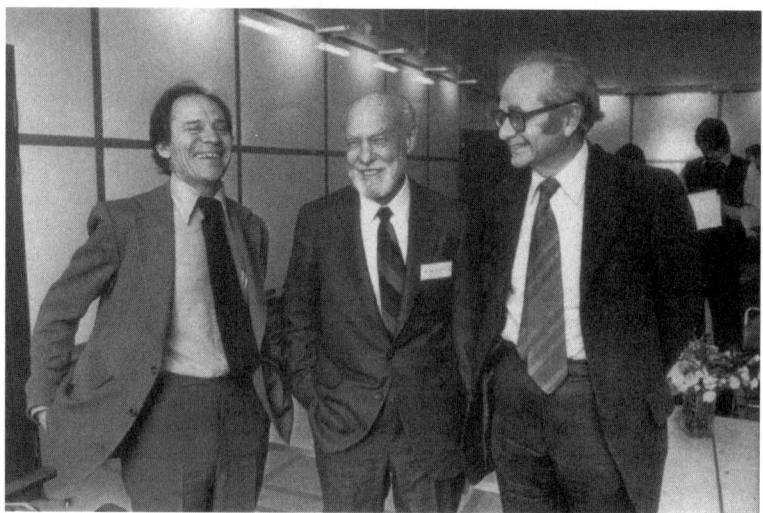

Fig. 27A.1: Torsten Wiesel, Roger Sperry, and David Hubel in Stockholm, 1981.

two entirely different art forms: to tape-record a lecture, transcribe it and publish just as it was spoken, full of "aws" and "ums", hesitations, repetitions, and backtracking, makes for terrible reading; and to prepare a manuscript for publication and then read it was, if anything, worse. We had gotten into the habit of winging our lectures and saw no reason to change when we gave our talks at the Karolinska in Stockholm.

We worked hard over the final versions of the lectures and sent them in to *Science,* where Nobel lectures are traditionally published. Word came back one day from the chief editor, that the essays were unfortunately too long, and should be shortened, mine by 30% and Torsten's by 50%. I immediately lifted the phone and called Torsten, and found that his reaction, one of fury, was the same as mine, and that our solutions to the problem were identical. We called *Nature* in England and told them our story. They answered that of course they could not guarantee to publish our lectures sight unseen but would be happy to look at them. I suggested that we call *Science* and ask them to send the manuscripts over to the *Nature* office in Washington—but the *Nature* editor quickly said "Oh that would be a bit harsh; please just send us a new printout"—which we did. That is how our lectures came to be published in *Nature*, in all their great length.

Evolution of Ideas on the Primary Visual Cortex, 1955–1978: A Biased Historical Account

DAVID H. HUBEL • *Harvard Medical School, Department of Neurobiology, Boston, Massachusetts*

INTRODUCTION

In the early spring of 1958 I drove over to Baltimore from Washington, D.C. and in a cafeteria at Johns Hopkins Hospital met Stephen Kuffler and Torsten Wiesel, for a discussion that was more momentous for Torsten's and my future than either of us could have possibly imagined.

I had been at Walter Reed Army Institute of Research for three years, in the Neuropsychiatry Section headed by David Rioch, working under the supervision of M.G.F. Fuortes. I began at Walter Reed by developing a tungsten microelectrode and a technique for using it to record from chronically implanted cats, and I had been comparing the firing of cells in the visual pathways of sleeping and waking animals.

It was time for a change in my research tactics. In sleeping cats only diffuse light could reach the retina through the closed eyelids. Whether the cat was asleep or awake with eyes open, diffuse light failed to stimulate the cells in the striate cortex. In waking animals I had succeeded in activating many cells with moving spots on a screen, and had found that some cells were very selective in that they responded when a spot moved in one direction across the screen (e.g. from left to right) but not when it moved in the opposite direction (1) (Fig. 1). There were many cells that I could not influence at all. Obviously there was a gold mine in the visual cortex, but methods were needed that would permit the recording of single cells for many hours, and with the eyes immobilized, if the mine were ever to begin producing.

I had planned to do a postdoctoral fellowship at Johns Hopkins Medical School with Vernon Mountcastle, but the timing was awkward for him because he was remodeling his laboratories. One day Kuffler called and asked if I would like to work in his laboratory at the Wilmer Institute of Ophthalmology at the Johns Hopkins Hospital with Torsten Wiesel, until the remodeling was completed. That was expected to take about a year. I didn't have to be persuaded; some rigorous training in vision was just what I needed, and though Kuffler himself was no longer working in vision the tradition had been maintained in his laboratory. Torsten and I had visited each other's laboratories and it was clear that we had common interests and similar outlooks. Kuffler suggested that I come over to discuss plans, and that was what led to the meeting in the cafeteria.

It was not hard to decide what to do. Kuffler had described two types of retinal ganglion cells, which he called "on-center" and "off-center". The receptive field of each type was made up of two mutually antagonistic regions, a center and a surround, one excitatory and the other inhibitory. In 1957 Barlow, FitzHugh and Kuffler had gone on to show that as a consequence retinal ganglion cells are less sensitive to diffuse light than to a spot just filling the receptive-field center (2). It took me some time to realize what this meant: that the way a cell responds to any visual scene will change very little when, for example, the sun goes behind a cloud and the light reflected from black and white objects decreases by a large factor. The cell virtually ignores this change, and our subjective assessment of the objects as black or white is likewise practically unaffected. Kuffler's center-surround receptive fields thus began to explain why the appearance of objects depends so little on the intensity of the light source. Some years later Edwin Land showed that the appearance of a scene is similarly relatively independent of the exact color composition of the light source. The physiological basis of this color independence has yet to be worked out.

From *Les Prix Nobel en 1981*, pp. 221–256 and *Nature*, 1982, 299: 515–524.

Nobel lecture, 8 December 1981

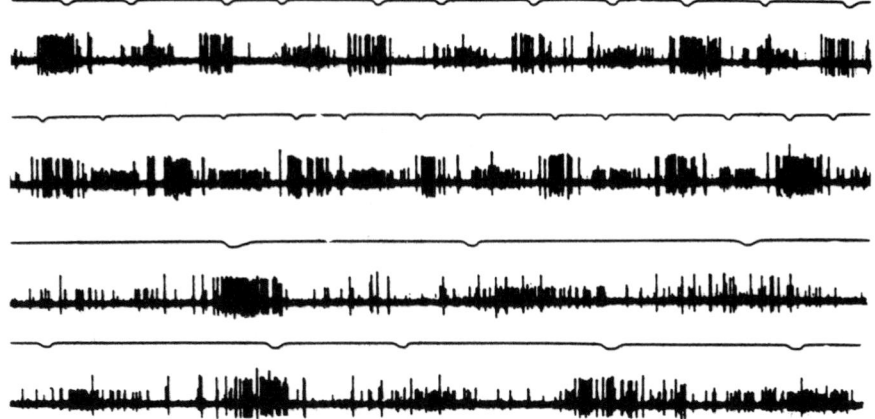

Fig. 1. Continuos recording from striate cortex of an unrestrained cat. In each dual trace the lower member shows the microelectrode oscilloscope recording from two cells, one with large impulses, the other smaller ones. The stimulus was small to-and-fro hand movements in front of the cat. Each movement interrupted a light beam falling on a photoelectric cell, producing the notches in the upper beam. The upper two pairs of records represent fast movements, the lower ones slower movements. Each line represents 4 seconds. (1)

The strategy (to return to our cafeteria) seemed obvious. Torsten and I would simply extend Stephen Kuffler's work to the brain; we would record from geniculate cells and cortical cells, map receptive fields with small spots, and look for any further processing of the visual information.

My reception in Kuffler's office the first day was memorable. I was nervous and out of breath. Steve at his desk, rotated around on his chair and said "Hi, David! Take off your coat. Hang up your hat. Do up your fly." His laboratory was informal! But it took me a month, given my Canadian upbringing, to force myself to call him Steve. For the first three months no paycheck arrived and finally I screwed up the courage to go in and tell him. He laughed and laughed, and then said "I forgot!"

Torsten and I didn't waste much time. Within a week of my coming to Hopkins (to a dark and dingy inner windowless room of the Wilmer Institute basement, deemed ideal for visual studies) we did our first experiment. For the time being we finessed the geniculate (at Walter Reed I had convinced myself that geniculate cells were center-surround) and began right away with cortex. The going was rough. We had only the equipment for retinal stimulation and recording that had been designed a few years before by Talbot and Kuffler

(3). A piece of apparatus resembling a small cyclotron held the anesthetized and paralyzed cat with its head facing almost directly upwards. A modified ophthalmoscope projected a background light and a spot stimulus onto the retina. The experimenter could look in, see the retina with its optic disc, area centralis and blood vessels, and observe the background light and the stimulus spots. Small spots of light were produced by sliding 2 cm × 5 cm metal rectangles containing various sizes of holes into a slot in the apparatus, just as one puts a slide into a slide projector. To obtain a black spot on a light background one used a piece of glass like a microscope slide, onto which a black dot had been glued. All this was ideal for stimulating the retina and recording directly from retinal ganglion cells, since one could see the electrode tip and know where to stimulate, but for cortical recording it was horrible. Finding a receptive field on the retina was difficult, and we could never remember what part of the retina we had stimulated. After a month or so we decided to have the cat face a projection screen, as I had at Walter Reed and as Talbot and Marshall had in 1941 (4). Having no other head holder, we continued for a while to use the ophthalmoscope's head holder, which posed a problem since the cat was facing directly up. To solve this we brought in some bed sheets which we slung between the pipes and cobwebs that graced the ceiling of the Wilmer basement, giving the setup the aura of a circus tent. On the sheets we projected our spots and slits. One day Vernon Mountcastle walked in on this scene, and was horror struck at the spectacle. The method was certainly inconvenient since we had to stare at the ceiling for the entire experiment. Then I remembered having seen in Mountcastle's laboratory a Horsley-Clarke head holder that was not only no longer being used but also had the name of the Wilmer Institute engraved on it. It was no other than the instrument that Talbot had designed for visual work when he and Marshall mapped out visual areas I and II in the cat, in 1941 (4). For years Vernon had used it in his somatosensory work, but he had recently obtained a fancier one. Torsten and I decided to reclaim the Wilmer instrument, not without some trepidation. To give ourselves confidence we both put on lab coats, for the first and last times in our lives, and looking very professional walked over to Physiology. Though Mountcastle was his usual friendly and generous self, I suspect he was loath to part with this treasure, but the inscription on the stainless steel was not to be denied and we walked off with it triumphantly. It is still in use (now at Harvard: we literally stole it from the Wilmer), and has probably the longest history of uninterrupted service of any Horsley-Clarke in the world.

A short while before this adventure we had gone to a lecture by Vernon (this was a few years after his discovery of cortical columns) (5) in which he had amazed us by reporting on the results of recording from some 900 somatosensory cortical cells, for those days an astronomic number. We knew we could never catch up, so we catapulted ourselves to respectability by calling our first cell No. 3000 and numbering subsequent ones from there. When Vernon visited our circus tent we were in the middle of a 3-unit recording, cell Nos. 3007, 3008, and 3009. We made sure that we mentioned their identification numbers. All three cells had the same receptive-field orientation but neither Vernon nor we realized, then, what that implied.

At times we were peculiarly inept. Our first perfusion of a cat was typical. One morning at about 2:00 a.m. we had arranged two huge bottles on an overhead shelf, for saline and formalin, and were switching over from saline to formalin when the rubber tubing came off the outlet of the formalin bottle and gave us an acrid early morning cold

shower. We did not relish being preserved at so young an age! The reference to 2:00 a.m. perhaps deserves some comment, because neurophysiologists, at least those who study animals, have the reputation of doing experiments that last for days without respite. We soon found that such schedules were not for us. I knew we were losing traction in an experiment when Torsten began to talk to me in Swedish; usually this was around 3:00 a.m. The longest experiment we ever did was one in which I arrived home just as my family was sitting down for breakfast. I had almost driven off the road on the way back. At the risk of becoming what Mountcastle termed "part-time scientists" we decided to be more lenient with ourselves, giving the deteriorating condition of the animal as the official reason for stopping early.

Our first real discovery came about as a surprise. We had been doing experiments for about a month. We were still using the Talbot-Kuffler ophthalmoscope and were not getting very far; the cells simply would not respond to our spots and annuli. One day we made an especially stable recording. (We had adapted my chronic recording system, which made use of Davies' idea of a closed chamber (6), to the acute experimental animals, and no vibrations short of an earthquake were likely to dislodge things.) The cell in question lasted 9 hours, and by the end we had a very different feeling about what the cortex might be doing. For 3 or 4 hours we got absolutely nowhere. Then gradually we began to elicit some vague and inconsistent responses by stimulating somewhere in the midperiphery of the retina. We were inserting the glass slide with its black spot into the slot of the ophthalmoscope when suddenly over the audiomonitor the cell went off like a machine gun. After some fussing and fiddling we found out what was happening. The response had nothing to do with the black dot. As the glass slide was inserted its edge was casting onto the retina a faint but sharp shadow, a straight dark line on a light background. That was what the cell wanted, and it wanted it, moreover, in just one narrow range of orientations.

This was unheard of. It is hard, now, to think back and realize just how free we were from any idea of what cortical cells might be doing in an animal's daily life. That the retinas mapped onto the visual cortex in a systematic way was of course well known, but it was far from clear what this apparently unimaginative remapping was good for. It seemed inconceivable that the information would enter the cortex and leave it unmodified, especially when Kuffler's work in the retina had made it so clear that interesting transformations took place there between input and output. One heard the word "analysis" used to describe what the cortex might be doing, but what one was to understand by that vague term was never spelled out. In the somatosensory cortex, the only other cortical area being closely scrutinized, Mountcastle had found that the cells had properties not dramatically different from those of neurons at earlier stages.

Many of the ideas about cortical function then in circulation seem in retrospect almost outrageous. One has only to remember the talk of "suppressor strips", reverberating circuits, or electrical field effects. This last notion was taken so seriously that no less a figure than our laureate-colleague Roger Sperry had had to put it to rest, in 1955, by dicing up the cortex with mica plates to insulate the subdivisions, and by skewering it with tantalum wire to short out the fields, neither of which procedures seriously impaired cortical function (7, 8). Nevertheless the idea of ephaptic interactions was slow to die out. There were even doubts as to the existence of topographic representation, which was viewed by some as a kind of artifact. One study, in which a spot of light projected anywhere in the retina evoked potentials all over the visual cortex, was interpreted as a refutation of topographic representation, but the result almost certainly came from working with a dark-adapted cat and a spot so bright that it scattered light all over the retina. It is surprising, in retrospect, that ideas of nonlocalization could survive in the face of the masterly mapping of visual fields onto the cortex in rabbit, cat and monkey done by Talbot and Marshall far back in 1941 (4).

It took us months to convince ourselves that we weren't at the mercy of some optical artifact, such as anyone can produce by squinting one's eyes and making vertical rays emanate from street lights. We didn't want to make fools of ourselves quite so early in our careers. But recording in sequence in the same penetration several cells with several different optimal orientations would, I think, have convinced anyone. By January we were ready to take the cells we thought we could understand (we later called them "simple cells") and

write them up. Then as always what guided and sustained us was the attitude of Stephen Kuffler, who never lectured or preached but simply reacted with buoyant enthusiasm whenever he thought we had found something interesting, and acted vague and noncommittal when he found something dull. Neither of us will ever forget writing our first abstract, for the International Congress of Physiology in 1959 (9). We labored over it, and finally gave a draft to Kuffler. The following day when I came in Torsten was looking more glum than usual, and said "I don't think Steve much liked our abstract". It was clear enough that Kuffler wasn't quite satisfied: his comments and suggestions contained more words than our original (Fig 2)! Writing, it may be added, did not come easy to either of us at the beginning, and our first paper, in 1959, (10) went through eleven complete reworkings.

HIERARCHY OF VISUAL CELLS

During the years 1959–62, first at the Wilmer Institute and then at Harvard Medical School, we were mainly concerned with comparing responses of cells in the lateral geniculate body and primary visual cortex of the cat. In the lateral geniculate we quickly confirmed my Walter Reed finding that the receptive fields are like those of retinal ganglion cells in having an antagonistic concentric center-surround organization. But now we could compare directly the responses of a geniculate cell with those of a fiber from an afferent retinal ganglion cell, and we found that in geniculate cells the power of the receptive-field surround to cancel the input from the center was increased. This finding was subsequently confirmed and extended in a beautiful set of experiments by Cleland, Dubin and Levick (11), and for many years remained the only known function of the lateral geniculate body.

In the cat striate cortex it soon became evident that cells were more complex than geniculate cells, and came in several degrees of complexity (12). One set of cells could be described by techniques similar to those used in the retina by Kuffler; we called these "simple". Their receptive fields, like the fields of retinal ganglion cells and of lateral geniculate cells, were subdivided into antagonistic regions illumination of any one of which tended to increase or decrease the rate of firing. But simple cells differed from retinal ganglion cells and lateral

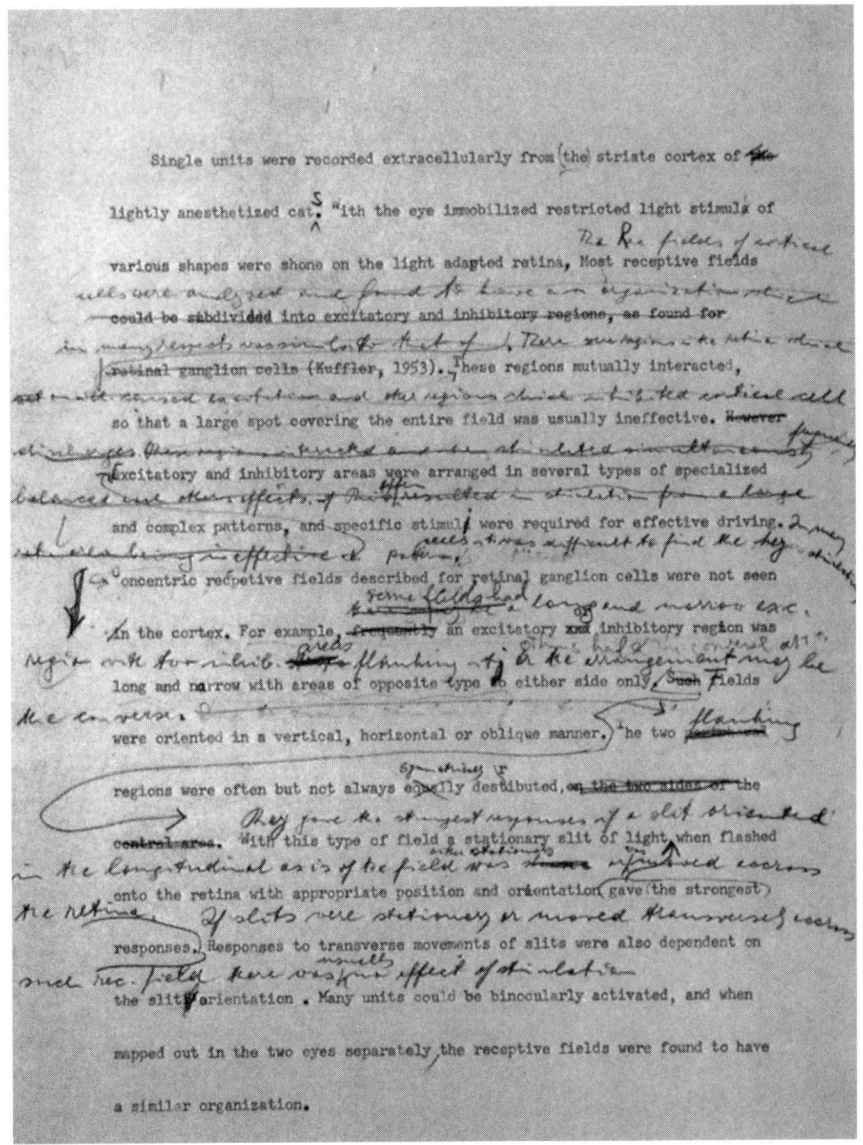

Fig. 2. First draft our first abstract (8), showing comments by Kuffler.

geniculate cells in the striking departure of their receptive fields from circular symmetry; instead of a single circular boundary between center and surround the antagonistic subdivisions were separated by parallel straight lines whose orientation (vertical, horizontal or oblique) soon emerged as a fundamental property (Fig. 3a). The optimal stimulus, either a slit, dark bar or edge, was easily predictable from the geometry of the receptive field, so that a stationary line stimulus worked optimally when its boundaries coincided with the boundaries of the subdivisions (Fig. 3c), and displacing the line to a new position parallel to the old one generally resulted in a sharp decline in the response. Perhaps most remarkable of all was the precise nature of the spatial distribution of excitatory and inhibitory effects: not only did diffuse light produce no response (as though the excitatory and inhibitory effects were mutually cancelling with the precision of an acid-base titration), but any line oriented at 90° to the optimal was also without effect, regardless of its position along the field, suggesting that

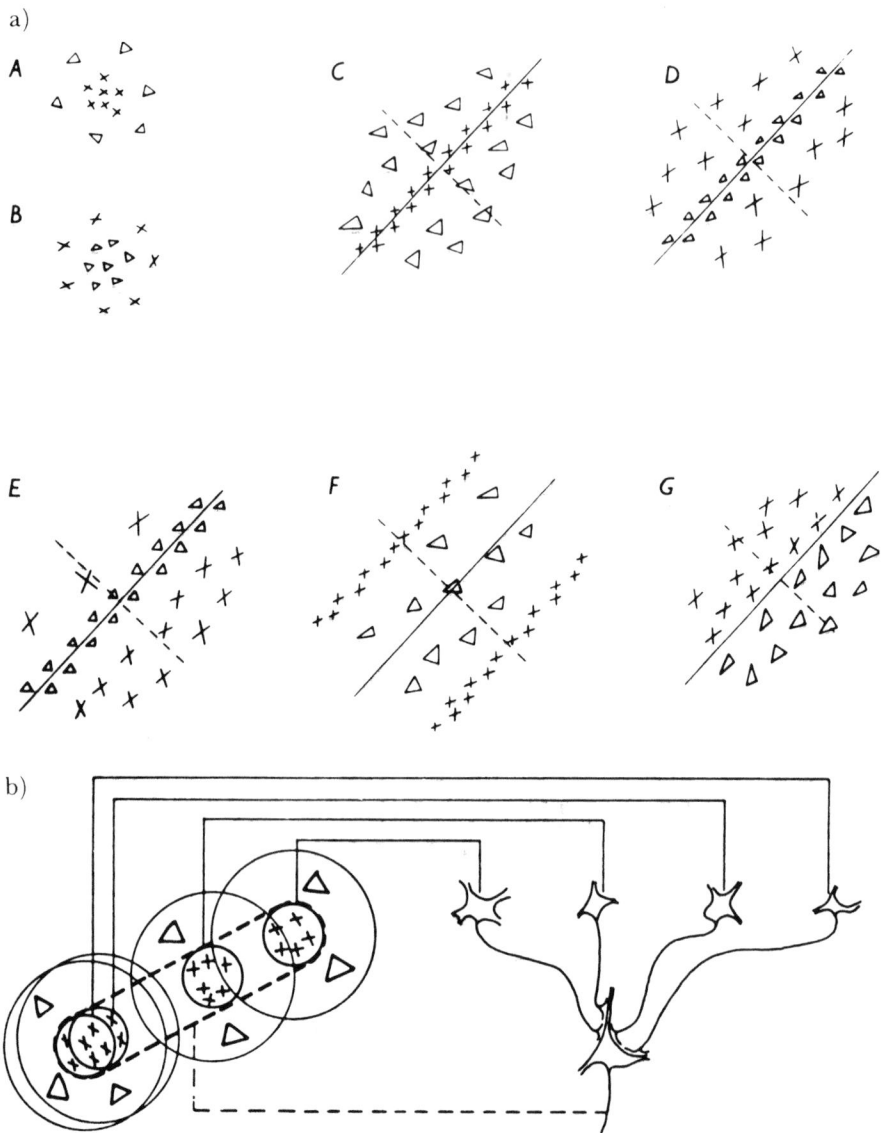

Fig. 3. a) *Common arrangement of lateral geniculate (A and B) and simple cortical (C–G) receptive fields. X, areas giving excitatory responses ('on' responses); △, areas giving inhibitory responses ('off responses). Receptive-filed orientations are shown by continuous lines through field centers; in the figure these are all oblique, but each arrangement occurs in all orientations (Figure 2 (12)).*

b) Possible scheme for explaining the organization of simple receptive fields. A large number of lateral geniculate cells, of which four are illustrated in the right in the figure, have receptive fields with 'on' centers arranged along a straight line on the retina. All of these project upon a single cortical cell, and the synapses are supposed to be excitatory. The receptive field of the cortical cell will then have an elongated 'on' center indicated by the interrupted lines in the receptive-field diagram to the left of the figure (Figure 19 (12)).

c) Responses to shining a rectangular slit of light 1 × 8°, so that center of slit is superimposed on center of receptive field, in various orientations, as shown. Receptive field is of type C (see part (a) of this figure), with axis vertically oriented (Figure 3 (10)).

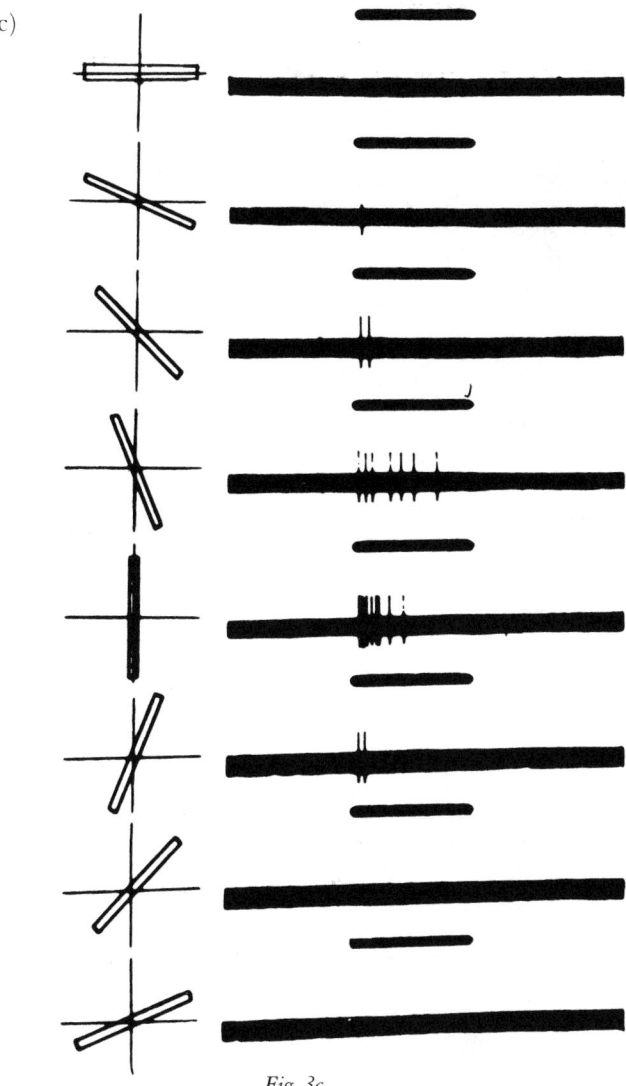

c)

Fig. 3c

the subpopulations of receptors so stimulated also had precisely mutually cancelling effects.

In the cat, simple cells are mostly found in layer IV, which is the site of termination of the bulk of the afferents from the lateral geniculate body. The exact connections that lead to orientation specificity are still not known, but it is easy to think of plausible circuits. For example, the behavior of one of the commonest kinds of simple cells may be explained by supposing that the cell receives convergent excitatory input from a set of geniculate cells whose on-centers are distributed in overlapping fashion over a straight line (Fig. 3b). In the monkey, the cells of Layer IVc (where most geniculate fibers terminate) seem all to be concentric

center-surround, and the simple cells are probably mainly in the layers immediately superficial to IVc. No one knows why this extra stage of center-surround cells is intercalated in the monkey's visual pathway.

The next set of cells we called "complex" because their properties cannot be derived in a single logical step from those of lateral geniculate cells (or, in the monkey, from the concentric cells of layer IVc). For the complex cell, compared to the simple cell, the position of an optimally oriented line need not be so carefully specified: the line works anywhere in the receptive field, evoking about the same response wherever it is placed (Fig. 4a). This can most easily be explained by supposing

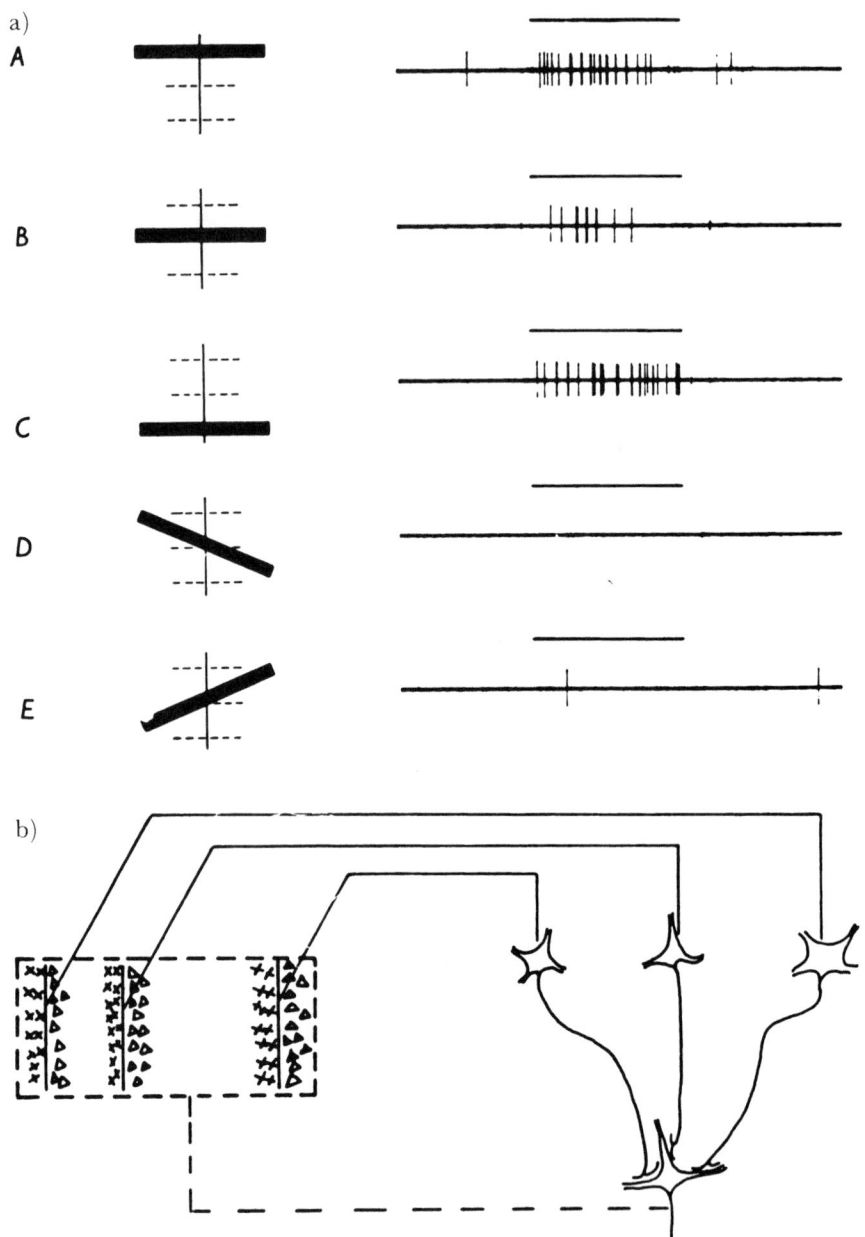

Fig. 4. a) *Complex cell responding best to a black horizontally oriented rectangle placed anywhere in the recep-*
tive field (A–C). Tilting the stimulus rendered it ineffective (D, E).

b) *Same cell, showing response to a moving horizontal bar, downward movement better than upward (A),*
and no response to a moving vertical bar (B). Time 1 sec. (Figures 7 and 8 (12)).

c) *Possible scheme for explaining the organization of complex receptive fields. A number of cells with sim-*
ple fields, of which three are shown schematically, are imagined to project to a single cortical cell of higher order.
Each projecting neuron has a receptive field arranged as shown to the left: an excitatory region to the left and an
inhibitory region to the right of a vertical straight-line boundary. The boundaries of the fields are staggered
within an area outlined by the interrupted lines. Any vertical-edge stimulus falling across this rectangle, regard-
less of its position, will excite some simple-field cells, leading to excitation of the higher-order cell. (Figure 20
(12)).

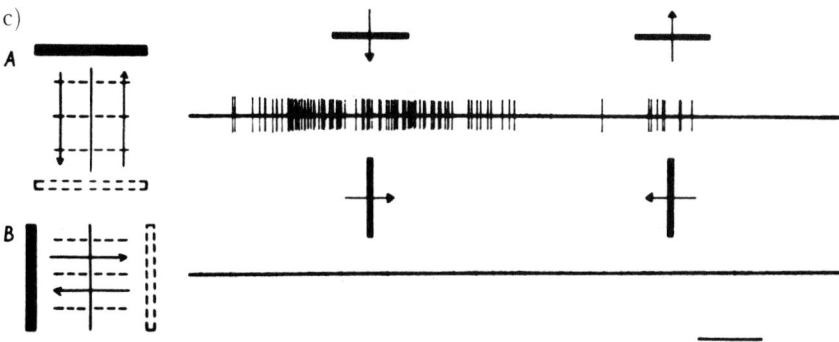

Fig. 4c

that the complex cell receives inputs from many simple cells, all of whose receptive fields have the same orientation but differ slightly in position (Fig. 4b). Sharpness of tuning for orientation varies from cell to cell, but the optimal orientation of a typical complex cell in layer II or III in the monkey can be easily determined to the nearest 5–10°, with no more equipment than a slide projector.

For a complex cell, a properly oriented line produces especially powerful responses when it is swept across the receptive field (Fig. 4c). The discharge is generally well sustained as long as the line keeps moving, but falls off quickly if the stimulus is stationary. About half of the complex cells fire much better to one direction of movement than to the opposite direction, a quality, called "directional selectivity", which probably cannot be explained by any simple projection of simple cells onto complex cells, but seems to require inhibitory connections with time delays of the sort proposed by Barlow and Levick for rabbit retinal ganglion cells (13).

HYPERCOMPLEX CELLS

Many cells, perhaps 10–20% in area 17 of cat or monkey, respond best to a line (a slit, edge or dark bar) of limited length; when the line is prolonged in one direction or both, the response falls off. This is called "end stopping". In some cells the response to a very long line fails completely (Fig. 5) (14). We originally called these cells "hypercomplex" because we looked upon them as next in an ordered hierarchical series, after simple and complex. We saw hypercomplex cells first in areas 18 and 19 of the cat, and only later in area 17. Dreher subse-

quently found cells, in all other ways resembling simple cells, that showed a similar fall-off in response as the length of the stimulus exceeded some optimum (15). It seems awkward to call these cells hypercomplex; they are probably better termed "simple end-stopped" in contrast to "complex end-stopped".

Complex cells come in a wide variety of subtypes. Typical cells of layer II and III have relatively small receptive fields, low spontaneous activity, and in the monkey may not only be highly orientation selective but also fussy about wave length, perhaps responding to red lines but not white. They may or may not be end-stopped. Cells in layers V and VI have larger fields. Those in V have high spontaneous activity and many respond just as well to a very short moving line as to long one. Many cells in layer VI respond best to very long lines (16). These differences are doubtless related to the important fact, first shown with physiologic techniques by Toyama, Matsunami and Ohno (17) and confirmed and extended by anatomical techniques, that different layers project to different destinations—the upper layers mainly to other cortical regions, the fifth layer to the superior colliculus, pons and pulvinar, and VI back to the lateral geniculate body and to the claustrum.

In the last 10 or 15 years the subject of cortical receptive-field types has become rather a jungle, partly because the terms 'simple' and 'complex' are used differently by different people, and undoubtedly partly because the categories themselves are not cleanly separated. Our idea originally was to emphasize the tendency toward increased complexity as one moves centrally along the visual

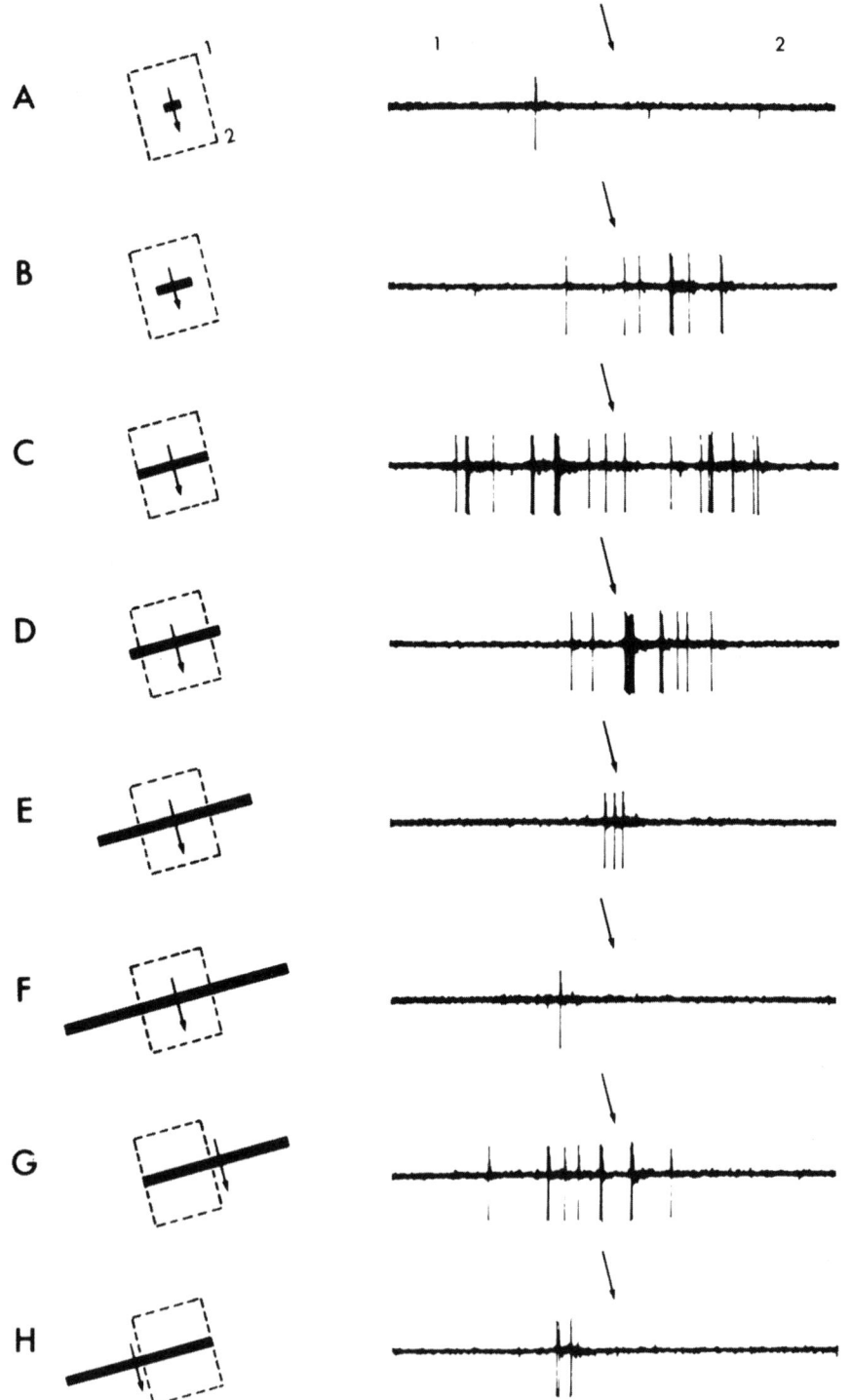

Fig. 5. Hypercomplex cell, responding to a black bar oriented 2:30–8:30, moving downward. Optimum response occurred when stimulus swept over area outlined (C); stimulating more than this region (D–H) or less (A, B) resulted in a weaker response. Sweep duration 2.5 sec. (Figure 19 (14)).

path, and the possibility of accounting for a cell's behavior in terms of its inputs. The circuit diagrams we proposed were just a few examples from a number of plausible possibilities. Even today the actual circuit by which orientation specificity is derived from center-surround cells is not known, and indeed the techniques necessary for solving this may still not be available. One can nevertheless say that cells of different complexities, whose receptive fields are in the same part of the visual field and which have the same optimal orientation, are likely to be interconnected, whereas cells with different optimal orientations are far less likely to be interconnected. In the monkey a major difficulty with the hierarchical scheme as outlined here is the relative scarcity of simple cells, compared with the huge numbers of cells with concentric fields in IVc, or compared with the large number of complex cells above and below layer IV. The fact that the simple cells have been found mainly in layer IVb also agrees badly with Jennifer Lund's finding that layer IVcβ projects not to layer IVb but to layer III. One has to consider the possibility that in the monkey the simple-cell step may be skipped, perhaps by summing the inputs from cells in layer IV on dendrites of complex cells. In such a scheme each main dendritic branch of a complex cell would perform the function of a simple cell. All such speculation serves only to emphasize our ignorance of the exact way in which the properties of complex cells are built up.

Knowing how cortical cells respond to some visual stimuli and ignore others allows us to predict how a cell will react to any given visual scene. Most cortical cells respond poorly to diffuse light, so that when I gaze at a white object on a dark background, say an egg, I know that those cells in my area 17 whose receptive fields fall entirely within the boundaries of the object will be unaffected. Only the fields that are cut by the borders of the egg will be influenced, and then only if the local orientation of a border is about the same as the orientation of the receptive field. A slight change in position of the egg without changing its orientation will produce a dramatic change in the population of activated simple cells, but a much smaller change in the activated complex cells.

Orientation-specific simple or complex cells "detect" or are specific for the direction of a short line segment. The cells are thus best not thought of

as "line detectors": they are no more line detectors than they are curve detectors. If our perception of a certain line or curve depends on simple or complex cells it presumably depends on a whole set of them, and how the information from such sets of cells is assembled at subsequent stages in the path, to build up what we call "percepts" of lines or curves (if indeed anything like that happens at all), is still a complete mystery.

ARCHITECTURE

When I began my training in neurophysiology at Walter Reed I was lucky enough to be influenced by new and vigorous traditions of experimental neuroanatomy, represented by Walle Nauta, and by a new blend of neuroanatomy and neurophysiology represented at Walter Reed, Johns Hopkins, and the National Institutes of Health by (among others) Jerzy Rose, Vernon Mountcastle, and Robert Galambos. One day very near the beginning of my term at Walter Reed, Jerzy Rose, on the steps of the Research Institute, very sternly told me that I had better make it my business to know exactly where my recording electrode was. I subsequently began to use the Hopkins—Walter Reed technique of making one electrode track or several parallel tracks through cortex, recording as many cells as possible in each track and then reconstructing the tracks from the histology. This made it possible to work out the response properties of single cells and also to learn how they were grouped. It was put to use most dramatically by Vernon Mountcastle, whose discovery of columns in the somatosensory cortex was surely the single most important contribution to the understanding of cerebral cortex since Cajal. Our addition to the reconstruction technique was the strategy of making multiple small (roughly 100 μm diameter) electrolytic lesions along each track by passing small currents through the tungsten electrodes. I worked out this method at Walter Reed by watching the coagulation produced at the electrode tip on passing currents through egg white. The lesions made it possible to be sure of the positions of at least several points along a track; other positions were determined by interpolating depth readings of the microelectrode advancer.

By the early 1960s our research had extended into four different but overlapping areas. Closest to conventional neurophysiology was the working out of response properties (i.e. receptive fields) of single cells. We became increasingly involved with architecture, the grouping of cells according to function into layers and columns, studied by track reconstructions. This led in turn to experiments in which single-cell recording was combined with experimental anatomy. It began when one day James Sprague called to tell us that his chief histological technician, Jane Chen, was moving to Boston and needed a job: could we take her? Luckily we did, and so, despite our not possessing anatomical union cards, we acquired an expert in the Nauta method of making lesions in nervous tissue and selectively staining the degenerating axons. It seemed a terrible waste not to use this method and we soon got the idea of working out detailed pathways by making microelectrode lesions that were far smaller than conventional lesions and could be precisely placed by recording with the same electrodes. It became possible to make lesions in single layers of the lateral geniculate body, with results to be discussed shortly. Finally, still another phase of our work involved studies of newborn animals' postnatal development, and the effects of distorting normal sensory experience in young animals. This began in 1962 and grew steadily. Torsten Wiesel will discuss these experiments.

Having mentioned Jane Chen, this is perhaps as good a place as any to acknowledge our tremendous debt to many research assistants who have helped us over the past 22 years, especially to Jane and to Janet Wiitanen and Bea Storai, and also to Jaye Robinson, Martha Egan, Joan Weisenbeck, Karen Larson, Sharon Mates, Debra Hamburger, Yu-Wen Wu, Sue Fenstemaker, Stella Chow, Sarah Kennedy, Maureen Packard and Mary Nastuk. For photographic assistance I am grateful to Sandra Spinks, Carolyn Yoshikami and Marc Peloquin. In electronics and computers David Freeman has continued to amaze us with his wizardry for 12 years. And for secretarial help and preservation of morale and sanity I want to thank Sheila Barton, Pat Schubert and Olivia Brum.

ORIENTATION COLUMNS

What our three simultaneously recorded cells, Nos. 3009, 3010 and 3011, mapped out on the overhead sheet in September 1958, with their parallel orientation axes and separate but overlapping field positions, were telling us was that neighboring cells have similar orientations but slightly different receptive-field positions. We of course knew about our visitor Mountcastle's somatosensory columns, and we began to suspect that cells might be grouped in striate cortex according to orientation; but to prove it was not easy.

Our first indication of the beauty of the arrangements of cell groupings came in 1961 in one of our first recordings from striate cortex of monkey, a spider monkey named George. In one penetration, which went into the cortex at an angle of about 45° and was 2.5 mm long, we were struck right away by something we had only seen hints of before: as the electrode advanced the orientations of successively recorded cells progressed in small steps, of about 10° for every advance of 50 μm. We began the penetration around 8:00 p.m.; five hours later we had recorded 53 successive orientations without a single large jump in orientation (Fig. 7). During the entire time, in which I wielded the slide projector and Torsten mapped the fields, neither of us moved from our seats. Fortunately our fluid intake that day had not been excessive! I have shown this illustration many times. So far only one person, Francis Crick, has asked why there was no interruption in layer IVc, where according to dogma the cells are not orientation-specific. The answer is that I don't know.

In the cat we had had occasional suggestions of similar orderliness, and so we decided to address directly the problem of the shape and arrangement of the groupings (18). By making several closely-spaced oblique parallel penetrations we convinced ourselves that the groupings were really columns in that they extended from surface to white matter and had walls that were perpendicular to the layers (Fig. 8). We next made multiple close-spaced penetrations, advancing the electrode just far enough in each penetration to record one cell or a group of cells. To map a few square mm of cortex this way required 50–100 penetrations, each of which took about 10–15 minutes. We decided it might be better to change careers, perhaps to chicken farming. But although the experiments were by our standards exhausting they did succeed in showing that orientation columns in the cat are not generally pillars but parallel slabs that intersect the surface either as straight parallel stripes or swirls (Fig. 9).

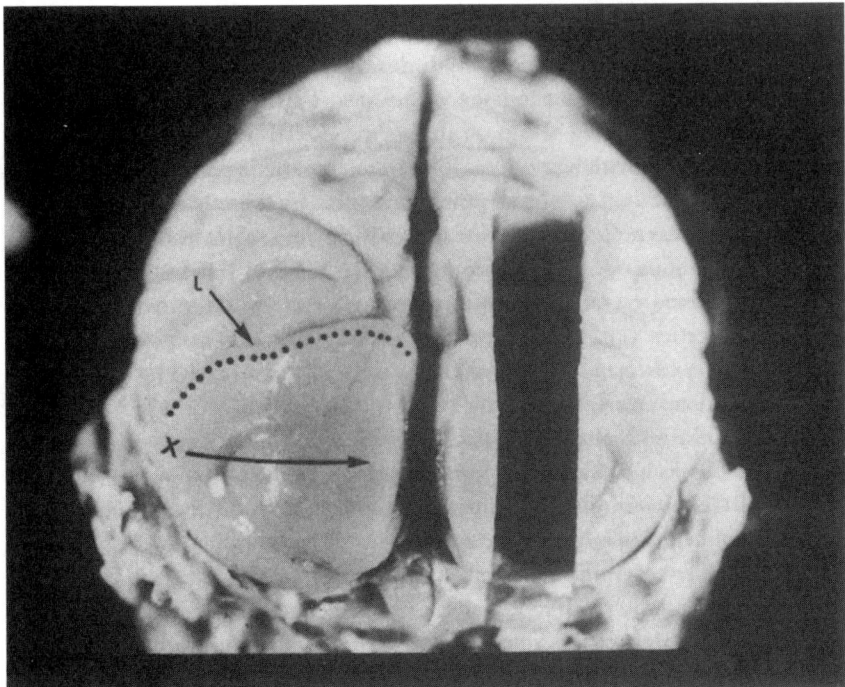

Fig. 6. a) *Brain of a macaque monkey, perfused with formalin, viewed from above and behind. The occipital lobe is demarcated in front by the lunate sulcus (L) and consists mainly of the striate cortex, area 17, which occupies most of the smooth surface, extending forward to the dotted line (the 17–18 border). If followed medially area 17 curves around the medial surface of the brain and continues in a complex buried fold, a part of which lies underneath the convexity and parallel to it. X marks the projection of the fovea; movement in the direction of the arrow corresponds to movement along the horizon; movement along the dotted line, to movement down along the vertical midline of the visual field. The brain on removal from the skull does not, of course, look exactly like this: the groove in the right hemisphere was made by removing a parasagittal block of tissue to produce the cross section of Figure 6b. (Figure 6a (29)).*

6b) Low power Nissl-stained section from a parasagittal block such as that of Figure 6a. It is what would be seen if one could stand in the groove of 6a and look to the left. A marks the outer convexity; B the buried fold, and arrows indicate the 17–18 borders, the upper right one of which is indicated by the dotted line in Figure 6a. (Figure 6b (29)).

6c) Cross section through monkey striate cortex showing conventional layering designations. W, white matter. Deeper layers (VI, V) of the buried fold of cortex are shown in the lower part of the figure (compare Figure 6b). Cresyl violet. (Figure 10 (29)).

Reversals in direction of orientation shift, like those shown in Fig. 7, are found in most penetrations. They occur irregularly, on the average about once every millimeter, and not at any particular orientation such as vertical or horizontal. We still do not know how to interpret them. Between reversals the plots of orientation vs. electrode position are remarkably linear (19). I once, to exercise a new programmable calculator, actually determined the *coefficient of linear correlation* of such a graph. It was 0.998, which I took to mean that the line must be very straight indeed.

For some years we had the impression that regular sequences like the one shown in Fig. 7 are rare—that most sequences are either more or less random or else the orientation hovers around one angle for some distance and then goes to a new angle and hovers there. Chaos and hovering do occur but they are exceptional, as are major jumps of 45–90°. It took us a long time to realize that reg-

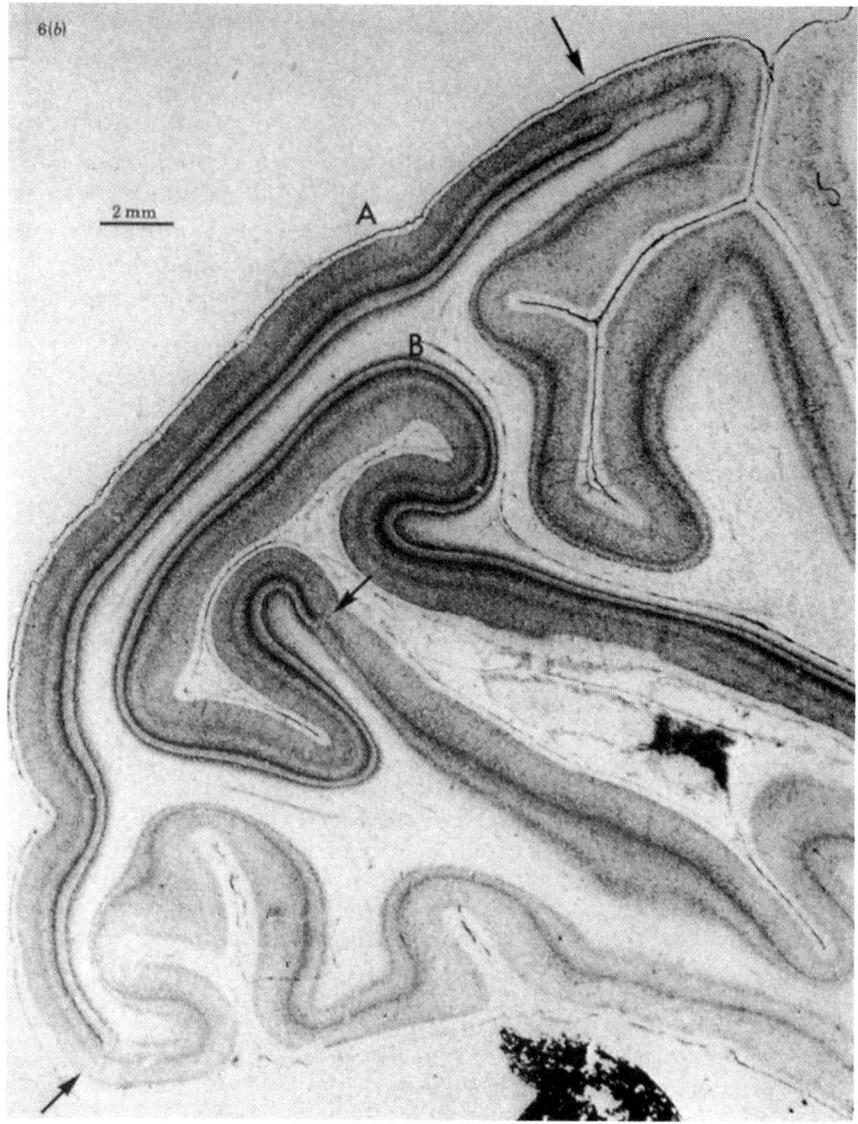

Fig. 6b

ularity is the rule, not the exception, probably because only around the mid-1970s did we begin making very oblique or tangential penetrations. Also for these experiments to be successful requires electrodes coarse enough to record activity throughout a penetration, and not simply every 100 μm or so. Such electrodes look less aesthetically pleasing, a fact that I think has happily tended to keep down competition.

Our attempts to learn more about the geometry of orientation columns in the monkey by using the 2-deoxyglucose technique (20) suggest that iso-orientation lines form a periodic pattern but are far from straight, being full of swirls and interruptions. Experiments done since then (21) suggest that the deoxyglucose is possibly also labelling the cytochrome blobs (see below). Similar work in the tree shrew by Humphrey (22) has shown a much

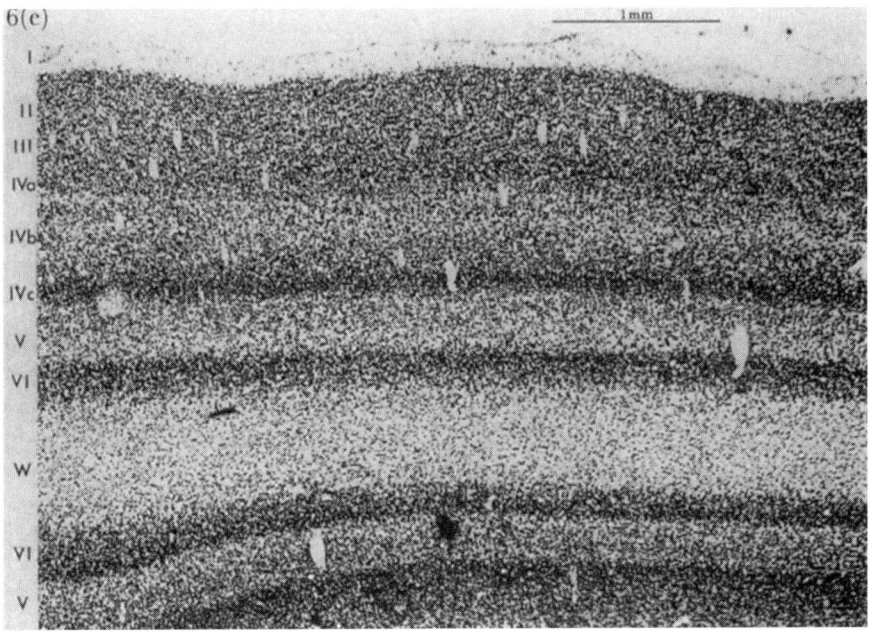

Fig. 6c

more regular pattern and Stryker, Wiesel and I have seen more regularity in the cat (unpublished). Both tree shrew and cat lack the cytochrome blobs.

OCULAR DOMINANCE COLUMNS

A major finding in our 1959 and 1962 papers (10, 12), besides the orientation selectivity, was the presence in the striate cortex of a high proportion of binocular cells. Since recordings from the lateral geniculate body had made it clear that cells at that stage are for all practical purposes monocular, this answered the question of where, in the retino-geniculocortical pathway, cells first received convergent input from the two eyes. More interesting to us than the mere binocularity was the similarity of a given cell's receptive fields in the two eyes, in size, complexity, orientation and position. Presumably this forms the basis of the fusion of the images in the two eyes. It still seems remarkable that a cell should not only be wired with the precision necessary to produce complex or hypercomplex properties, but should have a duplicate set of such connections, one from each eye. (That this is hard wired at birth will form some of the material for Torsten Wiesel's lecture.) Though the optimum stimulus is

the same for the two eyes, the responses evoked are not necessarily equal; for a given cell one eye is often better than the other. It is as if the two sets of connections were qualitatively similar but, for many cells, different in density. We termed this relative effectiveness of the two eyes "eye preference" or "relative ocular dominance".

In the macaque it was evident from the earliest experiments that neighboring cells have similar eye preferences. In vertical penetrations the preference remains the same all the way through the cortex. Layer IVc, in which cells are monocular, is an exception; here the eye that above and below layer IV merely dominates the cells actually monopolizes them. In penetrations that run parallel to the layers there is an alternation of eye preference, with shifts roughly every 0.5 mm. The conclusion is that the terminals from cells of the lateral geniculate distribute themselves in layer IVc according to eye of origin, in alternating patches about 0.5 mm wide. In the layers above and below layer IV horizontal and diagonal connections lead to a mixing that is incomplete, so that a cell above a given patch is dominated by the eye supplying that patch but receives subsidiary input from neighboring patches (Fig. 10).

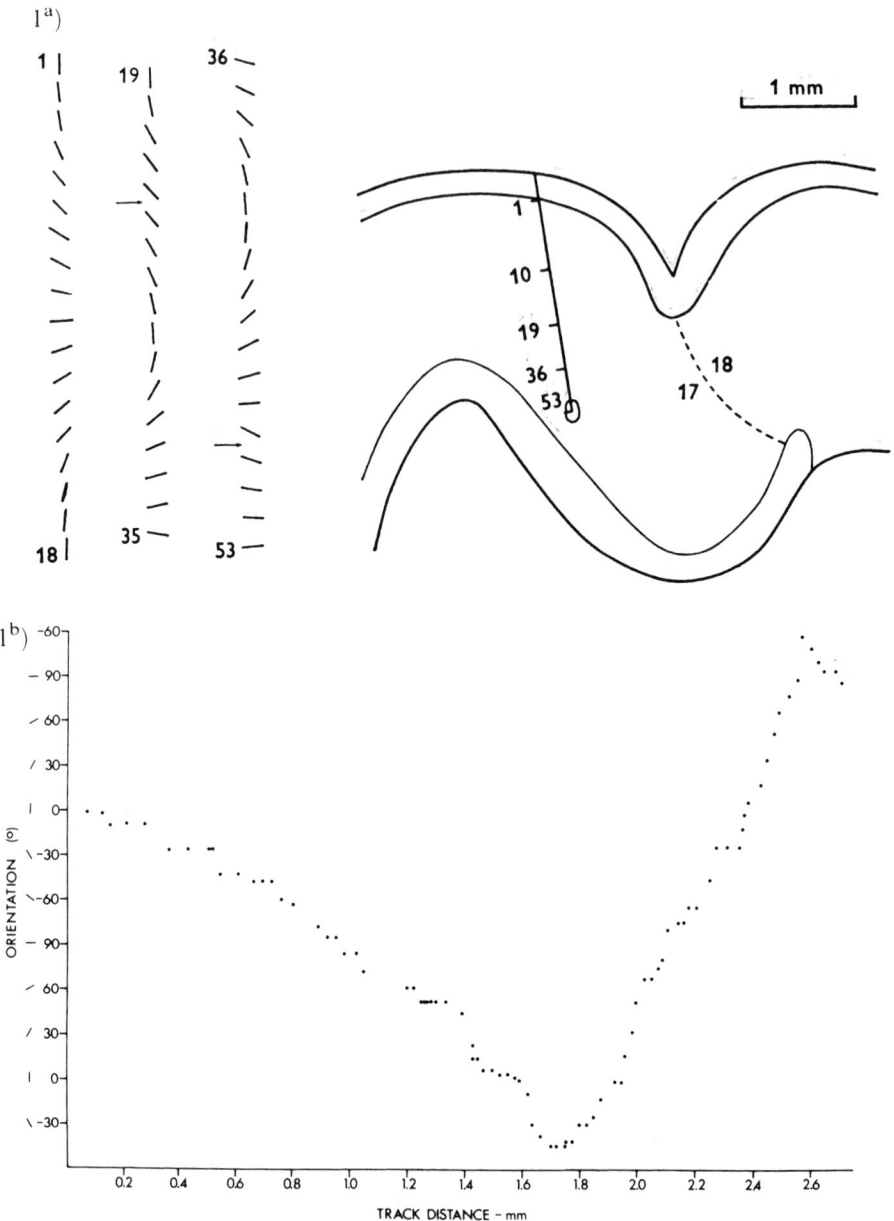

Fig. 7. a) *Reconstruction of a penetration through striate cortex about 1 mm from 17–18 border, near occipital pole of a spider monkey called George. To the left of the figure the lines indicate receptive-field orientations of cells in the columns traversed; each line represents one or several units recorded against a rich unresolved background activity. Arrows indicate reversal of directions of shifts in orientation (32).*

b) *Graph of stimulus orientation in degrees vs. distance along electrode track in mm, in the experiment shown in (a). Vertical is taken as 0°, clockwise is positive, anticlockwise negative.*

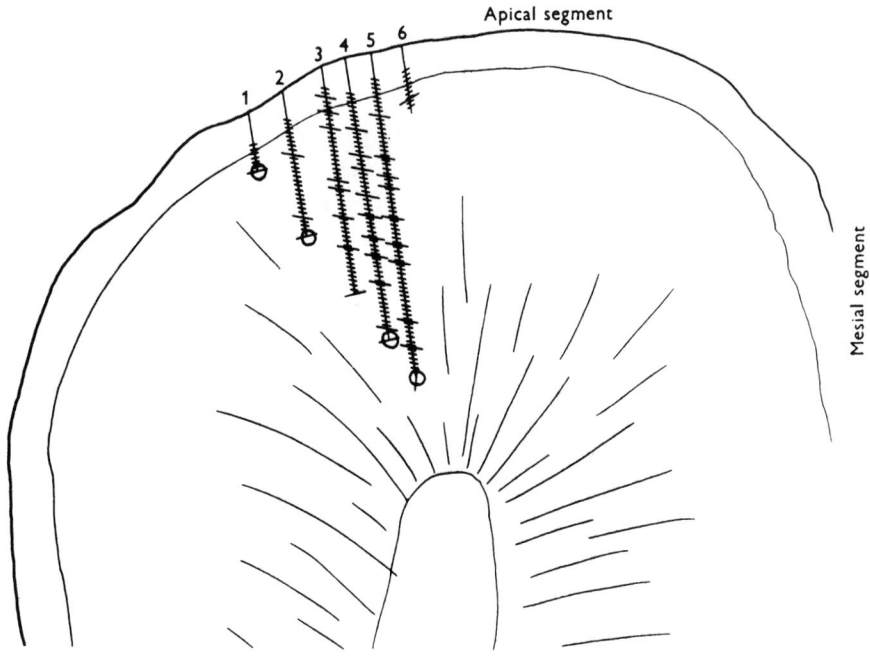

Fig. 8. Coronal section through cat visual cortex showing reconstructions of 6 parallel microelectrode penetrations. (Nos. 1, 2, 4 and 5 end with lesions shown as circles.) Short lines perpendicular to tracks indicate receptive-field orientation; lines perpendicular to tracks represent horizontal orientation. (The longer of these lines represent single cells, the shorter ones, multiple unit recordings). Most of the territory traversed by penetrations 2–5 is in one orientation column, whose left hand border lies at the ends of tracks 2–4. Scale 1 mm. (Figure 2 (18)).

The geometry of these layer-IV patches interested us greatly, and was finally determined by several independent anatomical methods, the first of which involved the Nauta method and modifications of the Nauta method for staining terminals worked out first by Fink and Heimer and then by a most able and energetic research assistant, Janet Wiitanen (23). By making small lesions in single geniculate layers we were able to see the patchy distribution of degenerating terminals in layer IV, which in a face-on view takes the form not of circumscribed patches but of parallel stripes. We also showed that the ventral (magnocellular) pair of layers projects to the upper half of IVc, (subsequently called IVc α by Jennifer Lund), whereas the dorsal 4 layers project to the lower half (IVc β), and that the line of Gennari (IVb), once thought to

receive the strongest projection, is actually almost bereft of geniculate terminals.

While the Nauta studies were still in progress we read a paper in which Bernice Grafstein reported that after injecting a radioactive aminoacid into the eye of a rat, radioactive label could be detected in the contralateral visual cortex, as though transneuronal transport had taken place in the geniculate (24). (The rat retinogeniculocortical pathway is mainly crossed.) It occurred to us that if we injected the eye of a monkey we might be able to see label autoradiographically in area 17. We tried it, but could see nothing. Soon after, while visiting Ray Guillery in Wisconsin, I saw some aminoacid transport autoradiographs which showed nothing in light field but in which label was perfectly obvious in dark field. I rushed back, we got

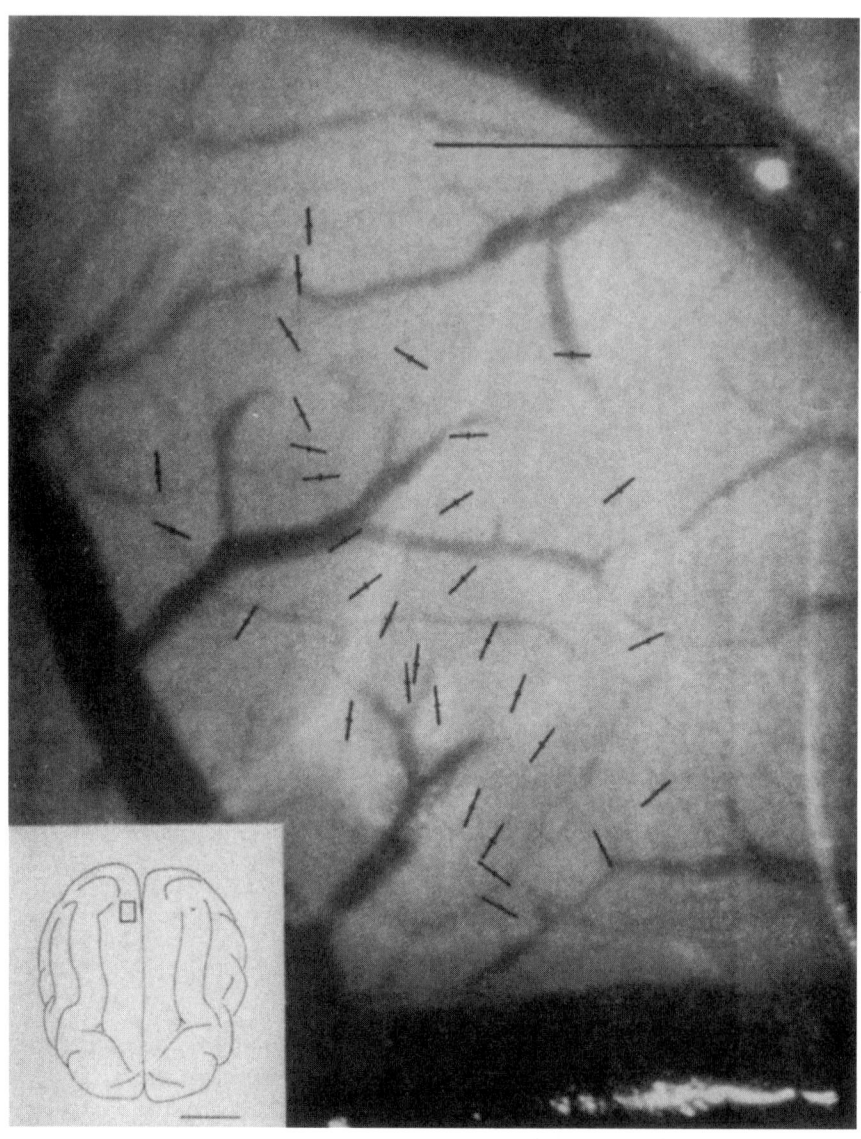

Fig. 9. Surface map of a small region of cat visual cortex. Receptive field orientations are shown for 32 superficial penetrations. Regions of relatively constant orientation run more or less right-to-left in the figure, or mediolateral on the brain (see inset). Going from above down, in the figure, or from posterior to anterior of the brain, is associated with anticlockwise rotation. Scale 1 mm; inset scale 1 cm. (Plate 2 (18)).

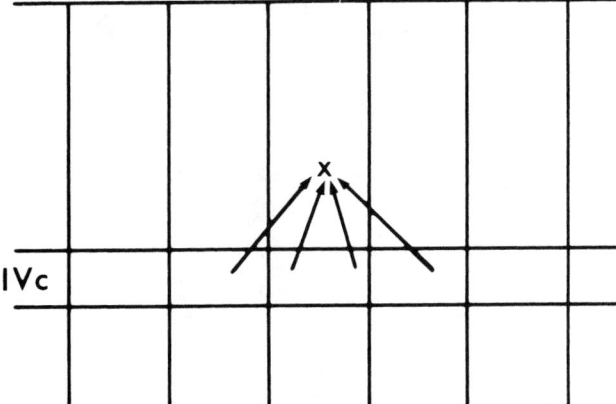

Fig. 10. Scheme to illustrate the wiring of a binocular cell in a layer above (or below) layer IVc. The bulk of the afferents to the striate cortex from the lateral geniculate body, themselves monocular, are in the macaque monkey strictly segregated by eye affiliation in layer IVc, and thus the cells in this layer are strictly monocular. A cell outside of IVc, labelled X in the diagram, receives its input connections, directly or indirectly by one or more synapses, from cells in IVc (to some extent also, perhaps, from layers IVa and VI). Cells in IVc will be more likely to feed into X the closer they are to it; consequently X is likely to be binocular, dominated by the eye corresponding to the nearest patch in IVc. The degree of dominance by that eye is greater, the closer X is to being centered in its ocular dominance column, and cells near a boundary may be roughly equally influenced by the two eyes. (Figure 12 (29)).

out our slides, borrowed a dark-field condenser, and found beautiful alternating patches throughout all the binocular part of area 17 (25) (Fig. 11). This method allowed us to reconstruct ocular dominance columns over much wider expanses than could be mapped with the Nauta method (Fig. 12). It led to a study of the pre- and postnatal visual development of ocular dominance columns, and the effects of visual deprivation on the columns, which Torsten will describe.

RELATIONSHIP BETWEEN COLUMNS, MAGNIFICATION AND FIELD SIZE

To me the main pleasures of doing science are in getting ideas for experiments, doing surgery, designing and making equipment, and above all the rare moments in which some apparently isolated facts click into place like a Chinese puzzle. When a collaboration works, as ours has, the ideas and the clicking into place often occur simultaneously or collaboratively; usually neither of us has known (or cared) exactly where or from whom

ideas came from, and sometimes one idea has occurred to one of us, only to be forgotten and later resurrected by the other. One of the most exciting moments was the realization that our orientation columns, extending through the full thickness of the cat cortex, contain just those simple and complex cells (later we could add the hypercomplex) that our hierarchical schemes had proposed were interconnected (12). This gave the column a meaning: a little machine that takes care of contours in a certain orientation in a certain part of the visual field. If the cells of one set are to be interconnected, and to some extent isolated from neighboring sets, it makes obvious sense to gather them together. As Lorente de Nó showed (26), most of the connections in the cortex run in an up-and-down direction; lateral or oblique connections tend to be short (mostly limited to 1 to 2 mm) and less rich. These ideas were not entirely new, since Mountcastle had clearly enunciated the principle of the column as an independent unit of function. What was new in the visual cortex was a clear function, the transformation of information from circularly symmetric

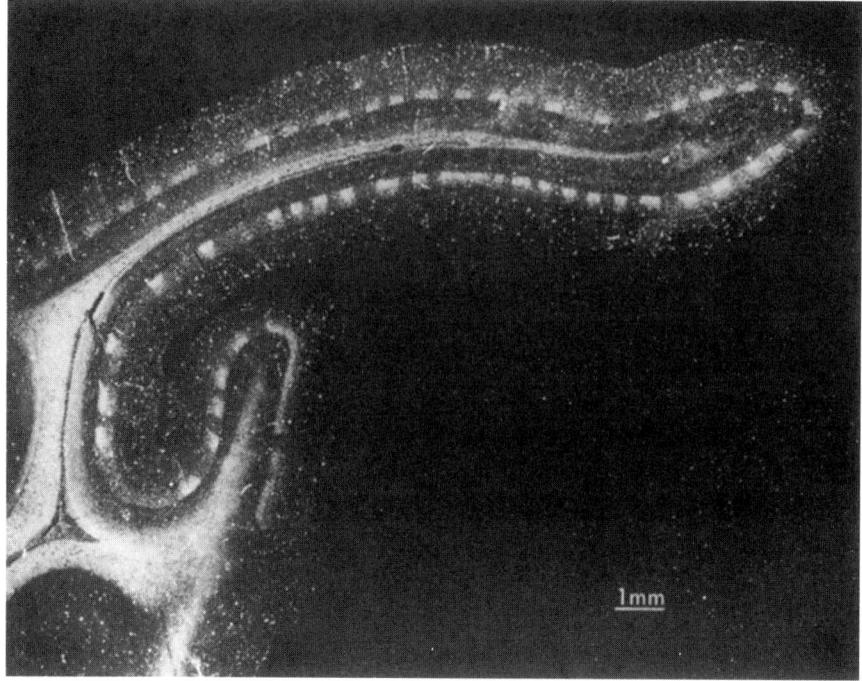

Fig. 11. Dark-field autoradiograph of striate cortex in an adult macaque in which the ipsilateral eye had been injected with tritiated proline-fucose 2 weeks before. Labelled areas show as white. Section passes in a plane roughly perpendicular to the exposed surface of the occipital lobe, and to the buried part immediately beneath (roughly, through the arrow of Figure 6a). In all, about 56 labelled patches can be seen. (Figure 22 (29)).

form to orientation-specific form, and the stepwise increase in complexity.

A similar argument applies to the ocular dominance columns, a pair of which constitutes a machine for combining inputs from the two eyes—combining, but not completely combining, in a peculiar grudging way and for reasons still not at all clear, but probably related in some way to stereopsis. (Whatever the explanation of the systematically incomplete blending, it will have to take into account the virtual but not complete absence of dominance columns in squirrel monkeys.) If the eyes are to be kept functionally to some extent separate, it is economical of connections to pack together cells of a given eye preference.

To my mind our most aesthetically attractive and exciting formulation has been the hypercolumn (not, I admit, a very attractive term!) and its relation to magnification. The idea grew up gradually, but took an initial spurt as a result of a question

asked by Werner Reichardt during a seminar that I gave in Tübingen. I had been describing the ordered orientation sequences found in monkeys like George, when Werner asked how one avoided the difficulty arising from the fact that as you move across the cortex visual field position is changing, in addition to orientation. Could this mean that if you looked closely you would find, in one small part of the visual field, only a small select group of orientations represented? The answer seemed obvious: I explained that in any one part of the visual field all orientations are represented, in fact probably several times over. Afterwards the question nagged me. There must be more to it than that. We began to put some seemingly isolated facts together. The visual fields map systematically onto the cortex but the map is distorted: the fovea is disproportionately represented, with 1 mm about equivalent to 1/6° of visual field. As one goes out in the visual field the representation falls off, logarithmically, as Daniel

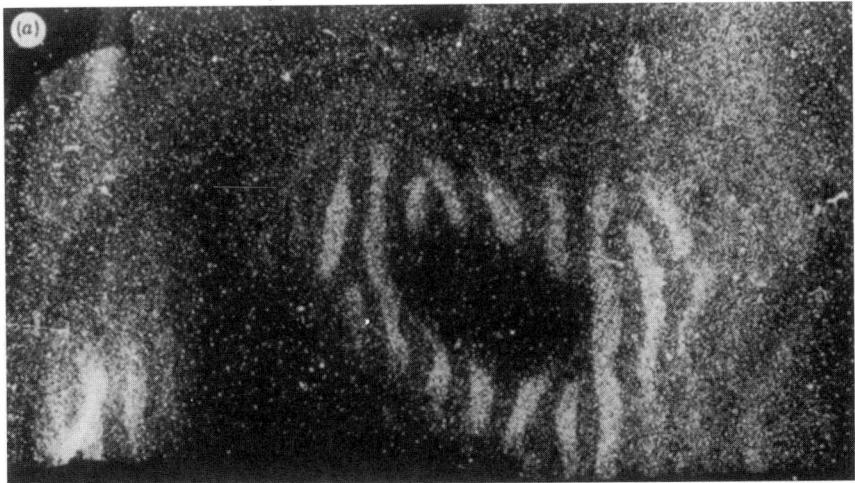

Fig. 12. Autoradioagraphs from the same (normal) animal as Figure 11, but hemisphere contralateral to the injected eye (dark field).

a) A section tangential to the exposed dome-like surface of the occipital lobe, just grazing layer V, which appears as an oval, surrounded by layer IVc, which appears as a ring containing the labelled parallel bands; these appear as light against the dark background.

b) A composite made by cutting out layer IVc from a number of parallel sections such as the one shown in (a), and pasting them together to show the bands over an area some millimeters in extent.

c) Reconstruction of layer IVc ocular dominance columns over the entire exposed part of area 17 in the right occipital lobe, made from a series of reduced-silver sections (33). The region represented is the same as the part of the right occipital lobe shown in Figure 6a. Dotted line on the left represents the midsagittal plane where the cortex bends around. Dashed c-shaped curve is the 17–18 border, whose apex, to the extreme right, represents the fovea. Every other column has been blackened in, so as to exhibit the twofold nature of the set of subdivisions. Note the relative constancy of column widths.

and Whitteridge had shown (27), so that in the far periphery the relationship is more like 1 mm = 6°. Meanwhile the average size of receptive fields grows from center of gaze to periphery. This is not unexpected when one considers that in the fovea our acuity is very much higher than in the periphery. To do the job in more detail takes more cells, each looking after a smaller region; to accommodate the cells takes more cortical surface area. I had always been surprised that the part of the cortex representing the fovea is not obviously thicker than that representing the periphery: the surprise, I suppose, comes from the fact that in the retina near the fovea the ganglion cell layer is many times thicker than in the periphery. The cortex must be going out of its way to keep its uniformity by devoting to the detailed tasks more area rather than more thickness.

We decided to look more carefully at the rela-tionship between receptive-field size and area of cortex per unit area of visual field (28). When an electrode is pushed vertically through the cortex and encounters a hundred or so cells in traversing the full thickness, the receptive fields vary to some extent in size, and in a rather random way in posi-tion, so that the hundred maps when superimposed cover an area several times that of an average receptive field (Fig. 13a). We call this the "aggre-gate receptive field" for a particular point on the cortex. On making a penetration parallel to the surface there is a gradual drift in field position, superimposed on the random staggering, in a direction dictated by the topographic map (Fig. 13b). We began to wonder whether there was any law connecting the rate of this drift in aggregate position and the size of the fields. It was easy to get a direct answer. It turned out that a movement of about 2 mm across the cortex is just sufficient to

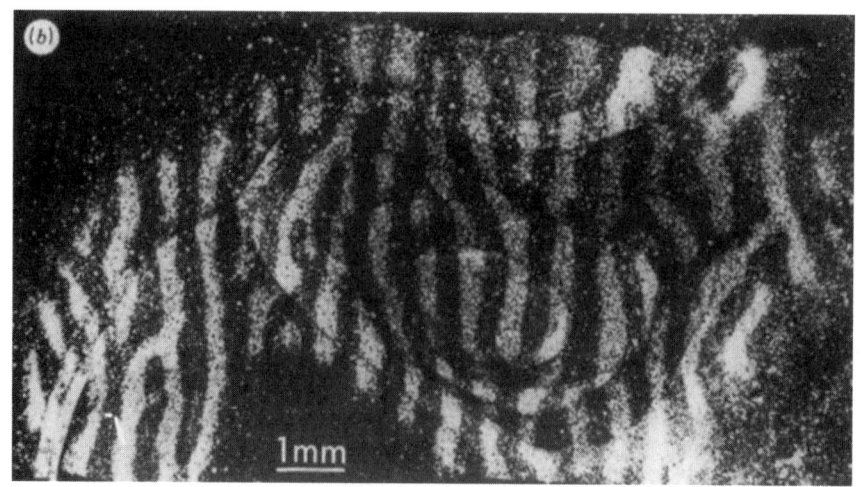

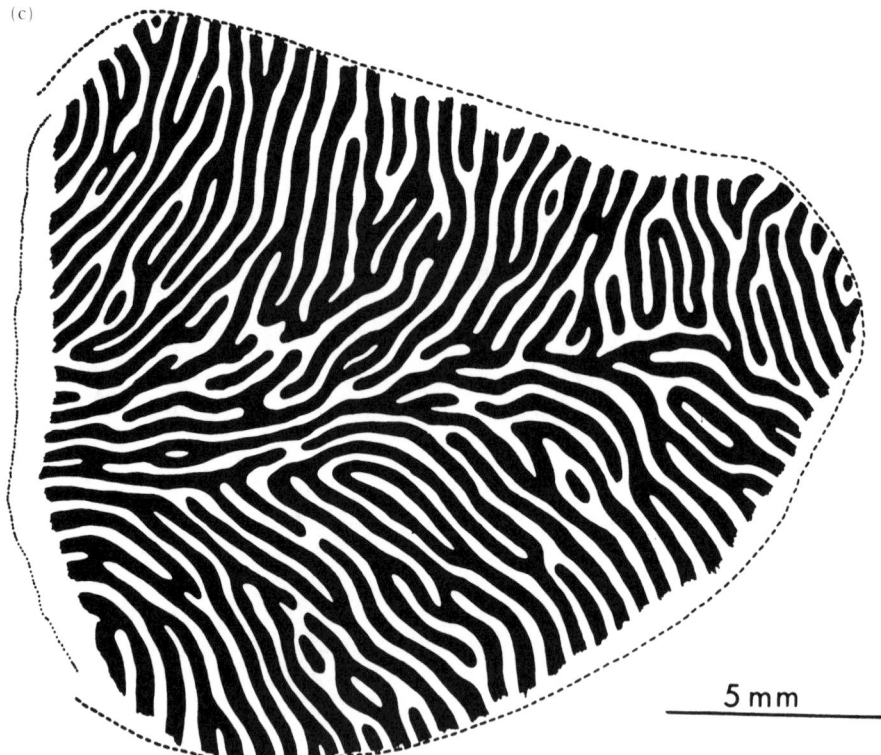

Fig. 12 b & c

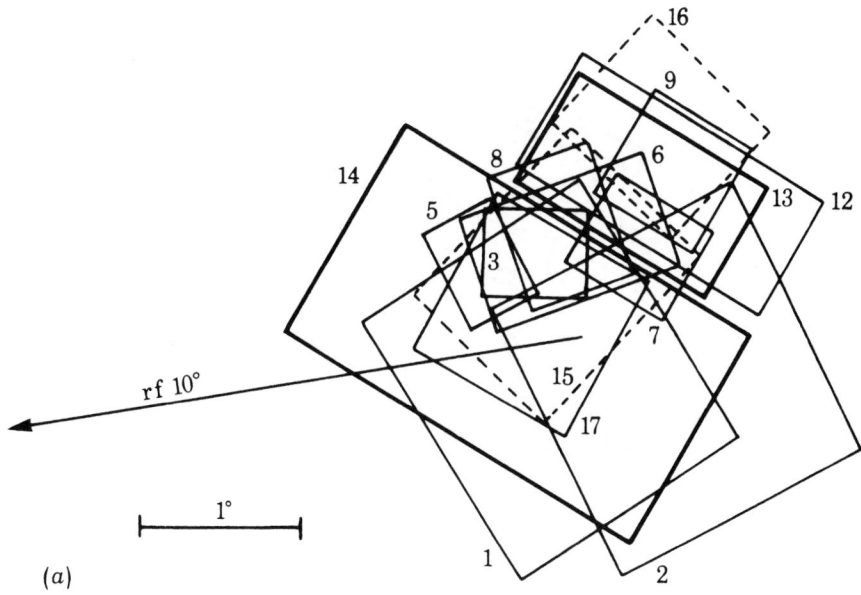

Fig. 13. a) *Receptive-field scatter: Receptive-field boundaries of 17 cells recorded in a penetration through monkey striate cortex in a direction perpendicular to the surface. Note the variation in size, and the more or less random scatter in the precise positions of the fields. The penetration was made in a part of the cortex corresponding to a visual field location 10° from the center of gaze, just above the horizontal meridian. Fields are shown for one eye only. Numbers indicate the order in which the cells were recorded. (Figure 1 (28)).*

b) See p. 682. Receptive-field drift: Receptive fields mapped during one oblique, almost tangential penetration through striate cortex, in roughly the same region as in (a). A few fields were mapped along each of four 100 μm segments, spaced at 1 mm intervals. These four groups of fields are labelled 0, 1, 2 and 3. Each new set of fields was slightly above the other, in the visual field, as predicted from the direction of movement of the electrode and from the topographic map of visual fields onto cortex. Roughly a 2 mm movement through cortex was required to displace the fields from one region to an entirely new region. (Figure 2 (28)).

produce a displacement, in the visual field, out of the region where one started and into an entirely new region. This held everywhere across the striate cortex (and consequently in the visual field). In the fovea the displacement was tiny and so were the fields. As one went out, both increased in size, in parallel fashion (Fig. 14). Now things indeed seemed to mesh. George and other monkeys had taught us that a 1–2 mm movement across cortex is accompanied by an angular shift in receptive-field orientation of 180–360°, more than one full complement of orientations. We have termed such a set of orientation columns (180°) a "hypercolumn". Meanwhile, the ocular dominance shifts back and forth so as to take care of both eyes every millimeter—a hypercolumn for ocular dominance. Thus

in one or two square millimeters there seems to exist all the machinery necessary to look after everything the visual cortex is responsible for, in a certain small part of the visual world. The machines are the same everywhere; in some parts the information on which they do their job is less detailed, but covers more visual field (Fig. 15).

Uniformity is surely a huge advantage in development, for genetic specifications need only be laid down for a 1–2 mm block of neural tissue, together with the instruction to make a thousand or so.

We could, incidentally, have called the entire machine a hypercolumn, but we did not. The term as we define it refers to a complete set of columns of one type. I mention this because uniformity has

(b)

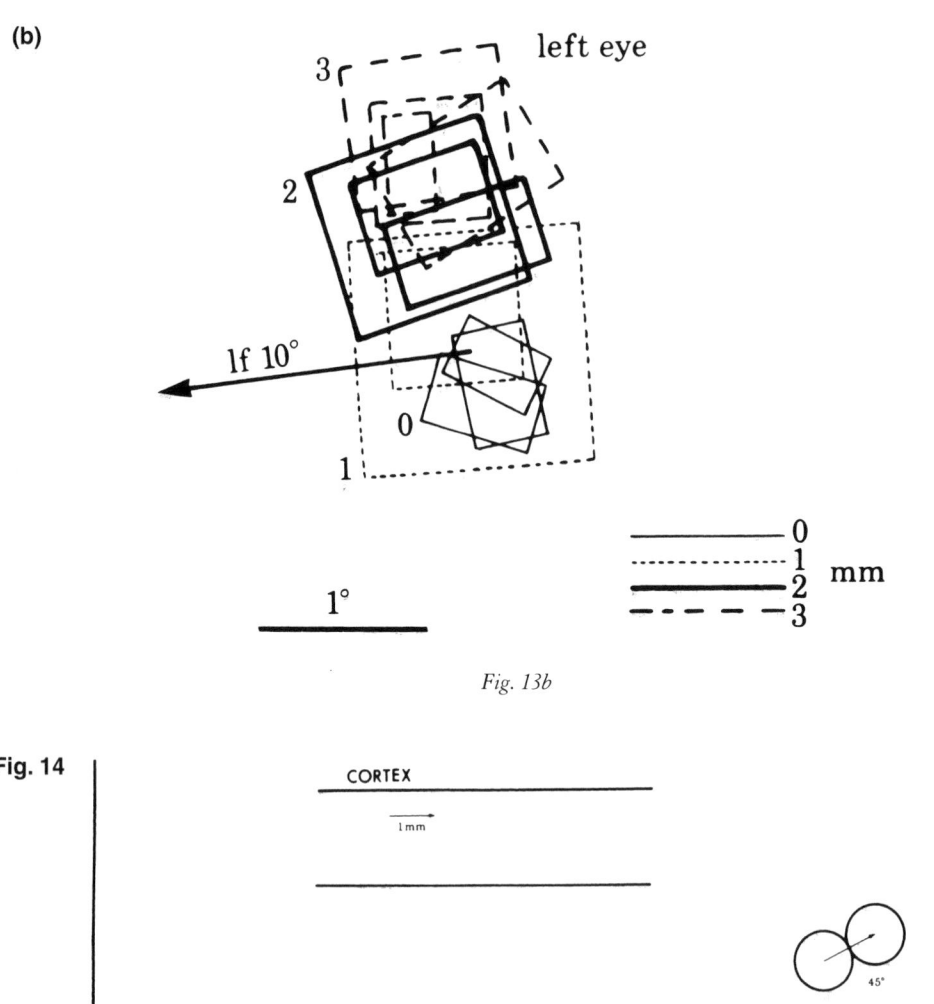

Fig. 13b

Fig. 14

Fig. 14. Variation of receptive-field drift with eccentricity: The diagram represents one quadrant of the field of vision, and the circles represent aggregate receptive fields, the territory collectively occupied by respective fields of cells encountered in a microelectrode penetration perpendicular to the cortical surface. Each pair of circles illustrates the movement in aggregate receptive field accompanying a movement along the cortex of 1–2 mm. Both the displacement and the aggregate field size vary with distance from the fovea (eccentricity), but they do so in parallel fashion. Close to the fovea the fields are tiny, but so is the displacement accompanying a 1–2 mm movement along the cortex. The greater the distance from the fovea, the greater the two become, but they continue to remain roughly equal (28).

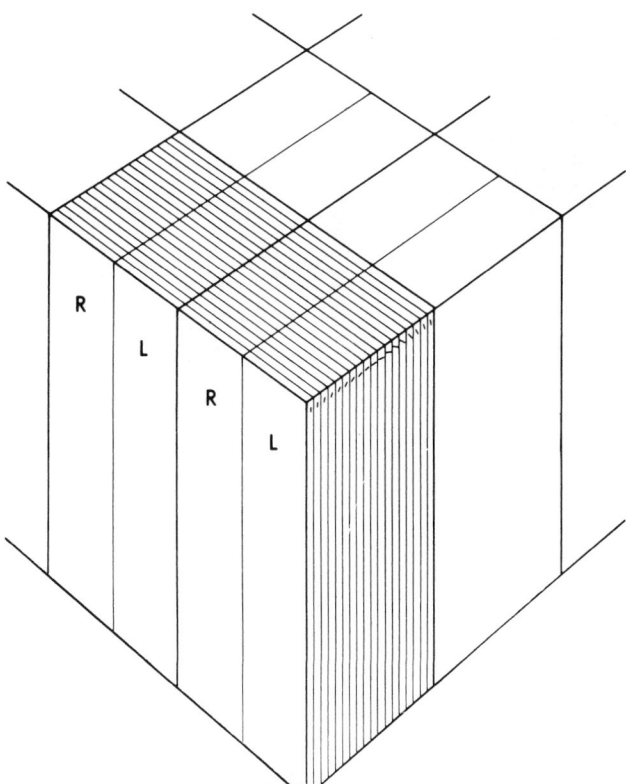

Fig. 15. Model of the striate cortex, to show roughly the dimensions of the ocular dominance slabs (L,R) in relation to the orientation slabs and the cortical thickness. Thinner lines separate individual columns; thicker lines demarcate the two types of hypercolumn: two pairs of ocular dominance columns and two sets of orientation columns. The placing of these hypercolumn boundaries is of course arbitrary; one could as well begin the orientation hypercolumn at horizontal or any of the obliques. The decision to show the two sets of columns as intersecting at right angles is also arbitrary, since there is at present no evidence as to the relationship between the two sets. Finally, for convenience the slabs are shown as plane surfaces, but whereas the dominance columns are indeed more or less flat, the orientation columns are not known to be so, and may when viewed from above have the form of swirls. (Figure 27 (29)).

obvious advantages, not just for the cortex but also for terminology. Perhaps one could use "module" to refer to the complete machine.

There are two qualifications to all of this. I do not mean to imply that there need really be 2,000 separate definable entities. It need not matter whether one begins a set of orientation columns at vertical, horizontal or any one of the obliques; the decision is arbitrary. One requires two dominance columns, a left and a right, and it makes no difference which one begins with. (In fact, as I will soon point out, it now looks as though the blocks of tissue may really be discrete, to a degree that we could not have imagined two years ago.) Second, there may well be some differences in cortical machinery between the center and periphery of the visual field. Color vision and stereopsis, for example, probably decline in importance far out in the visual fields. I say this not to be obsessively complete but because in the next few years someone will probably find some difference and pronounce the con-

cept wrong. It may of course be wrong, but I hope it will be for interesting reasons.

I should perhaps point out that the retina *must* be nonuniform if it is to do a more detailed job in the center. To have more area devoted to the center than to the periphery is not an option open to it, because it is a globe. Were it anything else the optics would be awkward and the eye could not rotate in its socket.

A few years ago, in a Ferrier Lecture (29), Torsten and I ended by saying that the striate cortex is probably now (was, then) in broad outline, understood. This was done deliberately: one did not want the well to dry up. When one wants rain the best strategy is to leave raincoat and umbrella at home. So the best way to guarantee future employment was to declare the job finished. It certainly worked. Two years ago Anita Hendrickson and her coworkers and our laboratory independently discovered that monkey striate cortex, when sectioned parallel to the surface and through layers II

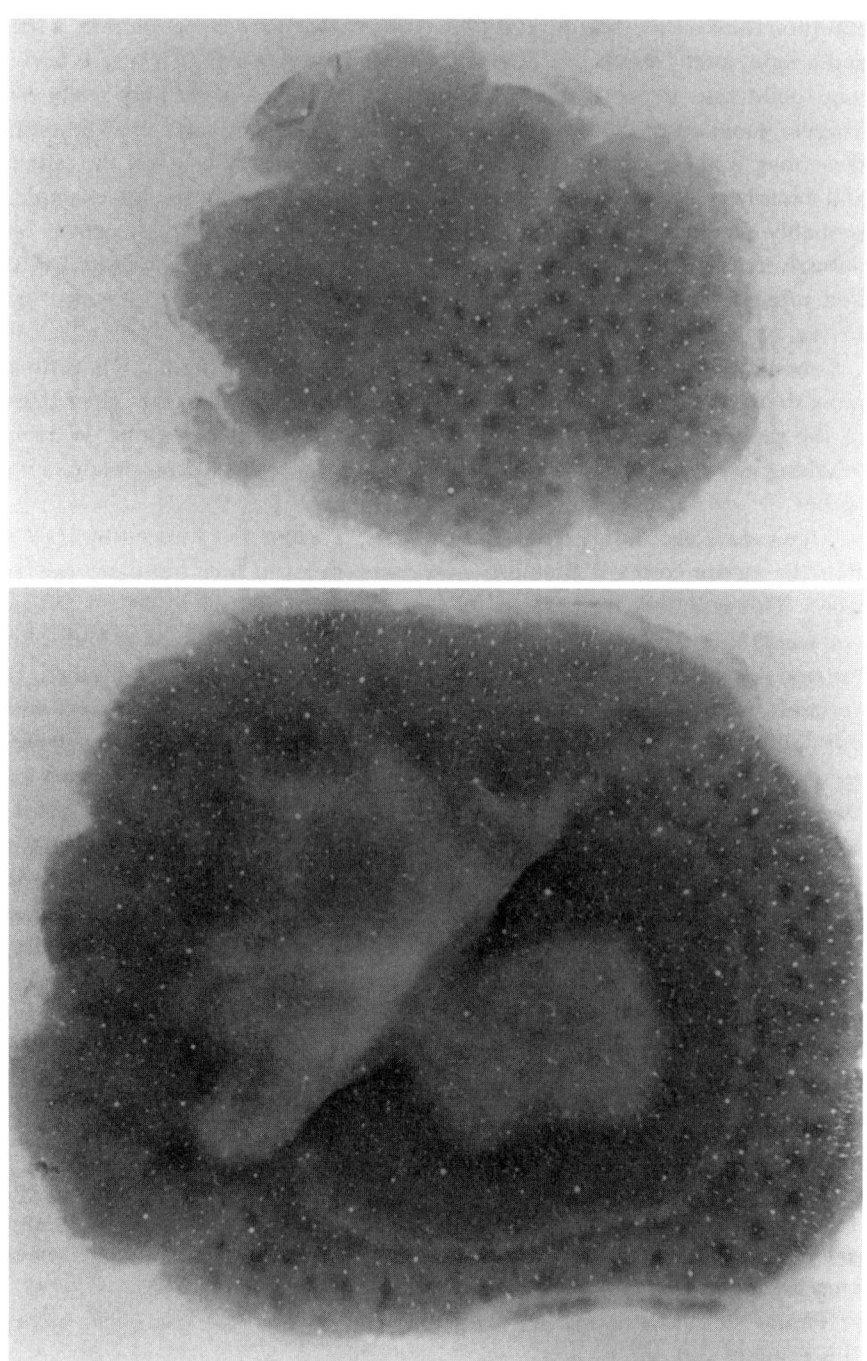

Fig. 16. Tangential sections through the visual cortex of the squirrel monkey; cytochrome oxidase stain. The sections pass through the 17–18 border, which runs obliquely in the figure with area 17 below and to the right and 18 above and left. (Hubel and Livingstone, unpublished) The left-hand section passes through layer III, and the blobs can be seen easily in area 17. The right-hand section is tangential to layer V where blobs can be again seen, though faintly; these lie in register with the upper-layer blobs. The coarse pattern in area 18 is now under study and promises to be interesting.

and III and stained for the enzyme cytochrome oxidase, shows a polka-dot pattern of dark blobs quasi-regularly spaced 1/2–1 mm apart (Fig. 16) (30,21). It is as if the animal's brain had the measles. The pattern has been seen with several other enzymatic stains, suggesting that either the activity or the machinery is different in the blob regions. The pattern has been found in all primates examined, including man, but not in any nonprimates. In macaque the blobs are clearly lined up along ocular dominance columns (19). Over the past year Margaret Livingstone and I have shown that the cells in the blobs lack orientation selectivity, resembling, at least superficially, cells of layer IVc (31). They are selectively labeled after large injections of radioactive proline into the lateral geniculate body, so it is clear that their inputs are not identical to the inputs to the rest of layers II and III. Thus an entire system has opened up whose existence we were previously quite unaware of and whose anatomy and functions we do not yet understand. We are especially anxious to learn what, if any, the relationship is between the cytochrome blobs and the orientation columns.

Things are at an exciting stage. There is no point leaving the umbrella home; it is raining, and raining hard.

References

1. Hubel, D. H., (1958) Cortical unit responses to visual stimuli in nonanesthetized cats. Amer. J. Ophthal. 46: 110–122.
2. Barlow, H. B., FitzHugh, R. and Kuffler, S. W., (1957) Dark adaptation, absolute threshold and Purkinje shift in single units of the cat's retina. J. Physiol. 137: 327–337.
3. Talbot, S. A. and Kuffler, S. W., (1952) A multibeam ophthalmoscope for the study of retinal physiology. J. Opt. Soc. Am. 42: 931–936.
4. Talbot, S. A. and Marshall, W. H., (1941) Physiological studies on neural mechanisms of visual localization and discrimination. Am. J. Ophthal. 24: 1255–1263.
5. Mountcastle, V. B., (1957) Modality and topographic properties of single neurons of cat's somatic sensory cortex. J. Neurophysiol. 20: 408–434.
6. Davies, P. W., (1956) Chamber for microelectrode studies in the cerebral cortex. Science 124: 179–180.
7. Sperry, R. W., Miner, N., and Meyers, R. E., (1955) Visual pattern perception following subpial slicing and tantalum wire implantations in the visual cortex. J. Comp. Physiol. Psych. 48: 50–58.
8. Sperry, R. W. and Miner, N., (1955) Pattern perception following insertion of mica plates into visual cortex. J. Comp. Physiol. Psych. 48: 463–469.
9. Hubel, D. H. and Wiesel, T. N., (1959) Respective field organization of single units in the striate cortex of cat. XXI Int. Congr. Physiol. Sci., Buenos Aires, p. 131.
10. Hubel, D. H. and Wiesel, T. N., (1959) Receptive fields of single neurones in the cat's striate cortex. J. Physiol. 148: 574–591.
11. Cleland, B. G., Dubin, M. W., and Levick, W. R., (1971) Simultaneous recording of input and output of lateral geniculate neurones. Nature New Biol. 231: 191–192.
12. Hubel, D. H. and Wiesel, T. N., (1962) Receptive fields, binocular interaction and functional architecture in the cat's visual cortex. J. Physiol. 160: 106–154.
13. Barlow, H. B. and Levick, W. R., (1965) The mechanism of directionally selective units in rabbit's retina. J. Physiol. 178: 477–504.
14. Hubel, D. H. and Wiesel, T. N., (1965) Receptive fields and functional architecture in two non-striate visual areas (18 and 19) of the cat. J. Neurophysiol. 28: 229–289.
15. Dreher, B. (1972) Hypercomplex cells in the cat's striate cortex. Invest. Ophth. 11: 355–356.
16. Gilbert, C. D. (1977) Laminar differences in receptive field properties of cells in cat visual cortex. J. Physiol. 268: 391–421.
17. Toyama, K., Matsunami, K., and Ohno, T., (1969) Antidromic identification of association, commissural and corticofugal efferent cells in cat visual cortex. Brain Res. 14: 513–517.
18. Hubel, D. H. and Wiesel, T. N., (1963) Shape and arrangement of columns in cat's striate cortex. J. Physiol. 165: 559–568.
19. Hubel, D. H. and Wiesel, T. N., (1974) Sequence regularity and geometry of orientation columns in the monkey striate cortex. J. Comp. Neur. 158: 267–294.
20. Sokoloff, L., Reivich, M., Kennedy, C., DesRosiers, M. H., Patlak, C. S., Pettigrew, K. D., Sakurada, O. and Shinohara, M., (1977) The [^{14}C] deoxyglucose method for the measurement of local cerebral glucose utilization: theory, procedure, and normal values in the conscious and anesthetized albino rat. J. Neurochem. 28: 897–916.
21. Horton, J. C. and Hubel, D. H., (1981) Regular patchy distribution of cytochrome oxidase staining in primary visual cortex of macaque monkey. Nature 292: 762–764.
22. Humphrey, A. L., Skeen, L. C., and Norton, T. T., (1980) Topographic organization of the orientation column system in the striate cortex of the tree shrew (*Tupaia glis*). II. Deoxyglucose mapping. J. Comp. Neur. 192: 549–566.
23. Hubel, D. H. and Wiesel, T. N., (1972) Laminar and columnar distribution of geniculocortical fibers in the macaque monkey. J. Comp. Neur. 146: 421–450.
24. Grafstein, B. (1971) Transneuronal transfer of radioactivity in the central nervous system. Science 172: 177–179.
25. Wiesel, T. N., Hubel, D. H., and Lam, D. M. K., (1974) Autoradiographic demonstration of ocular-dominance columns in the monkey striate cortex by means of transneuronal transport. Brain Res. 79: 273–279.
26. Lorente de Nó, R. (1949) Cerebral cortex: architecture, intracortical connections, motor projections. Chapt. 15 in Fulton, J. F.: *Physiology of the Nervous System,* 3rd edition, Oxford University Press, New York and London.
27. Daniel, P. M. and Whitteridge, D., (1961) The representation of the visual field on the cerebral cortex in monkeys. J. Physiol., Lond. 159: 203–221.
28. Hubel, D. H. and Wiesel, T. N., (1974) Uniformity of monkey striate cortex: a parallel relationship between field size, scatter, and magnification factor. J. Comp. Neur. 158: 295–306.
29. Hubel, D. H. and Wiesel, T. N., (1977) Ferrier Lecture. Functional architecture of macaque monkey visual cortex. Proc. R. Soc. Lond. B. 198: 1–59.

30. Hendrickson, A. E., Hunt, S. P., and Wu, J.-Y., (1981) Immunocytochemical localization of glutamic acid decarboxylase in monkey striate cortex. Nature 292: 605–607.

31. Hubel, D. H. and Livingstone, M. S., (1981) Regions of poor orientation tuning coincide with patches of cytochrome oxidase staining in monkey striate cortex. Neurosci. Abst. 11th Ann. Meeting, Los Angeles, 118.12.

32. Hubel, D. H. and Wiesel, T. N., (1968) Receptive fields and functional architecture of monkey striate cortex. J. Physiol. 195: 215–243.

33. LeVay, S., Hubel, D. H., and Wiesel, T. N., (1975) The pattern of ocular dominance columns in macaque visual cortex revealed by a reduced silver stain. J. Comp. Neur. 159: 559–576.

The Postnatal Development of the Visual Cortex and the Influence of Environment

TORSTEN N. WIESEL • *Harvard Medical School, Department of Neurobiology, Boston, Massachusetts*

INTRODUCTION

In the early sixties, having begun to describe the physiology of cells in the adult cat visual cortex,[1] David Hubel and I decided to investigate how the highly specific response properties of cortical cells emerged during postnatal development. We were also interested in examining the role of visual experience in normal development, a question raised and discussed by philosophers since the time of Descartes. The design of these experiments was undoubtedly influenced by the observation that children with congenital cataracts still have substantial and often permanent visual deficits after removal of the cataract and proper refraction.[2] Also, behavioral studies had shown that animals raised in the dark or in an environment devoid of contours have a similar impairment of their visual functions,[3,4]

Because of the difficulties associated with raising kittens in total darkness, we decided to fuse the lids by suture. This procedure prevented any form vision without completely light depriving the animal. We expected this to be an effective procedure because cortical cells respond to contours and are insensitive to changes in levels of diffuse light.[5] Initially we raised kittens with only one eye closed, using the other eye as a control. This design turned out to be fortunate, because—as shown below—

the effects of single eye closure on the visual cortex are more dramatic than the results obtained from animals raised with both eyes occluded or kept in the dark.

Our initial findings were that kittens with an eye occluded by lid suture during the first three months of life were blind in the deprived eye, and that in the striate cortex the majority of the cells responded only to stimulation of the normal eye.[6] This defect appeared to be localized to the visual cortex, perhaps at the site of interaction between geniculate afferents and cortical cells.[7] From another series of experiments, we found that the properties of orientation specificity and binocularity developed through innate mechanisms.[8] This result, taken together with the monocular deprivation experiment, indicated that neural connections present early in life can be modified by visual experience. Such neural plasticity was not observed in the adult cat, but existed only during the first three postnatal months.[9]

The early experiments were done in the cat, but we soon turned our attention to the rhesus macaque monkey. After having demonstrated that cells in the monkey visual cortex also respond selectively to lines of different orientations and often are binocular[10] we showed that the monkey was also susceptible to visual deprivation,[11] a finding subse-

From *Les Prix Nobel en 1981,* pp. 261–283 and *Nature,* 1982, 299: 583–591.

Nobel lecture, 8 December 1981

quently confirmed and extended.[12,13,14,15] Further advances in our understanding of the nature of and mechanism underlying the deprivation phenomena depended on working out some of the functional architecture of the visual cortex. This was done through further physiological experiments in the normal animal and by using newly developed anatomical methods.[16,17,18,19,20] Over the years we have pursued the normal and developmental studies in parallel, and this has accelerated our progress in both areas. For example, while the deprivation experiments depended on the understanding of the functional architecture of the normal adult animal, we were alerted to the existence of ocular dominance columns in the cat by experiments we had done in strabismic animals.[21]

In this lecture I will present our current understanding of the development of the monkey visual cortex and the role of visual experience in influencing neural connections. Rather than attempting to discuss in any detail the now very extensive literature in the field, my emphasis will be on the work carried out in our laboratory (for reviews see references 22, 23 and 24). David Hubel and I did much of this work in collaboration with Simon LeVay.

MONOCULAR DEPRIVATION

The procedure of suturing a monkey's eyelid shut creates a condition similar to a cataract, since though the light reaching the retina through the closed lid is only slightly attenuated (by factor of 3), the forms of objects are no longer visible. As mentioned above, when the deprived eye is opened after months of deprivation, the animal is unable to see with it; there are no obvious changes in ocular media, the retina or the LGN that can explain this deficit; instead marked changes have occurred at the level of the primary visual cortex (striate cortex). Even if the ocular media are clear, the occluded eye develops with time a marked axial length myopia (5–12 D over a 1 year period).[25]

One way of seeing the change is to record from cells in the striate cortex and determine their ocular preference.[7] In the monkey there is normally a fairly even balance between cells driven preferentially by one eye and cells driven preferentially by the other.[10] In layer IV most cells are strictly monocular, and outside of layer IV they are usually binocular, though they still tend to respond more strongly to stimulation of one eye than to the other. There are about as many cells preferring stimulation of the left eye as cells preferring stimulation of the right (Fig. 1, left). Under conditions of monocular deprivation, however, the great majority of cortical cells are driven exclusively by the nondeprived eye (Fig. 1, right).[11,12,13] One could ask whether this can be accounted for in terms of changes occurring at the level of the lateral geniculate nucleus. Although the cells lying in the geniculate layers that receive input from the deprived eye are smaller than those in the non-deprived layers (Fig. 2), they are present in normal numbers, respond briskly to stimulation of the deprived eye and have normal receptive fields. Since geniculate cells are functionally normal and the cortical cells are altered in their properties there must be some change in the effectiveness of the geniculocortical connections. We were interested in investigating whether there were any structural changes associated with this abnormality.

The first aspect of cortical organization to be examined is the pattern of input of the geniculate afferents to the cortex. This can be done using the autoradiographic technique for tracing neuronal connections, transsynaptically from the eye[18,20] or by a fiber stain[19] (see also lecture of David Hubel). When in the normal monkey the input from the lateral geniculate nucleus reaches layer IV of the cortex, the information from the two eyes is still segregated. The input from each eye is distributed into a series of branching and anastomosing bands, which are about 0.5 millimeter wide, and alternate with similar bands serving the other eye (Fig. 3A). This pattern of innervation forms the anatomical basis for ocular dominance columns. Cells in the superficial and deep layers, while tending to be more binocular than cells in layer IV, still are more strongly influenced by the eye that provides input to the column in which they reside. The relative influence of the two eyes is shown by making tangential electrode penetrations through different cortical layers. Such penetrations in the normal monkey show regular changes in eye preference as expected from the columnar arrangements (Fig. 3A; Fig. 4, top).

In an animal that has undergone monocular deprivation, the geniculate terminals with input from the non-deprived eye take over much of the

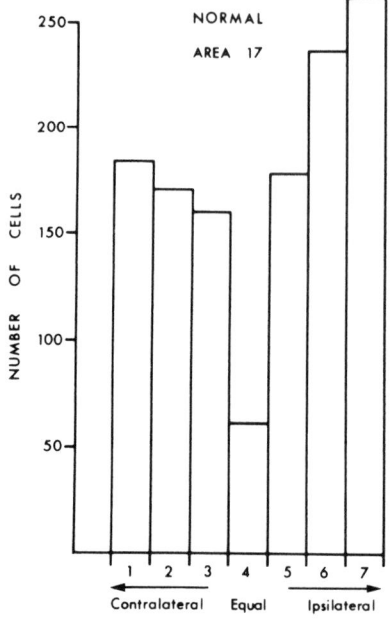
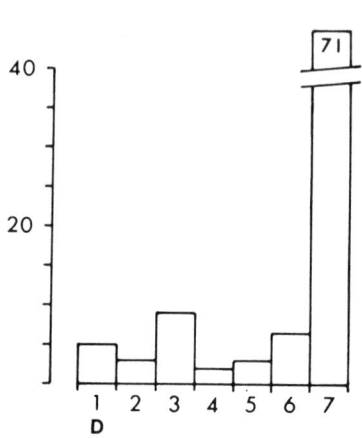

Fig. 1. Ocular dominance histograms in normal and monocularly deprived rhesus macaque monkeys.
   Left histogram: *1256 cells recorded from area 17 in normal adult or juvenile rhesus monkeys.*[13]
   Right histogram: *obtained from a monkey in which the right eye was closed at 2 weeks for 18 months.*[15]
It shows the relative eye preference of 100 cells recorded from the left hemisphere. The letter D indicates the side of the histogram corresponding to dominance by the deprived eye.
   Cells in layer IVC are excluded in this figure and in histograms of all other figures. Cells in group 1 are driven exclusively from the contralateral eye, those in group 7 from the ipsilateral eye, group 4 cells are equally influenced, and the remaining group are intermediate.

space that would normally have been occupied by terminals from the deprived eye (Fig. 3B).[13,15] The deprived eye input has shrunken down to occupy the small strips lying between the terminals of the non-deprived eye input. Tangential electrode penetrations through cortical layers reveal long expanses of cells driven by the non-deprived eye interrupted by small patches of cells that are either unresponsive or driven by the deprived eye (Fig. 4, middle). As will be shown later in this paper, this expansion of the input from the non-deprived eye occurs at the level of single geniculate afferents. Cells in the deprived layers of the geniculate are smaller than normal. One reason for this is that their shrunken cortical arbors may require a smaller soma to maintain them, as originally proposed by Guillery and Stelzner (1970).[26]

   Morphological examination of the lateral geniculate nucleus in these animals showed that there is a good relationship ($_r$ = 0.91) between the relative size of normal and deprived cells and the relative size of normal and deprived ocular dominance columns in layer IVC.[15] Thus measuring geniculate cell sizes is yet another means of evaluating the effects of monocular closure.

   From the histogram shown in Figure 1 one cannot tell whether many cells have changed allegiance from the deprived to the non-deprived eye or have simply become unresponsive. The autoradiographic labelling of the afferents in layer IV (Fig. 3B) shows that a greater proportion of the cells in layer IV receive direct input from the non-deprived eye. The consequence of this change is that cells at later stages have shifted their allegience from the deprived to the nondeprived eye, rather than becoming unresponsive. This conclusion is supported by the physiological findings that the large majority of cells in superficial and deep layers

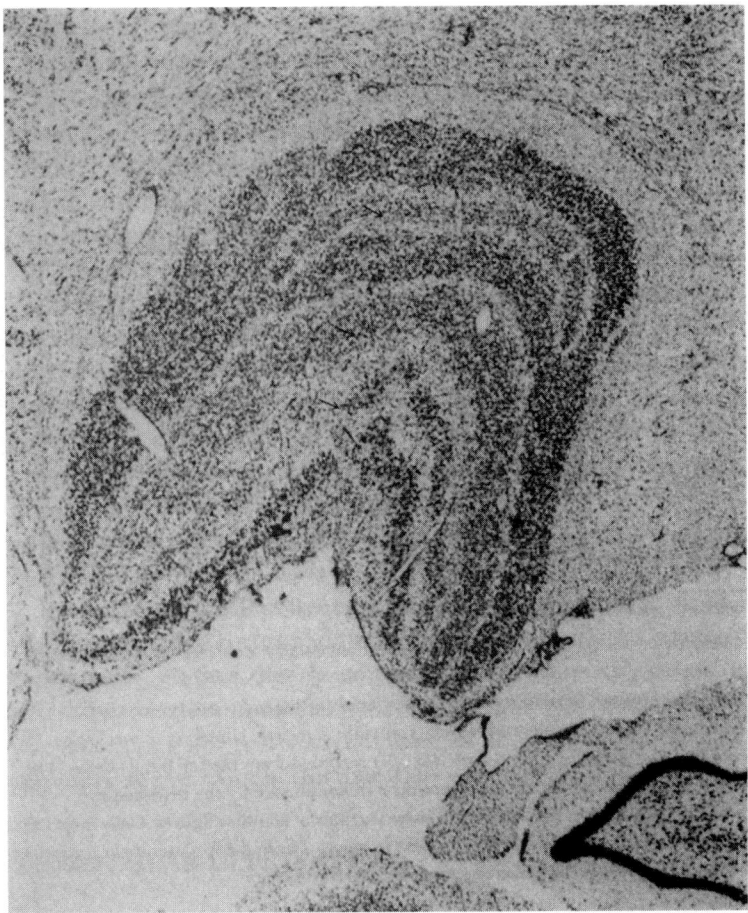

Fig. 2. *Coronal section through the right lateral geniculate nucleus of the monkey with right eye closed at 2 weeks for 18 months (fig. 1, right). Note the atrophy in the layers receiving input from the deprived eye (indicated by arrows). Stained with cresyl violet; frozen section.*[13]

respond only to the stimulation of the normal eye (Fig. 4 middle).

THE CRITICAL PERIOD

Having observed these dramatic effects of monocular suture early in an animal's life, we wanted to determine if there was a period over which the cortex retained its plasticity.

Our experiments in adult cats and monkeys[6,15] showed that long periods of monocular lid suture did not result in the sort of changes in the visual cortex described above. Instead, we found that there is a definite period of time, early in life, during which the visual system shows this lability. We termed this the "critical period." The perma-

nent visual deficits observed in children with congenital cataracts are therefore most likely a result of changes in the visual cortex that occurred during the critical period. Adult humans suffering from cataracts for many years will have normal vision when the cataracts have been removed presumably because they are well past their critical period at the onset of the disease.

The critical period in the monkey was estimated by closing one eye at different ages and keeping it closed for several months or longer.[15] The deprivation effect was gauged by the relative influence of the two eyes on single cortical cells (ocular dominance distribution), by the distribution of the input from the two eyes in layer IV (using the autoradiographic technique shown in

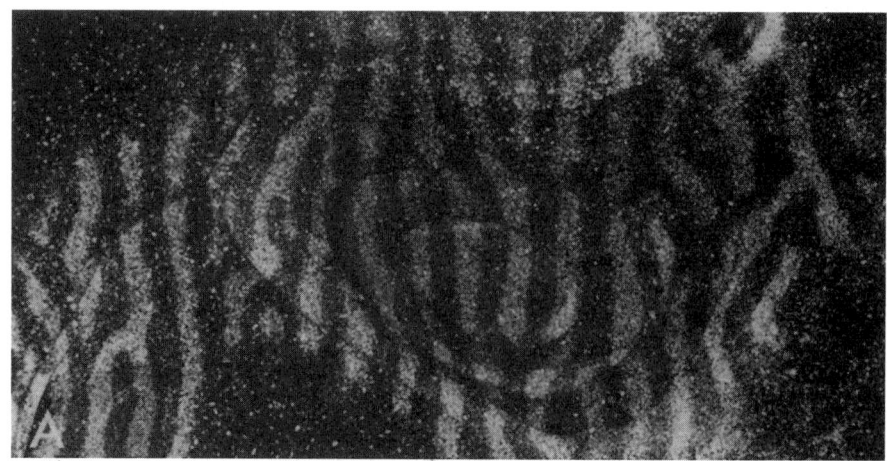

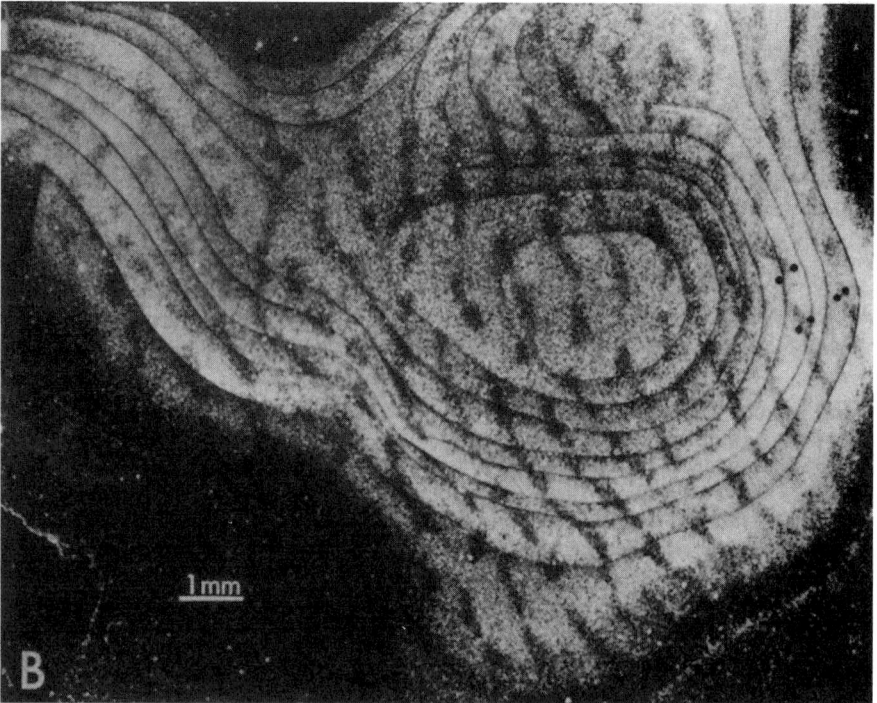

Fig. 3. Dark field autoradiographs of monkey striate cortex following injection of ³H-Proline in the vitreous of one eye 2 weeks before.

A: Normal monkey, a montage of a series of tangential sections through layer IVC. The light stripes, representing the labelled eye columns, are separated by gaps of the same width representing the other eye. B: Monocularly deprived monkey, again a montage from a series of tangential sections through layer IVC. Same monkey as in Fig. 1, right, and Fig. 2, which had the right eye closed at 2 weeks for 18 months. The input from the normal eye is in form of expanded bands which in places coalesce, obliterating the narrow gaps which represent the columns connected to the closed eye.

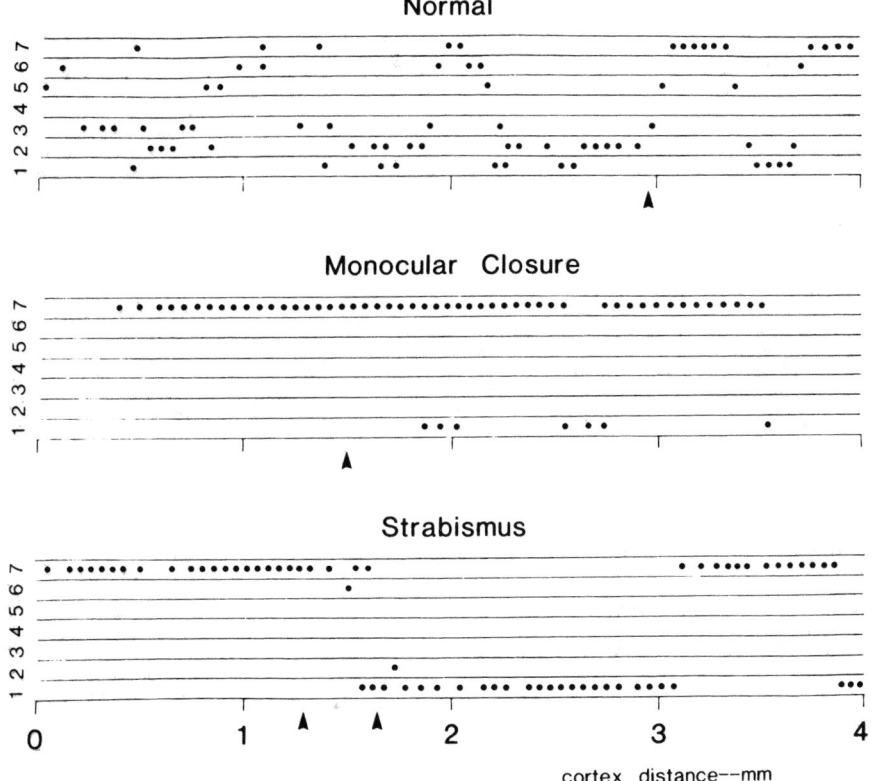

Fig. 4. *Eye preference of cells recorded in oblique penetrations through the cortex in a normal monkey, a monocularly deprived monkey, and a monkey raised with strabismus. Ocular dominance categories (1–7) are shown
relative to the distance the electrode penetrated through the cortex.*

*Top: Penetration in a normal monkey which shows the sinusoidal shift in eye preference with distance. The
arrowhead indicates that the electrode entered layer IVC, in which cells are monocular, and there are abrupt
shifts of dominance from one eye to the other.*

*Middle: Oblique penetration in a monkey raised with monocular closure (same monkey as in Figs. 1–3).
Note that outside layer IV all cells are driven only by normal eye (7), and in layer IVC (see arrow) there are only
short stretches of cells with input from the deprived eye. The observed overlap of input from left and right eye is
not present in the normal monkey.*

*Bottom: A monkey with a 10° convergent squint produced by sectioning of the lateral rectus at three weeks.
(Same animal as in Fig. 11, left histogram). The illustration shows the result of oblique penetration through the
striate cortex made when the animal was 3½ years old. Even outside of layer IV cells were monocular, with
equal stretches of cortex dominated by either eye.*

Fig. 3), and by comparing the cell sizes in deprived
and non-deprived layers of the LGN. The physiological results in monkeys with one eye closed at 2
weeks, 10 weeks, 1 year of age, and in the adult are
illustrated in terms of ocular dominance histograms in Figure 5. The earliest closure produced
the most severe shift of preference toward the normal eye. The same degree of shift could be seen up
to an age of 6 weeks. At that age the animal's sus-

ceptibility to monocular deprivation began to
decline, but as is shown in the figure, it was still
pronounced at 10 weeks and was detectable at one
year. As indicated above, there were no cortical
changes when the closure was done in the adult.

The changes occurring in the geniculo-cortical innervation were in general agreement with the
physiology, though the time course was somewhat
different (Fig. 6). Animals with a closure at 2 and

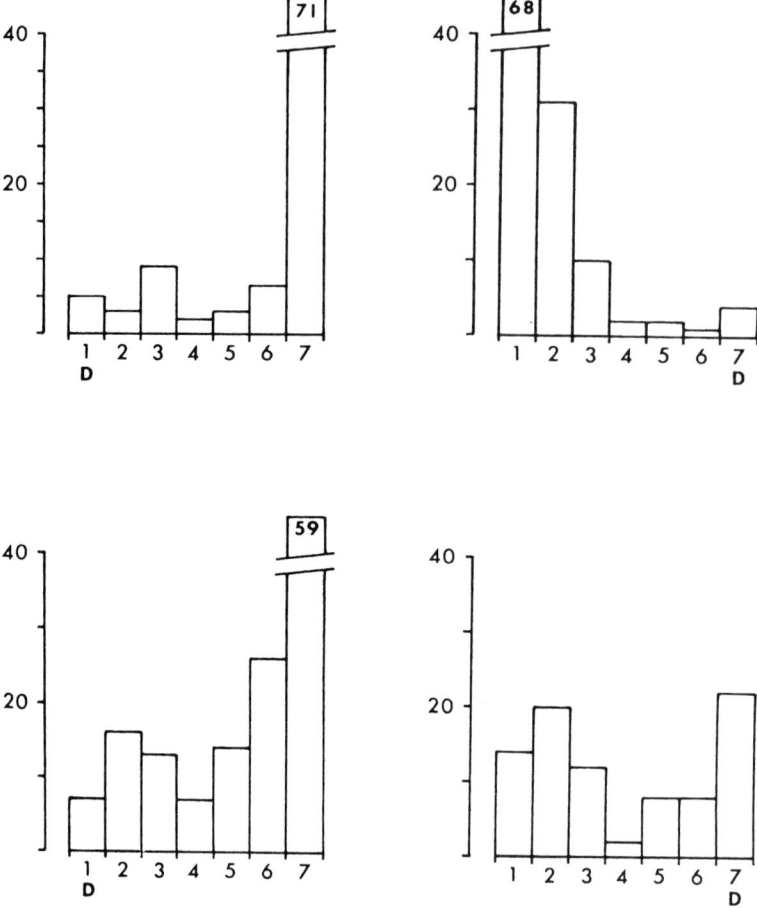

Fig. 5. *Ocular dominance histograms of monkeys with one eye occluded by lid suture at different ages and examined after relatively long periods of closure.*[15]

Upper left: *Same monkey as in figs 1–4. Right eye closed at 2 weeks for 18 months (cf. Fig. 1, right).*

Upper right: *A monkey with right eye closed at 10 weeks for 4 months. Strong dominance of normal eye but not as pronounced as at earlier closure. Duration of deprivation relatively short, but our experience is that at this age the main changes in eye preference occur within the first few months of closure.*

Lower left: *A monkey with right eye closed at 1 year for a period of 1 year. A moderate shift in preference toward the non-deprived eye. This was particularly true for cells in layers II and III.*

Lower right: *Adult monkey (6 years old) with one eye occluded for 1½ years. There was no obvious difference in eye preference from that observed in the normal monkey.*

5½ weeks showed the expected expansion of the non-deprived geniculate terminals; closure at 10 weeks showed a more moderate expansion, and at one year the pattern was indistinguishable from that in the adult. Geniculate cell sizes in the deprived layers changed in a parallel fashion, showing marked shrinkage at early closures, moderate reduction in closure at 10 weeks and no change when closed at one year. Since in the clo-

sure at one year we observed physiological changes in the absence of a change in the pattern of geniculate innervation, there must presumably be changes occurring at subsequent levels in the cortical circuit.[13,14] At any rate, in the adult even this "higher level" of plasticity disappears.

The high degree of susceptibility to deprivation at early ages is also apparent from experiments in which one eye in monkeys was closed for short

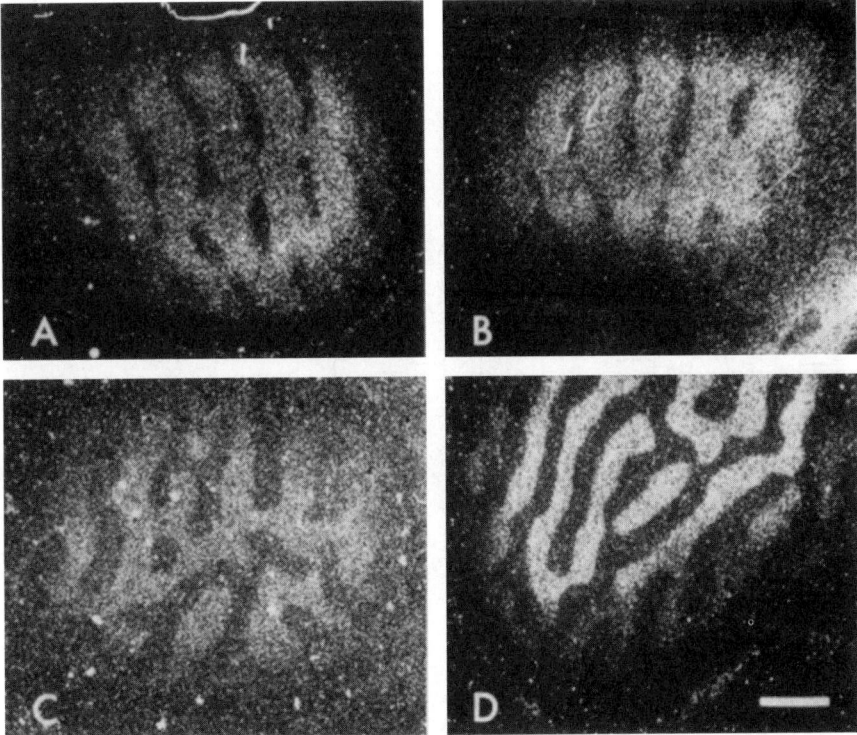

Fig. 6. *Autoradiographic labelling patterns from the striate cortex of four monocularly deprived monkeys illustrating the distribution of geniculate terminals in layer IVC after closures at different ages. In all cases the normal (left) eye was injected with ³H Proline thereby labelling the nondeprived geniculate terminals.¹⁵*

A: *Right eye closed at 2 weeks for 18 months. Same animal as in Fig. 1 (right), Fig. 4 (middle) and Fig. 5 (upper left).*

B: *Right eye closed at 5½ weeks for 16 months.*

C: *Right eye closed at 10 weeks for 4 months. Same animal as in Fig. 5 (upper right).*

D: *Right eye closed at 14 months for 14 months. The unlabelled bar is 1 mm.*

periods. Before 6 weeks of age, it was sufficient to close an eye for a few days to obtain substantial change in eye preference. The ocular dominance histogram from a monkey with one eye closed for 12 days is shown in Fig. 7 (left). During the subsequent several months a marked change required several weeks of closure, and during the second year any change required months of closure.

From these and similar experiments by us[13,15] and others[14,27] we conclude that the macaque monkey is highly susceptible to monocular deprivation during the first six weeks of life, at which age the sensitivity declines progressively, so that at 1½ to 2 years the monkey loses this type of neural plasticity. The length of the critical period varies between species. In cats it is 3 to 4 months,[9,28] and from clinical observations in humans it may extend up to 5–10 years, though the susceptibility to deprivation appears to be most pronounced during the first year and declines with age.[29,30,31]

RECOVERY FROM DEPRIVATION

Monocular closure during the entire critical period in cats and monkeys leads to permanent blindness.[32,33,34] Presumably there is no recovery of vision after the eye is opened because the pattern of geniculate innervation and the eye preference of cortical cells can no longer be modified. During the period of high susceptibility partial recovery of

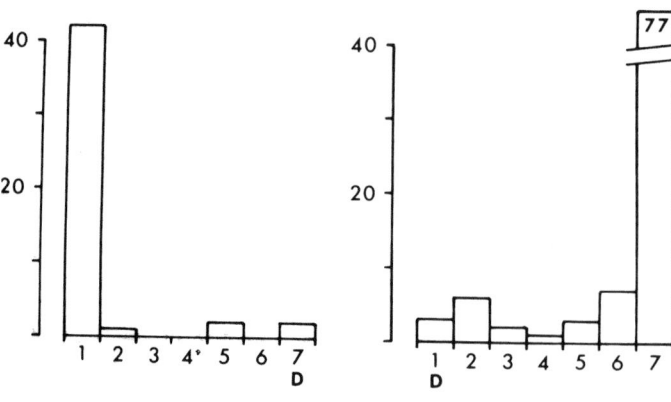

Fig. 7. Left: *Ocular dominance histogram for 47 neurons recorded in a 20-day-old monkey whose right eye had been closed since 8 days of age. The physiological picture is similar to that seen after months of deprivation.*[15]

Right: *Ocular dominance histogram of 99 cells recorded in a monkey whose right eye was closed from 21 to 30 days of age. In spite of a subsequent 4 years of binocular vision, most cortical neurons were still unresponsive to stimulation of the right eye.*[15]

vision in the deprived eye is possible after brief periods of monocular closure.[15,34,35,36] This was shown in a monkey with one eye closed between days 21–30, after which the monkey lived with both eyes open for a period of 4 years. Initially the animal appeared blind in the deprived eye but, with time, it slowly regained the use of the eye and the final acuity was 20/80–100 as compared to 20/40 in the non-deprived eye. The recordings from the striate cortex showed a marked dominance of the non-deprived eye (Fig. 4, right). If there was an increase in the number of cells driven by the once deprived eye, it was not very obvious. There was a marked narrowing of the deprived columns and a corresponding widening of the non-deprived ones. Thus even if there had been some behavioral recovery, these results demonstrate that a few days of monocular closure had caused clear physiological and anatomical changes in the striate cortex.

These results are relevant to observations in children who have been monocularly deprived for short periods of time. When tested later, some children were found to have reduced acuity in the once patched eye and the degree of deficit depended on how young the child was at the time of patching.[38,39] The experience in children with cataract removal indicates that surgery must be performed very early in the critical period in order to prevent the appearance of any deficit.[40,41]

A procedure commonly used in children with strabismic amblyopia is to place a patch over the good eye to improve vision in a weak eye. In monocularly deprived animals it was possible to open the sutured eye and close the normal eye, 9 here termed "reverse suture." Both in the cat and monkey, reverse suture led to a complete switch in eye preference if it was done within the early part of the critical period.[15,27,28,37] The geniculate innervation of layer IVC also reversed so that the shrunken regions controlled by the initially closed eye expanded at the expense of the other eye, and consequently the cortical cells switched eye preference in favor of the eye closed first.[15,37,42] An example is shown in Figure 8 (top) in which the eye reversal was done at 3 weeks, and the recordings done 8 months later. The ocular dominance histogram shows that the initially closed eye, which at the time of eye reversal would have influenced very few cortical cells, now became strongly dominant. The autoradiography (Fig. 9A) shows a marked expansion in layer IVCβ of the initially deprived geniculate terminals. When reversal was done at 6 weeks the physiology indicated a complete reversal, with a strong dominance of the initially deprived eye. (Fig. 8, lower left) Such a marked shift was not reflected in the innervation of layer IV, in which the initially deprived eye had succeeded only in regaining its normal territory (Fig. 9C). This indicates that a significant part of the changes were occurring at the level of intrinsic cortical connections. Finally, reversing at one year failed to produce any restoration of the function of the initially deprived eye (Fig. 8, lower right; Fig. 9D). Though it is possible to cause changes by

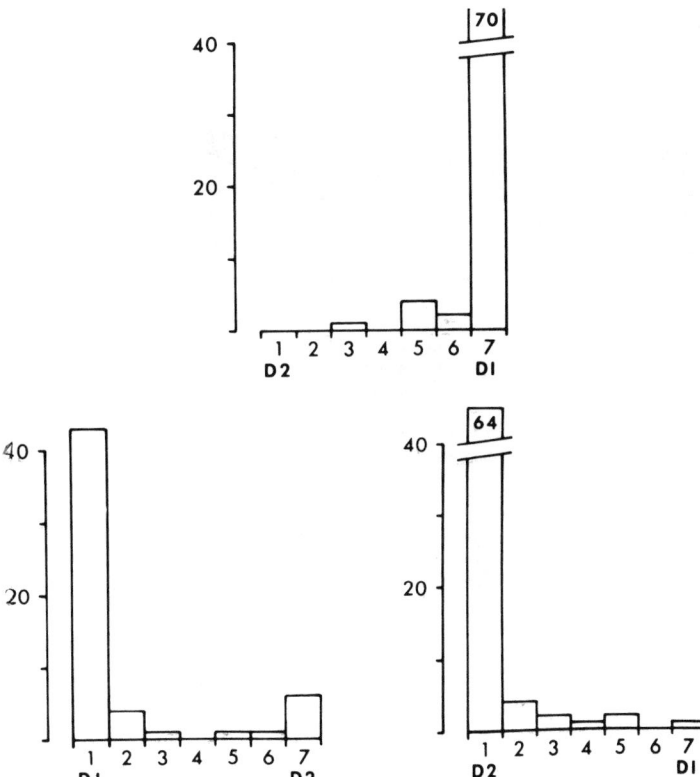

Fig. 8. Ocular dominance histograms of cortical cells recorded in three monkeys in which reversed suture was done at various ages.[15]

Upper histogram: 77 cells recorded from the right striate cortex of a monkey with the right eye (D_1) closed at 2 days for 3 weeks and the left eye (D_2) closed at 3 weeks for about 8 months. Nearly all neurons responded only to the initially deprived right eye (D_1).

Lower left: 56 neurons recorded from the left striate cortex. Right eye (D_1) closed at 3 days for 6 weeks; left eye (D_2) closed at 6 weeks for 4½ months. Again nearly all neurons were driven exclusively by the initially deprived right eye (D_1).

Lower right: 74 neurons recorded from the left striate cortex. Right eye (D_1) was closed at 7 days for 1 year; left eye (D_2) was closed at 1 year for 2½ years. In this case there was no effect of the reversal; nearly all the cells responded only to the initially open eye.

monocular deprivation at one year (Fig. 5, lower left), it appears to be more difficult to repair connections that have already been changed once.

Looking more closely at the autoradiography of the geniculate input to layer IVC in the monkey with the reversal at 3 weeks (Fig. 9 A and B), one sees a surprising result. The initially deprived eye took over much of the area of innervation of the lower part of layer IVC (IVCβ), but failed to reverse the dominance of the other eye in the upper part of layer IVC (IVCα). Apparently, the eye preference of the majority of cortical cells is determined primarily by the cells in IVCβ (Fig. 8 top, 9A and B). Layer IVCβ is innervated by cells in the dorsal part of the lateral geniculate nucleus (parvocellular layers) and IVCα by cells in the ventral part of the same nucleus (magnocellular layers). The result of the eye reversal experiment indicates that the critical period is different for the two cell types. Whereas the critical period is over for the magnocellular input at 3 weeks, the parvocellular input apparently begins to lose its ability to expand

at 6 weeks (Fig. 9C), a time when intracortical connections still show considerable plasticity. This suggests that throughout the brain each functional unit has a unique program of development.

MECHANISM: DISUSE VERSUS COMPETITION

These experiments demonstrate that when a binocular cortical cell is not stimulated by a given eye, then the input from that eye drops out. Other forms of visual deprivation have shed some light on the mechanism of the effect of monocular deprivation. For example, if disuse were an important factor, one might expect that with both eyes closed, cortical cells would not be driven by either eye. Experiments in cats and monkeys raised under conditions of binocular deprivation showed, however, that cells were readily driven by the two eyes.[28,43,44] The cortex in the monkey was nonetheless altered in a very substantial way, in that very few cells were binocularly responsive.[44] This is

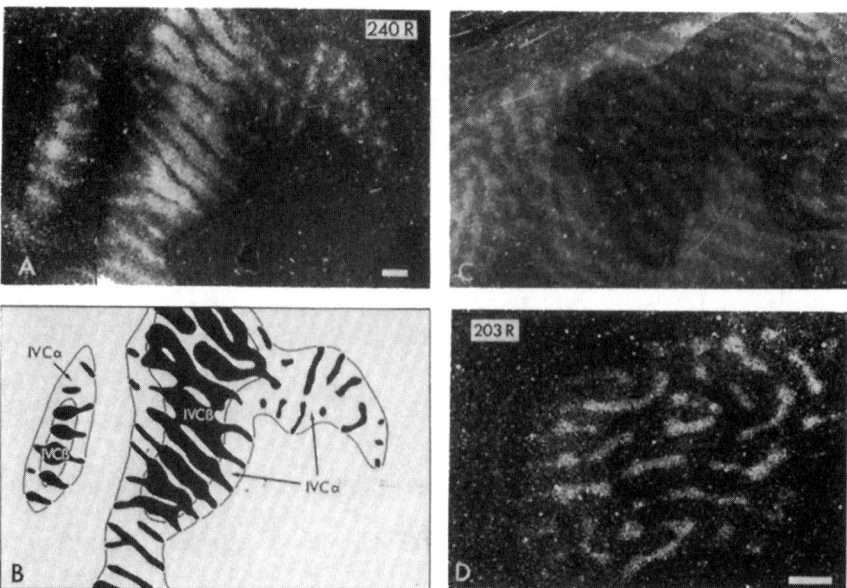

Fig. 9. Effect of reversed suture at various ages on the labelling pattern of geniculate terminals in layer IVC.

A: Same monkey as in the upper part of Fig. 8, in which reversed suture was done at 3 weeks of age. The initially deprived (right) eye was injected with ³H Proline. A single tangential section. In the central region the labelled bands are expanded. In the surrounding belt the bands are contracted. These two regions correspond to the β and α sublaminae of layer IVC. Unlabelled bar is 1 mm.

B: Key to A, showing the distribution of label (in black) and the boundaries of the sublaminae IVCα and IVCβ, traced from an adjacent section stained with cresyl violet. Note that the thin labelled bands in IVCα run into the centers of the enlarged bands in IVCβ, meaning that the two sets of bands, though of very different width, are still in register with each other just as they are in normal animals.

C: The autoradiographic montage of the labelling pattern in monkey with reversed suture at 6 weeks (cf. lower left, Fig. 8). The initially deprived right eye was injected. The labelled bands are of about normal width indicating a recovery from the effects of the early deprivation, but not a complete reversal. Most of the montage shows layer IVCβ. In layer IVCα the labelled columns remained shrunken (not illustrated).

D: Autoradiographic montage from the monkey with reverse suture at 1 year of age (Fig. 8, lower right). The labelled columns (for the initially deprived right eye) remain shrunken, indicating that the late reversal did not permit any anatomical recovery. Scalemarker = 1 mm.

illustrated in figure 10, in which a monkey had both eyes sutured from birth to 4 weeks of age. Except for the obvious lack of binocular cells, the cortex seemed quite normal. The cells were briskly responsive, showed a high degree of orientation selectivity, and had regular sequences of shifts in orientation preference. From tangential electrode penetrations we were also able to see a clear segregation of the cells into unusually distinct ocular dominance columns, even outside of layer IV. When monkeys are kept in the binocularly deprived condition for many months a considerable fraction of the cells are unresponsive or respond only sluggishly, and often show lack of orientation

preference. Binocular closures in kittens had a similar effect except that neither short nor long term deprivation led to an obvious loss of binocular cells.[28,43]

Evidence for competitive mechanisms has also been found by measurements of geniculate cell sizes in an ingenious set of experiments.[26,45,46] First it was demonstrated in monocularly occluded kittens that deprived cells in the monocular segment of the nucleus were of normal size, whereas those in the binocular segment showed marked shrinkage.[26] Next Guillery produced a monocular region in the zone of binocular overlap by making a local retinal lesion in the normal eye of monocularly

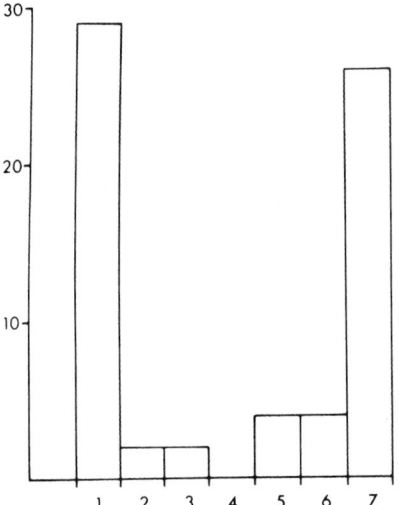

Fig. 10. Ocular dominance histogram of a monkey with binocular lid suture from birth to 30 days of age. Note the low number of binocular cells.[44]

occluded kittens.[45] Again the deprived geniculate cells with no competitive input from the other eye were of normal size, and those outside the topographical area corresponding to the retinal lesion showed the usual shrinkage. Finally, it could be demonstrated that binocular closure in kittens apparently did not lead to a reduction in geniculate cell size[46] as originally reported by us.[43] These experiments lend strong support to the hypothesis that competitive mechanisms rather than disuse are prime factors in producing the changes observed under conditions of monocular deprivation.

Because many cortical cells are binocular from birth, the loss in the monkey of binocular cells at early times after closure suggests that in order for cortical cells to sustain a binocular input the two eyes must work together. Another situation that interrupts coordinated activity from the two eyes is strabismus.[47] One way of producing experimental strabismus is to section an extraocular muscle. Sectioning the lateral rectus causes the eye to deviate inward (convergent strabismus), whereas sectioning the medial rectus produces an outward deviation of the eye (divergent strabismus). After surgery the sectioned muscle usually reattaches behind the original site, so that except for the misalignment, normal eye movements are restored. In

four monkeys with convergent strabismus the operation was performed between 3–5 weeks.[48] When the animals were examined after a year or more, three of them had normal acuity in both eyes but lacked the ability to fuse the images in the two eyes. The striate cortex of these animals had normal single unit activity, but there was a striking absence of binocular cells (Fig. 11, left). Tangential penetrations showed that the monocular cells were grouped in the usual regular columnar pattern (Fig. 4, bottom), suggesting that binocular cells had lost the input from the nondominant eye. The fourth monkey had low acuity in one eye and fewer cortical cells were driven from that eye than from the normal eye (Fig. 11, right). When in five additional monkeys a strabismus was produced at later times during the critical period, there was an increase in the proportion of binocularly driven cells. From these results and experiments in cats and monkeys reported ear lier[49,50,51] it seems that the period during which the cortex can be influenced by the artificially induced strabismus is comparable in duration and sensitivity to that observed with monocular deprivation.

The binocular deprivation and strabismus experiments support the notion that competition, rather than disuse, is the main cause of the observed changes.[43] The right circumstances must exist, however, for the competition to occur, since cells in the normal monkey tend to be dominated by one eye or the other,[10] and the dominant eye does not take over the cell completely. The difference between normal and deprived animals is that under normal conditions a cell receives input synchronously from the two eyes, whereas in monocularly deprived, strabismic, or binocularly deprived animals the two eyes do not act together. The maintenance of a given input may depend on the rate of firing of the postsynaptic cell while that input is active[3] so that in normal animals the nondominant input is maintained by the activity of the dominant input. Carefully designed experiments by Singer et al[52] and Wilson et al[53] have provided support for the notion that it is crucial to activate the postsynaptic cell in order to change ocular dominance (for a more general discussion of synapse formation and stabilization see references 54 and 55).

In addition to providing insight into the mechanisms of development and plasticity in the

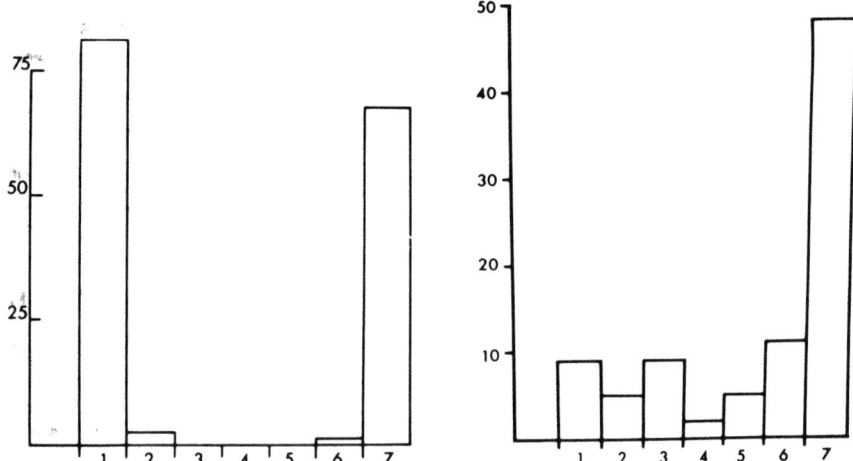

Fig. 11. Ocular dominance histograms of cells recorded in the striate cortex of two strabismic rhesus monkeys.[48]

Left: Histogram shows the eye preference of cells recorded in a 3 year old monkey in which the lateral rectus of the right eye was sectioned at 3 weeks of age. There is a nearly complete absence of binocular cells; the cells are driven exclusively either by the right or the left eye. As shown in Fig. 4 (lower) cells are clustered in a columnar fashion. The monkey had a 10° convergent strabismus, normal acuity in both eyes, but could not fuse images presented separately to the two eyes.

Right: A monkey with lateral rectus muscle of the right eye sectioned at 3 weeks. The animal had a convergent strabismus. Behavioral testing showed normal acuity in the left eye (20/30) and lower acuity in right eye (20/60 to 20/120). There was no difference in refraction between the two eyes. The histogram shows that the amblyopic eye influenced fewer neurons in the superficial and deep layers of the striate cortex. The ocular dominance columns in layer IVC had normal appearance when examined in tangential sections stained with a reduced silver method (Liesegant).[19]

visual cortex, the strabismus experiments may be of direct clinical relevance. A common situation in children with strabismus is that they have good vision in both eyes, but cannot fuse the images in the two eyes. These children often use the two eyes alternately, fixating and attending first with one eye and then with the other. The lack of binocular cells in strabismic animals is perhaps the physiological basis of this condition.[47,12] Another common consequence of strabismus in children is a loss of acuity in one eye (strabismic amblyopia). The physiological mechanism of this condition is less well understood, even if our experiments (Fig. 11, right) and those of others[12,56] indicate that one eye has been weakened in its ability to drive cortical cells, as is seen in monocular deprivation.

As mentioned above, late monocular deprivation in the monkey (see Fig. 5, lower left) and reversal experiments (Fig. 8, lower left, and Fig. 9C) caused alterations in the cortical circuit at stages subsequent to the input from the lateral geniculate nucleus. Another series of experiments illustrated this point quite dramatically. The approach is a variation of the original experiments by Hirsch and Spinelli[57] and by Blakemore and Cooper[58] in which kittens were raised viewing only stripes of one orientation. In our experiments we allowed a monkey to see vertical stripes through one eye only.[59] The other eye was deprived by lid suture. This effectively produced a different condition of deprivation for different populations of cortical cells: those with vertical orientation preference were monocularly deprived, and those with horizontal orientation preference were binocularly deprived. We recorded from the striate cortex after 57 hours of exposure (between days 12–54 after birth) and found normal levels of activity and cells of all orientations with their usual regular columnar arrangement.[17] There was an overall dominance of the open eye, but when we produced sep-

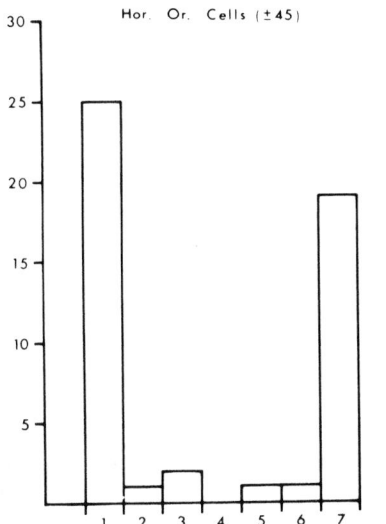
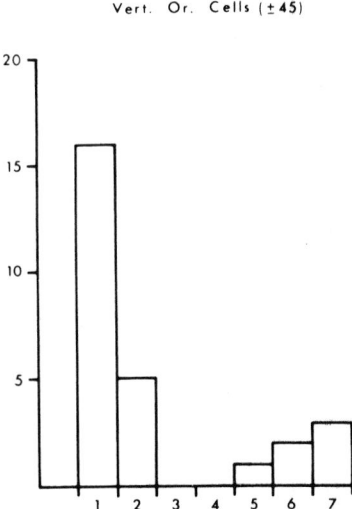

Fig. 12. *Ocular dominance histograms of cells recorded from a monkey with the right eye closed at 12 days of age, then dept in the dark except for 57 hours of self-exposure to vertical stripes during the subsequent 42 days.*

Left histogram: *48 cells recorded in the right striate cortex with preferred orientation within ±45° of the horizontal axis. There were few binocular cells and a good number of monocular cells responding to stimulation of either the left or the right eye. Similar distribution of eye preference to that seen in binocularly deprived animals (cf. Fig. 10).*

Right histogram: *27 cells with preferred orientation within ±45° of the vertical axis. Majority of the recorded cells responded to the open eye producing a histogram similar to that seen after monocular deprivation.*[59]

arate ocular dominance histograms for vertically and horizontally oriented cells (Fig. 12), it became clear that horizontally oriented cells tended to be driven monocularly by either eye (a picture typical of binocular deprivation), and vertically oriented cells tended to be driven monocularly by the exposed eye only (a picture typical of monocular deprivation). Thus these findings again demonstrate that in addition to influencing the thalamo-cortical input, deprivation can alter the connections in the cortex without causing changes in that input. This question has also been addressed in the kitten by somewhat different approaches but with essentially the same results.[60,61]

In looking at the effects of various forms of deprivation one gets certain insights into the processes that govern the balance between different inputs, enabling the visual cortex to integrate information in the appropriate manner. We have learned that competition and synchronization of inputs are important factors in forming and main-

taining this balance. If these processes are disturbed early in life, the system can be permanently altered.

NORMAL DEVELOPMENT

We cannot properly evaluate the experiments on visual deprivation without having detailed knowledge about the normal development of the visual system. To assess the relative importance of the genetic program and the visual environment, it is necessary to evaluate the capabilities of the visual cortex at birth. The monkey is visually alert at or very soon after birth and cells in the visual cortex show orientation preference and binocularity, as in the adult monkey. This was shown by single cell recordings in neonatal monkeys with no experience of contours or forms.[44]

Compared to the monkey, the kitten is far less well developed at birth; the eyes do not open until the second week and kittens tend to spend their first three weeks mainly eating and sleeping. In the visual cortex cells tend to give weak or erratic responses during the early postnatal period and come to respond like adult cells at about 3–4 weeks of age.[9,28,62] During the same time period cortical cells differentiate and active synapse formation takes place.[63,64] Whether cells in the cat visual cortex develop normally without visual experience, as was originally reported for binocularly sutured kittens,[8] was questioned at first[65] but subsequently confirmed in several studies.[62,66,67,68] Whether in the kitten all cortical cells can develop fully through innate mechanisms is not entirely clear, since animals raised in the dark or with binocular lid closures seem to have a certain fraction of unresponsive or unoriented cortical cells.[62,66,68]

The newborn animal does differ from the adult in one significant respect, relating to the segregation of the afferents from the two eyes in layer IVC. In the newborn monkey we were able to show by eye injection of ^{3}H-proline that the inputs from the two eyes are strongly overlapping with only a mild fluctuation in eye dominance in a band-like pattern.[13] Sokoloff and his colleagues[69] confirmed this observation using the 2-deoxyglucose method. In the monkey foetus Rakic showed that initially the left and right-eye afferents overlap completely, and not until a few days before birth do they begin to sort out into ocular dominance columns.[70] We followed this process of segregation postnatally; it was completed by 4–6 weeks of age (Fig. 13).[13] Recordings also indicated an initial overlap, followed by separation of the inputs from the two eyes in layer IVC and the time course of the events were similar. The process of segregation did not require visual experience, since it also occurred in an animal raised in the dark.[15] In kittens ocular dominance columns are formed much as they are in monkeys, showing a sequence of initial overlap and segregation during the first few months of life,[71] even though in this species visual experience appears necessary for their normal development.[72]

In the kitten it has been possible to examine the segregation of ocular dominance columns at a single cell level. In the early postnatal period, a single geniculate afferent gives off numerous branches innervating without interruption an area covering several future ocular dominance columns without interruption (Fig. 14, top).[73] As the axon matures,

there appears to be a selective loss of branches, so that ultimately it innervates ocular dominance columns serving one eye and leaves gaps for the columns serving the opposite eye (Fig. 14, middle).[74,76] In a cat monocularly deprived during its critical period, a geniculocortical afferent with input from the normal eye is shown in the bottom of Fig. 14.[77] It appears to have innervated an area that normally would have been occupied by the other eye.

Both the autoradiography (Fig. 3) and the single cell reconstructions (Fig. 14) suggest a mechanism for the expansion and contraction of ocular dominance columns in monocular closure. The terminals with input from the normal eye continue to occupy the territory which normally they would have relinquished, while the deprived terminals are trimmed to an abnormal extent. Another mechanism appears to operate at slightly later stages: when the ocular dominance columns are fully segregated (at six weeks of age in the monkey), monocular closure still causes an expansion and a contraction of the columns similar to that seen after earlier closure (Fig. 6B). This argues for a mechanism of sprouting by one axon into the territory originally occupied exclusively by the deprived eye. Perhaps sprouting occurs from the axon branches that traverse the ocular dominance columns for the other eye (see Fig. 14, middle). Reverse suture experiments also indicate that both trimming and sprouting are involved in plastic changes of the geniculocortical pathway (Fig. 9A, B, C). We know little of the biochemical mechanisms underlying these changes, except for the intriguing observation of the possible role of norepinephrine in neural plasticity.[78] Since the critical period seems to vary in onset and duration between different brain regions and even between layers of an individual cortical area (cf. IVCα and IVCβ in monkey striate cortex,[15] Fig. 9A and B) the control of plasticity appears to be specific and localized, not a phenomenon controlled by diffuse processes.

CONCLUSIONS

Innate mechanisms endow the visual system with highly specific connections, but visual experience early in life is necessary for their maintenance and full development. Deprivation experiments demonstrate that neural connections can be modulated

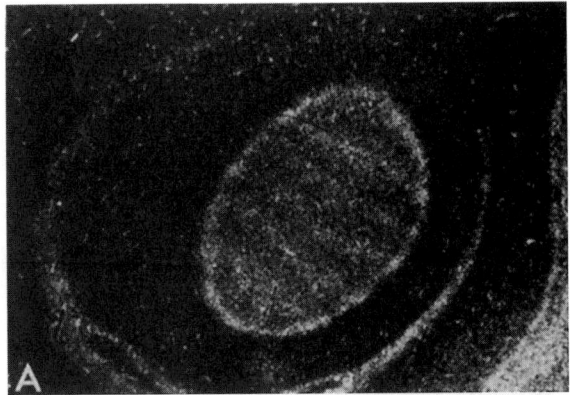

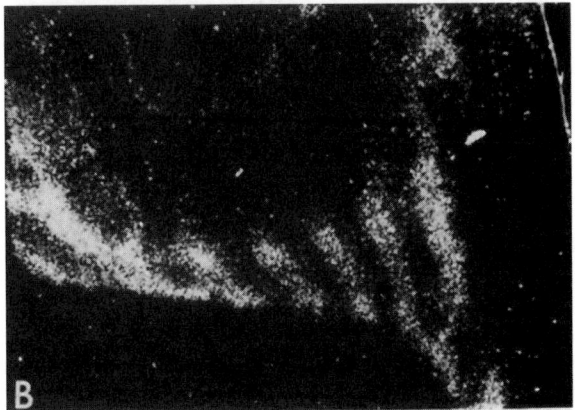

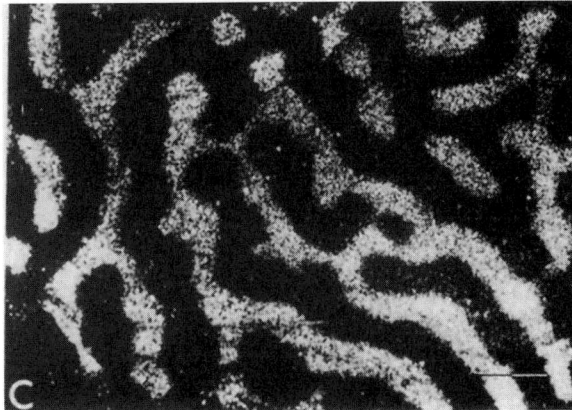

Fig. 13. Darkfield autoradiographs of geniculate afferent terminals in the striate cortex of normal neonatal monkeys in which the right eye had been injected with a radioactive tracer 1–2 weeks earlier.[15]

A: A normal 6-day-old monkey; single section from the left hemisphere that graces IVC tangentially in the central oval region. Silver grains are distributed continuously over layer IVC, but there are bands of alternating higher and lower grain density, indicating that afferents for the two eyes are in the process of columnar segregation.

B: A normal 3-week-old monkey; a single section through layer IVC of the left hemisphere which shows a clear columnar pattern but with a slight blurring of the margin of labelled bands, suggesting a modest intermixing of left and rigth eye afferents at the borders of ocular dominance columns.

C: A 6-week-old normal monkey; autoradiographic montage of the geniculate labelling pattern in layer IVC of the right striate cortex. The ocular dominance columns appear as sharply defined as in the adult monkey. The unlabelled bar is 1 mm. Adapted from Reference 15.

by environmental influences during a critical period of postnatal development. We have studied this process in detail in one set of functional properties of the nervous system, but it may well be that other aspects of brain function, such as language, complex perceptual tasks, learning, memory and personality, have different programs of development. Such sensitivity of the nervous system to the effects of experience may represent the fundamental mechanism by which the organism adapts to its environment during the period of growth and development.

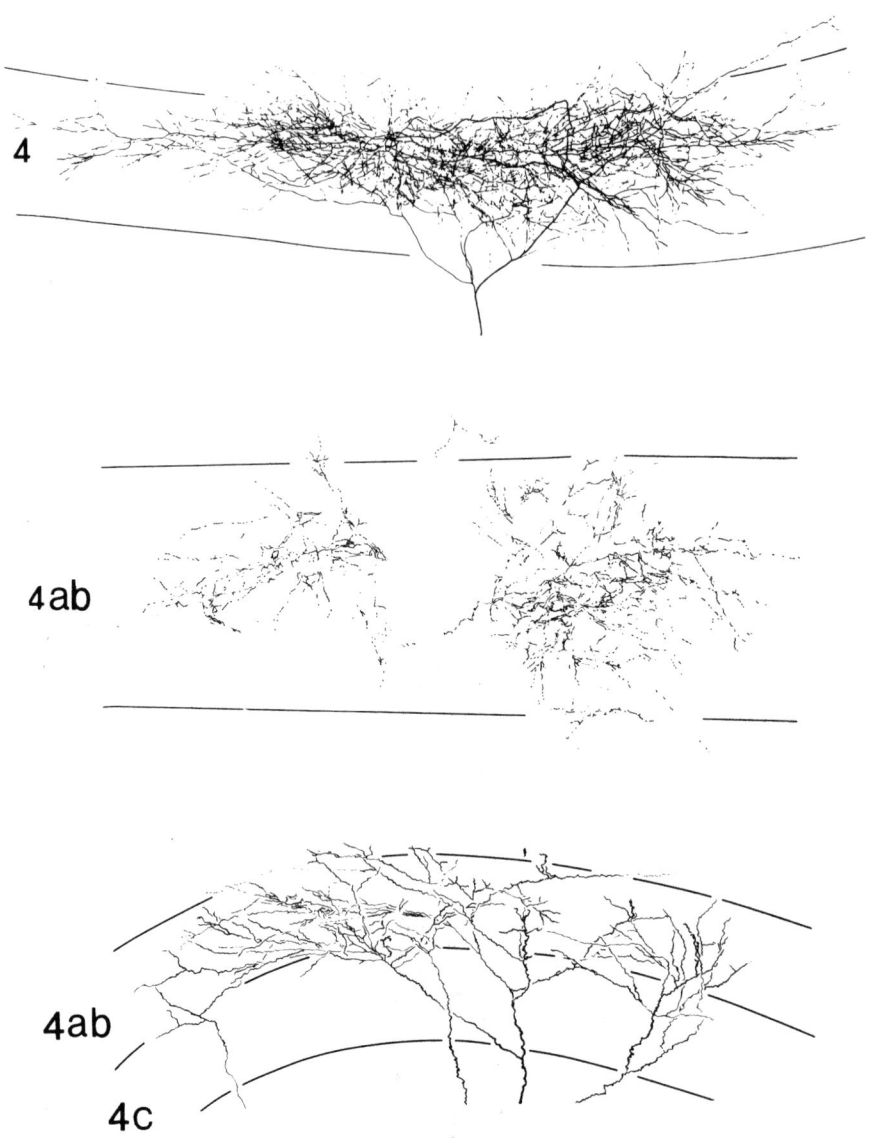

Fig. 14. Patterns of aborization of single geniculate axons in layer 4 of cat visual cortex.

Upper: *A 17-day-old kitten; the arborization of a single afferent is shown at an age prior to the columnar segregation.[71] The axon, impregnated in its entirety with the Rapid Golgi method, arborizes profusely and uniformly over a disc-shaped area that is more than 2 mm in diameter. The use of this illustration is gratefully acknowledged (LeVay, S. and Stryker, M.P.).[73]*

Middle: *Normal adult cat; off-center geniculate afferent (Y-type)[75] injected intra-axonally with horse radish peroxidase (HRP) in the striate cortex. The arborization is entirely within layer 4 ab and forms two patches separated by a terminal-free gap. Presumably this pattern corresponds to the segregation of the input from the two eyes in a columnar fashion.[76]*

Lower: *Monocularly deprived cat (2 weeks—more than 1 year); a non-deprived Y-type afferent with an on-center receptive field injected intra-axonally with HRP. The arborization is primarily within layer 4 ab but does not have the normal patchy distribution of terminals. The absence of a terminal free region indicates that non-deprived geniculate branches are present in the territory that normally belongs only to the other eye.[77]*

ACKNOWLEDGMENTS

I wish to express my gratitude and affection to the staff, faculty and students in the Department of Neurobiology. For over two decades this has been a unique place because of its blend of scientific excellence and compassion. The late Stephen Kuffler played a very special role in the creation of this environment and his spirit and attitude will always serve as an inspiration. My scientific career began in a serious way at Johns Hopkins Medical School and developed further during the past twenty years at Harvard Medical School. I am indebted to both of these institutions for providing me with invaluable opportunities for scientific training and research. I want also to recognize Robert Winthrop who generously provided the resources for my endowed professorship. It is obvious that our work could not have been carried out all these years without federal support; it is a pleasure to acknowledge the steady and generous support from the National Eye Institute. Finally I wish to thank Drs. Anne Houdek and Charles Gilbert for their help in preparing the manuscript.

References

1. Hubel, D. H. and Wiesel, T. N., J. Physiol. 160: 106–154 (1982).
2. von Senden, M., Space and Sight. The Free Press, Glencoe, 1960.
3. Hebb, D. O., The Organization of Behavior. Wiley, New York, 1949.
4. McCleary, R. A., Genetic and Experiential Factors in Perception. Scott Foresman and Company, Glenview, 1970.
5. Hubel, D. H. and Wiesel, T. N., J. Physiol. 148: 574–591 (1959).
6. Wiesel, T. N. and Hubel, D. H., T. N., J. Neurophysiol. 26: 1003–1017 (1963).
7. Wiesel, T. N. and Hubel, D. H., J. Neurophysiol. 26: 978–993 (1963).
8. Hubel, D. H. and Wiesel, T. N., J. Neurophysiol. 26: 994–1002 (1963).
9. Hubel, D. H. and Wiesel, T. N., J. Physiol. 206: 419–436 (1970).
10. Hubel, D. H. and Wiesel, T. N., J. Physiol. 195: 215–243 (1968).
11. Wiesel, T. N. and Hubel, D. H., Int. Union of Physiol. Sciences (I.U.P.S.) ABSTRACTS P. 118–119 (1971).
12. Baker, F. H., Grigg, P. and von Noorden, G. K., Brain Res. 66: 185–208 (1974).
13. Hubel, D. H., Wiesel, T. N. and LeVay, S., Phil. Trans. Soc. London B. 278: 377–409 (1977).
14. Blakemore, C., Garey, L. J. and Vital-Durand, F., J. Physiol. 283: 223–262 (1978).
15. LeVay, S., Wiesel, T. N. and Hubel, D. H., J. Comp. Neurol. 191: 1–51 (1980).
16. Hubel, D. H. and Wiesel, T. N., J. Comp. Neurol. 146: 421–450 (1972).
17. Hubel, D. H. and Wiesel, T. N., J. Comp. Neurol. 158: 267–294 (1974).
18. Wiesel, T. N., Hubel, D. H. and Lam, D., Brain Res. 79: 273–279 (1974).
19. LeVay, S., Hubel, D. H. and Wiesel, T. N., J. Comp. Neurol. 159: 559–576 (1975).
20. Hubel, D. H. and Wiesel, T. N., Proc. R. Soc. Lond. B. 198: 1–59 (1977).
21. Hubel, D. H. and Wiesel, T. N., J. Neurophysiol. 28: 229–289 (1965).
22. Barlow, H. B., Nature 258: 199–204 (1975).
23. Pettigrew, J. D. In: Neuronal Plasticity, ed. C. Cotman. pp. 311–330, New York, Raven (1978). Symposium presentation, Berlin.
24. Movshon, J. A. and van Sluyters, R. C., Ann. Rev. Psychol. 32: 477–552 (1981).
25. Wiesel, T. N. and Raviola, E., Nature 266:66–68 (1977).
26. Guillery, R. W. and Stelzner, D. J., J. Comp. Neurol. 139: 413–422 (1970).
27. Crawford, M. L. J., Blake, R., Cool, S. J. and von Noorden, G. K., Brain Res. 84:150–154 (1975).
28. Blakemore, C. and van Sluyters, R. C., J. Physiol. (London) 237: 195–216 (1974).
29. Arden, G. B. and Barnard, W. M., Trans. Ophthalmol. Soc. U. K. 99: 419–431 (1979).
30. Vaegan, and Taylor, D., Trans. Ophthalmol. Soc. U. K. 99: 432–439 (1979).
31. von Noorden, G. K., Am. J. Ophthalmol. 92: 416–421 (1981).
32. Dews, P. B. and Wiesel, T. N., J. Physiol. 206: 437–455 (1970).
33. Ganz, L., Hirsch, H. V. B. and Tieman, S. B., Brain Res. 44: 547–568 (1972).
34. Wiesel, T. N., Unpublished results.
35. Mitchell, D. E., Cynader, M. and Movshon, J. A., J. Comp. Neurol. 176: 53–64 (1977).
36. Olson, C. R. and Freeman, R. D., J. Neurophysiol. 41:65–74 (1978).
37. Blakemore, C., Vital-Durand, F. and Garey, L. J., Proc. R. Soc. Lond. B 213: 399–423 (1981).
38. Awaya, S., Sugawara, M. and Miyake, S., Trans. Ophthalmol. Soc. U. K. 99: 447–454 (1979).
39. Odom, J. V., Hoyt, C. S. and Marg, E., Arch. Ophthalmol. 99: 1412–1416 (1981).
40. Beller, R., Hoyt, C. S., Marg, E. and Odom, J. V., Amer. J. Ophthal. 91(5): 559–565 (1981).
41. Jacobson, S. G., Mohindra, I. and Held, R., Brit. J. Ophthalmol. 65: 727–735 (1981).
42. Swindale, N. V., Vital-Durand, F. and Blakemore, C., Proc. R. Soc. Lond. B 213: 435–450 (1981).
43. Wiesel, T. N. and Hubel, D. H., J. Neurophysiol. 28: 1029–1040 (1965).
44. Wiesel, T. N. and Hubel, D. H., J. Comp. Neurol. 158: 307–318 (1974).
45. Guillery, R. W., J. Comp. Neurol. 144: 117–130 (1972).
46. Guillery, R. W., J. Comp. Neurol. 148: 417–422 (1973).
47. Hubel, D. H. and Wiesel, T. N., J. Neurophysiol. 28: 1041–1059 (1965).
48. Wiesel, T. N. and Hubel, D. H., Unpublished results.
49. Yinon, U., Exp. Brain Res. 26:151–157 (1976).
50. Crawford, M. L. J. and von Noorden, G. K., Invest. Ophthalmol. 18: 496–505 (1979).
51. Jacobson, S. G. and Ikeda, H., Exp. Brain Res. 34: 11–26 (1979).
52. Singer, W., Rauschecker, J. and Werth, R., Brain Res. 134: 568–572 (1977).
53. Wilson, J. R., Webb, S. V., Sherman, S. M., Brain Res. 136: 277–287 (1977).
54. Stent, G. S., Proc. Natl. Acad. Sci. U.S.A. 70: 997–1001 (1973).
55. Changeux, J.-P. and Danchin, A., Nature 264: 705–712 (1976).
56. Ikeda, H. and Wright, M. J., Exp. Brain Res. 25: 63–77 (1976).
57. Hirsch, H. V. B. and Spinelli, D. N., Science 168: 869–871 (1970).

58. Blakemore, C. and Cooper, G. F., Nature 228: 477–478 (1970).
59. Wiesel, T. N., Carlson, M. and Hubel, D. H., In preparation.
60. Cynader, M. and Mitchell, D. E., Nature 270: 177–178 (1977).
61. Rauschecker, J. P. and Singer, W., Nature 280: 58–80 (1979).
62. Buiserret, P. and Imbert, M., J. Physiol. 255: 511–525 (1976).
63. Marty, R., Archiv. D'Anatomie Microscopique et de Morphologie Experimentale 52: 129–264 (1962).
64. Cragg, B. G., J. Comp. Neurol. 160: 147–166 (1975).
65. Pettigrew, J. D., J. Physiol. 237: 49–74 (1974).
66. Blakemore, C. and von Sluyter, R. C., J. Physiol. 248: 663–716 (1975).
67. Sherk, H. and Stryker, M. P., J. Neurophysiol. 39:63–70 (1976).
68. Singer, W. and Tretter, F., J. Neurophysiol. 39: 613–630 (1976).
69. Des Rosiers, M. H., Sakurada, O., Jehle, J., Shinohara, M., Kennedy, C. and Sokoloff, L., Science 200: 447–449 (1978).
70. Rakic, P., Philos. Trans. R. Soc. London, Ser. B. 278: 245–260 (1977).
71. LeVay, S., Stryker, M. P. and Shatz, C. J., J. Comp. Neurol. 179: 223–244 (1978).
72. Swindale, N. V., Nature 290: 332–333 (1981).
73. LeVay, S. and Stryker, M. P., Soc. Neurosci. Symp. 4: 83–98 (1979).
74. Ferster, D. and LeVay, S., J. Comp. Neurol. 182: 923–944 (1978).
75. Enroth-Cugell, C. and Robson, J. G., J. Physiol. 182: 923–944 (1966).
76. Gilbert, C. and Wiesel, T. N., Nature 280: 120–125 (1979).
77. Gilbert, C. and Wiesel, T. N., Unpublished observations.
78. Kasamatsu, T. and Pettigrew, J. D., J. Comp. Neurol. 185: 139–162 (1979).

Chapter 28 • Epilogue: Summing Up •

Perhaps the most remarkable thing about our collaboration is the fact that it continued for 25 years, much longer than most collaborations. Ours had the special quality that it was between equals, in age and in seniority. Our two abilities were not identical but were complementary. An analogy might be Gilbert and Sullivan (Steve Kuffler once jokingly compared us to Huntley and Brinkley). Rosencrantz and Guildenstern also come to mind. As we look back, what stands out is the almost total absence of disagreements. When, late at night, should we finally quit and go home? Whom among fellow scientists did we revere or otherwise? What should we do next? We never quite knew or even discussed where our ideas came from: they presumably arose in the long discussions that went on during our interminable experiments, and once an idea was hatched by one of us it was often forgotten, only to be resurrected months later by the other.

Almost absent from our way of working and thinking were hypotheses, at least explicit ones. We regarded our work as mainly exploratory, and although some experiments were done to answer specific questions, most were done in the spirit of Columbus crossing the Atlantic to see what he would find. Today our grant proposals would surely be criticized as not being "hypothesis driven", as not following the rules of Science as taught in high school and as exemplified especially in physics. We believe that such rules as to how Science (with a capital S) is done, or should be done, are largely fiction, an attempt to retrospectively codify a process that often amounts to groping. There simply are no rules as to how to do science. Looking back, we can recognize times when we must have had something vaguely resembling a "hypothesis". Probably we could have dressed up our thought processes in those terms, but we would have found it dishonest to do so, even for grant-application purposes. Similarly, the way scientific papers are written usually represents a kind of fiction in rearranging the order in which ideas occur and the work is done, to form a logical sequence that may have little basis in reality. Papers written in the 1800s are often more open and honest (if that is the right word) in saying how ideas developed. In our papers we tried to preserve some of that and even succeeded in inserting a few jokes, if only to prove that the reviewers had occasional lapses of attention. Above all we tried to make our papers easy to read. With almost religious determination we avoided abbreviations, with the sole exceptions of LGB and EPSP. That avoidance probably cost the publishers all of three extra lines at the end of some of our papers, but it must have saved our readers many minutes of searching back to find what the letters stood for. We tried to make our illustrations easy to read by resisting the temptation to combine eighteen small figures into one large one, a custom perhaps started by Eccles and perpetuated by Eric Kandel. We tried to avoid figure-legends in which the a's, b's and c's are buried in text instead of being separated by paragraphs, so that the poor reader has to search for the tiny letters with a dissecting microscope. We were often unsuccessful because of the puzzling resistance of editors. All this was in attempts to make our papers less tiring and tiresome to read: we hope we succeeded.

How do we find our field today, in comparison with its state when we set out on this adventure in 1958? We set out at a perfect time. Virtually nothing had been done with microelectrodes in the visual cortex—or in the cortex in general, except for Mountcastle's marvelous beginning in the somatosensory cortex. We had the necessary techniques—or we had the leisure to develop them ourselves. A little earlier and we might have ended up studying impulses and synapses, or possibly the spinal cord, which was very popular in the 1950s. In the visual cortex we had little competition for about ten years, perhaps because it was generally felt that our type of work was too arduous, or perhaps because it was assumed that you had to understand the retina perfectly before going more centrally. Something like that certainly happened in the auditory system, in which the research got hung up on the end organ, and the auditory cortex was, and still is, relatively neglected.

Today we have some concerns about the present state of our field. One unfortunate development is the fading of neuroanatomy. Our work, at least much of it, involved a close coupling of physiology and neuroanatomy, and in the 1970s we were doing about as much of one as of the other. We certainly were lucky in inheriting techniques like the Nauta method and autoradiography—or one might say we were good at ignoring those who said that only the experts should attempt them. Typically we used a monkey each week, often doing separate physiological and anatomical studies in the same monkey. That allowed us to work out much of the structural and physiological relationships that are so important in understanding the cortex. We were also lucky in working at a time before the animal rights groups had made it so much harder to do research involving animals—harder in the sense of expenses and the hoops to be jumped through to get past all the layers of red tape that exist today. Monkeys are now many times more expensive, and the hoops are more numerous. To use monkeys today at the rate we used them in the 1970s and 1980s would be almost impossible.

We were lucky in having youth on our side. Today we certainly would not have the stamina to stay up all night, even once a week. For all these reasons the field has turned increasingly to the use of awake-behaving chronically implanted monkeys, in which one monkey can be recorded from for months or years, and one can work for four hours each day and then go home to dinner. The catch is that parallel anatomical studies are practically impossible because the brain becomes available only after many months, and has been recorded from so many times that it resembles a pincushion.

A second, in some ways unfortunate, trend in visual-cortex physiology is its increasing popularity, with hundreds of labs working in dozens of the known visual cortical areas. So the competition is greater, by orders of magnitude. We do not fully understand why, in the realm of systems physiology, vision should have become so dominant, relative to other systems. To some extent it probably is a bandwagon effect: when a field becomes trendy, people stream in from all sides, as happened many years ago in the case of the bolo-bat and the hula hoop. When we started out, the most dynamic branch of sensory neurophysiology was somatosensory, thanks to Clinton Woolsey and especially Vernon Mountcastle. The switch over to vision, while hard to explain, could have been related to the high information content of vision, relative to touch and joint position. If that is the reason, then it is hard to see why the central auditory path is so neglected.

A third problem represents to us an example of illnesses that scientific fields can be subject to. In neurophysiology this is the increasing popularity of theory, sometimes called *computation*. No one familiar with developments in physics in the past century or so could possibly deny the importance of theory in that branch of science. But it seems to us that the chances of theory ever assuming a comparable importance in biology (and in particular, neurobiology) may be slim. One indeed has the impression that the main proponents of theory in neurophysiology may be scientists who have trained in mathematics and, having gone into biology, are reluctant to give up the mathematics. I can understand that, having had some training in mathematics and once having expected to use it in neurophysiology. In the best hands (and one thinks of people such as David Marr, Horace Barlow, Werner Reichardt, Terry Sejnowski, Christof Koch and Francis Crick), our field has certainly benefited. But in the case of such subjects as "linear systems analysis," the emphasis seems either puzzling or wrong. No one with much experience with cortical cells could think of them in any real sense as *linear*. Our feelings concerning the use of sine-wave gratings, already referred to here and there in this book, always in a pejorative way, will come as no surprise to readers who have put up with our dogmatism thus far. Another hot topic in recent years has been "multiplexing", the notion that a cell's responses can reflect its involvement with a multitude of variables, and that few if any cells are highly specialized. Visual scientists who are in any way burdened with a familiarity with cells in the visual cortex of higher mammals will be astonished at the idea that all cells carry information about all variables (such as orientation, movement direction, color, spatial frequency, and stereopsis). What has struck us from the very first was the increasing degree of specialization of cells as one goes from level to level in the central nervous system, and the specialization already apparent in most cells in V-1. We have double-opponent cells with their color and center-surround selectivity and their lack of orientation selectivity; the sharp orientation selectivity of most other cells in V-1 (outside layer 4) along with their frequent movement–direction selectivity, but with an almost total lack of concern with color; cells that respond to black slits but not to white, or the reverse; or those that respond to both black and white; or those that respond to red slits, but neither black nor white. Multiplexing seems to imply a small amount of specialization for many variables, with the sorting out presumably being left to later stages in the nervous system, if it occurs at all. The idea is ingenious but seems not to be used very much by the brain. Of course we have many examples of a cell's encoding more than one variable: cells involved with stereopsis seem always to be orientation selective; most V-1 color-coded cells have center-surround fields, but to lack orientation selectivity. Most cells indeed seem to encode an assortment of variables, but a very limited assortment. What we do not see is a small degree of specialization for many or all possible variables.

The field of molecular biology, which we regard as more successful as a science than our field, seems largely to have avoided being beset with computation. In *The Molecular Biology of the Gene* I look in vain for equations. No one has tried to fit a protein molecule to a Gabor function, as far as I know. One could be terribly wrong about such things, and it will be interesting to see how our field develops. I do sense that fields of science, like biological organisms, can become sick, and I hope that does not happen to neurophysiology.

Why did we at last stop collaborating, around 1980? The prize came in 1981, so that event must have been unrelated. Forces promoting our separation had been present from an early time—even our staunchest supporter, Steve Kuffler, repeatedly and gently suggested we might be wise to split and each take on postdoctoral collaborators and different projects. But always in the end we had complete support from Steve to go on stubbornly working together. As time went on, the main force towards separation was increasing pressure to do administration and teaching that we could not entirely avoid. I had had a dose of being a department head, and stood it for a year, giving up when it became clear that the installation of a pencil-sharpener in the physiology department secretary's office required me to discuss the matter over coffee with each of the other tenure department members. In 1973 Steve Kuffler, having been leader of our group since its inception at Johns Hopkins and chairman since the neurobiology department's founding in 1966, decided to step down. A successor had to be found; I had learned my lesson, but Torsten was a sitting duck and too conscientious to refuse. While the department was still young and small, the administration was relatively light, but as it got bigger, with more faculty and graduate students, the drain on his time increased. It got so that our customary Tuesday experiments were being done without prior planning and with little subsequent discussion. In the end we felt like two horses continuing to drag the same plough over the same terrain year after year, with constant guilt feelings that we were neglecting one or another committee or were getting behind in letters of recommendation.

We are nevertheless grateful at having had so many years of uninterrupted research. We were wise enough, perhaps, to avoid the usual trap of taking on many dependent postdocs and graduate students, gradually letting them do more and more of the research we enjoyed, while we spent more and more time at the desk writing papers, grant requests and letters of recommendation, and losing our feel for the research. We did have small numbers of postdocs and graduate students, but made them independent, giving advice gently and rarely, as Steve had done with us. That way, we felt, we did not deprive them of the main thing a beginning scientist needs to learn: to get one's own ideas and try them out. The strategy worked, for our trainees (if that is the right word!) have done well.

From 1980 to 1990 I collaborated with Margaret Livingstone, who had begun as a graduate student in our department, in a study of color and stereopsis in V-2. We carried on a regular dialogue with Edwin Land, whom Torsten and I had gotten to know in the 1970s and 1980s. I greatly admired his inventiveness, and his death, in 1991, came as a severe blow.

I then collaborated with Stephen Macknik and Susana Martinez-Conde on a study of microsaccadic eye movements and the bursts of firing they produce in cells in the primary visual cortex. Finally, with a fellow Canadian, Kevin Duffy, I have been looking at receptive fields in the striate cortex of dark-adapted monkeys.

Today I run a class for 12 freshman Harvard College undergraduates, with weekly discussions and a lab. In their first semester at college their enthusiasm over starting college has not yet worn off, and these seminars have been my best teaching experience in 45 years of university life. The program was founded years ago by Edwin Land, motivated by his disaffection over having had so little contact with his professors when he was a student at Harvard.

We must end by saying words of thanks to the society that supported us. We were most fortunate that the National Institutes of Health existed and that the Eye Institute came into being at just about the time we started. And especially that the members of the NIH Eye Institute were so supportive and such a pleasure to work with. The other piece of luck was everything about the university system of the United States, especially the relative freedom from domination by department heads, particularly in handling one's finances; the freedom to move to some other place if not satisfied, and perhaps above all the wonderful enthusiasm and overall quality of the students. These are all things that explain the success of biological research in this country, and to a large extent explain its lack of success in other countries, even wealthy ones. We have, and do, complain loudly about many problems this country has had and still has—the swings in politics such as the McCarthy and Nixon eras, Vietnam, and prevailing attitudes to the Kyoto Accord, the World Court, Iraq, the gun lobby, and so on. But about the handsome way our research and our fellow biologists' research has been supported we have only gratitude.

LIST OF PAPERS INCLUDED

Normal Physiology and Anatomy

1. Hubel DH and Wiesel TN (1959) Receptive fields of single neurones in the cat's striate cortex. *J Physiol* 148:574–591.
2. Hubel DH and Wiesel TN (1960) Receptive Fields of Optic Nerve Fibres in the Spider Monkey. *J Physiol* 154:572–580.
3. Hubel DH and Wiesel TN (1961) Integrative action in the cat's lateral geniculate body. *J Physiol* 155:385–398.
4. Hubel DH and Wiesel TN (1962) Receptive fields, binocular interaction and functional architecture in the cat's visual cortex. *J Physiol* 160:106–154.
5. Hubel DH and Wiesel TN (1965) Receptive fields and functional architecture in two nonstriate visual areas (18 and 19) of the cat. *J Neurophysiol* 28:229–289.
6. Wiesel TN and Hubel DH (1966) Spatial and chromatic interactions in the lateral geniculate body of the Rhesus monkey. *J Neurophysiol* 29:1115–1156.
7. Hubel DH and Wiesel TN (1967) Cortical and callosal connections concerned with the vertical meridian of visual fields in the cat. *J Neurophysiol* 30:1561–1573.
8. Hubel DH and Wiesel TN (1968) Receptive fields and functional architecture of monkey striate cortex. *J Physiol* 195:215–243.
9. Hubel DH and Wiesel TN (1969) Visual area of the lateral suprasylvian gyrus (Clare-Bishop area) of the cat. *J Physiol* 202:251–260.
10. Hubel DH and Wiesel TN (1970) Cells sensitive to binocular depth in area 18 of the macaque monkey cortex. *Nature* 225:41–42.
11. Hubel DH and Wiesel TN (1972) Laminar and columnar distribution of geniculo-cortical fibers in the macaque monkey. *J Comp Neurol* 146:421–450.
12. Wiesel TN, Hubel DH, and Lam D. (1974) Autoradiographic demonstration of ocular-dominance columns in the monkey striate cortex by means of transneuronal transport. *Brain Res* 79:273–279.
13. Hubel DH and Wiesel TN (1974a) Sequence regularity and geometry or orientation columns in the monkey striate cortex. *J Comp Neurol* 158:267–293.
14. Hubel DH and Wiesel TN (1974b) Of monkey striate cortex: a parallel relationship between field size, scatter, and magnification factor. *J Comp Neurol* 158:295–306.

Deprivation and Development

15. Wiesel TN and Hubel DH (1963) Effects of visual deprivation on morphology and physiology of cells in the cat's lateral geniculate body. *J Neurophysiol* 26:978–993.
16. Hubel DH and Wiesel TN (1963) Receptive fields of cells in striate cortex of very young, visually inexperienced kittens. *J Neurophysiol* 26:994–1002.
17. Wiesel TN and Hubel DH (1963) Single-cell responses in striate cortex of kittens deprived of vision in one eye. *J Neurophysiol* 26:1003–1017.
18. Wiesel TN and Hubel DH (1965) Comparison of the effects of unilateral and bilateral eye closure on cortical unit responses in kittens. *J Neurophysiol* 28:1029–1040.
19. Hubel DH and Wiesel TN (1965) Binocular interaction in striate cortex of kittens reared with artificial squint. *J Neurophysiol* 28:1041–1059.
20. Wiesel TN and Hubel DH (1965) Extent of recovery from the effects of visual deprivation in kittens. *J. Neurophysiol* 28:1060–1072.
21. Hubel DH and Wiesel TN (1970) The period of susceptibility to the physiological effects of unilateral eye closure in kittens. *J Physiol* 206:419–436.
22. Hubel DH and Wiesel TN (1971) Aberrant visual projections in the Siamese cat. *J Physiol* 218:33–62.
23. Wiesel TN and Hubel DH (1974) Ordered arrangement of orientation columns in monkeys lacking visual experience. *J Comp Neurol* 158:307–318.
24. Hubel DH, Wiesel TN, and LeVay S (1977) Plasticity of ocular dominance columns in monkey striate cortex. *Phil Trans R Soc Lond B* 278:377–409.(?)
25. LeVay S, Wiesel TN, and Hubel DH (1980) The development of ocular dominance columns in normal and visually deprived monkeys. *J Comp Neurol* 191:1–51.

Three Reviews

26. Hubel DH and Wiesel TN (1977) Functional architecture of macaque monkey visual cortex. *Proc R Soc Lond B* 198:1–59, Ferrier Lecture.
27. Hubel, D.H. (1982) Evolution of Ideas on the Primary Visual Cortex, 1955–1978. A Biased Historical Account. In: *Les Prix Nobel en 1981*, pp. 221–256.(x).
28. Wiesel, Torsten N. The Postnatal Development of the Visual Cortex and the Influence of Environment. In: *Les Prix Nobel en 1981*, pp. 261–283. (x)

GLOSSARY

ABSTRACT Short summary of a paper or poster to be presented at a scientific meeting, usually published in advance of the meeting. Usually only one or several paragraphs in length.

ADRIAN, LORD (E. D.) (1889–1977) Neurophysiologist at Trinity College, Cambridge, England, famous for work in the central nervous system, especially cortical encephalography, sleep mechanisms, vision, and motor system. Nobel prize [1932], shared with C. S. Sherrington "for their discoveries regarding the functions of neurons".

ADVANCER, MICROELECTRODE The apparatus that moves a microelectrode forward through the brain or other tissue in small controlled steps, by means of a piston-cylinder arrangement, a stepping motor, or a screw.

AFFERENT Of nerve fibers, input, etc., carrying impulses to a structure (cf. *efferent*).

ANESTHESIA In the animal experiments described here, the anesthetics most used were barbiturates, either Pentothal (sodium thiopental) or Nembutal (sodium pentobarbital), administered in intermittent intramuscular injections or by continuous intravenous injection. Towards the end of the 1970s we began to use inhalation anesthetics, especially halothane.

ARTERIOVENOUS SHUNT Abnormality in which an artery is directly connected to a vein, bypassing a capillary bed. Can occur as a congenital abnormality, in certain tumors, or as a result of surgical joining of an artery to a vein for hemodialysis.

AUTORADIOGRAPHY *See* p. 317 for description.

BARLOW, HORACE (born 1921). Neurophysiologist and psychophysicist, noted for studies of frog retinal ganglion cell physiology (originated the idea of "trigger features"); studies of dark adaptation and spontaneous firing of retinal ganglion cells in cats (with Stephen Kuffler); responses to movement in rabbit retinal ganglion cells; responses of cat cortical cells to binocular (stereoscopic) cues; and for psychophysical studies in vision.

BAUMGARTNER, GÜNTER (1924–1991) Neurologist and neurophysiologist. Collaborated with Richard Jung in early recordings from visual cortex. Later head of neurology in Zurich.

BÉKÉSY [1899–1972] Auditory neurophysiologist, noted for work on hair cells. Nobel prize physiology or medicine, 1961.

BLAKEMORE, COLIN (born 1944) Professor of Physiology, Oxford University. Research in visual neurophysiology includes visual cortex, especially binocular depth mechanisms, studies of postnatal development, and many psychophysical topics. Main research has been in cats and monkeys.

BLASDEL, GARY (born 1949) Neurophysiologist, best known for studies of neuroanatomy and neurophysiology of mammalian visual system, and for developing optical methods for surface mapping of cerebral cortex, especially striate cortex of macaque monkeys, using voltage-sensitive dyes.

BLOBS A term causing some annoyance to colleagues in neuroanatomy and neurophysiology, referring to groups of cells in visual cortex (V-1) of primates and perhaps cats, visible on tangential and transverse sections stained for the enzyme cytochrome oxidase (and other enzymatic stains). In macaques they are centered on ocular dominance columns, about ½ mm apart and about 0.2 mm in diameter. First noted in cross-sections by Margaret Wong Riley.

Shown by Jonathan Horton, Margaret Livingstone and Hubel to contain center-surround cells (lacking orientation selectivity), frequently double-opponent. Also called *dots, puffs, spots,* etc.

BOWDITCH, HENRY P. First chairman of physiology, Harvard Medical School, from 1883 to 1893.

CANNON, WALTER B. (1871–1945) Celebrated for work in general physiology, especially regulatory mechanisms and homeostasis. Second chairman of physiology at Harvard Medical School.

CHIASM, OPTIC Site of crossing of optic nerve fibers in mammals. On arriving at the chiasm, somewhat more than half (in primates) of the fibers from each eye cross and proceed to the lateral geniculate body on the other (contralateral) side; the rest stay on the same (ipsilateral) side. The fibers that cross are those that come from the nasal (inner) half of each retina, corresponding to the temporal halves of the visual fields.

COLOR CONSTANCY The stability of the color (or hue) of an object despite variations in the spectral content of the light source. The neural circuits responsible for this are not clear, but our guess is that double-opponent cells are involved.

COLUMN Term coined by Vernon Mountcastle, who was the first to describe cortical columns in the somatosensory cortex. It refers to a group of cells extending from the cortical surface to the white matter, more or less cylindrical, with a cross-sectional area of up to several square millimeters. In the primary visual cortex, columns are of two types, subserving ocular dominance and orientation (the system of blobs might also be considered columnar), and they take the form of sheets rather than pillars, as the term *column* might seem to suggest.

COMPOUND ACTION POTENTIAL Response recorded from a whole nerve containing many fibers, initiated usually by electrical stimulation, and usually seen as a deflection or set of deflections on an oscilloscope. The shape of the response is determined by the shapes of the impulse deflections of the individual nerve fibers, and by the conduction velocities of the fibers that make up the nerve.

CONWAY, BEVIL (born 1974) Postdoctoral fellow, neurobiology, Harvard Medical School from 2003. First to confirm the presence of cortical double-opponent cells in macaque cortex through the combined use of cone-isolation techniques and reverse-correlation receptive-field mapping.

CORPUS CALLOSUM Large band of myelinated fibers crossing from one cerebral hemisphere to the other. An example of a commissure (the anterior commissure and posterior commissure being two others).

DAW, NIGEL W. (born 1933) Postdoctoral student in our lab with Alan Pearlman (1967–1969). The first to describe double-opponent cells, in retinas of goldfish.

DILATION AND CURETTAGE Procedure in gynecology consisting of dilating the cervix and scraping the inner wall of the uterus, for treating incomplete miscarriage or bleeding.

DOUBLE-OPPONENT CELLS Cells with opponent center-surround receptive fields in which centers are fed by two sets of opponent cones and the surrounds by two sets. For example, a cell's receptive field center might receive excitation from long wavelength cones, and inhibition from middle wavelength cones, and its surround receive excitation from middle wavelength cones and inhibition from long wavelength cones. First described in goldfish retina by Nigel Daw (1968), and subsequently observed in striate cortex of macaques by Hubel and Wiesel (1968) and shown to be present in blobs by Margaret Livingstone and Hubel (1984). Double-opponent cells were studied with cone isolating stimuli by Conway (2001).

ECCENTRICITY Distance, usually expressed in degrees, between some retinal point and the fovea.

ECCLES, SIR JOHN CAREW (1903–1997) Neurophysiologist, Australian, Rhodes Scholar from Melbourne, worked with Sherrington in England, then moved to Sydney Australia, then to Otago University in New Zealand (1944–1951). He returned to Australia in 1952 (the National University, Canberra, where he remained until 1966, when he came to the United States of America (Chicago and Buffalo). He worked on synaptic mechanisms, especially in the spinal cord of cats, where he established the importance of inhibitory synaptic transmission (and originated the terms *EPSP* and *IPSP*). In the cerebellum, he worked out the main circuit and its physiology. Nobel prize in Medicine or Physiology, 1963, shared with Alan Hodgkin and Andrew Huxley.

EEG (ELECTROENCEPHALOGRAM) Record of cortical slow waves made by gross (1 mm or larger) electrodes placed on scalp. Used in research and clinical diagnosis.

EFFERENT Of nerve fibers, carrying impulses away from a structure (cf. afferent).

ELECTROCORTICOGRAM. (ECG). Record of cortical slow waves made by gross (1 mm or larger) electrodes placed on cortical surface. Used clinically and in research.

ELECTRODE (see also **microelectrode**). For *recording* neural activity: usually a metal wire placed in or on the tissue being studied. Also used to *stimulate* neural structures by injecting current, or to *destroy* (coagulate) neural tissue in order to identify recording sites, to trace pathways by observing the course of degenerating fibers, or to study the effects (behavioral or physiological) of the destruction.

ELECTROLYTIC LESION Means of destroying neurological tissue by passing electric current through an electrode. Small electrolytic lesions can be used to identify microelectrode recording sites in the brain on histological examination, or to produce degeneration of axons for tracing pathways.

EPSP: EXCITATORY POST-SYNAPTIC POTENTIAL Transient change in membrane potential, usually depolarizing, in response to an impulse or impulses arriving over an excitatory presynaptic fiber or fibers.

EXCITATION In neurophysiology, a process leading to impulse generation, or increase in frequency of impulses, or a depolarization of the membrane of a nerve cell—and consequent increase in the release of transmitter by the cell.

EXTRACELLULAR RECORDING The recording of electrical activity of a cell, usually a nerve cell, in which the electrode remains in close proximity to, but outside the cell. Often used to record action potentials, with signals that are generally many times smaller than those recorded intracellularly. The most commonly used electrodes are metallic, because of their low impedance.

FIXATION, VISUAL The act of positioning the eyes so that a visual target is made to fall on the fovea.

FOVEA Usually defined as a region of retina subtending about 1 degree of visual field, where acuity is highest, and rods are absent.

FOWLER, H.G. Author of *Modern English Usage* (Oxford, 1926).

FUORTES, M.G.F. Italian, worked mainly at Walter Reed Army Institute of Research, Washington, D.C., collaborated with Karl Frank on mammalian spinal cord, and worked independently on mammalian vision.

GALAMBOS, ROBERT (born 1914) Auditory neurophysiologist, worked at Harvard on sonar system in bats. Then at Walter Reed Army Institute of Research, in the 1950s and 1960s, and later at Madison, Wisconsin, studied responses of cochlear nuclei and other brain stem nuclei, in cats.

GOLGI METHOD OR STAIN Methods of staining nervous tissue, in which a very small number of nerve cells (or glia cells) are stained, often in their entirety.

GRANDMOTHER CELL Jocular term conveying the idea of a single cell that fires impulses only in response to one's grandmother, presumably the sight of her, the recollection of her, or the idea of her.

GRANIT, RAGNAR (1900–1991) Swedish neurophysiologist known for research on mammalian visual system and cerebellum. Nobel prize, in medicine or physiology 1967.

GRAY MATTER Regions of brain and spinal cord that contain nerve cell bodies, together with their axons, dendrites, and synapses. "Gray" refers to the appearance of freshly cut sections.

GUILLERY, RAYNOR (born 1929) Madison, Wisconsin, and Oxford, England. Neuroanatomist, contributed mainly to mammalian visual system anatomy, especially lateral geniculate body and cortex.

HEBB, DONALD (1904–1985) Canadian Psychologist, born in Nova Scotia, head of Psychology Dept, McGill University, noted especially for proposing a synaptic mechanism for learning, in what became known as the *Hebb Synapse*.

HEMIPARESIS Weakness of face, arm, and leg on one side, generally caused by damage to the motor cortex or the fiber tracts descending from cortex to spinal cord. It is associated with brisk deep tendon reflexes and increased muscle tone on the side contralateral to a brain lesion.

HODGKIN, ALAN (1914–1998) Neurophysiologist best known for his work, with Andrew Huxley, on the ionic basis of the nerve impulse, for which they shared the Nobel prize in 1963 with Sir John Eccles. Worked in Cambridge, England.

HUDSPETH, JAMES ALBERT Graduate student at Harvard Medical School with Wiesel and Hubel, 1967–1973. Noted for his work on auditory hair cells.

HUXLEY, SIR ANDREW (born 1917) Neurophysiologist best known for his work, with Alan Hodgkin, on the ionic basis of the nerve impulse, for which they shared the Nobel prize in 1963 with Sir John Eccles.

IMPULSE (NERVE) Term signifying an all-or-nothing propagated event, the main means by which most nerve cells communicate. Consists of a reversal of the potential between the inside and outside of the nerve cell that lasts about

1 millisecond and is propagated along the fiber at rates up to many meters/second. When an impulse reaches the terminals of the nerve fiber, it generally causes the release of a neurotransmitter and subsequent depolarization, hyperpolarization, or lowering of the impedance, of the postsynaptic membrane.

INHIBITION In neurophysiology, suppression of impulse activity of a neurone, or lessening of the neurotransmitter that the neurone releases. Usually associated with hyperpolarization, or a lowering of membrane impedance, either of which will tend to counteract any excitatory influences.

INTEGRATION Term used by Sherrington. In this book we use it to refer to the summing up, by a single cell, of all its excitatory and inhibitory inputs.

INTRACELLULAR RECORDING Electrical recording from a nerve or muscle cell, of resting potentials, impulses, or excitatory or inhibitory synaptic events; made by inserting a microelectrode (usually a micropipette filled with a conducting solution—KCl, NaCl, etc.) through the cell membrane into the cytoplasm.

IPSP Inhibitory post-synaptic potential. Transient change, usually hyperpolarization, in membrane potential in response to an impulse arriving in an inhibitory presynaptic fiber.

JASPER, HERBERT H. (1906–1999) Neurophysiologist, contributed to developing the electroencephalogram (EEG) as a diagnostic tool in neurology. Close collaborator of the neurosurgeon Wilder Penfield. Worked at the Montreal Neurological Institute 1938–65, and the University of Montreal (1965–1999).

JOHNS HOPKINS HOSPITAL Baltimore, Maryland. Opened in 1889, situated close to Johns Hopkins Medical School (founded 1893), and associated with Johns Hopkins University.

JOURNAL OF PHYSIOLOGY Founded 1878 by the Physiological Society, London. The first journal devoted entirely to physiology. A leading journal publishing research articles in all areas of physiology, with headquarters in Cambridge, England.

JUNG, RICHARD (1911–1986) Neurologist and neurophysiologist, head of neurology in Freiberg, Germany; one of the first to record single cells from the cortex in cats. Many of Germany's leading post-World War II neurophysiologists trace their research ancestry to Jung.

KANDEL, ERIC R (born 1929) Neurobiologist. Contributed to the synaptic basis of learning. Nobel Prize for Medicine or Physiology, with Paul Greengard, "for their discoveries concerning signal transduction in the nervous system".

KATZ, SIR BERNARD (1911–2003) Neurophysiologist best known for his work, with Sir John Eccles and Stephen Kuffler, on synaptic transmission. Was the first to describe, with Ricardo Miledi, quantal mechanisms of synaptic release. Worked in Sydney, Australia, and at University College, London. Nobel prize in 1970, shared with Ulf Von Euler and Julius Axelrod, "for their discoveries concerning the humoral transmitters in the nerve terminals and the mechanism of their storage, release and inactivation."

KUFFLER, STEPHEN (1913–1980) Neurophysiologist with an immense range that included synaptic transmission, mammalian vision, spinal cord in cats, studies of glia, and chemical synaptic modulators. Born in Austria-Hungary, he worked in Sydney, Australia (1940–1945, with Katz and Eccles), Chicago (1945–1947), the Wilmer Institute of Ophthalmology at Johns Hopkins Hospital in Baltimore (1947–1959), and at Harvard Medical School in Boston, where he founded the Department of Neurobiology in 1966 and was chairman from 1966 to 1973.

LATERAL GENICULATE NUCLEUS Peanut-size collection of cells that forms part of the thalamus. Receives its main input from the optic tract, and hence from retinal ganglion cells. Like other thalamic nuclei, it sends its axons to the cerebral cortex and receives projections back from the cortex. In primates it projects to the primary visual (striate) cortex.

LESION In the context of neurology, the destruction of neural tissue—a fiber pathway or part or all of a group of cells. In research, the purpose of producing a lesion can be to study the effects of destruction by using physiological or behavioral techniques, or to trace neuronal pathways by staining the degenerating fibers or terminals, or to determine the position of an electrode tip.

LETTVIN, JEROME Y. Neurophysiologist, at MIT. Noted especially for work with Humberto Maturana on optic nerve fibers of the frog, and among the first to describe their complex response properties.

LIVINGSTONE, MARGARET (born 1950) Graduate student in laboratory of Edward Kravitz, Harvard Medical School. Now Professor of Neurobiology, Harvard Medical School. Noted for research on lobster nervous system, studies of neurochemistry of the brain of drosophila (fruit fly), and monkey visual neurophysiology. Collaborated with Hubel (1980 to 2000).

LUND, JENNIFER Neuroanatomist, noted for studies of the visual cortex, especially striate cortex, of monkeys. The leading authority on visual cortex anatomy studied by the Golgi method.

MAGNIFICATION Relation between distance along a structure such as the visual cortex and distance in the visual field, usually expressed as millimeters/degree. In the cortex, it varies as a function of eccentricity, being maximal in the fovea and falling off with eccentricity.

MAGNOCELLULAR LAYERS In macaque and human lateral geniculate bodies, the two ventral (lower) large-cell layers, separated from each other and from the dorsal layers by interlaminar leaflets. Cells have center-surround receptive fields, mainly type 4 (see pp. 215–216).

MARSHALL, WADE Head of neurophysiology at NIH in Bethesda, Maryland, in the 1950s. Known for work on vision (with Samuel Talbot) and for his studies of spreading depression.

MATURANA, HUMBERTO Neurophysiologist, at MIT in the 1950s and. Noted especially for work with Jerome Y. Lettvin on optic nerve fibers and the tectum of the frog, and among the first to describe their complex response properties.

MICROELECTRODE In neurophysiology, usually a micropipette filled with a conducting solution (KCl, NaCl, etc.), or a wire tapered to a fine tip and coated with insulating material such as glass or a lacquer. Used to record electrical activity, from outside a cell or small group of cells (extracellular recording), or from inside a single cell (intracellular recording).

MODULE see pp. 364–365.

MONTREAL GENERAL HOSPITAL One of the two leading English hospitals in Montreal.

MONTREAL NEUROLOGICAL INSTITUTE Institute devoted to neurology, neurosurgery, and neurological research, associated with the Royal Victoria Hospital and McGill University, founded by the Rockefeller Institute in 1934.

MOUNTCASTLE, VERNON (born 1918) Pioneer in recording from a variety of brain structures in cats and monkeys. Worked at Johns Hopkins Medical School. Best known for studies of somatosensory cortex, and for his discovery of cortical columns in 1957.

MT (Middle temporal) A visual area in occipital lobes of monkeys, first described in New World monkeys, called V-5 in macaques by Zeki, probably homologous with the Clare-Bishop area (PMLS) of cats. The cells have large receptive fields and show striking direction selectivity to movement.

MYELIN Wrapping, like a jelly-roll, of nerve axons by many layers of lipid-containing glial membranes that serve to increase resistance and lower capacitance between outside and inside of an axon, resulting in increased speed of conduction.

NATIONAL EYE INSTITUTE (NEI) One of the institutes of the National Institutes of Health centered in Bethesda, Maryland. The NEI was founded in 1968. Like other institutes of the NIH, it supports research through an intramural component, located in Bethesda, and an extramural program that awards grants to individual investigators or groups, mainly at universities in the United States of America.

NAUTA, WALLE J. H. (1916–1994) Neuroanatomist, who introduced a new era by developing methods for tracing neural pathways by making lesions and staining the degenerating fibers with silver stains.

NEUROPHYSIOLOGY The study of the function of the nervous system, in contradistinction to neuroanatomy (the study of the morphology of the nervous system) and neurochemistry (the study of its chemistry). It is a branch of physiology (which also includes studies of the function of cells, or organs such as heart, kidney and so on) or, depending on how one cuts the cake, a branch of neurobiology, which includes neuroanatomy and neurochemistry. The term *electrophysiology* implies a type of neurophysiology in which the tools are electrical stimulators and recording devices.

NISSL SUBSTANCE Basophilic organelles contained in cytoplasm of neuronal cell bodies and dendrites. Stained by cresyl violet, methylene blue, and toluidine blue.

OFF-RESPONSE In vision, an increase in impulse rate produced when light is turned off or made dimmer. When an off-response occurs, one often sees a suppression of impulse activity (or a hyperpolarization of the cell membrane) during the time the light was on. Thus an off-response is often an indication of an inhibitory process.

OLFACTORY BULB A collection of cells at the base of the brain that receives input from olfactory receptors in the nose, which mediate the sense of smell.

ON-RESPONSE In vision, an increase in impulse rate produced when light is turned on or made brighter.

OPHTHALMOSCOPE Instrument for viewing the retina. Direct ophthalmoscope (the common type) consists of a light to illuminate the retina and a set of lenses to bring the retina to a focus in the eye of the viewer. Used in clinical examinations (the retina being the only part of the central nervous system visible from the outside), and in our experiments for fitting contact lenses to the animal, in order to bring the projection screen to a focus, and to determine the positions of the optic disc and fovea by training a light spot on them, locking the position of the instrument and projecting a second small spot back onto the projection screen.

OPTIC DISC Region of vertebrate retina where the optic nerve originates. In cats, macaque monkeys, and humans, it is located just below the horizontal meridian about 18 degrees medial, on the retina, to the fovea.

PARVOCELLULAR LAYERS In macaque and human lateral geniculate bodies, the four dorsal (upper) small-cell layers, separated by interlaminar leaflets. Most cells have center-surround receptive fields, mostly color coded (type 1), but some are broad-band (type 3). Some have receptive fields with two overlapping opponent-color components (type 2).

PENFIELD, WILDER (1891–1976) Neurosurgeon, director of Montreal Neurological Institute from the time of its founding (1934) until his retirement (1960). Important in developing neurosurgical approaches to treatment of epilepsy, and for his contributions to the mapping of the human cerebral cortex.

PIGMENT EPITHELIUM Layer of cells containing the dark pigment, melanin, lying just behind the retinal photoreceptors. It serves to mop up the light that has passed by the receptors, and is the site of reconstitution of the visual purple that has been bleached by light. The pigment is lacking in albinos and Siamese cats.

PREPOTENTIAL See pp. 92, 96–98 for our use of this term.

PRIMARY VISUAL CORTEX See *visual cortex*. Also called *striate cortex* and *V-1*.

QUEEN SQUARE Nickname for Institute of Neurology of University College, London. A leading hospital and center for neurology in England.

RAKIC, PASCO (born 1933) Neurobiologist noted for emphasizing the importance of Bergmann glial fibers in determining growth pathways of neurones in the cerebral cortex, and for his studies of prenatal development of ocular dominance columns in monkeys.

RAMON Y CAJAL (1852–1934) Spanish, the most eminent of neuroanatomists, who used mainly the Golgi method to establish the neurone doctrine (that neurones are separate entities and do not form a syncytium), and to describe the wealth of neuronal cell types and interconnections in a variety of species, especially mammals. His most famous work was the *Histologie du Système Nerveux,* in two volumes, translated into French from the original Spanish. Nobel Prize (1906), shared with Camillo Golgi "in recognition of their work on the structure of the nervous system".

RECEPTIVE FIELD The area of a sensory surface from which sensory receptors converge on a single nerve cell, directly or by way of intermediate nerves. The cell may be any neuron in the central nervous system that is connected to the receptors, perhaps over many synapses. A receptive field is thus defined in terms of a sensory surface (skin, retina etc.), and in terms of a single cell in the nervous system. In the case of vision, it consists of the population of rods and cones, and consequently the area on the retina that connects to any given cell in the retina or to some more central structure, such as the lateral geniculate body or the visual cortex. The term can also be defined physiologically, as the region of retina (or visual field) over which a cell can be influenced by visual stimuli. Given the richness of interconnections in the central nervous system, the extent of a cell's receptive field may be hard to define precisely, and will often depend on the stimuli employed. (The term was first used for somatic sensation by Sherrington, and for vision by Hartline.)

RECEPTOR Used in neurophysiology in two entirely different ways. *(1)* The term can refer to a cell or part of a cell that reacts to sensory information, such as light, mechanical deformation, or a chemical. Examples are rods and cones of the retina; skin mechanoreceptors or hair cells of the inner ear; and olfactory receptors in the nose. *(2)* The term is also used to refer to a protein molecule contained in the membrane of a cell, which reacts to specific chemicals in the extracellular fluid, such as neurotransmitters.

RESPIRATOR An "iron lung" used to provide artificial respiration to animals during physiological experiments and to humans whose respiration is paralyzed. In many of the experiments described in this book, animals received systemic curare-like drug injections to paralyze the eye muscles, and artificial respiration had to be used because the diaphragm and intercostals muscles were paralyzed along with most other voluntary muscles.

RETINA Neural apparatus in the eye, responsible for converting light into electrical signals. It is located on the inside of the eyeball, covering its posterior half, about ¼ mm thick, and consists of three layers of cell bodies separated by two layers of axons and dendrites and synapses. The outermost layer, closest to the sclera, consists of the light-sensitive receptors, the rods and cones. The retina is, strictly speaking, part of the central nervous system.

RETINAL GANGLION CELLS Cells lodged in the innermost layer of the retina, which receive their input from rods and cones with one or more cell types intervening, and which send their axons to the brain. There are about one million in each eye, in humans and monkeys. In the brain, they end in the lateral geniculate nucleus of the thalamus, the superior colliculus (optic tectum), and several other small nuclei in the brainstem.

RUSHTON, WILLIAM (1901–1980) Trinity College, Cambridge. Known for his work on the nerve impulse, and for contributions to visual psychophysics, especially dark adaptation and color vision. Originated the terms *dark light* and *chlorolabe, erythrolabe,* and *cyanolabe* for the three cone pigments whose spectral sensitivities he was the first to determine.

SALK INSTITUTE Biomedical laboratories located in La Jolla, California, founded in 1963 by Jonas Salk, who developed the first vaccine against the polio virus in 1955.

SHATZ, CARLA J. (born 1947) Graduate student with us from 1971 to 1976, noted especially for her work on the neurodevelopment of the mammalian visual system. Chairperson of the neurobiology department at Harvard Medical School, 2000 to present.

SHERRINGTON, SIR CHARLES SCOTT (1857–1952) Neurophysiologist who worked at the Universities of London, Liverpool, and Oxford. Most famous for studies of spinal reflexes and sensory and motor systems. Author of Integrative Action of the Nervous System (1906) and Reflex Activity of the Spinal Cord (1932). Originator of the terms *neuron, synapse* and *receptive field* (in the context of the skin surface from which a single sensory nerve fiber could be influenced). Nobel prize (1932), shared with E. D. Adrian "for their discoveries regarding the functions of neurons".

SINEWAVE GRATING Parallel stripes whose intensities vary as a sinusoidal function of distance perpendicular to the orientation of the stripes. When used as a visual stimulus, the stripes are often moving. Frequency of firing may vary with phase of stripes and as a function of their spatial frequency.

SOCIETY FOR NEUROSCIENCE Founded in [1970] with a membership now (2003) numbering over 25,000, with membership not confined to the United States of America. Annual meetings, usually in November, are held in the few American or Canadian cities with facilities large enough to accommodate the members who wish to attend.

SOMATOSENSORY CORTEX Part of the cerebral cortex devoted to somatic sensation, especially touch and joint position. Located in the parietal lobes of primates.

SPIKE Term loosely used in neurophysiology to refer to the record of an impulse or action potential.

STEREOPSIS The process of combining the slightly different images in the two eyes to achieve depth perception.

STEREOTAXIC APPARATUS (also called Horsley-Clarke apparatus) A means of locating any part of the brain (for electrode placement, for example), using a Cartesian coordinate system in which (0, 0, 0) is usually arbitrarily chosen to be 10 mm above a plane passing through the inferior orbital margins and the two bony external ear canals. Stereotaxic *atlases* have been prepared for brains of many species, such as cats, mice, and macaque monkeys, usually with one page devoted to a given plane, such as the frontal, sagittal, or horizontal planes.

STRABISMUS; SQUINT As used here, the terms are synonymous. Faulty alignment of the two eyes, frequently, resulting in double vision or suppression of vision and possibly blindness in one eye. Termed *divergent,* when the two eyes look outwards, *convergent,* when they look inwards. May be congenital, or acquired through injury to an eye muscle or nerve supplying it.

STRIATE CORTEX See *visual cortex.* Also called *V-1*, area 17, and *primary visual cortex.*

STRUNK, WILLIAM, AND WHITE, E. B. Authors of *The Elements of Style* (New York: Macmillan Co., 1959).

SUPERIOR CERVICAL GANGLION Groups of cells in the cervical (neck) region of mammals, serving autonomic functions.

SYNAPSE Junction between two neurones, comprising a presynaptic portion from which neurotransmitter is released (in the case of a chemical synapse), and a postsynaptic portion with receptors that react to the transmitter in a way that leads to excitation or inhibition of the postsynaptic cell. Any given synapse is either excitatory or inhibitory, depending on the neurotransmitter and the postsynaptic receptors. An *electrical synapse* is one in which the currents associated with the presynaptic ending are sufficient to influence the postsynaptic cell.

TALBOT, SAMUEL Neurophysiologist at Johns Hopkins Medical School. Worked in vision, with Kuffler and Wade Marshall.

THOMPSON, BENJAMIN (later Count Rumford) (1753–1814) Physicist noted especially for his contributions to the study of heat.

TOPOGRAPHY As used in neurobiology: the mapping of a neuronal structure in terms of its sensory, motor, or other physiological characteristics. In vision, in the case of the cerebral cortex, this refers to the mapping, on the cortex, of the visual fields; in somatic sensation, the skin surface and limb joints; in audition, the optimal frequency of sounds or the direction of origin of sounds.

TRINITY COLLEGE, CAMBRIDGE UNIVERSITY Founded 1546 by Henry VIII. Largest and wealthiest of the Cambridge colleges. Masters of Trinity have included Lord Adrian, Alan Hodgkin, and Andrew Huxley.

VISUAL CORTEX The part of the cerebral cortex of mammals devoted to vision. It is located in the occipital lobes, and in primates comprises perhaps over a dozen subdivisions. The largest of these, variously known as *striate cortex, primary visual cortex,* or *V-1,* receives its main input directly from the lateral geniculate body of the thalamus, which in turn receives its input from the eye.

WALD, GEORGE (1906–1997) Noted for his work on visual pigment chemistry. Nobel Prize in Medicine or Physiology 1967 with Granit and Hartline "for their discoveries concerning the primary physiological and chemical visual processes in the eye".

WALTER REED Walter Reed Army Medical Center, located in Washington, D.C. Includes the Walter Reed Army Institute of Research.

WHEATSTONE, SIR CHARLES English physicist (1802–1975). Popularized the Wheatstone Bridge, a device for measuring electrical resistance; discovered stereopsis; invented the stereoscope.

WHITE MATTER Regions of brain and spinal cord that consist mainly of myelinated nerve fibers, in contrast to grey matter, which consists of cell bodies, fibers, dendrites, synapses, and glia. The myelin covering the nerve axons produces the white appearance in freshly cut sections. *Subcortical white matter* refers to white matter below the cortex, consisting mainly of nerve fibers leaving from or arriving at the cortex.

WILMER INSTITUTE OF OPHTHALMOLOGY Part of the Johns Hopkins Hospital, devoted to clinical ophthalmology and related research. In the 1950s Stephen Kuffler headed a small group at the Wilmer, working on visual neurophysiology, synaptic physiology, spinal cord physiology, the physiology of glial cells, and so on.

ZEKI, SEMIR Neuroanatomist and neurophysiologist, at University College, London. Noted especially for defining the numerous prestriate visual areas that lie anterior to the primary visual cortex.

ACKNOWLEDGMENTS

I am embarrassed to say how many people and hours went into reading over this manuscript. Beata Zolovska read and criticized it more than a half dozen times, from many standpoints, praising the parts she found amusing and protesting over the boring parts. Her comments were enormously helpful, especially in preventing my sarcasms from offending more people than absolutely necessary. Bevil Conway read it once, closely, and repeatedly asked for "more juice". (He will be shocked and disappointed if this last sentence ends with the full stop followed by the closed quote, in the illogical, American order. I have pled with Oxford and can only hope for the best.) Also thanks to Antonio Damasio, Pierce Howe, Joyce and Richard Tedlow, Elio Raviola, and Ruth, my wife, for valuable comments. Ruth especially for putting up with all the lost weekends. To Jennifer Wilson, who helped prepare many of the photographs. And to Lyn Feeney, for help in preparing the manuscript and for enduring all my temper tantra over that fearsome obstacle course, Microsoft Word.

TODAY, FORTY-SIX YEARS AFTER STARTING

After leaving the presidency of Rockefeller University in 1998, Torsten Wiesel was named director of the Shelby White and Leon Levy Center for Mind, Brain, and Behavior. In 2000, he was appointed secretary general of the Human Frontier Science Program Organization (HFSP), which supports international and interdisciplinary collaboration between investigators in the life sciences as well as the training of students in top laboratories. He is the president of the International Brain Research Organization (IBRO) and chair of the Board of Governors of the New York Academy of Sciences. Since 1994, he has also served as chair of the Committee on Human Rights for the National Academies of Sciences and Engineering and Institute of Medicine. Dr. Wiesel is a board member of the Hospital for Special Surgery,

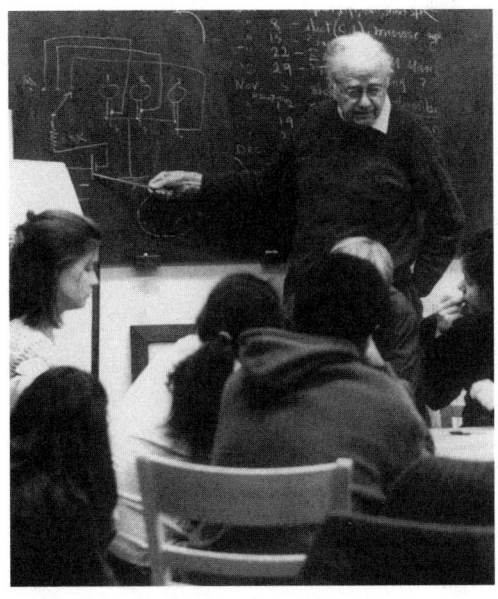

David Hubel, teaching first-year Harvard college students, 2001.

the Population Council, and the Pew Center on Global Climate Change, and he has continued to chair the review committee of the Pew Scholars and Pew Latin American Fellows programs. In addition, Dr. Wiesel is a member of scientific advisory boards in the United States, Brazil, China, Italy, and Japan.

David Hubel retired in 2000 from his University Professorship at Harvard, but continues to do full-time research and teaching at Harvard Medical School. His research at present is on the subject of steropsis in pre-striate cortical regions in monkeys. He teaches a full course each fall term to a groups of twelve Harvard first-year undergraduate students, and is advisor to several graduate students and postdoctoral fellows. He continues to be successful in avoiding any kind of administration. He spends spare time playing the piano, and on electronics, languages, tennis, and on vacations on Cape Breton Island in Canada.

INDEX

Page numbers that are underscored indicate figures